Mechanisms of Neurological Disease

Mechanisms of Neurological Disease

Anthony J. Lewis
M.B., B.S., F.R.C.P. (C.)
Associate Professor, Department of Pathology,
University of Ottawa Faculty of Medicine;
Neuropathologist, Ottawa Civic Hospital, Ottawa

Little, Brown and Company Boston

First Edition

Library of Congress catalog card No. 75–25160

ISBN 0–316–52336–4

Printed in the United States of America

To Judith McKenna, who made the climate in which it was possible to write this book and put up with it (and the writer) for the past two years. Who said women have no patience?

Contents

Preface

I have gathered a posy of other men's flowers, and nothing but the thread that binds them is my own.
—Montaigne

I hope that this book will be useful, and better still interesting, to nonspecialists in neuropathology whose activities bring them into contact with neurological problems and who seek an introduction to the abnormalities of function and structure that are clinically manifest in their patients. More specifically, it is offered with senior medical students and residents in the clinical neurological specialties and general pathology in mind. There is brief presentation of some important areas in the basic neurological sciences, since I have found this to be almost always necessary in teaching both medical students and residents. However, familiarity with material taught in the first year or two of medical studies is presupposed. The book does not set out to be either sufficiently comprehensive or detailed to serve trainees in the specialty of neuropathology itself, except in an introductory role.

Insofar as abnormal function and structure constitute the proper field of study of pathology, this book is largely an account of neuropathology. Relevant anatomy, biochemistry, and physiology are introduced in relation to disease groupings whenever possible, rather than being isolated at the beginning of the book, although some introductory chapters appeared unavoidable. A conscientious attempt has been made to include current research and concepts wherever possible, even though some of the data and deductions may be contentious or even speculative and may require rethinking as new information becomes available. Such material is called to the attention of the reader as it occurs. I feel that its inclusion is strongly justified because it demonstrates the pace of research in neurological disease and the many intrinsic fascinations in the study of neurology. Much of this newer material comes from the fields of physiology and biochemistry. This appreciably dilutes the amount of descriptive morphology (morbid anatomy) hitherto often regarded as the sum total of "pathology" by students and residents. A moderate deemphasis of purely morphological details is very desirable for nonspecialists, since functional studies not only are more fundamental, but also offer better prospects for discovering effective methods of therapy.

To keep size within reasonable bounds, selection of material has been unavoidable. The primary consideration was adequate coverage of common clinical problems, and so attention has been focussed on head injury, stroke, edema, and the reactions of the central nervous system to general bodily disease. With somewhat less common entities, such as the degenerative diseases, an attempt has been made to extract as many generalizations as possible about the whole group and to place these early in the chapter, to avoid repetitious detail and, I hope, to facilitate learning. However, I have not been completely consistent, and some of the rare neurological diseases, like the inborn errors of metabolism, are reviewed at moderate length because of their academic rather than their clinical importance.

The general approach and emphasis have evolved over twenty years of teaching groups that have varied in their enthusiasm, from conscripted medical officers to residents on the eve of examination, and from trying to answer the questions of students and residents over this period. An American professor, apparently not in medicine, is credited with the remark that "teaching without research is like confession without sin." Lacking confession, I cannot make a direct comparison, but my experience does not validate the pejorative implications; most of my professional life has been spent working fulltime in a service hospital environment, with many excellent teachers among my colleagues. Such teaching background has not seemed to be a disadvantage vis-à-vis more academically inclined men, since even the research-oriented teacher, instructing in a field much wider than his own research interests, is necessarily drawing on the work of others. Accordingly, the limits of my ambition have been to gather material together with enthusiasm and, it is hoped, with a reasonable degree of discrimination, and to present it in an accessible, readable, and useful form, as a neurobiological *other men's flowers.*

Correspondingly, I owe an incalculable debt to workers in all fields of neurobiology and clinical neurology. This debt is very incompletely expressed in the bibliographies at the ends of the chapters, which principally list recent reviews of the subject and draw attention to articles based on current investigations that are in a particularly exciting and important phase. From these sources, the interested student can easily compile full bibliographies. If significant reviews or articles have been omitted, this merely reflects the limited hours in each day and not any lack of interest or appreciation.

Over and above the general indebtedness, some specific thanks are due. Manuscript chapters have been read and many errors noted and suggestions made by Drs. G. Siegel, University of Michigan Medical Center, and K. Marshall, University of Ottawa Faculty of Medicine; E. Atack, B. Benoit, and W. Poznanski, Ottawa Civic Hospital; L. Heffernan and H. McDonald, Dalhousie University, Halifax; and G. Watters, Montreal Children's Hospital. Residual errors and misrepresentations are my sole responsibility, the more so as I did not accept all suggestions offered. From the publishers, great help, encouragement, and enthusiasm have been received from Lin Richter, Cynthia Chapin, and Clifton Gaskill, and I am grateful also for the patience and (presumed) equanimity of the copyeditors. The immense job of typing and retyping was carried out with true Scandinavian "cool" by Seija Murray, and a great deal of expert, extra laboratory work was done by the chief neuropathology technologist of the Ottawa Civic Hospital, Alistair Gregor. Thanks are also due to members of the Audiovisual Unit of the Ottawa Civic Hospital, who prepared most of the illustrations. My colleagues in the Department of Laboratory Medicine have shown great forbearance in the face of brain reports that are late, even by the normally relaxed neuropathological standards.

Finally, especial and deep personal thanks to two people: Norbert Kerenyi of Toronto and Charles Winship of Halifax, whose constant encouragement, confidence, and assistance in so many ways have been a source of often much needed sustenance. I earnestly hope that the results will measure up to their expectations.

A. J. L.

Ottawa

Anatomy and Physiology of the Central Nervous System

I

The Brain at Autopsy

1

The teaching of neuroanatomy normally relies heavily on specially prepared dissections and on the use of large sections stained to demonstrate some structural feature, usually myelin. Some of the features thus demonstrated are not of great significance in the proper evaluation of clinically diseased brains, toward which it seems that medical knowledge of neuroanatomy should be oriented. This chapter is therefore based on standard autopsy methods, that is, examining the brain externally and in serial gross section in the frontal plane (hemispheres) or transversely (cerebellum and brain stem). Structures of clinical importance that cannot be seen in this manner will be shown in Chapters 5 to 8, in the context of their functional interrelationships. Thus, this chapter should be regarded as an orientation in the major structures for use in the autopsy room and as an introduction to later, more detailed considerations.

Except when there is urgency, as in certain medicolegal cases, brains are fixed, usually in formalin, for a period of two to three weeks before being cut. The texture of fresh brain, especially in some diseases, makes adequate examination very difficult, though occasionally it may be necessary to take a small, unfixed sample for special methods of examination. Fixed gray matter has a cream or creamy-brown appearance and except in infant brains is readily distinguishable from the white matter. The autopsy brain includes the leptomeninges, which cover its surface, together with the intracranial arteries and those draining veins running within the brain or on its surface. (Details of vascular anatomy will be considered in a later chapter.) Occasionally, pieces of dura are left in situ superiorly.

LEPTOMENINGES AND SUBARACHNOID SPACE

The outermost and thickest meninx, the dura, which includes the venous sinuses, usually remains largely adherent to the inside of the skull. The two inner layers, collectively known as leptomeninges, are removed with the brain. Between them is the subarachnoid space, which varies in width. Major arteries and draining veins run in the subarachnoid space, with numerous branches that penetrate the brain.

The outer layer of the leptomeninges is the arachnoid, which only approximately follows the contours of the brain and is more closely apposed to the dura. It does not dip down into the cerebral sulci, so that the subarachnoid space is wider over them. It is only loosely reflected from the undersurface of the cerebellum to the dorsal surface of the medulla, and from the ventral surface of the midbrain and pons to the inferior surface of the forebrain, so that in these and similar areas the subarachnoid space is especially wide, forming cisterns (such as the cisterna magna beneath the cerebellum and the interpeduncular cistern at the base of the brain).

The arachnoid is a translucent membrane with a smooth outer surface except over the superior frontal and parietal areas near the midline, where it is frequently torn in removing the brain, and shows thick, whitish plaques with a nodular surface. These are the pacchionian bodies, which are from a few millimeters up to 1 cm in diameter and project into the dural blood spaces for the reabsorption of cerebrospinal fluid (Chap. 4). The arachnoid is pierced by arteries entering the subarachnoid space and by veins and cranial nerves leaving it. Torn ends of veins are often seen in the same region as the pacchionian bodies, although in life they cross the subdural space to enter venous sinuses. Similar torn veins may be seen in other regions. In elderly persons, an area of slight thickening and opacity of the arachnoid spreads laterally from the midline over the upper surfaces of the hemispheres; in the absence of associated changes, this is not considered to be abnormal.

The inner layer of the leptomeninges is the pia, which follows every contour of the brain surface and can be detached from it only with some difficulty. The outer pial surface is not smooth, since strands of delicate tissue connect pia and arachnoid, the subarachnoid space thus being like a sponge rather than an unobstructed fluid layer. The pia is perforated by small arteries entering the brain and by cranial nerves and veins leaving it.

EXTERNAL APPEARANCES

The brain consists of a forebrain, mostly made up of the cerebral hemispheres, and a cerebellum and brain stem, which are attached to the basal surface of the forebrain, a little behind the midpoint. For examination, the cerebellum and brain stem are detached by an oblique, transverse incision through the midbrain, just behind the mamillary bodies.

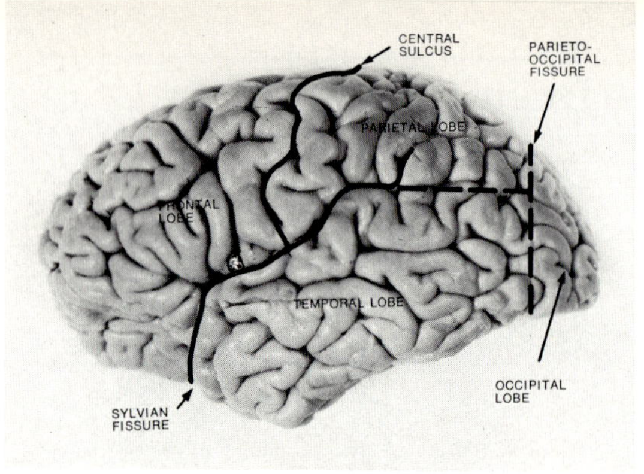

A

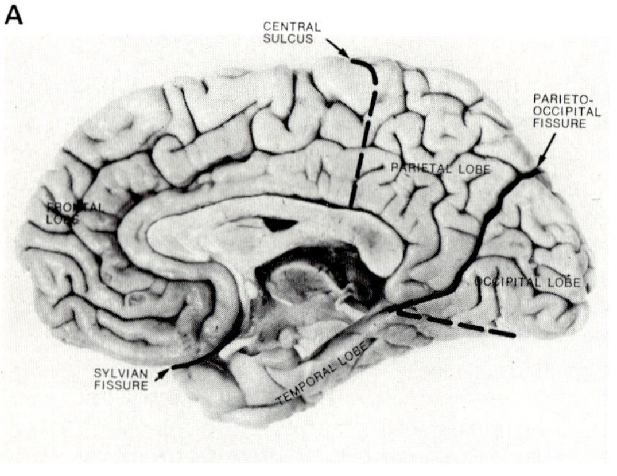

B

Fig. 1-1. Lateral (top) and medial (bottom) views of cerebral hemispheres showing the lobes.

Division of the Cerebral Hemispheres into Lobes

The forebrain consists largely of the two cerebral "hemispheres" (Fig. 1-1), which are in reality more quarter-spheres, with a temporal lobe projecting below the basal surface. Across the midline they are connected by a broad transverse band, the corpus callosum, which may be seen by separating the upper surfaces of the hemispheres. The corpus callosum has an anteroposterior extent one-third or slightly greater than that of the hemispheres and a little toward the front; thus, the occipital lobes project farther posterior to the corpus callosum than the frontal lobes do anterior to it. The hemispheres are also connected by hypothalamic structures at the base of the brain. Each hemisphere has a flattened medial surface and a convex superolateral surface. The inferior (basal) surface is more irregular; the posterior third is made slightly concave by the upper surface of the cerebellum, and its anterior portion becomes continuous with the temporal lobe, which slopes downward and forward to the rounded temporal pole. The pole is separated by the deep sylvian fissure from the anterior third of the basal surface, which is flat, with a slope downward toward the midline. The entire hemispheric surfaces are thrown into folds (*gyri*) separated by troughs (*sulci*). Although these can be seen through the leptomeninges, they are better appreciated by removing the arachnoid and subarachnoid vessels.

The sylvian fissure, already seen running laterally on the basal surface, turns backward and slightly upward on the lateral surface, reaches about two-thirds of the way toward the occipital pole, and terminates by turning briefly up toward the superior margin. The *frontal and parietal lobes* lie above the sylvian fissure, and the *temporal lobe* lies below it. A relatively deep and constant central sulcus extends from the superior margin of the hemisphere, about two-thirds of the way back from the frontal pole, downward and forward on the superolateral surface, to reach the sylvian fissure. It separates the *frontal lobe* in front from the *parietal lobe* behind. A third constant landmark is the parieto-occipital fissure on the medial surface, extending from below the posterior end of the corpus callosum, obliquely upward and backward to the superior margin, separating the *parietal lobe* in front from the *occipital lobe* behind.

The other boundaries of the cerebral lobes are arbitrary. On the lateral aspect, a vertical line drawn down from the upper tip of the parieto-occipital fissure separates the *parietal and temporal lobes* in front from the *occipital lobe* behind. A horizontal line, drawn backward from the sylvian fissure (at the point where it turns upward) to meet the vertical line, separates the *parietal lobe* above from the posterior end of the *temporal lobe* below. On the medial sur-

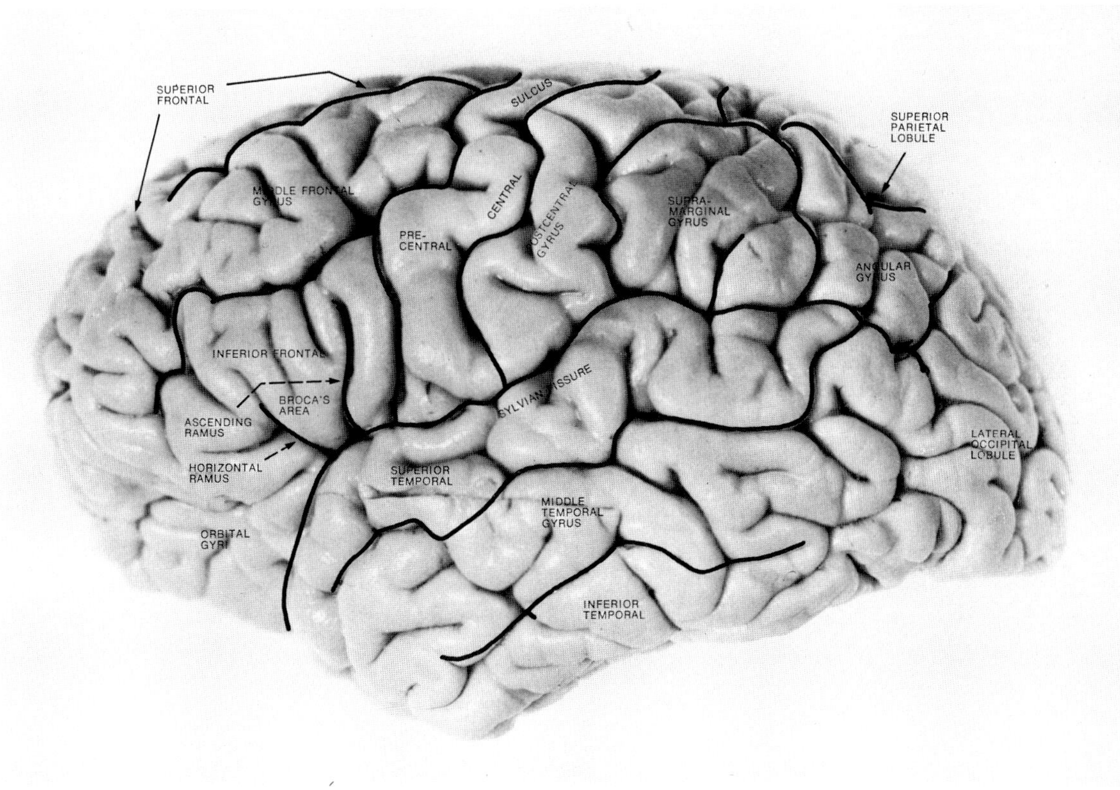

Fig. 1-2. Lateral view of left cerebral hemisphere showing major gyri.

face, a line drawn from the upper end of the central sulcus perpendicular to the corpus callosum separates the *frontal lobe* anteriorly from the *parietal lobe* posteriorly. On the inferior surface, a line drawn from the lower (anterior) end of the parieto-occipital fissure to join the lateral vertical line separates the *temporal lobe* anteriorly from the *occipital lobe* posteriorly. It is apparent that division of the cerebral hemisphere into four lobes is merely a device for approximate localization and may be in no way related to the morphology or function of the cortex.

Gyri of the Frontal Lobe

The superolateral surface of the frontal lobe is divided into four gyri. The pattern, as in other areas, is often obscured by the dividing sulci being variable and incomplete, or by prominent development of secondary sulci. The most constant is the precentral sulcus, which runs approximately parallel to the central sulcus, between 1 and 2 cm anterior to it, but may be irregular or even incomplete. Between it and the central sulcus lies the *precentral gyrus.* The remaining cortex is divided by superior and inferior frontal sulci into three unequal bands parallel to the superior margin. These are the *superior, middle, and inferior frontal gyri,* the former overlapping into the medial surface of the hemisphere and including most of the frontal pole (Fig. 1-2). The short inferior gyrus is divided by small branches of the sylvian fissure, the anteriormost passing almost horizontally forward (*horizontal ramus*) and the other passing vertically (*ascending ramus*). Between the two rami is *Broca's*

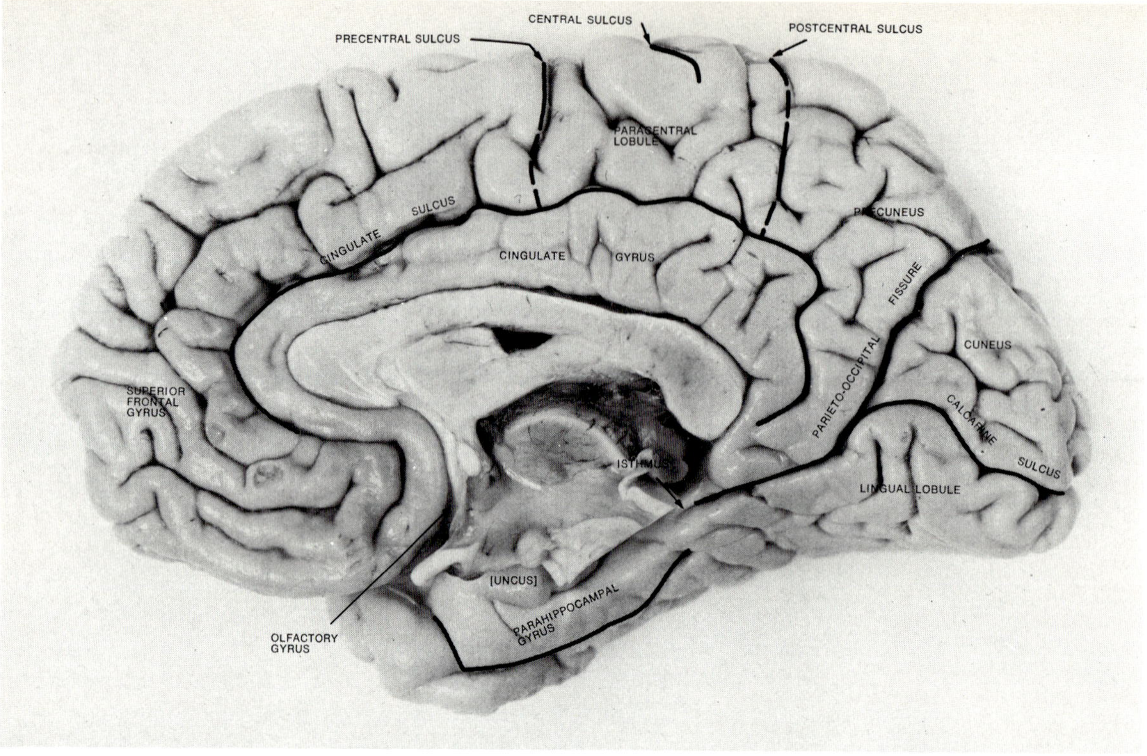

Fig. 1-3. Medial view of right cerebral hemisphere showing major gyri.

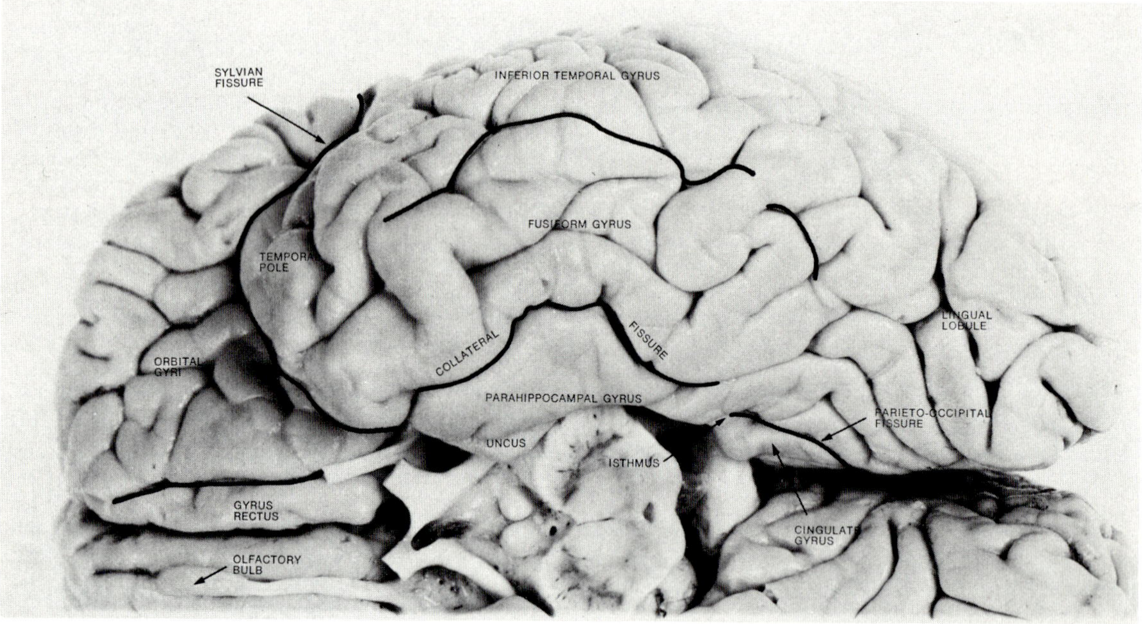

Fig. 1-4. Basal view of left cerebral hemisphere showing major gyri.

area, though usually the eponym is applied only to the left hemisphere in right-handed persons and to the right hemisphere in left-handed persons. The medial surface of the frontal lobe (Fig. 1-3) shows the constant cingulate sulcus, parallel to the corpus callosum, separating the superior frontal gyrus above and anteriorly from the *cingulate gyrus* (adjacent to the corpus callosum). The medial extension of the precentral gyrus forms a part of the *paracentral lobule.* The inferior (orbital) surface of the frontal lobe (Fig. 1-4) shows irregular, shallow *orbital gyri*, with a constant *gyrus rectus* along the medial edge, the olfactory tract and bulb lying lateral to this gyrus.

Gyri of the Parietal Lobe

The superolateral aspect of the parietal lobe (Fig. 1-2) is intersected by irregular sulci. The most constant is the postcentral sulcus, which runs approximately parallel to the central sulcus, 1.5 to 2.0 cm behind it. Between the postcentral and central sulci lies the *postcentral gyrus*. The posterior parietal cortex is more arbitrarily divided into the *supramarginal gyrus*, which lies around the termination of the sylvian fissure, the *angular gyrus* lying behind it (around the termination of the superior temporal sulcus), and the *superior parietal lobule*, demarcated inferiorly by irregular folds, the intraparietal sulcus. The supramarginal and angular gyri together form the *inferior parietal lobule.* The medial aspect of the lobe (Fig. 1-3) is small and includes the posterior cingulate gyrus, the posterior half of the paracentral lobule (a median extension of the postcentral gyrus), and the *precuneus,* a posterior area extending as far as the parieto-occipital fissure.

Gyri of the Occipital Lobe

The lateral aspect of the occipital lobe (Fig. 1-2) is small, intersected by irregular, shallow sulci and is called the *lateral occipital lobule.* The medial and inferior surfaces of the lobe (Figs. 1-3 and 1-4) are continuous and approximately bisected by the calcarine fissure, which branches from the midpoint of the parieto-occipital fissure and extends downward and back to the occipital pole. The area above this is the *cuneus;* below, mainly on the inferior surface, lies the *lingual lobule.*

Gyri of the Temporal Lobe

The lateral surface of the temporal lobe (Fig. 1-2) is horizontally divided by the superior temporal sulcus, below and parallel to the sylvian fissure, which turns upward at its posterior end to enter the parietal lobe (angular gyrus). Above, lies the *superior temporal gyrus*, and the *middle temporal gyrus* lies below. At about the junction of the lateral and basal surfaces of the temporal lobe, the middle temporal sulcus separates the middle temporal gyrus (above) from the *inferior temporal gyrus* (medially). On the basal surface (Fig. 1-4), a deep collateral fissure separates a narrow strip of cortex running alongside the midbrain, the *parahippocampal gyrus,* from a more lateral area that includes the inferior temporal gyrus and *fusiform gyrus,* incompletely separated by an inferior temporal sulcus. The anterior end of the parahippocampal gyrus bears a medially facing swelling, the *uncus* (Fig. 1-3), which lies anterior to the midbrain. Its posterior end curves upward onto the medial surface of the hemisphere, toward the posterior end of the corpus callosum, where it is separated from the cingulate gyrus by the parieto-occipital fissure.

Optional Fifth (Limbic) Lobe

Some prefer to divide the cerebral cortex into five lobes, detaching portions of the frontal, temporal, and parietal lobes to form the *limbic lobe,* on the medial and basal hemispheric surfaces (Figs. 1-3 and 1-4). This is evolutionarily older cortex lying in a ring round the corpus callosum, hypothalamus, and brain stem. It includes the cingulate gyrus (in front of, above, and behind the corpus callosum) and the parahippocampal gyrus (lateral to the hypothalamus and brain stem). These are connected anteriorly by a narrow vertical *olfactory gyrus,* below the corpus callosum and in front of the third ventricle, and posteriorly by a narrow prolongation of the cingulate gyrus, the *isthmus,* which runs downward and forward between the parieto-occipital fissure and the choroidal fissure (where vascular pia is invaginated into the lateral ventricle to form the choroid plexus). Above the olfactory gyrus, anterior to the front wall of the third ventricle, lies an area of small (parolfactory) gyri, which, with small islands of underlying gray matter, constitutes most of the *septal region* (the other part is the septum pellucidum).

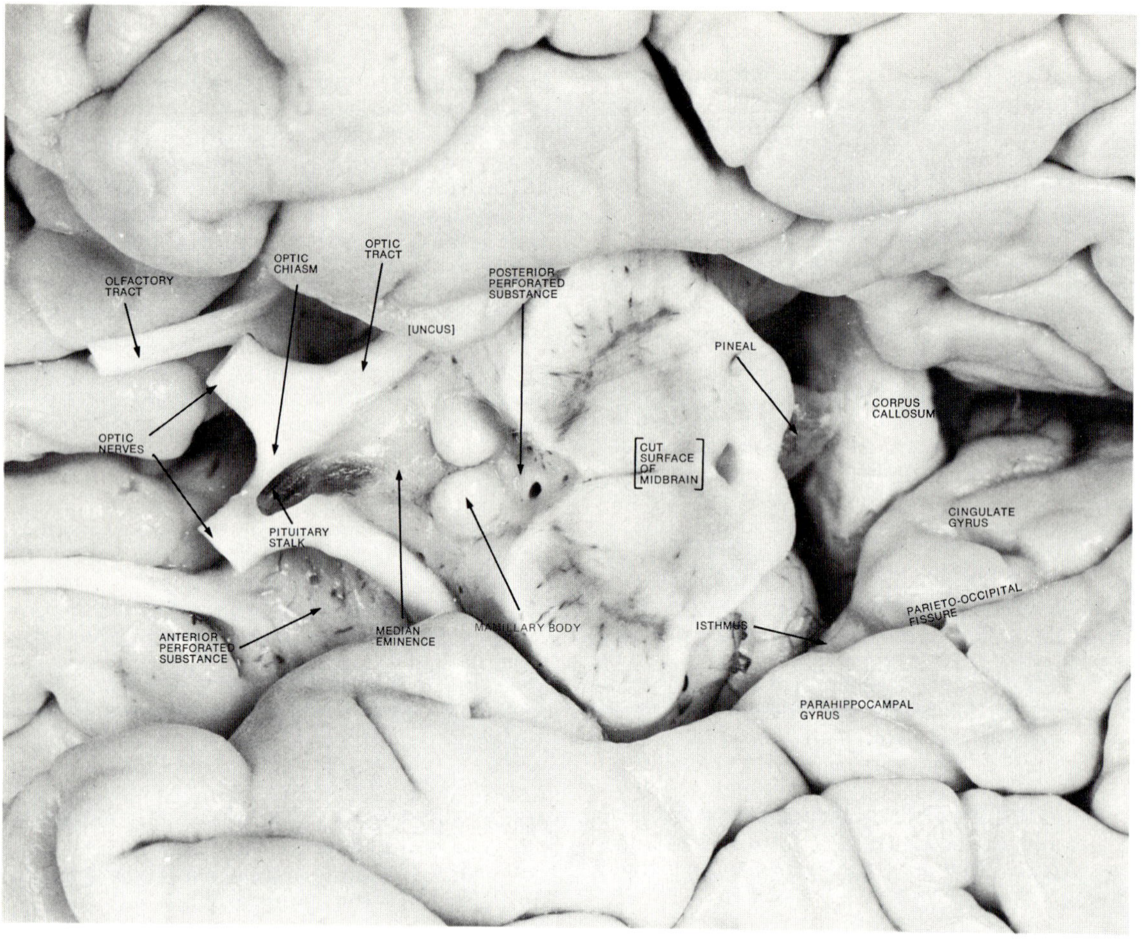

Fig. 1-5. Structures at the base of the brain, as seen after removal of the cerebellum and brain stem.

Base of the Brain

Other than the convoluted cortex and its meninges, the only forebrain structures externally visible are in the midline of the base (Fig. 1-5). Most prominent, about 1.5 cm anterior to the cut surface of the midbrain, are the cut ends of the two *optic nerves,* each about 4 X 2 mm on cross section, which join in the midline to form the *optic chiasm,* a substantial, transverse, white bar. Appearing from underneath the optic nerves and passing forward on the orbital surfaces of the frontal lobes, 0.5 to 1.0 cm from the midline, are the flattened, white *olfactory tracts,* 3 to 4 cm long, which end in slightly thicker structures, the *olfactory bulbs.* The tract and bulbs usually lie in a sulcus along the lateral border of the gyrus rectus. If the optic nerves are gently picked up and bent backward, two large vessels, the anterior cerebral arteries, are seen running forward toward the midline, where they disappear together between the hemispheres. If these arteries also are removed, it may be seen that the posterior end of the olfactory tract forms the faintly discernible *olfactory striae* (Fig. 1-6), one turning medially and disappearing in the midline to the olfactory gyrus and the other turning laterally into the sylvian fissure. The optic tracts, arising from the chiasm and winding posteriorly round the mid-

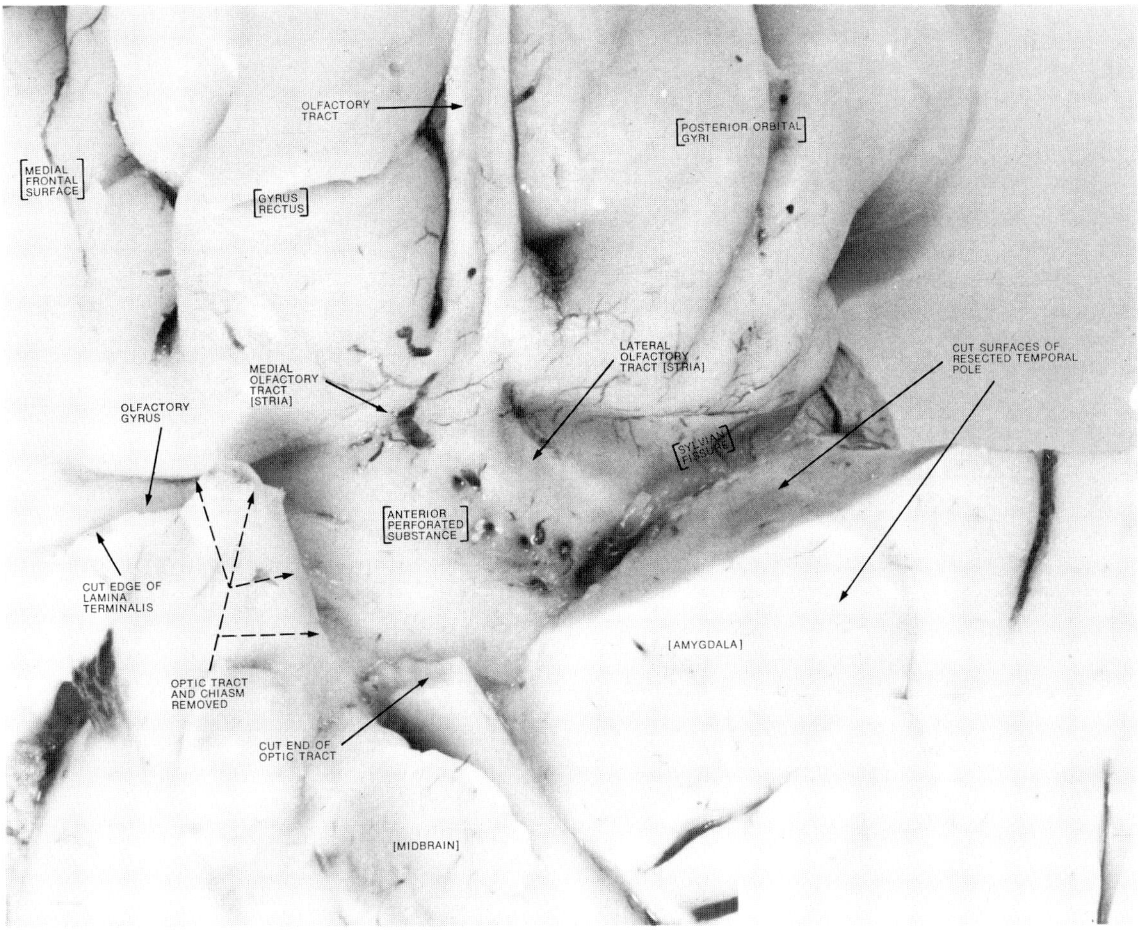

Fig. 1-6. Dissection of region of anterior perforated substance. (The optic chiasm and much of the temporal pole have been removed, and the view is from below and medially, the left edge of the photograph showing structures in the sagittal plane.)

brain, also become visible. Lying between the olfactory striae, anterolateral to the optic tract, is a pale, pitted area, the *anterior perforated substance* (substantia innominata), which extends laterally into the sylvian fissure toward the uncus. The anterior perforated substance is an olfactory input area and includes reduced remnants of the olfactory tubercles and prepyriform cortex that are so prominent in mammals for which olfaction has great survival value.

Immediately in front of the cut surface of the midbrain are the two *mamillary bodies,* small, rounded projections, 5 to 6 mm in diameter, one on either side of the midline. In the confined area behind the mamillary bodies and in front of the midbrain lies the *posterior perforated substance,* which is a single, midline structure. Also in the midline, between the optic chiasm and the mamillary bodies, is the *median eminence,* a small projecting, slightly brownish area, terminating in a slender, ruptured stalk (in life, the pituitary gland is attached to the stalk).

Midline (Sagittal) Section Separating the Hemispheres

Occasionally, it may be necessary to separate the hemispheres by a midline incision through the corpus callosum and other midline structures. (This is also helpful in visualizing deeper structures and the ventricular

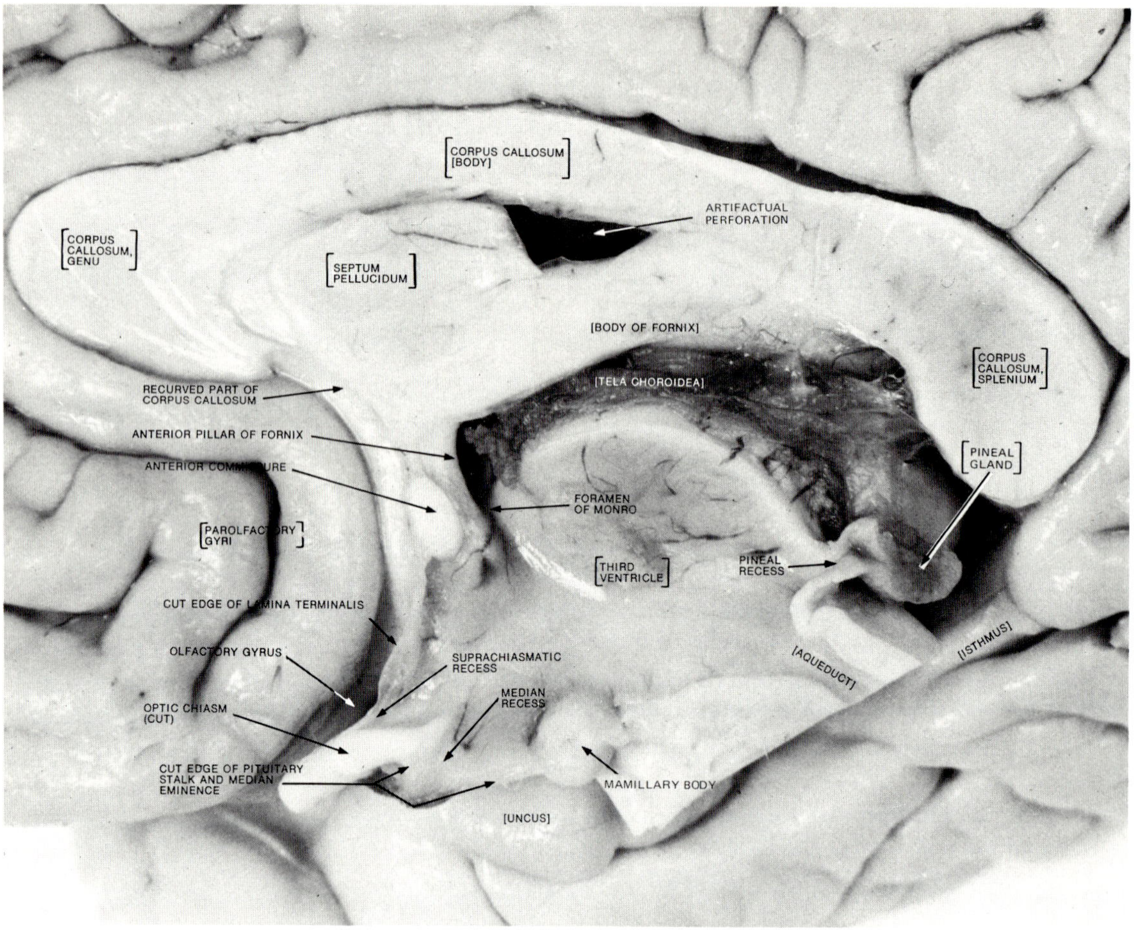

Fig. 1-7. Medial view of structures related to the third ventricle and corpus callosum.

system.) The gyral pattern on the medial surface, which includes parts of all four (or five) cerebral lobes, has been described. The most massive bisected structure is the *corpus callosum,* which has about one-third the anteroposterior extent of the hemispheres, averages 0.4 to 0.6 cm in thickness and is largely surrounded by the cingulate gyrus (Fig. 1-7). The round, thickened anterior end (genu) turns downward and then backward in a hook shape to join the *lamina terminalis,* a very thin membrane running across the midline behind the olfactory gyri. This passes down (and sometimes slightly forward) to join the upper surface of the cut optic chiasm. Near its upper end is a cut bundle of transversely running fibers, the *anterior commissure,* about the same size as the chiasm. The lamina terminalis separates the interhemispheric subarachnoid space from the third ventricle, of which it forms the anterior wall. Between the chiasm and the mamillary body is the thin, brown membrane, peaked downward, of the median eminence, continuous with the pituitary stalk. The posterior margin of the mamillary body is continuous with the midbrain.

The cut midline surface of the midbrain is divided by a shallow, narrow channel, the *aqueduct,* 2 to 4 mm wide, into a thick anterior and a somewhat thinner posterior portion, both of which form part of the posterior wall of the third ventricle. The posterior extremity of the third ventricle is continued by a thin membrane, arising dorsally from the midbrain and passing backward to the brown, triangular *pineal gland,* usually measuring about 5 X 8 mm.

The wall of the third ventricle, seen from the midline, may be indistinctly divided into a lower and upper part. The lower part is the medial boundary of the *hypothalamus* (below a line from foramen of Monro to aqueduct); the upper part is the medial boundary of the *thalamus.* Above the thalamus may be seen meningeal tissue, passing forward between the pineal gland and the posterior corpus callosum and containing a large vessel, the internal cerebral vein. This tissue is continuous across the midline to form the roof of the third ventricle, or *tela choroidea,* but is so delicate that it is usually not obvious in midline sections; thus, the ventricle appears to have no

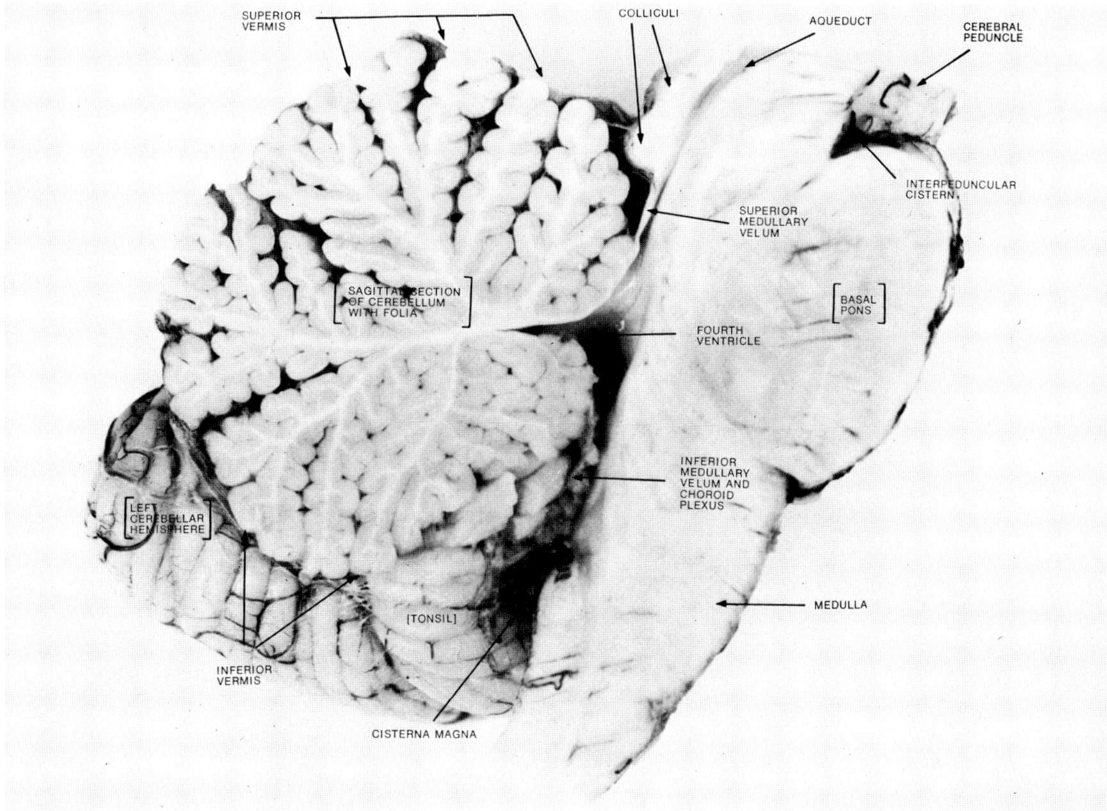

Fig. 1-8. Sagittal section through cerebellum, fourth ventricle, and brain stem.

roof. The tela choroidea is bounded anteriorly by a band of white tissue, the *fornix*, issuing from the wall of the third ventricle immediately behind the anterior commissure and curving upward and backward (above the thalamus and tela choroidea) to the undersurface of the corpus callosum. If the posterior thalamus is gently lifted away from the hemisphere and the overlying meninges are cleared away, the fornix may be seen to curve downward and then forward, passing along the parahippocampal gyrus. At the anterior end of the tela choroidea is a small tuft of pale, brownish choroid plexus, marking the position of the *foramen of Monro*, through which a probe may be passed into the lateral ventricle. Posteriorly, the tela choroidea is continuous with the choroidal fissure, marking the inner edge of the posterior cingulate gyrus, isthmus, and parahippocampal gyrus, through which the meninges invaginate the body and inferior horn of the lateral ventricle to form the choroid plexus. Note that the fornix and parahippocampal gyrus form parallel structures external (i.e., above, then behind, then below) to the choroidal fissure.

Although the fornix is attached to the undersurface of the corpus callosum posteriorly, further forward it slopes downward between the foramen of Monro and the lamina terminalis, and a large, approximately triangular space is left between the upper and anterior margin of the fornix and the anterior corpus callosum. This is closed by a thin membrane, the *septum pellucidum*, often containing prominent small vessels. The septum pellucidum is usually a midline structure and separates the anterior horns of the two lateral ventricles. Occasionally, it consists of two vertical parallel lamellae with a small intervening space, the cyst of the septum pellucidum, but this is of no clinical significance.

The Cerebellum

The cerebellum and brain stem, although containing vital structures, are considerably smaller than the combined forebrain. They represent only 6% of the total brain weight at birth, a figure that rises to around 12% by the age of 2 years and remains roughly constant thereafter.

The cerebellum lies dorsal to the brain stem (Fig. 1-8) and beneath the inferior surfaces of the posterior temporal and occipital lobes, normally extending posteriorly almost as far as the occipital pole. Its surface is covered by very narrow sulci in approximately parallel arrays, which run generally horizontally, 1.5 to 3.0 mm apart. Although some of the sulci are more important developmentally than others, none is clearly distinguishable externally. The cere-

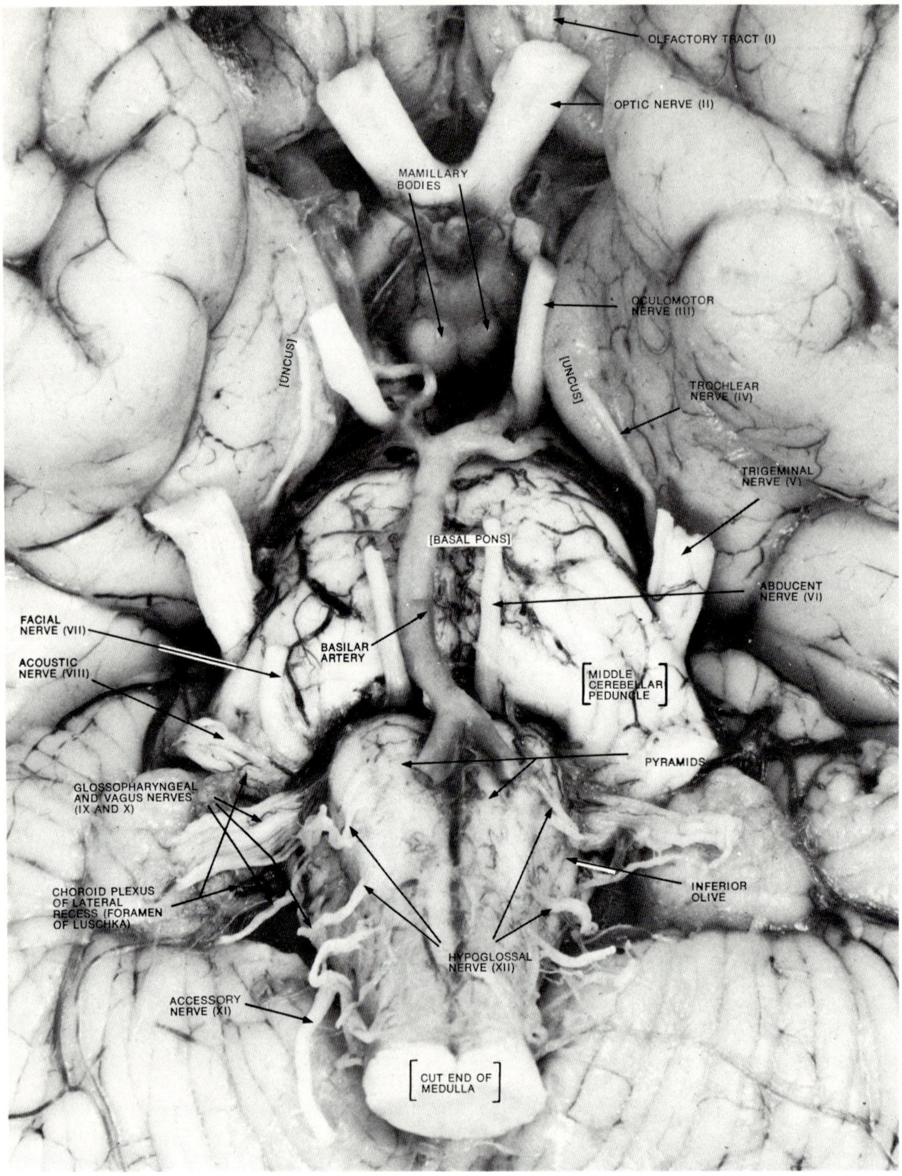

Fig. 1-9. Cranial nerves (basal view of brain).

bellum has a superior surface that is approximately flat but somewhat peaked in the midline and a posteroinferior surface that consists of two hemispheres, separated in the midline by a deep cleft. The two surfaces are indistinctly separated by a blunt margin around the posterior and lateral extremities. The midline (sagittal) part is the *vermis*, and it is apparent from the preceding description that the vermis is clearly visible on the superior surface but hidden by the cerebellar hemispheres on the posteroinferior surface, where it lies at the bottom of a midline cleft. The *cerebellar tonsils* lie in the cleft, facing one another across the midline and immediately dorsal to the medulla.

The Brain Stem

The most conspicuous structure of the brain stem (Figs. 1-8, 1-9) is the base of the *pons*, a broad strand applied transversely across the ventral and lateral surfaces of the brain stem. It is about 2 cm wide ventrally, but narrows laterally where it passes dorsally to the anterior surface of the cerebellum as the middle cerebellar peduncle, the largest of the three paired cerebellar attachments to the brain stem. There is usually a shallow midventral groove running in the midline of the pons and carrying the basilar artery. The fifth cranial nerve arises from the lateral aspect of the basal pons as a conspicuous

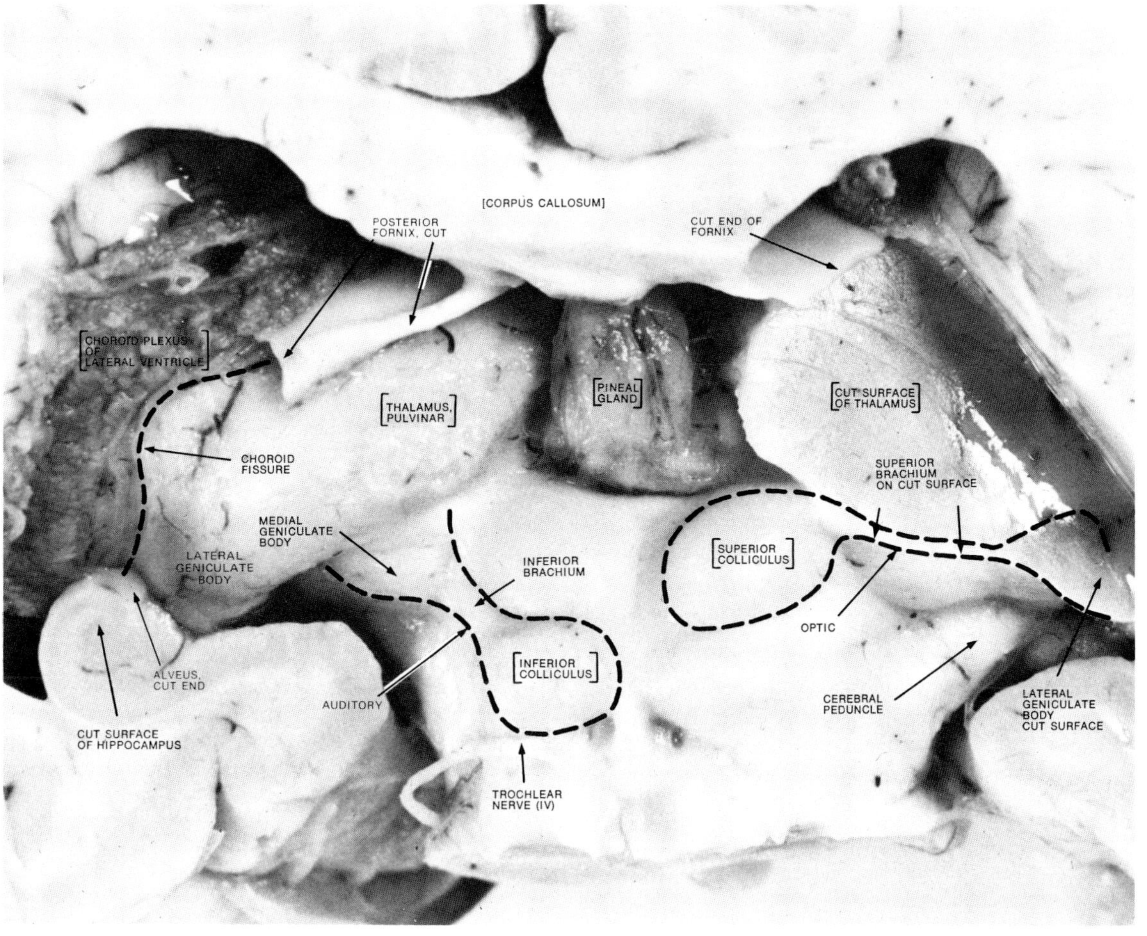

Fig. 1-10. Posterior view of midbrain and adjacent structures, showing the colliculi and geniculate bodies and the line of the choroid fissure of the lateral ventricle. (The pulvinar has been cut in the frontal plane on the right, but is intact on the left. A part of the left fornix has been removed to display the choroid fissure. The trochlear nerve was accidentally torn on the right.)

bundle of closely set rootlets. The dorsal pons is not externally visible.

On the ventral aspect of the intact brain (before severing the cerebellum and brain stem) the cerebral peduncles may be seen diverging slightly from the midline as they pass upward from the upper border of the pons to enter the cerebral hemispheres (the zone of entry partly encircled by the optic tracts). Since the midbrain, of which the cerebral peduncles are a part, is only about 1 cm long, the mamillary bodies and the posterior perforated substance lie close to the upper border of the pons. The third cranial nerves arise in the cleft between the cerebral peduncles, just above the pons. On the cut surface of the midbrain (Fig. 1-20 *F*), after brain stem and cerebellum are detached, the cerebral peduncles may be seen as broad, flat, uniformly white ventrolateral projections, with a band of gray pigment, the substantia nigra, lying deep to them. The cut surface also shows the aqueduct, lying more dorsally in the midline, and paired, rounded dorsal projections, representing either the inferior or superior colliculi (according to the plane of section). The two superior and two inferior colliculi are not readily seen in examination of the intact brain, or even of the separated cerebellum and brain stem, since they are completely covered by the superior cerebellum. Together, they make up the collicular plate dorsal to the aqueduct (Fig. 1-10). Below the inferior colliculi, near the mid-dorsal line, arise the slender fourth cranial nerves, which therefore have to wind round the midbrain to reach the ventral surface.

The medulla, or lowest part of the brain stem, emerges beneath the base of the pons (and usually shows an oblique lower cut end, where the brain has been separated from the spinal cord during removal). It has a midventral groove on either side of which run the pyramids, two prominent longitudinal ridges. Below the lower margin of the pons and lateral to the pyramids, extending downward for about 1 cm, a slight, rounded projection on each side represents the site of the inferior olivary nucleus. Between pyramids and olives arise the small rootlets which make up the twelfth cranial nerve. Lateral to the olives arises another, longer series of rootlets, which make up the ninth, tenth, and eleventh (accessory) nerves – in descending order. At the lower border of the base of the pons, above the pyramids, arise the sixth cranial nerves and, more laterally, the seventh and then eighth nerves, separated by a thin root representing the sensory division of the seventh nerve (facial nerve).

The medulla also has a less conspicuous middorsal groove, which widens under the inferior cerebellum to form the lower part of the diamond-shaped fourth ventricle. Small, indistinct swellings near the lower tip (obex) of the ventricle and lateral to its lower edges represent the positions of the gracilis and cuneate nuclei, and the edges then continue to form the inferior cerebellar peduncles. The arachnoid membrane is loosely reflected from the undersurface of the cerebellum to the dorsal surface of the medulla, leaving a substantial space (the cisterna magna) between the arachnoid and the pia that forms the roof of the lower fourth ventricle. This region is almost inevitably torn during removal of the brain, but there is probably a midline deficiency in the pial roof of the fourth ventricle, the foramen of Magendie, through which cerebrospinal fluid (CSF) may pass from the ventricular system into the subarachnoid space of the cisterna magna. Immediately anterior to the cerebellum at the lower margin of the middle cerebellar peduncle will usually be seen a small, brownish tuft of choroid plexus, the free end of a lateral projection of the fourth ventricle on each side, which terminates as an opening, the foramen of Luschka, also allowing egress of CSF into the subarachnoid space. (The foramina of Luschka and Magendie are the only natural openings through which fluid can leave the ventricular system.) Adjacent to the tuft of choroid plexus, a minute tag of cerebellar tissue, just two or three small folia, is often seen; this is the flocculus, the most primitive (vestibular) part of the cerebellum.

THE SPINAL CORD

The spinal cord, infrequently given routine examination at autopsy, could profitably be looked at more often. It extends, in the adult, from the foramen magnum to the level of the first or second lumbar vertebra. It has layers of meninges similar to those of the brain, but the dura, instead of being tightly attached to the inside of the vertebral canal, is separated from it by a layer of epidural fat and is therefore usually removed with the cord, except at the extreme upper end, where it becomes attached to the margin of the foramen magnum. Between the arachnoid and pia lies a subarachnoid space, continuous with that surrounding the brain.

The cord shows two slight fusiform enlargements, one representing approximately segments C-3 to T-1 (the cervical enlargement) and the other representing segments L-2 to S-2 (the lumbosacral enlargement). The width in these areas is about 0.9 to 1.1 cm, compared with 0.7 to 0.8 cm in the intervening thoracic region. Below the lumbosacral enlargement, the cord tapers rapidly to a thin thread, the terminal filament (filum terminale), which is usually not noticed since it is surrounded by the lumbosacral nerve roots (cauda equina). The cross sections of the cord are all oval, the width being slightly greater than the anteroposterior measurement. This disparity is most marked in the the cervical enlargement and thoracic cord, but the lumbosacral enlargement is almost round.

The anterior (ventral) surface of the cord may be recognized by a small midline vessel, the anterior spinal artery. The posterior surface shows an irregular plexus of vessels, representing a part of the venous drainage. The anterior (motor) roots arise from the ventrolateral aspect, forming an almost continuous longitudinal series of rootlets, which combine to form a smaller number of discrete ventral roots, one to each cord segment. The posterior (sensory) roots similarly arise on the dorsolateral aspect. At any given level, the size of the anterior and posterior roots is approximately equal. In the two enlargements, the nerve roots are larger and the segments are shorter. At the lower end of the cervical enlargement, there is usually an abrupt transition from large to small anterior roots, the lowest large root being generally taken as C-8 (occasionally as T-1) and serving as a reference point for segmental localization. Because the cord is considerably shorter than the vertebral canal, only the upper roots are approximately horizontal. Lower ones become progressively more vertical with a longer intraspinal course, so that those arising from the lumbosacral enlargement form the cauda equina, which occupies the vertebral canal below the termination of the cord. The dorsal root ganglia are usually situated close to the vertebral canal, sometimes even within the intervertebral foramen, and are not always present when the cord is removed. Sometimes a few spindle-shaped ganglia up to 0.5 or 0.6 cm in diameter are found to be attached to sensory roots of the cauda equina.

INTERNAL STRUCTURES IN THE FOREBRAIN

The internal structures in the forebrain will be described as they are seen during normal autopsy cutting in frontal (vertical transverse) sections at intervals of 1.25 to 1.5 cm. The sections are illustrated and described as viewed from their anterior aspects.

Sections Anterior to the Insula

Sections anterior to the level of the corpus callosum (not illustrated) show no connection between the hemispheres, which consist entirely of cerebral white matter, covered by a layer of cortex that is between

0.2 and 0.4 mm thick. The cortex shows numerous folds in toward the center of the white matter that correspond with sulci and secondary sulci seen on the surface. The cortex is sharply demarcated from the underlying white matter, which is uniform except for occasional small radial vessels, just discernible to the naked eye. Sections through the anterior genu of the corpus callosum are similar in appearance, except that the cortex on the medial aspect is interrupted by the broad band of the corpus callosum, similar in appearance and consistency to the hemispheric white matter.

A little further back, at the level of the temporal poles (Fig. 1-11), the corpus callosum is considerably broader and on either side of the midline fans out above and below a crescent-shaped cavity, the anterior tip of the lateral ventricle. Indenting this cavity laterally lies an oval mass of gray matter, the head of the *caudate nucleus*. The succeeding section (Fig. 1-12) shows two parts of the corpus callosum separated by the vertical septum pellucidum in the midline; the upper broader band is the callosum proper, and the lower narrow band is the recurved portion on its way back to join the lamina terminalis. Gray matter lateral to the ventricles is now divided by an incomplete, oblique band of white matter, the *anterior limb of the internal capsule*, into the head of the caudate nucleus medially (in the wall of the ventricle) and the anterior part of the *putamen* laterally, separated from the frontal cortex by a thin, indistinct, gray band, the *claustrum*.

Sections through the Anterior Part of the Insula, Anterior to the Thalamus

A large additional area of cortex, not visible externally, now becomes apparent (Fig. 1-13). Earlier sections showed that the sylvian fissure (above the temporal lobe and below the frontal lobe) is lined by cortex. The upper and lower bands of cortex become continuous at the posterior termination of the fissure (Fig. 1-13, right) and its lateral end turns posteriorly as the floor of a very deep lateral extension. This floor widens posteriorly, so that the fissure, as seen from the lateral surface, is bounded by two bars of cortex and white matter, the *opercula*, which hide its floor, the *insula*. The insula lies lateral to the putamen, separated from it by the claustrum and two thin layers of white matter (the band between the claustrum and the putamen is the external capsule). The folds that hide the insula from external view are, below, the temporal operculum (superior temporal gyrus on the surface); above, the frontal operculum anteriorly (formed by the inferior frontal and lower end of the precentral gyri); and, posteriorly, the parietal operculum (formed by the lower end of the postcentral and the supramarginal gyri).

In passing posteriorly, the putamen enlarges, and the caudate nucleus becomes smaller. The lower recurved layer of the callosum becomes thin and angulated upward to the septum pellucidum, so that it envelopes a thin layer of cortex on each hemisphere (the olfactory gyrus).

A section through the optic chiasm (Fig. 1-14) shows the increased complexity of the internal structures, although the general pattern of the cortex, now including the insula, is well maintained. The area of junction of the lower frontal and upper temporal cortex shows large arteries in the subarachnoid space (the middle cerebral artery and its branches). Here, the undersurface of the frontal lobe is made up of an irregular layer of gray matter, with no white matter beneath it, bounded medially by the medial division of the olfactory tract and laterally by its lateral branch (as seen externally). These can usually not be seen on the coronal sections and have to be assumed. Further back, the area is bounded by the optic tract medially and is therefore the anterior perforated substance. Above it runs a horizontal white band, the *anterior commissure*, and in the midline, between the two anterior perforated areas and below the anterior commissure, is the lamina terminalis, a translucent transverse membrane, joining the optic chiasm. Close to the midline, above the anterior commissure, are two thick, white tracts, the anterior pillars of the fornix, which run toward the undersurface of the callosum. On either side lies the lateral ventricle, approximately triangular in section, the medial surface being the fornix, the upper surface the corpus callosum, and the oblique inferolateral surface the much-reduced caudate nucleus. Lateral to the caudate lies the thick, white anterior limb of the internal capsule, inclined downward and medially. Lateral to the angle formed by the internal capsule and the anterior commissure is a triangular wedge of gray matter, divided into a small, paler medial part, the pallidum, and a larger lateral part, the putamen. The claustrum is conspicuous at this level, its lower edge thickened and often blending with the anterior perforated substance.

Sections through the Posterior Part of the Insula and Thalamus

A section through the median eminence (Fig. 1-15) also passes through the foramina of Monro, which are communicating channels between the lateral and third ventricles. At this level, well behind the transverse part of the sylvian fissure, the white matter of the temporal and frontal lobes is continuous on either side of the claustrum. An irregular thickening extends deeply from the medial cortex of the temporal lobe. This is the *amygdala*, which blends superiorly with the reduced anterior perforated substance (lateral to the optic tract) and the pallidum. The latter is now divided into a lateral and a medial division by an approximately vertical, slightly curved line, parallel to that separating pallidum and putamen. The third ventricle is a thin midline slit, which splits at its upper margin to form the foramina of Monro, separated by the fornix, which there curves forward and downward. The lateral ventricles remain approximately triangular; the caudate nuclei have become even smaller. Below the caudate nuclei, the *thalamus* appears in the inferolateral wall of the lateral ventricle and in the wall of the third ventricle. At this level it appears as a small, raindrop-shaped, gray mass (the *anterior nucleus*) below the foramen of Monro, with a less well-defined

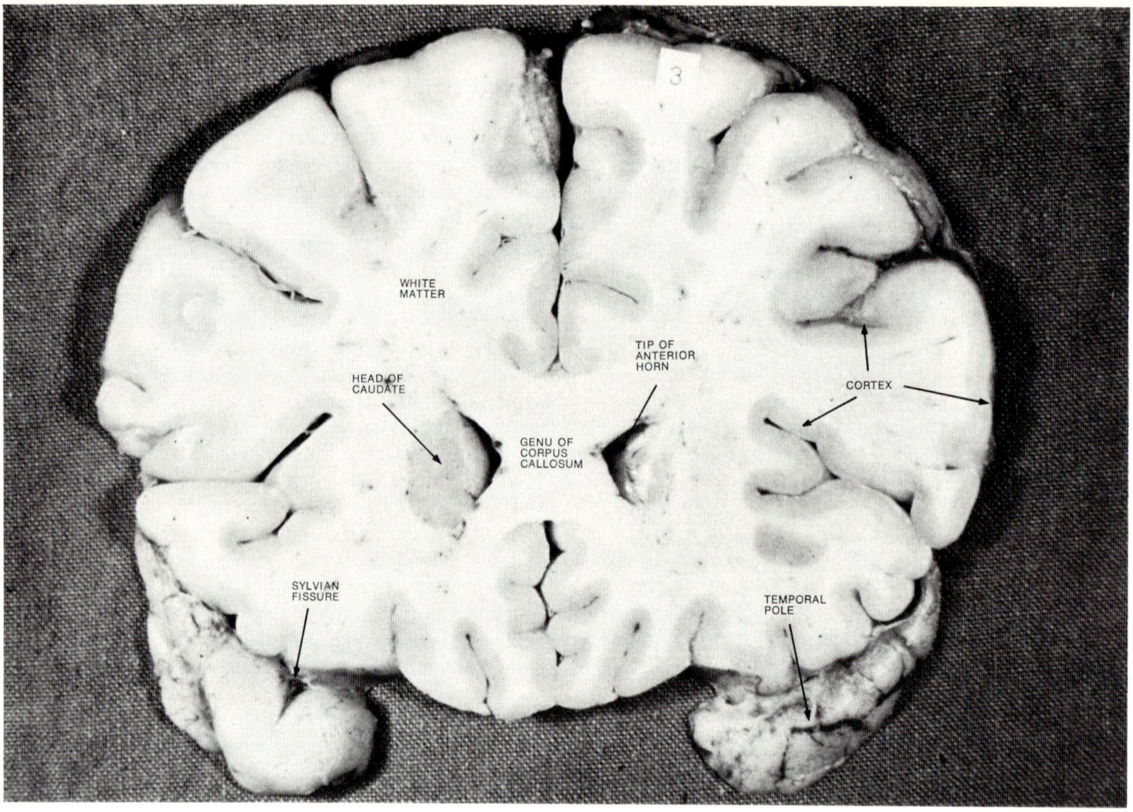

Fig. 1-11. Frontal section at level of tip of temporal pole.

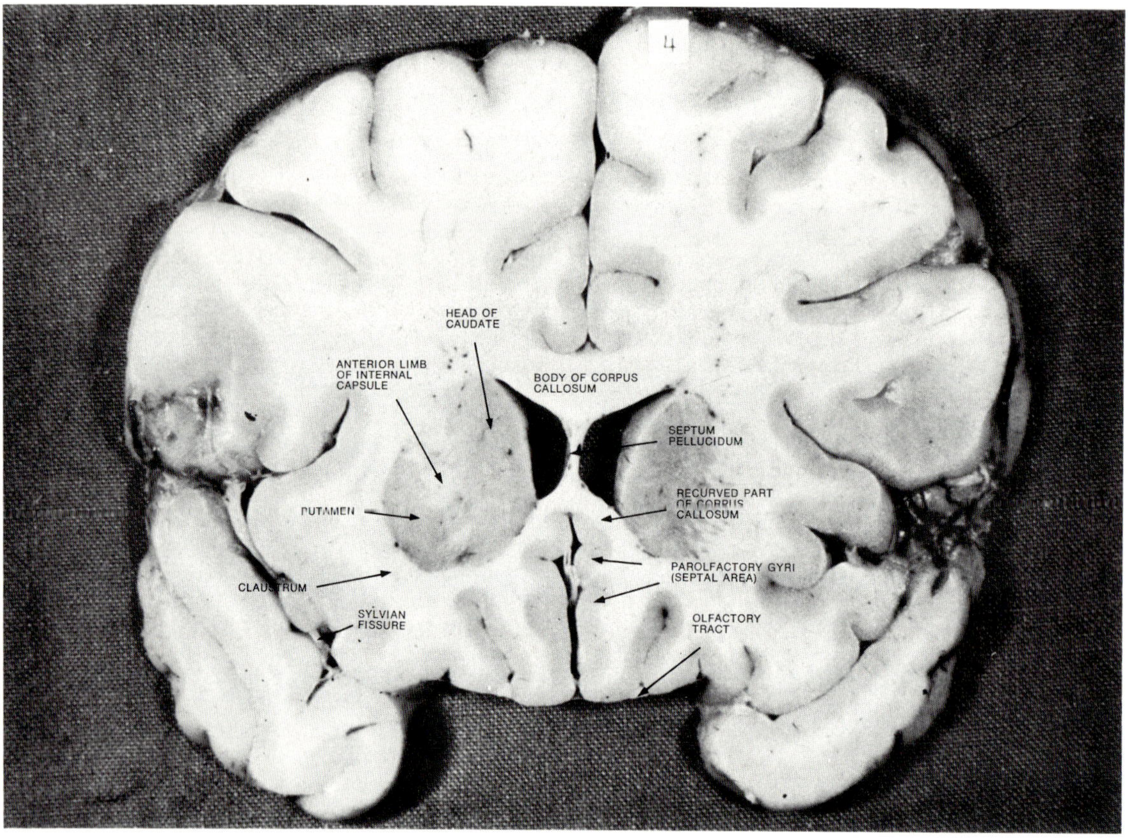

Fig. 1-12. Frontal section at level of the anteriormost part of the septum pellucidum.

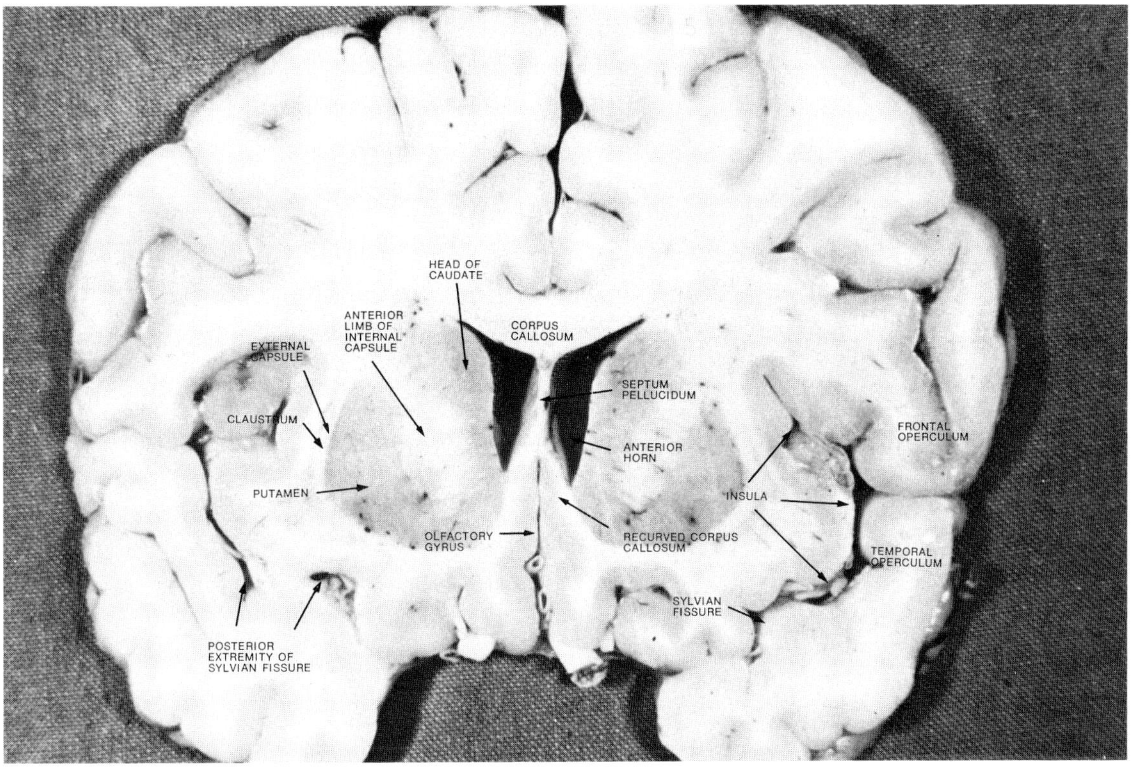

Fig. 1-13. Frontal section at level of anterior septum pellucidum and posterior reflection of transverse part of sylvian fissure.

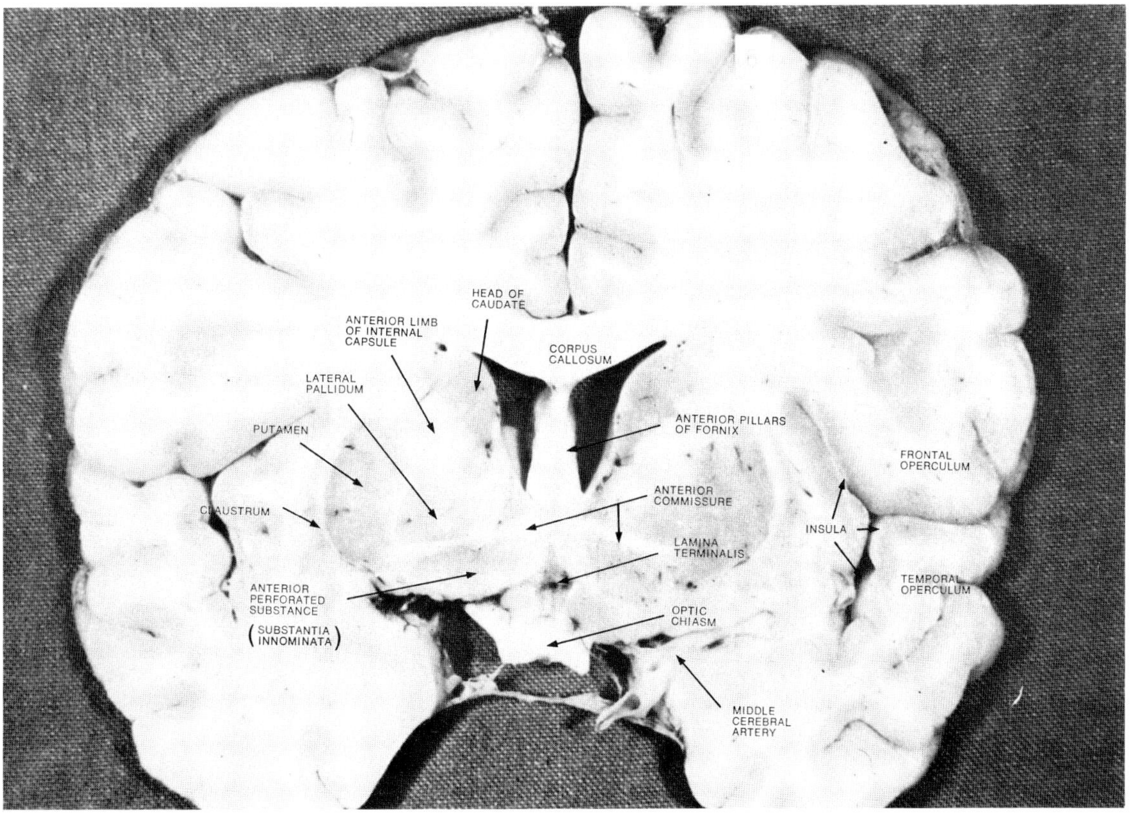

Fig. 1-14. Frontal section at level of optic chiasm, lamina terminalis, and anterior commissure.

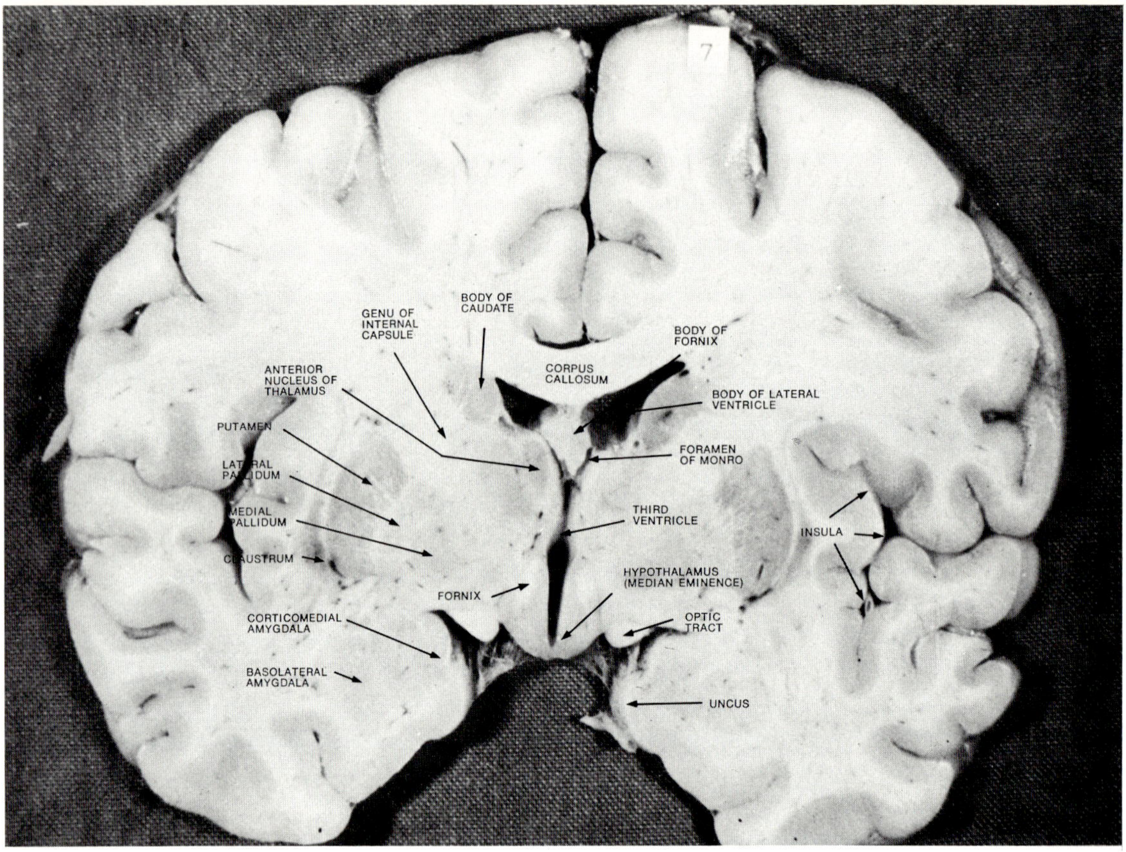

Fig. 1-15.

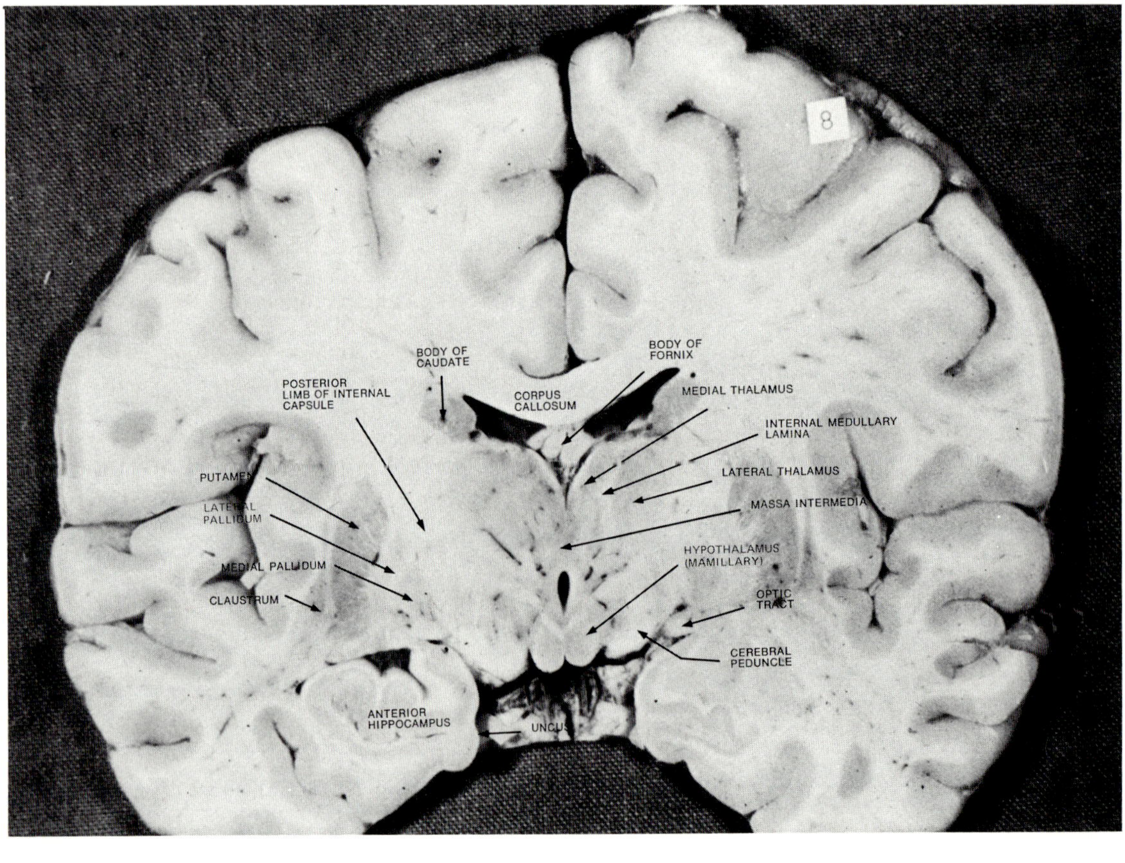

Fig. 1-16.

Fig. 1-15. Frontal section at level of median eminence and foramen of Monro.

Fig. 1-16. Frontal section at level of mamillary bodies.

lateral area. The lower wall of the third ventricle is formed by gray matter, the anterior *hypothalamus*, within which may be seen the continuation of the fornix on its way to the mamillary body. The internal capsule now separates putamen and pallidum (laterally) from the caudate and thalamus (medially). At this point it bends when viewed in horizontal section. Thus, the area is known as the *genu (knee) of the internal capsule.*

A section through the mamillary bodies (Fig. 1-16) shows a similar pattern. The basal ganglia (claustrum, putamen, and pallidum) are displaced further laterally. The internal capsule (*posterior limb*, behind the genu) reaches the base of the brain and becomes continuous with the midbrain *cerebral peduncles.* Between the peduncles are the mamillary bodies and adjacent gray matter, which form the posterior hypothalamus. Laterally, wedged between peduncles and temporal lobes, are the optic tracts. The most medial cortex of the temporal lobes (anterior hippocampus) has a convoluted appearance; the whole medial temporal projection in front of the midbrain is the *uncus*. The third ventricle at this level may be divided by the two thalami joining across the midline, the massa intermedia. The upper part may appear continuous (underneath the fornix) with the lateral ventricles, but is really separated by the delicate tela choroidea attached to the superomedial aspect of the thalamus on each side. The lateral ventricle at this level (the body) is flattened horizontally, with the corpus callosum above, the upper surface of the thalamus below, the fornix medially, and the much reduced body of the caudate nucleus lateral to it. Two small internal cerebral veins may be seen in the tela choroidea. The thalamus is much larger than in the preceding section but is not sharply defined, either from the internal capsule laterally or from the hypothalamus below. Although it consists of many subdivisions, both functionally and microscopically, on gross examination these are difficult or impossible to distinguish. Sometimes, a faint, pale line, the *internal medullary lamina*, may be seen running vertically through the thalamus.

In a section through the anterior part of the midbrain (Fig. 1-17), the cortex and white matter are much as before. The pattern of the hippocampus becomes more simple, and a mass of choroid plexus may be seen above it in the inferior horn of the lateral ventricle (a curved, slitlike area, above and lateral to the hippocampus). The plexus enters the ventricle through the choroidal fissure between the optic tract and hippocampus. In the roof of the inferior horn lies a small gray mass, the tail of the caudate nucleus; followed forward, this merges with the amygdala at the tip of the inferior horn; followed backward, it passes upward (around the posterior end of the thalamus) to join the body of the caudate. The insula is deeper, so that the opercula are broader. The temporal operculum is covered by gyri, which run from the lateral surface in toward the insula (*transverse temporal gyri*). The white matter of the temporal lobe is continuous with the frontoparietal white matter (on either side of the claustrum) and also with the posterior limb of the internal capsule (beneath the putamen and pallidum and above the optic tract: the sublenticular internal capsule). The putamen, pallidum, and claustrum have become smaller, and the medial division of the pallidum is no longer present. The posterior and sublenticular limbs of the internal capsule run directly into the peduncle. The fornix has become wider and flatter, but the shape and relationships of the lateral ventricles are little changed. The thalamus has become more rounded and blends inferiorly with the subthalamus. The *subthalamus* is a poorly defined, horizontal shelf of tissue projecting forward from the upper end of the midbrain and containing, in addition to white and gray matter (Forel's fields and zona incerta), a well-defined, lens-shaped mass, the *subthalamic nucleus*, which lies obliquely below the thalamus, immediately internal to the internal capsule. Between the subthalamic nuclei are the anterior edges of the *red nuclei*, and below and lateral to both is the oblique and pigmented upper end of the *substantia nigra*, also in direct contact with the internal capsule.

In a section through the center of the midbrain (not illustrated), the hippocampal gyrus has become simplified in cross section and shows a conspicuous "sickle" of white matter attached to its upper medial surface. This is the dentate fascia, which becomes continuous posteriorly with the laterally expanded fornix. The inferior horn retains the same slitlike contour and is closed medially by a pial membrane, from which the choroid plexus originates. The insula is now deeper and smaller, and the transverse temporal gyri are well marked. Claustrum, putamen, and pallidum have virtually disappeared, and there is continuity between temporal and frontoparietal white matter. That part of the white matter lying immediately lateral to the posterior thalamus (behind the putamen) is sometimes termed the *retrolenticular portion of the capsule*. The posterior margin of the sublenticular internal capsule is marked by the geniculate bodies, which lie inferolateral to the thalamus (without intervening white matter) and are generally considered part of it. The medial geniculate body is poorly defined from the thalamus proper. The lateral geniculate body, which lies in lateral contact with the medial geniculate body, has a yellowish-brown color and a "Napoleon's hat" shape, which makes it readily distinguishable. At this level, the thalamus is related inferiorly to the midbrain rather than the subthalamus, and the rounded red nuclei lie below it. The substantia nigra and cerebral peduncles are present. In the back of the third ventricle may be seen a horizontal bar (below the plane of section), which is the upper end of the dorsal midbrain (collicular) tissue. Below this bar the third ventricle becomes continuous with the aqueduct, and above the aqueduct it forms the pineal recess.

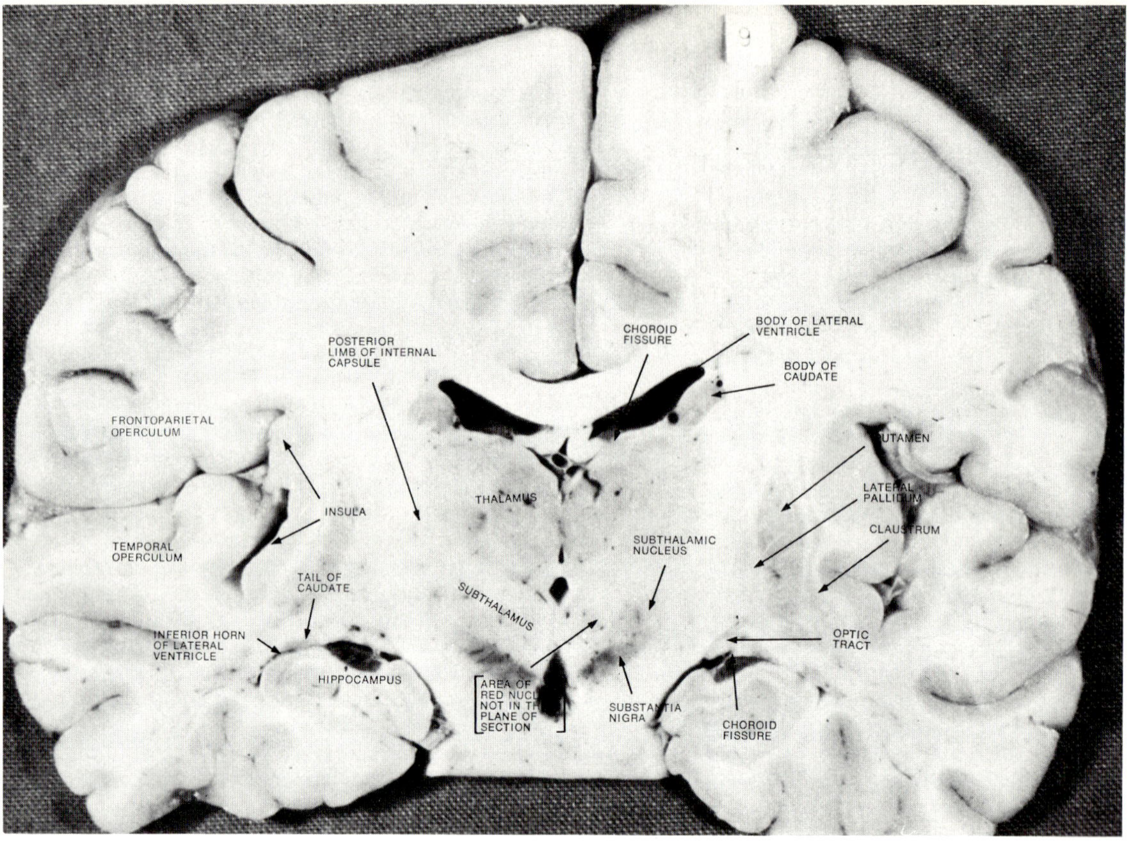

Fig. 1-17.

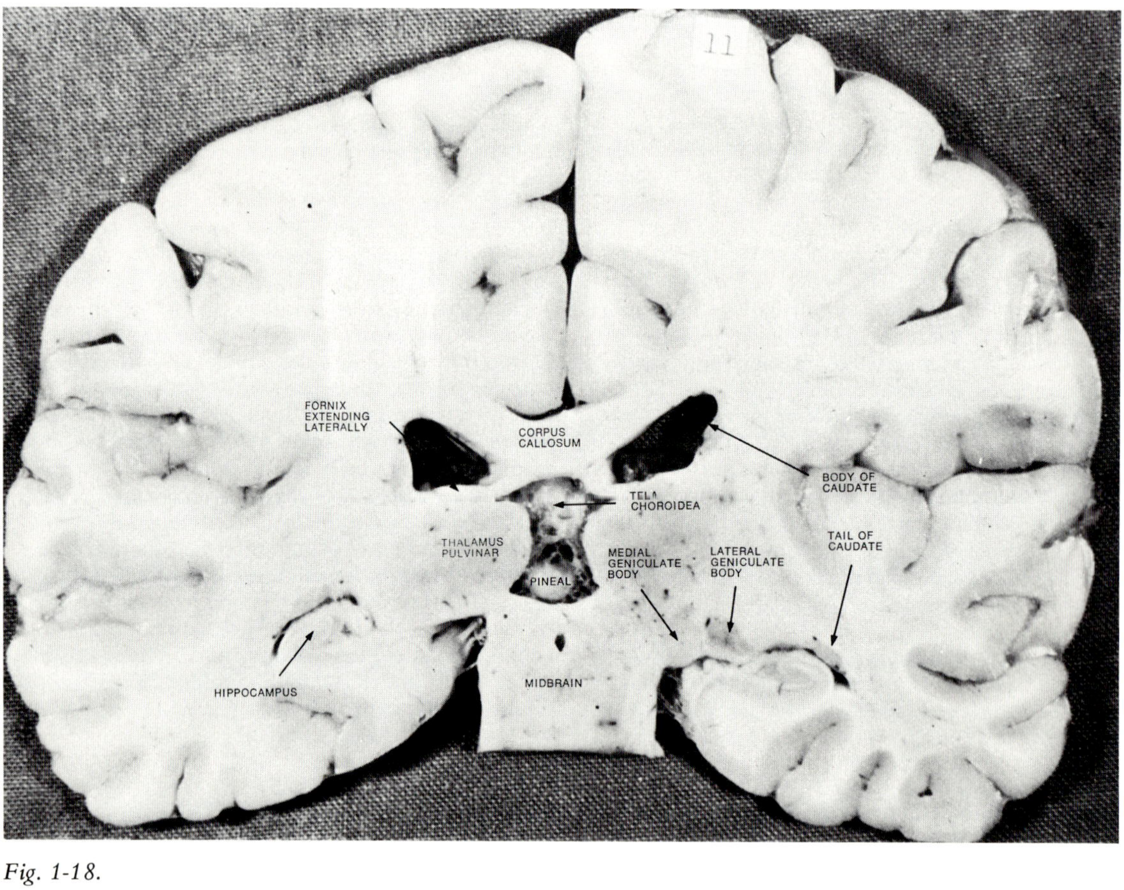

Fig. 1-18.

Fig. 1-17. Frontal section at level of posterior perforated substance and subthalamic nucleus.

Fig. 1-18. Frontal section at level of lateral geniculate body, pulvinar, and pineal gland.

In a section through the posterior edge of the midbrain (Fig. 1-18), the only deep gray matter remaining is the posterior end of the thalamus (pulvinar). This is attached inferomedially to the collicular region of the midbrain, with a wide intervening space formed by the expanded posterior end of the tela choroidea and containing the pineal gland below and the great cerebral vein (vein of Galen), formed by confluence of the internal cerebral and other veins above. The lateral ventricles are now more widely separated, as the fornices have moved laterally, and the caudate nucleus, both in the ventricle body and inferior horn, is small and inconspicuous. The insular floor has almost disappeared, though a deep sylvian fissure remains. At the posterior end of the thalamus the lateral ventricle abruptly changes in cross section from a horizontal to a large, oblique shape, inclined from the corpus callosum downward and laterally over the hippocampus and fornix. There it becomes continuous with the inferior horns and, passing posteriorly, becomes smaller, retaining the same shape, to become continuous with the posterior (occipital) horn.

At more posterior levels (not illustrated), only cortex and white matter are seen, with the progressively diminishing posterior horn situated ventromedially. The horn is indented from the medial aspect by the deep calcarine sulcus noted externally.

INTERNAL STRUCTURE OF THE CEREBELLUM, BRAIN STEM, AND SPINAL CORD

Much of the internal structure of the brain stem is not visible to naked eye examination but requires histological and even electrophysiological studies. This is because of the small size of the brain stem, in spite of the numerous structures it contains and a phylogenetically ancient lack of distinction between gray and white matter. A relatively brief description of the cerebellum, brain stem, and cord is therefore in order.

Structure of the Cerebellum

The cerebellum externally shows closely packed, narrow sulci, arranged approximately horizontally. The convolutions (*folia*) of the cerebellar cortex are therefore best seen by vertical or parasagittal sectioning. When cut in this way (Fig. 1-8), the cerebellum shows a thin, highly convoluted cortex, 1.0 to 1.5 mm in thickness, with finely branching white-matter cores and a relatively small mass of central white matter (corpus medullare), continuous with the middle cerebellar peduncles ventrally and the smaller superior and inferior peduncles above and below. If the cerebellum is cut transversely, it is seen that most of the white matter is laterally situated in the hemispheres, with a relatively thin layer in the midline (vermis), which is excavated by the tent-shaped fourth ventricle with a midline peak. A conspicuous structure within the lateral cerebellar white matter is a markedly folded, walnut-shaped gray layer, the *dentate nucleus,* which has an opening directed medially and upward. On transverse section the dentate nuclei are seen to be obliquely arranged on either side of the fourth ventricle roof, inclined ventrally and laterally. Between them, also in the roof of the fourth ventricle (Fig. 1-19), are several less distinct, older but smaller cerebellar nuclei. (Unfortunately, the cerebellar nuclei are not quite in alphabetical order; from lateral to medial they are the dentate, emboliform, globose, and fastigial.) The cerebellum is anatomically divided into lobes, but these seem to be of minimal clinical importance in the current state of knowledge.

Structure of the Brain Stem

Structure of the Midbrain

Transverse sections of the midbrain (Fig. 1-20 *E* and *F*), a short structure, show a butterfly shape, broader rostrally (*F*) (because the cerebral peduncles diverge as they enter the forebrain). The aqueduct, which is 2 or 3 mm in diameter, is situated dorsally in the midline; it expands at its upper end into the third ventricle and at its lower end into the fourth ventricle. Dorsolateral to the aqueduct the low, rounded colliculi project from the midbrain surface, two superior and two inferior, but little internal structure can be made out. The aqueduct is surrounded by the periaqueductal gray matter, somewhat heart-shaped; broader dorsally, it extends beneath the colliculi and then has concave, ventrolateral borders, which rapidly converge to the ventral midline. In some brains it can be clearly distinguished. In the upper midbrain, the rounded red nuclei (which are somewhat pink in the fresh brain, but tan in color after formalin fixation), 6 to 8 mm across, lie ventrolateral to the periaqueductal gray matter, surrounded by thin capsules of white matter that coalesce in the midline. The cerebral peduncles, broad, flattened bands, project ventrolaterally, separated in the ventral midline by a deep cleft. Separating the peduncle from the central midbrain is the slightly curved, irregular, pigmented substantia nigra, gray or black in appearance. The peduncles consist of uniform white tissue. (If the sections are very high, the lower tip of the medial geniculate body may be present in the groove between the dorsal edge of the cerebral peduncle and the superior colliculus.)

Structure of the Pons

The shape of transverse sections through the pons varies with the level (Fig. 1-20 *C* and *D*) partly because the middle cerebellar peduncles slope downward as they pass back into the cerebellum.

Sections through the upper pons (Fig. 1-20 *D*) take the shape of an extremely fat pear, the broad part being the basal pons and the narrow part the tegmentum or dorsal pons. The basal pons is streaky

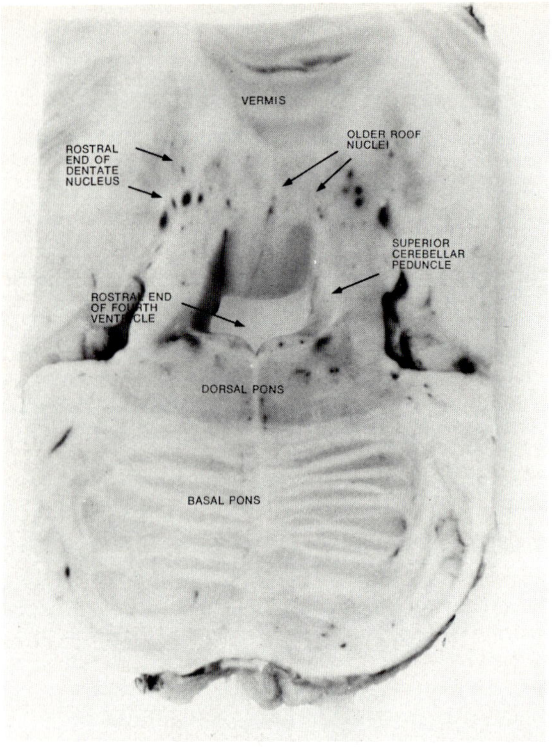

Fig. 1-19. Slightly oblique transverse section of pons and cerebellar white matter to show deep cerebellar nuclei.

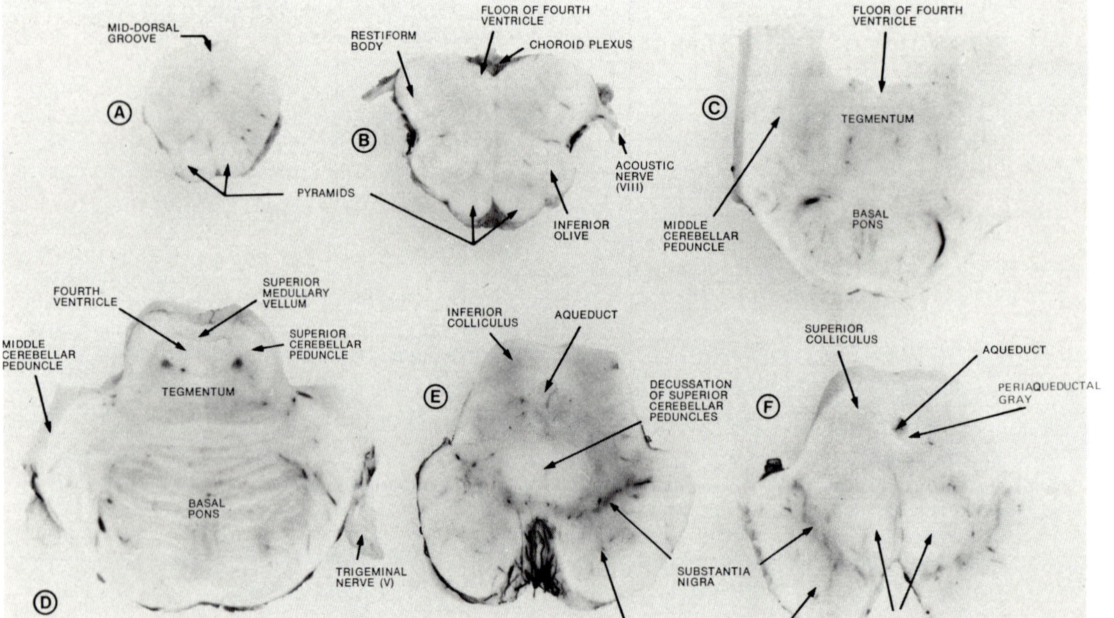

Fig. 1-20. Transverse sections of brain stem at representative levels. A and B = medulla; C and D = pons; E and F = midbrain – all in ascending order.

in appearance, showing horizontal, narrow white bands interspersed with irregular gray areas. The bands are myelinated fibers that run to the middle cerebellar peduncle or through the pons to the medulla and cord. The gray areas are the pontine nuclei. In the tegmentum, the aqueduct has widened to form the triangular upper end of the fourth ventricle, covered on its dorsal aspect only by a very thin layer of tissue (anterior medullary velum). Its two ventrolateral boundaries are the periventricular gray matter, continuous with periaqueductal gray matter above and sometimes distinguishable by the naked eye. This part of the tegmentum contains the superior cerebellar peduncles cut transversely, appearing as well-defined, round white areas, one on either side in the tegmentum or joined in the midline as they cross over.

The middle (Fig. 1-20 *C*) and lower pons are wider than the upper pons and are continuous dorsolaterally with the middle cerebellar peduncles. Of the middle pons, approximately two-thirds is the base; this is similar in appearance and structure to the corresponding part of the upper pons. The dorsal one-third is the tegmentum, which lies in the floor of the widened fourth ventricle. The tegmentum is bounded both ventrally and laterally by the base and middle cerebellar peduncles, and no clear structures may be seen within it. The fourth ventricle is widest at the junction of the pons and medulla, and here are situated the lateral recesses and foramina of Luschka.

Structure of the Medulla

Sections through the upper medulla (Fig. 1-20 *B*) show its dorsal part to be slightly wider than its ventral part. Most ventral are the pyramids, consisting of triangular or crescentic fields of white matter, partially separated in the midline by the ventral groove. Immediately dorsal to the pyramids and projecting slightly from the surface are the inferior olivary nuclei, consisting of convoluted laminae of gray matter, open medially. The dorsal part of the section shows two dorsolateral masses, which are continuous above with the inferior cerebellar peduncles. Between these, forming the floor of the wide fourth ventricle, is an area with no obvious internal structure. A median raphe is usually apparent, running from the midline of the fourth ventricle to the midventral cleft between the pyramids. The fourth ventricle is roofed by a thin tela choroidea, similar to that of third ventricle, bearing tufts of choroid plexus (but this is almost invariably ruptured during handling of the brain).

Sections through the lower medulla (Fig. 1-20 *A*) below the tip of the fourth ventricle, are approximately round, with two ventral projections corresponding to the pyramids. A much more shallow mid-dorsal groove is apparent, which does not represent a continuation of the fourth ventricle, but rather of the mid-dorsal groove of the spinal cord from below. No other structures are readily discernible on the cut surface.

Structure of the Spinal Cord

Transverse sections of the spinal cord show the same general structure throughout, although the size and proportions of the central gray and peripheral white matter vary. The central gray is approximately H-shaped, with a thin bar extending across the midline; two dorsal horns project dorsolaterally, nearly to the surface of the cord; and two anterior horns project anteriorly and somewhat less laterally, approaching less closely to the cord surface. The gray matter is more bulky in the cervical and lumbosacral enlargements, especially in the anterior horns, which are wider and blunter than in other regions. In the upper cervical and thoracic regions, the anterior and dorsal horns are of approximately the same size. Since much of the white matter is composed of fibers connecting all levels of cord to the brain, it becomes progressively thicker at higher levels. This is particularly noticeable in the dorsal (posterior) columns between the dorsal horns, which are represented by a narrow rectangular area in the lumbosacral region, but have a broad, triangular contour in the cervical area. The posterior (sensory) roots enter the cord opposite and slightly medial to the tips of the dorsal horns. The anterior (motor) roots originate in small branches over a somewhat wider anterolateral segment of the cord circumference. A small lateral horn may be seen in the thoracic region, projecting between the anterior and dorsal horns, but is not present in cervical or lumbosacral cord.

THE VENTRICULAR SYSTEM

It is possible at this stage to try and synthesize from the preceding observations the shape of the cerebral ventricular system, though this is more easily appreciated in horizontal and parasagittal cuts (Fig. 1-21). Each cerebral hemisphere contains a lateral ventricle (the *first* and *second* ventricles), consisting of a central region (the body) with three projections of unequal size, resembling a wishbone or spur. The anterior (frontal) horn is the largest projection and merges with the body. The body tapers backward as the occipital (posterior) horn and also gives off an inferiorly recurved temporal (inferior) horn.

The anterior horns are triangular in section, separated in the midline only by the septum pellucidum. Their upper surface is the corpus callosum, and their concave inferolateral surface is the head of the caudate nucleus. Arbitrarily, the anterior horn becomes the body at the level of the foramen of Monro. The anterior part of the body is, in cross section, a horizontally flattened rectangle, the medial margin being the fornix, the corpus callosum lying above, the caudate nucleus laterally, and the upper surface of the thalamus inferiorly. It contains an expansion of the tela choroidea of the third ventricle, which enters between thalamus and fornix, forming a choroid plexus (which is absent from the anterior horn). At the posterior end of the thalamus, the body of the ventricle becomes deeper, and the choroid plexus is thickest in this area. The choroid

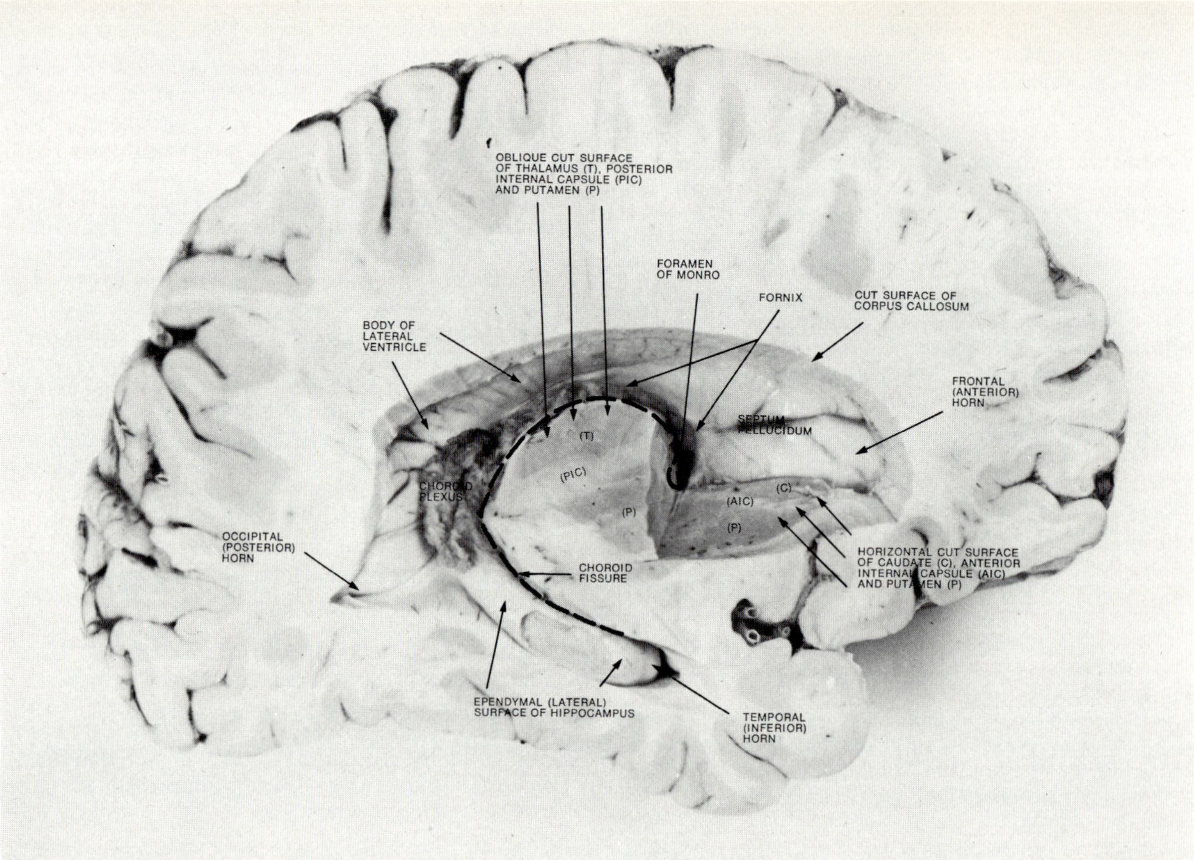

Fig. 1-21. Parasagittal section of right cerebral hemisphere viewed from the lateral aspect, to show lateral ventricle. (Much of the thalamus, internal capsule, and basal ganglia, a little occipital white matter, and part of the corpus callosum have been removed.)

fissure continues to separate the thalamus and midbrain from the fornix and dentate fascia, admitting the choroid plexus of the inferior horn. The inferior horn is a narrow, curved, slitlike cavity, above and lateral to the hippocampus, with the tail of the caudate nucleus running in its roof and terminating at the amygdala. The posterior horn is a progressively narrowing, backward extension of the body of the ventricle, maintaining the same oblique orientation in the ventromedial part of the occipital lobe and indented from its medial or inferomedial aspect by the calcarine cortex and white matter.

Cerebrospinal fluid formed in the lateral ventricles has only one route of egress, namely, through the foramina of Monro into the third ventricle. The third ventricle is a vertical midline structure, whose roof is formed by tela choroidea, and it has its own choroid plexus. Fluid produced in the lateral and third ventricles passes through the aqueduct to reach the fourth ventricle. The fourth ventricle is diamond-shaped when viewed from behind and triangular in transverse sections. Its floor is relatively flat, but has several shallow markings, indicating underlying structures. The upper roof of the fourth ventricle, between the superior cerebellar peduncles, is a glial membrane without choroid plexus. The roof of the lower part is tela choroidea with choroid plexus and probably contains a midline foramen (of Magendie). From the widest part of the ventricle there are two lateral, open recesses emerging between the cerebellum and the middle cerebellar peduncle as the foramina of Luschka. Although in fetal life the fourth ventricle was continuous with the central canal of the spinal cord, the latter is completely obliterated, and the inferior angle of the fourth ventricle becomes a blind end. Thus, the only route of flow for cerebrospinal fluid is from lateral ventricles to third ventricle, through the aqueduct to the fourth ventricle, and out into the subarachnoid space of the posterior fossa.

Cells of the Central Nervous System

2

The central nervous system (CNS) includes two classes of cells, of which the most thoroughly investigated have been the neurons, the primary functional elements. These are elongated, branching cells with definite polarity (conducting in one direction only), which by making functional (not syncytial) connections with one another, form complex cell networks. They receive sensory information from the body, and (indirectly) from the environment, process the data thus made available, compare them with stored data, and issue appropriate instructions (via the motor nerves, autonomic system, or neuroendocrine systems) directed toward favorably modifying the internal milieu, the environment, or both. The second category comprises the glial cells, long regarded merely as space-fillers or the "skeleton" for the neurons and much less intensively investigated. Four types of glial cells are recognized, although one type, the microglia, are actually mesenchymal (reticuloendothelial) cells, resident within the CNS, and another type, ependymal cells, are found only in relation to the ventricles and central canal of the cord. The other two types, astrocytes and oligodendroglia, are present in all parts of the CNS, intimately mixed with the neurons. They have functions beyond the mere filling of interstitial space. Thus, they are probably concerned with the entry of water and solutes into the CNS, control of the extracellular space, formation and maintenance of myelin sheaths, possibly metabolism of the neurons themselves, and reaction to damage or loss of neurons.

HISTOGENESIS

Except for microglial cells, these diverse types of cells originate in a columnar epithelium (Fig. 2-1), visible in the dorsal axis of the human embryo by 20 days as a deep midline groove. By the twenty-third day, the edges have fused to form the closed neural tube, except at the extreme anterior and posterior ends. This tube is rapidly separated by mesenchyme from the overlying epithelium. In the process of separation, dorsolateral longitudinal bands of cells, the neural crests, are formed. These are important in developing the peripheral nervous system (except for somatic motor and autonomic preganglionic fibers), the meninges, the accessory cells of peripheral nerves, and melanocytes.

Epithelium in the neural groove is already pseudostratified, mitoses being restricted to the free surface. This arrangement is continued in the closed neural tube, so that mitoses occur adjacent to the lumen, in conspicuous rounded cells interspersed among the columnar epithelium (ependymal zone). The mantle zone, composed of closely packed nuclei, is rapidly formed around the ependymal zone, and beyond this (adjacent to mesenchyme) is a relatively anuclear marginal zone. In spite of the three-layered appearance, electron microscopy shows that all cells are radial, with one process attached to the external limiting membrane and the other attached to its fellows and to the luminal surface by terminal bars.

Experiments with colchicine or vincristine, which arrest mitosis, show that mitotic figures accumulate in both ependymal and mantle zones. Estimation of nuclear DNA content indicates accumulation in the mantle zone, presumably preparatory to mitotic division. The conclusion (Fig. 2-2) is that cells in both zones are capable of mitosis, their nuclei moving to the ependymal zone for this process. Mitotic spindles are arranged parallel to the lumen, so that each daughter cell retains its terminal bar attachment to the luminal surface. Confirmation of this nuclear migration has been obtained by injection of tritiated thymidine. This disappears from the circulation within an hour of injection and can therefore be incorporated in DNA only during this period. Examination of neuroepithelium 1 hour after injection shows labeling of DNA in the mantle zone, 4 hours after injection most of the DNA is adjacent to the lumen in dividing cells, and about 4 hours after this it has reverted to the mantle zone. Thus, at this stage, there is a uniform cell population (neuroepithelial cells), without recognizable differentiation of neuronal and glial precursors, and there is no essential distinction between mantle and ependymal zones.

However, shortly after the neural groove closes, a layer of rounded cells appears adjacent to the external limiting membrane. This layer does not take up tritiated thymidine, so the cells are not synthesizing DNA. These cells have a rounded nucleus with a small, prominent nucleolus and are considered to be neuron precursors (neuroblasts). Five to six hours after thymidine injection they are joined by more cells of similar morphology but containing radioactive DNA; these have arisen from the previously undiffer-

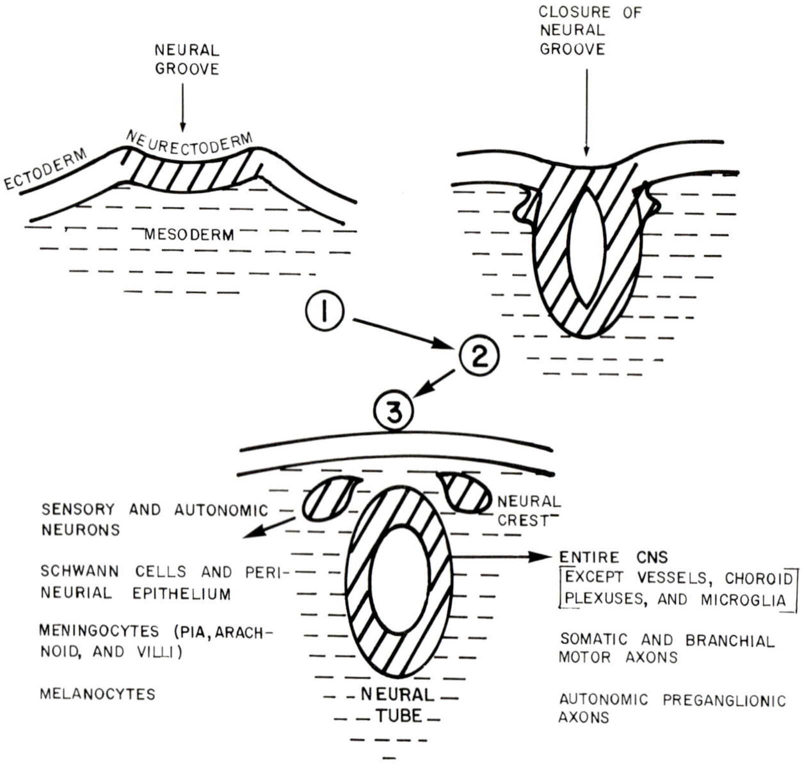

Fig. 2-1. Transverse sections through dorsal axial region (1) of embryo early in fourth week, showing closure of neural groove (2), separation of neural crests (3), and their adult derivatives.

entiated neuroepithelial cells. For a short period, neuroblasts retain their connection with the ependymal surface by a fine process, the *transient dendrite.* When they lose this process, they become rounded cells adjacent to the external limiting membrane, incapable of further division. In the spinal cord and brain stem they remain relatively central and mature to form the nuclei of the gray matter (Fig. 2-3). Neurons of the cerebellum are formed partly from neuroepithelial cells lining the rostral edges of the fourth ventricle (rhombic lip) and partly from similar displaced cells that migrate from the rhombic lip, over the surface of the developing cerebellum, to form the external granular layer (which is neuroepithelial, not neuronal, in nature). In the cerebral hemispheres, newly formed neuroblasts from the region of the lateral ventricles migrate outward to form the cerebral cortex. Later-maturing neuroblasts migrate through the earlier layers, so that the cerebral cortex is formed, as it were, from within outward, the superficial cells being those most recently formed.

In summary, the lineage of neurons is reasonably well understood. They are the first cells to differentiate from the neuroepithelium and are then incapable of further division, merely migrating as necessary to take up their position in the mature CNS. The only recognized precursal form is the rounded neuroblast, with relatively short, inconspicuous cell processes.

Little comparable experimental work has been done on the derivation of glial cells. Their origin from undifferentiated neuroepithelial cells has been demonstrated by tritiated thymidine, which first labels a proportion of neuroblasts and only some

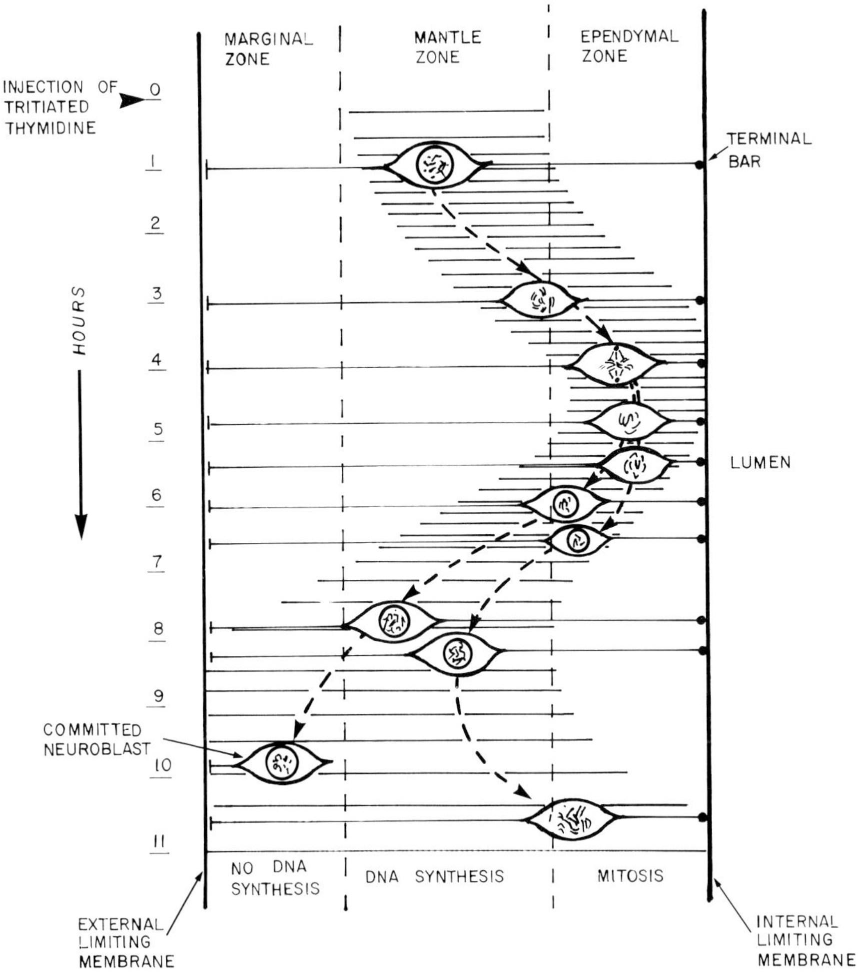

Fig. 2-2. Cycle of nuclear migration in the primitive neural epithelium demonstrated by injection of ^{3}H-thymidine. The shaded area represents radioactivity, as determined by autoradiography. At first confined to premitotic cells synthesizing DNA in the mantle zone, activity moves into the ependymal zone, where mitoses occur, then back again. Activity in the marginal zone is due to the differentiation of committed (unipotential) neuroblasts.

days later labels mature astrocytes and oligodendroglia. The morphology of the intermediate stages is by no means clear, though immature glial cells, with either a single process running to the external limiting membrane or with no long processes, are clearly recognized and are designated *spongioblasts.* Unlike neuroblasts, these cells remain capable of division by mitosis, up to at least the fourth or fifth month in the human embryo and perhaps later in CNS damage. It appears probable that the spongioblast is a common ancestor for both astrocytes and oligodendroglia and that a number of these undifferentiated cells persist after birth (Fig. 2-3), since they would be required for the postnatal production of oligodendroglia with continuing myelination. The lack of clear lines of development in glial formation is reflected in the confusion in glial tumor nomenclature (see Chap. 25).

NEURONS

The neuron is the functional element of the CNS, and whatever new importance may be ascribed to the glial cells, it is generally assumed that they function in a supportive, not a conductive, role. Each neuron has a cell body (perikaryon, or soma) that contains the nucleus, is 5 to 75μ in diameter and may be

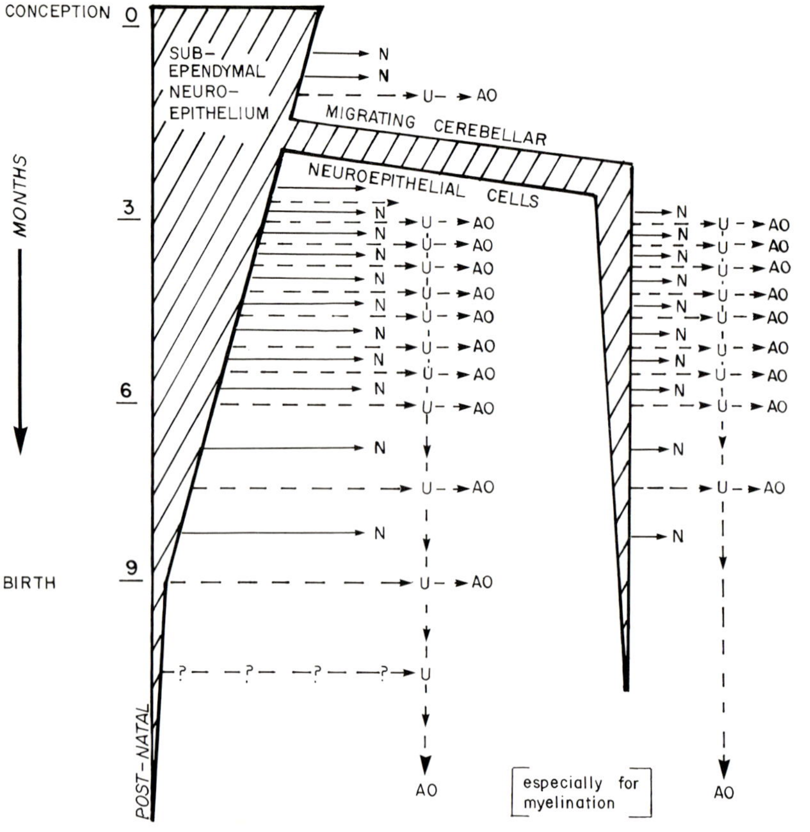

Fig. 2-3. Differentiation of CNS cells. The shaded area represents multipotential (neuroepithelial) cells either remaining adjacent to the ependyma (left) or migrating over the cerebellum (right). Neuroblasts (N) can only migrate and mature, whereas glial precursor cells (U) can also undergo mitotic division, ultimately differentiating as astrocytes (A) and oligodendroglia (O). Some precursor cells may persist in postnatal life, and serve as a source of new oligodendroglia accompanying myelination.

rounded, polygonal, or elongated (pyramidal) (Fig. 2-4). From the cell body arise several or many dendrites, which are frequently branching processes that may extend as much as 1 mm from the cell body and resemble it in function and ultrastructure. Conduction is afferent, toward the cell body. With a few minor exceptions, there is only one axon, or efferent process, varying tremendously in length from 200μ up to 1 meter. At its origin the axon is thinner than the dendrites and it divides much less often except at its termination, where it forms numerous branches (telodendria). In some neurons the axoplasm may have a thousand times the volume of the cell body.

Each neuron (cell body and processes) is completely enclosed by a continuous plasmalemma and has no cytoplasmic continuity with other neurons. However, close functional continuity is established at the synapses, which usually occur between axonal branches on the one hand and dendrites or cell bodies on the other. (There are other types of synapses.) Conduction across the synapse is unidirectional, from axon to dendrite or soma. Because of the extremely complex branching of dendrites and axons, a single axon may form synapses with thousands of nerve cells, and a single nerve cell may have synaptic connections with thousands of axons. Thus, neural networks too complex for visualization are built up. The overall shape of a neuron, including the density and distribution of its processes, is the key to its function but unfortunately is very difficult to determine.

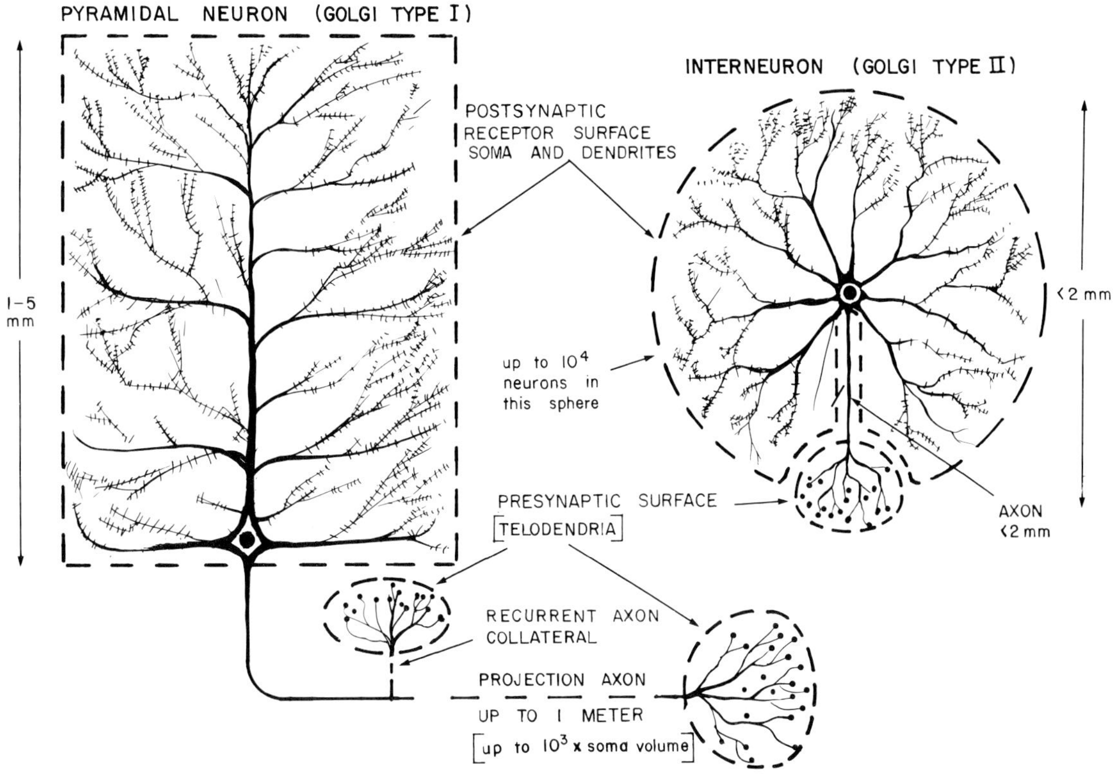

Fig. 2-4. Two types of neuron from the cerebral cortex. The Golgi type I cells (pyramidal, polymorphic) have long axons leaving the cortex (projection fibers), whereas the type II (granule) cells are locally distributed. Large numbers of these type II interneurons are responsible for the voluminous cortex of primates, especially man.

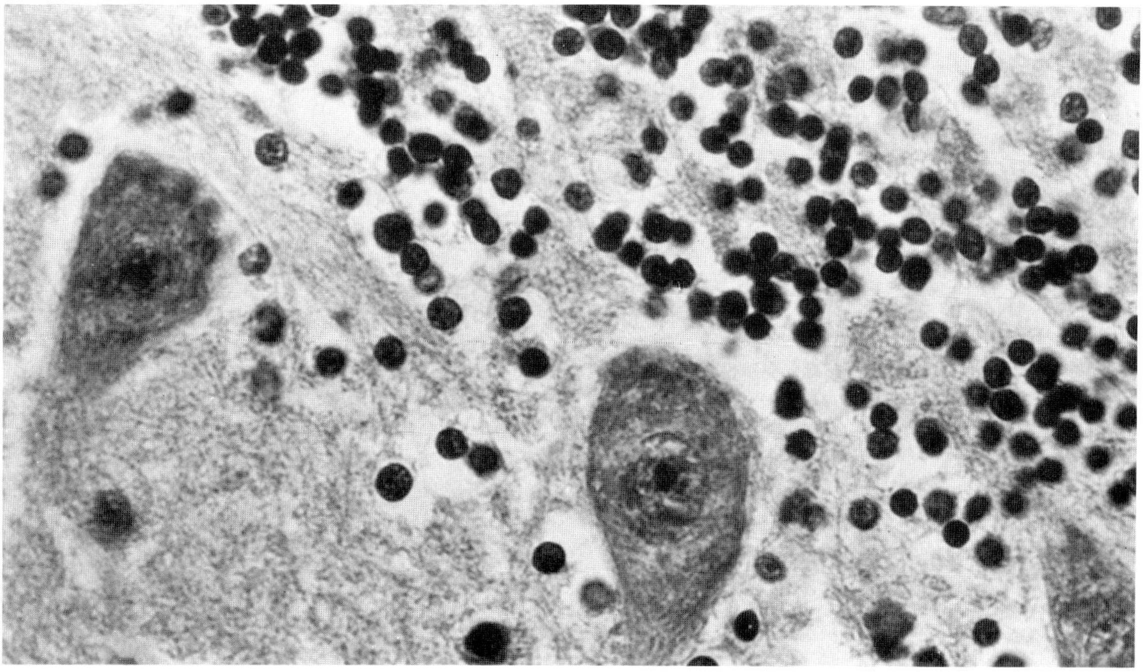

Fig. 2-5. Extremes in the morphology of normal neurons; Purkinje's cells and internal granular cells. (H & E, X750.)

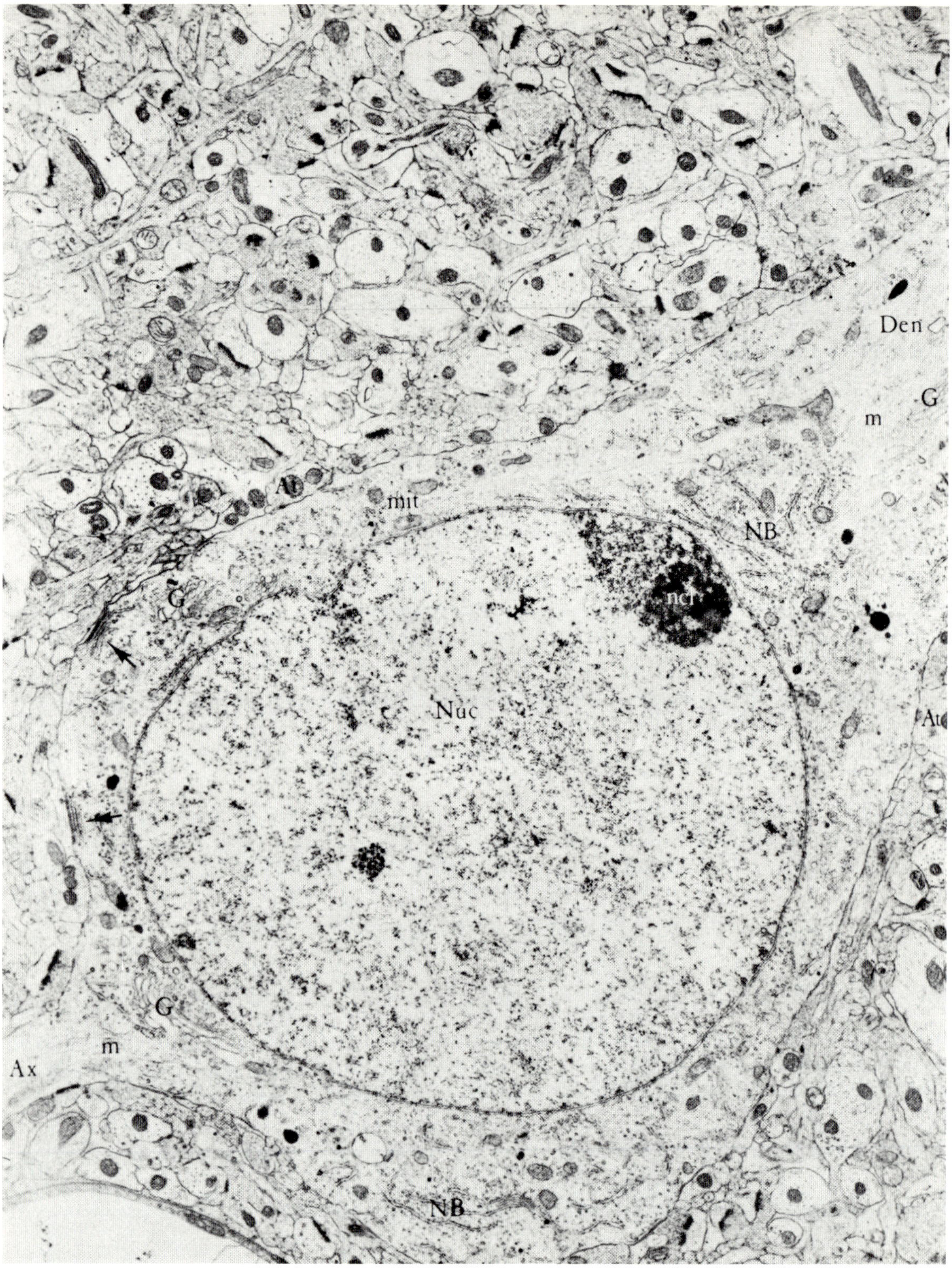
Den
G
m
At
mit
NB
ncl
G
Nuc
At
G
m
Ax
NB

Fig. 2-6. Cell body of a cortical pyramidal neuron (rat). Nuc = nucleus; ncl = nucleolus; NB = Nissl bodies; G = Golgi apparatus; mit = mitochondria; m = microtubules; Ax = axon; Den = apical dendrite; At = axon terminals forming synapses. (X12,000.) (From Peters, Palay, and Webster.)

Since microscopic sections are 5 to 20μ thick, a complete neuron is never seen. Instead, cell bodies with short segments of attached dendrites and axons, and many isolated segments of dendrites and axons from cell bodies elsewhere, are included in the section. It is therefore legitimate to describe the morphology of the cell body, dendrite, and axon separately, although of course they represent only parts of a single cell. Further justification for separate treatment lies in the fact that they are usually demonstrated by different staining techniques, and that in the minute fragments of tissue used for electron microscopy pieces of cells can only be identified by variations in their ultrastructure (and then often not with total certainty).

Cell Body

Some neurons are only 5 to 6μ in diameter, usually rounded, with little cytoplasm. Medium-sized and larger neurons may be rounded, elongated or pyramidal, and as large as 70 to 80μ (Fig. 2-5). In small neurons the nucleus is dark and uniform, with clumped chromatin; in larger cells it is pale, usually central, with a conspicuous nucleolus, and, while usually round, may show flattening or even creases. The cytoplasm contains variable numbers of irregular, triangular, or dustlike basophilic particles (Nissl bodies), which are particularly prominent in motoneurons, but have varying distribution, often specific to different cell types. Nissl bodies are reduced or absent near the origin of the axon (axon hillock). By silver impregnation, neurofibrils may be seen within the cell body as straight, unbranched structures entering dendrites and axons.

The cell body (Fig. 2-6) is surrounded by a typical three-layered plasmalemma, 75 to 80 A thick, the inner dark layer being thicker. The nucleus is enveloped in a double membrane. Each layer is about 75 A thick and the layers are separated by 150 A. The inner membrane is smooth but the outer is continuous with part of the endoplasmic reticulum (even a few ribosomes may be attached externally). The entire membrane shows pores about 700 A across, closed by a slightly thickened plate with a central electron-dense area, and has an underlying fibrous membrane. The nucleus contains a prominent electron-dense nucleolus without a membrane, partly granular and partly fibrillary in structure. The nuclear matrix is more electron-lucent and contains irregular chains of granules, whose visibility depends on fixation.

Neuronal cytoplasm contains extensive endoplasmic reticulum, largely granular, which presumably correlates with the high rate of protein synthesis. It forms closed, linear profiles of irregular shape and extent (Nissl bodies consist of closely set, parallel arrays of such membranes), occasionally with small cisterns just internal to the plasmalemma but not communicating with it. Associated with the granular endoplasmic reticulum are polysomes, clusters of free ribosomes in rosette, spiral, or linear formation.

Golgi's complex is a special part of the nongranular reticulum, forming packed, flat, often fenestrated cisterns or vesicles, 200 to 600 A wide, around the cell nucleus. Some vesicles have 150 A projecting spines on the outer surface, representing septa separating hexagonal compartments on the outside of the vesicle (alveolate or coated vesicles). These either bud from, or coalesce with, cisterns of Golgi's complex and include hydrolases (acid phosphatase among others). Larger (1000-A) alveolate vesicles originate from the plasmalemma by pinocytosis, and possibly both types empty their contents into multivesicular bodies, converting them to lysosomes. Other lysosomes contain granular or mixed granular-fibrillary material and (possibly) also are derived from Golgi's complex.

Other cell organelles include mitochondria and usually lipofuscin granules. Microtubules and neurofilaments, less conspicuous than in the cell processes, form interlacing bundles, perhaps representing routes of movement for lysosomes and mitochondria. It is probably clumping of microtubules and neurofilaments that forms the neurofibrils seen on light microscopy.

Dendrites

Each neuron has multiple branching dendrites, arising from the apex, apex and base, or even the entire surface of the cell body (Fig. 2-7). They are relatively broad, tapering processes, which branch freely at acute angles and show short lateral projections (dendrite spines). Spines are usually more numerous in the intermediate and distal parts of the dendrite, have a narrow neck and a bulbous tip that forms the postsynaptic membrane, and are about 2μ in length. Their morphology is variable, even on a single dendrite. Dendrites, unlike axons, rarely extend more than 1 mm from the cell body and are not myelinated. Light microscopy on routine sections shows only the bases of dendrites attached to cell bodies, containing Nissl bodies and filamentous structures. The full complexity of dendritic branching can only be seen in special preparations. This development is a late stage in neuronal maturation, probably not complete for almost two years after birth in the human being and responsible for the decreased packing density of neurons (cell bodies) in the primate cortex as compared with subprimates and also for the progressive reduction of packing density during the first year or two of life. In the human neonate the cerebral cortex contains 60,000 to 440,000 neurons per cubic millimeter, whereas at 2 years of age these figures are reduced to 6,000 to 35,000. A mature dendritic tree may have a hundred times the surface area of its parent cell body.

Under the electron microscope (Fig. 2-8), dendrites are seen to contain large numbers of micro-

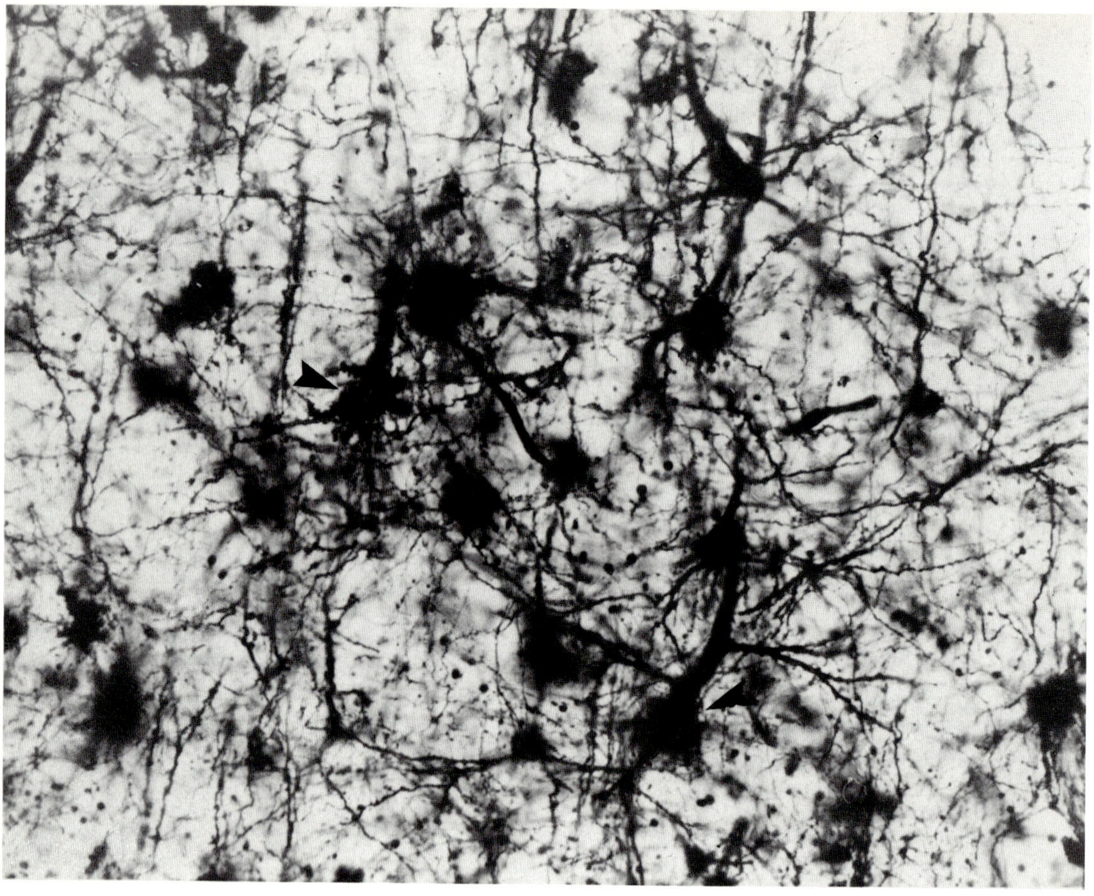

Fig. 2-7. Dendrites in cerebral cortex, pyramidal (arrows) and granular cells. Note the short spines on many dendrites. (Golgi-Cox method, X300.)

tubules (180 to 240 A across), but few neurofilaments. Mitochondria and nongranular endoplasmic reticulum are often elongated along the cell process; granular reticulum and ribosomes are present at the base, but diminish distally. As in the cell body, the plasmalemma is modified to form postsynaptic membranes, especially on the spines; these do not contain tubules or filaments, but show a characteristically "fluffy" cytoplasm, possibly due to small fibrillae. In the cerebral cortex only, there is often a *spine apparatus*, consisting of two or three flattened cisterns with intervening dense material.

Although present in almost all cells of the body, microtubules are especially numerous in neuronal cell bodies, dendrites, and axons. They are hollow, unbranched structures of indefinite length, and transverse sections show a circular arrangement of 12 to 13 subunits, often with a central electron-dense area. Side arms may be seen, forming cross bridges if the tubules are less than 400 A apart (as in the initial segment of the axon). Microtubules are an essential constituent of cilia, flagella, tails of spermatozoa, and mitotic spindles, but their role in the neuron is not clear. They may be associated with the formation of neuronal processes, maintenance of neuronal shape, or with axoplasmic flow (see Chap. 3). Microtubules are dissociated by colchicine and vincristine into protein subunits with a molecular weight of 100 to 130,000.

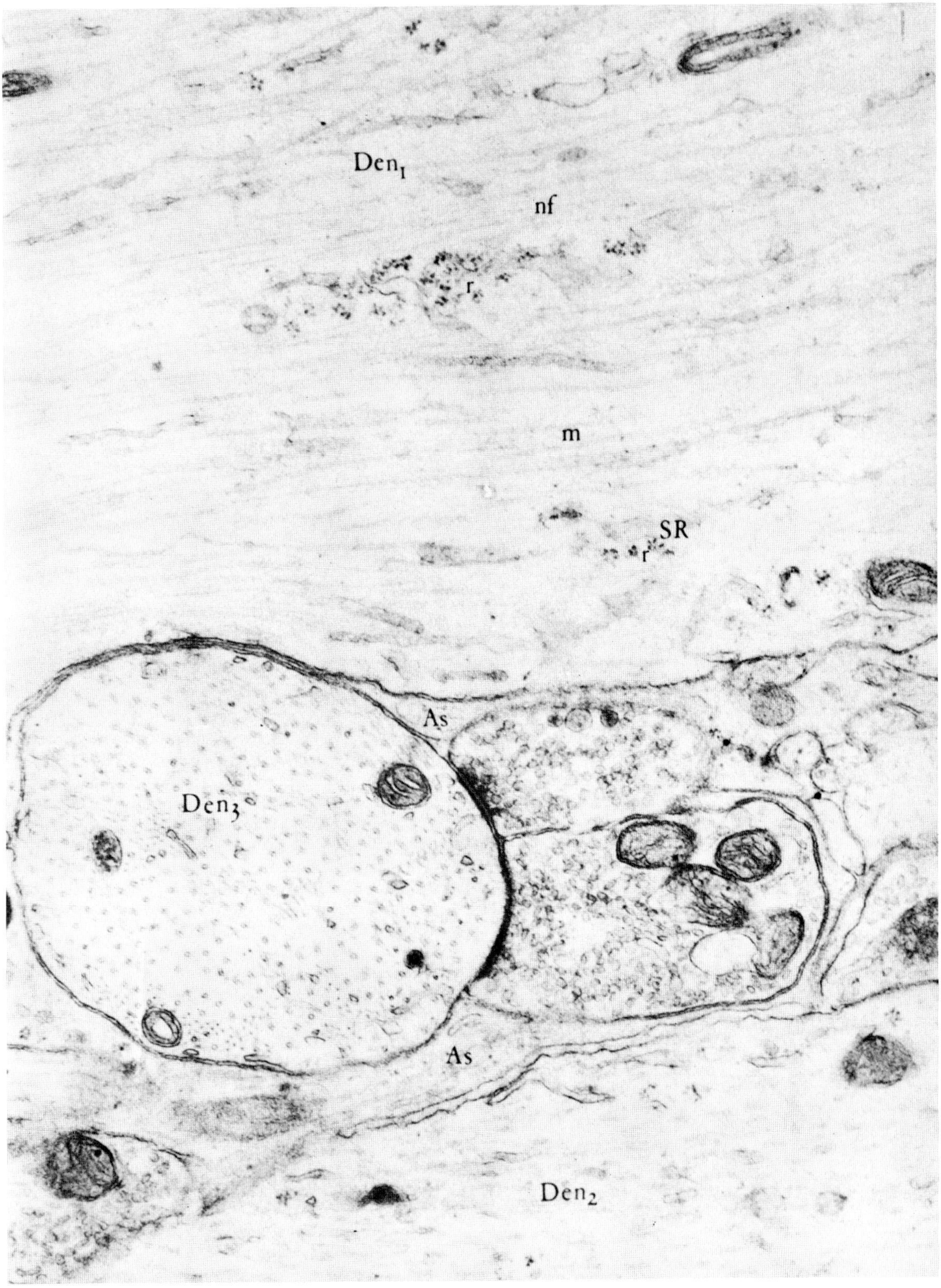

Fig. 2-8. Dendrites from spinal cord in longitudinal and transverse section (rat). Den_1 and Den_2 are cut longitudinally, Den_3 transversely; m = microtubules; nf = neurofilaments; SR = nongranular endoplasmic reticulum; r = ribosomes. Two synaptic terminals synapse on the right side of Den_3, and the synapses show an astrocytic sheath (As). (X41,000.) (From Peters, Palay, and Webster.)

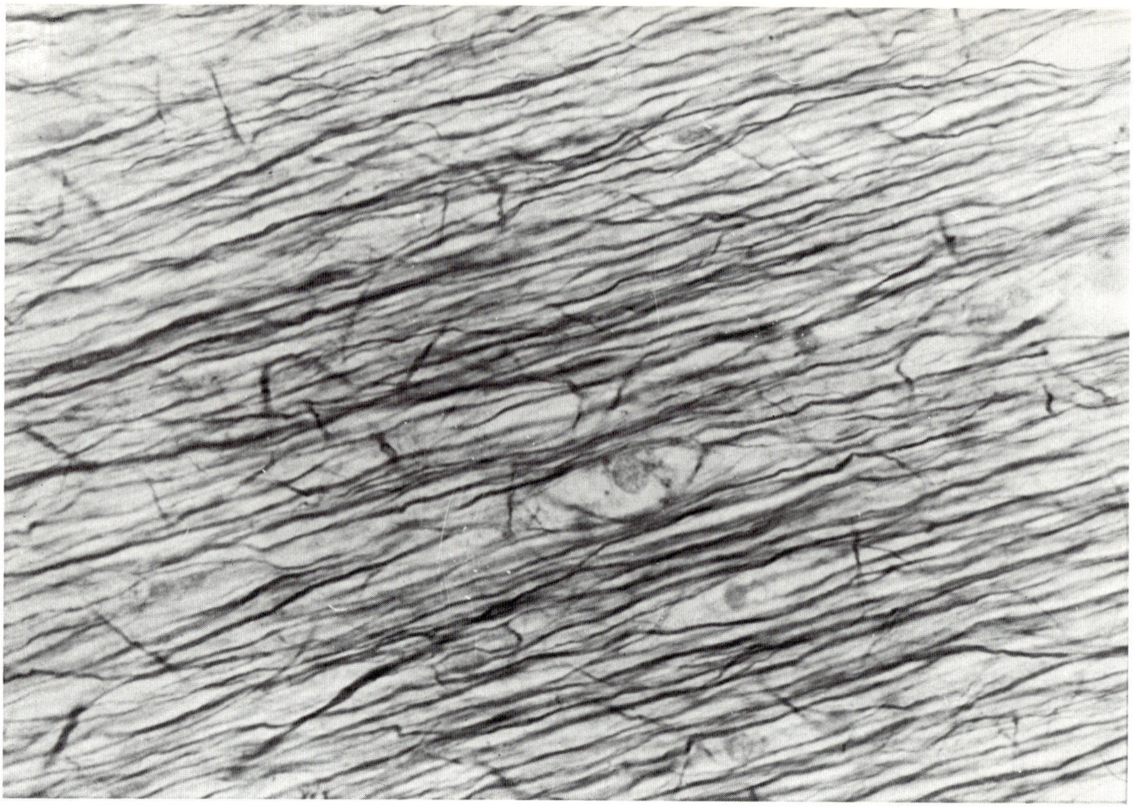

Fig. 2-9. Normal axons from the cerebellar white matter in longitudinal section. (Silver, X750.)

Axons

A nerve cell produces only one axon, which is narrow at its origin (initial segment), but then remains of uniform caliber as far as its terminal branches. A few branches of the main stem arise at right angles, and the length varies from less than 1 mm up to 1 meter. In routine sections, axons cannot be seen, though their origin from larger cells may be located by the absence of Nissl bodies. Such axon hillocks are not present in medium-sized and small neurons. Special techniques demonstrate axons under light microscopy, but show no internal structure (Fig. 2-9). Many axons have a concentric lipid and protein (myelin) sheath of variable thickness (see p. 36).

Axons contain microtubules and neurofilaments. Tubules are conspicuous during development and in nonmyelinated forms, but mature, myelinated axons contain more neurofilaments. Microtubules are conspicuous in the constricted initial segment of the axon (Fig. 2-10), where they may be only 250 A apart and show cross bridging. Neurofilaments are only 80 to 90 A across and seem to be composed of subunits in either linear or helical array. They rarely show side arms. These subunits (molecular weight 75,000) may be different from those of tubules, but there is experimental evidence for the interchangeability of these two organelles. Axons contain few mitochondria (often elongated), small (300 to 500 A) vesicles, and scanty longitudinal cisterns (probably nongranular reticulum). They are generally considered not to contain granular endoplasmic reticulum or ribosomes. The axonal mem-

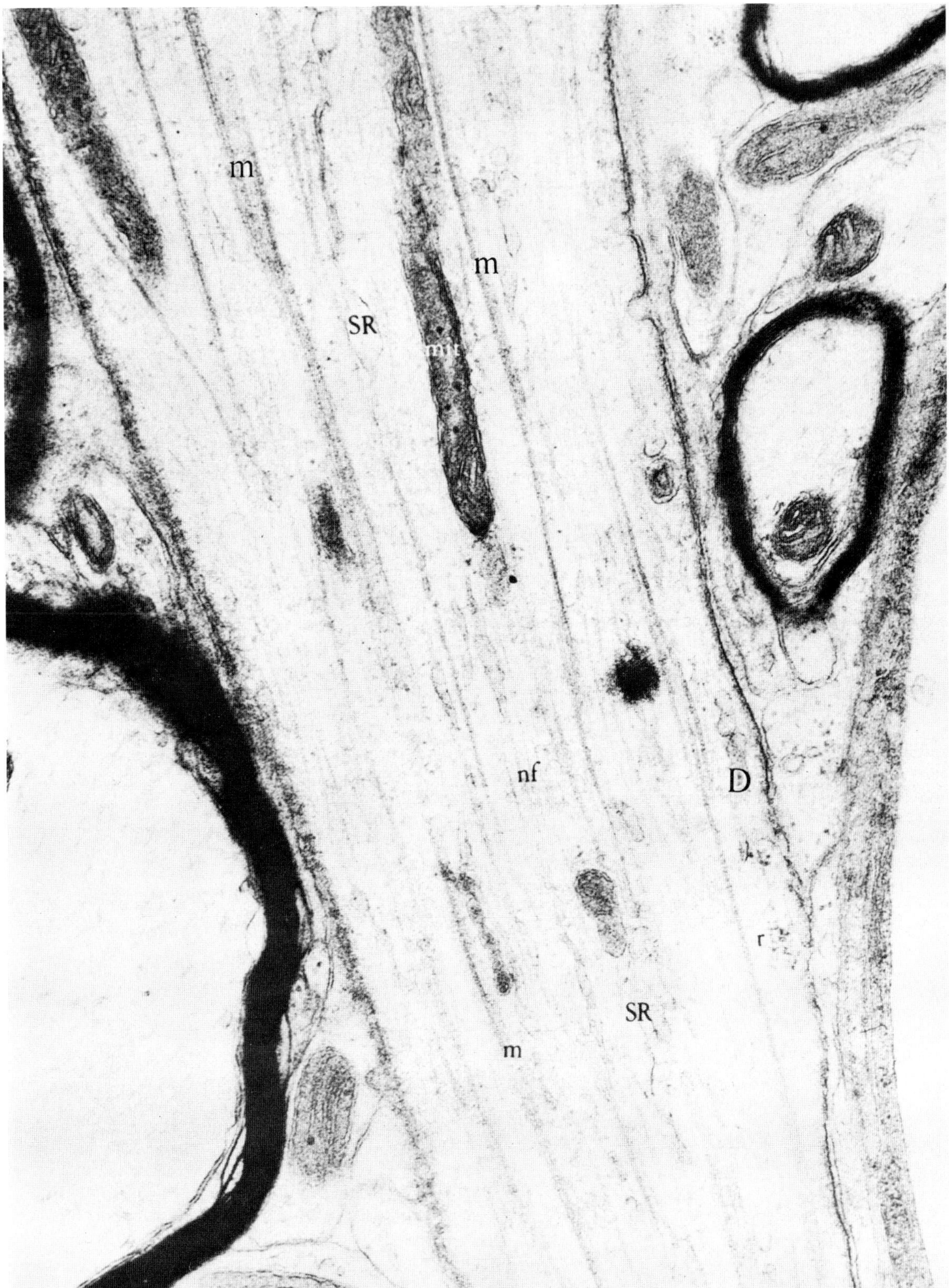

Fig. 2-10. Initial segment of an anterior horn motoneuron (rat), cut longitudinally. m = Microtubules; nf = neurofilaments; mit = mitochondrion; SR = nongranular endoplasmic reticulum; D = dense granular layer beneath axolemma. (×45,000.) (From Peters, Palay, and Webster.)

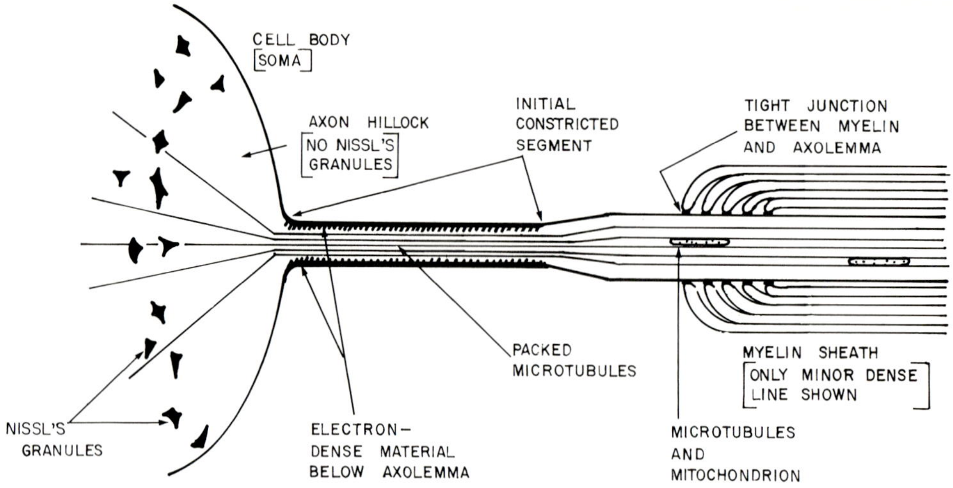

Fig. 2-11. Origin of the axon from a neuronal cell body. Note the initial constricted segment without myelin and the sealing of individual myelin lamellae to the axolemma by tight junctions, effectively closing off the myelinated part of the axon from the extracellular space.

brane (axolemma), continuous with the cell body, is a typical three-layered unit membrane, with the inner dense layer thicker than the outer. At the initial segment (Fig. 2-11), the bare areas between myelin segments (nodes of Ranvier), and where axons form the postsynaptic membrane (axoaxonal synapse), a granular, electron-dense (250 A) layer lies immediately beneath the axolemma. Above and below the nodes of Ranvier (paranodal regions), where terminal myelin loops overlie the axon, axolemma and myelin form parallel, electron-dense rings around the axon, sealing the internodal regions from the extracellular space. Branching occurs only at the nodes of Ranvier, where synaptic terminals with local accumulation of vesicles (axodendritic or axosomatic synapses) may also be seen.

Synapses

Although synapses may occasionally be seen or inferred in good light-microscope preparations, especially if degenerated, knowledge of their structure is only available from the electron microscope. Synapses generally occur between an axon that forms the presynaptic terminal (bouton terminale or bouton en passant) and the receptive surface (postsynaptic membrane) of a dendrite or cell body. These are the typical axodendritic and axosomatic synapses. However, synapses between two axons (axoaxonal) are well documented, and, more recently, dendrodendritic, somatosomatic, and somatodendritic synapses have been found. All have the features of chemically transmitting synapses (notably, asymmetry of the membrane and synaptic vesicles on one side) and appear to be distinct from the junctional zones that may connect dendrites and cell bodies, apparently as stabilizing mechanisms. Junctional zones and synapses may occur close together. The overall significance of these complexes requires further elucidation.

The synapse (Figs. 2-12, 2-13) is an area of close approximation between two plasma membranes, that of the presynaptic and that of the postsynaptic cell. The membranes are separated by a 200- to 400-A cleft, containing granular material of undetermined nature. In addition to mitochondria and occasional microtubules, the presynaptic process contains vesicles or dense-core bodies, 300 to 500 A across, which probably store transmitter substances. The postsynaptic membrane is characteristically thickened, but this is not a constant feature, and the membrane may be symmetrical or even show presynaptic thickening. The spine apparatus, apparently confined to neurons in the primate cortex, was previously mentioned. Synapses will be discussed in greater detail in Chapter 3.

Myelin

Myelin is a spirally wound, lipid membrane surrounding some axons in central and peripheral nervous tissue (Fig. 2-14). In myelinated axons, myelin starts

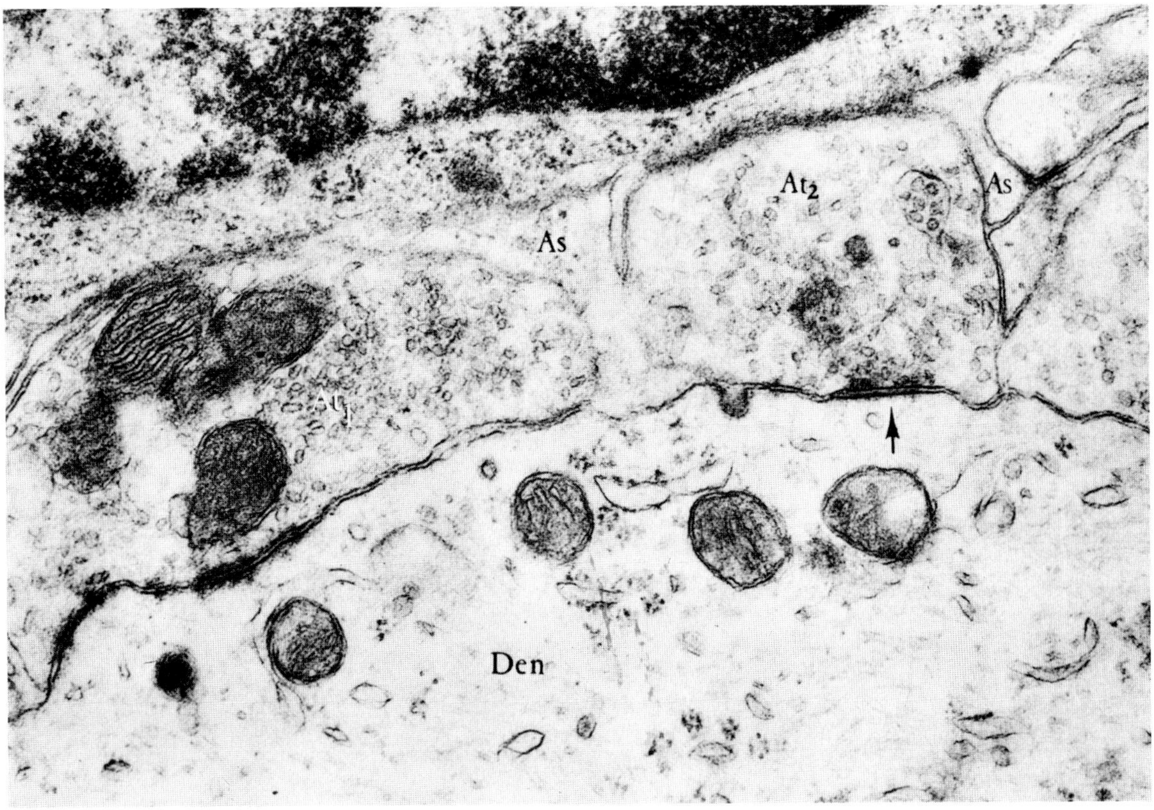

Fig. 2-12. Two axodendritic synapses from the spinal cord (rat). The presynaptic terminals (At_1 and At_2) contain mitochondria (on left, At_1) and many small vesicles. The postsynaptic dendrite (Den) contains mitochondria and large irregular profiles of nongranular endoplasmic and lysosomal character. Both membranes show areas of dense granular material that are more marked postsynaptically. The synapses are covered by astroglial processes (As). (X43,000.) (From Peters, Palay, and Webster.)

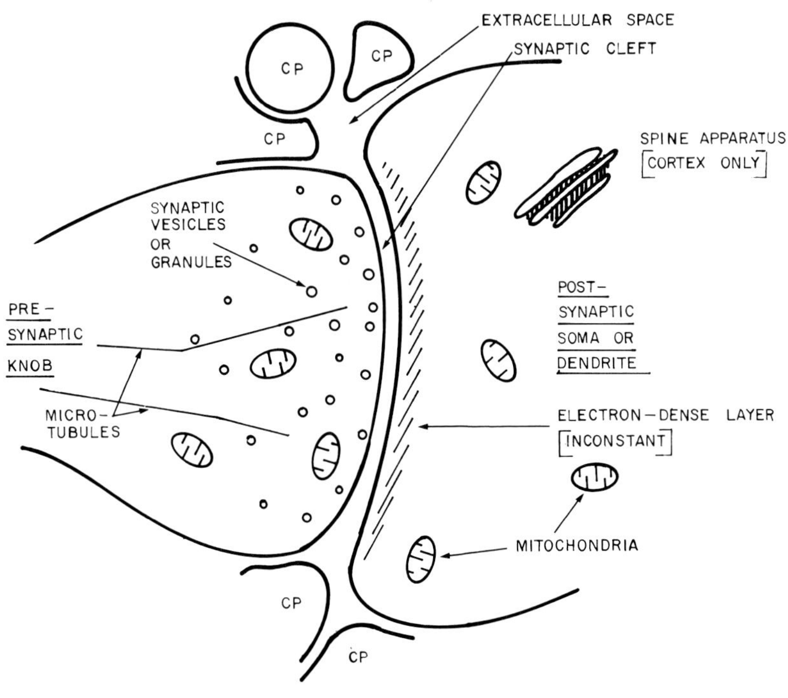

Fig. 2-13. Essential features of a synapse. Compare with Figure 2-12. CP = glial cell process.

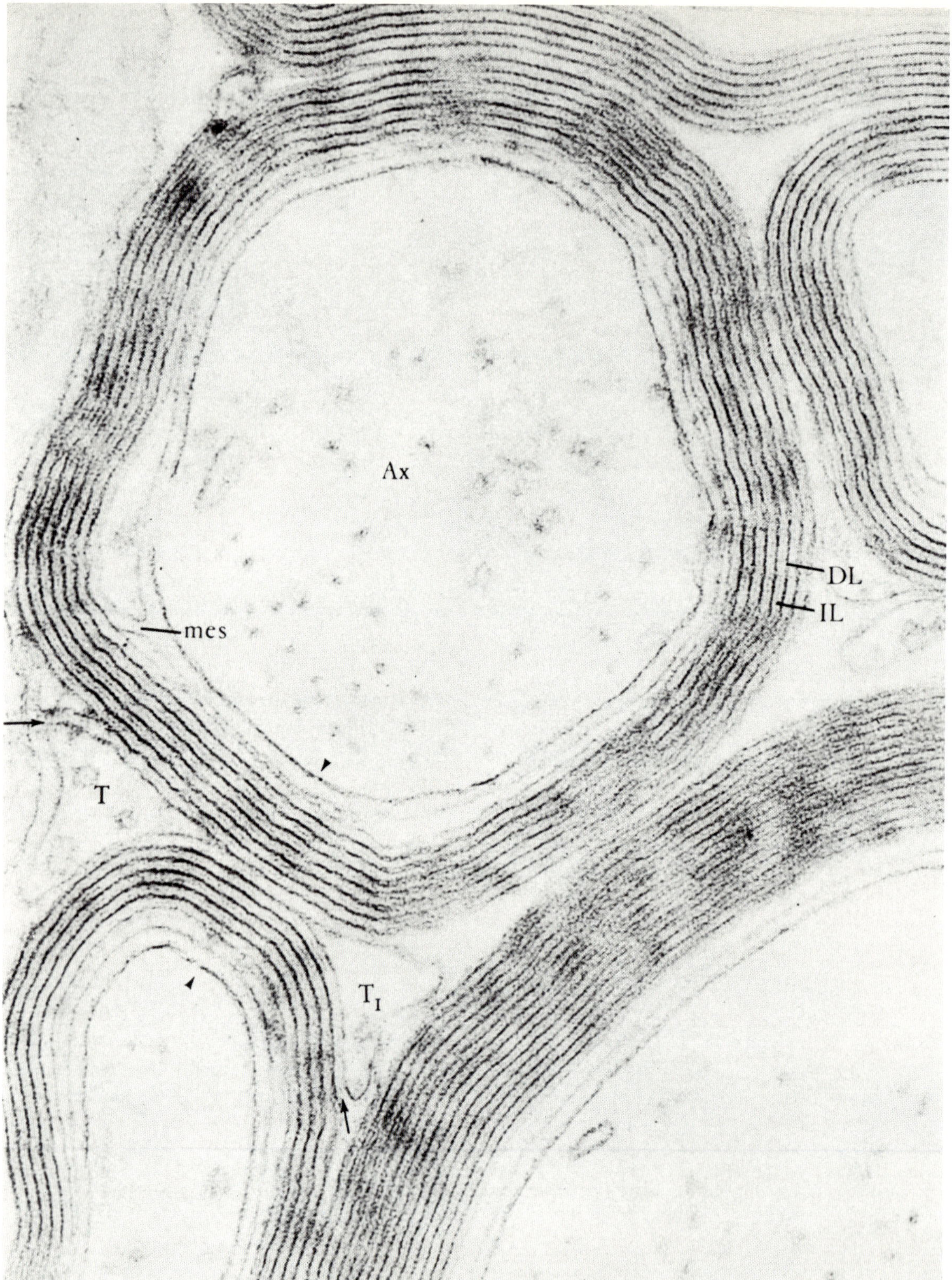

Fig. 2-14. Myelinated axons of the optic nerve in transverse section (rat). Ax = axon; DL = major dense line; IL = minor dense or intra-period line; T and T_1 = external longitudinal cytoplasmic tongues; mes = mesaxon with internal tongue above. (×187,000.) (From Peters, Palay, and Webster.)

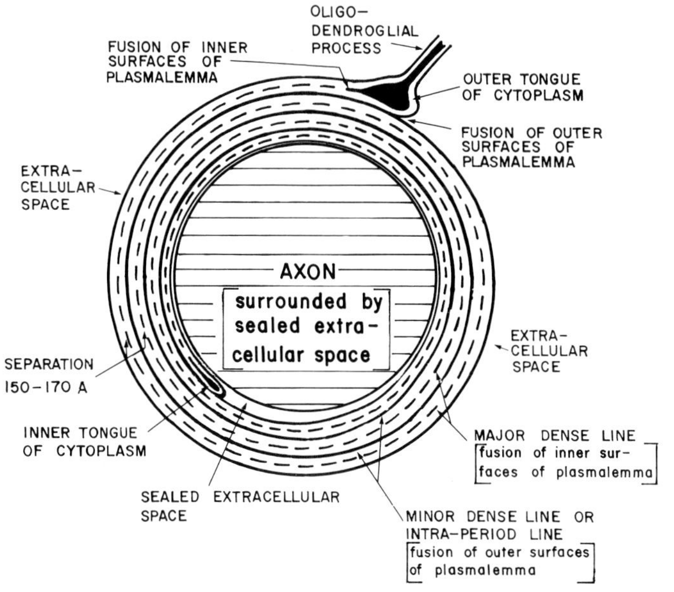

Fig. 2-15. Transverse section of myelinated axon. Compare with Figure 2-14.

immediately beyond the initial segment and continues along branches and telodendria almost to the terminal synaptic ramifications, interrupted by the nodes of Ranvier. It is usually formed from processes of oligodendroglial cells, although a role for astrocytes has not been conclusively disproved. A single oligodendroglia must form processes on several nearby axons, as there are many more internodes than glia in the CNS. A thin tongue of cytoplasm (Fig. 2-15) is present at the inner edge of the spiral adjacent to the axon and a second thin, longitudinal tongue at the outer edge, covering only a small part of the circumference. Where the sheath is interrupted at the nodes, these two longitudinal tongues are connected by a spiral of cytoplasm in the free edges of the individual myelin lamellae. Each internode (myelin segment) is formed by a single cell process, and the nodes of Ranvier are the intervals between adjacent internodes. In the paranodal regions (Fig. 2-16), the myelin sheaths gradually become thinner, the inner lamellae disappearing first, so that the outer are the longer. The bare axon at the node of Ranvier is freely open to the extracellular space. Branching may occur at nodes, or a small lateral presynaptic projection may form an axodendritic synapse. Each lamella is about 170 to 180 A thick, and electron microscopy shows alternating major dense lines, formed by fusion of the cytoplasmic surfaces of plasma membranes, and minor dense (intra-period) lines, formed by fusion of external surfaces. The incisures of Lanterman (Fig. 2-17), persistent cytoplasmic channels running spirally from the outer to the inner edge of myelin sheath within the internodes, splitting the major dense lines, are either less frequent or less readily seen in the central than in the peripheral nervous system. A more detailed account of myelin and its formation is given in Chapters 4 and 21.

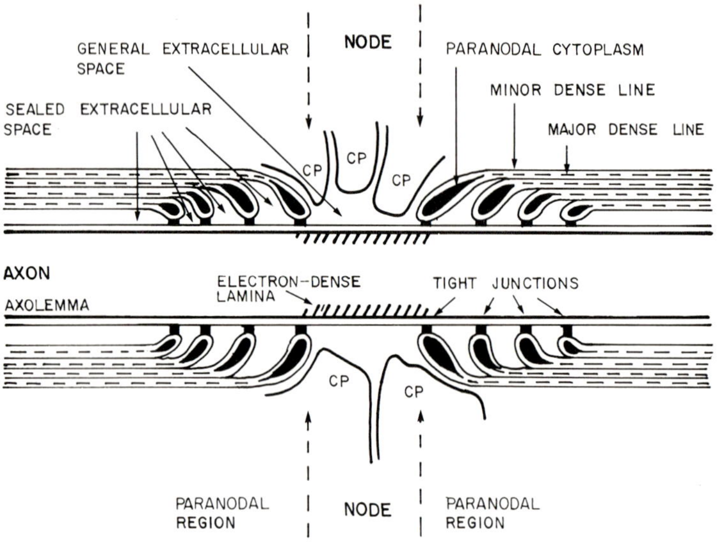

Fig. 2-16. Longitudinal section through node of Ranvier. Note the sealing of the myelin lamellae to the axolemma by tight junctions, closing off the internodes from the extracellular space. Also note the relatively wide extracellular space around the nodal (bare) axon. Dense granular material is present below the axolemma at the node, as in the initial segment. CP = cytoplasmic process.

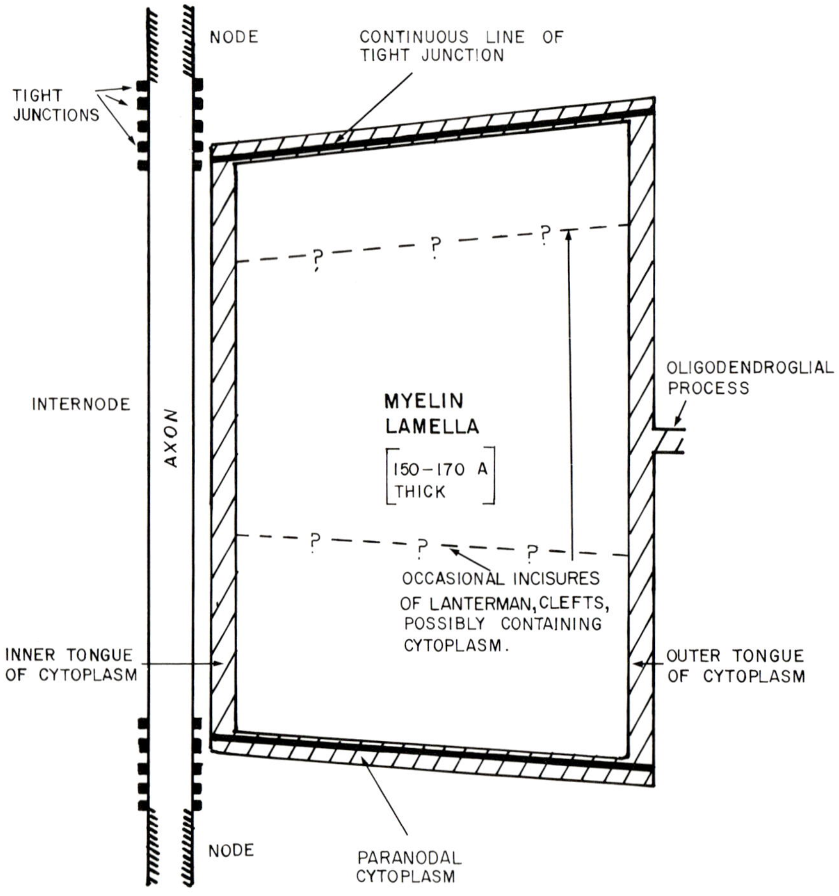

Fig. 2-17. Myelin internode "unrolled" to form a single sheet one lamella thick. Note residual cytoplasm at the edges of the sheet. Also note the presence of a continuous line of tight junction along each end, applied in spiral fashion to the axolemma.

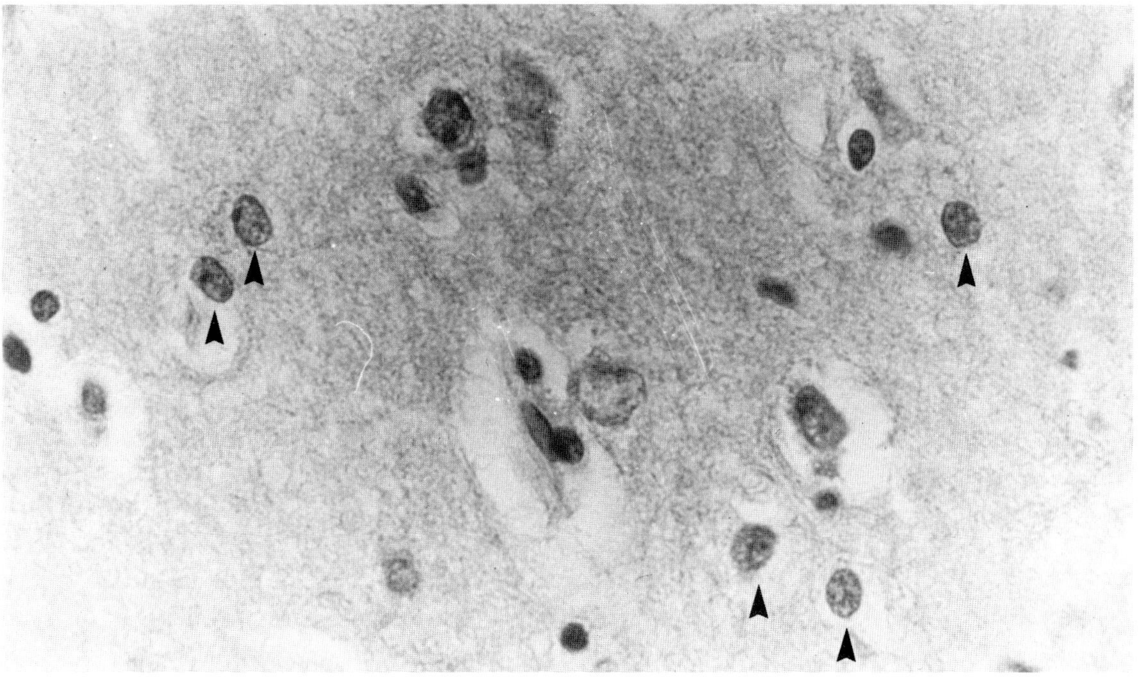

Fig. 2-18. Astrocytes (arrows). Only the nucleus is seen in routine preparations. (H & E, X750.)

ASTROCYTES

The astrocyte is the largest glial cell, having a cell body 20 to 35μ in diameter. It has a rounded, oval, or slightly irregular nucleus with a light chromatin pattern and without a clearly visible nucleolus (Fig. 2-18). The cell body gives rise to numerous, branching processes, one of which is frequently thicker than the others; this terminates either in a flattened expansion on a capillary or other small blood vessel (the foot process) (Fig. 2-19) or beneath the pia, to contribute to the pial-glial layer. In fibrous astrocytes the processes are longer and branch less often, but at acute angles; the cell body and processes contain numerous glial fibrils. In protoplasmic astrocytes the processes branch more frequently and at less acute angles, giving a somewhat "mossy" appearance; they contain fewer or no visible fibrils. Astrocytes are present throughout the central nervous system. Those in the deep gray matter and the deeper layers of the cerebral and cerebellar cortex are mostly protoplasmic. It seems probable that fibrillary and protoplasmic astrocytes are interchangeable and that both have the potential of forming glial fibers. These fibers are a feature in some parts of the normal CNS, notably in the subependymal and subpial regions (including the molecular layer of the cerebral cortex), the median raphe of the brain stem and spinal cord, and the region of the inferior olivary nuclei. Glial fibers are usually present around blood vessels.

With hematoxylin and eosin staining, only the nuclei of astrocytes can be recognized. It is often difficult to distinguish them from the nuclei of oligodendroglia or even of small neurons. Suitable staining methods show glial fibers within the filamentous processes. Electron-microscopically (Fig. 2-20), cell bodies and processes have a light (but not watery)

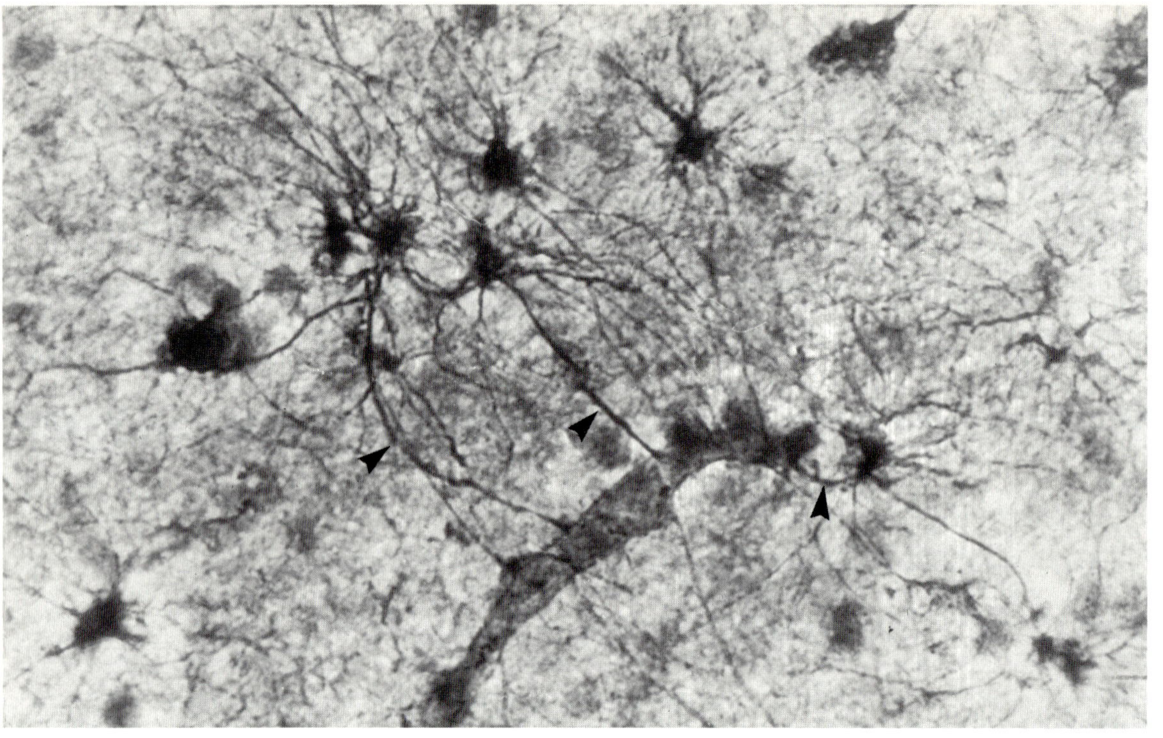

Fig. 2-19. Astrocytes in white matter (fibrillary), showing the processes. The foot processes (arrows) make close contact with a capillary. (Cajal method, X750.)

cytoplasm, and a somewhat irregular nucleus, often with a folded nuclear membrane. The cytoplasm contains some mitochondria, scanty granular endoplasmic reticulum but very few ribosomes, a well-developed Golgi's complex, typical lysosomes, and characteristic osmiophilic bodies (200 to 400 A) that contain glycogen. Glial filaments are 60 to 100 A wide, hollow, and form parallel arrays up to 1 to 2μ in diameter (visible on light microscopy) in the cell body and processes (especially in fibrillary forms). They are composed of globular subunits different from those of neurofilaments and probably do not form side arms or cross branches, in spite of a slightly irregular outline. Neurofilaments are absent. The processes of fibrous astrocytes are cylindrical and smooth. By contrast, the processes of protoplasmic astrocytes adapt to surrounding cells and often form very thin lamellae (e.g., around synapses). Both may show junctional zones, but so far, these appear to have no coherent pattern.

OLIGODENDROGLIA

Oligodendroglia are somewhat smaller than astrocytes and characteristically appear as small, oval cells with a rounded, darkly staining nucleus. The cell body produces a small number of delicate, branching processes, less branched and shorter than those of astrocytes. Oligodendroglia are widely distributed in the CNS and typically occur in rows within white matter (interfascicular oligodendroglia) and in relation to neurons in gray matter (perineuronal satellite cells).

With routine stains (Fig. 2-21), only the small, dark nuclei of oligodendroglia cells can be visualized.

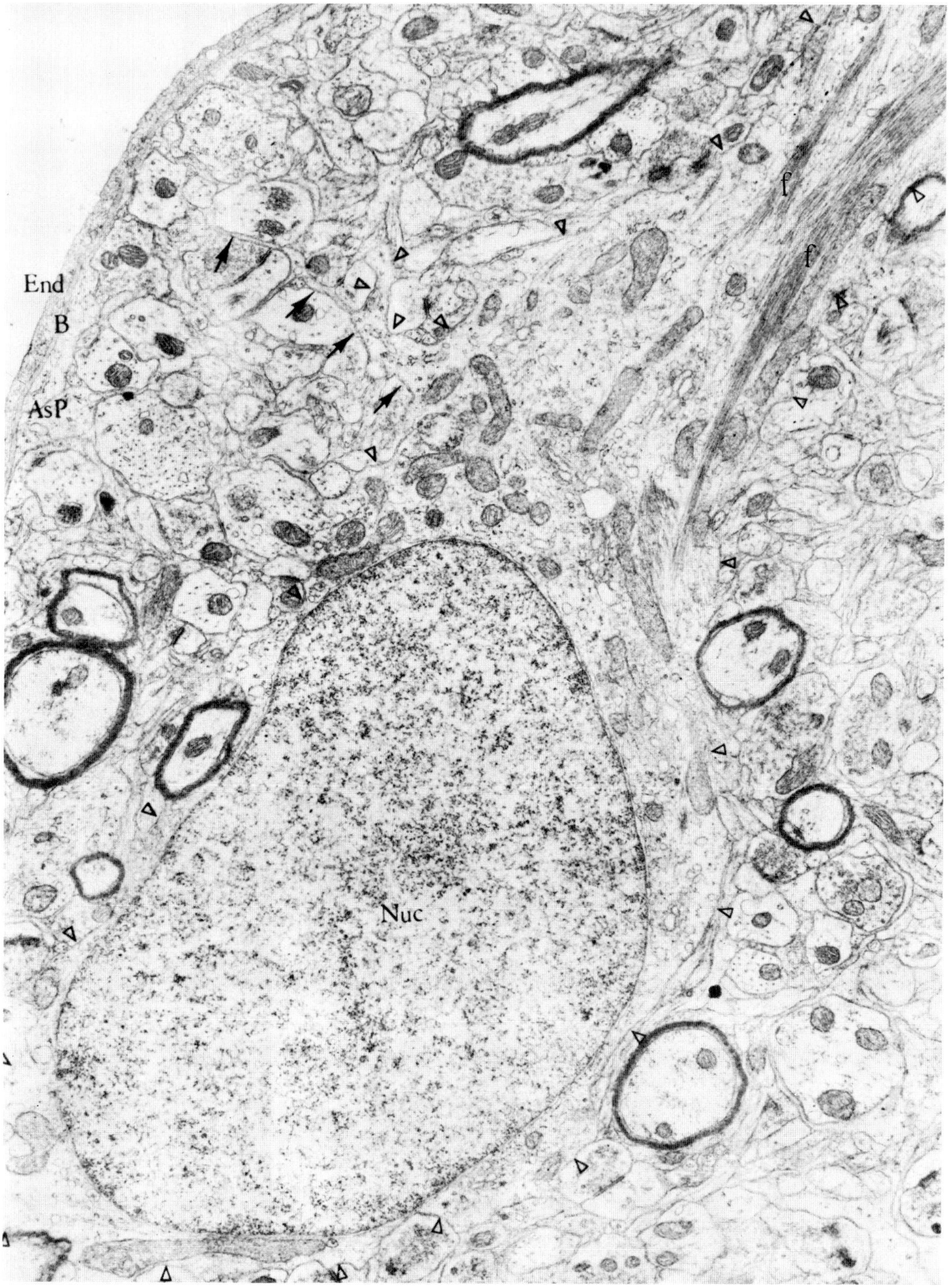

Fig. 2-20. Protoplasmic astrocyte (triangles) and fine process (arrows) with irregular cell body from cerebral cortex (rat). Nuc = nucleus; f = glial fibrils. Capillary wall (End) shows a continuous layer of subjacent foot processes (AsP) with an intervening basement membrane (B). (X19,000.) (From Peters, Palay, and Webster.)

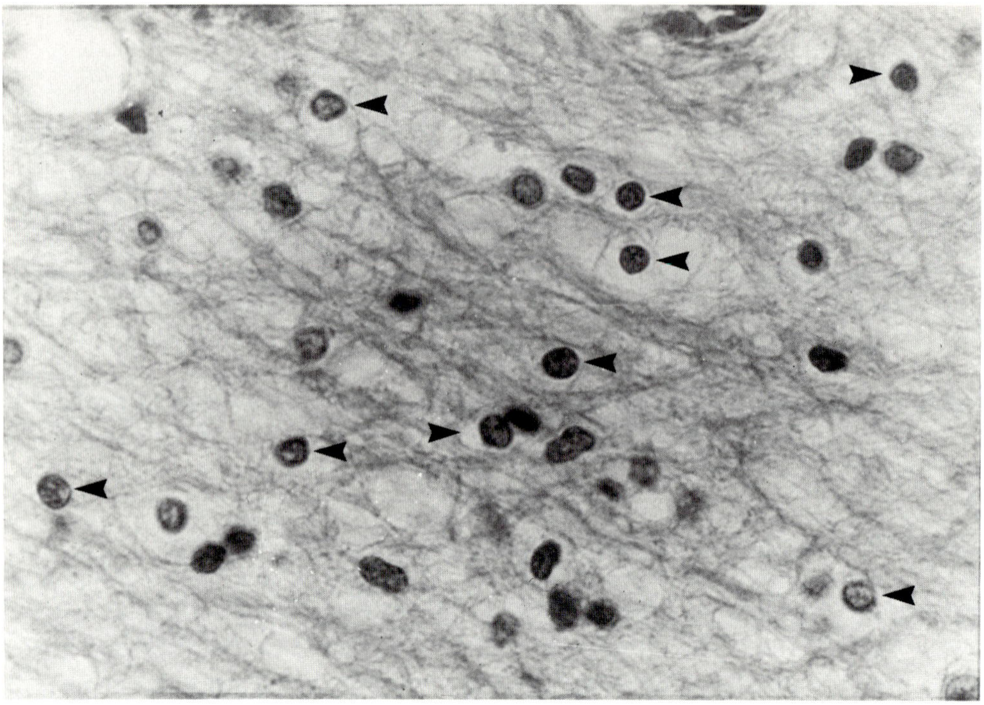

Fig. 2-21. Oligodendroglial cells (arrows) in white matter. They are not always readily distinguishable from astrocytes. (H & E, ×750.)

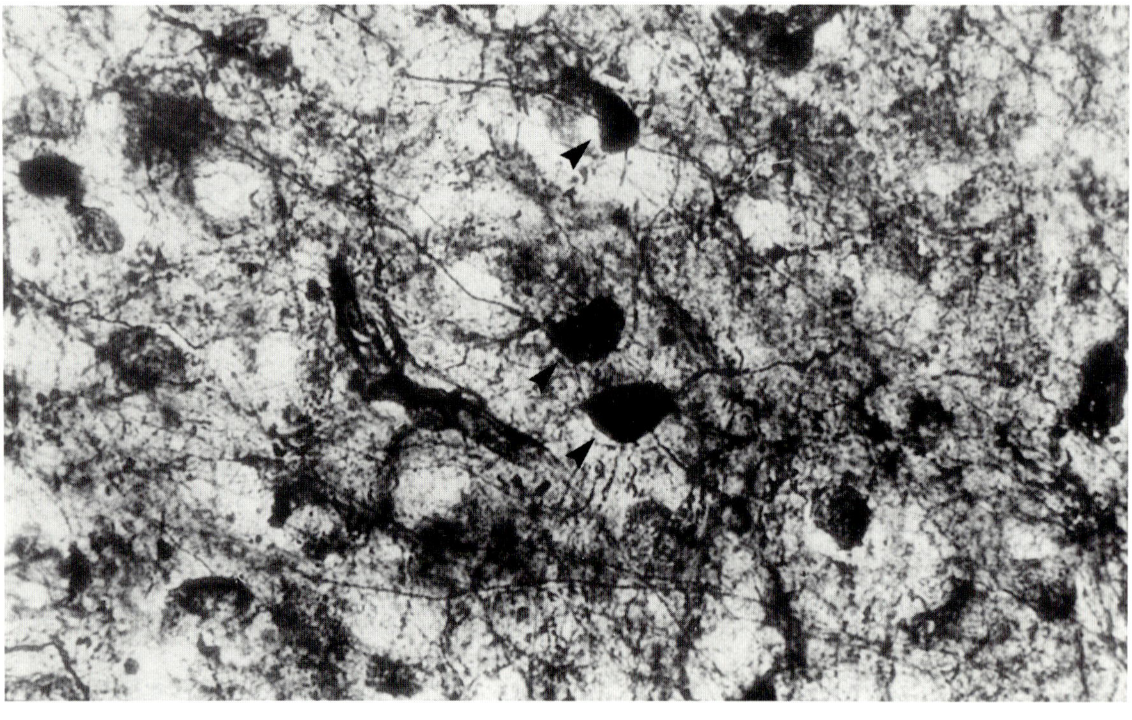

Fig. 2-22. Oligodendroglial cells (arrows) in white matter, showing oval body and short branched processes, often thickened at branch points. (Weil-Davenport method, ×750.)

Metallic impregnation methods show the cell body and processes (Fig. 2-22). Electron-microscopically (Fig. 2-23), the round, oval, or occasionally irregular nucleus shows a well-marked nucleolus as well as peripherally clumped, only occasionally diffuse, chromatin. Nuclear membranes, often widely separated, contain pores. The cytoplasm is more electron-dense than that of any other CNS cell and contains abundant, closely packed ribosomes, polyribosomes, and granular endoplasmic reticulum. There is a well-developed Golgi's complex surrounding the nucleus, and moderate numbers of mitochondria are present. In addition there are numerous microtubules and occasional fine filaments as in astrocytes, together with lysosomes and a few glycogen granules.

There is no conclusive electron-microscopic evidence for intermediate cells in the normal CNS, although in reactive conditions, cells with dense cytoplasm but large numbers of glial fibrils, sharing some characteristics of oligodendroglial and astroglial types, have been observed.

EPENDYMAL CELLS

The ependyma consists of a layer of cells, varying from low cuboidal to columnar (Fig. 2-24), which lines spaces derived from the central canal of the neural tube; namely, the ventricular system, the lateral pouches of the fourth ventricle, and the (often incomplete) central canal of the cord. Since maturation of the CNS includes a reduction in the size of most central cavities by fusion of the walls, ependymal cells may be seen entrapped in glial tissue in such areas, most often adjacent to the occipital and frontal horns of the lateral ventricles and in the gray commissure of the spinal cord. Where the leptomeninges have invaginated the ventricular system to form choroid plexus, the ependymal lining is modified to become choroidal epithelium.

Because of their location, ependymal cells are readily recognized in the mature nervous system since there are no residual neuroepithelial cells. The nuclei are round, or oval at right angles to the ventricular surface, and show moderately dense, granular staining. Cytoplasm is pale and on occasion shows small vacuoles, and cilia may be seen on the free surface. The characteristic nuclear pattern makes these cells easily recognizable, even where they have lost contact with the ventricular surface.

Seen electron-microscopically, the cytoplasm contains moderate numbers of mitochondria, granular and nongranular endoplasmic reticulum, and a well-developed Golgi's complex, especially at the apex (free surface). Glial filaments, 70 to 80 A across, similar to those in astrocytes, are present, and there are moderate numbers of microtubules at the apex. The nucleolus is prominent, chromatin is diffusely distributed, and the nuclear membrane may show indentations. The ventricular surface of the cell carries not only cilia but also an irregular pattern of microvilli (less regular than those of intestinal mucosa). Laterally, plasma membranes of adjacent cells interdigitate, and there are spotty cell junctions near the ventricular surface. The base of the cell may be flat or rounded, but in primates there are probably no processes resembling those seen in astrocytes. There is no basement membrane.

Particularly in primates there is a subependymal glial layer, which consists of fibers from astrocytes with a regular arrangement that varies from region to region. Microglial cells are present, and there is often a layer of subependymal astrocytic cell bodies, frequently with a small nucleolus and diffuse chromatin pattern, lying between the subependymal glia and the neuropil. At least in the hypothalamus (infundibular recess), the presence of nerve cell processes and other structural modifications suggest possible neuroendocrine functions.

MICROGLIA

The microglial cells are derived from neither the neural tube nor crest, but are reticuloendothelial cells derived from mesenchyme, which enter the CNS with blood vessels. As inactive "fixed macrophages" in the CNS, they have a peculiar, branched conformation, unlike that seen in phagocytic cells elsewhere, probably occupying interstices in the neuropil.

In routinely stained sections (Fig. 2-25), only small numbers of microglial nuclei can be seen, and they may be difficult to distinguish from those of glial cells. Characteristically, they are elongated or slightly oval, hyperchromatic with no distinct internal structure, and distributed especially in the subependymal and subpial zones and around vessels. By staining techniques involving silver (Fig. 2-26), scanty, short, irregular, slightly branched processes may be visualized.

Electron-microscopic identification is uncertain, perhaps because oligodendroglial and microglial cells have a similar appearance. However, it has been suggested that the light-microscopic features previously noted as typical of microglia may simply be those of somewhat atypical glia (probably oligodendroglia), in which case all reticuloendothelial cells seen in CNS disease would be derived from vascular adventitia or the circulation. A cell has been described in the optic nerve, cortex, and cord that has electron density between that of astrocytes and oligodendroglia and shows few microtubules, fibrils, or glycogen granules, a somewhat open granular endoplasmic reticulum, dense laminar bodies, and droplets. Such cells are more numerous in the immature CNS and may represent spongioblasts that persist in the adult as precursor (not intermediate) cells, accounting for the low residual level of mitotic activity manifested in reactive glia. They appear to be phagocytic, but otherwise do not resemble microglial cells. The entire question of the electron-microscopic identification of glia (other than typical astrocytes, oligodendroglia, and ependyma) appears to need clarification.

GRAY AND WHITE MATTER

Neuronal cell bodies are not evenly distributed throughout the CNS but collect in functional units that are present within typical gray matter and

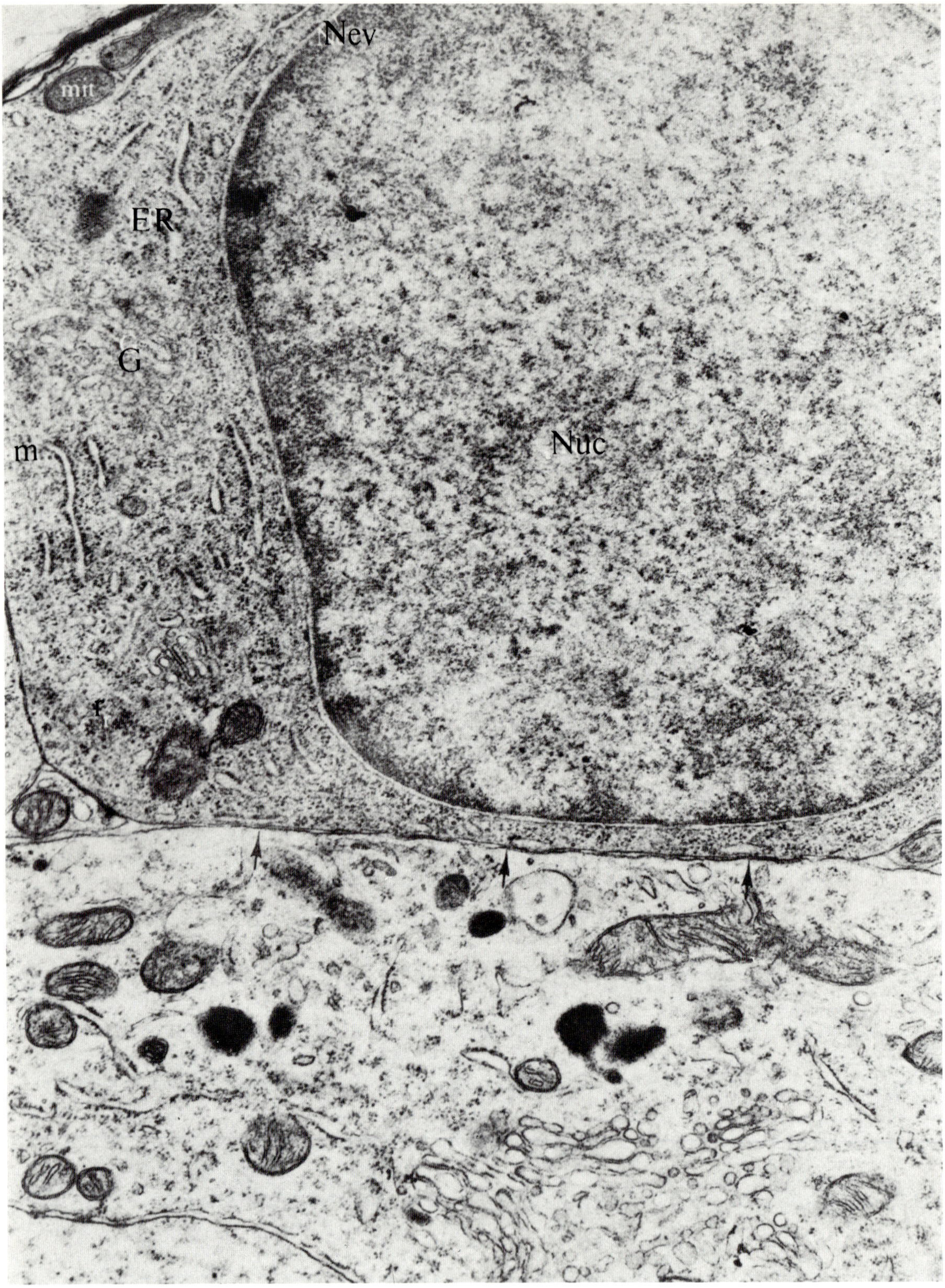

Fig. 2-23. A satellite oligodendroglia of the spinal cord (rat) adjacent to an anterior horn cell (below, arrows mark adjacent membranes). Nuc = nucleus; Nev = nuclear envelope; G = Golgi apparatus; ER, r = granular endoplasmic reticulum and ribosomes; mit = mitochondria; m = microtubules. (X33,000.) (From Peters, Palay, and Webster.)

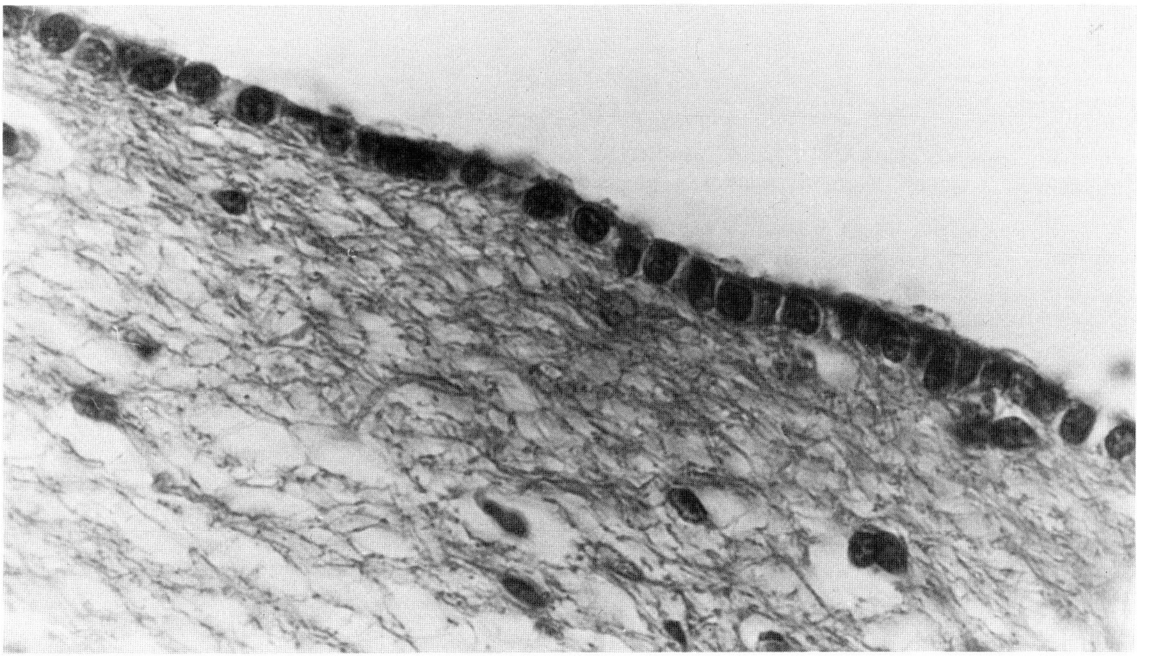

Fig. 2-24. Ependymal lining of ventricles. (H & E, ×750.)

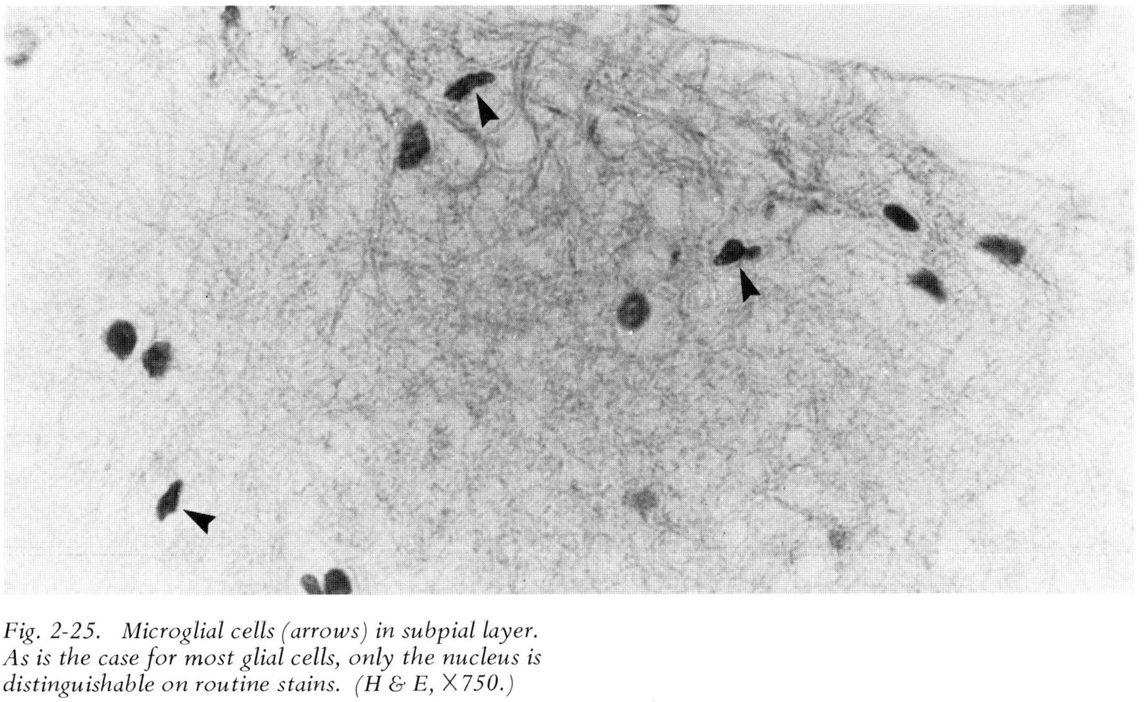

Fig. 2-25. Microglial cells (arrows) in subpial layer. As is the case for most glial cells, only the nucleus is distinguishable on routine stains. (H & E, ×750.)

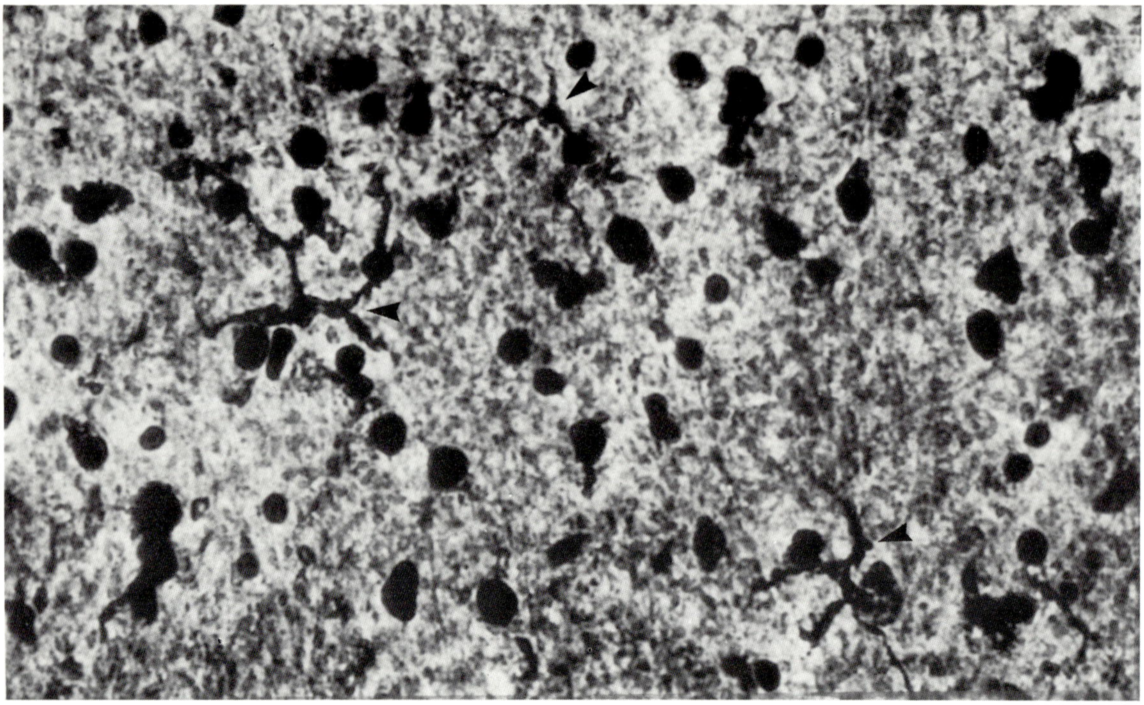

Fig. 2-26. Microglial cells, showing stunted, irregular processes and elongated cell bodies (arrows). (Weil-Davenport method, X750.)

absent from white matter. White matter has a high content of myelinated axons, which gives the tissue its typical appearance, seen in the peripheral parts of the spinal cord, in descending and ascending tracts in the brain stem, and in the core of the cerebral and cerebellar hemispheres. These areas contain no neuronal cell bodies, and their population is largely oligodendroglia, with some astrocytes and elements of the mesenchymal-vascular framework. Gray matter contains much less myelin than does white matter, though it is rarely completely absent. It consists largely of neuronal cell bodies, nonmyelinated dendritic ramifications, and axon terminals, mingled with glial cells. Examples are the cortex of the cerebrum and cerebellum, the central gray matter of the hemispheres (basal ganglia and thalamus), and the central gray matter of the cord.

The intrinsic structures of the brain stem (i.e., excluding the long ascending and descending tracts) are made up of functional units that are much smaller than those in the hemispheres and cord and usually not grossly distinguishable. These areas are called reticular formation rather than gray or white matter and contain a complex mixture of neuronal cell bodies and dendrites, small bundles of myelinated and unmyelinated axons, and glial cells.

The role of myelin in differentiating gray from white matter is shown in the neonatal human brain, which has little or no myelin in the cerebral hemispheres, in which the cortex, white matter, basal ganglia, and thalamus are much more difficult to distinguish than in the adult brain. It is important to understand that many nuclei of clinical importance, including the cranial nerve nuclei and subdivisions of the reticular formation and thalamus, are not visible on gross examination, but have been defined as a result of extensive histological, and sometimes electrophysiological, work. Similarly, a number of myelinated fiber tracts of clinical importance, such as the ansa lenticularis and the optic or auditory radiations, are not grossly distinguishable.

NEURONAL CIRCUITS

Although an understanding of the organization of neuronal networks is a prerequisite for interpretation of CNS function, the interrelationships between individual neurons, even in a small area, are obscure. The structural organization of the cerebellar cortex is known in some detail, but much less is known about the cerebral cortex. Any neuronal pool modifies its input, and the term *relay nucleus*, applied, for example, to the gracilis or cuneate nucleus or to nuclei of the ventrolateral thalamus, is an incomplete, although convenient, designation.

Although no complete categorization of neural networks is possible, there are certain basic patterns (Fig. 2-27).

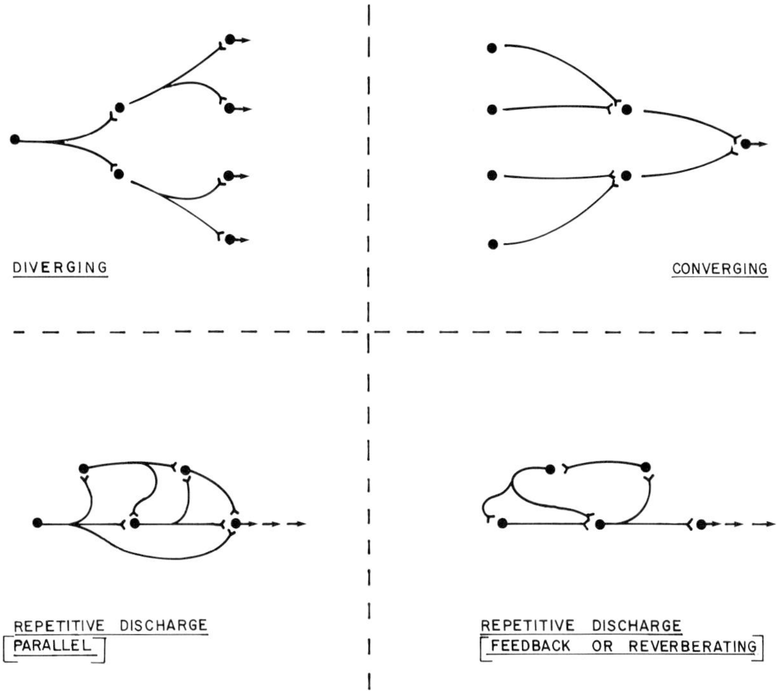

Fig. 2-27. Highly oversimplified representations of a few basic types of neuronal circuits.

Diverging Circuits

Neural activity originating in a single neuron or pool diverges within the CNS in such a fashion that it reaches many neurons or pools. An example of the former is the relationship between a single Betz's cell of the motor cortex and the multiple anterior horn cells it stimulates. Similarly, dorsal root ganglia form neuronal pools, and the incoming dorsal root afferent fibers branch to reach spinal cord gray matter in the same and adjacent segments and to join several ascending tracts reaching various parts of the hindbrain.

Converging Circuits

Multiple influences may be brought to bear on a single neuron or neuronal pool. An example of the former is the simultaneous influence of myelinated and nonmyelinated dorsal root fibers on individual neurons in the dorsal horn. An example of the latter is the influences from higher and lower centers that reach the Purkinje's cells of the cerebellar cortex.

Repetitive Discharge Circuits

The duration of output considerably exceeds the duration of input and theoretically might be infinite, were not other competitive or inhibitory afferent impulses continually arriving. These repetitive discharge circuits occur in at least two forms. One consists of approximately parallel, interconnecting pathways, in which transmission is essentially in one direction. The reticular formation of the brain stem is an example. The other is associated with axonal branching and feedback to an earlier neuron in the chain, thus forming circular or reverberating circuits, in which the neurons may continually stimulate one another. Duration of output from reverberating circuits is longer than from parallel circuits. Such reverberating mechanisms are probably operant within the cerebral cortex and other regions and also between different areas of the brain, such as the thalamus and cerebral cortex. In addition to other functions, they originate rhythmic activity, such as the cardiac and respiratory cycles. In our present state of knowledge it does not appear feasible to connect them with longer rhythms of the circadian type (see Chap. 8).

ARCHITECTURE AND ORGANIZATION IN THE CEREBRAL CORTEX

The cerebral cortex is 1.5 to 4 mm thick and weighs 500 to 600 g, which is 40% of total brain weight. The most primitive is the allocortex (archipallium and paleopallium), which either shows no lamination or has fewer than six layers and originally subserved the sense of smell; it includes the hippocampus, anterior perforated substance, olfactory gyrus, and small associated areas. Related to this functionally, although more typical in structure, is the mesocortex (juxtallocortex), which includes the cingulate, isthmic, and parahippocampal gyri. These areas correspond to the fifth (limbic) lobe, described in Chapter 1. All other cerebral cortex is neocortex, the mesocortex and neocortex together making the neopallium. This is stratified into six layers, which may or may not be readily distinguishable. These are numbered from the pial surface inward:

Layer I (molecular) contains relatively few cell bodies and is composed mainly of ascending axons and dendrites from deeper layers.
Layer II (external granular) contains variable numbers of small, round cells and a few pyramidal cells, both with dendrites rising to the molecular layer.
Layer III (external pyramidal) is similar to layer II, from which it may be hard to distinguish, but has a higher proportion of small pyramidal cells.
Layer IV (internal granular) is almost entirely composed of small, multipolar, granular (Golgi type II) cells.
Layer V (deep pyramidal) is composed of medium- to large-sized pyramidal cells (including the Betz's cells of the main motor cortex).
Layer VI (fusiform, spindle-shaped, or pleomorphic) is composed of variably shaped medium-sized to large cells, with a few granular cells and includes some pyramidal components.

Where all six of these layers are relatively evenly represented, the cortex is termed *homotypic*. In some areas, such as the precentral and postcentral gyri, certain layers are reduced or exaggerated, and the cortex is then termed *heterotypic*. Although this stratification is the more readily apparent, of equal functional importance is the formation of vertical columns (cylinders or prisms), which is established for the sensorimotor area and probably exists elsewhere (see Chap. 7).

Types of Neurons

There is much architectural diversity in the cerebral cortex, based on the layers and the vertical organization. Nonetheless, there are fundamentally only four types of neurons present (Fig. 2-28).

Pyramidal Cells. In sections, pyramidal cells appear triangular, with a flat base facing inward and a pointed apex directed at the surface. From the apex, a long, branching dendrite reaches the molecular layer, and both it and the cell body have numerous horizontal dendrites. This extensive "tree" is heavily covered with dendritic spines. The cell body is 15 to 70μ long, and most of these cells occur in layers III, V, and VI. Their axons pass into the underlying white matter, with at least one recurrent branch back into the cortex. Such axons form *projection fibers* to subcortical centers, *commissural fibers* to the opposite hemisphere (largely through the corpus callosum), or *association fibers* to other parts of the same hemisphere. They make up much of the hemispheric white matter. The polymorphic cells in layer VI have the same type of dendritic pattern and axonal projection as pyramidal cells and are more properly regarded as variants of these cells than as a separate cell type.

Granular (Golgi Type II) Cells. These occur in all cortical laminae, but are concentrated in layers II and IV. They are small, round, or star-shaped cells with numerous highly branched dendrites and a short, branching axon that is 1 mm or even shorter in length (Fig. 2-28). This axon does not leave the cortex. An enormous increase in numbers of this type of cell has resulted in enlargement of the brain in primates, especially in man.

Martinotti's Cells. These occur mainly in layers V and VI as medium-sized cells of variable shape, with short, branching dendrites and a myelinated axon directed toward the surface and with horizontal branches in all cortical layers.

Horizontal (Cajal) Cells. These occur only in the superficial layer I of the cortex, and both axon and dendrites run in a horizontal plane.

Circuitry

Little is currently known about the circuitry of the cortex, but it certainly includes arcs and loops. Thalamic afferents synapse mainly with pyramidal cell bodies or their proximal dendrites (either directly or through Golgi's cells), whereas afferent fibers from the ascending reticular activating system connect mainly with the more distal dendrites.

ARCHITECTURE AND ORGANIZATION OF THE CEREBELLAR CORTEX

The cerebellar cortex, unlike that of the cerebral hemispheres, is of uniform structure in all areas, irrespective of phylogenetic antiquity, and of even thickness (about 1 mm). Three layers are distinguishable.

1. The *molecular layer* is the most superficial and makes up about half the total thickness. It contains few cells, but has an extensive intersecting network of axons and dendrites derived from cells in the lower layers.
2. The *Purkinje's cell layer* is a single layer of conspicuous cells separating the molecular and internal granular layers.
3. The *internal granular layer* is the deepest of the three and of about the same thickness as the molecular layer. It is densely cellular, consisting of small close-packed cells with occasional small areas free of nuclei (which contain the glomeruli, see below).

Types of Neurons

There are at least five cell types in the cerebellar cortex, despite its apparent simplicity relative to cerebral cortex (Fig. 2-29).

1. *Purkinje's cells* are among the largest in the brain. They are flask- or pear-shaped with a large outwardly directed apical dendrite which branches very extensively in the molecular layer in a plane

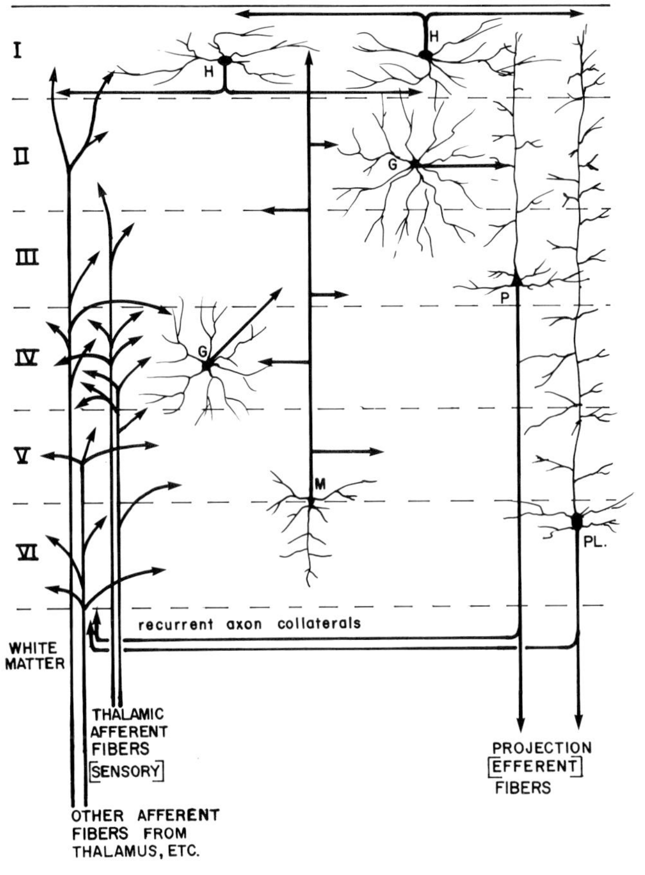

Fig. 2-28. Neuronal types in the cerebral cortex (axons represented by thick lines; dendrites by thin, less regular lines). The layers from which efferent fibers originate, and in which afferent fibers terminate, are apparent. G = Golgi type II cell; H = horizontal cell of Cajol; M = Martinotti's cell; P = pyramidal cell; PL = pleomorphic cell.

at right angles to the folia. The axons run to deep cerebellar nuclei, except for a few fibers passing directly to vestibular nuclei.

2. *Granule cells* contribute more than half the number of cells in the internal granular layer, and are small and dark with little apparent cytoplasm. Their dendrites ramify locally, forming complexes with the terminals of afferent (mossy) fibers and Golgi cell axons, which are called *glomeruli.* The granule cell axons pass radially into the molecular layer and bifurcate in a T-shape, each branch running along a folium; they are therefore called *parallel fibers.*
3. *Golgi's cells* are slightly fewer and larger than the granule cells, and are mixed with them in the internal granular layer. Their dendrites pass into the molecular layer where they ramify both parallel and perpendicular to the folia: a few remain in the granular layer. Their axons are profusely branched and remain in the granular layer.
4. *Stellate cells* are few in number and present in the outer molecular layer. Their dendrites branch in the molecular layer perpendicularly to the folia, and their T-shaped axons also run in the molecular layer in the same plane.
5. *Basket cells* are also rather sparse and occur in the deeper molecular layer. The distribution of dendrites and axons is similar to that of stellate cells.

Circuitry

Two types of fiber afferent to the cerebellar cortex may be distinguished. Climbing fibers almost entirely originate in the inferior olives. They are thin fibers branching only in the molecular layer, where each forms myriad synaptic contacts with one Purkinje's cell and probably a few adjacent stellate or basket cells. Mossy fibers seem to represent all other afferent sources and are thick, extensively branching fibers forming synapses with large numbers of granule cells over a wide area, and also with some Golgi's cells (and perhaps basket and stellate cells). Both types of afferent fiber, and the granule cells, are excitatory, so that Purkinje's cells may be excited

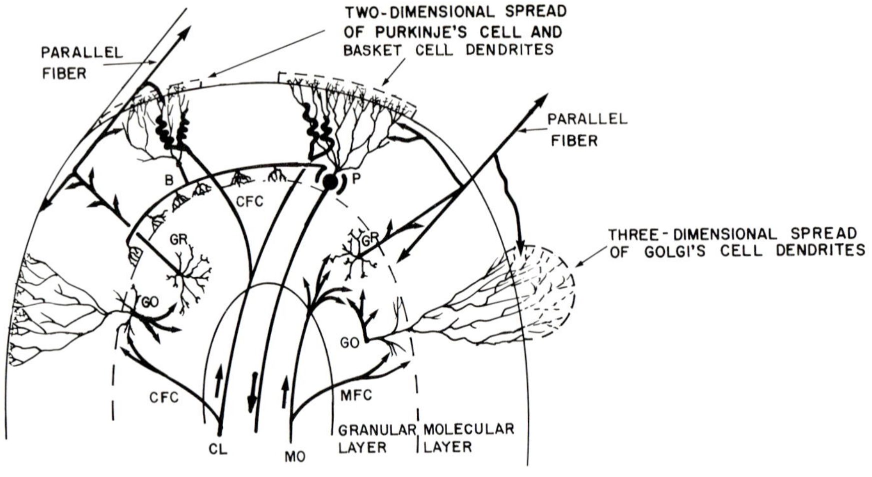

Fig. 2-29. Section across a cerebellar folium showing the cortical layers (the Purkinje's cell layer lies between the molecular and granular layers). Axons are represented by thick lines, and dendrites by thin, less regular lines. Stellate cells (see text) are omitted for clarity. CL = climbing (afferent) fiber; CFC = climbing fiber collateral; MO = mossy (afferent) fiber; MFC = mossy fiber collateral; B = basket cell; GO = Golgi's cell; GR = granule cell; P = Purkinje's cell.

locally and directly by climbing fibers, or much more diffusely by mossy fibers via the granule cells. Both types of excitation are limited in time and space by extensive inhibitory networks (Fig. 2-30) which use Golgi, basket, and stellate cells. Thus the climbing fibers excite stellate and basket cells which in turn inhibit the Purkinje's cells, and the mossy fibers excite Golgi's cells which inhibit the granule cells. The two pathways are also interconnected and can inhibit one another. The geometrical and extensive interaction possible in the molecular layer implies coordination of large areas of cerebellar cortex, but the functional aspects of this remain for future exploration.

So far as is known the only efferent fibers from the cortex are the Purkinje's cell axons, which also send recurrent collaterals back to molecular and granular layers, presumably to the inhibitory cells. Most of these axons pass to the deep nuclei and are thought to be inhibitory. Whether *some* of them are excitatory, or whether there is some other pathway excitatory to the neurons of the deep nuclei (e.g., collaterals of the climbing and mossy fibers) remains to be determined.

EXTRACELLULAR SPACE

The extracellular space (ECS) in the brain is narrow and tortuous, being represented by the interstices between the cell bodies and the processes of both neuronal and glial elements. In a normal brain, no ECS can be distinguished on light microscopy. Electron microscopy shows CNS cellular elements and processes closely apposed, although this apposition is somewhat lessened if care is taken to avoid asphyxial and postmortem changes during the preparation of the tissue, and if the type, concentration, and sequence of fixing and processing reagents are carefully selected. Under these circumstances there seems to be a perceptible ECS in white matter, presumably slightly wider at the nodes of Ranvier, where the axolemma is directly continuous with extracellular spaces. In gray matter the ECS appears to be represented by a uniform interval of approximately 200 A between adjacent plasma membranes, though some studies have indicated wider spaces in the vicinity of synapses. Early calculations of ECS volume were as low as 3 to 5% of total brain volume, but with the precautions previously mentioned, it is now calculated to be 15 to 20% of total brain volume. Estimations by other methods (see Chap. 4) suggest a range of 13 to 23% of total brain volume. Since the ECS seems to contain faintly granular material, and glial cells in culture produce mucopolysaccharides (which can be detected in normal brain), it appears likely that these mucopolysaccharides are at the cell surfaces. It then becomes a matter of semantics as to whether the normal "ECS" is truly intercellular or is a permeable outer zone of the cell membrane.

Morphologically, the ECS is internally limited by the ependymal cells and their intercellular junctions. Externally, beneath the pia, it is limited by expanded astrocytic processes, usually separated only by a 200-A interval and frequently showing incomplete intercellular junctions. Around vessels, with or without a meningeal or mesenchymal investment, there is a similar layer of astrocytic processes (foot processes), which form a more or less continuous boundary and show some intercellular junctions. The internodal regions of myelinated axons are sealed off from the ECS by membrane fusion (zonulae occludentes), formed between the axolemma and successive layers of the myelin sheath.

In summary, the ECS covers neuronal cell bodies and dendrites (except at the synaptic clefts), the

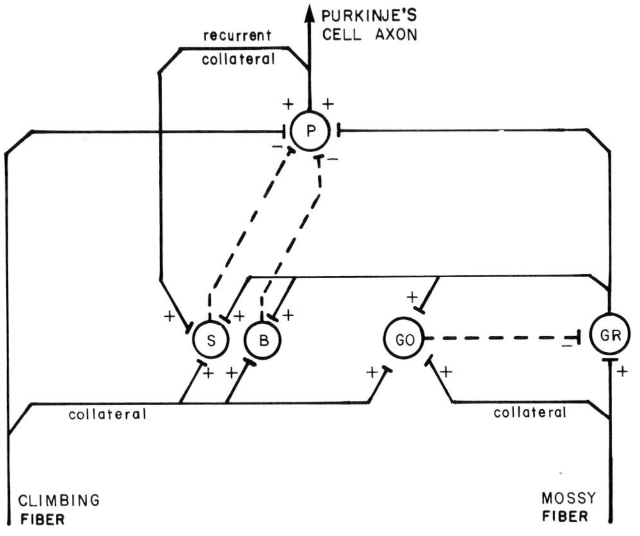

Fig. 2-30. Simplified circuit diagram of cerebellar cortex. B = basket cell; GO = Golgi cell; GR = granule cell; P = Purkinje's cell; S = stellate cell. + = excitatory synapse; – = inhibitory synapse.

initial segments and nodal regions of myelinated axons, the entire length of unmyelinated axons, and the cell bodies and processes of glial and microglial cells, except at the irregular and "spotty" intercellular junctions.

Because the permeability of cerebral vessels to many substances is much lower than that of vessels of other parts of the body, a barrier system has been postulated, prompting an intensive search for unusual morphological features. Capillaries in the brain do show unusual features. The endothelium exhibits little or no pinocytosis and does not contain the localized, extremely thin areas seen in some other parts of the body (fenestration). Moreover, intercellular junctions between endothelial cells seem to be complete, unlike those in capillaries elsewhere. The basement membrane is thick, and moderate numbers of pericytes are present.

The pericapillary region is unique in that it contains no mesenchymal elements, such as collagen fibers, but instead is formed by a ring of astrocytic foot processes, almost or completely covering the vessels and sharing a basement membrane with the endothelial cells. The margins between the foot processes show many intercellular junctions, and since this appears to be one unique feature of vascular complexes in the CNS, it had been surmised that it was the site of the barrier. However, the sealing of the foot processes one to the other is not complete, and it now appears that the ECS can reach the capillary basement membrane at some points. Further discussion of the blood-brain barrier in its functional aspects will be found in Chapter 4.

BIBLIOGRAPHY

Brightman, M. W., and Palay, S. L. The fine structure of ependyma in the brain of the rat. *J. Cell Biol.* 19:415-439, 1963.

Duncan, D. and Hild, W. Embryogenesis of the Nervous System. In J. Minckler (Ed.), *Pathology of the Nervous System.* New York: McGraw-Hill, 1968. Vol. 1, pp. 77-90.

Glees, B. and Meller, K. Morphology of Neuroglia. In G. H. Bourne (Ed.), *The Structure and Function of Nervous Tissue.* New York: Academic, 1968. Vol. 1, pp. 301-323.

Langman, J. Histogenesis of the Central Nervous System. In G. H. Bourne (Ed.), *The Structure and Function of Nervous Tissue.* New York: Academic, 1968. Vol. 1, pp. 33-65.

Luse, S. Microglia. In J. Minckler (Ed.), *Pathology of the Nervous System.* New York: McGraw-Hill, 1968. Vol. 1, pp. 531-538.

Luse, S. The Neuron. In J. Minckler (Ed.), *Pathology of the Nervous System.* New York: McGraw-Hill, 1968. Vol. 1, pp. 553-585.

Olmstead, J. B., and Borisy, G. G. Microtubules. *Annu. Rev. Biochem.* 42:507-540, 1973.

Peters, A. The Morphology of Axons of the Central Nervous System. In G. H. Bourne (Ed.), *The Structure and Function of Nervous Tissue.* New York: Academic, 1968. Vol. 1, pp. 142-186.

Peters, A., Palay, S. L., and Webster, H. de F. *The Fine Structure of the Nervous System.* New York: Harper & Row, 1970.

Schadé, J. P., and Ford, D. M. *Basic Neurology.* Amsterdam: Elsevier, 1965.

Shelanski, M. L., and Feit, H. Filaments and Tubules in the Nervous System. In G. H. Bourne (Ed.), *The Structure and Function of Nervous Tissue.* New York: Academic, 1972. Vol. 6, pp. 47-80.

Tennyson, V. M., and Pappas, G. D. Ependyma. In J. Minckler (Ed.), *Pathology of the Nervous System.* New York: McGraw-Hill, 1968. Vol. 1, pp. 518-531.

Neuronal Function

3

CELL MEMBRANES

Structure

All cells, including those of the central nervous system, are bounded by a plasmalemma (cell membrane), with a thickness of 75 to 90 A. Under the electron microscope (depending on method of fixation) the plasmalemma is usually seen to have three layers; the central layer is relatively electron-lucent and the outer two layers are electron-dense. The inner (cytoplasmic) dense layer often appears thicker than the external layer. Occasionally, the central zone appears to be crossed by faint, transverse striations, giving a "railroad-track" appearance. It is possible that the central zone consists of two layers of elongated, lipid molecules, with their hydrocarbon chains (hydrophobic) directed to the center of the membrane and polar (hydrophilic) ends directed toward the cytoplasm and extracellular fluid. Each side is probably covered by protein molecules, forming a thicker layer adjacent to the cytoplasm than adjacent to the exterior.

Although the protein-lipid-protein arrangement is generally accepted, other models have been postulated, especially to account for ionic permeability (pores). A particularly attractive possibility is a micellar (globular) arrangement of lipids (Fig. 3-1), especially if this can alternate with the lamellar arrangement previously noted, depending on the ratio of monovalent and divalent cations (see p. 60). In other models, the protein layers are discontinuous, and it has even been suggested that the entire membrane is an artifact. As noted in Chapter 2, there are membrane modifications (presently of uncertain significance) at synaptic junctions and in the initial segment and nodes of myelinated axons.

Relationship of Ion Concentrations in Extracellular and Intracellular Fluid with Membrane Potential

The plasmalemma separates extracellular and intracellular fluids of widely different ionic composition. The largest differences are between the high concentrations of Na^+ and Cl^- outside the cell and of K^+, N-acetylaspartate, and protein (the latter functioning as anion) inside the cell. The concentration gradients of these ions across the membrane, combined with differing membrane permeabilities, are probably mainly responsible for the internal negative potential (membrane potential), which varies from about −70 mv in the neuronal cell body to about −90 mv in the axon. Other ions make minor contributions. Transient alterations in permeability to the major ions, and consequent ionic shifts across the membrane, are associated both with the action potential (axonal conduction) and with postsynaptic potentials (synaptic transmission).

The evolutionary origin of the widely differing ionic concentrations is unknown, but it is generally conceded that these concentration differences are responsible for the membrane potential, not vice versa. The membrane is considered completely impermeable to N-acetylaspartate and protein, which represent the main intracellular anions. Thus, attention has been largely directed to Na^+, K^+, and Cl^-. For each one of these in isolation, in the presence of different concentrations across a membrane of limited permeability, such as the plasmalemma, diffusion rapidly creates a (trans) membrane potential opposing flow along the concentration gradient, such that net flow (flux) of that ion across the membrane is zero (Fig. 3-2). If either concentration is varied, this *equilibrium potential* must also vary. For monovalent ions, the equilibrium potential can be calculated by the simplified Nernst equation (strictly applicable only at 27°C):

$$E = 60 \cdot \log_{10} \frac{C_o}{C_i} \text{ mv}$$

E is the equilibrium potential, C_i the concentration inside the cell and C_o the concentration outside. For Na^+, with an external concentration of 109 mEq per liter and an internal concentration of 10.4 mEq per liter, the equilibrium potential is approximately +60 m (i.e., inside-positive). For K^+, with an outside concentration of 2.25 mEq per liter and an inside concentration of 124 mEq per liter, the equilibrium potential is −95 mv (i.e., inside-negative), and for Cl^- with an outside concentration of 77.5 mEq per liter and an inside concentration of 1.5 mEq per liter, the equilibrium potential is about −70 mv. Since the actual intracellular potential is between −65 and −90 mv, it follows that if the cell membrane were completely permeable to all three ions (Fig. 3-3), there would be a moderate efflux of K^+, a slight influx or efflux of Cl^-, and a massive influx of Na^+.

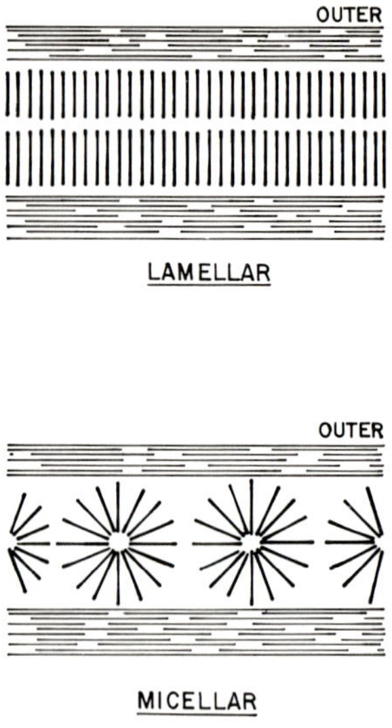

Fig. 3-1. Orientation of lipid molecules (thick lines) in lamellar and micellar membrane conformations.

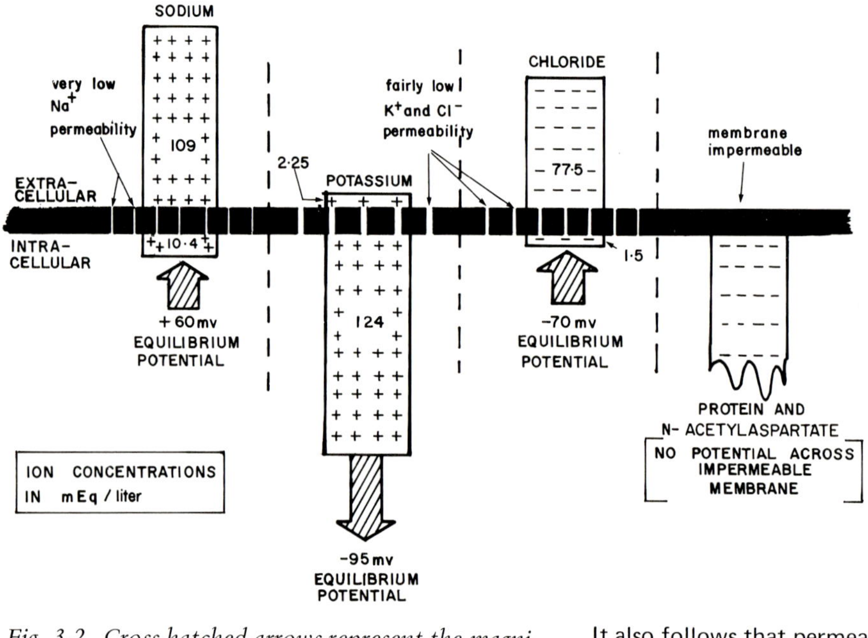

Fig. 3-2. Cross-hatched arrows represent the magnitude of the transmembrane potentials (equilibrium potentials), which can be calculated as necessary to maintain the observed internal and external ion concentrations across a permeable membrane. (Each ion is considered here in isolation, and the direction of the arrow indicates the effect of the equilibrium potential, having regard to the change of the ion).

It also follows that permeability to Na^+ is very low, since there is a great difference – about 140 mv – between the actual and the equilibrium potentials for Na^+.

In fact, the resting cell membrane has only a slight permeability to Na^+, which is also pumped out of the cell by an energy-dependent membrane mechanism. Permeability of the resting membrane to K^+ and Cl^- is about fifty times its permeability to Na^+ (although it is still low), and loss of potassium is balanced partly by the internal negativity of the cell (opposing loss of positively charged ions) and partly by the active influx of potassium in exchange for pumped-out sodium. As a result of the membrane permeabilities, the resting potential is relatively close

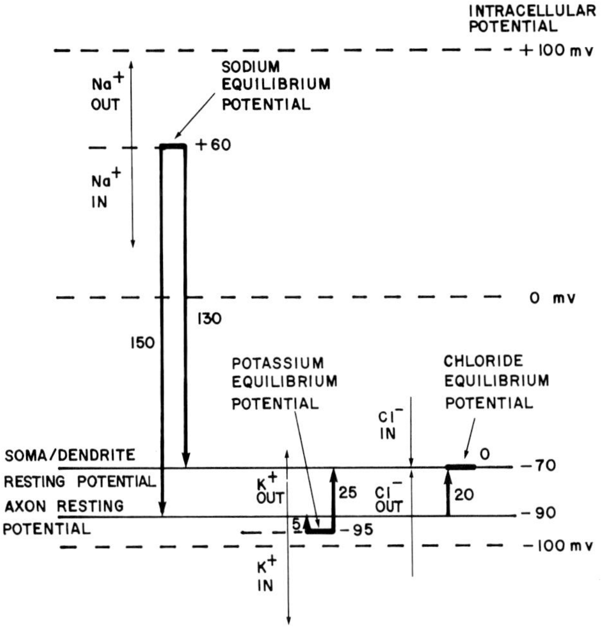

Fig. 3-3. Length and direction of the heavy vertical arrows indicate the magnitude and direction of the movement of the respective ions if the membrane suddenly became freely permeable to them, *either in the soma and dendrite, or in the axon. Such movement would of course be proportional to the difference between the actual and equilibrium potentials and might be in or out, according to the direction of this difference and the change on the ion. Obviously, the "disequilibrium" for Na^+ is much greater than for K^+ or Cl^-.*

to the equilibrium potentials for K^+ and Cl^-, and it is the tendency of K^+ to diffuse from the cell, unaccompanied by anion, which is believed largely responsible for the resting membrane potential. The lack of exact correspondence is due to some permeability to Na^+, Cl^-, and minor ions.

Both Na^+ efflux and K^+ influx are temperature-dependent. Both fluxes are abolished by agents (e.g., ouabain) known to inhibit (Na^+ + K^+)-activated adenosine triphosphatase (ATPase), an enzyme located in cell membranes and believed responsible for utilizing chemical bond energy in adenosine triphosphate (ATP) to drive the sodium-potassium pump. Although the precise molecular mechanism is unknown, this enzyme complex appears to mediate appropriate exchanges of Na^+ and K^+ at the inner and outer membrane surfaces. It is estimated that about 15% or more of the cellular energy metabolism is utilized by the pump.

PASSIVE MEMBRANE POTENTIALS

Within limits, the membrane potential may be modified by applied current (Fig. 3-4), using intracellular and extracellular electrodes or two external electrodes (for quantitation, the former must be used). If the internal electrode is positive, the membrane potential is reduced (depolarization), and if negative, it is increased (hyperpolarization). With a depolarization of more than about 25 mv, a self-propagating action potential is produced in excitable membranes such as the axolemma and sarcolemma. With these exceptions, passively induced changes in membrane potential are localized within 1 to 2 mm of the tip of the internal electrode; they decrease in amplitude with increasing distance from the electrode and also rise and fall more slowly with such increasing distance. These phenomena of attenuation, both in time and in space, are called *electronic decay* and depend on

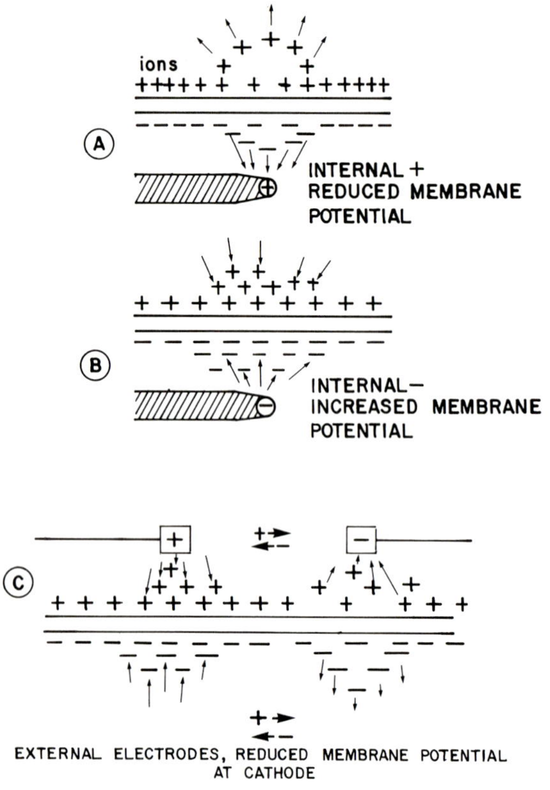

Fig. 3-4. Alteration of membrane potential by electrodes. A = Depolarization (hypopolarization) by internal anode. B = Hyperpolarization by internal cathode. C = Hyperpolarization by external anode and depolarization (hypopolarization) by external cathode.

the membrane resistance and capacitance. (For a detailed treatment and mathematical analysis, appropriate texts should be consulted.)

Using two external electrodes, hyperpolarization occurs beneath the positive electrode (anode) and depolarization beneath the negative electrode (cathode). Current flow in solutions is carried by ions; cations move from positive to negative, and anions move from negative to positive. Since membrane permeability is low, cations pile up externally at the anode, attracting anions internally, causing hyperpolarization. On the other hand, cations from the external surface are attracted to the cathode, releasing anions from the inner surface and causing depolarization (strictly speaking, hypopolarization). The released internal anions flow to the membrane under the anode, with an opposite flow of cations.

ACTION POTENTIAL

All animal membranes have a membrane potential (resting potential), which may be modified by the application of current as described. A further characteristic, possessed only by *excitable membranes,* is that depolarization (hypopolarization) beyond a certain degree (about 25 mv) causes propagation of an electrical impulse over the entire cell membrane, called an *action potential* (Fig. 3-5).

Changes in Ionic Permeability

Study of the membrane during passage of an action potential shows a sudden depolarization, or even

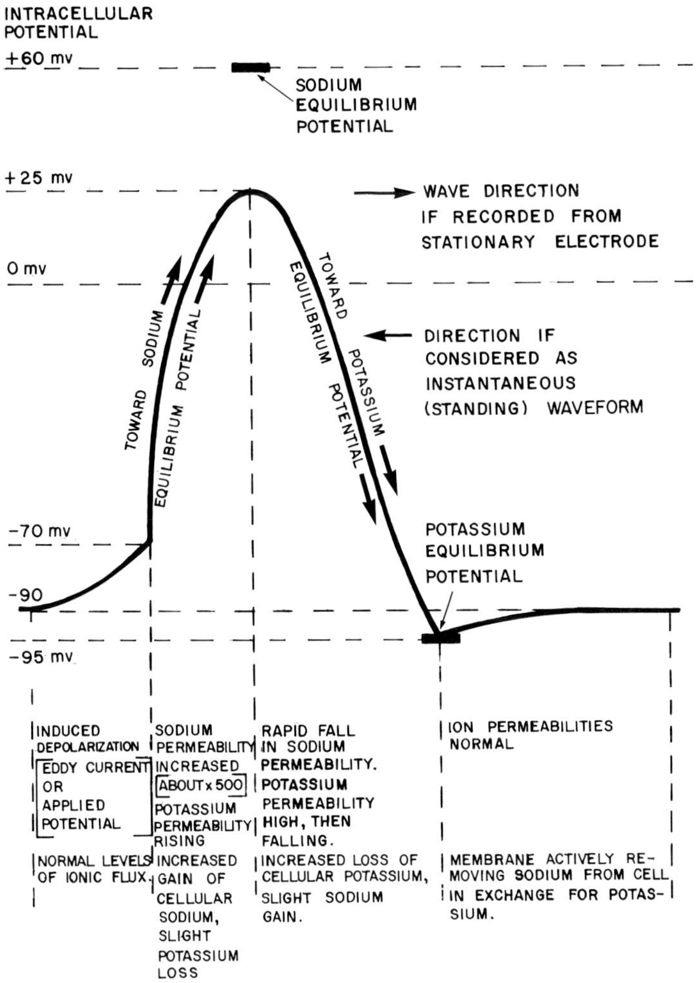

Fig. 3-5. Membrane potential changes (thick line) and alterations in membrane ion permeability (indicated below) during an action potential. Note that the alterations in ion flux, though large proportionately, are small in relation to toal intra- and extracullular ion pools and have little effect on ion concentrations.

reverse polarization to about +25 mv. During this period Na^+ permeability is transiently increased at least 500-fold over that of the resting membrane, an increase that ceases almost as suddenly as it starts. As Na^+ permeability falls back to normal there is a somewhat slower rise in K^+ permeability, so that the membrane repolarizes and even overshoots the resting potential by 5 or 10 mv, reaching about −95 mv, very close to the K^+ equilibrium level. There is then a slow return to the resting level as the K^+ permeability falls to normal. This sequence is intrinsic in excitable membranes and, once initiated (artificially by applied current or physiologically by postsynaptic potentials in the cell body or dendrite), is self-completing. Physiologically, where the internal and external ion concentrations are virtually constant, the action potential has constant amplitude and duration (0.2 to 0.5 milliseconds) and is therefore an all-or-nothing response. However, it is temperature-dependent, with delayed development and reduced amplitude in hypothermia.

Propagation

Since the initial point of depolarization is in contiguity with membrane carrying a normal resting potential, currents are set up that cause depolarization of adjacent membrane (Fig. 3-6). Thus, spread over the whole cell occurs by means of a continuous series of eddy currents and an advancing front of depolarization. Behind the front, the membrane is repolarized. The necessity for progressive depolarization imposes a limit on the speed of conduction, since it is induced by a capacitative current (ions do not cross the membrane until the threshold of massively increased Na^+ permeability is reached). For a short period following the action potential, the membrane is refractory and cannot be restimulated. Although the changes in potential are

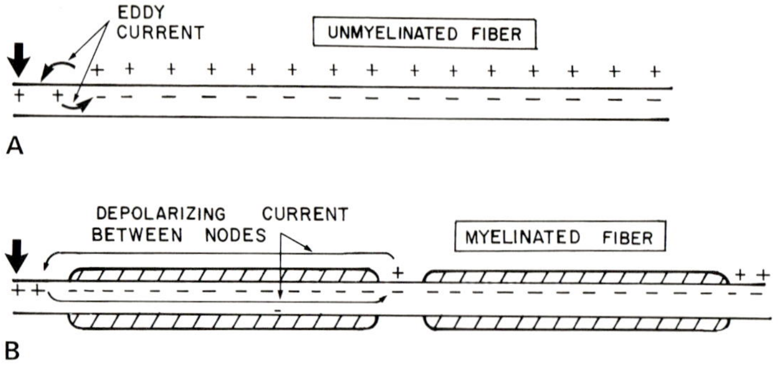

Fig. 3-6. Propagation of axon depolarization (action potential) in (A) unmyelinated and (B) myelinated fibers. Note the much smaller total length to be depolarized in B.

dramatic, the actual numbers of ions crossing the membrane is small. Even in a fine, unmyelinated fiber only 0.1μ in diameter, one action potential raises the internal [Na^+] only by about 10%.

The speed of conduction could be markedly increased, were it possible to decrease the area of axonal membrane to be depolarized. This effect is achieved in myelinated fibers in which the axon is covered by lengths of myelin (internodes) about one thousand times the fiber diameter, separated by nodes 0.5 to 2.5μ wide. An axolemma with a myelin sheath has markedly greater electrical resistance than naked axolemma, so that following the path of least resistance, eddy currents bypass the myelinated areas and are conducted between adjacent nodes of Ranvier. Since conduction is much faster than depolarization, this increases the speed of fiber conduction by a factor of 20 to 25. This is termed *saltatory conduction.* Resistance to current flow in the axoplasm decreases with an increasing cross-sectional area, so that larger fibers, even without myelin, conduct more rapidly than smaller ones.

Effective Stimuli

Experimental depolarization by current pulses of known shape, intensity, and duration has shown not only that there is a minimum strength of applied current (the threshold or rheobase) necessary to induce an action potential but that there is also a minimum duration. Thus, for any nerve fiber, a strength-duration curve may be plotted (Fig. 3-7). The *chronaxy* is the minimum time in which a stimulus of twice threshold strength will produce an action potential and is proportional to the product of resistance and capacitance for the membrane. Since alterations in membrane polarization persist for a finite time, two stimuli, each slightly subthreshold but applied in close succession, may summate to produce an action potential. Following an action potential, the threshold is raised to infinity for about 0.5 milliseconds (absolute refractory period), followed by a progressively decreasing threshold down to normal levels (partial refractory period). Thus, the maximum rate of impulse conduction is about 1000 per second. The mechanism of refractoriness is unknown.

Changes in Membrane Structure

The mechanism of changes in membrane permeability that accompany the action potential is not understood, but it may depend on altered conformation of macromolecules (Fig. 3-8) that is due to an exchange of ions within the membrane itself. Current work indicates that the membrane in the resting stage is largely occupied by calcium ions, which induce a conformation, perhaps lamellar, with some properties of a water-in-oil emulsion, including low permeability and high resistance. Depolarization may be accompanied by an increased rate of K^+ leakage, with replacement of the divalent ions (Ca^{++}) in the membrane by monovalent ions (K^+), and a consequent alteration in some membrane properties suggesting a change from a water-in-oil to an oil-in-water conformation. The latter may be micellar, and there is a marked increase in permeability and lowering of resistance. Apparently all excitable membranes require a divalent external cation, which can occupy the ion-binding sites; the majority also require a univalent external ion, such as Na^+.

Experimental work on the effect of Ca^{++} on macromolecules and artificial lipid membranes strongly supports the preceding concept. Protein on the two sides of the axolemma is markedly different in function, since the external application of proteases has little or no effect on the action potential, whereas internal application abolishes or otherwise alters it. Perhaps protein not only is responsible for maintaining mechanical integrity but in some way also controls the permeability. The macromolecular and ionic theories of nerve excitation are not mutually contradictory, but represent successive phases in the induction of an action potential. The progressive membrane replacement of divalent ion (presumably Ca^{++}) by internal K^+ ultimately produces a change in emulsion form and permeability, which is then followed by the ionic shifts accompanying (and causing) the action potential.

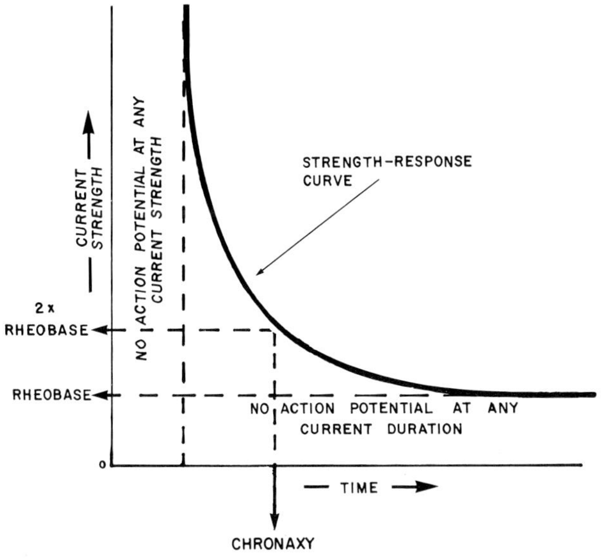

Fig. 3-7. Strength-duration curve for production of an axonal action potential. Note the necessity for a finite time of stimulation as well as a minimum current strength.

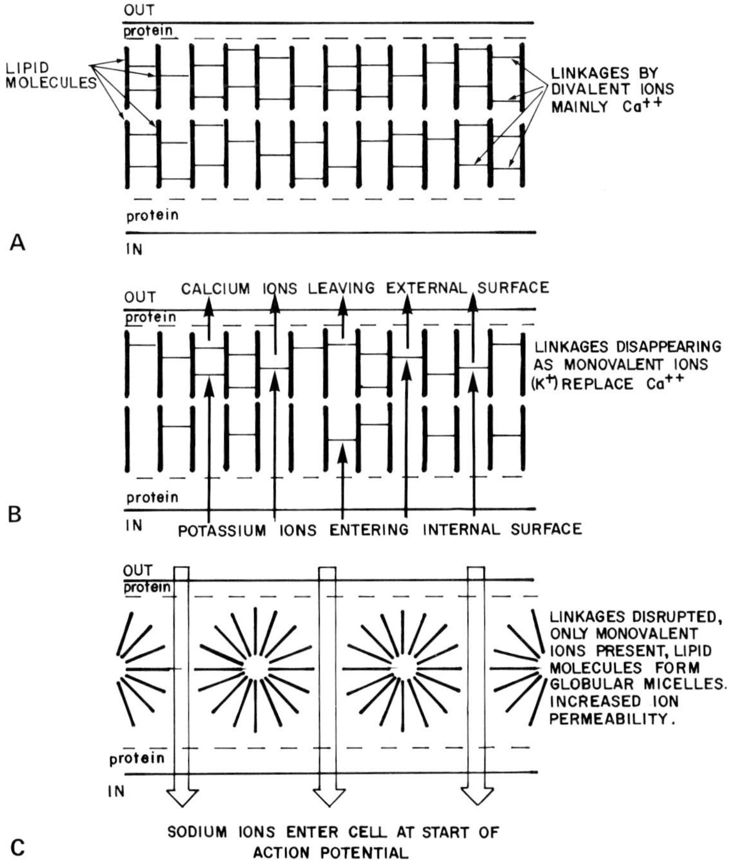

Fig. 3-8. A postulated mechanism for increasing membrane permeability to ions. In the resting lamellar stage, parallel lipid molecules are cross-linked by Ca^{++} (A), but reduction of potential (depolarization) permits K^+ to enter from the intracellular fluid (B), disrupting the Ca^{++} linkages and leading to micellar conformation (C). Na^+ can now more readily enter the cell (axon) between the lipid micelles.

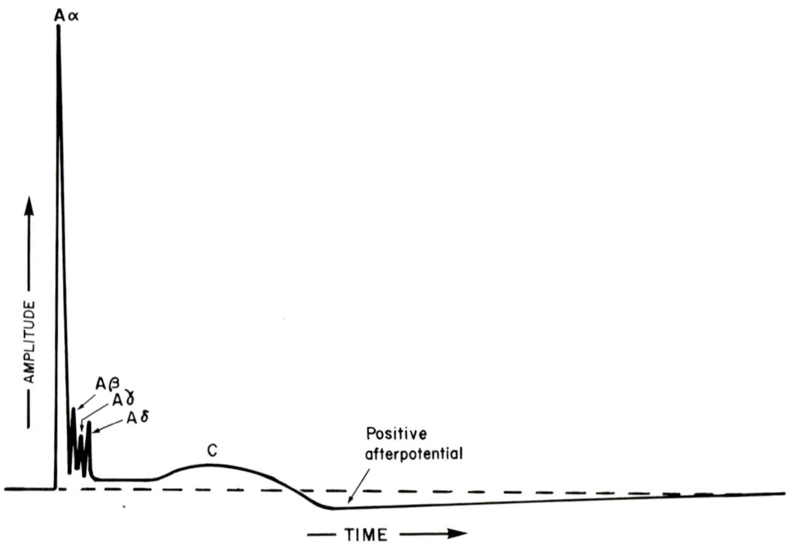

Fig. 3-9. Compound action potential recorded from a mixed (sensory and motor) peripheral nerve.

COMPOUND ACTION POTENTIALS

In clinical practice it is not generally feasible to use intracellular electrodes or to study conduction in a single axon, but rather to study groups of axons that make up peripheral nerves. If such a nerve is stimulated by applied current, the resulting electrical activity recorded at a distance is the *compound action potential* (CAP), resulting from all axons for which the stimulus is effective (threshold or higher). The CAP is not an all-or-nothing phenomenon, since it includes large numbers of individual action potentials, some elicited by low stimuli, others by high. Each nerve therefore has a threshold stimulus, producing the least observable response, an intermediate (suprathreshold or submaximal) stimulus range (during which the amplitude and duration of the CAP increase to a maximum), and a maximum stimulus, above which there is no further change.

The form of the CAP varies with the type of nerve. In a motor nerve, composed mainly of large fibers, it is essentially a single, large, early spike, followed by a long minor *after potential,* first in the same direction as the spike (negative) and then opposite (positive). These low-amplitude potentials may last, all told, about 45 seconds. Their origin is not clear. In a mixed or sensory nerve, the axon potential is much more complicated (Fig. 3-9). Earliest is a complex peak (*A*), which has four components (α, β, γ, δ) and then, after some delay, a diffuse peak (*C*). The *A* potentials are from myelinated fibers (of decreasing diameter from α to δ), and the *C* potentials are from unmyelinated fibers; this dramatically indicates the difference in conduction velocities. For *A* fibers, velocity in meters per second is four to five times the external diameter in microns, whereas for *C* fibers the factor is only about 1.7. All fibers exhibit afterpotential, being hyperexcitable in the first (negative) phase and hypoexcitable in the second (positive) phase. (*B* fibers are preganglionic, sympathetic, and myelinated; they have only a negative afterpotential, with reduced excitability.)

SYNAPTIC CONDUCTION

The synapse is the site of conduction of excitation from one neuron to another and is described in Chapter 2. Presynaptic and postsynaptic membranes are separated by a synaptic cleft, and impulse conduction is due to release of a chemical, the neurotransmitter, from the presynaptic terminal, thus ensuring that conduction can only be in one direction. However, electrical transmission has not yet been conclusively ruled out in the vertebrate CNS and certainly occurs in invertebrates.

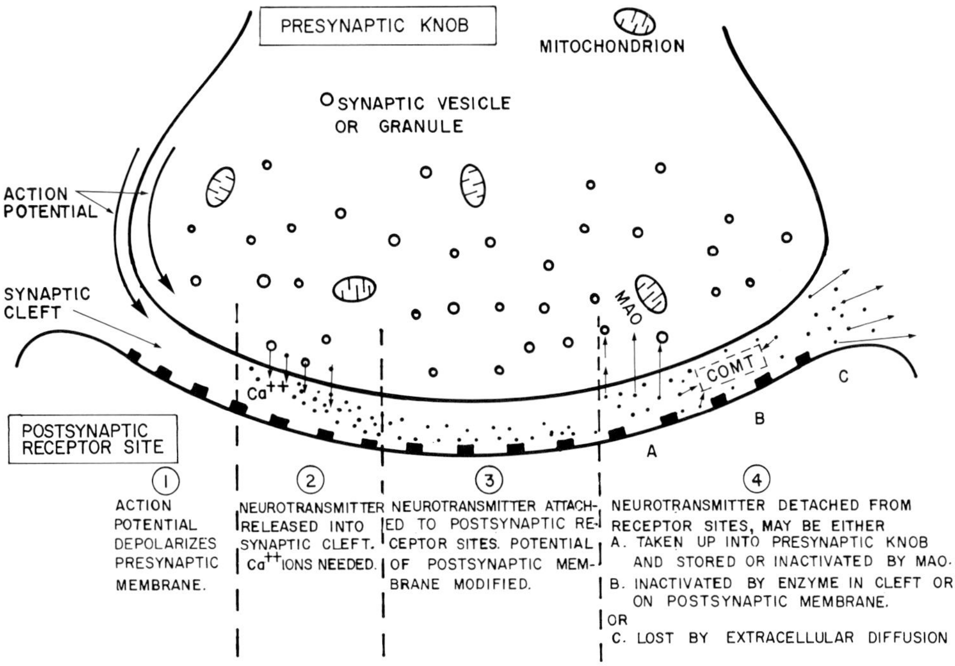

Fig. 3-10. Sequence of events (1-4) occurring during synaptic transmission. The mechanism of action of transmitter on postsynaptic receptor sites is not known, but the net effect may be alteration or stabilization of postsynaptic membrane potential. COMT = catechol-O-methyltransferase; MAO = monoamine oxidase.

Transmission begins (Fig. 3-10) when the presynaptic membrane is depolarized by arrival of the action potential, which facilitates release of the transmitter substance present in vesicles or granules (and possibly also free) in the presynaptic cytoplasm. Release requires the presence of Ca^{++} and is inhibited by Mg^{++}. The mechanism by which the action potential releases transmitter is unknown, but the amount released is proportional to the net amplitude of the action potential. The transmitter diffuses across the synaptic cleft and, presumably through combination with postsynaptic receptor sites (although, again, little is known of the chemical mechanism), produces permeability changes in the postsynaptic membrane. The arrival of a single impulse at a presynaptic terminal does not necessarily, and indeed may only rarely, suffice to generate an action potential in the postsynaptic cell. Functionally, there are at least three types of synapses, though they have not been clearly differentiated under the electron microscope. They are:

1. Excitatory synapses, in which there is some depolarization of the postsynaptic membrane.
2. Inhibitory synapses, in which the transmitter causes either slight hyperpolarization, or no change in potential, of the postsynaptic membrane.
3. Presynaptic inhibitory (axoaxonal) synapses, in which the inhibitory terminal is on another presynaptic terminal and not on the soma-dendrite receptor surface. The arrival of the inhibitory action potential at the first terminal reduces the membrane potential of the second terminal and therefore decreases transmitter release from the latter.

Excitatory Postsynaptic Potential

The excitatory postsynaptic potential (EPSP) is a depolarization up to 10 mv at the postsynaptic membrane (potential down to −60 mv), with correspondingly lesser change with increasing distance over the receptor area. If the membrane potential is artificially altered (by an internal electrode), the EPSP changes both in sign and in size (Fig. 3-11). When the membrane potential is set at zero, the EPSP is also zero. If the membrane potential is reversed, so that the inside of the cell is positive, the EPSP is reversed, becoming a hyperpolarization. It appears that the EPSP is tending toward a membrane potential of 0 mv, which physiologically represents depolarization, and that it may be due to an increase in permeability to all ions. At physiological potentials and concentrations, this would have little effect on Cl^- flux, causing mainly increased Na^+ influx and K^+ efflux. Studies on the motor end-plate of muscle suggest a similar mechanism, the change in permeability for

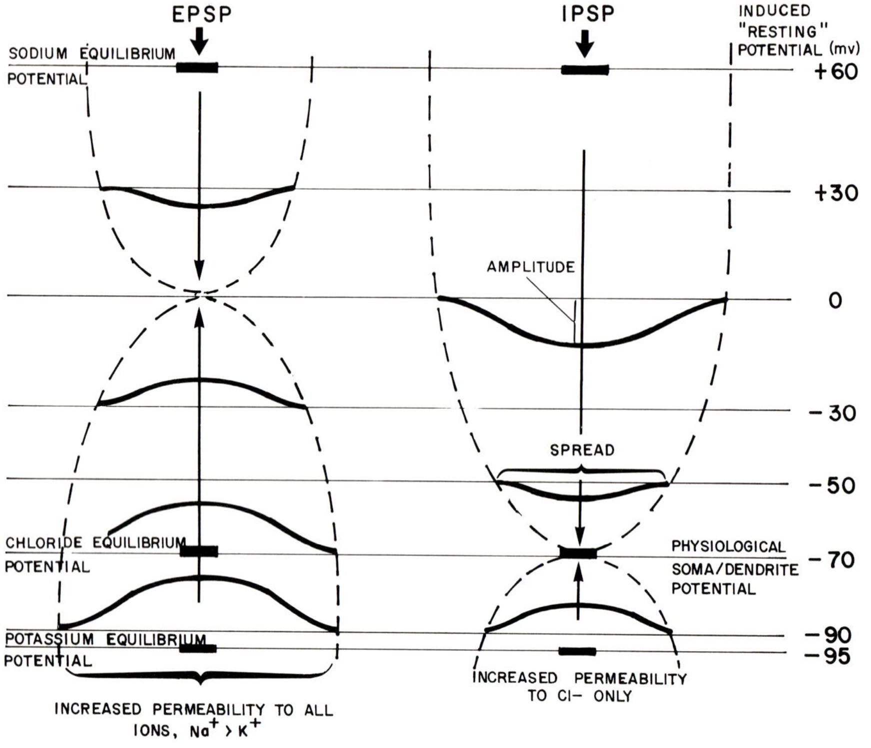

Fig. 3-11. Postsynaptic membrane potential changes at excitatory (EPSP) and inhibitory (IPSP) synapses. Note the effect of altering the resting membrane potential on the amplitude, spread, and direction of potential changes.

Na^+ being larger than for K^+. Measured changes in Na^+ permeability following passively changed axonal membrane potential are also consistent.

Inhibitory Postsynaptic Potential

The inhibitory postsynaptic potential (IPSP) is limited to the central nervous system in vertebrates. At resting potential, no postsynaptic potential change is produced by an inhibitory synapse (Fig. 3-11), but if the membrane is partially depolarized, a change toward the resting value (repolarization) occurs. Experimentally, inhibitory stimuli tend to reduce artificial (passive) hyperpolarization, so that the tendency is toward maintenance of, or restoration to, the resting potential (i.e., the inhibitory stimulus acts as a "membrane clamp"). Clearly, Na^+ permeability (equilibrium potential +60 mv) is unaltered, and it appears that permeability to Cl^- (and, possibly, to K^+ or to both) is principally involved, since the resting potential is close to the equilibrium potential of Cl^- (−70 mv).

Presynaptic Inhibitory Potential

The existence of "synapses on synapses" (Fig. 3-12) has been shown by the electron microscope in most of the CNS, though apparently rarely in the cortex. Presynaptic inhibition is not associated with any change in postsynaptic membrane potential, even if the latter is passively altered, and there is no change in the threshold of the postsynaptic cell to direct stimulation. Drugs affect the IPSP and presynaptic inhibitory potential (PSIP) differently. Thus,

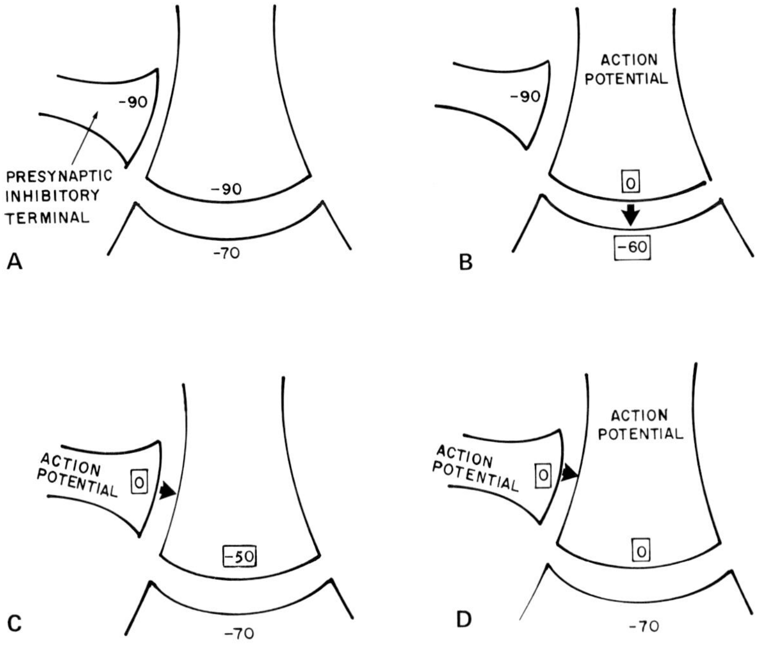

Fig. 3-12. Presynaptic inhibition. A = Resting state; B = excitatory action potential causes EPSP; C = inhibitory action potential alone does not affect postsynaptic membrane; D = combined action potentials show blockage of the normal EPSP. Arrows represent release of neurotransmitter. Figures representing membrane potentials (in mv) are approximations only.

strychnine depresses IPSP but enhances PSIP, and picrotoxin depresses PSIP with no effect on IPSP. Barbiturates may increase and prolong the PSIP. It is assumed that PSIPs, through an unidentified neurotransmitter, reduce the presynaptic membrane potential (depolarization) and so reduce release of neurotransmitter. Thus, although the amplitude of the axonal action potential is constant, it can be modulated at the synapse by changes in the synaptic knob resting potential. If this is reduced by a PSIP, the amplitude of the presynaptic action potential is correspondingly reduced.

Slow Synaptic Potentials

Slow postsynaptic potentials, with gradual onset and several seconds' duration, have been described and are apparently *not* due to continued transmitter activity but to activation of an electrogenic pump in the postsynaptic membrane. There is no change in ionic permeability, and potential may be raised or lowered. The function of slow synaptic potentials is speculative and might include modulation of activity of neural networks.

Interaction of Postsynaptic Potentials

The complete system of dendrites attached to a cell body, together with the cell body itself and the initial (constricted) segment of the axon, may be considered as a unit (Fig. 3-13). This unit receives hundreds or thousands of impulses through synapses on the dendrites or soma (not the initial segment); each impulse effects only a small change in membrane potential. Since individual postsynaptic changes are nonpropagated, they have many of the properties (including electrotonic decay) of the passively induced potentials previously discussed; and since the

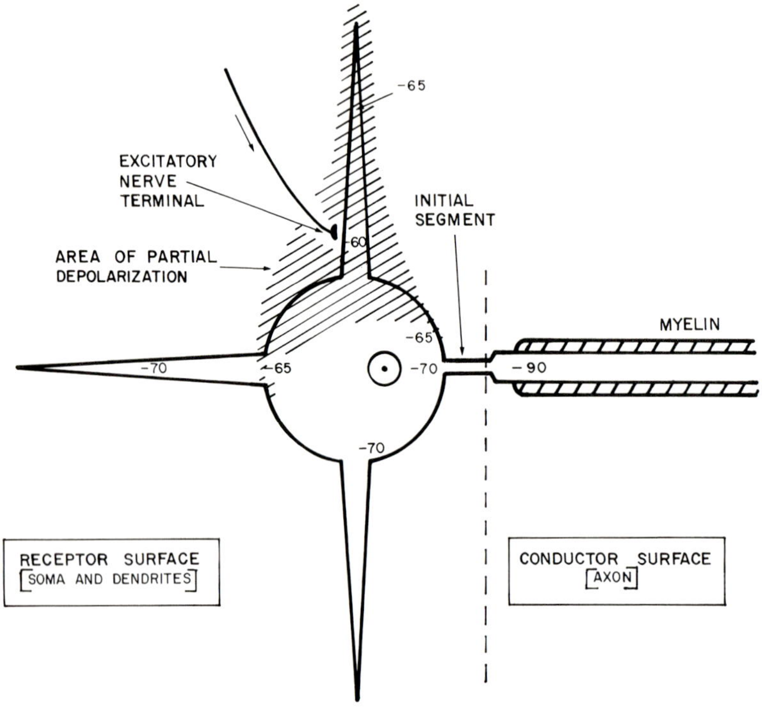

Fig. 3-13. Receptor surface of a neuron (soma and dendrites), showing the spread and the attenuation of the EPSP produced by excitation at a single synapse.

total diameter of a neuron with its dendritic field rarely exceeds 2 mm, it may be assumed that the potential changes produced at any postsynaptic membrane are propagated over much of the receptor surface (cell body plus dendrites) and initial segment and have a finite time of persistence.

The net potential change of the receptor surface and initial segment is the algebraic sum of the depolarizations produced by excitation and the hyperpolarizations produced by inhibition (Fig. 3-14). The receptor surface therefore has the ability of summation, and its potential changes in no way resemble the all-or-nothing response of the axon. Summation may occur in space, due to excitatory impulses arriving through different synapses concurrently; or in time, with excitatory impulses enhanced by residual depolarization due to slightly earlier arrivals. Both effects are commonly termed *facilitation.* If the receptor surface is effectively depolarized by about 20 mv (i.e., the membrane potential is reduced from –70 to –50 mv), electrotonic spread ensures depolarization of 10 mv or more in the initial segment, sufficient to initiate an action potential. This is propagated along the axon (the conducting or effective action potential), retroactively over the cell, and over at least the proximal parts of the dendrites. Retrograde spread is slow, at under 1 meter per second. The cell body and dendrites have a refractory period during which they cannot initiate an action potential, however large the stimulus.

The term *facilitation* is applied not only to summation in an individual neuron, but also to a neuron pool. Stimulating a small afferent nerve bundle may cause action potentials (firing) in 100 neurons but lesser depolarization of, say, a further 1000 in the surrounding area. Stimulation of a second afferent bundle may fire 100 different neurons and partly depolarize another 1000. If the neurons fired are largely different groups but the partly depolarized groups overlap, then simultaneous stimulation of both nerve bundles will fire not only the original 200 neurons but also some others that are partly depolarized by each stimulus and are able to summate both. Thus, instead of 200, perhaps 500 or even more neurons may fire. This is an example of facilitation. If the distribution of the two afferent nerve bundles is closely similar (e.g., 90 of the 100 neurons fired may be fired by either bundle separately), then simultaneous stimulation may actually result in fewer than the expected number of firings, a phenomenon termed *occlusion.*

Facilitation of an individual neuron has a time course similar to that of electrotonic decay, falling to half its initial value in about 4 milliseconds. Inhibition requires about 0.5 milliseconds to reach its maximum, whereas facilitation is virtually immediate. The difference is not explained, though an interneuron has been suggested. Transmission across a synapse shows perceptible delay, probably not exceeding 0.5 milliseconds, and is much slower than axonal conductions. The maximum frequency of synaptic

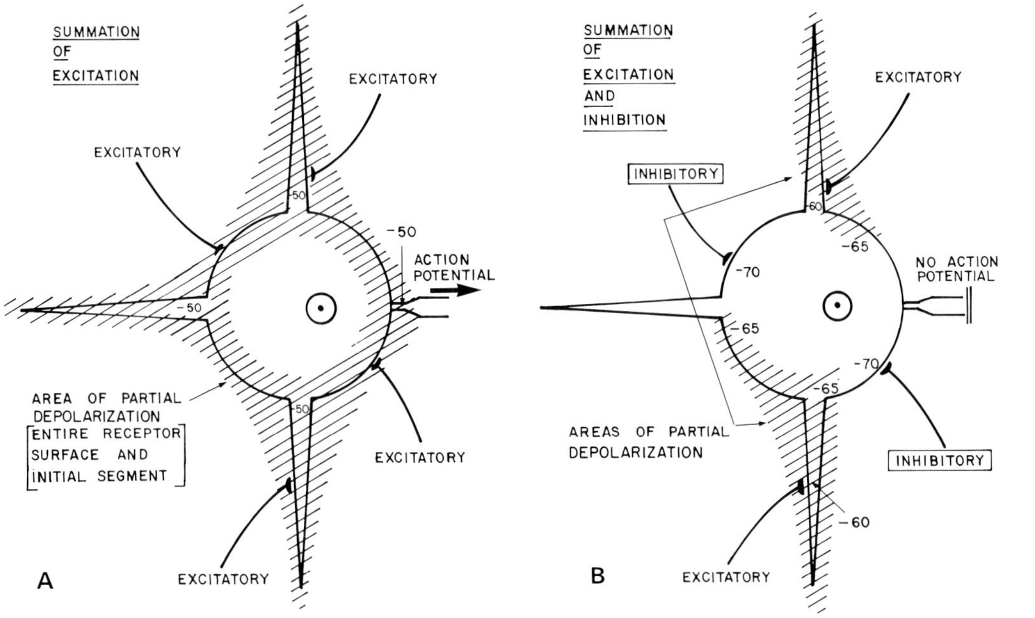

Fig. 3-14. Representation of summation (A) produced by activation of four excitatory synapses and (B) produced by two excitatory and two inhibitory synapses. In A, an action potential is produced. In reality, not four but probably several hundred synapses are activated on any neuron at any given time.

transmission is only about 100 per second compared with 1000 per second for axons.

Synaptic transmission is metabolically more vulnerable than axonal conduction. Ischemia or anesthetic agents more readily depress transmission than conduction and therefore have an earlier effect on networks consisting of many neurons (e.g., the reticular activating system) than on those with only a few.

Reasons for the lower membrane potential in the receptor area, as compared with the axon, are unknown, though it could reflect continual excitatory bombardment. One result of this lower resting potential is that Cl^- is very close to its equilibrium potential. Alterations in ionic permeabilities associated with postsynaptic potentials (see pp. 63 and 64) are less well defined than those associated with the action potential.

NEUROTRANSMITTERS

Synaptic transmission in vertebrates appears to be exclusively chemical and unidirectional, although in some evolutionarily earlier forms electrical transmission, which is bidirectional, occurs. Several chemical mediators of synaptic transmission are known and others suspected. It is probable that such variability assists localization of function within the CNS.

Release and Reuptake of Transmitters

Presynaptic cytoplasm contains vesicles or granules, 300 to 500 A in diameter, which tend to be clustered adjacent to the presynaptic membrane, along with mitochondria and sometimes other organelles. Since neurotransmitters are released in small packages (quanta), and electron microscopy has revealed no substrate for these other than synaptic vesicles or granules, it may well be that they are the sites from which transmitters are released, by a process of exocytosis into the synaptic cleft. This is well established for granules of the adrenal medulla, because the same proportions of transmitter (epinephrine), adenosine triphosphate (ATP), and a specific protein (chromagranin A) are released as are present in the granules. However, evidence that one quantum is the content of one vesicle or granule is circumstantial for synapses and neuromuscular junctions. The evidence is equivocal because the transmitter not only is present in vesicles and granules, but also is free in the cytoplasm and often seems to form two separate pools, one relatively stable and one labile; the most recently synthesized is the earliest released. This could be adduced as evidence that the cytoplasmic labile component is readily released, with the vesicles acting as storage sites; alternatively, if the vesicles nearest the presynaptic membrane discharge and then resynthesize or take up transmitter, on the arrival of the next action potential they may again discharge (the transmitter most recently synthesized). If a synapse is repetitively stimulated, an initial high rate of transmitter release (labile component) falls to a sustained lower rate, presumably from the stable pool.

The presynaptic cytoplasm is the ultimate destination of materials carried by *axoplasmic flow* from the cell body. Such flow has at least two forms: a slow bulk movement, largely of protein, at 1 to 6 mm per day, and a much faster particulate movement, perhaps in both directions, at 100 to 2800 mm per day. The mechanisms are unknown, but may involve microtubules or neurofilaments. Flow is energy-dependent, though continuing for a short time in severed axons. The fast flow includes vesicles or granules seen by electron microscopy in small numbers in axons and may be the major, or only, source of such structures in presynaptic cytoplasm. However, a limited capacity for protein synthesis is found presynaptically, and some vesicles may be formed locally. Much neurotransmitter is known to be synthesized in the cell body and passed down the axon to synapses, but the latter also possess the necessary enzymes for synthesis in situ, and the relative importance of the two sites may vary with the individual transmitters. (Since the cytoplasmic bulk transported down the axon each day may be several times the volume of the cell body, axoplasmic flow presumably has additional functions, such as axonal maintenance, nutrition, and even RNA transport to effect structural synaptic changes if such prove to be involved in memory.)

Released in the synaptic cleft, the transmitter reacts reversibly with postulated receptor sites on the postsynaptic membrane, in some way altering ionic permeability as previously discussed. It is essential that it be rapidly cleared before the next arriving stimulus. Therefore, mechanisms for its instantaneous inactivation must exist. At least three such mechanisms are known. Probably the most important is *reuptake* of transmitter back through the presynaptic membrane. This mechanism rapidly removes transmitter from the cleft and thus from its activity on the postsynaptic membrane. A second important mechanism is *inactivation* by appropriate enzymes; for well-established transmitters, such enzymes are invariably present, either in the cleft and adjacent extracellular space, or in the cytoplasm, or both. A third mechanism – and a less prompt and less effective one – is the simple *diffusion* of the neurotransmitter through the extracellular space. As noted in Chapter 2, this extracellular space is more extensive around synaptic junctions than around most other gray matter components and frequently consists of several channels radiating away from the cleft between adjacent cell processes.

Identification of Transmitters

Although neurotransmitters in relatively simple tissues (muscle, sympathetic ganglia) can usually be readily identified by their concentration, the presence of synthesizing and inactivating enzymes, and reproduction of their effects by application of exogenous transmitter, the situation in the CNS is more complex. There is no mass of tissue with only one potential transmitter, and concentrations of many amines and aminoacids are relatively high. Local application of transmitter at the synaptic junction is virtually impossible because of the structural complexity. So many substances have been proposed as neurotransmitters, including acetylcholine, monoamines (such as epinephrine, norepinephrine, and serotonin), neutral amino acids (such as γ-aminobutyric acid [GABA], which are probably inhibitors), and acidic amino acids (which are probably excitors) that there are relatively long lists of (often indirect) criteria that a proposed substance must meet in order to be generally acceptable as a transmitter. These include:

1. The presence of the suspected transmitter with its synthesizing enzymes (inactivating enzymes may be less important, because of other mechanisms of inactivation).
2. The collectibility of the transmitter on stimulation.
3. Reproducibility of all physiological effects when the suspected transmitter is applied exogenously (this requires at least the techniques of microiontophoresis and intracellular recording).
4. Pharmacological identity (meaning that other agents, such as strychnine or picrotoxin, have the same effects both on physiological transmission and on the action of exogenous transmitter).

Because of technical difficulties, such rigid criteria are rarely met for CNS transmitters. On more or less circumstantial evidence, it seems that the following substances function as central neurotransmitters: acetylcholine, norepinephrine, dopamine, and serotonin. Less certain candidates are histamine, GABA, and glycine, among others. Whereas the first group (and possibly histamine) are released at synaptic terminals of restricted groups of neurons and are not general metabolites, amino acids such as GABA and glycine are present in most or all cells and could not meet strict criteria for neurotransmitters. Only a substance which is released from axon terminals as a result of an action potential and which modulates the excitability of the postsynaptic membrane is a transmitter. A substance involved in general metabolic activity, which alters the excitability of several or many neighboring cells perhaps by simple diffusion, is a "regulator" or "modulator," and some amino acids may fall into this group.

Acetylcholine

Localization

Acetylcholine seems to be a transmitter for the ascending reticular activating system (ARAS) and excites some 25% of cortical neurons, especially in layer V. Within the ARAS, appropriate enzymes for synthesis and inactivation are present. Cortical cells excited by stimulation of the ARAS do not respond to stimulation of thalamic relay nuclei. Possible additional functions of acetylcholine that have been proposed are that it acts as a cortical inhibitor (in intracortical neurons originating arcuate fibers) and that it acts as an excitatory transmitter at the cortical terminations of the auditory and optic radiations (cell

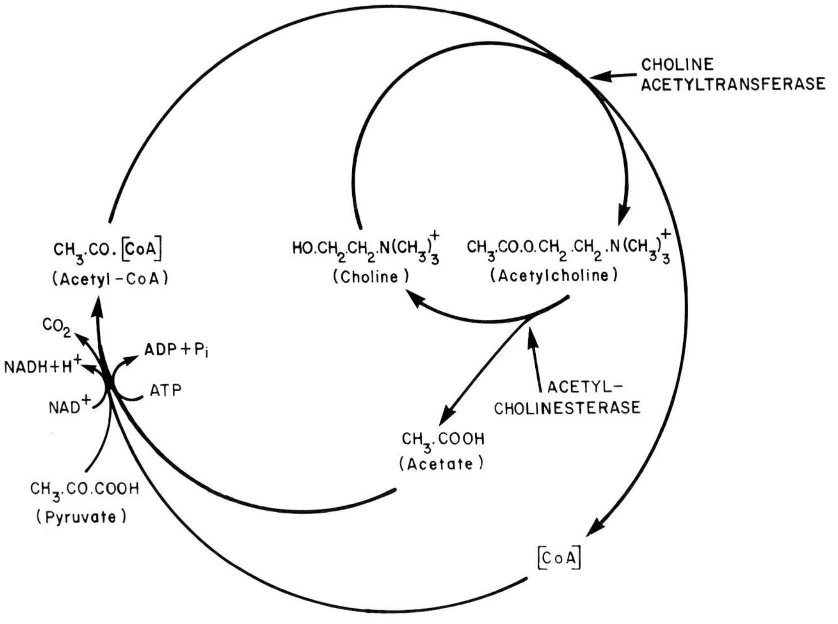

Fig. 3-15. Acetylcholine metabolism. CoA = coenzyme A; ADP = adenosine diphosphate; P_i = inorganic phosphate; ATP = adenosine triphosphate; NAD^+ and NADH = oxidized and reduced nicotinamide adenine dinucleotide.

bodies in the lateral and medial geniculate bodies). However, recent evidence does not support this hypothesis. Some excitatory cholinergic fibers terminate in the basal ganglia, but their origin is not clear. Peripherally, acetylcholine is the transmitter for all preganglionic autonomic fibers, both sympathetic and parasympathetic, all postganglionic parasympathetic fibers, some sympathetic fibers (e.g., those of the sweat glands), and motor fibers to skeletal muscle (neuromuscular junctions).

Concentrations of acetylcholine and its synthesizing enzyme, choline acetyltransferase (CAT), are approximately parallel and range from 1 to 7 ppm, with high levels in the upper brain stem and basal ganglia and low levels in the cord, cerebellum, medulla, and hypothalamus. (The concentration is 9 to 18 ppm in ventral roots, 0 to 0.25 in dorsal roots, 4 to 6 in mixed nerves such as the sciatic, and 18 to 44 in the superior cervical ganglion.) The inactivating enzyme, acetylcholinesterase, is at a uniformly high level in all parts of the CNS, not correlating well with acetylcholine or CAT. The significance of this is not clear. It could suggest a vestigial pattern in which most neurons were originally cholinergic; or it could indicate other, more generalized functions for acetylcholine, such as increased phosphate incorporation in membrane lipids (including phosphatidic acid) or depolarization by activation of a Cl^- pump (of unknown function).

Metabolism

Although the enzymes CAT and acetylcholinesterase (AChE) are largely synthesized in the cell body, acetylcholine itself seems to be formed mainly in the presynaptic cytoplasm. No effective inhibitors for CAT are known. Acetylcholine (Fig. 3-15) is formed in the cytoplasm, rather than in the vesicles, by the combination of acetylcoenzyme A (acetyl-CoA) (or acetate and coenzyme A) with choline (or possibly phosphatidylcholine); choline concentrations are rate-limiting although avidly taken up from the extracellular space. Once formed, an appreciable but uncertain proportion of acetylcholine remains in the cytoplasm, and the remainder is stored in clear vesicles, each thought to contain 300 to 3000 molecules. It is unknown whether release into the synaptic cleft is from the cytoplasmic or vesicle fraction, but it appears to occur in discrete "units."

Following release into the synaptic cleft and reaction with the postsynaptic membrane, acetylcholine is rapidly destroyed by AChE, which is present within the cleft and other extracellular space and is apparently attached to most neuronal and glial membranes. In addition to AChE, which is present in most parts of the body, other enzymes are present that split choline esters (pseudo-cholinesterases) but have only a slow action on acetylcholine. The two may be distinguished by synthetic substrates, since AChE rapidly breaks down acetyl-β-methylcholine (methacholine) but has little effect on the benzoyl, butyryl, or propionyl esters of choline. Pseudo-cholinesterase has opposite effects. AChE is a very rapidly acting enzyme with four active centers on each molecule and splits acetylcholine into free choline and acetic acid. Neural tissues are generally

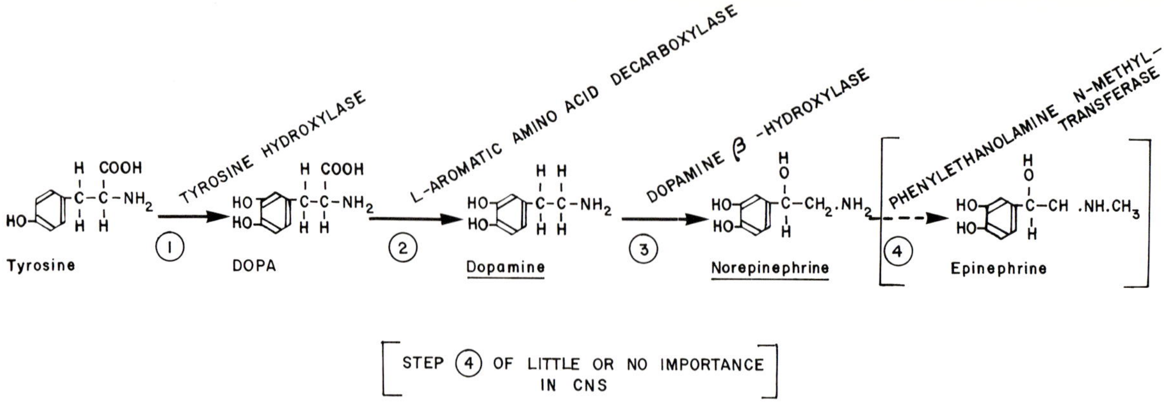

Fig. 3-16. Catecholamine (dopamine, norepinephrine, and epinephrine) synthesis.

low in pseudo-cholinesterase, except for sympathetic ganglia.

Some acetylcholine receptors in the CNS are muscarinic and specifically blocked by atropine, but the latter also appears to exert a nonspecific local anesthetic action when injected iontophoretically, complicating the interpretation of results. The effects of acetylcholine in the cortex (presumably ARAS) are measured in seconds both at onset and duration. Some receptors may be nicotinic.

Catecholamines: Norepinephrine and Dopamine

Localization

Derived from the amino acid tyrosine, norepinephrine and dopamine are found in separate anatomical pathways of the CNS. In both, much of the transmitter is synthesized in the cell body and reaches the terminal by axoplasmic flow. Such cell bodies are largely situated in the older parts of the brain.

Noradrenergic cells (i.e., producing norepinephrine) are present mainly in the ventral brain stem and give rise to descending fibers to the gray matter of the spinal cord, local fibers to brain stem nuclei, and ascending fibers to the hypothalamus and (mainly limbic) cortex. Lesions in the ventrolateral midbrain tegmentum decrease norepinephrine levels in the forebrain, presumably by severing the ascending axons. *Dopaminergic* cells are chiefly in the substantia nigra, with fibers passing to the neostriatum and olfactory tubercles. The majority of dopaminergic and noradrenergic systems are inhibitory, but some ascending noradrenergic fibers to the cortex may be excitatory, forming part of the ARAS. Fibers to the cord may be inhibitory to interneurons.

Concentrations of norepinephrine (in parts per million) range from a high of about 1.15 in the hypothalamus, through 0.2 to 0.5 in the brain stem and inferior head of caudate and 0.04 to 0.2 in the cortex, to such low levels as 0.01 in white matter. Concentrations of a synthesizing enzyme, L-amino acid decarboxylase (dopa decarboxylase), are roughly parallel. Dopamine levels are very low in the cortex, cerebellum, and white matter but reach 4 to 6 ppm in the caudate and putamen, with lower values in the midbrain, thalamus, and hypothalamus. Epinephrine has very low concentrations in the CNS, about 10% of those of norepinephrine. However, the olfactory bulb and tubercle contain the enzyme phenylethanolamine-N-methyltransferase, necessary for the synthesis of epinephrine and absent from other parts of the brain.

Metabolism

Norepinephrine and dopamine do not penetrate the blood-brain barrier, although a precursor, dopa, does so readily if blood levels are raised. Catecholamines are therefore synthesized (Fig. 3-16) within the CNS from tyrosine (itself largely formed from phenylalanine in the liver). The enzyme tyrosine hydroxylase, which converts tyrosine to dopa, is confined to the CNS in the cell bodies and terminals of dopaminergic and noradrenergic cells. L-amino acid decarboxylase (dopa decarboxylase) converts dopa to dopamine and is widely spread in most tissues of the body; it is in no way specific for dopa. In the noradrenergic cells, dopamine is further converted to norepinephrine by a third enzyme, dopamine-β-hydroxylase, which is present in synaptic granules; the other two enzymes appear to be cytoplasmic.

The rate of catecholamine formation is limited by the low activity of tyrosine hydroxylase; L-amino acid decarboxylase and dopamine-β-hydroxylase have at least 10^2 to 10^3 more capacity. Therefore, attempts to reduce catecholamine formation are logically directed at inhibiting tyrosine hydroxylase. Both catecholamines are stored in synaptic granules with dense cores — norepinephrine, at least, in combination with ATP and chromogranin A, as in the adrenal medulla. Similar granules in dopaminergic terminals probably contain dopamine. Both epinephrine and norepinephrine resemble acetylcholine in that there seem to be at least two pools within the synaptic terminal, possibly representing granular and cytoplasmic locations.

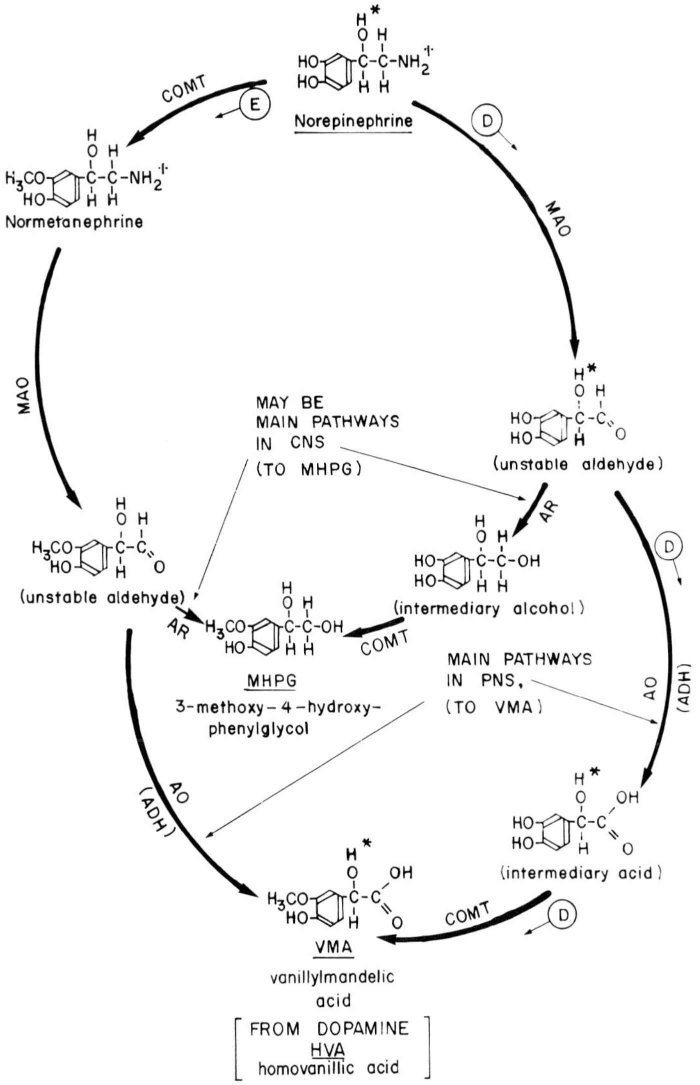

*Fig. 3-17. Inactivation pathways of catecholamines. The pathways and structural formulas shown are for norepinephrine. Note that MHPG may be a major end product in the CNS, but not in the PNS. Dopamine preferentially follows the path marked D, and the structural formulas differ only in the replacement of – OH by – H at *. Epinephrine differs only in the replacement of – NH_2 by – $NH.CH_3$ at '/' and preferentially follows pathway E (to VMA in the PNS). AR = aldehyde reductase; AO (ADH) = aldehyde oxidase (dehydrogenase); COMT = catechol-O-methyltransferase; MAO = monoamine oxidase.*

As with acetylcholine, little is known about the release of catecholamines into the synaptic cleft, or about how they react with the postsynaptic membrane to produce appropriate permeability changes. Once released, they are rapidly removed from the synaptic cleft; an energy-dependent reuptake across the presynaptic membrane is the major mechanism. An enzyme, catechol-O-methyltransferase (COMT), is present in extracellular fluid (including the synaptic cleft) and inactivates catecholamines by inserting a methyl side chain. Once resorbed into the presynaptic terminal, amine may be transferred back to granules or destroyed by monoamine oxidase (MAO), a mitochondrial enzyme which oxidatively deaminates the side chain of both norepinephrine and dopamine. Further enzyme activity (Fig. 3-17) produces several end products, including 3-methoxy-4-hydroxy-phenylglycol (MHPG) and vanillylmandelic acid (VMA) from norepinephrine, and homovanillic acid (HVA) from dopamine. Removal of such metabolites across the barrier system (at least the blood-CSF barrier) is energy-dependent (active).

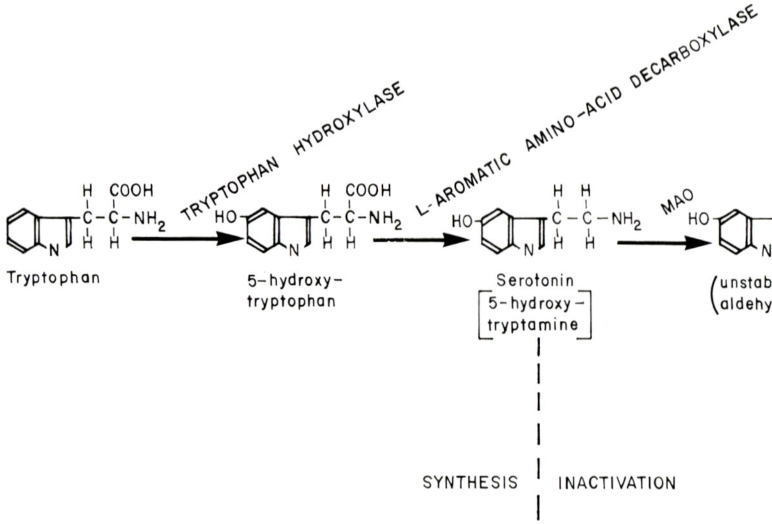

Fig. 3-18. Serotonin metabolism (inactivation pathways are not certain, but a major end product is 5-HIAA). AO (ADH) = aldehyde oxidase (dehydrogenase); MAO = monoamine oxidase.

Serotonin

Serotonergic cell bodies are mainly in the lower brain stem raphe, with fine fibers passing to other brain stem nuclei and to the spinal cord. There are probably some in the midbrain reticular formation, with fibers passing to the forebrain, especially the hypothalamus. Serotonin levels are highest in the pineal gland, moderate in the substantia nigra (1 ppm), 0.4 to 0.8 ppm in the cord, brain stem, hypothalamus, and striate body, and up to 0.2 ppm in the limbic cortex. Only 1 to 2% of total body serotonin is in the CNS.

Serotonin does not penetrate the blood-brain barrier. It is formed in the CNS (Fig. 3-18) from tryptophan by successive hydroxylation and decarboxylation, reactions analogous to those producing dopamine from tyrosine. Tryptophan hydroxylase is rate-limiting because of low concentration. Both it and L-amino acid decarboxylase are free cytoplasmic enzymes. On ultracentrifugation, serotonin appears to be within synaptic granules, but, as for dopamine, the granules are fragile and serotonin is readily lost. There appear to be two synaptic pools, as for the catecholamines. As is the case for other neurotransmitters, little is known about serotonin's release or effect on the postsynaptic membrane. Its mechanisms of inactivation are not established, but probably it can be actively taken up into the synaptic terminal. It is inactivated by MAO and other enzymes, producing 5-hydroxyindoleacetic acid (5-HIAA), which may be actively excreted by the choroid plexus.

In the pineal gland, serotonin is converted to melatonin by successive acetylation (using acetyl-CoA as donor, not specific to pineal tissue) and methylation (using S-adenosylmethionine, and the enzyme hydroxyindole-O-methyltransferase [HIOMT], which is specific to pineal tissue). Melatonin is not a neurotransmitter, but it may be a pineal hormone (see Chap. 8).

Histamine

Histamine as a potential neurotransmitter is less well investigated than the other neurotransmitters. It seems to have the same general distribution as the catecholamines and serotonin, largely in the brain stem and hypothalamus and probably in the pineal gland. There is some evidence of binding (granules?) in synaptic terminals, but little is known of its fiber connections.

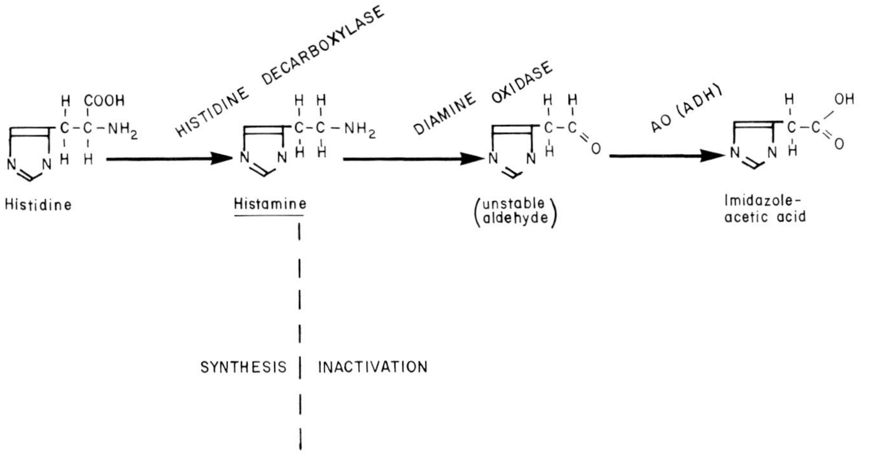

Fig. 3-19. Probable metabolism of histamine in the CNS. AO (ADH) = aldehyde oxidase (dehydrogenase).

Like other biogenic amines, histamine barely crosses the blood-brain barrier and is presumably synthesized in the brain. The maximum concentration is 0.9 ppm found in the hypothalamus, with about half as much in the midbrain, thalamus, and limbic cortex. Brain tissue has the necessary enzyme (histidine decarboxylase) to form histamine from the amino acid histidine (Fig. 3-19), although the enzyme distribution is not well documented. Inactivation is probably by MAO, to produce imidazoleacetic acid, with or without methylation.

Neutral Amino Acids

γ-Aminobutyric Acid

Well-established neurotransmitters may be either inhibitory or excitatory. However, some neutral amino acids, including GABA and glycine, are also known to inhibit spinal and cortical neurons and could be released at inhibitory synapses. It first appeared that they might differ from physiological inhibitors in failing to produce hyperpolarization. More recent work has shown that GABA (Fig. 3-20) causes hyperpolarization, at least in cortical and vestibular neurons, which, like some physiological inhibition, is not blocked by strychnine. Both types of inhibition are reversed by intracellular injection of Cl^- and by picrotoxin. Bicuculline antagonizes the hyperpolarizing effects of GABA both in the cortex and vestibular nucleus and also blocks physiological inhibition, at least in the latter. GABA and its producing enzyme, glutamic decarboxylase, are present only in CNS tissue, including the retina, and GABA has been demonstrated in synaptic vesicles. However, GABA levels fall in oxygen-induced convulsions and rise in hypoxemia, probably as part of a general metabolic response that affects the whole cell membrane. It is possible that GABA has a dual role in the CNS, both as a modulater and as a true neurotransmitter.

Glycine

Although glycine (Fig. 3-21) was originally considered a less potent inhibitor than GABA or other neutral amino acids such as taurine or β-alanine, it has since been shown in high concentration in the cord, especially in the ventral gray matter where interneurons are present; levels of GABA and taurine in the cord are uniformly lower. If interneurons are destroyed by ischemia, GABA and taurine levels are scarcely altered, whereas glycine and aspartate are significantly reduced, apparently in proportion to loss of neurons. Glycine has been found to produce hyperpolarization, and its action is blocked by strychnine. It may therefore be the inhibitor produced by some descending spinal tracts. It has little effect in the cortex.

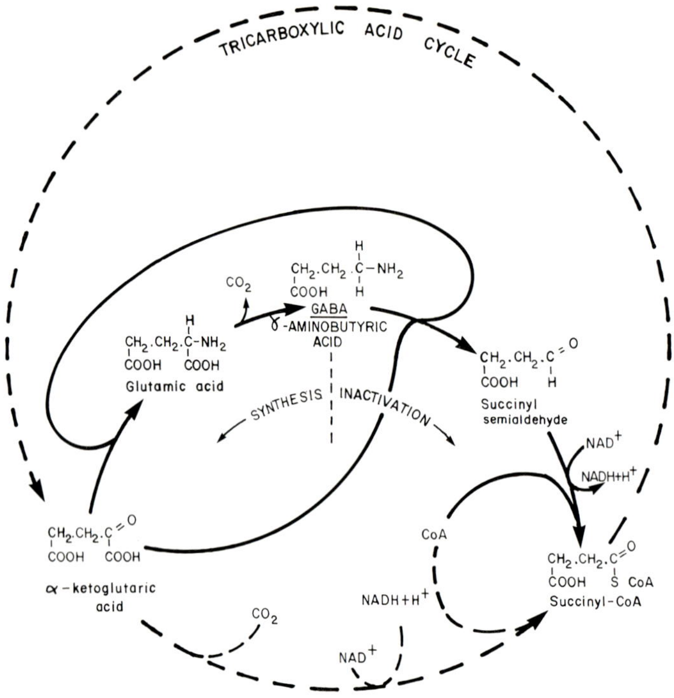

Fig. 3-20. Probable metabolic pathways of GABA (γ-aminobutyric acid) in the CNS and relationship to the tricarboxylic acid cycle (GABA shunt). For details of tricarboxylic acid cycle, see Chapter 13.

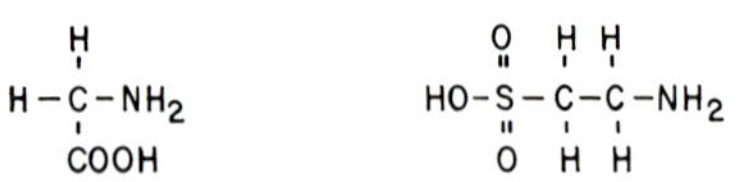

GLYCINE TAURINE

Fig. 3-21. Glycine and taurine, two neutral amino acids with a possible neurotransmitter role.

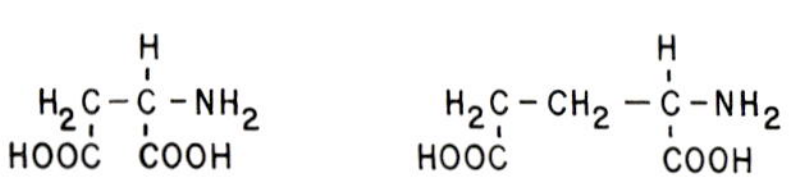

ASPARTIC ACID GLUTAMIC ACID

Fig. 3-22. Glutamic and aspartic acids, two acidic amino acids with a possible neurotransmitter role.

Taurine

Taurine (Fig. 3-21) is an acidic (sulphated) amine of relatively high concentration in the brain, highest in the frontal and occipital lobes. In mammals it is formed from cysteine by oxidation and decarboxylation, the necessary enzymes being present in human brain but not in other tissues. Taurine levels in cerebrospinal fluid are 20% higher than those in the serum. Although taurine inhibits neurotransmission, it is less effective than glycine or GABA, and so far no specific role for it has been discovered.

Acidic Amino Acids

It is apparent that acetylcholine and the monoamines are only some of the central excitatory agents, largely confined to the ARAS. The search for other agents has pointed to glutamic and aspartic acids. Glutamic acid (Fig. 3-22) is a powerful excitant in the brain and cord but appears to excite in all areas and may therefore have a metabolic rather than a transmitting role. Recently, it has been found to excite only about half the neurons of the gracilis and cuneate nuclei and to depolarize neurons but not glial cells. Spinal dorsal nerve roots contain more glutamic acid than do ventral roots, and application of glutamic acid reproduces the natural firing pattern of the gracilis and cuneate nuclei, for which it could be the natural excitatory transmitter. Aspartic acid (Fig. 3-22) appears to be associated with interneurons in the gray matter of the spinal cord, where it may oppose glycine by acting as an excitatory transmitter.

Other Possible Neurotransmitters

There is no good evidence for specific transmitter roles for the prostaglandins, substance P, or ergothioneine, although the latter is present in high concentration in the cerebellum, where other (known) transmitters are singularly lacking.

BIBLIOGRAPHY

Albers, R. W., Siegel, G. J., Katzman, R., and Agranoff, B. W. *Basic Neurochemistry.* Boston: Little, Brown, 1972.

Axelsson, J. Catecholamine functions. *Annu. Rev. Physiol.* 33:1-30, 1971.

Baldessarini, R. J., and Karaboth, M. Biochemical physiology of central synapses. *Annu. Rev. Physiol.* 35:273-304, 1973

Brazier, M. A. B. Electrical Activity of the Nerve Cell. In G.H. Bourne (Ed.), *The Structure and Function of Nervous Tissue.* New York: Academic, 1968. Vol. 2, pp. 393-408.

Brazier, M. A. B. Electrical Activity of the Nerve Fiber and Propagation of the Nerve Impulse. In G. H. Bourne (Ed.), *The Structure and Function of Nervous Tissue.* New York: Academic, 1968. Vol. 2, pp. 409-421.

Cooper, J. R., Bloom, E. E., and Roth, R. H. *The Biochemical Basis of Neuropharmacology.* New York: Oxford University Press, 1970.

DuPraw, E. J. *Cell and Molecular Biology.* New York: Academic, 1968.

Eyzaguirre, C. *Physiology of the Nervous System.* Chicago: Year Book, 1969.

Hall, Z. W. Release of neurotransmitters and their interaction with receptors. *Annu. Rev. Biochem.* 41:925-952, 1972.

Hebb, C. CNS at the cellular level: Identity of transmitter agents. *Annu. Rev. Physiol.* 32:165-192, 1970.

Hebb, C., and Morris, D. Identification of Acetylcholine and Its Metabolism in Nervous Tissue. In G. H. Bourne (Ed.), *The Structure and Function of Nervous Tissue.* New York: Academic, 1969. Vol. 3, pp. 25-60.

Hornykiewicz, O. Dopamine and Its Physiological Significance in Brain Function. In G. H. Bourne (Ed.), *The Structure and Function of Nervous Tissue.* New York: Academic, 1972. Vol. 6, pp. 367-415.

Johnston, P. V., and Roots, B. I. *Nerve Membranes.* New York: Pergamon, 1972.

McIlwain, H., and Bachelard, H. S. *Biochemistry and the Central Nervous System.* Edinburgh and London: Churchill/Livingstone, 1971.

Otsuka, M. γ-Aminobutyric Acid in the Nervous System. In G. H. Bourne (Ed.), *The Structure and Function of Nervous Tissue.* New York: Academic, 1972. Vol. 4, pp. 249-289.

Page, I. H. Serotonin and the Brain. In G. H. Bourne (Ed.), *The Structure and Function of Nervous Tissue.* New York: Academic, 1969. Vol. 3, pp. 289-307.

Phillis, J. W. The Pharmacology of Synapses. New York: Pergamon, 1970.

Roberts, E., and Matthysse, S. Neurochemistry: At the crossroads of neurobiology. *Annu. Rev. Biochem.* 39:777-820, 1970.

Ruch, T. C., Patton, H. D., Woodbury, J. W., and Towe, A. L. *Neurophysiology* (2nd ed.). Philadelphia: Saunders, 1966.

Schadé, J. P., and Ford, D. H. *Basic Neurology.* Amsterdam: Elsevier, 1965.

Shore, P. A. Transport and storage of biogenic amines. *Annu. Rev. Pharmacol.* 12:209, 1972.

Vogt, M. Functional aspects of the role of catecholamines in the central nervous system. *Br. Med. Bull.* 29:168-178, 1973.

Von Euler, U. S. Adrenergic Neuroeffector Transmission. In G. H. Bourne (Ed.), *The Structure and Function of Nervous Tissue.* New York: Academic, 1968. Vol. 2, pp. 423-462.

Watanable, A. Macromolecules and Excitation. In G. H. Bourne (Ed.), *The Structure and Function of Nervous Tissue.* New York: Academic, 1972. Vol. 6, pp. 335-366.

Whittaker, V. P. The Subcellular Fractionation of Nervous Tissue. In G. H. Bourne (Ed.), *The Structure and Function of Nervous Tissue.* New York: Academic, 1969. Vol. 3, pp. 1-24.

Functions of Supporting Cells

4

Central nervous system cells that support the function of neurons include the glia (astrocytes, oligodendroglia, ependymal cells), cells derived from the neural crest and forming leptomeninges (arachnoid and pia), and cells of the vascular-mesenchymal framework. The latter will only be dealt with in so far as this framework relates to functional boundaries of or within the CNS. The functions of glial cells have been less investigated than those of the neurons, presumably because it was realized early that they do not perform a primary information processing role. Indeed, they were often regarded merely as a skeleton within the central nervous system, increasing the rigidity of the brain and cord and acting as a filler between cell bodies, dendrites, and axons.

Since it was realized that myelin sheaths were applied to axons rather than forming an integral part of them, it became necessary to look for a cell responsible for the production and maintenance of myelin (analogous to Schwann's cells in the peripheral nervous system). It is now generally accepted that oligodendroglial cells form and maintain myelin, although photographic documentation is much less copious than for peripheral nerves.

A glial and leptomeningeal function receiving increasing attention is that of modifying the milieu of neurons and their processes by controlling the formation, composition, and removal of extracellular fluid (ECF) (within the brain and cord) and cerebrospinal fluid (CSF) (adjacent to the internal and external linings of the brain parenchyma). This is of particular significance in the central nervous system, because the ionic composition of the ECF affects synaptic and axon potentials, and because within the brain or cord there is nothing morphologically similar to a lymphatic system. This control may also involve the channeling of electrical current within the ECF. Other roles discussed for the glial cells include direct nutritional or other metabolic support for neuronal activity, over and above that mediated in a general way through the composition of the ECF. The mechanical effects of glia in stabilizing CNS tissue are probably of little or no importance, and the same results could certainly be achieved by much less specialized and complex cells.

CENTRAL MYELINATION

The structure of the myelin sheath (see Chap. 2), especially the residual cytoplasm, and analogy with the known formation of myelin by Schwann's cells in the peripheral nervous system (PNS), make it clear that CNS myelin represents a spirally wrapped, condensed cytoplasmic process, completely covered by ECF except for a narrow cytoplasmic strip at the outer edge, which is presumably connected to the myelin-forming cell. Myelin-axonal junctions exclude the axon from the ECF except at the nodes.

Oligodendroglia in Formation of Myelin

Electron microscopy has shown occasional myelin internodes to be connected to an oligodendroglial cell by processes as long as 10 to 12μ, which pass from about the center of the outer cytoplasmic strip. Continuity of the plasma membrane of the cell and the outer layer of myelin has been seen in the CNS of both fetus and adult. It is probable that one internode is formed by one oligodendroglial process (although this has not been unequivocally demonstrated), but one glial cell may provide several internodes on adjacent axons. This conclusively indicates that CNS myelin cannot be formed by the cell rotating around the axon, but presumably is formed by intercalated growth throughout the spiral, particularly at its inner edge. Immature myelin lamellae are actually thin layers of oligodendroglial cytoplasm enclosed in a plasma membrane, and this "loose myelin" persists in some lower evolutionary forms, and occasionally as a single layer around neurons even in mammals. Development to true myelin consists in extrusion of cytoplasm (except at the extreme edges as previously noted), with apposition of the inner surfaces of the plasmalemma to form the major dense line. Similarly, the ECF between the layers is extruded, and apposition of the external surfaces of the membranes forms the minor dense line.

Since the electron-microscopic distinction of oligodendroglia from astrocytes is difficult in immature animals (i.e., during myelination), some properties of the oligodendroglia may be noted that

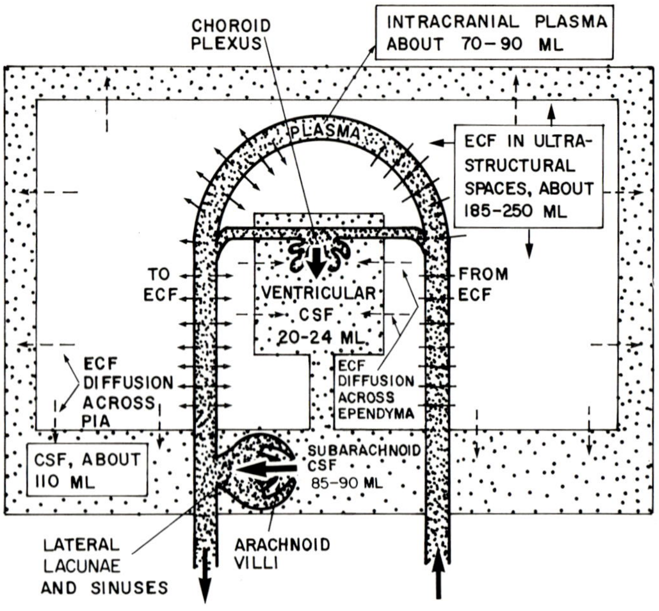

Fig. 4-1. Extracellular fluid compartments in the craniospinal cavity include the plasma (dark stipple), from which CSF is produced in the ventricles and to which it returns from the subarachnoid space (heavy arrows); the cerebrospinal fluid (light stipple); and the extracellular fluid, which is not illustrated except for its diffusion into the CSF (dashed arrows).

make them more likely candidates than the astrocytes for myelin production. They are said to have a higher RNA content than the astrocytes, to incorporate RNA precursors more actively, and to contain higher concentrations of enzymes for the hexose monophosphate pathway, producing nicotinamide-adenine dinucleotide phosphate (NADPH) for lipid synthesis. Such enzyme activity is locally raised before and during myelination.

Oligodendroglial cells have been classified into four types, all but the first closely related to myelination. *Type 1* cells are found in gray, white, and reticular matter. Characteristically, they are perineuronal cells, 15 to 20μ in diameter, with a moderate number of fine, rarely branching processes. *Types 2 through 4* cells are found in white matter only. They are large cells 20 to 40μ in diameter, with a few stout, flattened, or fine processes that are often seen in relation to myelin sheaths.

Maintenance of Myelin

It has been noted that the appearance of large numbers of oligodendroglial cells in the CNS precedes myelination and that disease processes involving oligodendroglia are accompanied by lack of myelin or demyelination. Persistent oligodendroglial cells in demyelinated areas may be of type 1, perhaps related to the maintenance of axons.

The presumed function of myelin sheaths (see Chap. 3) lies in their increasing the resistance and decreasing the capacitance of the axon membrane in the internodes, causing saltatory conduction. This depends on compaction and dehydration of the myelin lamellae, and oligodendroglia presumably maintain such a state. Individual lipid and protein components of myelin are being continually replaced — again, presumably by oligodendroglial cells, although their half-lives differ. Much of the oxygen consumption in white matter is probably due to oligodendroglial cells, since histopathologically they are only slightly less vulnerable to hypoxemia and ischemia than are neurons.

CONTROL OF FLUID MILIEU

The fluid milieu of the brain (Fig. 4-1) includes ECF between the cells and CSF in the ventricular and subarachnoid cavities. *Cerebrospinal fluid* is produced by the choroid plexuses in the ventricles. After entering the subarachnoid space, it is reabsorbed into dural venous sinuses. It represents bulk fluid, with relatively rapid formation and removal, in which diffusion of solutes can readily take place. *Extracellular fluid,* on the other hand, although probably in free communication with CSF, is restricted to spaces of ultramicroscopic dimensions, does not exhibit bulk movement, and is less likely to be of similar composition at all points than is CSF. Plasma is the third fluid compartment in the cranial cavity,

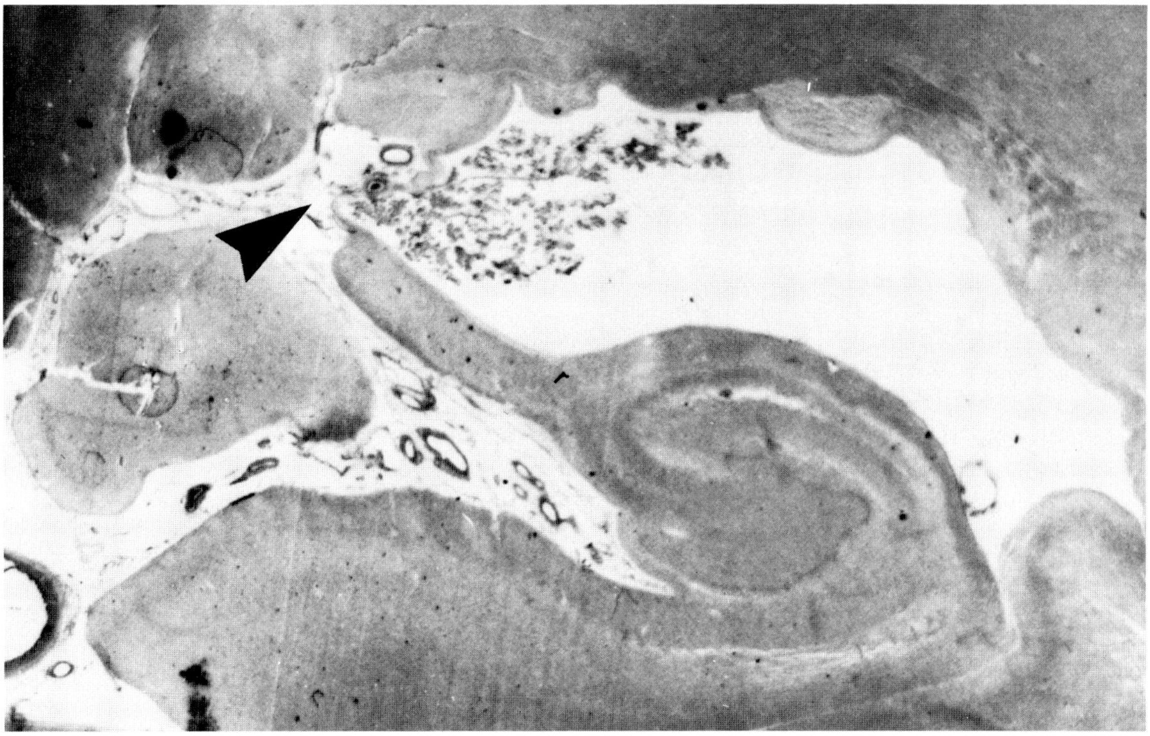

Fig. 4-2. Choroid fissure of the inferior horn (arrow), showing the continuity of the meninges and the choroid plexus. (H & E, ×6.)

and a major role of the supporting cells is production of CSF (and probably ECF) from plasma filtrate.

Ventricles and Cerebrospinal Fluid Production

The ventricles are a system of cavities within the brain (see Chap. 1), which, although they communicate with one another, are completely shut off from the subarachnoid spaces, except through foramina in the roof of the fourth ventricle. They are entirely surrounded by brain parenchyma, except for the narrow choroidal fissures of the lateral ventricles and the tela choroidea in the roof of the third and fourth ventricles. In such areas the ventricle is invaginated by slightly modified, highly vascular meninges to form choroid plexuses.

Ependyma

The ventricles are derived from the lumen of the neural tube, and except where invaginated by meningeal tissue, they are lined by single-layered columnar ependyma, recognizably a remnant of the original neuroepithelium. Although in the primate brain the ependymal cells do not have basal processes, there is no basement membrane, and they rest directly on a layer of subependymal astrocytes. They are connected near the free surface by cell junctions, but these are spotty and do not form complete occlusive bands between the cells. The apical surfaces carry irregular folds and projections and sometimes cilia. The height of the ependymal layer is variable; it is generally greater overlying gray matter and low over subjacent myelinated tracts.

Choroid Plexus

The choroid plexuses consist of invaginated meningeal tissue of striking vascularity, covered by a single layer of columnar cells, which at the edges is continuous with the ependymal layer. The largest plexuses are in the bodies and inferior horns of the lateral ventricles (Fig. 4-2); the inferior parts are supplied by the anterior choroidal artery and the superior parts by the posterior choroidal arteries passing forward in the roof of the third ventricle. The venous drainage converges on a thickened area in the body, whence a single vein runs forward to the region of the foramen of Monro. Smaller tufts of plexus are present in the upper part of the third ventricle and the caudal part of the fourth ventricle. The choroid plexuses have a branching structure, and the total area may be 200 cm^2. Numerous large, thick-walled capillaries run close to the overlying epithelium; they appear fenestrated, but electron microscopy indicates that their pores are closed by a very thin membrane. Between the vessels and the epithelium lies an exceedingly thin layer derived from the pial cells and the basement membrane of the columnar epithelium. Spaces in the choroid plexus stroma contain branching pial cells.

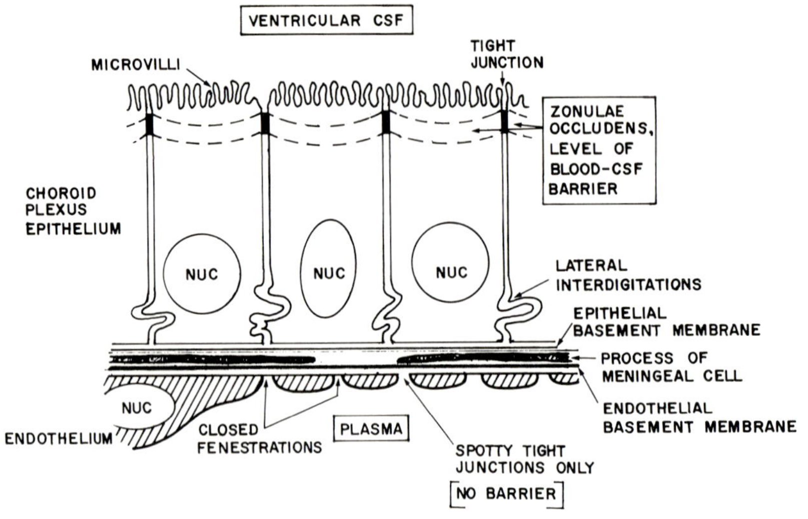

Fig. 4-3. Interface between plasma and CSF at the choroid plexus. Note the complete barrier of tight junctions at the apical ends of the plexus epithelial cells. Another plasma-CSF interface is present at the arachnoid villi (see Fig. 4-8).

The choroidal epithelium (Fig. 4-3) is usually higher than the ependyma and shows a few specializations often associated with secretory activity. The apical surfaces carry microvilli, which, although less regular than those in the intestine, are more regular than the projections on ependymal cells. They may also be ciliated. The lateral surfaces show intercellular junctions including circumcellular zonulae occludentes at the apex and relatively complex interdigitations nearer the base, which is flat and rests on a thin basement membrane. Cellular organelles show no striking departure from normal, with moderate numbers of mitochondria, a well-developed apical Golgi's complex, and endoplasmic reticulum which is largely agranular.

Cerebrospinal Fluid Formation

There is both direct and indirect evidence of formation of CSF by the choroid plexuses, and in man the rate of secretion is probably about 0.5 ml per minute, which, assuming a total volume of about 140 ml, corresponds to a turnover time of 4.5 or 5 hours. Contributions made by the individual choroid plexuses have not been established. Evidence for production of CSF includes hemoconcentration in the plexus venous blood and collection of secretion from exposed plexus under oil. Evidence for the active nature of secretion of CSF is noted later. There is no evidence of active (i.e., metabolically dependent) secretion or absorption by *ependymal cells,* though the composition of freshly secreted CSF is modified by passive equilibration with ECF through both ependymal and pial surfaces.

Cerebrospinal Fluid Escape to Subarachnoid Space

It is generally accepted that the foramen of Magendie truly exists, at least in the human being, averaging between 10 and 15 mm^2 in area. (It is probably also present in the anthropoid apes but not in subprimates.) The two foramina of Luschka appear to be present in all species. Through these openings, CSF enters the subarachnoid space of the posterior fossa. Total ventricular volume in the adult is 20 to 24 ml, representing only about 15% of the CSF volume.

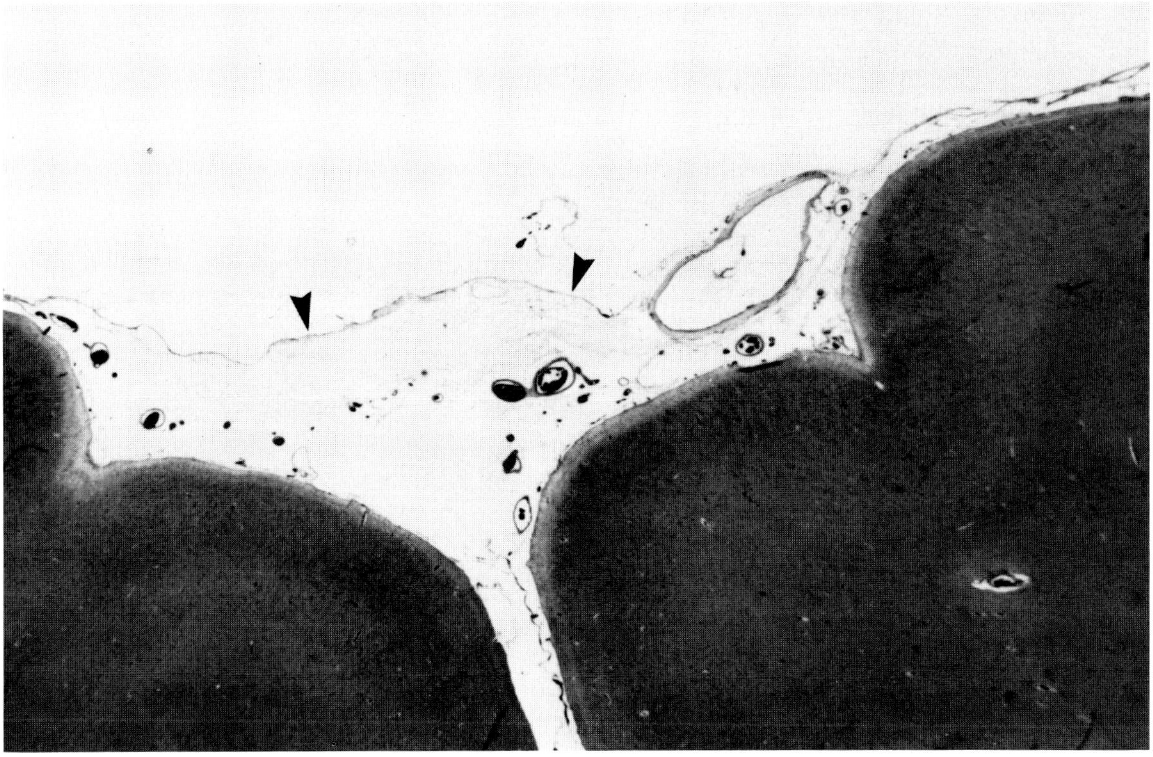

Fig. 4-4. Subarachnoid space between the crowns of adjacent gyri. The pia is a delicate layer attached to the brain surface, whereas the arachnoid (arrows) bridges the space. (H & E, ×6.)

Subarachnoid Space and Cerebrospinal Fluid Absorption

Boundaries of Subarachnoid Space

The subarachnoid space is an actual, CSF-filled space (Fig. 4-4) covering the entire surface of the brain and cord, bounded internally by the pia, a single layer of flattened cells with a tendency to overlap and possibly also to leave small gaps in a few areas. The pial cells rest on a glial sheet, apparently a continuous, intact layer formed by the expanded processes of subpial astrocytes. The pial cells and the glial processes are separated by a basement membrane that appears more closely related to the contours of astrocytes than of pial cells; where pial cells have been reported as absent, basement membrane was still present. This "external limiting layer" of the brain is commonly referred to as the *pia-glia layer* (Fig. 4-5).

The outer border of the subarachnoid space is formed by the arachnoid, which is thicker than the pia and conforms more closely to the contours of the cranial cavity than of the underlying brain. The width of the subarachnoid space therefore varies markedly; it forms dilatations (cisterns) in some regions, but is very narrow over the convexities. The arachnoid membrane consists of several layers of large cells with pale cytoplasm and branching processes, which tend to interlock. There is no basement membrane, and there appear to be no intercellular junctions, so that the membrane contains irregular intercellular channels potentially communicating between subarachnoid and subdural spaces. Arachnoid and pia are connected by delicate bundles of collagen fibers,

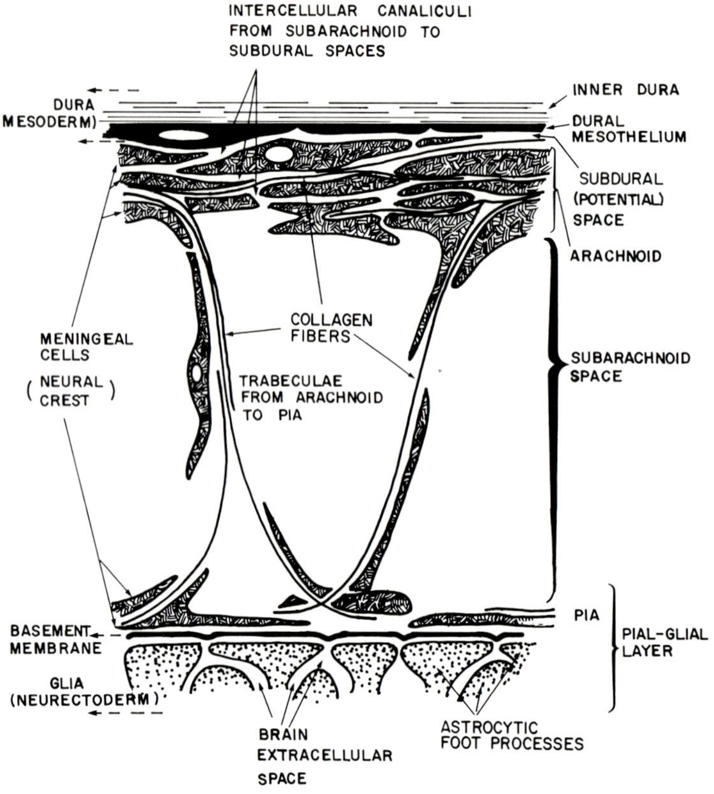

Fig. 4-5. As shown, the subarachnoid space is bounded externally by the arachnoidal layer and internally by a thin, even incomplete layer of pial cells. Some collagen fibers are present.

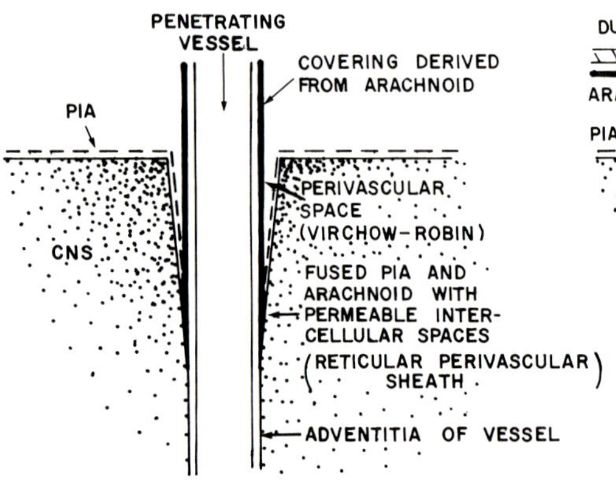

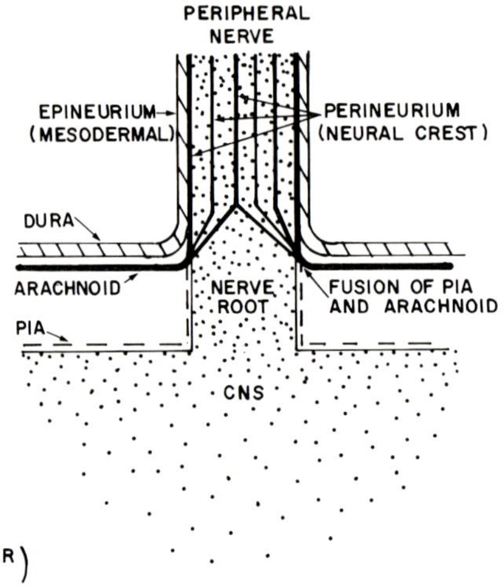

Fig. 4-6. Relationships of pia, subarachnoid space, and arachnoid to vessels penetrating the brain surface (left) and to cranial or spinal nerve roots (right). Note the early fusion of pia and arachnoid in both cases.

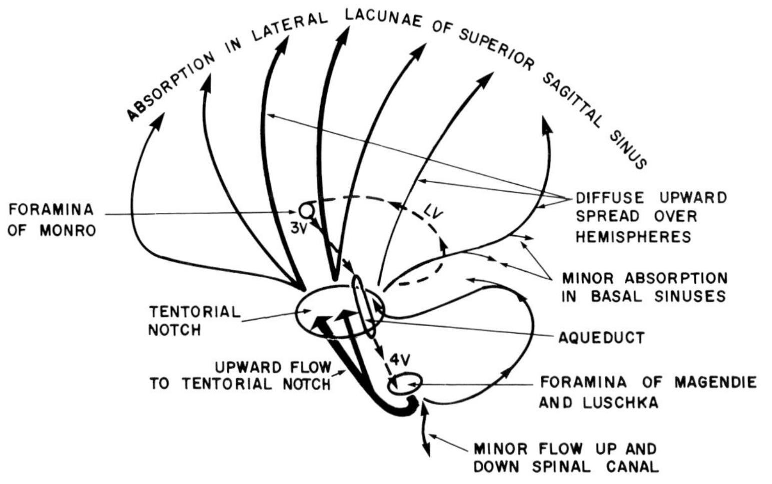

Fig. 4-7. Schematic representation of CSF flow, viewed from the left side. Dashed arrows = ventricular flow; solid arrows = subarachnoid flow. LV = lateral ventricle; 3V = third ventricle; 4V = fourth ventricle.

often covered with leptomeningeal cells; similar fibers may be found within the arachnoid itself. The subarachnoid space contains large and medium-sized arteries and veins, but apparently has no capillary network; it is traversed by veins, arteries, and nerve roots.

The pia and the arachnoid apparently derive from the neural crest and are not mesenchymal. The nearest mesenchymal layer to the brain and cord is the flattened mesothelium that lines the inner surface of the dura; electron-microscopically, these mesothelial cells are smaller, darker, and contain fewer mitochondria than the leptomeningeal cells.

Extensions of Subarachnoid Space

Possible extensions of the subarachnoid space along cranial and spinal nerve roots and nerves have occupied much attention because they might imply communication between the subarachnoid and lymphatic spaces. Such communication appears to be best established in respect to the olfactory nerves, where perineural spaces, piercing the cribriform plates, have been shown to be continuous with lymphatic spaces in the olfactory mucosa. A sleeve of the subarachnoid space surrounds the optic nerves (which are extensions of the brain), but does not appear to communicate with lymphatic channels in the orbit. Other cranial and spinal nerves have relatively short sleeves of subarachnoid space, their covering layers of pia and arachnoid being fused (Fig. 4-6). No anatomical continuity has been demonstrated between the subarachnoid space (surrounding nerve roots) and the lymphatic spaces of the peripheral nerves, although in some experiments, small amounts of colloidal material, injected into the subarachnoid space, have been found in lymph nodes adjacent to the vertebral columns. If true communications exist, it may reasonably be concluded that they are quantitatively insignificant.

Controversy has also been generated concerning possible prolongation of the subarachnoid space into the CNS parenchyma (around arteries and veins). Such prolongation (Virchow-Robin space) certainly exists at the point of perforation (Fig. 4-6). Although claims were made that it reaches precapillary arterioles, it now appears that the pia and arachnoid layers fuse shortly below the surface of the brain (much as they do when covering nerve roots) to produce a combined layer of leptomeningeal cells, which gradually becomes thinner. Since leptomeningeal cells are not closely juxtaposed and have no intercellular junctions, canaliculi between the cells may provide a considerable degree of permeability. This layer of leptomeningeal cells, the *reticular perivascular sheath,* differs from the true adventitia, which is mesenchymal. Both are absent from capillaries.

Cerebrospinal Fluid Flow in Subarachnoid Space

Circulation of CSF after emergence from the fourth ventricle has been studied by the use of radioisotopes and, less successfully, by the use of dyes. Studies confirm the long-standing impression (Fig. 4-7) that the major flow is anteriorly round the brain stem and through the tentorium to the base of the brain, together with a diffuse slow spread over the cerebral hemispheres toward the falx. There is no conclusive evidence for substantial flow either up or down the spinal canal. Of the 115 to 120 ml of CSF present in the subarachnoid space, about 30 ml are in the spinal canal, where circulation appears to depend largely on respiration, coughing, and general bodily movements. Relative stagnation may account for differences in chemical composition between fluids from the lumbar and cisternal regions (see p. 89).

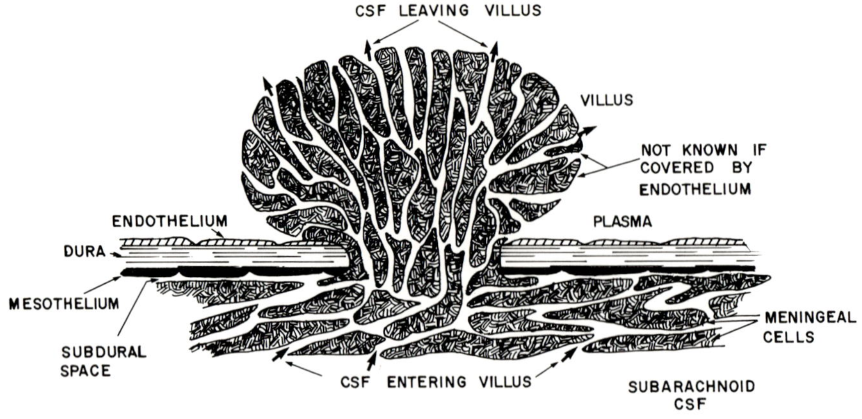

Fig. 4-8. Arachnoid villus projecting into a lateral lacuna or dural venous sinus. The route of CSF flow is the intercellular spaces between the meningeal cells.

Cerebrospinal Fluid Absorption

Thus, CSF is continuously being produced, and the bulk flow appears to be upward to the region of the falx. Correspondingly, structures responsible for CSF absorption are found in the parasagittal regions (and to a lesser extent elsewhere) in connection with dural venous sinuses. These are the arachnoid villi (Fig. 4-8), small tuftlike projections of arachnoid tissue that have penetrated the dura, their tips lying either in dural sinuses or in lateral branches of the sinuses (lateral lacunae). Villi are masses of arachnoid cells, sometimes with a hollow core continuous with the main subarachnoid space and probably not covered by sinus endothelium. Like other leptomeningeal cells, those of the villi have intercellular channels, 4 to 12μ in width, following a branching course from the subarachnoid space to the lumen of the vessel. There appear to be no structural valves, and it is presumed that when CSF pressure exceeds that in the vessel, these channels are opened; should vascular pressure be in excess, compression of the tip of the villi closes the channels and prevents reflux of blood into the subarachnoid space.

In many species (and in human infants), only arachnoid villi are available for CSF absorption. During early childhood, and probably progressively through life, larger, grossly visible structures, similar histologically, develop in the parasagittal regions, opening into the lateral lacunae of the superior sagittal sinus. These *arachnoidal (pacchionian) granulations* presumably serve the same function as the much smaller villi, and their growth is accompanied by increased size of lateral lacunae. Villi and granulations are present (in decreasing order of frequency) in the walls of the superior sagittal, transverse, cavernous, and superior petrosal sinuses, medial meningeal veins, and sphenoparietal and straight sinuses. Small extrusions of arachnoidal tissue into or through the dura are present in spinal nerve root pouches; occasionally, they enter small intradural veins. However, these root "villi" are small, irregular in distribution, and frequently do not make contact with vessels. They can be of little significance in the absorption of CSF (corresponding with the absence of a demonstrable, significant flow down the spinal canal).

Extracellular Space

In many body tissues, such as muscle, the extracellular space appears to be 12 to 15% of the total tissue volume and is easily seen on light or electron microscopy in the mesenchymal stroma. It contains collagen and other extracellular fibers, fibroblasts, macrophages, and lymphatic vessels. The extracellular space may be estimated by injection of substances, such as inulin or sulfate, to which cell membranes are (virtually) impermeable. Such substances distribute themselves entirely between the plasma water and the ECF water, and (assuming no cell penetration and that concentration in ECF is equal to concentration in plasma) it is a matter of simple proportion to calculate what percentage of the total tissue water is extracellular. This percentage is the *inulin space, sulfate space,* and so on, depending on the marker used, and as the value varies slightly with different markers, there is probably some degree of cell penetration. Thus, in muscle, the inulin and sulfate spaces are about 13.5%, whereas the sodium and chloride spaces are 17%.

Morphology

In the CNS, the extent of the extracellular space has only recently been appreciated. By light microscopy no spaces are visible in the parenchyma, background material between the cells being a uniform, eosinophilic *neuropil* made up of the processes of neurons and glial cells. Electron microscopy at first showed structures within the CNS separated only by a minimum interval of approximately 200 A between adjacent plasma membranes, and there was then thought to be essentially no extracellular space. Later work showed slightly wider, irregular spaces, particularly in gray matter in the region of synaptic junctions

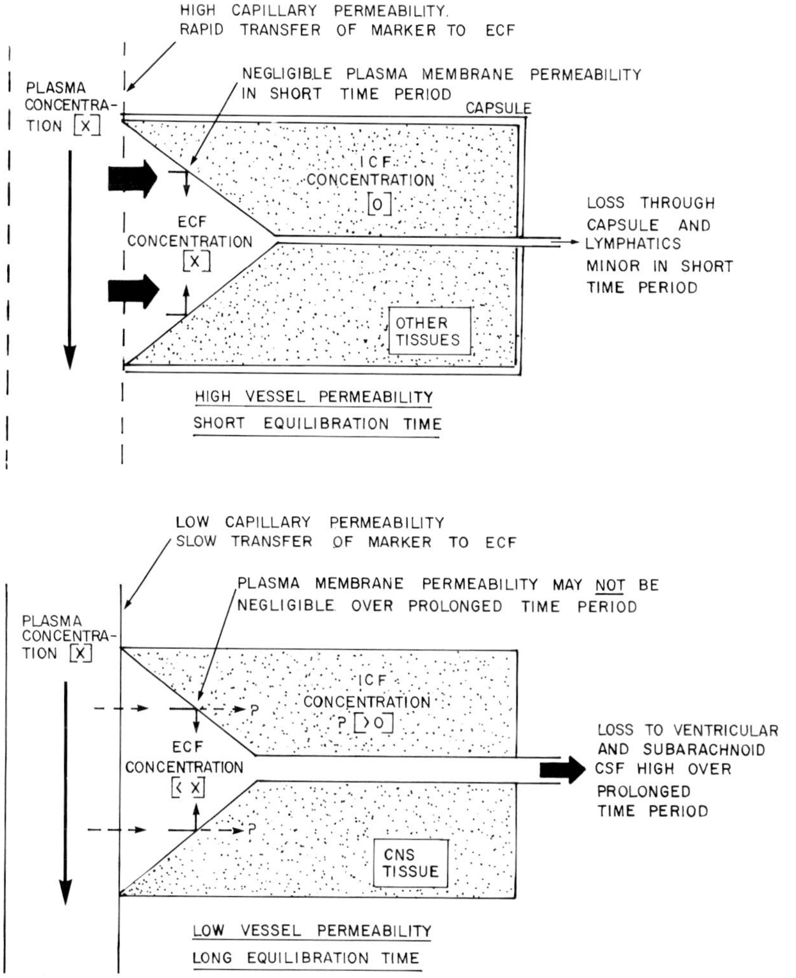

Fig. 4-9. Comparison of the value of markers in estimating extracellular volume in general body tissues (above) and in CNS (below). In the CNS, markers cross the blood-brain barrier slowly, and equilibration is delayed. Because of this, there may be appreciable entry of markers into cells and loss to surrounding CSF. Both introduce inaccuracies in estimates of extracellular volume. ICF = intracellular fluid.

and in white matter near the nodes of Ranvier. It has been demonstrated that large molecules, such as protein, can move readily even in a 200-A space. Sucrose diffuses only about 15% more slowly than in bulk solution, and Na^+ and K^+ are even less hampered.

If all processes were separated by a 200-A gap, the percentage of extracellular space would depend on the average diameter of cellular elements. Thus, if the average diameter were 0.1μ, extracellular space would be calculated as 30%; if it were 0.5 to 0.75μ, this figure would be reduced to 5 to 7%. Direct measurements from photographs first suggested a space of approximately 5%. Probably these measurements reflected unduly tight packing of the cellular elements with reduction of the extracellular space because of asphyxia, which causes a very rapid absorption of extracellular water and Cl^- into neuronal and glial processes. Attempts to avoid such artifacts by ultra-rapid fixation have raised the estimated extracellular space from about 5% to 10 to 12%.

Estimation of Volume by Physiological Methods

Intravenous injection of markers only partially resolves the problem, as the effective permeability of CNS capillaries is much less than in other parts of the body because of the blood-brain and blood-CSF barriers (see pp. 87–88). Although these barriers do not exclude markers from the brain, they make equilibration time between the plasma and brain much longer than in other tissues. Consequences of these long equilibration times (Fig. 4-9) include diffusion between the brain and CSF (lowering brain concentration) and possible entry of the marker into cells. A further complication of these calculations is that the water content of the CNS

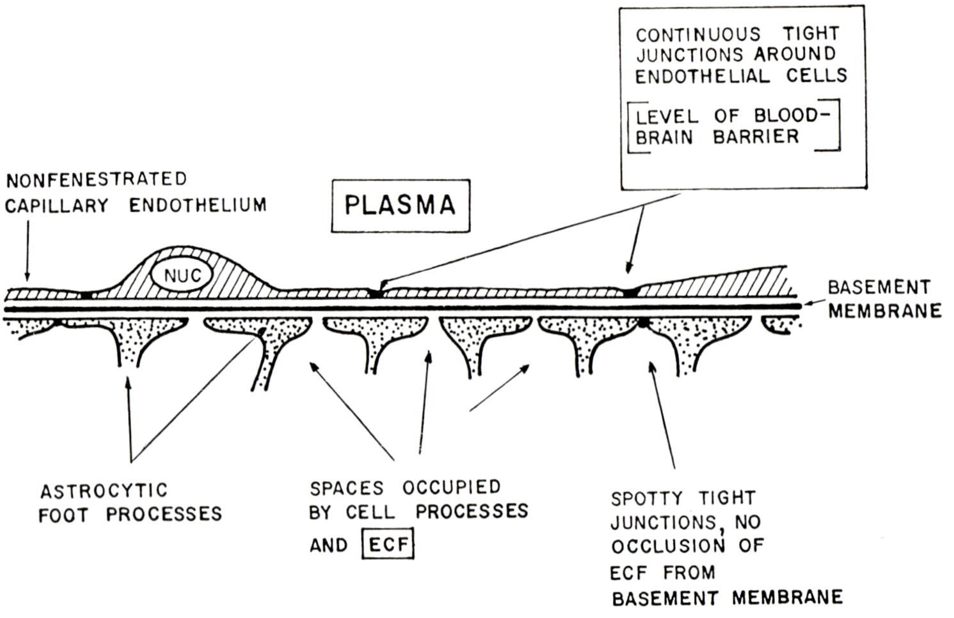

Fig. 4-10. Interface between plasma and brain ECF. This is the blood-brain barrier, which, according to current views, is largely due to the continuous tight junctions surrounding and joining endothelial cells and to the lack of endothelial fenestration.

(79%) is lower than that of other tissues. Drainage into CSF can be circumvented by presenting the marker at the same concentration simultaneously in CSF and plasma. Then, *if it is assumed* that the permeability of plasma membranes is so low that even during a long equilibration time there will be no intracellular leakage, currently available data suggest a space of 15 to 20%, similar to that in other tissues.

With sophisticated technology and (disputed) mathematical theory the electrical resistance of the CNS may also be used to calculate the extracellular space. It is assumed that resistance to current flow is much lower in the extracellular space than where (lipid) plasma membranes have to be crossed. A resultant figure around 25% is higher than that given by other methods, and the theory currently being applied may not be adequate. Nonetheless, serial measurements may have some comparative value, for they show a markedly increased resistance following asphyxia and a reduction in cerebral edema.

Intracranial Fluid Compartments

It is apparent that there are three extracellular fluid compartments in the craniospinal cavity: plasma, CSF, and ECF. Exchanges are obviously of fundamental importance to the maintenance of CNS function, not only mechanically, in terms of intracranial volume, but also for supply of oxygen and nutrients, removal of metabolic products, and possibly for protection of the CNS against deficiencies in body homeostasis. The boundaries or interfaces between each compartment have been studied both morphologically and physiologically, and there appears to be a considerable barrier to diffusion between plasma on the one hand and CSF and ECF on the other.

The morphological features of compartmental barriers may be summarized as follows:

1. *Between plasma and ECF (blood-brain barrier).* The interface (Fig. 4-10) consists of nonfenestrated, tightly joined endothelial cells and a relatively complete layer of flat foot processes derived from astrocytes, with an intervening basement membrane that appears to be shared (see p. 53).

2. *Between plasma and CSF (blood-CSF barrier).* The interface at the *choroid plexus* consists of two cytoplasmic layers (Fig. 4-3) separated by a basement membrane and occasionally containing fragments of meningeal cell cytoplasm. The endothelial layer differs from that in the brain in having fenestrations or pores, although electron microscopy indicates that these are really closed by an attenuated membrane 60 to 70 A thick. The choroidal epithelium is a high columnar layer, with cell junctions at the apical ends, apparently completely occluding the intercellular spaces between them. A second interface between the CSF and plasma is *at the arachnoid villi and granulations* (Fig. 4-8). Here, the intervening layer is composed of branched leptomeningeal cells with relatively wide intercellular channels of 4 to 12 A across.

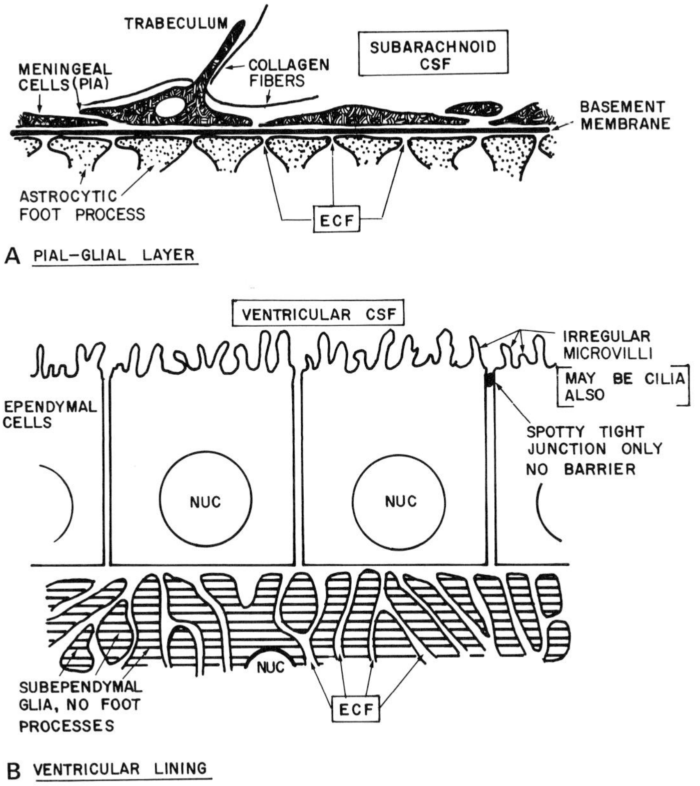

Fig. 4-11. Interfaces between CSF and ECF at the brain surface (above) and at the ventricular lining (below). Note the absence of continuous tight junctions in both situations, correlating with absence of a physiological barrier.

3. *Between CSF and ECF.* This boundary is present in the ventricles and on the surface of the brain and therefore has two morphological forms (Fig. 4-11). *In the ventricles,* the interface is a layer of columnar epithelial cells with intercellular junctions that do not occlude intercellular channels (leading from the extracellular space to the ventricular space). This ependyma does not have a basement membrane and rests on a layer of subependymal glia lacking the flattened, contiguous processes of the subpial astrocytes. *On the surface of the brain* is the pial-glial layer, consisting of expanded astrocytic processes and a more or less continuous layer of pial cells, separated by a basement membrane. No intercellular junctions are apparent, so there is theoretical continuity of intercellular spaces from the extracellular to the subarachnoid compartments.

Fluid Exchange between Extracellular Compartments

Demonstration of Barriers between Plasma and Other Compartments

The concept of restricted exchange between plasma and other extracellular compartments of the CNS dates from observations that intravenous dyes do not stain the CSF or brain (except in a few restricted areas) and that solute concentrations in normal CSF differ from those in plasma. While many vital dyes are bound to plasma proteins, which could restrict their diffusion, nonetheless they still equilibrate freely with ECF in other parts of the body. The terms *blood-brain barrier* and *blood-CSF barrier* date from such observations. Later, it was considered that the blood-brain barrier might be due to the lack of ECF in the brain, and therefore reside in the plasma membranes of CNS cells themselves rather than at the capillaries. The demonstration of an extracellular space probably similar in volume to that in other tissues, together with inferences that may be drawn about the solute composition of brain ECF by studying the CSF (see pp. 91–92), indicate that the blood-brain barrier is as real a physiological phenomenon as the blood-CSF barrier.

Material to which plasma membranes are impermeable (ECF markers) enter the brain and CSF slowly, presumably because some type of membrane is involved in the barrier phenomenon. Substances such as urea, generally considered freely and rapidly diffusible and readily entering cells, still equilibrate slowly with intracranial contents, as compared with other fluids and tissues. Urea equilibrates slowly in

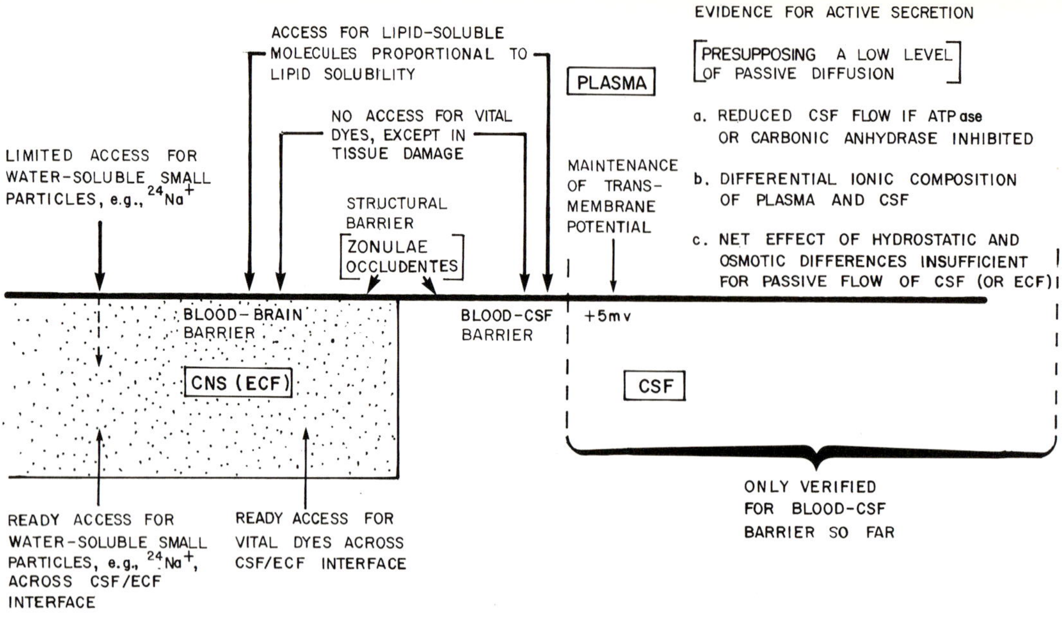

Fig. 4-12. Summary of evidence for the existence of blood-brain and blood-CSF barriers (thick black line). The physiological and structural evidence (left two-thirds of diagram) of such restricted diffusion supports the existence of active secretion across the barriers (right one-third of diagram). At present, direct evidence is available only with respect to the blood-CSF barrier.

gray matter and more slowly in white matter and generally takes longer in the brain than in the cord. Greater lipid solubility increases the rate of uptake and equilibration; ethylthiourea equilibrates much faster than thiourea, and lipid-soluble barbiturates (thio derivatives) also equilibrate rapidly (thiobarbital compared with barbital). In calculating CNS concentrations, mathematical allowance must be made for the unusually low water content of the brain and cord.

Further evidence for the existence of the blood-brain barrier is the rapid rate of uptake of materials into the brain from the CSF, compared with the rate from plasma. Thus the isotope $^{24}Na^+$ diffuses into the brain three times faster through the small area of ependyma than through a vastly greater area of capillaries, indicating that the blood-brain barrier is a great deal more effective than the ependymal barrier. In areas of damaged brain (e.g., by inflammation), uptake of $^{24}Na^+$ from the blood rises, whereas that from CSF remains unchanged.

A few restricted areas in the brain stain with plasma dyes and appear to lack a blood-brain barrier (the neurohypophysis, median eminence, wall of the optic recess, pineal gland, and the vascular area postrema at the lower end of the fourth ventricle). Paradoxically, if dye is injected *into the CSF,* these areas accumulate less of it than the rest of the brain, because dye absorbed from the CSF can be taken up by their vessels. (Elsewhere, vascular uptake of dye occurs slowly if at all, showing that the blood-brain barrier is bidirectional.) Vessels in these areas have a perivascular space containing connective tissue, with both inner and outer basement membranes and, unlike other brain capillaries, show considerable pinocytosis.

Evidence for Active Secretion of Cerebrospinal Fluid (and Probably Extracellular Fluid)

The existence of physiological barriers between plasma on the one hand and CSF and ECF on the other (Fig. 4-12) poses problems for brain nutrition. To overcome the osmotic pressure exerted by protein within vessels, a vascular hydrostatic pressure of + 25 to + 30 mm Hg compared to the surrounding tissue is necessary for normal plasma filtration. It is questionable whether such a vascular pressure exists in the cranial cavity, which itself has a slight positive pressure. Furthermore, the plasma-CSF concentration ratios for individual solutes are widely variable, clearly indicating a semipermeable membrane with differing rates of solute flux across it. Thus, it does not appear that any *wholly passive* diffusion process could account either for the formation or for the observed composition of CSF, and it is necessary to postulate active (energy-dependent) secretion.

Adenosinetriphosphatase (ATPase) inhibitors (e.g., ouabain) drastically reduce CSF secretion and so do carbonic anhydrase inhibitors (e.g., acetazolamide), though the mechanisms of action of either enzyme are unclear. Active transport of selected ions may be responsible for membrane potential across the plexus (+5 mv on the CSF side); if Na^+ were actively transported across the membrane, the CSF would tend to become positive with respect to plasma, enhancing passive diffusion of chloride in the same direction and setting up of an osmotic gradient to "drag" water across the barrier. Such a mechanism is not proved, but might also account for the lower concentrations in CSF of nonionized solutes such as glucose and urea. Alternatively, it might be assumed that the membrane is impermeable to such solutes and that they cross by active transport. At present, there appears to be no conclusive evidence to elucidate the precise mechanism of CSF (or ECF) formation, though both are undoubtedly active processes, at least in part.

Fluid Exchange Between Cerebrospinal Fluid and Extracellular Fluid

Although there are definite barriers between plasma and CSF and between plasma and ECF, it is clear that there is no comparable barrier between CSF and ECF compartments, and they may be regarded as a single, passively diffusing compartment. There is no evidence of active secretory activity by the ependyma, and there is no significant transependymal potential. Barriers to free diffusion of large molecules (e.g., protein) between ECF and CSF are incomplete and purely mechanical, due to the narrow and tortuous nature of the extracellular space. Inferences as to the composition of ECF, which cannot be sampled directly, are based on the assumption of some degree of passive exchange between the two fluids. Lack of ependymal or pial barriers also has pharmacological implications, since it enables the blood-brain and blood-CSF barriers to be circumvented by intraventricular injection. It also permits the use of CSF, at least semiquantitatively, to estimate metabolic processes within the brain (e.g., determination of the metabolic products of transmitter amines in parkinsonism).

Composition of the Cerebrospinal Fluid

Relationship of Major Solute Concentrations to Those in Plasma

The blood-CSF barrier is virtually impermeable to protein, the plasma concentration being about 6500 mg per kilogram H_2O, compared with 25 mg per kilogram H_2O in the CSF. Since protein acts as a significant anion in plasma, it may be expected that levels of the other major anion, Cl^-, would be significantly higher in CSF, and this is indeed so. However, there are other factors that might be expected to cause differences between plasma and CSF ion concentrations. These include the effects of the Donnan equilibrium, the potential across the membrane (5 mv + on the CSF side), the partial protein-binding of cations in plasma (mainly, the divalent Ca^{++} and Mg^{++}), and the higher water content of CSF (99% compared with 93% for plasma).

Therefore, in attempting to assess the comparative importance of passive (diffusional) and active (energy-dependent) processes in the formation of CSF, it is not enough to make raw comparisons of the plasma and CSF concentrations. Rather, it is necessary to consider the observed values in CSF in comparison with the calculated theoretical values derived from dialyzing plasma across a semipermeable membrane at the observed potential. Figure 4-13 demonstrates the significant differences in this comparison. All figures for absolute concentrations are approximate, since there is considerable variability in published results, depending on the species, site of CSF sampling, and technical methods. However, the general *trends* of the differences and their approximate magnitudes are generally agreed on. (Bicarbonate concentrations are considered in Chapter 11.)

1. *Sodium (Na^+).* The plasma concentration is about 150 mEq per kilogram H_2O, compared with about 148 mEq per kilogram H_2O in CSF. However, since the theoretical CSF (ultrafiltrate) value would be 125 to 130, there is actually an increase of about 20 above the calculated CSF level. This could be regarded as evidence for active Na^+ secretion, which is indeed likely to be a significant factor in controlling CSF production and volume. Although the barrier permeability to Na^+ is very low, the CSF concentration varies closely (following a time lag of one to several hours) with that of plasma, suggesting that the *rate* of Na^+ secretion can be controlled. This is an essential mechanism in the maintenance of normal intracranial volume in the face of changes in total plasma osmolality (see Chap. 11).

2. *Potassium (K^+).* Respective concentrations in plasma and CSF are about 4.5 and 2.9 mEq per kilogram H_2O, whereas a calculated value based on passive diffusion into the CSF is about 4.1 mEq per kilogram H_2O. Thus, there is a very significant restriction on K^+ entry to the CSF, and the value is held almost constant in the face of severe increases and decreases of plasma concentration, unlike the situation existing for Na^+. This implies mechanisms of active transport that are saturated at subphysiological plasma $[K^+]$. In subarachnoid hemorrhage with erythrocyte lysis, the CSF $[K^+]$ is still maintained within close limits, suggesting that active extrusion of K^+ can occur.

3. *Calcium (Ca^{++}).* Total plasma calcium is about 4.8 mEq per kilogram H_2O, but of this, up to one-half is protein-bound. Cerebrospinal fluid $[Ca^{++}]$ is constant at about 2.5 mEq per kilogram H_2O, a value close to that calculated for an ultrafiltrate. However, this appears to be merely coincidental, since, like K^+, CSF Ca^{++} levels are held constant in the face of wide plasma variations. Intraventricular Ca^{++} injection suggests that active extrusion is also possible. Transport mechanisms similar to those for K^+ are indicated.

4. *Magnesium (Mg^{++}).* Much of the plasma magnesium (totaling about 1.7 mEq per kilogram H_2O) is protein-bound, but the CSF $[Mg^{++}]$ is about 2.4 mEq per kilogram H_2O. This value is for the most part well maintained (not as closely as for K^+ or Ca^{++}) in the face of high or low plasma levels, suggesting similar mechanisms for secretion and possibly extrusion.

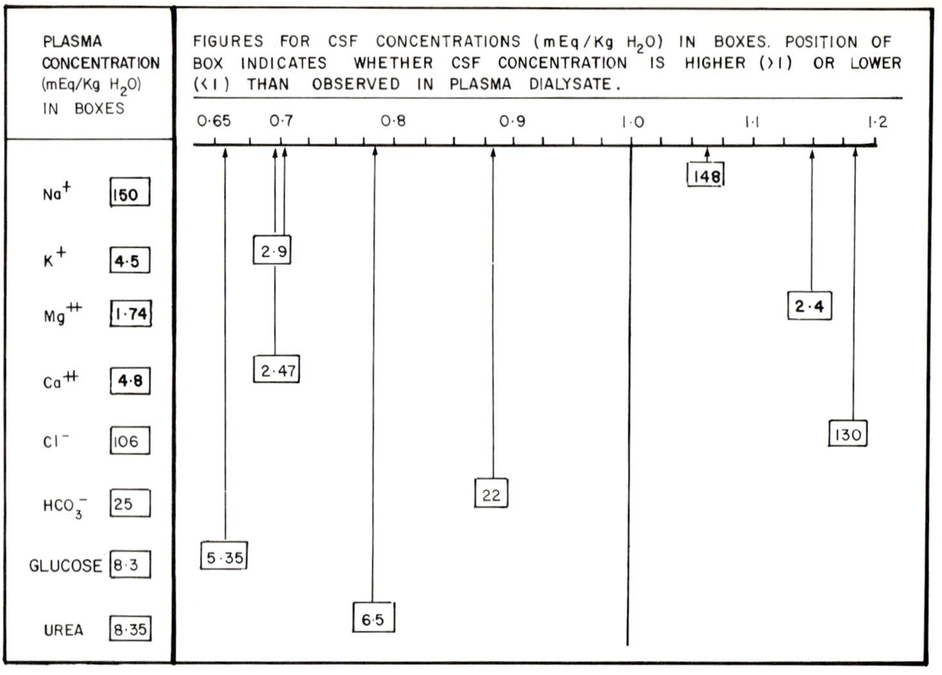

Fig. 4-13. Comparison of the composition of CSF with that of an ultrafiltrate derived from plasma dialyzed across a membrane bearing the barrier membrane potential.

5. *Chloride (Cl^-).* As noted, there is a considerable disparity between plasma [Cl^-] (about 106 mEq per kilogram H_2O) and CSF [Cl^-] (about 130 mEq per kilogram H_2O), much of it explicable by the need to substitute for anionic plasma protein and perhaps also by the positive potential of CSF relative to plasma. As do those of Na^+, CSF [Cl^-] values tend to reflect levels in plasma, though less closely. The question of active transport of Cl^- ions remains undecided.

Concentrations of most nonelectrolytes in the CSF (e.g., glucose and urea) are 20 to 30% lower than in plasma, but reflect plasma changes. Glucose is almost certainly actively transported into the CNS and probably therefore into the CSF also, but the rate is presumably dependent on plasma concentration within moderately wide limits. Probably, little CSF glucose is used in normal CNS metabolism, but CSF levels presumably serve to prevent diffusion from the cerebral tissues.

Cerebrospinal Fluid Clearance of Colloids and Particles

It is believed that the small amounts of protein in CSF are derived from the choroid plexus. The arachnoid villi and granulations seem freely permeable to protein since the level remains constant; experimentally, if blood is injected into the subarachnoid space, the resulting high CSF protein is reduced in a few hours, and even the red cells fall within a few hours or in one to two days. (In vitro, red cells may be seen to pass freely through the arachnoid membrane where villi are present.)

This behavior of the leptomeningeal cells toward plasma protein is different from their reaction to foreign colloids and particles, which are phagocytosed and remain within the intracranial and intraspinal spaces for a prolonged period (Fig. 4-14). Radioactive or fluorescent proteins or particles of ferritin injected into ventricular CSF enter the brain between the ependymal cells and may also be taken up by ependymal pinocytosis (there is no evidence of exocytosis at the base of the cells). Penetration is a little deeper over gray matter than over white, but in neither case extends much below the ependymal layer. This is presumably because of the narrowness and tortuosity of the extracellular spaces, since there appears to be no definable barrier. From the subarachnoid fluid, colloidal particles may penetrate the pia-glia layer very slightly, but particulate matter appears not to. It is clear that there is no bulk flow of colloids or particles across the ependyma or the pia, confirming that such material either escapes through the villi (plasma protein and red cells) or is phagocytosed by leptomeningeal cells (with a very minor loss via the olfactory nerves to nasal lymphatics).

Cerebrospinal Fluid Clearance of Small Molecules

Small molecules from CSF enter the extracellular space more freely than macromolecules in colloidal solution, but even here, because of the configuration and the absence of bulk flow, concentrations build

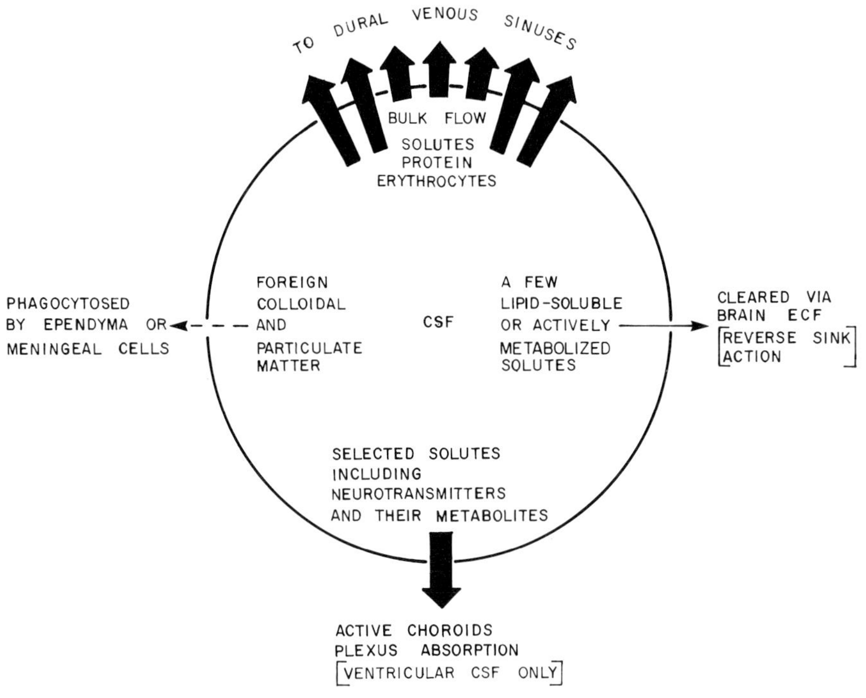

Fig. 4-14. Methods of removal (clearance) of particles, colloids, and solutes from the CSF.

up beneath ependyma and pia, so that diffusion is markedly slowed. Exceptions occur if the diffusing material can enter cerebral vessels or cells, especially if metabolized. If absorbed by vessels in the brain, they will also be cleared by choroid plexus vessels, crossing both barriers in the reverse direction; for lipid-soluble molecules, this may be a major method of clearance. It is possible to investigate bulk clearance (through the villi) separately from reabsorption clearance, either by maintaining high plasma concentration (which has no effect on bulk movement, but reduces diffusion into vessels), by reducing CSF secretion (e.g., with carbonic acid anhydrase) which reduces bulk flow, but does not affect diffusion, or by increasing CSF pressure (which increases bulk flow). A further method of CSF clearance is active absorption, which affects substances actively transported by the kidney (e.g., iodopyracet [Diodrast] and phenylsulfonphthalein [PSP], iodide, bromide, thiocyanate, quarternary bases, serotonin, and norepinephrine). These several methods of removal of solutes from CSF have complicated the interpretation of the relationship between CSF and ECF by equilibration studies.

Clearance differs between intraventricular and intrathecal injection, since in the latter, bulk flow is extremely sluggish. Diffusion between the cord ECF and spinal CSF is cumulatively greater than between the brain and intracranial CSF because of this absence of bulk clearance. Therefore, lipid-soluble substances may be cleared more rapidly from cord tissue than from the relatively stagnant spinal CSF. Conversely, lipid-insoluble substances such as $^{24}Na^{+}$, administered intravenously, diffuse from cord ECF to CSF and may accumulate in the lumbosacral fluid more than in cisternal CSF, giving a false impression of CSF production in the lower spinal canal.

Acetylcholine is present in very low levels, if at all, in normal CSF, presumably because of the presence of acetylcholinesterase. Detectable levels of acetylcholine occur in the CSF of epileptic persons, following electroshock therapy, and inconstantly in head injury. Serotonin is only detectable after head injury and is thought to be actively transported out by the choroid plexus. Epinephrine and norepinephrine are present at levels of 0.9 and 3μg per liter, about 25% of the levels in plasma, but in the same proportion. They are probably derived from plasma and are actively transported out by the plexus epithelium. Histamine levels in CSF are very low. The virtual absence of neurotransmitters from CSF, in spite of a constant, slow flow of ECF into the CSF, is doubtless due to the efficiency of synaptic reuptake mechanisms (see Chap. 3).

Composition of Extracellular Fluid

Since direct study of brain ECF has so far been impossible, only inferences about its nature can be drawn. For reasons already noted, it is considered to be at least in part a product of active secretion rather than a simple plasma ultrafiltrate. Solute concentrations in ECF will depend not only on the rate at which they cross the blood-brain barrier but also on rates of diffusional exchange between ECF and CSF, which are potentially high for small molecules and ions. Thus, if a concentration were initially higher in ECF, but the solute diffused rapidly into the CSF to be removed by bulk flow, or active absorption, or both, the level in ECF would fall rapidly. This is the *sink action* of CSF, a mechanism tending to equilibrate the two fluids. Theoretically, ECF could act as a sink for CSF. Since there is no bulk removal of ECF (only a slow flow into the CSF), buildup of high subependymal concentration limits sink action in this direction. If the solute is involved in active metabolism (e.g., glucose, phosphate), subependymal concentration is prevented. Calculation of sink action (in either direction) for such solutes is difficult.

Some solute concentrations of CSF differ in the ventricles and cisterna magna. In the absence of evidence for ependymal secretion, the most reasonable explanation would be diffusion between ECF and CSF. Measurements of such differences might then give at least a semiquantitative measure of solute concentrations in ECF, excluding metabolites. Intrathecal fluid cannot be used for such estimations, since it is relatively stagnant.

In comparison with ventricular or choroid plexus CSF, fluid from the cisterna magna shows even higher Cl^- concentration, unchanged Na^+ concentration, and lower levels of K^+, Ca^{++}, and Mg^{++}. Where it has been possible to collect CSF from the cortical subarachnoid space, Na^+, Ca^{++}, Mg^{++}, and Cl^- concentrations show little further change, but K^+ levels are even lower. Except for Mg^{++}, the changes in CSF ion concentrations along its flow path are not back in the direction of plasma ultrafiltrate, but represent increasing departures from such levels. It is assumed that CSF is adjusting by passive diffusion to the ionic composition of the ECF, which must therefore have a similar concentration of Na^+, must be higher in Cl^-, and must be lower in Ca^{++}, Mg^{++}, and (especially) K^+. In spite of the differences known to exist between the two fluids, CSF may be accepted as a much closer approximation to ECF than is the plasma and is commonly used when information about ECF levels is required. Cisternal CSF is a better indicator than ventricular CSF.

OTHER POSSIBLE GLIAL FUNCTIONS

A few potential further roles for the glia, less well documented experimentally, are discussed next.

Determining the Configuration of Extracellular Pathways

The extracellular pathways are narrow, branching, and interconnecting channels, often only 200 A wide, with a very high surface to volume ratio. However, the system is not entirely uniform. Around capillaries, at the pial-glial junction, and around neurons, the extracellular space is very narrow, but at the nodes of Ranvier and around synapses the extracellular space may form larger lacunae by convergence of fine channels. At least occasionally, CNS neurons are covered by a single membrane resembling compact myelin. More often, they are covered by attenuated glial sheets of the loose-myelin type (i.e., still including some cell cytoplasm); parallel lamellae of such loose myelin may be closely apposed or actually fused. Electric current might then be selectively channeled through the gaps that are present around synaptic junctions, and the current flow across any part of a neuronal membrane would be a function of the number of extracellular spaces opening close to it. (The principle is much the same as the channeling of current through nodal regions of myelinated axons.) The presence of loose or compact myelin around neurons could reduce variability in extracellular ionic concentrations, thus cutting down "noise." This would be of particular importance in the soma-dendrite region, since the integrative function depends on algebraic summation of very small membrane potential changes. Such a mechanism would be a third line of defense for ionic homeostasis, following the general body mechanisms and the barrier system. It is at least theoretically possible that such attenuated glial lamellae might separate functionally different neuron pools, isolating them from nonspecific afferent influences. The insulation would be equally effective with respect to neurotransmitters or ionic shifts.

Maintaining Ionic Homeostasis

Reported ionic concentrations and membrane potentials of glial cells leave it uncertain as to whether they affect local ion concentrations (e.g., by taking up K^+ lost through active neuronal membranes). Glial cells have been reported with internal potential varying from −50 to −65 mv. Perforated by microelectrodes, they show a constant potential with no dependence on neural activity, suggesting that they do not take up K^+ liberated from active neurons. Since their membrane potential varies with external K^+ concentration, as it does for neurons, there appears to be little evidence that they are cells with a high internal Na^+ level, as has been suggested. They appear to be depolarized by acetylcholine and by GABA, but the significance of this is unclear. Some observers have reported slow variations in glial potential of unknown significance. A relationship to contractility has been suggested, the latter having been observed in tissue cultures.

Support of Neuronal Metabolism

Of the total volume of a nerve cell, with a perikaryon 50μ in diameter and with 5μ processes totaling 100 cm in length, 99.7% is in the processes, so that even the large nucleus and nucleolus and considerable endoplasmic reticulum (Nissl bodies) must be functioning at near their maximum metabolic activity for the mere maintenance of cell integrity. In many invertebrates, satellite cells (including astrocytes) carry large quantities of glycogen and lipid, and their processes may invaginate the neuronal perikaryon; however, the vascular supply is usually much less. In the vertebrate CNS, vascularity is rich and glycogen stores are low, but glial cells may still have a role in the direct transfer of metabolites in and out of neurons.

It is of interest that the number of satellite cells (perineuronal oligodendroglia) appears to rise with the size of the animal (i.e., with the average length of axons). In layer VI of the cortex, the glia-to-neuron ratio is 4.5 in the whale, 1.9 in man, 1.6 in the horse, 0.47 in the rabbit, 0.46 in the chicken, and 0.25 in the frog. In some species the number of satellite cells varies along the thoracic nucleus of Clarke's column, from 5.6 ± 3 in the cervical portion of the cord up to 18.2 ± 6 in the sacral portion. In the cerebellar Purkinje's cells, the perikaryon volume rises only logarithmically with the size of the animal, whereas the length of the axon rises linearly; hence, there is a fall in the perikaryon to axon volume ratio. Correspondingly, associated glial cells rise from 9 per neuron in the rat to about 50 in the cow. The number of glia around anterior horn cells has been said to rise for about 3 hours following severe muscular exercise, then gradually reverse during the succeeding 4 to 5 hours, without evidence of mitotic or amitotic division. In several rodent species, crushing of the seventh or twelfth cranial nerves raises the number of glia in the corresponding motor nuclei for the period of axon regeneration.

In mammals, no interpenetration of neuronal and glial cells, as seen in invertebrates, has been noted, so any transfers occur across the normal tangential interfaces. It has been proposed that the cytoplasmic incisures of Lanterman in myelin may represent a route of nutrient transfer directly from oligodendroglial cell to axon, though the well-documented axoplasmic flow perhaps makes such a hypothesis unnecessary. Scattered reports have suggested that oxidative enzyme activity is higher in glial than in neuronal cells, but it is almost impossible to achieve separation of the two types, and reaction to oxygen-lack would suggest the contrary. Other reports propose alternation of enzyme activities, RNA synthesis, and so on, between neurons and oligodendroglia, depending on the activity of the former.

Clearly, the hypothesis of direct metabolic interdependence is highly speculative. It remains for future investigators to establish definitely the significance of the many structural and ultrastructural specializations of glial cells and their proportionately higher numbers in more advanced evolutionary forms.

BIBLIOGRAPHY

Bailey, O. T., and Smith, D. E. (Eds.) *The Central Nervous System* (Int. Acad. Pathol. Monogr. No. 9). Baltimore: Williams & Wilkins, 1968.

Broman, T., and Steinwall, O. The Blood-Brain Barrier. In J. Minckler (Ed.), *Pathology of the Nervous System.* New York: McGraw-Hill, 1968. Vol. 1, pp. 406-416.

Bunge, R. P. Glial cells and the central myelin sheath. *Physiol. Rev.* 48:197-251, 1968.

Davson, H. *Physiology of the Cerebrospinal Fluids.* London: Churchill, 1970.

Davson, H. The Blood-Brain Barrier. In G. H. Bourne (Ed.), *The Structure and Function of Nervous Tissue.* New York: Academic, 1972. Vol. 4, pp. 321-445.

Fleischhauer, K. Ependyma and the Subependymal Layer. In G. H. Bourne (Ed.), *The Structure and Function of Nervous Tissue.* New York: Academic, 1972. Vol. 6, pp. 1-46.

Katzman, R., and Pappius, H. M. *Brain Electrolytes and Fluid Metabolism.* Baltimore: Williams & Wilkins, 1973.

Lasansky, A. Function at the cellular level: Glia. *Annu. Rev. Physiol.* 33:241-256, 1971.

Mettler, F. A. Fluid Exchanges. In J. Minckler (Ed.), *Pathology of the Nervous System.* New York: McGraw-Hill, 1968. Vol. 1, pp. 417-424.

Siesjö, B. K., and Sørensen, S. C. *Ion Homeostasis of the Brain.* New York: Academic, 1971.

Slager, U. T. The Meninges. In J. Minckler (Ed.), *Pathology of the Nervous System.* New York: McGraw-Hill, 1968. Vol. 1, pp. 477-486.

van Harreveld, A. The Extra-cellular Space in the Vertebrate Central Nervous System. In G. H. Bourne (Ed.), *The Structure and Function of Nervous Tissue.* New York: Academic, 1972. Vol. 4, pp. 447-511.

Brain Pathways

5

Gross examination of the brain at autopsy fails to disclose many internal structures. These can be visualized only by special techniques, usually involving the use of myelin stains. In discussing the brain pathways in this and subsequent chapters, the description of the appearance of the brain on gross examination given in Chapter I will be augmented as necessary by illustrations of myelin-stained sections. No attempt is made to provide an atlas of myelination but only to illustrate structures, unseen in fixed, whole brain, which appear to have clinical relevance.

It has become commonplace to compare the brain with a computer, but except for the mathematically inclined reader, this analogy is of doubtful utility. Both in the CNS and the computer, it is relatively easy to analyze input and output. Beyond this point, the two problems are considerably different. The computer employs data processing, which is programmed and therefore comprehensible (to the initiate). While the same may be true of the brain, the nature of the program is unknown – and complex beyond the imagination. Furthermore, the CNS has capabilities of choice that amount to infinite modifications of its own program and are beyond the present and (hopefully) future ability of any computer.

Superficially, it is possible to analyze descriptively the data processing parts of the CNS on a phylogenetic basis. There is an ancient core of suprasegmental structures that comprises the reticular formation, hypothalamus, and limbic system and contains structures concerned with homeostasis, integration of early forms of environmental input, and mechanisms for the execution of appropriate rhythmical muscular responses. This core is susceptible to conditioning and capable to some degree of other kinds of learning and of memory. The original environmental inputs to this core (it has since acquired others) were spatially poorly discriminative and included coarse touch, pain, smell, taste, and balance. Output was through the pituitary, the autonomic nervous system, and motor fibers to somatic musculature. As environmental pressures increased, the system became inadequate.

The core then became overlaid, but never supplanted, by newer suprasegmental structures (e.g., the thalamus, basal ganglia, cerebellum, and neocortex) that could receive much more discriminative environmental information (fine touch, hearing, vision, and enhanced muscle proprioception), enabling correspondingly more appropriate and accurate somatic motor responses, particularly vocalization and the use of distal musculature (often asymmetrical). In higher primates, a greatly enlarged neocortex has developed, culminating in the capacity for abstract thinking and tool-making. A characteristic of all these accretions to the core is the use of large-fiber, heavily myelinated, rapidly conducting pathways with few synapses and a recognizable degree of point-to-point (topographical) representation, both of the body and the environment. The new and the old structures remain equally important and intimately connected, so that the CNS, except in disease, is a functionally integrated, harmonious system.

This chapter is concerned with a general description of CNS pathways, including those of current clinical relevance or associated with recent conceptual advances. A few pathways of especial clinical importance are considered separately in Chapters 6, 7, and 8. It must be realized that pathways of unexplored significance today may become of burning importance tomorrow because of some new advance in diagnosis or therapy. Current knowledge in the neurological basic sciences is subject to revision on an almost day-to-day basis.

RETICULAR FORMATION

Structure

The reticular formation is a central area in the brain stem (Fig. 5-1), extending from the lower medulla to the subthalamus, with neurons only loosely grouped into nuclei. In addition to its intrinsic (nonmyelinated, fine) fibers, it is intersected by nerve roots and bundles of myelinated and unmyelinated fibers derived from phylogenetically more recent structures. It is separated from the ependyma of the fourth ventricle and aqueduct by a zone of subependymal (periaqueductal) "central" gray matter. In the lower medulla the reticular formation lies mainly ventral to the central canal, appears continuous dorsally with the gracilis and cuneate nuclei, and extends laterally almost to the spinal nuclei of

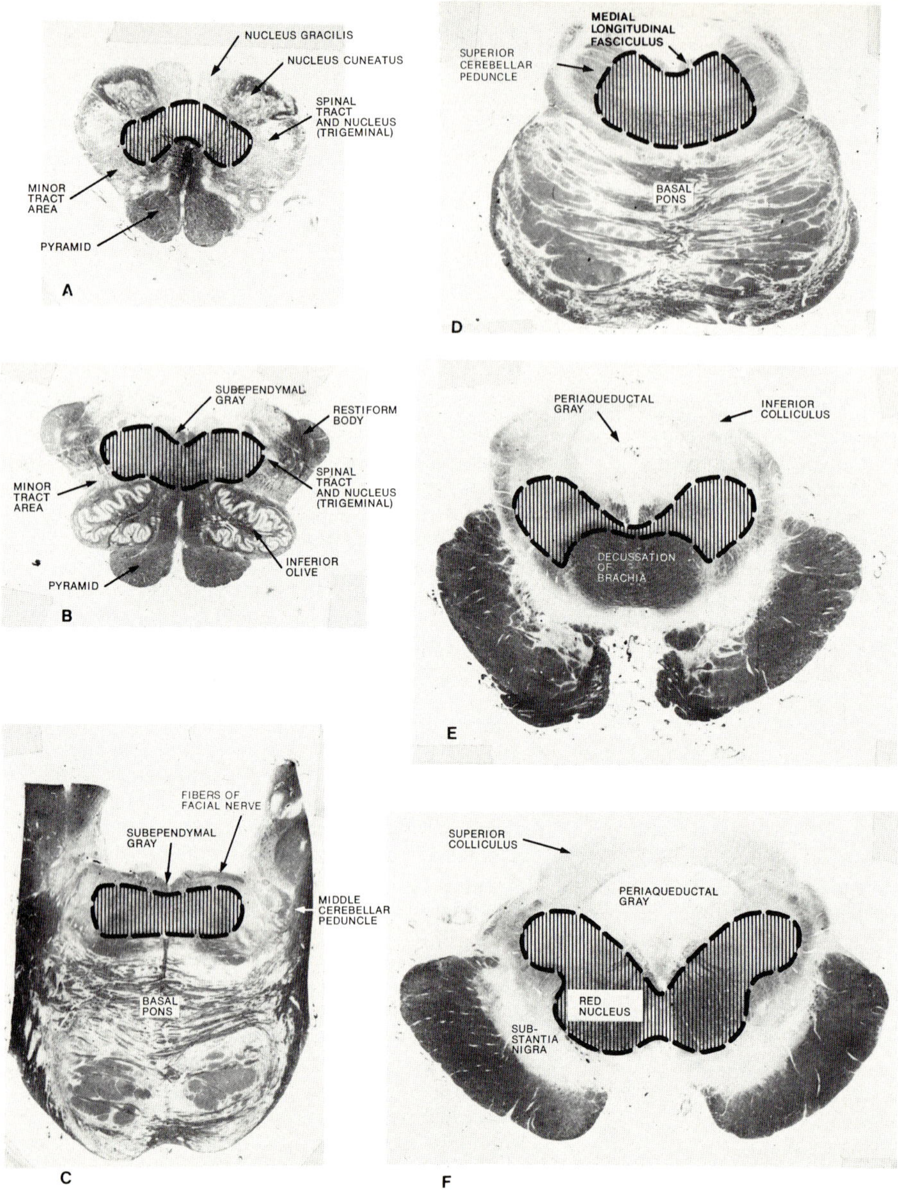

Fig. 5-1. Sections across the brain stem to show the approximate extent of the diffuse reticular formation. Levels A to F in ascending order. (Myelin stain, X3.)

the fifth (trigeminal) nerve. In the upper medulla, it lies between the central gray matter (dorsally) and the inferior and accessory olives (ventrally), extending laterally to the minor tract area and trigeminal spinal nucleus. In the pontine tegmentum, it intervenes between the subependymal gray matter and the lemnisci. In the midbrain it reaches its largest extent, extending from the periaqueductal gray matter ventrolaterally, to reach the substantia nigra and completely surround the red nuclei. It also extends anteriorly below the posterior part of the thalamus and is a major component of the subthalamus. More recently, it has become apparent that the brain stem reticular formation is only part of a continuous axial area that also includes some of the gray and adjacent white matter of the spinal cord, as well as nuclei of the thalamus lying either adjacent to the third ventricle (midline nuclei), ventrolateral to the thalamus proper (external laminar nuclei), or within the thalamus itself (intralaminar nuclei, including the centrum medianum).

Input

Input (Fig. 5-2) to the spinal and brain stem reticular formation is from all the spinal and cranial afferent

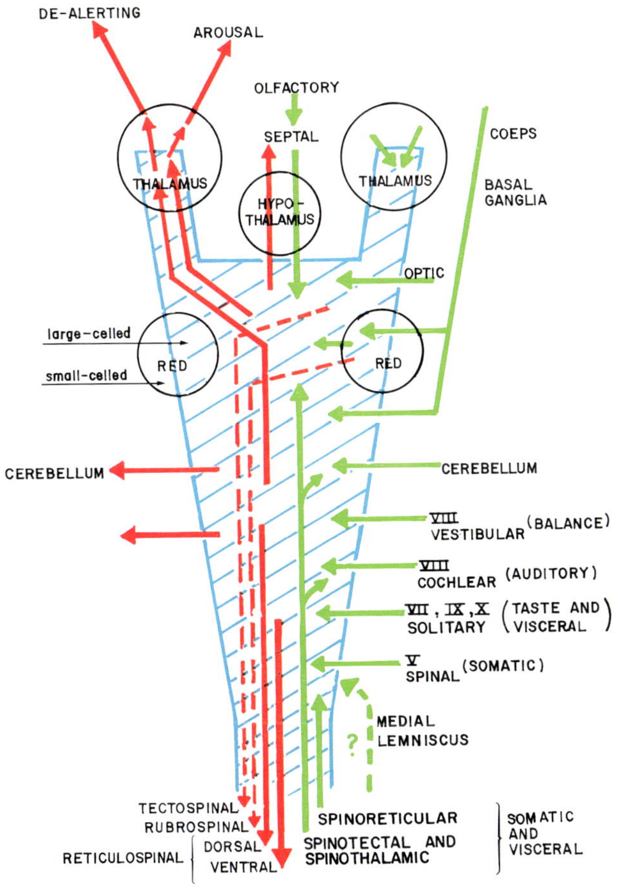

Fig. 5-2. Input to (green) and output from (red) the reticular formation. For the sake of clarity, each is represented on one side only, and internal connections along the length of the formation are omitted. COEPS = cortically originating extrapyramidal system.

nerves, both by collaterals and terminals. In addition to direct afferent input at the nerve root level, there are also ascending spinoreticular, spinotectal, and spinothalamic fibers; a considerable number of the latter reach the mesencephalic (midbrain) portion. In addition, the reticular formation receives collaterals from phylogenetically more recent afferent systems, probably including muscle proprioception and discriminative touch, certainly including hearing and vision. There are inputs from the cerebellum, basal ganglia, and cortex (the cortically originating extrapyramidal system [COEPS]). There is a massive input into the mesencephalic reticular formation from the hypothalamus, through the median forebrain bundle, mamillotegmental tract, and hypothalamo-interpeduncular bundle (as well as fibers to the closely related periaqueductal gray, running in the dorsal longitudinal fasciculus). The thalamic reticular formation receives fibers from the hypothalamus and from the limbic formation (particularly the hippocampus, via the fornix and anterior thalamic nucleus).

Output

The output (Fig. 5-2) from the brain stem reticular formation includes ascending and descending fibers, but many also run to adjacent structures within the brain stem and in the cerebellum, and there is a massive return flow through the median forebrain bundle to the hypothalamus. The descending fibers constitute the somewhat diffuse reticulospinal tract (part of the ventrolateral column of the spinal cord), and the ascending efferents consist of fibers that pass through, or synapse in, the thalamic reticular nuclei and are diffusely distributed to almost all the neocortex.

Circuitry

Many neurons of the reticular formation have dendrites that run at right angles to the neuraxis and an axon that branches to ascending and descending divisions (parallel to the neuraxis). Thus, a network with potentially enormous numbers of axodendritic and axosomatic synapses is formed. The reticular

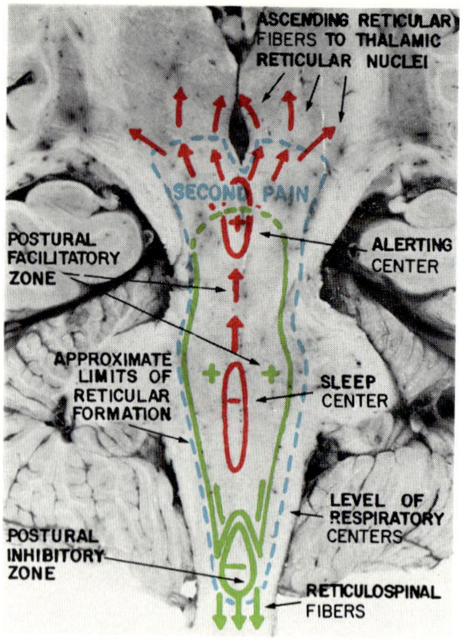

Fig. 5-3. Transverse section along the brain stem and posterior thalamus, indicating some of the localizations of function within the reticular formation, and its extent. Red = components of ascending reticular activating system; green = areas affecting postural tonus.

activating system shows high convergence and divergence, with necessarily imprecise topographical representation of body or environment. Many of the axons are short, so that passage through the cord and brain stem is largely by short paths connected by synapses and is relatively slow, especially as the intrinsic fibers are thin, with little or no myelin. This series of ascending and descending connections has been somewhat arbitrarily divided into spinospinal, spinoreticular, reticulospinal, and reticuloreticular tracts (the latter is the central tegmental bundle). In addition to these relays of axons, there are direct spinoreticular fibers, providing somewhat more rapid conduction.

Functions

Certain functions have been assigned with some confidence to the reticular formation, though localization within it is more dependent on physiological than on anatomical studies (Fig. 5-3). Fibers largely from the midbrain component ascend to the reticular thalamic nuclei and finally reach the neocortex. Some of these appear to be cholinergic and to cause desynchronization of the electroencephalogram (EEG) and cortical activation. This system is therefore termed the *ascending reticular activating system.* Other fibers originate more caudally (with other neurotransmitters such as norepinephrine, serotonin, or dopamine). These fibers also influence the neocortex but appear to inhibit it, with synchronization of the EEG and reduced wakefulness. Thus, the reticular formation probably includes an alerting center (rostrally) and a sleep center (caudally). It is not known whether the sleep center acts directly on forebrain structures or indirectly by inhibiting the alerting center (active and passive reticular deactivation respectively). The sleep center reduces the convulsive threshold of the cortex, which is raised by the alerting center. It seems that moderate activity of the alerting center is optimal; if activity is only moderate animals appear attentive and keenly aware of changes in the environment (orienting behavior). With excess activity, they become agitated, exhibit escape patterns of behavior, and respond less appropriately.

The descending reticulospinal fibers convey not only motor impulses originating in the reticular formation itself but also those from basal ganglia, which have no direct fiber connections with cord or brain stem motor nuclei. Functionally, the large-celled division of the red nucleus (vestigial in man) is part of the reticular formation, deriving its input largely from the intermediate cerebellum and originating the rubrospinal tract (closely related to the reticulospinal tract). Stimulation of neurons in the medial medullary part of the reticular formation

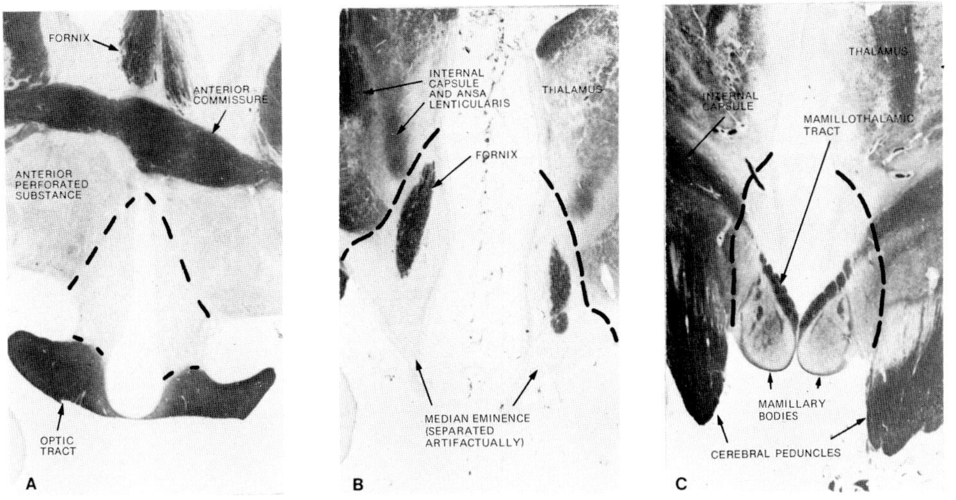

Fig. 5-4. Composite transverse sections through lower third ventricle and adjacent regions of the hypothalamus, showing its approximate extent. Levels A to C in anteroposterior sequence. (Myelin stain, ×3.)

inhibits the stretch reflex (see Chap. 7) of extensor (postural) muscles and facilitates flexor stretch reflexes via impulses descending in the ventral part of the reticulospinal tract. Stimulation of the lateral medullary, or more rostral, parts of the reticular formation causes converse extensor facilitation and flexor inhibition via impulses descending in the dorsal portion of the tract.

It seems probable that the brain stem reticular formation is the origin of primitive rhythmic or reciprocating movements, including pacing in lower mammals. Its autonomy has been markedly reduced by "corticalization" in primates. Physiological studies have shown inspiratory and expiratory centers at the level of the caudal end of the inferior olive, the former ventromedial and the latter dorsolateral. From these, a multisynaptic respiratory path descends in the ventrolateral column immediately deep to the spinothalamic fibers (where it may be injured in high cervical tractotomy).

The midbrain reticular formation appears to be particularly concerned in the appreciation of pain, since it receives afferents from the older spinothalamic tract (see Chap. 6). This pain is associated with affect, presumably by virtue of radiations through the thalamus to the cortex, including the limbic system.

HYPOTHALAMUS

Structure

The hypothalamus (Fig. 5-4) is an extremely small diencephalic structure in the walls of the lower half of the third ventricle, which forms its medial boundary on each side. It is bounded laterally by subthalamic structures, the internal capsule, and the anterior perforated substance; anteriorly by the lamina terminalis; and posteriorly by the midbrain. The thalamus lies above it, the line of demarcation being seen in the wall of the third ventricle as an indefinite hypothalamic sulcus that runs from the foramen of Monro to the upper end of the aqueduct. Rostrocaudally, the hypothalamus may be divided into anterior, middle, and posterior portions and mediolaterally, into periventricular, medial, and lateral parts, theoretically yielding nine areas (on each side). The periventricular part is continuous through the three divisions and forms a narrow layer lining the lower half of the third ventricle (Fig. 5-5). The anterior portion of the hypothalamus also contains the preoptic nucleus, which lies at the level of the lamina terminalis; the supraoptic nucleus, which lies over the origin of the optic tract; and the paraventricular nucleus, which represents a dorsal continuation

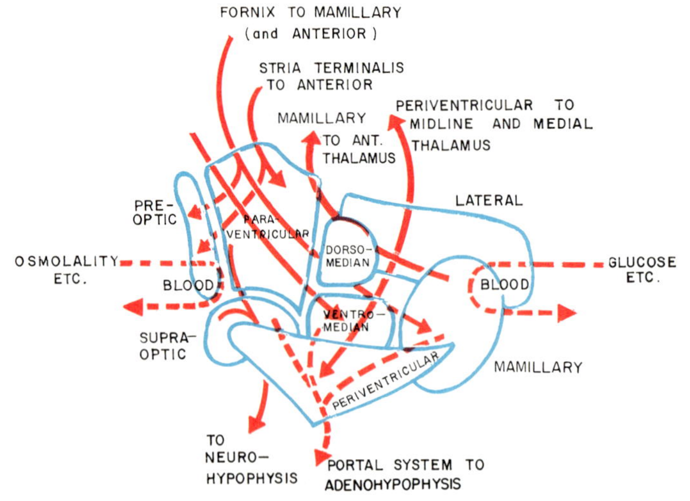

Fig. 5-5. Lateral, semischematic view of hypothalamus (anterior to left), showing its major component regions and some of their connections. (On histological sections, most of these areas cannot be recognized or clearly separated.)

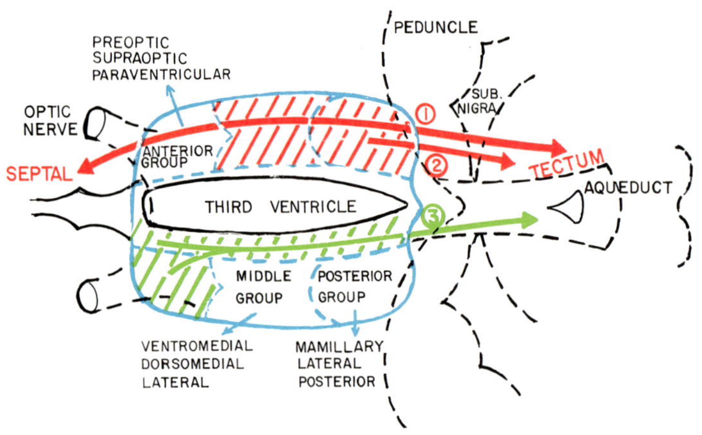

Fig. 5-6. Horizontal section through hypothalamus and midbrain, indicating some major fiber connections and an approximate division of the hypothalamus into predominantly sympathetic (red) and largely parasympathetic (green) areas. 1 = median forebrain bundle; 2 = mamillotegmental tract; 3 = dorsal longitudinal fasciculus.

of the supraoptic, deep to the periventricular layer. The middle portion contains two medial nuclei (dorsal medial and ventral medial) and a lateral nucleus. The posterior hypothalamus contains mamillary nuclei and, lying caudal to them, posterior nuclei adjacent to the midbrain tectum: there is also a lateral nucleus continuous with that of the middle portion. A few of these nuclei, such as the mamillary bodies and the supraoptic areas, may be distinguished easily, but generally the hypothalamus is seen to consist of a diffuse array of neurons separated by small, unmyelinated (or thinly myelinated) fibers. Several distinct fiber tracts traverse the area.

Input

Most of the input is from the reticular formation or the limbic system. Major tracts (Fig. 5-6) that communicate between the posterior hypothalamus and reticular formation are bidirectional. Thus, the median forebrain bundle can be regarded as input to and output from both areas, as can the dorsal longitudinal fasciculus, mamillotegmental tract, and other communications. The dorsal longitudinal fasciculus arises in the periventricular gray matter and passes

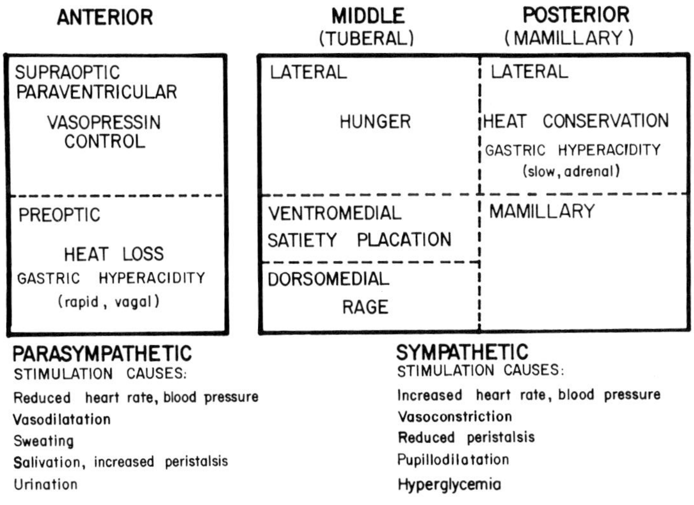

Fig. 5-7. Tabular representation of the allocation of some hypothalamic functions to various regions (horizontal section, right hypothalamus viewed from above).

back to the periaqueductal gray matter. The median forebrain bundle starts in the septal part of the limbic formation, passes backward and downward through the lateral hypothalamus, and terminates in the midbrain reticular formation. It is a pathway rather than a tract, since fibers are continually entering and leaving, and it serves as the major route of communication between all three core systems. Other input from the limbic system arrives via the stria terminalis from the amygdala, and via the fornix from the hippocampus. The fornix descends in front of the foramen of Monro and turns backward and slightly medially through the hypothalamus to reach the mamillary bodies. Some fibers from the fornix end in the preoptic region with those of the stria terminalis. The hypothalamus also receives input from the thalamus (by several thalamohypothalamic tracts, running chiefly between the medial thalamic nucleus and the periventricular hypothalamic nucleus).

Output

Hypothalamic output largely corresponds to input, since many of its connections are bidirectional. In addition, there is a conspicuous mamillothalamic tract running to the anterior nucleus of the thalamus, and a hypothalamo-hypophyseal tract running down the pituitary stalk to the neurohypophysis. An additional important output of the hypothalamus is neurosecretion into the pituitary portal system of vessels (see Chap. 8).

Functions

Most functions have been assigned to the hypothalamus on the basis of experiments involving stimulation, ablation, or both (Fig. 5-7). The function of two of its most striking connections, the fornix and the mamillothalamic tract, remains unknown.

The hypothalamus is closely concerned with autonomic function, appearing to integrate autonomic and neuroendocrine systems for body homeostasis. Overall, *the periventricular and anterior hypothalamus may be regarded as parasympathetic* and *the more caudal parts as sympathetic.* Stimulation of the preoptic nucleus appears to increase heat loss and change gastric acidity. Destruction of parts of the anterior hypothalamus has led to pulmonary edema and hemorrhage, possibly associated with constriction of veins and excess blood in the pulmonary circulation. Paraventricular and supraoptic neurons send axons to the neurohypophysis and appear to be neurosecretory. They are concerned with the control of osmolality, apparently by sensitivity to Na^+ or Cl^- levels (see Chap. 8). There seems to be a satiety center (associated with reduction or cessation of food intake) in the ventral median nucleus and a feeding center (associated with increased food intake) in the lateral nucleus. There is some evidence for centers controlling vasoconstriction and sphincter contraction in the lateral zone, stimulation of which also increases gastric acidity. Stimulation that is repeated or chronic may lead to gastric ulceration and hemorrhage. The posterior lateral nucleus appears to contain a heat-conservation center, opposing a loss center in the preoptic nucleus.

Stimulation of widespread areas in the middle and posterior hypothalamus apparently leads to pleasant or unpleasant sensations to such a degree that animals may be readily trained to apply or to discontinue such stimulation by activating simple electromechanical devices; these have been termed *pleasure centers* and *punishing centers.* Similar areas have been described in the limbic formation and the reticular formation of the midbrain, and they are presumably concerned in some way with the selection and reinforcement of appropriate responses to environmental stimuli.

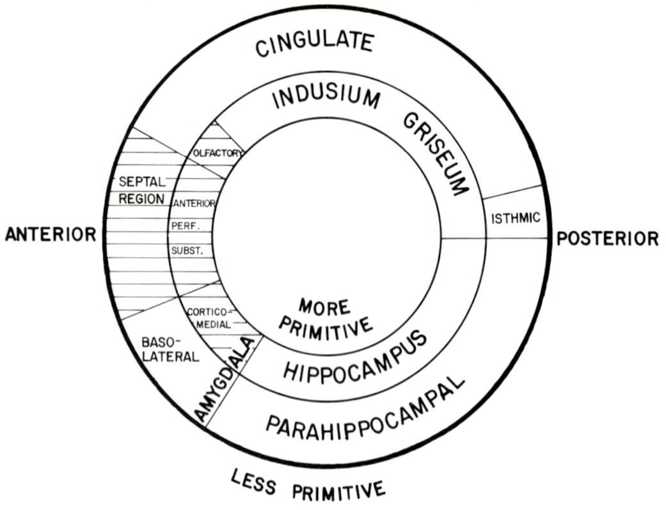

Fig. 5-8. Completely schematic representation of the components of the limbic formation, indicating an inner ring of more primitive parts (originally closer to the foramen of Monro) and an outer ring of less primitive parts. In the human being, some areas (e.g., the indusium griseum) are vestigial. Anterior perf. subst. = anterior perforated substance.

LIMBIC FORMATION

Structure

The limbic formation, or rhinencephalon, includes phylogenetically older parts of the cerebral hemispheres, originally concerned largely with olfaction. It consists of both cortex and subcortical masses of gray matter with intrinsic fiber tracts, and its nomenclature is confusing. Within the limbic formation itself, there are more and less primitive parts (Fig. 5-8).

The *more primitive parts* (archipallium and paleopallium) include the anterior perforated substance (with prepiriform cortex and olfactory tubercle), the corticomedial part of the amygdala and the periamygdaloid cortex, and the hippocampus. The cortex has fewer than the six layers typical of the neocortex and is often termed the *allocortex.* The *less primitive parts* are larger and include the parahippocampal, isthmic, cingulate, and olfactory gyri and a somewhat indefinite "septal region," lying anterior to the olfactory gyrus, including the parolfactory gyri. The septal region also includes the septum pellucidum and small gray masses beneath the cortex, collectively termed the *septal nuclei.* The basolateral part of the amygdala is also part of this less primitive limbic system.

Commissures

The limbic formation has two intrinsic commissures (Fig. 5-9): the anterior commissure runs in the upper margin of the lamina terminalis and connects the olfactory gyri, anterior perforated substance, olfactory tubercles, and amygdala; the commissure of the fornix connects the hippocampus and septal regions of each side. Fibers from some less primitive areas, such as the parahippocampal gyrus and cingulate cortex, may use the corpus callosum. Since the cerebral (telencephalic) vesicles originated by pouching of the ventricles through the foramina of Monro, the limbic structures were originally orientated around the foramen in a ring. Unfortunately, this simple relationship has been disrupted by development of the corpus callosum in the upper border of the lamina terminalis, so that many of the limbic pathways are now circuitous. By development of the temporal lobes, the hippocampus has been displaced from a superior to an inferior position.

Olfactory Pathways

Olfactory input (Figs. 5-8, 5-9 [left]) is direct to the anterior perforated substance and olfactory tubercle and indirect to the septal region and olfactory gyrus (via medial stria) and the corticomedial amygdala (via lateral stria). Structures of both sides are connected through the anterior commissure. Since fibers run from the tubercle and olfactory gyrus to the septal region, and since the major output from the corticomedial amygdala is via the stria terminalis (around the thalamus medial to the caudate) to the septal region, olfactory impulses converge in this area. They merge with other limbic input and cannot be distinguished further as a separate sense modality. The original path for olfactory sensation was from septal region to hypothalamus (with neuroendocrine output) and to the reticular formation (with reticulospinal output). There was probably a more direct olfactory pathway running from the septal region via the stria medullaris (along the medial border of the thalamus) to the habenula and thence in the

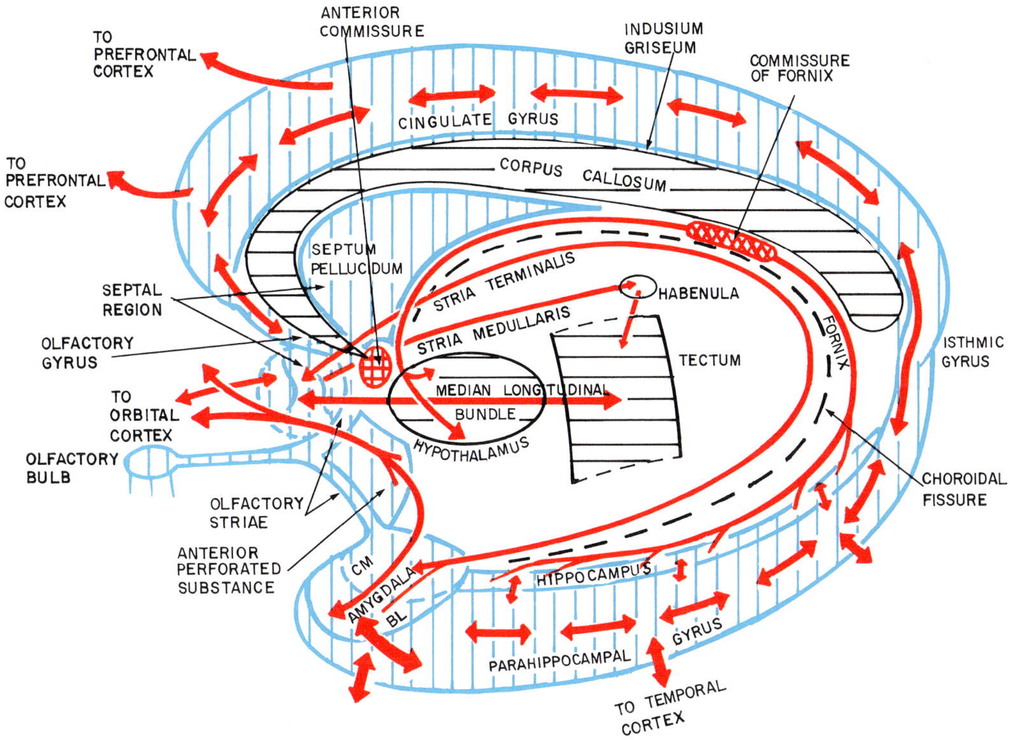

Fig. 5-9. Semischematic representation of the limbic formation (blue) and its internal and external connections (red). For details, see text. CM = corticomedial amygdala; BL = basolateral amygdala.

habenulopeduncular tract to the reticular formation, for appropriate motor responses. These pathways have now probably been subordinated to other functions, but the potency of olfactory input in causing changed affect remains very high.

Connections of Major Limbic Centers

The *basolateral amygdala* receives fibers from the hippocampus and parahippocampal gyrus, and there are also reciprocal connections with the orbital cortex. It sends some fibers to the medial column of thalamic nuclei.

The *hippocampus* receives fibers from the parahippocampal gyrus, temporal neocortex, basolateral amygdala, opposite hippocampus (via the commissure of the fornix), and septal region (via the fornix below the corpus callosum and the longitudinal striae above). The major efferent tract of the hippocampus is the fornix, which carries fibers to the opposite hippocampus, cingulate gyrus, septal region, and the anterior hypothalamus. The fornix also makes a major fiber contribution to the mamillary nucleus and supplies fibers to other hypothalamic nuclei and the mesencephalic reticular formation. A few hippocampal fibers pass (in the longitudinal striae) to the olfactory gyrus.

The *cingulate gyrus* communicates with adjacent neocortex (especially the frontal lobe), the caudate nucleus and putamen through the internal capsule, and the septum pellucidum and fornix by means of perforating fibers through the corpus callosum.

The connections of the *septal region* have in the main been described previously. It receives fibers from the amygdala, hippocampus, and olfactory tract and also from adjacent neocortex (especially orbital). It has a massive connection with the hypothalamus and brain stem reticular formation through the median forebrain bundle and sends a few efferent fibers (as the stria medullaris) to the habenula.

A summary of these diffuse, complex connections may be in order (Fig. 5-9). Within the limbic formation itself there is free bidirectional communication between virtually all areas. Efferent fibers pass to the hypothalamus and reticular formation (fornix, stria terminalis, and median forebrain bundle) and to adjacent neocortex, with a few to the thalamic reticular formation and possibly the caudate nucleus and putamen. Afferent fibers arrive from the olfactory tract, the hypothalamus and reticular formation (median forebrain bundle), and adjacent neocortex. Most of these external connections are also bidirectional.

Functions

It is apparent that the limbic system is intimately related to the hypothalamus and, through it, to the reticular formation, and that although originally an

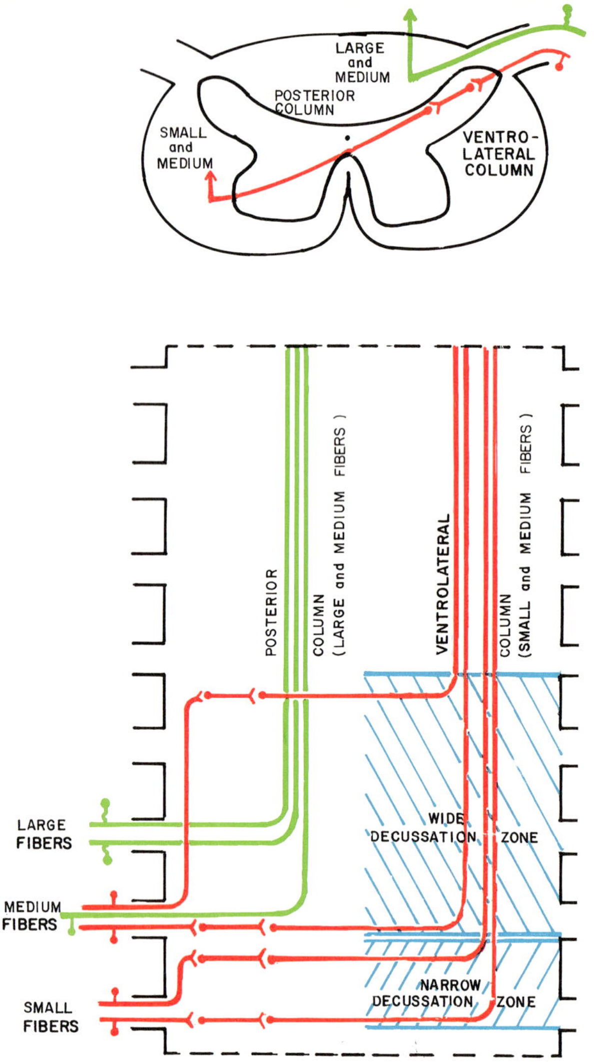

Fig. 5-10. Pathways followed by small, intermediate, and large afferent somatosensory fibers (cell bodies in dorsal root ganglia) on entering the spinal cord. Above, transverse section of cord. Below, transverse longitudinal section. Green = nondecussating posterior column fibers; red = synapsing primary and decussating secondary fibers; blue = zones of decussation.

olfactory receptor system, it now has many other functions. Pleasure and punishing centers have been identified in many parts of the limbic formation, and it is thought to be associated with the emotional overtones of experience, in which its widespread neocortical connections may play a part. It may thus act as a reinforcing or incentive system, which implies a degree of memory or storage. It is currently thought that the limbic formation is involved at least with recent memory (for which there is some clinical support). Its many connections would readily allow the establishment of reverberating circuits, including the postulated Papez circuit from the hippocampus, through the mamillary body, anterior thalamic nucleus, and cingulate gyrus, back to the hippocampus.

SOMATOSENSORY INPUT

General (skin) sensation is carried to the CNS by afferent fibers of varying size, from small nonmyelinated fibers to some of the largest myelinated fibers in the body. These groups of fibers are segregated within the posterior roots, cord, and brain stem (Fig. 5-10). The finest carry pain and temperature, the indefinite intermediate carry diffuse touch and pressure, and the largest carry highly localized touch. (The older nomenclature of these groups was protopathic, intermediate, and epicritic.)

Pathways in the Spinal Cord - Spinal Nerve Input

The *smallest fibers* (pain and temperature) enter the cord in the lateral divisions of the dorsal roots, pass across the dorsolateral (Lissauer's) bundle, and synapse in the substantia gelatinosa. After a possible further synapse within the dorsal horn (see Chap. 6), secondary (or tertiary) fibers cross the midline just ventral to the central canal and ascend in the lateral part of the ventrolateral column. There is only a narrow (single segment) zone of decussation immediately adjacent to the point of entry, so that fibers in any one root may all be interrupted by a localized, central expanding lesion, leading to segmental pain and temperature loss.

Fibers of medium size may follow a similar pathway, except that they tend to pass up the dorsal column ipsilaterally for a few segments and to decussate over a wider zone. They therefore are less susceptible to damage by localized central lesions. Other intermediate fibers continue to ascend (in the dorsal column of the same side) and synapse in the gracilis or cuneate nuclei.

The *largest fibers* all follow this route, ascending in the ipsilateral dorsal column to the lower medulla. They enter via the medial divisions of the dorsal roots, and their segmental collateral branches form a layer on the medial aspect of the dorsal horn, the medial root zone. Since incoming fibers accumulate from the lateral aspect of the dorsal column, it follows that (in the cervical or low medullary regions) the sacral fibers are medialmost, followed in order by the lumbar, thoracic, and cervical fibers. The medial part of the dorsal column is sometimes referred to as the fasciculus gracilis and the more lateral as the cuneate fasciculus. All afferent fibers, whichever paths they follow, give off collateral branches as they enter the CNS, and thus participate in segmental and intersegmental reflexes.

Pathways in the Brain Stem - Spinal Nerve Input

In the dorsal part of the lower medulla, dorsal column fibers terminate on neurons of the gracilis and cuneate nuclei, and secondary sensory fibers decussate

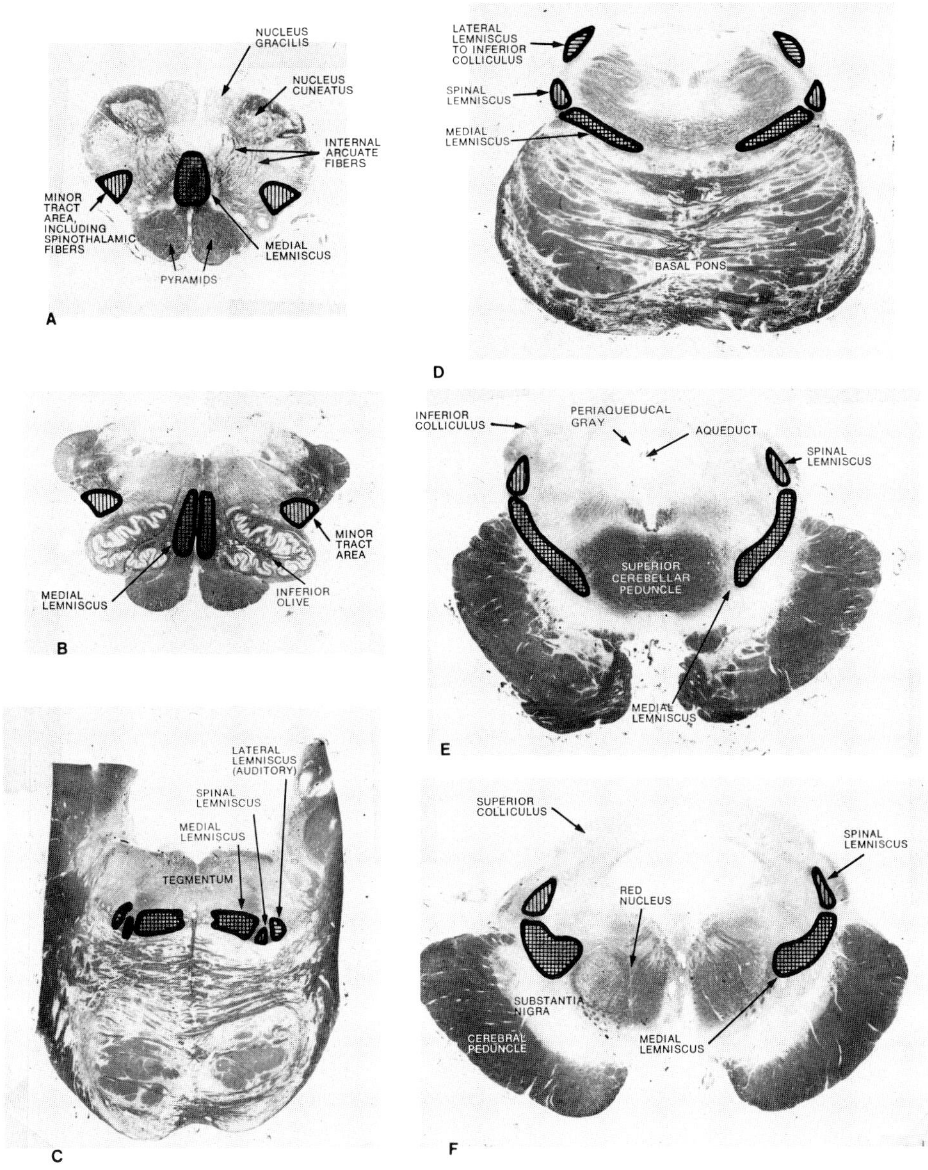

Fig. 5-11. Sections across the brain stem to show the positions of the sensory lemnisci (medial, spinal, and also the lateral lemniscus, composed largely of secondary auditory fibers). Levels A to F in ascending order. (Myelin stain, ×3.)

(as internal arcuate fibers) and turn upward adjacent to the median raphe, to form the medial lemniscus (Figs. 5-11, 5-12). In the medulla the lemniscus is parallel to the raphe, being adjacent to the pyramids ventrally and to the tectospinal tract and medial longitudinal fasciculus dorsally. In the pons, the fibers of the lemnisci spread laterally, so that the structure is parallel to the ventricular surface and separates the tegmentum from the base of the pons. Each is related to its fellow medially and to the spinal and lateral lemnisci laterally. In the midbrain there is further twisting, so that the lateral fibers come to lie more dorsally than the medial, and in this position they enter the inferior surface of the somatosensory thalamic relay nucleus. In the brain stem, lemniscal fibers are thought not to send collaterals to the reticular formation. Fibers in the medial lemniscus maintain topographical representation of the body surface. In the medulla, cervical fibers lie dorsally, lumbosacral fibers ventrally, and axial fibers medially; in the pons, the cervical fibers are medial, lumbosacral lateral, and axial fibers are ventral; and in the midbrain the cervical fibers are

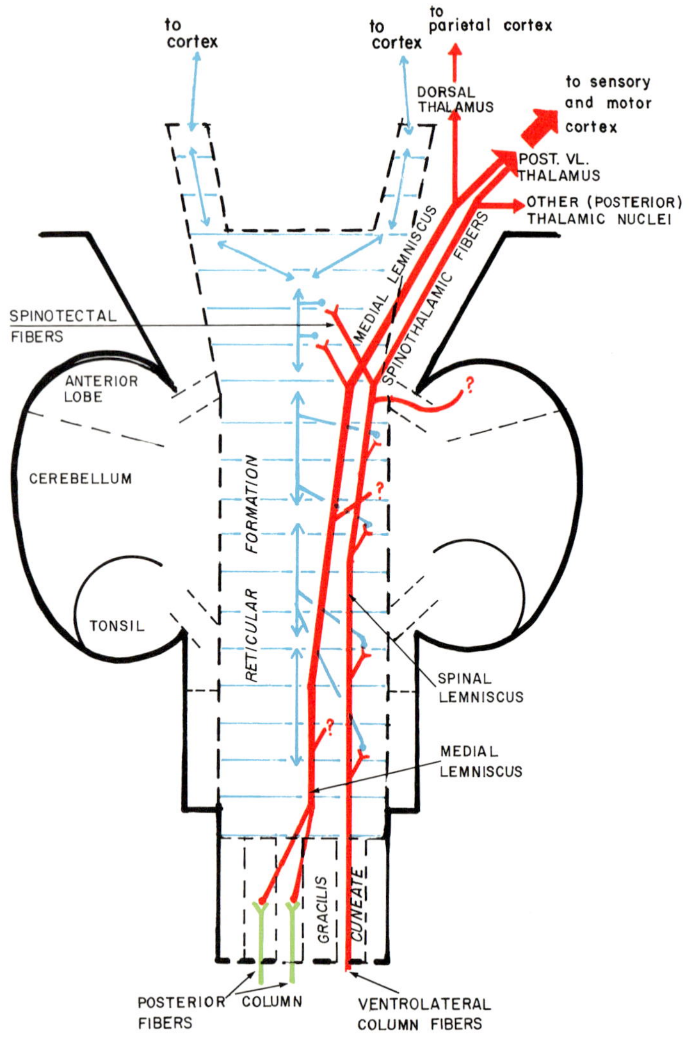

Fig. 5-12. Longitudinal brain stem and thalamic section, showing somatosensory pathways. Green = primary (undecussated) fibers; red = secondary and tertiary (decussated) fibers; blue = reticular formation and intrinsic connections. Post. vl. thalamus = posterior ventrolateral (somatosensory) thalamic nucleus.

ventromedial, the lumbosacral fibers dorsolateral, and axial fibers are ventrolateral.

The smaller fibers and intermediate fibers that have already decussated in the cord (Figs. 5-11, 5-12), ascend in the ventrolateral white matter and come together as a discrete tract in the lateral medulla, the spinal lemniscus. In the pons this lies between the medial and lateral lemnisci, and in the midbrain it lies dorsal to the medial lemniscus. Many of its fibers also enter the somatosensory thalamic nucleus. Smaller and less discrete than the medial lemniscus, it is probably not devoid of topographical representation, though this has been little studied. There is some evidence to indicate that a proportion of its fibers do not end in the somatosensory nucleus, but in other posteriorly situated thalamic nuclei, sometimes referred to as the *posterior group.* Further study of these terminals is in progress.

Pathways in the Brain Stem - Cranial Nerve Input

Somatosensory input from the face and head (Fig. 5-13) enters by the fifth cranial nerve and follows analogous pathways, with separation of the large (Aβ) and small (Aδ, C) fibers, the latter descending as the spinal trigeminal tract to the upper four seg-

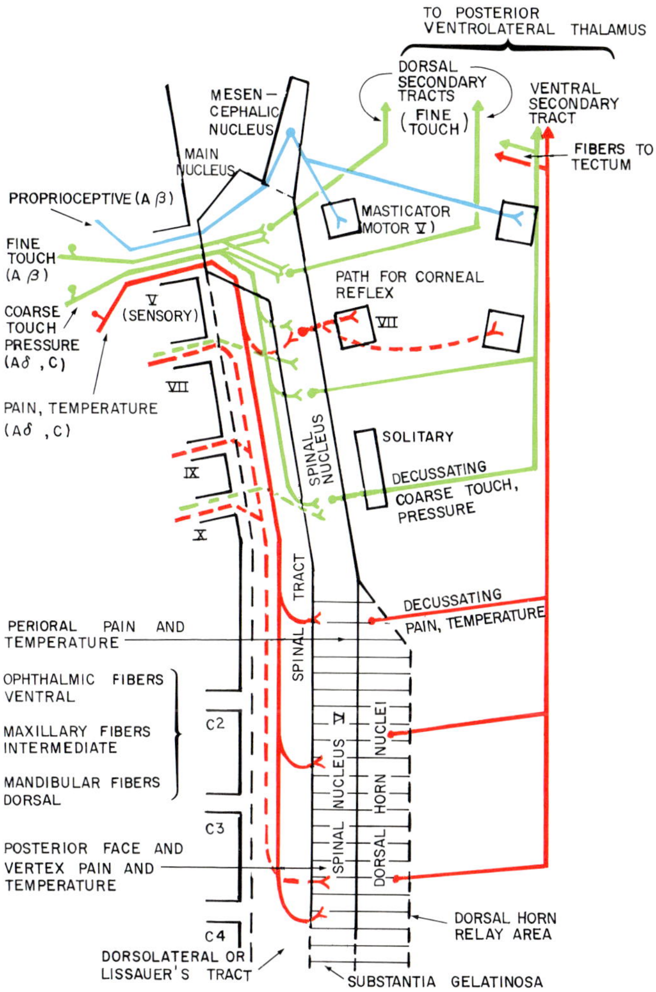

Fig. 5-13. Distribution and connections of somatosensory afferent fibers in cranial nerves (almost entirely trigeminal) (green = touch and pressure pathways; red = pain pathways; blue = proprioceptive pathways). (Note the cell body of the primary fiber within *the CNS.) The spinal nucleus and tract of the trigeminal nerve are continuous with the substantia gelatinosa and dorsolateral tract of Lissauer, respectively. Secondary fibers decussate as for the spinal somatosensory paths.*

ments of the cervical cord. Secondary fibers decussate and ascend to the thalamus, tectum, and other parts of the reticular formation.

PROPRIOCEPTIVE INPUT

Proprioceptive input (Fig. 5-14), derived from muscle spindles, tendon organs, and the pacinian corpuscles of the periosteum, joint capsules, and fascia, enters the CNS in large myelinated afferent fibers. It is distributed between the thalamus and cerebellum.

Thalamic Input

The thalamus receives information about joint position, and probably some muscle spindle input, through these direct fibers. Fibers destined for the thalamus follow the same course as the large somatosensory fibers. After giving off collaterals for segmental and intersegmental reflexes, they ascend in the dorsal columns (Fig. 5-15) to synapse in the lateral cuneate, gracile, and cuneate nuclei (Fig. 5-16) and then pass with the medial lemniscus to the somatosensory thalamic relay nucleus. Representation is contralateral, as it is for the somatosensory fibers.

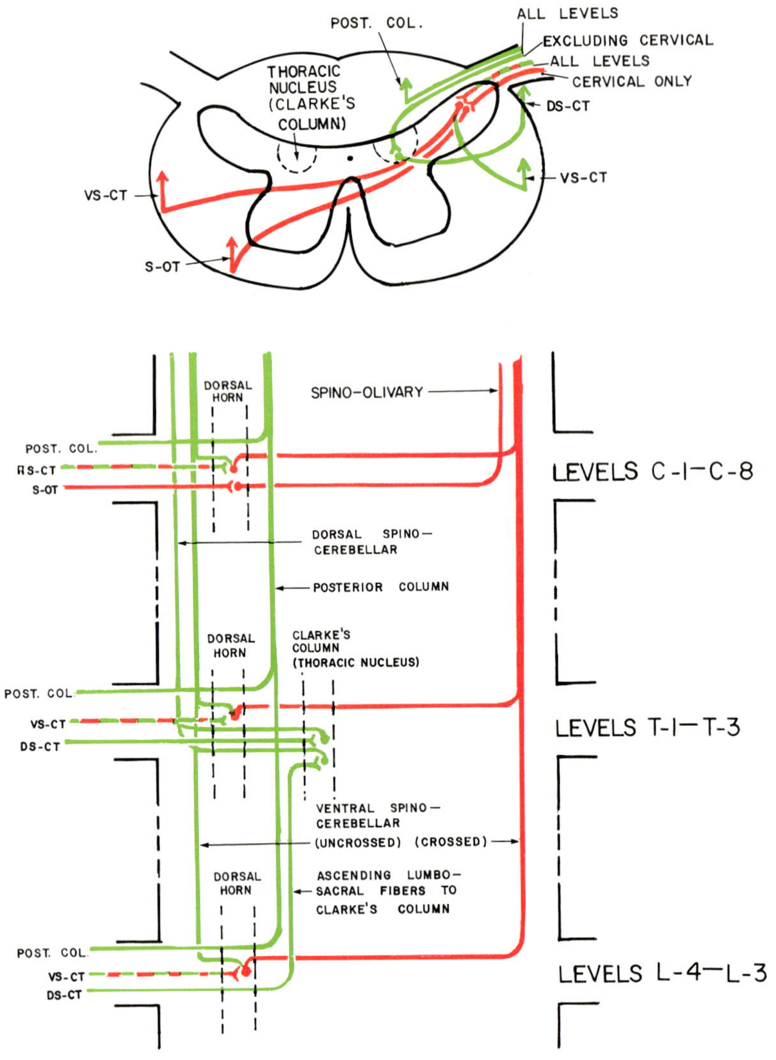

Fig. 5-14. Pathways followed by afferent proprioceptive fibers (cell bodies in dorsal root ganglia) on entering the spinal cord. (Above) transverse section of cord. (Below) transverse longitudinal section. Posterior column fibers (joint position sense) are destined for the thalamus and cortex, as are the large somatosensory fibers. Green = nondecussating primary and secondary fibers; red = decussating secondary fibers. Fibers entering the nerve roots are labeled according to their ascending connections, thus: DS-CT = dorsal spinocerebellar tract; VS-CT = ventral spinocerebellar tract; Post. Col. = posterior column; S-OT = spino-olivary tract; RS-CT = rostral spinocerebellar tract.

Cerebellar Input

Ventral and Rostral Spinocerebellar Tracts

Other fibers (Figs. 5-14, 5-15, 5-16), carrying largely information from tendon organs, synapse in the dorsal main nucleus of the spinal cord, secondary fibers ascending bilaterally as the *ventral (anterior) spinocerebellar tracts.* These pass upward through the minor tract areas of the medulla and dorsal pons, turning caudally to enter the cerebellum through the superior cerebellar peduncles. Decussated fibers again cross the midline within the cerebellum (so that most of the representation is ipsilateral) and are distributed to the vermal and paravermal regions of the cerebellar anterior lobe. Since the ventral spinocerebellar tract subserves largely the hindlimb and trunk areas, a physiologically detected but anatomically undefined "rostral spinocerebellar tract," performing similar functions for the forelimb and neck, is also present. Sites of relay are not yet described. Both tracts carry information from cutaneous afferents, especially pain receptors, as well as proprioceptive impulses.

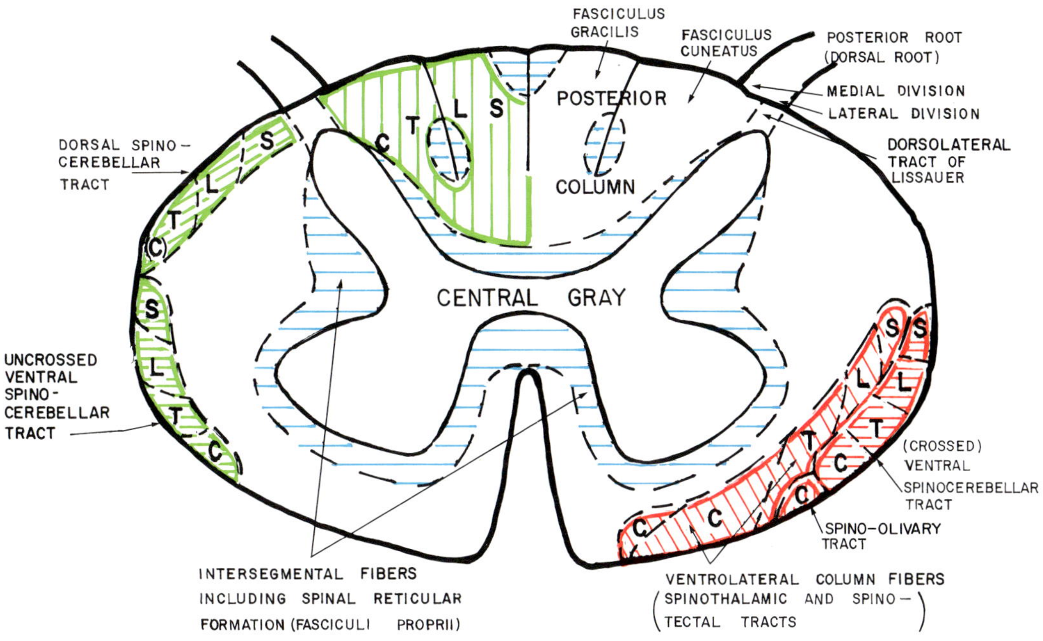

Fig. 5-15. Different trunk and limb areas (S = sacral; L = lumbar; T = thoracic; C = cervical) in ascending somatosensory and proprioceptive tracts. Green = undecussated fibers; red = decussated fibers; blue = intersegmental fibers, including spinal part of reticular formation.

Dorsal Spinocerebellar and Cervicocuneocerebellar Tracts

Fibers from the lumbosacral and thoracic regions (Figs. 5-14, 5-15, 5-16) synapse in the thoracic nucleus of Clarke instead of the dorsal main nucleus, and since this is only present from T-1 to L-3, lower lumbar and sacral fibers ascend in the dorsal column before synapsing. Secondary neurons ascend in the lateral white matter of the same side as the *dorsal (posterior, lateral) spinocerebellar tract,* pass through the minor tract area, and enter the cerebellum through the inferior peduncle for distribution to the tonsil and anterior lobe. Again, representation is mainly ipsilateral. The classic dorsal spinocerebellar tract largely represents the hindlimb and trunk and, for the forelimb and neck, there appears to be a *cervico-cuneocerebellar tract* relaying in the lateral cuneate nucleus (which is homologous with the thoracic nucleus of Clarke). This tract enters the cerebellum through the ipsilateral inferior cerebellar peduncle and has a distribution similar to that of the dorsal tract. Both of these tracts convey information largely from muscle spindles and tendon organs. In addition, they carry touch, pressure, and pain information from the skin.

Indirect Spinocerebellar Tracts

Some fibers in the cervical region, and fewer more caudally, synapse in the dorsal main nucleus, from which secondary fibers decussate to form the spino-olivary tract, ascending ventral to the ventral spino-cerebellar tract. This reaches the cerebellum by synapsing in the inferior olivary complex and decussating as the internal arcuate fibers, which enter through the inferior peduncle. Again, projection is mainly ipsilateral. Some fibers ascending in the ventrolateral column synapse in the lateral reticular

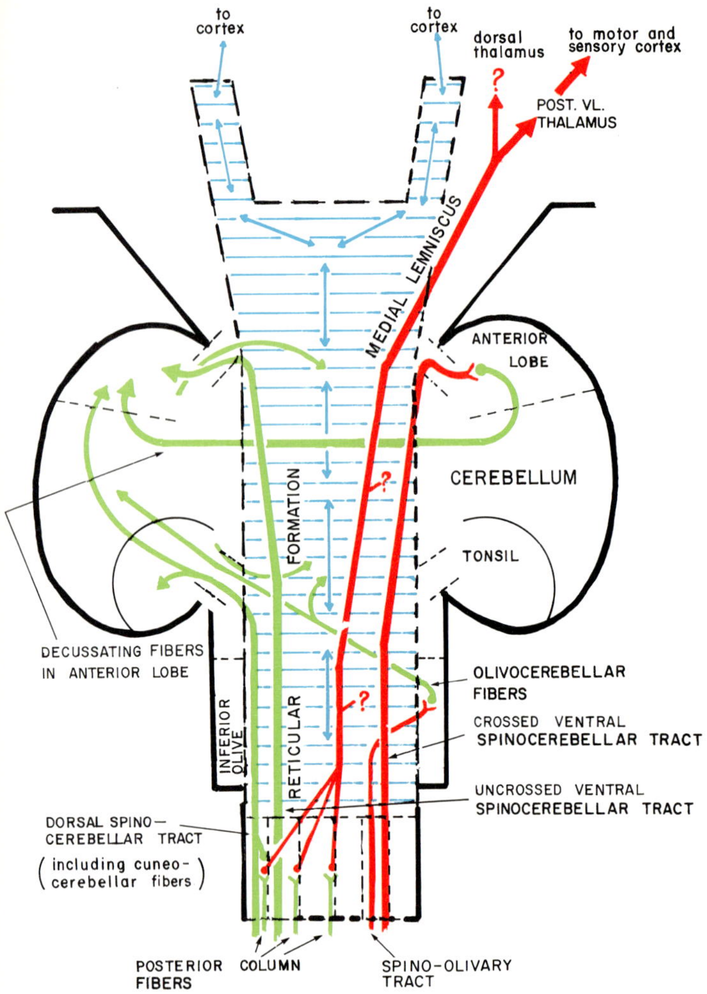

Fig. 5-16. Semischematic longitudinal brain stem and thalamic section, showing proprioceptive pathways. Green = pathways terminating on the same side at entry of the afferent impulse (in the cerebellum); red = pathways terminating contralaterally (in the thalamus). Post. vl. thalamus = posterior ventrolateral thalamus.

nucleus, from which fibers also pass to the cerebellum. Neither of these two systems is purely proprioceptive, cutaneous information also being conveyed.

Lesions involving both the spinocerebellar tracts and the spino-olivary tract on one side lead to ipsilateral hypotonia, with a tendency to fall to the same side. However, if the dorsal columns remain intact, good compensation takes place.

Cranial Nerve Input

Proprioceptive input from muscles of mastication appear unique, in that the neuronal cell bodies are within the CNS, where they form the mesencephalic trigeminal nucleus, whose efferent fibers are directed largely to the motor (masticator) trigeminal nucleus. The route for proprioceptive impulses from the facial muscles is not clear, though they presumably reach the brain stem with the facial nerve.

VESTIBULAR INPUT

The vestibular inflow is phylogenetically primitive, with only a small and (so far) clinically unimportant connection to the neocortex. Each incoming vestibu-

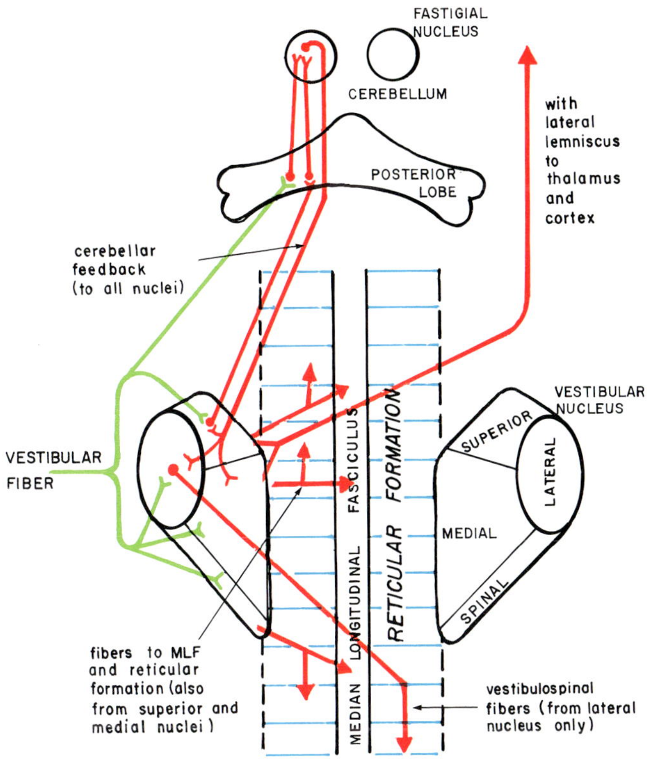

Fig. 5-17. Distribution and connections of vestibular afferent fibers. Green = primary fibers (cell body in vestibular ganglion); red = secondary and other connecting fibers; blue = reticular formation. MLV = median longitudinal fasciculus.

lar fiber divides into ascending and descending branches (Fig. 5-17). The *ascending branch* reaches the flocculonodular lobe of the cerebellum, either directly or through synapse in the superior vestibular nucleus; the *descending branch* synapses in one of the other three vestibular nuclei (lateral, medial, or spinal), whence most of the secondary fibers pass to the median longitudinal fasciculus or the reticular formation. A small component from the superior and medial nuclei crosses the midline to join the lateral lemniscus, which it leaves in the midbrain, to reach the posterior part of the somatosensory thalamic nucleus. There may be a connection between this nucleus and the temporal operculum just anterior to the auditory cortex. The vestibulospinal tract originates from the lateral nucleus only. All the vestibular nuclei receive a prominent cerebellar feedback, mostly from the fastigial nucleus but also including a direct cortical cerebellovestibular projection.

COCHLEAR INPUT

Each incoming cochlear fiber divides into two branches (Fig. 5-18), one passing to the dorsal and one to the ventral cochlear nucleus, disposed above and below the inferior cerebellar peduncle. From the ventral nucleus, most of the fibers decussate and ascend as the lateral lemniscus (lateral to the spinal and medial lemnisci) to reach the inferior colliculus. The *brachium of the inferior colliculus* passes to the medial geniculate body where synapse occurs, and the auditory radiation passes almost directly laterally as part of the sublenticular internal capsule to

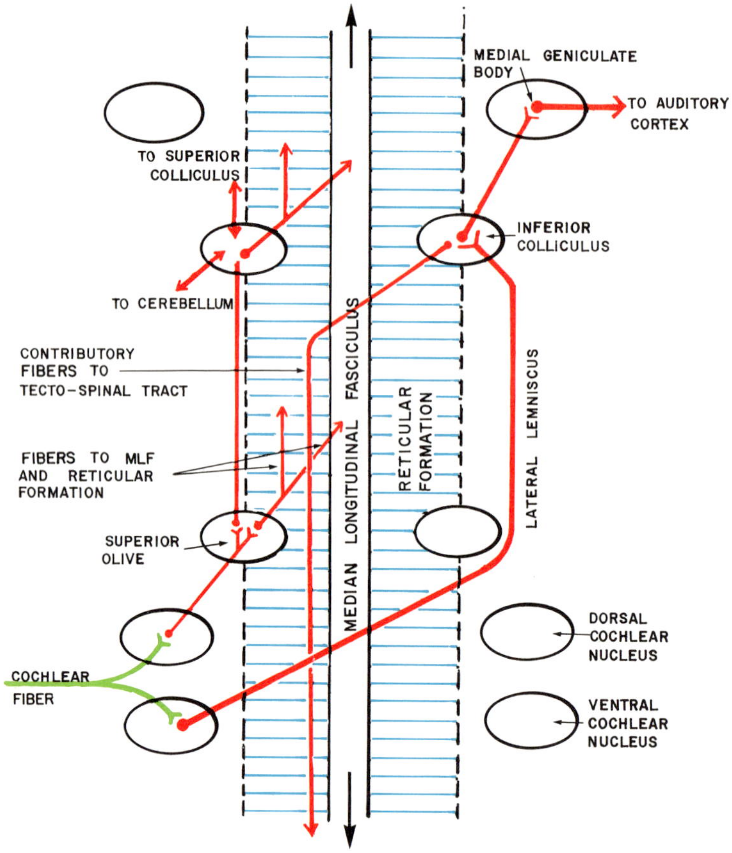

Fig. 5-18. Distribution and connections of cochlear afferent fibers. Green = primary fibers (cell body in cochlear ganglion); red = secondary and other connecting fibers; blue = reticular formation.

reach the posterior temporal operculum (Heschl's gyrus). Secondary neurons from the dorsal cochlear nucleus project to the superior olive, inferior colliculus, and thalamic reticular formation and thence diffusely to the cortex. Numerous collaterals pass to the medial longitudinal fasciculus and the reticular formation. The inferior colliculus makes a contribution to the tectospinal tract.

Because unilateral temporal cortical ablation does not cause unilateral deafness, an uncrossed auditory path has been suggested. However, recent work during stereotactic surgery failed to confirm it. Auditory paresthesias could only be elicited in the direct path of the lateral lemniscus, inferior colliculus, inferior brachium, medial geniculate body, and acoustic radiation and were always unilateral. The contradiction remains unexplained. These studies confirmed the presence of adjacent groups of vestibular and somatosensory fibers, though there appeared to be no overlap between the representation of different modalities. It should be noted that the effect of stimulation of secondary fibers, of whatever sensory modality, is the elicitation of paresthesias, not normal meaningful sensation. Thus, stimulation in the auditory pathway elicits low-pitched buzzing, humming, or clicking sounds; in the visual pathway, formless white flashes of light; and in the somatosensory pathway, typical paresthesias. In stimulation of the spinothalamic tract, perverted sensations of heat, pain, or burning (causalgia) are experienced.

The *inferior colliculus* consists of a central mass of gray matter (chief nucleus), connected to its fellow by intercollicular gray matter and surrounded by a capsule of mixed cells and fibers. The chief nucleus contains diffuse small- and medium-sized cells, and its major input is from the lateral lemniscus, probably with spatial representation of pitch. It also receives fibers from the superior colliculus and cerebellum. Its major efferent is the inferior brachium to the medial geniculate body, but efferent fibers also pass to the cerebellum (running in the anterior medullary velum and partially decussating), projecting auditory impulses to the vermis and paravermal region, and to the superior colliculus. The medial geniculate body (in primates) has a large-celled ventral part and a small-celled dorsal part. It receives afferents from the inferior colliculus (and possibly a few direct lemniscal fibers) and has bidirectional connections with the auditory cortex.

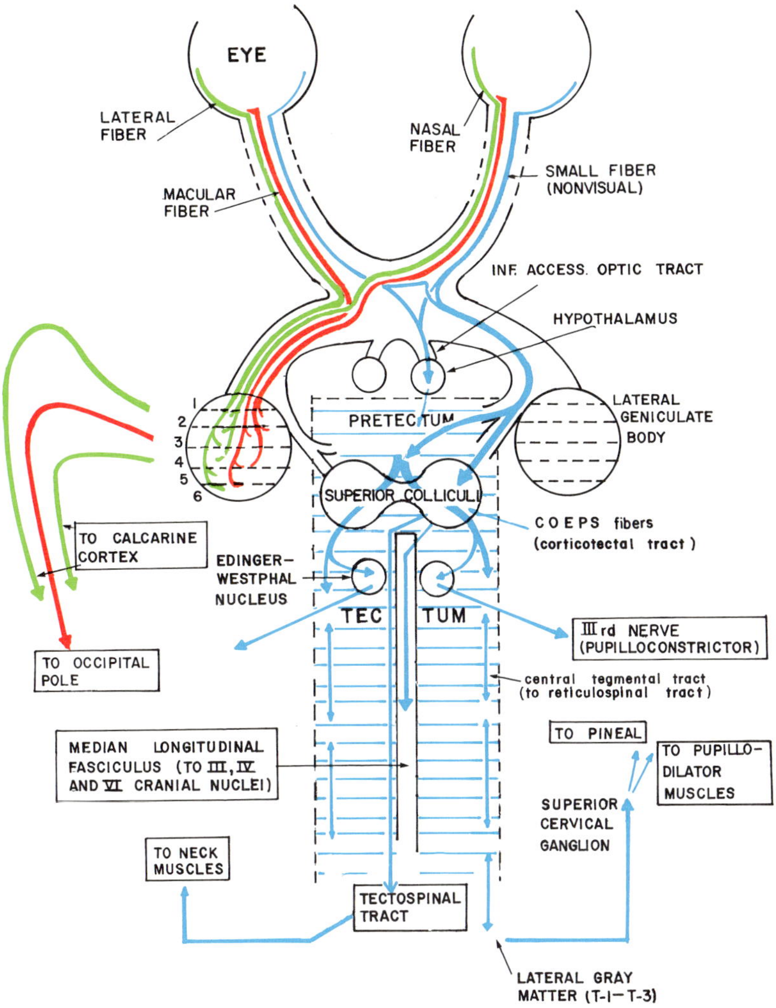

Fig. 5-19. Central connections of optic nerve fibers (schematic, viewed from above). Green = fiber paths for right half of field of vision; red = fiber paths for macular region; blue = small optic nerve fibers, their central connections, and the reticular formation (visual fibers for the left field of vision are not shown); I–VI = correspondingly numbered layers of the lateral geniculate body (see text).

VISUAL INPUT

Optic Nerve and Tract

Visual afferent fibers arise from the ganglion cells of the retina from rods (with a high degree of convergence) and from cones (with low convergence). Considerable information processing occurs within the retina but is beyond the scope of this discussion (see appropriate texts). Optic nerve fibers are topographically arranged according to their origin in the retina, with those from the macula in the center. Near the chiasm, the macular fibers tend to spread out as a horizontal band across the nerve, with superior retinal fibers lying dorsally and inferior fibers lying ventrally. At the chiasm (Fig. 5-19), fibers from the medial half of each nerve (from the nasal half of each retina) cross over to the opposite side and, in the process of doing so, first loop slightly forward into the opposite nerve. Each optic tract therefore consists of fibers from the temporal half of the ipsilateral retina and the nasal half of the contralateral retina, superiorly originating fibers lying above and inferior ones below. The optic nerve and tract up to this point contain a few small, thinly myelinated fibers. Just before reaching the lateral geniculate body these fibers separate as a small bundle, passing as the *superior brachium* to the superior colliculus of the midbrain. The remaining large, heavily myelinated fibers reach the lateral geniculate body.

Lateral Geniculate Body and Optic Radiation

The *lateral geniculate body* consists of a dorsal part, the relay nucleus for the visual pathway, and an extremely small ventral nucleus that is vestigial in man. The dorsal nucleus consists of six parallel bands of neurons, arranged one above the other and numbered from below. Layers I, II, and IV receive fibers from the nasal half of the opposite retina, and layers III, V, and VI receive ipsilateral temporal fibers. The topographical representation of the retina is as in the optic tract: fibers from the midline of the retina lie medially, and fibers from the ipsilateral edge lie laterally. Since there are five to six times more fibers in the optic radiation than in the tract, it is assumed that each fiber synapses with several geniculate neurons.

All efferent fibers from the lateral geniculate body pass to the visual cortex as the *optic radiation*; functional connections with the pulvinar appear to be mediated through the cortex. The optic radiation forms part of the sublenticular internal capsule, running laterally above and in front of the inferior horn of the lateral ventricle and spreading out forward in its roof. Thus, the lowermost fibers loop anteriorly, before the whole group turns posteriorly to reach the cortex of the calcarine sulcus and occipital pole. Topographical representation is of the contralateral visual field and is retained in the radiation and the cortex, the macular and midline fibers passing to the occipital pole, with more laterally originating fibers progressively farther forward on the medial surface of the hemisphere.

During the passage of visual impulses from retina to cortex, the proportional representation of the macula becomes progressively greater, and it occupies most of the occipital polar region. Fibers from the superior retina lie in the upper bank of the sulcus, and fibers from the inferior retina lie in the lower bank. Short afferent fibers from the visual cortex (area 17) pass only to the surrounding pericalcarine area (area 18), with further short relays to area 19, both of the latter being considered visual association areas. Area 17 probably sends no long projection fibers, but areas 18 and 19 project to many other regions, including the thalamic nuclei.

Visual Input to Brain Stem

Although a few of the small retinal fibers may pass to the pontomedullary reticular formation, most reach the superior colliculus and midbrain reticular formation. Originally a complex, coordinating structure, the colliculus is laminated. Spinotectal and bulbotectal fibers run to the deep layers (probably proprioceptive, from eye and neck muscles), small retinal fibers run to the intermediate layers (preserving topographical representation), and fibers from a large corticotectal tract run to the superficial parts. In man, the colliculus appears to be a reflex center, normally involved in such responses as tracking moving objects and startle reactions to a flash of light. It discharges through the medial longitudinal fasciculus and tectospinal tract (coordinating eye and neck muscles), and also has a retinotopic projection to posterior thalamus and parietal association cortex. This projection may be responsible for unconscious reaction to light and movement presented to the blind half-field in cortical hemianopia (often termed "blind sight").

Pupillomotor fibers originate mainly in the midbrain reticular formation (some may start in the superior colliculus), the two sides being coordinated through the posterior commissure. Pupilloconstrictor fibers (parasympathetic) originate in the Edinger-Westphal nucleus and pass with the oculomotor nerve to the ciliary ganglion, from which secondary fibers reach the iris and ciliary body through the long ciliary nerves. These fibers are also responsible for accommodation by contraction of the ciliary muscle. Pupillodilator fibers (sympathetic) originate in the midbrain reticular formation. They decussate and pass via the central tegmental and reticulospinal tracts to the thoracic lateral column and superior cervical ganglion. Secondary fibers accompany the carotid, internal carotid, and ophthalmic arteries. Impulses linking accommodation and pupilloconstriction may originate in the premotor cortex or superior colliculus, perhaps as a result of tension in the medial rectus muscle associated with convergence. Impulses linking fear and pupillodilatation are presumably part of a general sympathetic discharge that involves the midbrain reticular region and many other regions.

A third, unanalyzed component of the optic fibers (inferior accessory optic tract) apparently reaches the hypothalamus, from which fibers pass to the midbrain reticular formation (through the median forebrain bundle) and are distributed with the vascular sympathetic outflow to the pineal gland (see Chap. 8).

TASTE INPUT

Relatively little is known about the pathways of taste input. Fibers appear to enter the nucleus tractus solitarii in the medulla, probably its rostral part. Secondary fibers may join the medial lemniscus and pass to the medialmost part of the somatosensory nucleus of the thalamus. There is thought to be a relay to a cortical area at the extreme lower end of the postcentral gyrus.

THE THALAMUS

The thalamus is a conspicuous gray mass, situated in the upper lateral wall of the third ventricle and below the bodies of the lateral ventricles (Fig. 5-20). It extends back considerably from the foramen of Monro to overlap the midbrain, its posterior pole (pulvinar) being free and covered in pia. Laterally, it is defined by the internal capsule (posterior limb) and the external laminar (reticular) nucleus; inferiorly, it is related to the hypothalamus, subthalamus, and subarachnoid space (at the pulvinar). The only internal structure that may be visible grossly is a vertical, slightly myelinated *internal medullary lamina,* which splits anteriorly to enclose the anterior nucleus (at the posterior margin of the foramen of Monro). Cytoarchitecturally, the thalamus has been divided into many nuclei with resounding combinations of Latin names. In terms of afferent and efferent connections (and so, presumably, in terms of function), it is most easily considered as being made up of three "columns" running anteroposter-

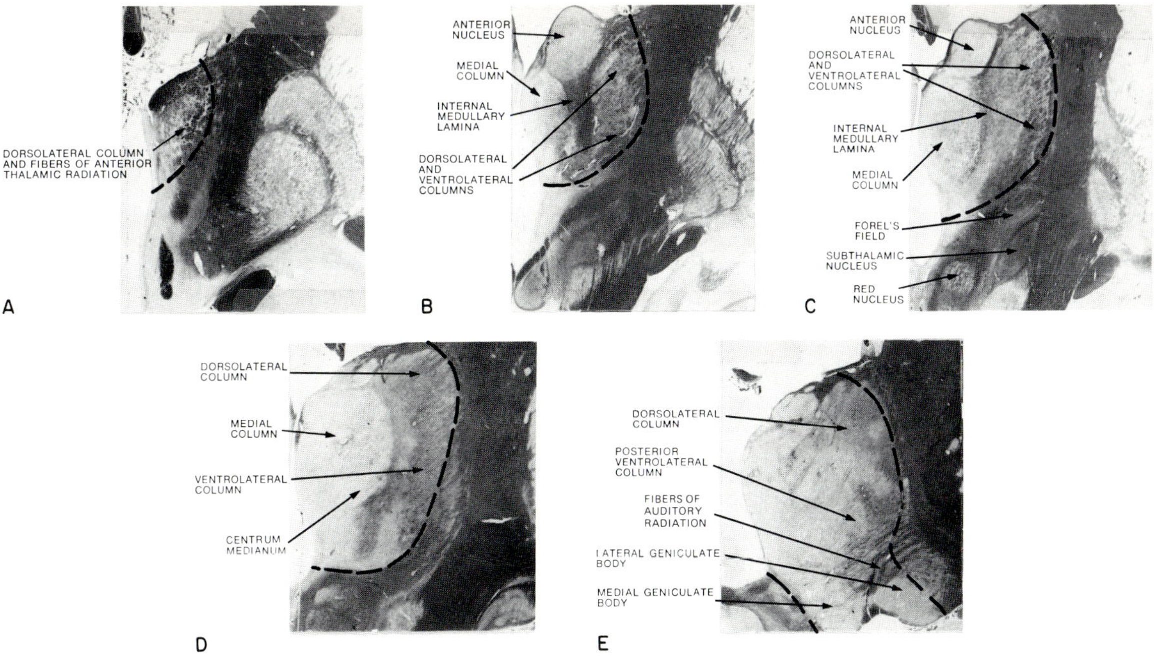

Fig. 5-20. Composite transverse sections through wall of third ventricle, showing the extent of the thalamus. Levels A to E in anteroposterior sequence. (Myelin stain, × 1.5.)

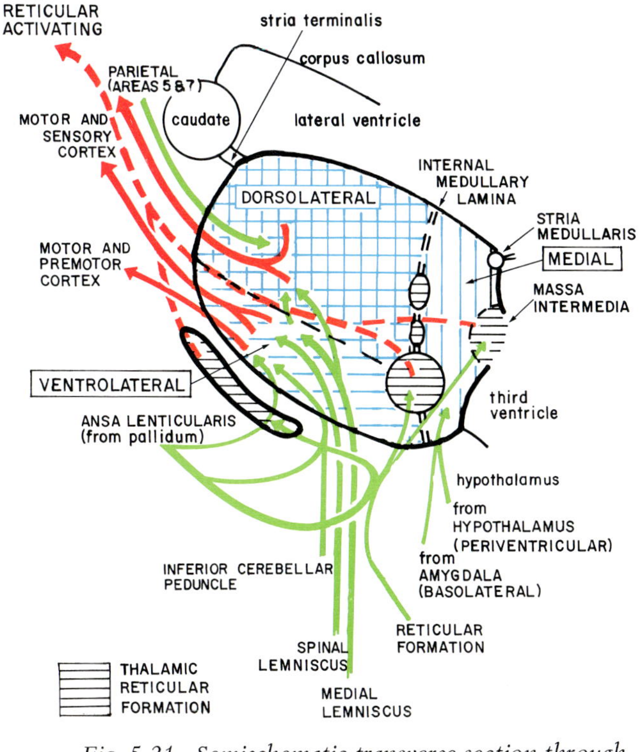

Fig. 5-21. Semischematic transverse section through thalamus, showing (blue) the three columns of nuclei (medial, vertically hatched; dorsolateral, cross-hatched; ventrolateral, horizontally hatched), the archithalamic components (black, horizontally hatched), and some afferent (green) and efferent (red) connections.

iorly, to which must be added the anterior nucleus and the reticular (archithalamic) nuclei noted previously (midline and intralaminar, including the centrum medianum and external laminar) (Figs. 5-21, 5-22).

Medial Thalamic Nuclei Associated with Frontal Lobe

The *medial column* (nuclei medialis dorsalis and medialis ventralis) is all of the thalamus medial to the internal medullary lamina, with the sole exception of the small midline reticular nuclei. It has its major, bidirectional connections with the frontopolar and premotor cortex and also receives some fibers from the basolateral amygdala and the periventricular nuclei of the hypothalamus.

Dorsolateral Thalamic Nuclei Associated with Parietal Lobe

The *dorsolateral column* (nuclei lateralis dorsalis, lateralis posterior, and pulvinar) lies outside the internal medullary lamina and under the body of the lateral ventricle, and includes the entire pulvinar. It has extensive reciprocal connections, primarily with the parietal cortex. The pulvinar, at least, has a considerable additional input in many sensory modalities, receiving fibers from the pericalcarine and auditory cortex and collaterals of lemniscal and trigeminal fibers that pass to the somatosensory nucleus. Its connections with the parietal cortex, especially areas 5 and 7, suggest involvement with fine sensory discrimination.

Ventrolateral Thalamic or Relay Nuclei

The *ventrolateral column* (nuclei ventralis anterior, ventralis lateralis, ventralis posterolateralis, and

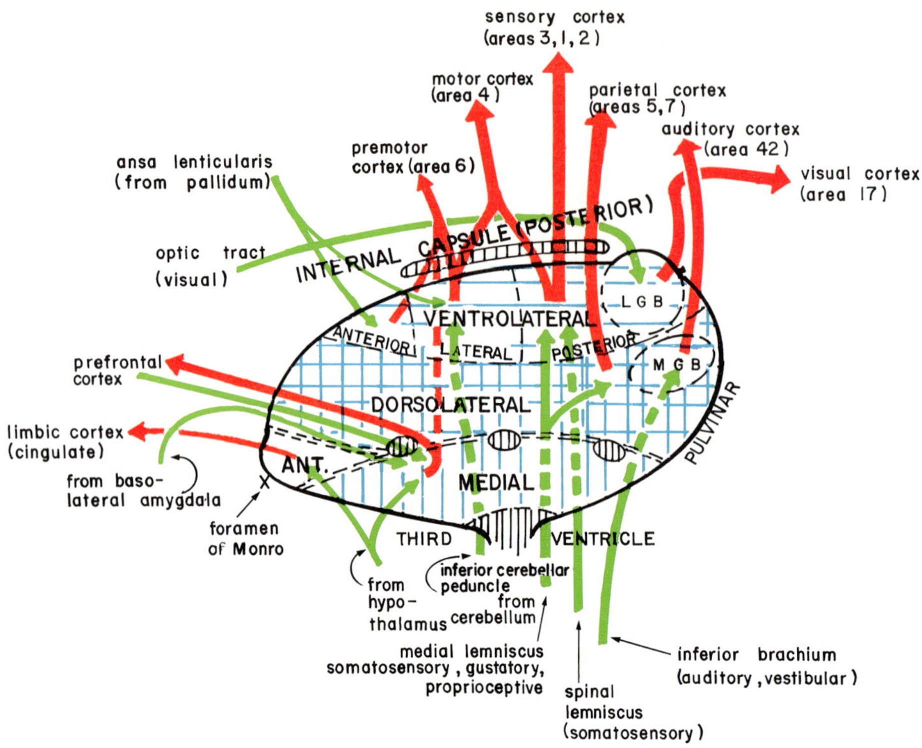

Fig. 5-22. Semischematic horizontal section through right thalamus (blue) viewed from above, showing the three main columns (see Fig. 5-21), the archithalamic nuclei (black, vertically hatched), and the anterior nucleus (not hatched). Some afferent (green) and efferent (red) connections are shown. LGB = lateral geniculate body; MGB = medical geniculate body.

ventralis posteromedialis) lies external to the internal medullary lamina below the dorsolateral column; it is shorter and less bulky than the latter. It faces down toward the midbrain and, instead of having the widespread cortical connections of the other columns, is a group of relay nuclei for input of a specific type (often sensory) to the cerebral cortex. It may be considered as divided into three parts (the smallest anterior and the largest posterior), namely, the anterior, lateral, and posterior (somatosensory) nuclei of the ventrolateral column, each with distinct afferent and efferent connections.

Anterior (Pallidal Relay) Nucleus

The small *anterior nucleus* (nucleus ventralis anterior) receives input from the pallidum and relays largely to the premotor cortex (area 6).

Lateral (Cerebellar Relay) Nucleus

The *lateral nucleus* (nucleus ventralis lateralis) receives its major input from the cerebellum (through the superior cerebellar peduncle), probably without relays in the small-celled red nucleus, but it also receives some fibers from the pallidum. There is thought to be somatotopic organization. Efferent fibers pass to areas 4 and 6 (motor and premotor cortex).

Posterior (Somatosensory Relay) Nucleus

The larger *posterior (somatosensory) nucleus* (nucleus ventralis posterior, lateralis et medialis) lies directly above the medial and spinal lemnisci in the midbrain and receives these as well as secondary trigeminal and possibly vestibular and taste fibers. It thus has input from the body surface, derived both from the large dorsal root afferents (via the medial lemniscus) and from at least some of the smaller, poorly myelinated fibers (via the spinal lemniscus). Proprioceptive fibers are included in the contribution from the medial lemniscus. Since there is topographical representation of the body, the head posteriorly and medially (pars medialis), and the limbs anteriorly and laterally (pars lateralis), presumably sensory modalities must be fused at this level. Major efferent fibers pass to the postcentral cortex (areas 3, 1, and 2), but there may be fibers to the pulvinar from this nucleus, as well as direct lemniscal collaterals.

Geniculate (Auditory and Visual Relay) Nuclei

Functionally, the *medial and lateral geniculate bodies,* whose afferent and efferent connections have been described, belong to the ventrolateral column, though, anatomically, they are isolated on the undersurface of the pulvinar.

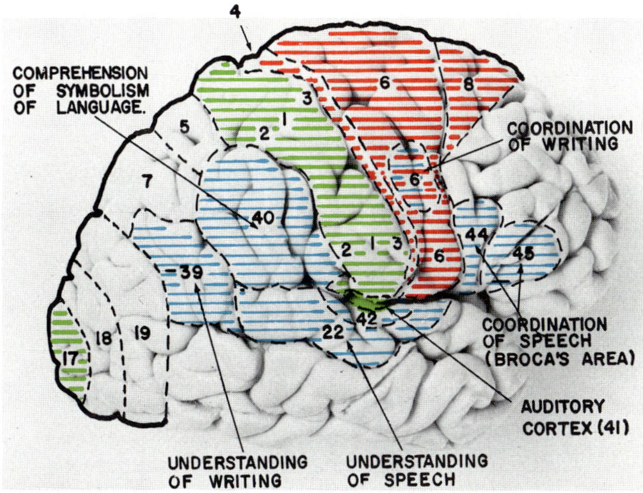

Fig. 5-23. Lateral view of right cerebral hemisphere, showing some important Brodmann's areas. Red = motor; green = sensory; blue and uncolored = association areas. Note: In right-handed people, the term Broca's area *is often restricted to the left hemisphere.*

Other Thalamic Nuclei

The small *anterior nucleus* (nucleus anterior), situated behind the foramen of Monro, receives the mamillothalamic tract and relays largely to the cingulate cortex.

As far as is known, there are also extensive connections within the thalamus, probably involving all constituent nuclei. Phylogenetically, the thalamus has developed in different epochs, the most primitive parts being the reticular and anterior nuclei.

CEREBRAL CORTEX

The cortex forms a layer 1.5 to 4.0 cm thick over the hemispheres, thrown into numerous folds (gyri) with a relatively constant basic pattern, which, however, bears no necessary relationship either to functional or even to cytoarchitectural units. It is therefore usual to designate areas of the cortex by number, a concept originally based on its architectural features. Several interpretations of these features have led to several systems of numeration. The Brodmann system is probably the most popular, and while many of the details are (at present) only of academic interest, perusal of the literature is facilitated by familiarity with at least some of the Brodmann areas. These differ not only in the relative cell populations of the constituent six layers but also in afferent and efferent connections.

Efferent fibers originate in the pyramidal (or polymorphic) cells of layers III, V, and VI in virtually all parts of the cortex, and each has a recurrent collateral back to the region of its parent cell body, with presumably a role in inhibitory feedback. The main efferent fiber may run to other parts of the hemisphere (association fiber), to a corresponding point in the opposite hemisphere (commissural fiber), or to a subcortical structure (projection fiber).

Afferent fibers may originate in other parts of the cortex or in subcortical structures. A majority, including those from the main thalamic nuclei and fibers crossing in the anterior commissure or corpus callosum, appear to terminate around granular cells in layer IV. Layer IV termination is especially developed in primates, probably reflecting extensive development of the granular cell network (see Chap. 2). However, ascending fibers of the reticular activating system pass as high as layer I, apparently effecting synapses in all layers. The sites of termination of association fibers are less well known but may also be predominantly in layer IV.

Not all parts of the cortex are equally supplied with *commissural fibers* (at least in monkeys). Callosal projections are especially dense in areas of the cortex corresponding to the midline of the body or the environment, at least in MsI, MsII, SmI, SmII (see Chap. 7), and the visual cortex, and they are appreciably fewer in areas that correspond to distal body surface or muscles or the edge of the field of vision. Association areas also show variation, though this cannot be topographically correlated. Commissural fibers for the anterior middle and inferior temporal gyri may traverse the anterior commissure.

Some of the functionally better defined Brodmann areas (Figs. 5-23, 5-24) include the following:

Areas 3, 1, and 2. These areas are arranged anteroposteriorly in thin, parallel strips that are not readily differentiated and together constitute the posterior wall of the central sulcus and the free surface of the postcentral gyrus, the *somatosensory cortex.* The granular cell layers (II and IV) are very prominent,

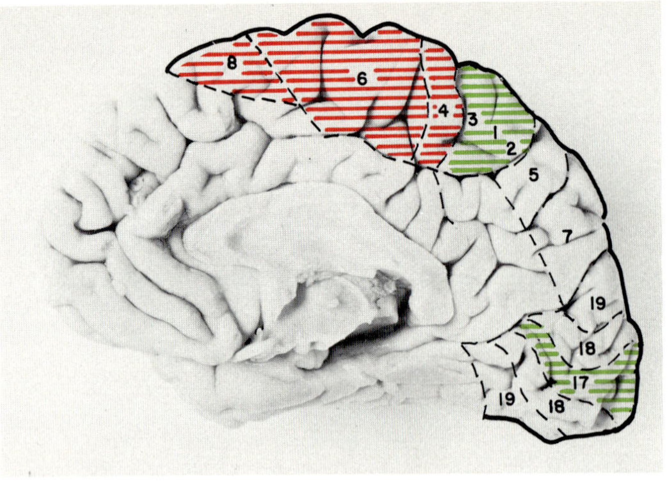

Fig. 5-24. Medial view of right cerebral hemisphere, showing some important Brodmann's areas. Red = motor; green = sensory; uncolored = association areas.

whereas pyramidal cells tend to be small. Areas 3, 1, and 2, especially area 3, are for input of somatosensory information, some of which is proprioceptive, and other sensory information including taste, via the somatosensory thalamic nucleus. However, since there is also direct motor output (not mediated through the main motor cortex), they are designated SmI (major sensory function, minor *m*otor function). There is clear topographical representation of the body, essentially a mirror image about the axis of the central sulcus of that in the main motor cortex. Thus, the head region rests above the sylvian fissure, and the legs and feet dangle over onto the medial surface. Axial (trunk) regions are represented posteriorly, and the hands, feet, face, and tongue are in the rear wall of the central sulcus (area 3). The measured surface area of cortical representation is proportional to the amount of sensory input and not to the size of the body part, so that the hands, feet, and face are seen grotesquely enlarged when a "homunculus" is superimposed on the cortex.

Area 4. This area constitutes the anterior wall of the central sulcus and a narrow strip of adjacent precentral gyrus. The granular cell layers are not especially well developed, but the pyramidal cells, especially of layer V, include the largest in the cortex (Betz's cells); pyramidal cells become gradually smaller as area 4 blends anteriorly with area 6. Area 4 is the major part of the *primary motor cortex,* but this also includes a variable strip of the bordering area 6, wherein are represented the trunk muscles. The whole area may be designated MsI by analogy with the main sensory cortex, since the motor cortex receives a significant direct sensory input in many modalities. Motor function is discussed further in Chapter 7.

Area 6. Often called the *premotor area,* area 6 occupies the remainder of the free surface of the precentral gyrus and the posterior ends of the middle and superior frontal gyri; it is much wider at the upper edge of the hemisphere than at the sylvian fissure. It has well-developed pyramidal cell layers (III and V) and is not distinct from area 4, with which its anterior part forms a functional unit (see Chap. 7).

Area 8. This area is an even less well-defined region anterior to area 6 and therefore lying in the middle parts of the middle and superior frontal gyri. The pyramidal layers are no longer unduly conspicuous, but stimulation causes somatic and visceral motor effects relating to the eyes (adversive head and eye movements, pupillary changes, and occasional lacrimation), and it is sometimes referred to as the *eye motor area.*

Areas 5 and 7. These areas approximately correspond to the superior parietal lobule (area 5 lying anteriorly) and are therefore part of the parietal association area. While their connections have not been completely defined, they certainly receive many fibers indirectly from the lemniscal system, via the dorsolateral thalamic nuclei and especially the pulvinar, concerned with discriminative touch. These connections, together with many clinical observations, suggest a role in such functions as stereognosis and other facets of fine tactile sensitivity.

Area 41. This area is almost completely buried in the posterior part of the sylvian fissure, where it forms part of the upward-facing surface of the posterior temporal operculum (transverse temporal gyri, or Heschl's gyrus), which is 2.0 to 2.5 cm wide at this point. Its outer extremity can be seen on the upper border of the superior temporal gyrus. Area 41 receives the fibers of the auditory radiation from the medial geniculate body, and there is probably topographical representation of sound frequency. Cortical representation of input from the labyrinths may lie in the same area.

Areas 42 and 22. Area 42 is a band around area 41 and in turn is surrounded by area 22, which makes up a large part of the superior temporal gyrus, at least of its posterior two-thirds (Wernicke's area). Clinical observations suggest that dominant hemisphere damage to this area results in inability to interpret spoken language, although such patients are not deaf. This condition, known as *word deafness,* suggests that 42 and 22 are part of an auditory association area concerned with investing auditory (speech) input with its symbolic significance.

Area 17. This area includes both the upper and lower walls of the calcarine sulcus and, on the free (medial) surface, an adjacent wedge-shaped area that is narrow anteriorly (near the parieto-occipital fissure), but broadens posteriorly to include the whole occipital pole. This is the calcarine or visual cortex, which receives fibers from (and probably only from) the lateral geniculate body, conveying visual information from the ipsilateral halves of both retinas (contralateral environment). The environment is topographically represented, the periphery of the field anteriorly and the center of the field (macula) in much greater detail at the pole. It is thought that efferent fibers from area 17 pass only to the adjacent areas 18 and 19, from which visual association fibers originate.

Areas 18 and 19. These areas form two concentric bands around the visual cortex. Areas 17, 18, and 19 together constitute the entire occipital lobe. The visual cortex appears to be much more protected, both in input and output, than are other cortical areas, perhaps reflecting the complexity of processing the very precise (and in primates, vitally important) visual input. Areas 17, 18, and 19 might be regarded as a single receptor area, even though direct visual input is confined to area 17.

Area 39. This region, approximately corresponding in extent to the angular gyrus, seems on clinical grounds to be necessary, at least in the dominant hemisphere, to invest written language with its symbolic meaning. Patients with lesions here need not be blind or have diminished visual acuity; rather, they suffer from *word blindness,* or alexia, not comprehending what they see perfectly well, just as most of us would not understand a page of Chinese script. Damage to areas 39 and 40 in the nondominant hemisphere causes abnormality in the patient's concept of body-image and space, with neglect both of contralateral visual stimuli and the contralateral side of the body.

Areas 44 and 45. These areas lie on the inferior frontal gyrus, primarily between the vertical and horizontal rami of the sylvian fissure, and in the dominant hemisphere correspond to Broca's motor speech area. Damage to this area causes loss of the ability to construct speech *(motor aphasia),* although there is no paresis of the laryngeal, tongue, or facial muscles. Interestingly, depending on the degree and perhaps the location of the damage, patients may retain speech with emotional content (swearing, singing) or may be able to utter one word, often the last they spoke before the lesion occurred. These areas might be regarded as motor association or motor assembly regions for the myriad muscular adjustments involved in speaking. When they are damaged, though each component speech movement remains possible, speech is uncoordinated.

Area 40. This area is, approximately, the supramarginal gyrus and so, with areas 39, 5, and 7, completes the lateral surface of the parietal lobe. Again, based on careful clinical observation, it appears, in the dominant hemisphere, to be concerned with language symbolism in all its aspects. Thus, lesions here commonly cause not only word deafness and word blindness but also inability to speak or write. Nondominant hemisphere lesions have the same effects as lesions in area 39. The two areas are frequently damaged together, both on the dominant and nondominant sides.

The involvement of large parts of the frontal, temporal, and parietal association areas in the sensory (receptive) and motor aspects of language is striking testimony to the significance of symbolic interpretation in the human brain. In addition to the areas that have been mentioned, clinicopathological studies indicate the existence of another dominant hemisphere center involved in the constructional aspects of writing, within the lateral part of area 6. Lesions in that area may be associated with inability to coordinate the movements of writing (agraphia). Thus, there are centers for the execution and for the interpretation of writing and speech, possibly all coordinated by area 40. Since execution and interpretation are not separable, patients with word blindness often cannot write, and those with word deafness often cannot speak normally. The converse need not apply, but it is clear that motor and sensory aphasias may not be sharply separable. The degree of bilaterality of all these centers is not yet clear, and the survival of emotive language, or of a language learned in childhood rather than one learned later, implies that dominance may not be complete even in right-handed persons and is probably still less so in the left-handed.

BIBLIOGRAPHY

Brodal, A. *Neurological Anatomy in Relation to Clinical Medicine* (2nd ed.). New York: Oxford University Press, 1969.

Donaldson, I. M. L. The properties of some human thalamic units: Some new observations and a critical review of the localisation of thalamic nuclei. *Brain* 96:419-440, 1973.

Elliott, H. C. *Textbook of Neuroanatomy* (2nd ed.). Philadelphia: Lippincott, 1969.

Hyvärinen, J. CNS: Afferent mechanisms with emphasis on physiological and behavioural correlations. *Annu. Rev. Physiol.* 35:243-272, 1973.

Karol, E. A., and Pandya, D. N. The distribution of the corpus callosum in the rhesus monkey. *Brain* 94:471-486, 1971.

Keele, C. A., and Neil, E. (Eds.). *Samson Wright's Applied Physiology* (12th ed.). London: Oxford University Press, 1971.

Ruch, T. C., Patton, H. D., Woodbury, J. W., and Towe, A. L. *Neurophysiology* (2nd ed.). Philadelphia: Saunders, 1966.

Tasker, R. R., and Organ, L. W. Stimulation-mapping of the upper human auditory pathway. *J. Neurosurg.* 38:320-325, 1973.

Wall, P. D., and Dubner, R. Somatosensory pathways. *Annu. Rev. Physiol.* 34:315-336, 1972.

Pain

6

Pain is essentially indefinable and cannot be quantitated. It is necessary to distinguish between *pain* as the perception of varied unpleasant stimuli and *suffering* as a person's total psychological reaction to this perception. All types of pain are unpleasant, projected with (more or less) precision to a part or parts of the body and associated with variable emotional reaction and autonomic response.

Exclusive of rare pain of CNS origin (e.g., thalamic pain), pain-producing stimuli are associated with potential or actual damage to peripheral tissues. The converse does not apply, and considerable tissue damage may be unaccompanied by pain. It is a clinical observation that a stimulus producing pain does so biphasically. There is a quick *first pain,* often described, for example, as "sharp." It is fairly well localized and without a heavy overlay of affect. A little later this is followed by *second pain,* less well localized and often qualified by adjectives such as "dull," "sickening," "aching," or "burning." If at all severe, it is often accompanied by a subjective emotional response and autonomic phenomena, such as dilatation of the pupils, tachycardia, and elevated blood pressure.

ADEQUATE STIMULI

Pain may be readily elicited from the skin and orificial mucosa, and there is no difference in capability for pain response between the skin (with or without hair), cornea, or mucous membranes of the nose and mouth. Other tissues can respond with a sensation of pain to various noxae, some of which are indicated in the following list:

1. *Subcutaneous tissue* is sensitive to pressure and chemical irritants.
2. *Muscle* is sensitive to pressure, cutting, and chemical irritants.
3. *The fascia and tendons* are sensitive to needle prick, pressure, and chemical irritants (as is the *periosteum* and, to a lesser degree, cancellous and compact bone).
4. *Articular cartilage* is insensitive, but *synovial lining* is very sensitive to mechanical and chemical irritants.
5. *Tooth enamel* is insensitive, but *dentine and pulp* are sensitive to changes in temperature or osmolality.
6. *Blood vessels* are sensitive to mechanical stimuli, such as needle prick or squeezing, and to chemical irritants. The arteries are more sensitive than veins, and sensitivity appears to reside in the adventitia. (Many sensory nerve fibers and endings in deep tissues and viscera lie close to vessels, and it may be that both deep and visceral pain are largely due to excitation of paravascular nerve fibers.)
7. *The brain and leptomeninges* are insensitive to electrical stimulation, cauterization, or incision.
8. *Sensory and mixed nerves* are sensitive to needle prick, cutting, heat, and chemical stimuli.
9. *The parietal pleura, parietal peritoneum,* and *parts of the parietal pericardium* (supplied by somatic nerves) are sensitive to needle prick, scratching, and chemical irritants, whereas the *visceral pleura, epicardium,* and *visceral peritoneum* are insensitive.
10. *The lung, liver, spleen, and kidney* (including the capsules of the latter three) are not sensitive to incision, pressure, or cauterization.
11. *The myocardium* is sensitive to chemical irritants (traction on the coronary arteries may also cause pain).
12. *The esophagus,* although said to appreciate cold and warmth, is considered insensitive to pain. *The healthy gut* is not sensitive to cutting, cautery, or clamping, but reacts to marked distention. (It is not clear whether intestinal colic is due to distension, muscular spasm, or traction on the mesentery.) Inflammation increases the sensitivity of the gastrointestinal tract, and the inflamed stomach, colon, and appendix are sensitive to squeezing or other mechanical pressure.
13. *The renal pelvis, ureter, base of the bladder, and urethra* are sensitive to squeezing, cutting, cauterization, and chemical irritants.
14. *The testis* is extremely sensitive to pressure, apparently due to nerve endings in the tunica vaginalis.
15. *The body of the uterus* is insensitive, but the *cervix* reacts to electrical stimulation and distention. (Muscular spasm during childbirth can cause pain.)

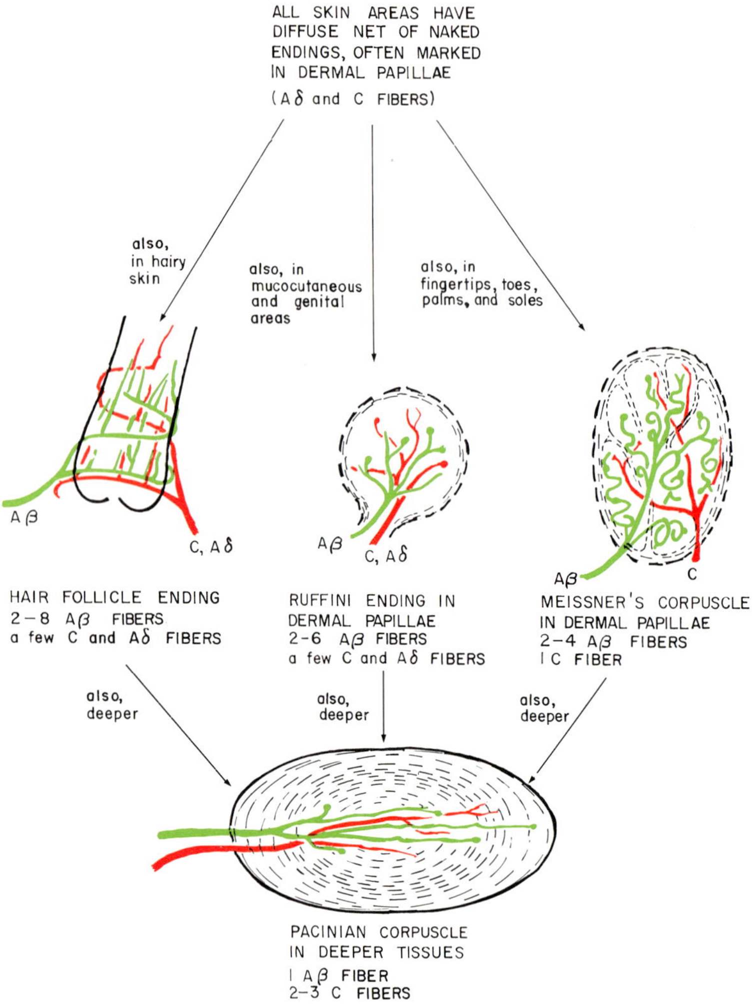

Fig. 6-1. Sensory receptors in skin and subcutaneous tissue. Green = thick myelinated (Aβ) fibers; red = fine myelinated and nonmyelinated (Aδ and C) fibers.

SOMATIC AND VISCERAL RECEPTORS

Morphology of Receptors

The primitive sensory receptors in the skin and subcutaneous tissue (Fig. 6-1) consist of a network of fine, unmyelinated, branching nerve fibers that increase in density toward the surface, with terminal branches that often penetrate between epidermal cells. This network exists as far back as invertebrates, but has developed certain specializations in hair-bearing animals and more in primates. Many nerve terminals show no apparent specialization, but others form small flat expansions (Merkel's discs) in relation to epidermal cells. The nerve network is particularly dense around hair follicles, each of which may also receive 5 to 10 myelinated fibers forming rings at the follicle base, with small vertical branches often ending in leaflike expansions resembling Merkel's discs. Both in hairless and hairy skin and at mucocutaneous junctions, papillae may contain complicated webs of naked nerve fibers devoid of a capsule; these are called *Ruffini endings* in the skin. In the mucocutaneous areas and genitalia, they may additionally receive 2 to 6 myelinated fibers, and loops of branching filaments as large as 0.1 mm in diameter may be formed.

Occasionally, the Ruffini or mucocutaneous endings, particularly the latter, show early condensation of perineurial epithelium, forming an indefinite capsule. Such endings probably are intermediate between the primitive naked network and truly capsulated endings. The most typical capsulated endings, *Meissner's* (tactile) corpuscles, occur only on hairless skin and only in primates. They are typically found in the palmar and plantar dermal papillae and increase in frequency toward the tips of the digits. Less well-developed tactile corpuscles are present on the sides of the palms, soles, and digits. The corpuscle is 0.03 to 0.08 mm in diameter,

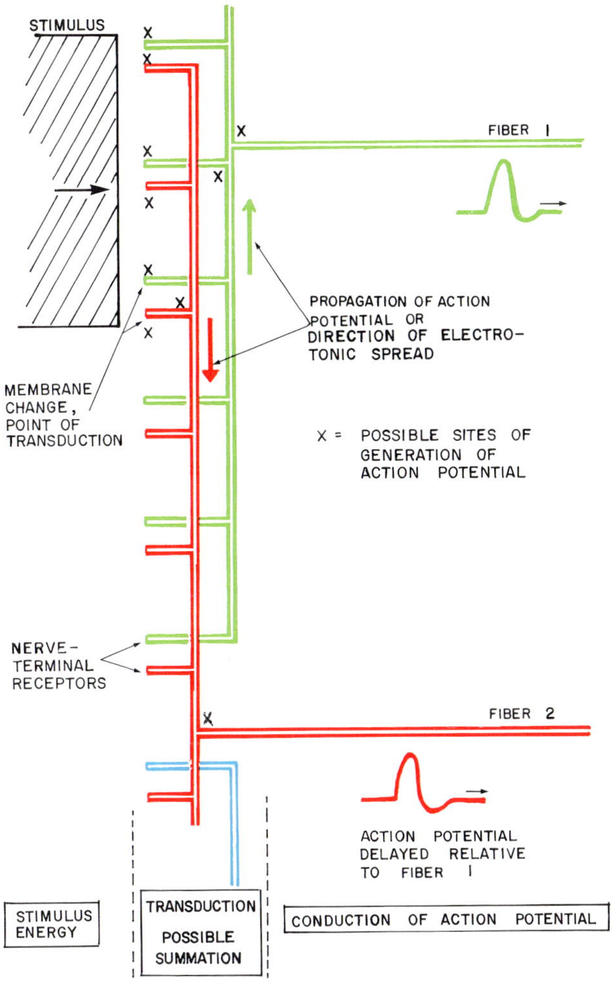

Fig. 6-2. Transduction of applied sensory stimuli to nerve impulses (action potentials). The site of summation of stimuli to produce an action potential is not known (see alternative sites [X]). Potentials in adjacent effectively stimulated fibers are not all in phase, and time differences may be one aid to CNS analysis of sensory input.

with a loose perineurial epithelial capsule, and it often appears deeply lobulated by similar cells of neural crest origin. Each is supplied by two to three (occasionally as many as nine) large myelinated fibers, which form complicated branches with beading and enlarged, sometimes spatulate, terminations. Each may also receive one small nonmyelinated fiber. Most tactile corpuscles are oval. Similar but round endings, principally in the cornea and mucocutaneous areas, may be referred to as bulboid (Krause's) corpuscles.

The structures described so far are all very superficial. *Pacinian corpuscles* are distributed in the deeper skin and subcutaneous tissue, particularly in relation to hairless areas of the hands, feet, and external genitalia, but are also present deeply, in association with tendons, fasciae, periosteum, and joint capsules. In fresh specimens as large as 0.5 $\times$ 2 mm, they are oval structures composed of concentric lamellae of perineurial epithelium. Each receives several finely myelinated or unmyelinated fibers and a single large myelinated fiber, which passes from end to end in the long axis, forming numerous side branches and terminal swellings. The only other sensory nerve endings in the deep dermis and subcutaneous tissue, or in any deeper somatic or visceral areas, are of the naked type, always associated with unmyelinated (or, at most, finely myelinated) small fibers.

Distribution of the various types of sensory endings indicates their probable functions. Hair follicle endings, Ruffini and mucocutaneous endings, and tactile corpuscles, restricted to the superficial dermis and epidermis, are thought to be associated with discriminative sensation. Tactile corpuscles, which increase rapidly in density at the extremities and are present only in primates, probably subserve finely discriminative touch especially. All these sensory endings are supplied by one or more large myelinated fibers, though some also have a fine unmyelinated fiber. Pacinian corpuscles are present in deep skin (especially hairless areas) and in association with the musculoskeletal system. They probably receive external pressure data and provide proprioceptive information. (Two other sources of proprioceptive information, the tendon organ and the muscle spindle, will be considered in Chapter 7.) The naked nerve endings are largely supplied by unmyelinated or fine myelinated fibers and are the only type of receptor present in every tissue capable of pain appreciation. Since specific thermoreceptors are not identified in man, it is possible that naked nerve endings also subserve cold and warmth. Relatively nondiscriminative touch and pressure may also be subserved by some of the naked endings, which are probably a mixed group.

Mechanisms of Receptor Activity

Transduction

Sensory stimulation involves the application of energy in some form – e.g., mechanical, thermal, electrical, or chemical. To convey information to the CNS, energy must be converted into a nerve fiber impulse by transduction. This is the function of sensory receptors (Fig. 6-2).

Receptors are the peripheral terminations of processes to which the concepts of axon and dendrite can only be applied with difficulty. Cell bodies, both for somatic and visceral sensory fibers, are present in dorsal root ganglia (or corresponding cranial nerve ganglia), and they have only a single process, which divides into a peripherally and a centrally directed fiber. The peripheral fiber forms multiple branches that end in the receptors, and the central fiber enters the cord in the posterior root. Electrophysiologically, the entire fiber is an axon, since the potential generated by the receptors passes centrally (in all-or-nothing fashion) to synapses within the CNS. However, it is possible that dendritic properties (summation of changes in membrane potential) may still be present in the distalmost branches, so that the likelihood of axonal discharge would be related to the number of the terminal receptors stimulated.

Allocation of Receptor Specificity

Sensory fibers show varying degrees of myelination, but any myelin sheath is lost at the sensory endings; these are separated from adjacent tissue by a capsule, or at least by a basement membrane derived from the Schwann's cell or perineurial epithelium.

There is nothing in the microscopic appearance of receptors to indicate their specificity, although certain inferences have been drawn from their distribution. Only physiological analysis enables the allocation of receptors to various sensory modalities. This is a formidable task, complicated by species variation. Complete specification of a receptor implies knowing its threshold to each mode of stimulation (with construction of a stimulus-response curve) and its rate of adaptation, after discharge, receptive field size, and central fiber connections.

In the human being, skin sensitivity to touch, pressure, pain, heat, and cold is punctate in distribution, inviting a search for the underlying receptor. Such studies, either in man or, hopefully, applicable to man, have shown several types of *touch, pressure, and vibration receptors* connected to large myelinated ($A\beta$) fibers (presumably the hair follicle, Ruffini and mucocutaneous endings, and tactile corpuscles). *Cold receptors* appear to be connected to large or small fibers ($A\beta$, $A\delta$, C). *Heat endings*, which appear to be few in man, have not been firmly identified, but may be connected to small fibers ($A\delta$, C). *Chemical stimulation,* which usually elicits pain, appears to be mediated through the $A\delta$ and especially the C fibers.

The characterization of sensory endings, and their identification with histological structures, is incomplete in man, partly because of the problems of identifying the stimulated spot histologically and especially because of the overlapping of receptive areas. A single sensory fiber may be distributed to 100 hairs over several square centimeters, and yet each hair is innervated by two to six sensory fibers. Localization is usually not dependent on the point-to-point representation of very small receptive fields, but is carried out somewhere in the CNS by analysis of responses from many overlapping fields.

Since pain may be elicited by the application of diverse forms of energy, it appears reasonable to search for a receptor with multiple specificity and a high threshold, since lesser amounts of the same forms of energy produce normal sensory information. Such receptors should be found among the naked nerve endings, but they have not been found there. It is not clear from current experimental work whether excessive stimuli directly cause pain via specific receptors or by spread of stimulation to adjacent pain receptors. The presence of both myelinated and small unmyelinated fibers in some touch and pressure endings suggests that, if excessively stimulated, they *could* originate pain.

Endogenous Pain-Producing Agents

The absence of a multispecific, high-threshold receptor points to the possibility that all painful stimuli activate a common mechanism, perhaps a receptor that is specific and of low threshold to some chemical or chemicals produced even by minor tissue damage. Pain may be investigated by the application of substances to the base of a skin blister (e.g., produced by cantharidin), or it can be investigated in experimental animals by the intra-arterial injection of substances stimulating the paravascular nerve endings (pain being inferred from the animal's reactions). By methods of this type it has been demonstrated that the following are potent pain producers at concentrations that are feasible even in minor tissue damage: a fall in pH to 6.2 or below, K^+ ions, acetylcholine, serotonin, histamine, plasma activated by glass or inflammatory exudate, angiotensin, substance P, and bradykinins. Even early inflammation is associated with liberation of bradykinins, activation of plasma, usually with an increase in K^+ levels (from damaged cells), and fall in pH. One or more of these changes could be the effective pain stimulus. Bradykinins may contain 9 to 11 amino acid residues (e.g., Arg-Pro-Pro-Gly-Phe-Ser-Pro-Phe-Arg·NH_2), and can produce pain in doses of less than 2μ. Intra-arterial injection produces pain (after a latent interval of 12 to 15 seconds) that is not affected by sympathectomy, but is prevented by dorsal root section.

Ischemic muscle produces pain (associated with impulses in the nonmyelinated afferent fibers) that is related to the work done and inversely related to the blood flow. If, with the circulation occluded, muscle is exercised until painful, pain will persist after exercise until the circulation is restored. Presumably, this pain, too, is on a chemical basis, K^+ ions being a likely cause, although a role for bradykinins cannot be excluded. There may be other endogenous agents acting directly to cause pain. The pain of peptic ulcer may depend on the presence of free acid. Injection of sodium urate crystals into a normal joint produces severe pain resembling gout (urates are known to activate the kinin-forming system).

Exogenous Pain-Producing Agents

Many exogenous pain-producing (algogenic) agents exist, although it is not clear whether they act directly on pain receptors or by damaging tissue. Stinging nettles produce acetylcholine, histamine, serotonin, and probably also a large molecular weight—poorly diffusible substance (perhaps a proteolytic enzyme), which might better account for the prolonged duration of pain and itch. Wasp venom contains high concentrations of serotonin, histamine, and a kinin, and hornet venom contains, in addition, a high concentration of acetylcholine. Bee stings produce pain

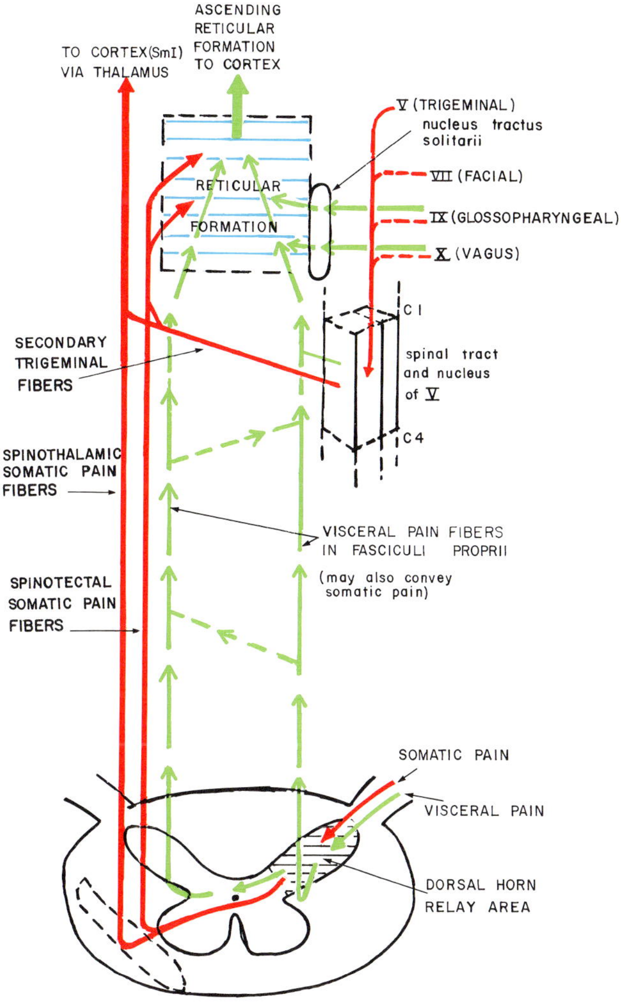

Fig. 6-3. Probable diagram pain pathway in the cord and from the trigeminal input (the diagram may be incomplete). Somatic pain (red) reaches the sensory cortex and reticular formation, but it is not clear whether the much more diffuse visceral pain pathways (green) relay to the cortex directly through the somatosensory nucleus or only through the ascending reticular system. Details of dorsal horn synapses are omitted (see Fig. 6-4).

by unidentified large molecules, including a basic polypeptide and a phospholipase that damages cell membranes. Ant bites inject formic acid in concentrations of 10 to 70%, according to the species. Bites of snakes are associated with many enzymes and toxins.

Although pain-producing agents are chemically diverse, many are cationic and could react with anionic receptor sites. Electron microscopy does not demonstrate any unusual features in receptor plasmalemma, but it is said to contain gangliosides of greater acidity (i.e., containing more N-acetylneuraminic acid) than other parts of the membrane. It is speculated that reaction of these groups with algogenic agents causes conformational changes, associated with altered ion permeability and membrane potential and ultimate generation of action potentials. Since the peripherally acting analgesics (e.g., aspirin) are also anionic, they must react with some other component of the plasmalemma, perhaps reducing enzyme activity.

PAIN PATHWAYS

Peripheral Nervous System

If a peripheral nerve is stimulated and a recording made proximally, a compound action potential with peaks is detected (see Chap. 3) due to rapidly conducting Aβ fibers, more slowly conducting Aδ fibers, and even more slowly conducting C fibers. Elicitation of pain is associated with Aδ and C conduction (small finely myelinated or unmyelinated fibers). These may be separated by progressive ischemia in a mixed nerve, which typically blocks conduction in larger fibers first. First pain disappears before second pain, suggesting that the former is carried in Aδ fibers and the latter in C fibers. Conversely, infiltration of a nerve with a local anesthetic blocks second pain earlier, since nonmyelinated fibers are the most susceptible to the action of local anesthetic agents. Pain fibers enter the cord (or brain stem) through the lateral divisions of posterior roots, which pass through the dorsolateral (Lissauer's) tract to enter the substantia gelatinosa.

Central Nervous System

Lemniscal Pathways

The incoming pain fibers (Fig. 6-3) end in the dorsal horn, where axons are said to originate that decussate ventral to the central canal within a short distance from the root of entry, and travel upward in the ventrolateral column as the lateral spinothalamic tract. This continues through the minor tract area of the lateral medulla and comes to lie lateral to the medial lemniscus in the pons, and dorsolateral to it immediately before entering the somatosensory (and other posterior) thalamic nuclei. Most of the decussating fibers are myelinated. However, extensive clinical experience indicates that pain is conveyed in a much wider zone than the classic lateral spinothalamic tract — indeed in almost a quarter circle from the lateral to near the midventral white matter — and it is more satisfactory to speak of "ventrolateral column fibers," rather than identifying specific tracts. Within this area, the sacral fibers are dorsolateral and superficial; the cervical fibers are ventromedial and deeper. The results of cutting the fibers for relief of intractable pain (tractotomy) suggest that they lie fairly near the surface, and that there may be partial segregation of pain-conducting from temperature-conducting fibers, which lie more deeply. A spinotectal tract, also formed from decussating fibers, has been described as running dorsally to the lateral spinothalamic tract. (It is reported that lateral spinothalamic fibers become fewer in number during their ascent through the pons and midbrain, which is equivalent to describing a spinotectal tract.)

Therefore, it seems desirable to modify slightly the classic conception of well-defined pain pathways as follows: Pain relay fibers cross the midline in the ventral commissure and turn rostrally to form one component of a diffuse area in the ventrolateral column, including what have been called ventral and lateral spinothalamic and spinotectal tracts. A considerable proportion of these fibers terminate in the midbrain (mesencephalic reticular formation), but many continue to the somatosensory and other nuclei of the thalamus and thence presumably to the postcentral cortex (SmI).

Pathways in Spinal and Brain Stem Reticular Formation

It is thought that visceral sensory fibers (which probably convey little except pain) also relay in the dorsal horn, probably at the lateral edge of the base adjacent to the intermediate horn (secondary visceral gray area). Ascending visceral fibers presumably form part of the fasciculi proprii of the cord lateral to the gray matter and are assumed to ascend in a multisynaptic, bilateral system, which joins the reticular formation of the brain stem. It is not known whether or not secondary visceral pain fibers ascend through the spinotectal or spinothalamic pathways.

Unfortunately, tractotomy for relief of intractable pain often produces only a temporary result, the pain recurring within a few months. Even bilateral tractotomy, which is customarily performed for visceral pain not responsive to narcotics, may not be permanently successful. This indicates an inherent plasticity in the pain pathways, best explained by assuming that not only the *visceral* afferent fibers, but also a proportion of *somatic* afferent fibers (possibly those arriving in the peripheral C fibers) ascend the cord in a bilateral multisynaptic system, which is a part of the spinal reticular formation. Internuncial neurons lie in the central gray matter and give rise to axons that form ascending and descending branches in the fasciculi proprii, synapsing with similar neurons at other levels. This ascending sensory system would be part of the spinospinal and spinoreticular formation (see Chap. 5) and be relatively immune to interruption by tractotomy.

It is likely that the more rapidly conducted, well-localized first pain travels through the spinothalamic (lemniscal) system to the thalamus, and that a diffuse, affect-inducing second pain is conducted through the spinotectal (lemniscal) and spinoreticular systems, reaching the mesencephalic reticular formation, limbic system, and hypothalamus (see Chap. 5), with autonomic effects and emotional overlay. (Other types of sensory input may have autonomic effects, including nausea, blood pressure changes, and fainting, but these are culturally acquired responses. The autonomic effects of pain are intrinsic.)

Cranial Nerve Input

A corresponding division of sensory fibers from the face and scalp occurs in the trigeminal nerve and its central connections. The Aδ and C fibers turn caudally as the spinal trigeminal tract and form synapses in the substantia gelatinosa of the spinal nucleus. (The spinal tract and nucleus of the trigeminal nerve are both homologous and physically continuous with the dorsolateral tract of Lissauer and the substantia gelatinosa of the cord respectively.) Relay fibers from the trigeminal gelatinosa directly enter the reticular formation of the brain stem and contribute to the crossed secondary trigeminal tracts, which reach the tectum and posterior thalamic nuclei. Somatic sensory fibers in the facial, glossopharyngeal, and vagal nerves also reach the spinal trigeminal tract and nucleus. General *visceral* sensory fibers of the vagus reach the nucleus tractus solitarii, from which no specific efferent tracts have been identified. Presumably, projection fibers directly enter the reticular formation.

MODULATION OF PAIN INPUT

Clinical Observations

Peripheral neuropathies, such as those associated with diabetes, alcoholism, or herpes, are often characterized by spontaneous, unpleasant sensations of pain (paresthesias), often burning in quality and resembling second pain. Crises of spontaneous pain may be present in tabes dorsalis, one of the manifestations of syphilis. In such conditions, or in normal pain due to injury, it has been observed that, within limits, other sensory stimuli such as touch or pressure, applied in the vicinity of painful foci, diminish perception of pain. It is a common observation that distraction by other stimuli or experiences readily leads to a temporary ignoring of mild pain; on the battlefield, even severe mutilating injuries may be temporarily disregarded. It appears that nonpainful environmental stimuli or variations in CNS activity can modulate pain perception. In the peripheral neuropathies and tabes dorsalis, there is a predominant destruction of large myelinated (Aβ) fibers. Since it is stimulation of just these fibers that seems to effect the modulation of pain, the hypothesis of an optimal balance between large and small fiber input has been advanced.

Gate Control Hypothesis (Dorsal Horn)

Modulation, or gating, could theoretically occur at any level of the CNS from the dorsal horn upward. Combined anatomical and physiological investigations of the dorsal horn area have suggested that it contains neural networks appropriate to the hypothesis (Fig. 6-4), though other areas are not excluded. The dorsal horn may be divided into six layers, labeled 1 through 6, starting with the substantia gelatinosa and finishing adjacent to the central gray matter. Small cells in the second and third layers send axons only as far as the deeper layers, where the cells of origin for ventrolateral column fibers are situated.

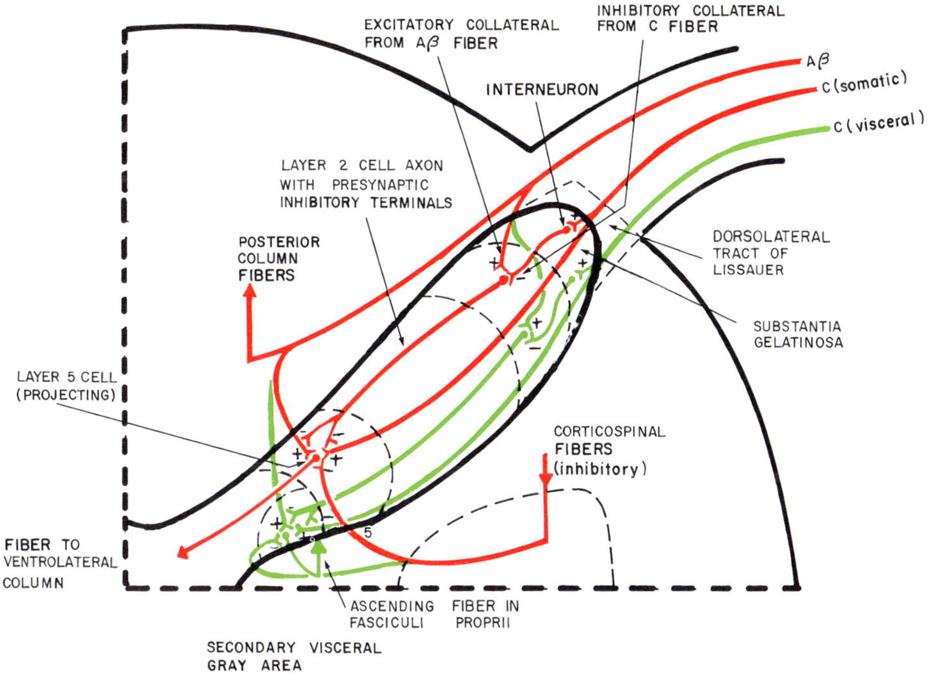

Fig. 6-4. Semischematic illustration of a pain-modulating (gate control) system in the dorsal horn (+ = excitation; – = inhibition). C fibers terminate by branches in layers 2 and 5, and posterior column fibers send collaterals to the same layers. The decussating secondary fibers originate in layer 5. For further details, see text.

The gate-control theory suggests that incoming fibers may form two groups of synapses; Aδ and C fibers send collaterals to the small cells in layer 2 and terminate on layer 5, whereas Aβ fibers send collaterals to both layers. All afferents are excitatory to layer 5 cells, but their effects on layer 2 cells are opposed, Aδ and C collaterals being inhibitory (presumably through an interneuron) and Aβ collaterals being excitatory. Fibers from layer 2 cells terminate in layer 5, causing presynaptic inhibition of the direct afferent impulses. In this system, incoming Aβ impulses may be either inhibitory or excitatory to the layer 5 cells, whereas Aδ and C impulses would be purely excitatory. Further, since afferent fibers are visceral as well as somatic, and since several or many fibers synapse on any single cell in the dorsal horn, the area integrates total sensory input from all the segmental structures (Fig. 6-5). The final activity in the ventrolateral columns represents a balance, which is dependent on the origin, modality, and intensity of sensory input.

Finally, it appears that direct cortical fibers sending collaterals to (or terminating in) the dorsal horn are inhibitory in nature and would reduce ventrolateral column discharge. Thus, Aβ impulses could act not only directly on the dorsal horn, but also (since ascending and descending pathways are oligosynaptic and rapidly conducting) indirectly via the cortex. The concept is equally applicable to cranial nerve sensory input to the spinal trigeminal nucleus.

Other Possible Sites of Modulation

The success of the gate-control theory in explaining many clinical and experimental observations does not preclude the possibility that inhibition or modulation of pain also occurs at other levels, or by other mechan-

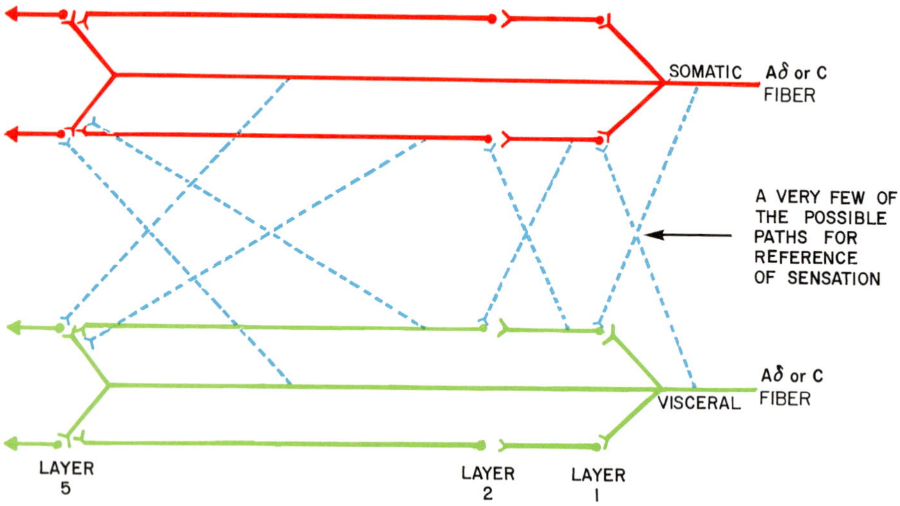

Fig. 6-5. Blue dashed lines represent just a few of the possible pathways for integration and reference of segmental sensory input.

isms, or both. Clinically, destruction of the posterior part of the dorsolateral thalamic column, including the pulvinar, frequently stops intractable pain, although again there is a tendency to recurrence. This part of the thalamus has a polysensory input and, with its extensive cortical projections, could well serve as a gating area. The cortex itself may be involved in inhibitory or modulatory activity. Prefrontal leukotomy, which destroys the connection between much of the frontal cortex and the medial nucleus of the thalamus, is effective in reducing the emotional and autonomic effects of pain, if not in reducing its perception.

HYPERALGESIA

Hyperalgesia is a state in which the normal threshold to pain is lowered, so that normally nonpainful stimuli produce pain, and painful stimuli produce more pain than usual. A related term is *hyperpathia,* in which the pain threshold is frequently normal, but pain, when produced, is more prolonged or more unpleasant than usual. Either or both these conditions may result from peripheral nerve disease or damage and would be a logical result if the gate-control theory is correct; since larger fibers are selectively destroyed, the balance at the gate is disturbed in favor of excitation.

Local Tissue Injury

The events following tissue injury are most easily seen on the skin (Fig. 6-6). Following pain at the site and time of injury, there is a short latent interval before the development of *primary hyperalgesia,* characterized by redness and swelling that extend a moderate distance around the area of tissue damage. This remains for several days, either concentrically, or extending in the direction of lymphatic drainage, which suggests release of some substance associated with hyperalgesia and vasodilatation, probably a kinin, by antidromic stimulation through collaterals of the damaged endings. The area of reddening and hyperalgesia represents the total receptive fields of all axons with a directly injured terminal, and it may extend if the liberated kinin enters the lymphatic drainage.

There is associated *secondary hyperalgesia* beyond the zone of reddening. The pain threshold is not lowered, so that, strictly speaking, it is hyperpathia, not hyperalgesia. It lasts only 36 to 48 hours and appears to represent referred pain secondary to convergence in the CNS, probably at the dorsal horn level.

Acute Nerve Injury

If a peripheral nerve is acutely sectioned (Fig. 6-7), the skin supplied only by that nerve becomes anesthetic and analgesic. The surrounding zone of overlap shows hypopathia, the raised pain threshold varying from infinity (in the sectioned autonomous zone) to normal (at the border of the adjacent normal autonomous zone). Within a few days of section, collaterals grow in from the adjacent nerves, and the anesthetic-analgesic area is replaced by a zone of hyperpathia and hyperalgesia. Pain sensation returns to normal after a few days and remains normal until the sectioned nerve regenerates and grows into the area, causing another short period of hyperalgesia and hyperpathia. These temporary periods are not well understood. They may reflect a greater degree of overlap of naked nerve terminals than of more specialized endings, together with a tendency for the smaller fibers to grow in (or mature) more rapidly than the larger. Imbalance of impulses at the gate-control area will result.

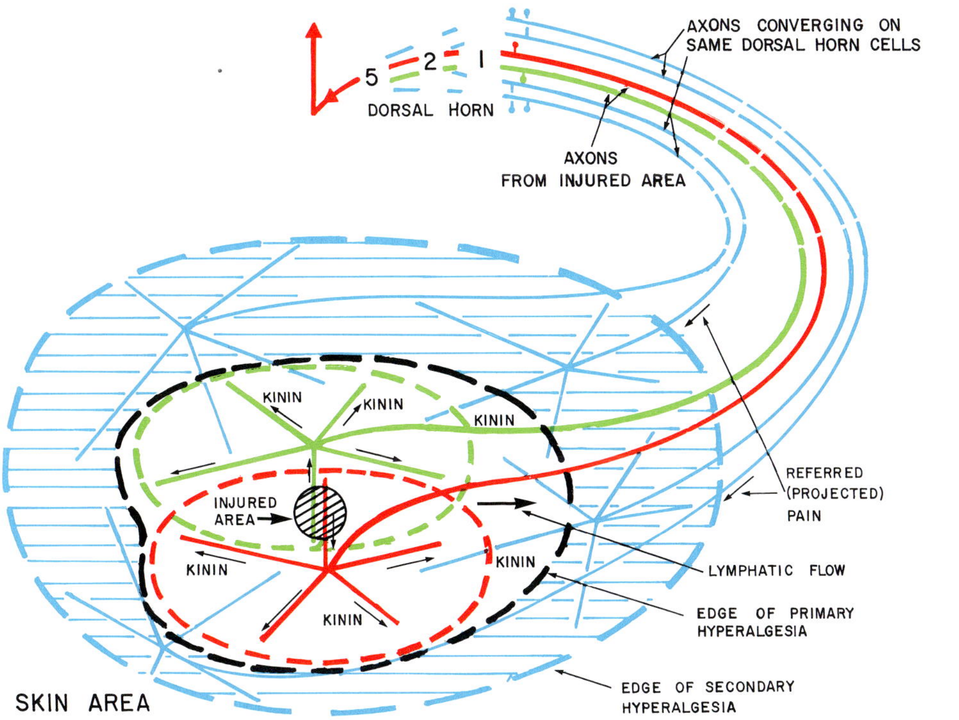

Fig. 6-6. Events following a focal skin injury (black hatched area). Any sensory fiber with a terminal branch in the injured area releases kinins from all its terminals, and these may spread within lymphatics. Kinins cause primary hyperalgesia (within black dashed line). Reference to adjacent sensory fibers at dorsal horn level causes secondary hyperalgesia (blue hatched area).

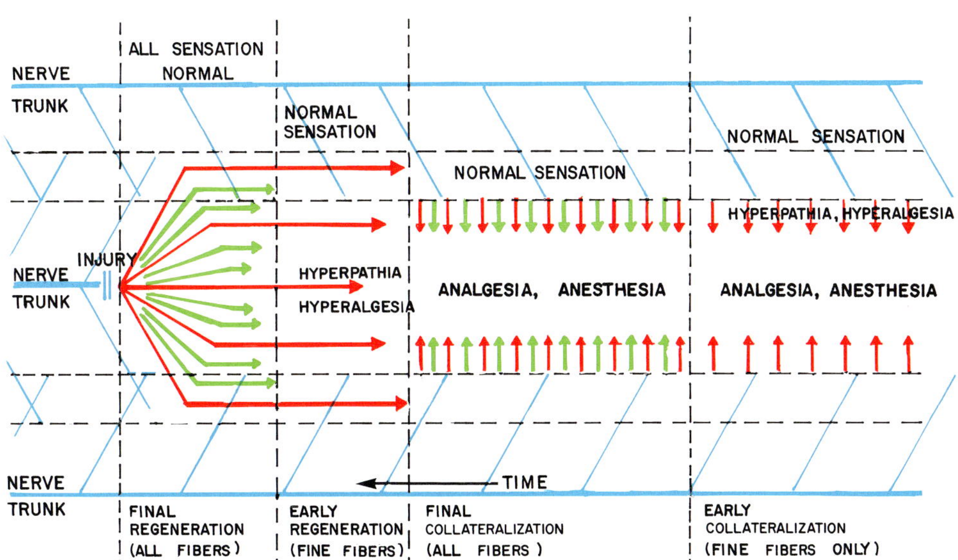

Fig. 6-7. Sequelae of acute injury to a peripheral nerve trunk (time sequence from right to left). Fine unmyelinated fibers (red) appear to grow faster than large myelinated fibers (green), zones of temporary imbalance of innervation causing hyperpathia and hyperalgesia. This occurs twice: first from collateral growth by adjacent uninjured fibers and later from regeneration of the injured nerve.

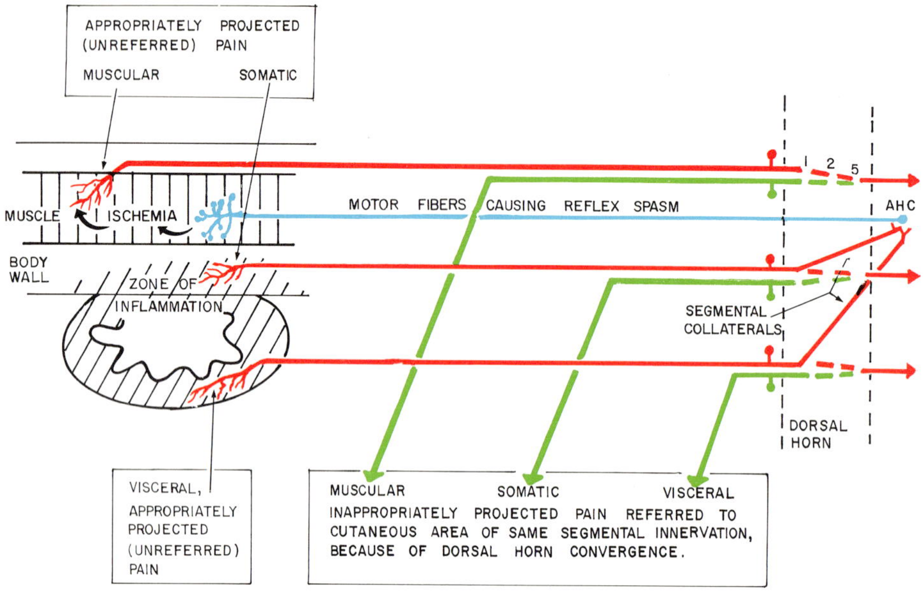

Fig. 6-8. Type and mechanisms of referred pain (in this case, from an inflamed viscus adjacent to the body wall, e.g., appendicitis). Three possible types of real pain, i.e., due to the stimulation of pain endings (red), and three of referred pain, i.e., due to convergence at the dorsal horn and peripheral assignation by the CNS (green) are seen.

REFERRED PAIN

Pain due to inflammation in deep and visceral structures is usually poorly localized, but it may be accompanied by cutaneous pain at a related or apparently remote area. *Referred pain* is pain perceived in an area other than that producing it.

Correlation of clinical and anatomical studies indicates that sensory afferents from inflamed deep somatic or visceral tissues reach the cord at the same level as afferents from cutaneous areas to which the pain is referred. Since, as previously noted, there is convergence of all segmental sources of sensory input on dorsal horn neurons, there must be extensive sharing of central paths between those visceral and somatic afferents that enter at one and the same segmental level. This does not explain why the CNS *habitually* refers pain to the cutaneous tissues rather than to the deep tissues. It is possible that localization in the skin is more accurate because it is usually facilitated by visual evidence and by concurrent stimulation of other modalities (e.g., touch) that are not available in deep tissues. It is also suggested that localization to the skin may be a form of habit reference. That is, since painful stimuli from the skin impinge on the CNS much more often than those from other tissues, it may have become a "habit" for painful stimuli passing through a group of dorsal horn neurons to be referred to the appropriate skin areas, irrespective of their peripheral pathway. There is some evidence in support of this hypothesis. One study has shown that patients with deep pain in the facial region, associated with tooth or sinus inflammation, refer it to the teeth much more often if they have had a great deal of dental work (and therefore presumably dental pain) than if they have had none.

Unfortunately, referred pain has even more complications (Fig. 6-8). Visceral inflammation may involve adjacent somatic structures, such as the peritoneum or pericardium, and these parietal structures may also give rise to diffuse local pain or to referred cutaneous pain. Furthermore, visceral inflammation, especially if there is somatic involvement, as above, may lead to reflex protective rigidity (spasm) of muscle, causing muscular ischemia, which itself may cause both local and referred pain. Thus, a given focus of visceral inflammation, if associated with local somatic irritation and muscle spasm, offers *six* possible pain projections.

1. *Visceral unreferred pain,* such as the substernal pain of angina and diffuse epigastric pain of peptic ulceration.
2. *Visceral referred pain,* as in the arm pain of angina and the groin pain of renal colic.
3. *Somatic unreferred pain,* such as the right lower quadrant pain of acute appendicitis.
4. *Somatic referred pain,* as when inflammation of the peripheral diaphragm is referred to the chest wall (intercostal nerves), or inflammation of the central diaphragm is referred to the neck and shoulder (phrenic nerve).

5. *Muscular unreferred pain,* which may be felt as local deep pain or at the bony attachments of muscle.
6. *Muscular referred pain,* which may be felt within areas of skin sharing the same afferent segmental level.

The problems of diagnosing visceral or other deep inflammation by studying patterns of pain may therefore be extremely confusing and may even appear to be illogical. They require extensive knowledge of the segmental innervation of body structures.

CENTRAL PAIN

Central pain is spontaneous pain, associated with an overreaction to stimulation and resulting from lesions confined to the CNS. It includes dysesthesias of a disagreeable type. Central pain may result from spinal cord lesions, such as syringomyelia, intramedullary tumors, multiple sclerosis, and trauma; from lower brain stem lesions, including vascular disease, neoplasms, syringobulbia, and multiple sclerosis; from thalamic lesions; and, much more rarely, from lesions involving the midbrain, basal ganglia, or cortex. All occur infrequently, but the most common type is thalamic pain (thalamic syndrome of Dejerine-Roussy), a rare complication of cerebrovascular disease in which the thalamogeniculate artery (see Chap. 14) is occluded and the posterior ventrolateral thalamic and adjacent nuclei are destroyed. The mechanism of central pain is unknown. However, one may speculate that there is usually loss of first-pain pathways without impairment of second-pain pathways, perhaps leading to diminished cortical stimulation and reduction of cortical descending inhibitory impulses to the dorsal horn gate control.

Central pain may be precipitated by virtually any sensory stimulus applied to any part of the body. It is often continuous, but is exacerbated in association with specific sensory events. The affected (contralateral) side of the body frequently shows hyperalgesia with severe hyperpathia (occasionally the pain threshold is normal, but hyperpathia is constant). These abnormalities may be present over an entire body half or sometimes over only a part. The acute incident is associated with contralateral hemiplegia that usually improves rapidly and with a contralateral hemianesthesia that persists and develops into the abnormal (hyperpathic) state after about a year.

ITCHING AND TICKLING

Itching originates from stimulation of superficial free nerve endings within or immediately beneath the epidermis, is conducted by small C fibers, and is relayed through the ventrolateral column. No chemical agent responsible for spontaneous itching has been isolated; however, experimentally, various agents, including proteolytic enzymes and liberators of histamine, appear to be effective.

Although itching and pain differ in the response they provoke (scratching versus evasion) and in their response to morphine, which often aggravates itching, it is not possible to dissociate them clinically. Thus, in complete analgesia, itching is absent, and in sensory dissociations, such as those due to an expanding lesion in the spinal cord, pain and itching are both lost. Itching is inhibited by painful stimuli, e.g., scratching.

Tickling may be regarded as itching produced by a light, external, moving stimulus. It resembles itch in that it evokes scratching behavior, is inhibited by pain, and is transmitted through the ventrolateral columns.

BIBLIOGRAPHY

Brodal, A. *Neurological Anatomy in Relation to Clinical Medicine* (2nd ed.). New York, London: Oxford University Press, 1969.

Casey, K. L. The neurophysiologic basis of pain. *Postgrad. Med.* 53:58-63, 1973.

Elliott, H. C. *Textbook of Neuroanatomy* (2nd ed.). Philadelphia: Lippincott, 1969.

Keele, C. A. Chemical causes of pain and itch. *Annu. Rev. Med.* 21:67-74, 1970.

Keele, C. A., and Neil, E. (Eds.). *Samson Wright's Applied Physiology* (12th ed.). London: Oxford University Press, 1971.

Melzack, R., and Wall, P. D. Pain mechanisms: A new theory. *Science* 150:971-979, 1965.

Meyer, G. A., and Fields, H. L. Causalgia treated by selective large fibre stimulation of peripheral nerve. *Brain* 95:163-168, 1972.

Ruch, T. C., Patton, H. D., Woodbury, J. W., and Towe, A. L. *Neurophysiology* (2nd ed.). Philadelphia: Saunders, 1966.

Schmidek, H. H., Fohanno, D., Erwin, F. R., and Sweet, W. H. Pain threshold alterations by brain stimulation in the monkey. *J. Neurosurg.* 35:715-722, 1971.

Sweet, W. H. Pain. *Ann. R. Coll. Phys. Surg. Can.* 3:223-233, 1973.

Thomas, P. K. The anatomical substrate of pain: Evidence derived from morphometric studies on peripheral nerve. *Can. J. Neurol. Sci.* 1:92-97, 1974.

Regulation of Muscle

7

All central nervous system influences on voluntary muscle are exerted through lower motoneurons, which include the anterior horn cells of the cord and the branchial and somatic motor nuclei of the brain stem. Each lower motoneuron, if it generates an action potential, causes contraction of a defined group of muscle fibers, the size of the group varying in different muscles. The combination of the lower motoneuron and the muscle fibers it innervates is a *motor unit.* Under normal circumstances there is no *spontaneous* firing of lower motoneurons, and *both* maintenance of muscle tone and execution of movement therefore are dependent on their adequate stimulation via the CNS. Pathways are extremely complicated and include:

1. Proprioceptive feedback from muscle and tendons and the joint capsules over which they operate, via the cord or brain stem.
2. Nonproprioceptive sensory input from all structures, especially skin, which are innervated at the same segmental level, via the cord or brain stem.
3. Feedback collaterals from the motor axons themselves (inhibitory).
4. Sensory input from other segments, including proprioceptive and nonproprioceptive components, via the cord or brain stem.
5. Pathways from the labyrinths (vestibulospinal and reticulospinal tracts).
6. Pathways originating in, or mediated by, the brain stem reticular formation (reticulospinal and rubrospinal tracts).
7. Indirect pathways from the cerebellum, operating through the reticular formation and cerebral cortex (reticulospinal and corticospinal tracts).
8. Pathways from an extensive area of the cerebral cortex, operating through the pyramidal tract and the cortically originating extrapyramidal system (COEPS) (corticospinal and reticulospinal tracts).

(Although, for convenience, tracts are designated spinal, homologous fibers pass to brain stem motor nuclei. Thus, "corticospinal tract" should be read "corticospinal-corticobulbar tracts.")

Thus, virtually the whole CNS is directly or closely involved in muscle control. As muscular activity represents almost the complete range of environmental responses of which an organism is capable, this is perhaps not surprising. As physiological research proceeds, the areas of the cerebral cortex apparently directly involved in motor activities become progressively larger, and the distinction between sensory and motor systems becomes blurred. To avoid constant reiteration, it should be noted here that as an increasing proportion of research is carried out on the primate brain, significant differences in CNS organization with ascent of the evolutionary scale are disclosed. This must be borne in mind when assessing the relevance of research carried out on subprimates.

Grossly oversimplifying, it may be said that skeletal muscle is caused to operate for three distinguishable reasons:

1. *Involuntary (reflex) movement in response to environmental stimuli,* presumably common to all forms of life with contractile tissues.
2. *Maintenance of position (posture),* including both orientation with respect to gravity (presumably common to all forms of life with axial orientation) and maintenance of stance against gravity (probably after emergence from water to air, with consequent lack of body support). Additional postural responses, necessitated by the upright posture, are only now becoming apparent.
3. *Execution of volitional movements,* organized or set in train by suprasegmental structures and not necessarily dependent on external stimuli.

To a considerable extent, the first of these activities is intrinsic to the segmental organization of the CNS (cord and parts of the brain stem), whereas the second and third require integration, initiation, or both, by suprasegmental parts of the brain. In the sections to follow, regulation of muscle activity will be discussed approximately in this sequence.

AFFERENT AND EFFERENT CONNECTIONS OF MUSCLE

Motor Fibers

Lower motoneurons are cells whose axons leave the CNS, and whose axon branches (telodendria) terminate as neuromuscular junctions (motor end-plates)

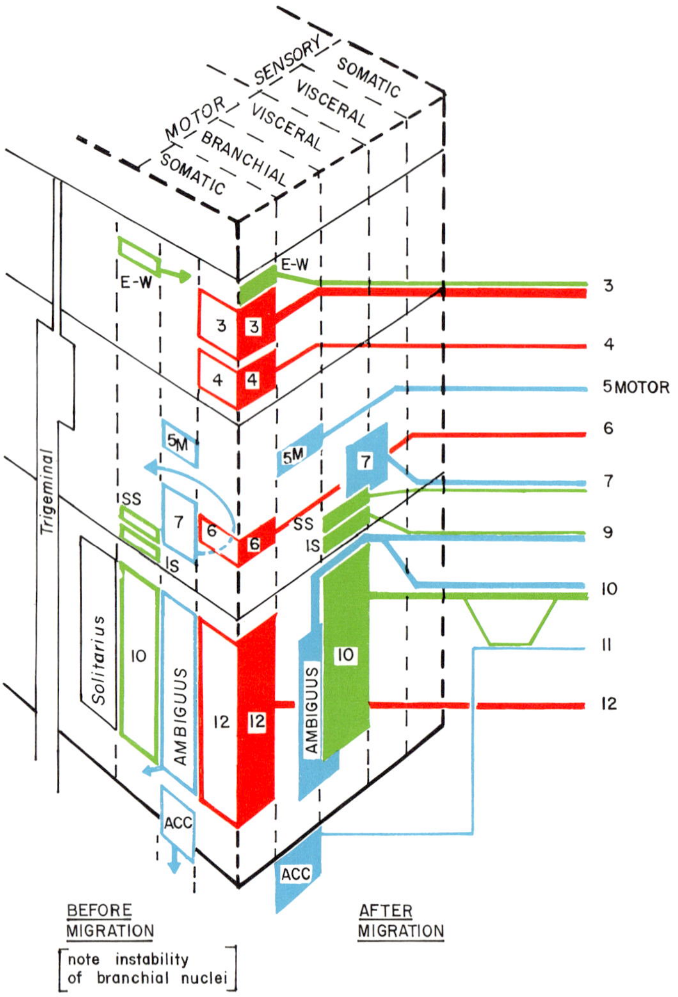

Fig. 7-1. Cranial motor nuclei before (left) and after (right) their fetal migrations, and their contributions to cranial nerves (right). The midbrain is represented at the top, followed in order by the pons and medulla. Red = somatic column; blue = branchial column; green = visceral column. The cranial sensory nuclei are represented on the left, uncolored. E-W = Edinger-Westphal nucleus; SS = superior salivatory nucleus; IS = inferior nucleus; ACC = accessory nucleus.

on skeletal muscle fibers, each of which has a single motor end-plate. The cell bodies are large and polygonal, with conspicuous Nissl bodies, and are situated in the branchial and somatic (Figs. 7-1, 7-2) brain stem motor nuclei (III, IV, motor V [masticator], VI, VII, ambiguus, accessory, XII) and in the anterior horns of the spinal cord (Fig. 7-3). Within motor nuclei, there are anatomically indistinct subgroupings that correspond to individual muscles, small muscle groups, or muscle actions. Thus, in the cord, flexor and adductor neurons lie deep to extensor and abductor neurons, and cells for the distal muscles lie lateral to those for the axial (trunk) structures. Each neuron has a dendritic field up to 1.5 mm across, with extensive overlap.

As it passes through the anterior white matter, each motor axon gives off a recurrent collateral, which passes back into the anterior horn to synapse with Renshaw cells. Motor axons are thick, heavily myelinated fibers, 10 to 20μ in diameter, which make up about 40% of the large fibers in a muscle nerve (the other 60% are large afferent fibers, mainly from spindles). When the axon reaches muscle, it branches extensively, supplying a group of muscle fibers with one motor end-plate each (Fig. 7-4). A

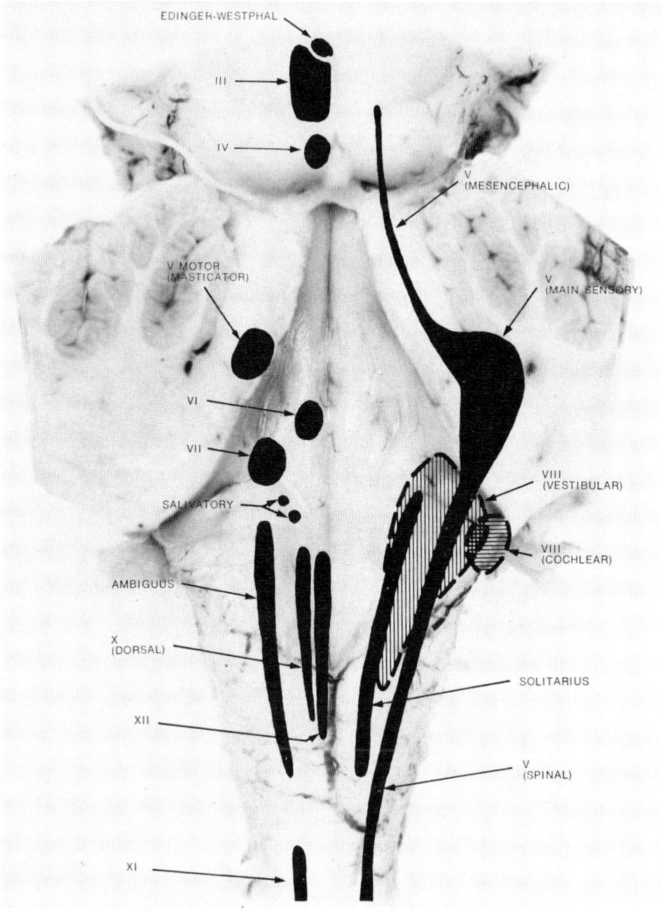

Fig. 7-2. Approximate positions of cranial nerve nuclei superimposed on a dorsal view of the brain stem.

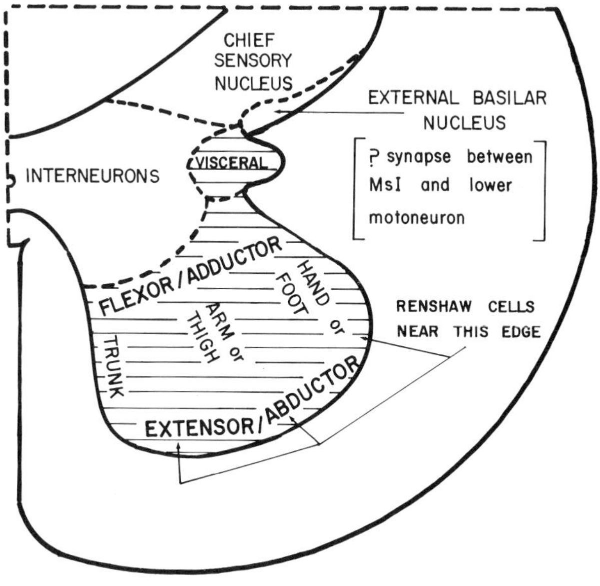

Fig. 7-3. Localization of motoneuron groups in the anterior and lateral horns of the spinal cord (hatched area). The positions of Renshaw cells and external basilar nucleus (see text) are also shown.

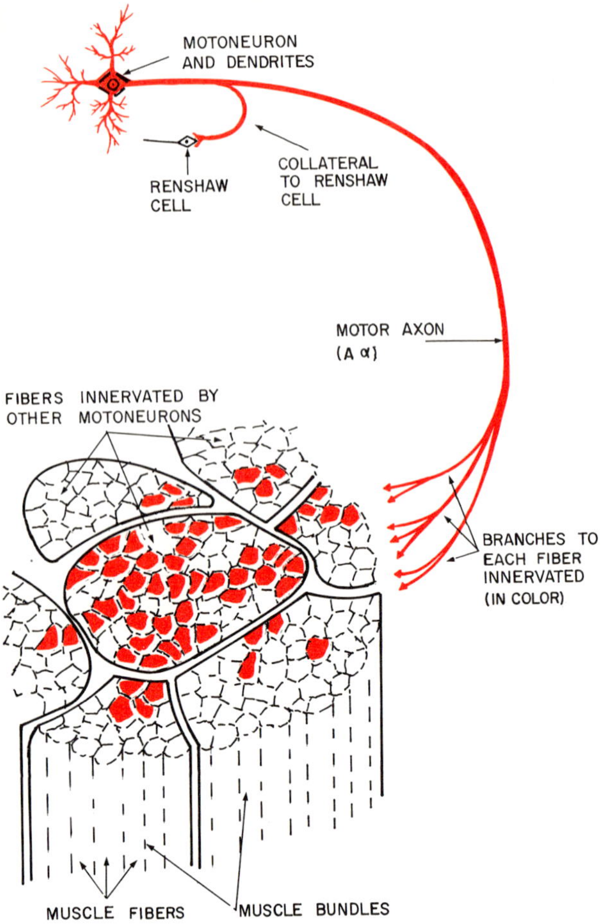

Fig. 7-4. Single motor unit (red). Note that the motor unit does not correspond to a single muscle bundle.

single axon may supply only 3 to 10 muscle fibers of small muscles that carry out delicate activities (e.g., extrinsic ocular muscles); or it may supply as many as 200 fibers of proximal muscles, concerned with postural or coarse, voluntary responses. The group of fibers innervated by one axon (motor unit) does not correspond to a muscle bundle but extends over adjacent bundles, with marked overlapping. Because of variation in the number of muscle fibers supplied, together with variation in the size of the fibers, the range of tension developed by a single motor unit varies from about 0.1 g in an external ocular muscle to about 50 g in a large limb muscle.

Sensory Feedback from Muscle and Tendon

Naked nerve endings in musculoskeletal tissues are believed to convey pain (see Chap. 6), which may lead to reflex muscle spasm as a response to inflammation (as in polymyositis) or ischemia (as in intermittent claudication). These nerve endings are probably of no importance in the regulation of normal muscle activity. Endings specifically concerned with proprioception are found in the joint capsule (joint organ), adjacent to attachments of the muscle to the periosteum or tendon (tendon organ), and within the muscle belly itself (muscle spindle).

Joint Organ

Of these three types of endings, the role of the *joint organ* has perhaps been least investigated. It is associated with a subjective sense of limb position, and its main central connections are through the thalamus to the sensory cortex rather than to the cerebellum.

Tendon Organ

The tendon organ (Golgi organ) is an encapsulated mechanoreceptor present at the ends of a muscle and stretched either by active contraction or passive lengthening of the muscle. Each tendon organ is supplied (Fig. 7-5) by one to two large (12 to 18μ) myelinated fibers (Aβ, group 1B), which branch on any fasciculi of the tendon included within the capsule. They exhibit little or no spontaneous firing in the absence of tension, but fire (without adaptation) if tension rises to, say, 100 to 200 g, the firing rate being proportional to the logarithm of the tension. One function appears to be protection against overstretching and rupture of the muscle, but there may be others not yet elucidated.

Muscle Spindle

The muscle spindle (Fig. 7-6) is a complex, encapsulated, elongated structure within the interstitial connective tissue of the muscle belly. Spindles probably are present in all skeletal muscle, but are less easy to find (perhaps less well capsulated) in branchial than in somatic musculature. Each spindle contains two types of muscle fibers, receives two types of motor axons, and originates two types of sensory fibers (Fig. 7-5). These muscle fibers are termed *intrafusal,* as opposed to the *extrafusal fibers* that make up the bulk of the muscle.

Each spindle contains one or two *bag fibers,* which are 7 to 8 mm long and about 25μ wide, with a central dilated, noncontractile "bag" containing several nuclei and not showing cross-striation (the rest of the fiber contains myofibrils and is striated). Each bag fiber is supplied by one to two medium-sized myelinated motor axons (2.5 to 4.5μ), and has one to six separate motor end-plates on the cross-striated regions. Each is surrounded by spiral receptor fibers (annulospiral endings) from which originate large (10 to 18μ) myelinated afferent fibers (Aβ, group IA). Small numbers of irregularly branching (flower-spray) endings, from which originate 4 to 10μ myelinated afferent fibers (Aβ, group II), are also present. The second type of intrafusal muscle fiber is the *chain fiber,* 4 to 5 mm long and about 12μ in diameter; there are four to eight in each spindle. Their motor axons are much smaller (1 to 2μ) and form irregular

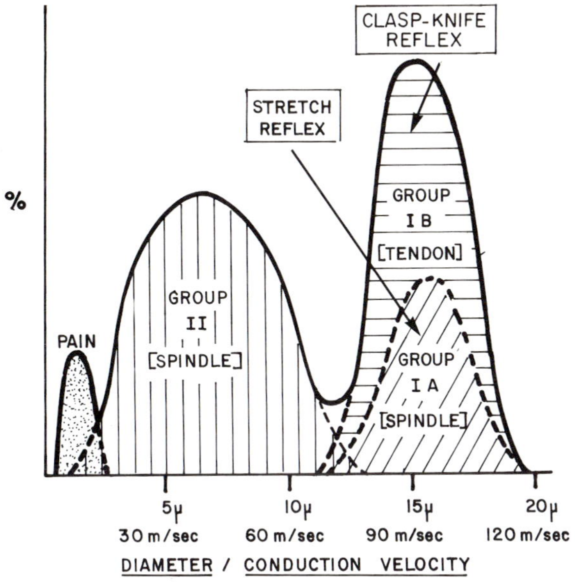

Fig. 7-5. Distribution of sensory (afferent) fibers in a muscle nerve (after degeneration of motor fibers due to anterior root section).

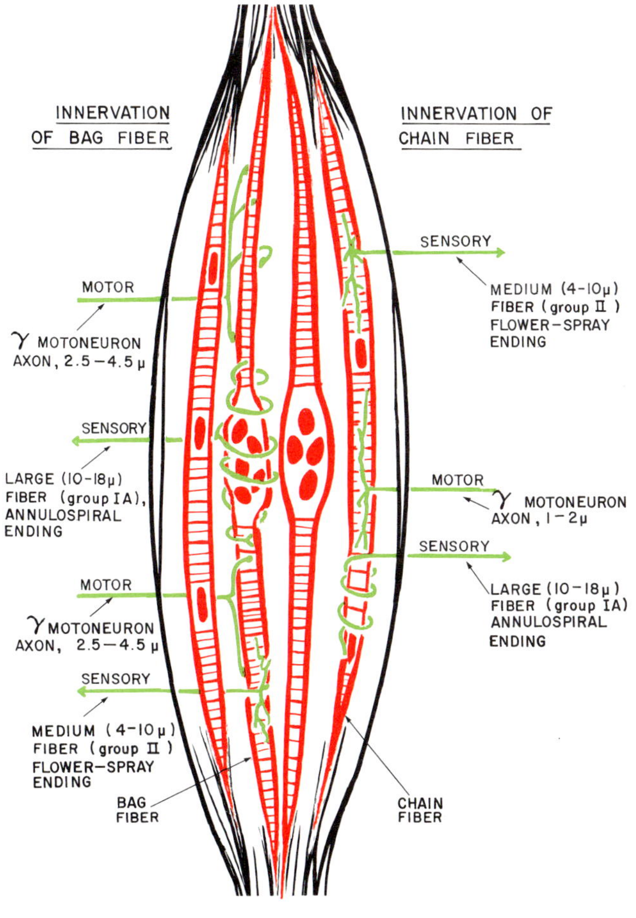

Fig. 7-6. Semischematic representation of a muscle spindle. Only four intrafusal fibers (red) are shown. Nerve fibers are shown in green. For details, see text.

networks (trail endings) rather than discrete motor end-plates. Both annulospiral and flower-spray endings are present on the chain fibers.

Much remains to be learned about the function and detailed structure of this complicated organ. Stimulation of the larger motor fibers presumably shortens the contractile ends of the bag fibers, increasing tension on the bag. Stimulation of the smaller motor fibers, which shortens the chain fibers, presumably reduces tension on the bag. The differential functions of the annulospiral and flower-spray endings are not clear. Even so, the general outlines of spindle function are discernible. Spindle afferent fibers (group IA) are excitatory mainly to motoneurons of the originating muscle, and this excitation involves only one synapse between the afferent fiber and the motor neuron (the only monosynaptic reflex arc known in man). Probably the facilitation of synergists, and certainly the inhibition of antagonists, acting across the same joint as the originating muscle and confined to the ipsilateral side, involve interneurons (it is a general principle that a single axon cannot be both inhibitory and excitatory). The CNS origin of the spindle motor fibers (gamma fibers) is in the same nuclear zone that originates the motor fibers (alpha fibers) to the main bulk of the muscle. It is probable that gamma motoneurons, like alpha motoneurons, are in clusters associated with individual muscles or movements; they resemble alpha motoneurons morphologically.

Since the spindle is situated within the muscle belly, it is stretched when the muscle is stretched (resembling the tendon organ in this respect). However, when the muscle *actively* contracts, the muscle spindle is shortened, whereas the tendon organ is stretched. Both are sensitive to stretching, but the spindle fires at much lower levels of tension, usually 1 to 2 g. The rate of firing is proportional to the logarithm of the tension, and the spindle is virtually nonadapting. It is common experience that within a wide range the position of a limb can be maintained irrespective of the load. In other words, the length of a muscle and its tension may vary independently. It appears that one function of the gamma neurons is to maintain a constant spindle firing rate by causing the spindle fibers to shorten as the muscle shortens, i.e., alpha and gamma motoneurons usually are firing at the same time. It is possible to discern a servomechanism for maintaining a given muscle length. If the muscle stretches, the spindle is stretched, the rate of spindle firing increases, alpha motoneurons are stimulated, and the muscle shortens. Muscle length can be altered directly by stimulating alpha motoneurons or indirectly by stimulation of gamma motoneurons (shortening the spindles, increasing the spindle firing rate, and thereby stimulating alpha motoneurons). The relative physiological importance of these two methods of provoking muscle contraction remains undetermined.

Inhibitory feedback is provided by the recurrent motor-axon collaterals that synapse with the Renshaw cells (interneurons in the margins of the anterior horn); the latter are directly inhibitory to alpha motoneurons.

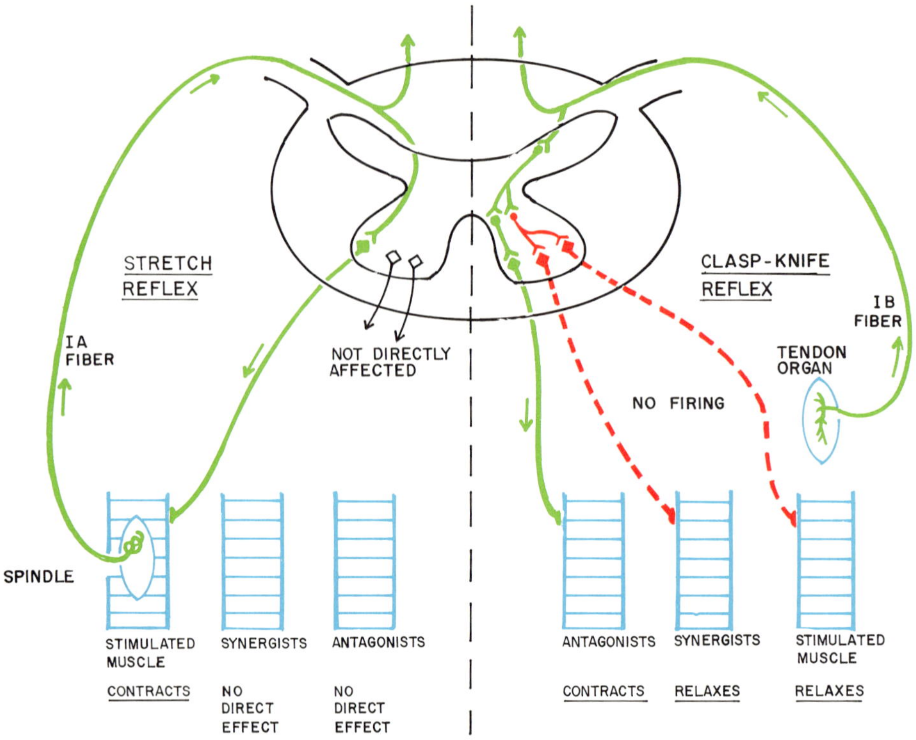

Fig. 7-7. Neural circuits involved in the stretch (left) and clasp-knife (right) reflexes. Green = activated circuits; red solid = inhibitory circuits; red dashed = inhibited circuits; blue hatched = skeletal muscle.

SEGMENTAL MUSCLE REFLEXES

Experimental study of segmental muscle reflexes requires the removal of all input to the anterior horn cell, other than that arriving via the posterior roots of the same segment, and imposes technical problems. Thus, knowledge of such reflexes is largely based on studies with subprimates in which suprasegmental reflexes have been eliminated by spinal section. However, available primate studies and clinical observations in human disease are broadly consistent with such knowledge. Following spinal section, all muscles innervated from segments below the section are flaccid (i.e., have no tonus), and movement does not occur in the absence of local sensory input, as from muscle spindles, tendon organs, and joint organs (proprioceptive), the skin (touch, pressure, temperature, or pain), or deep tissues (pain).

Stretch Reflex (Myotatic Reflex)

If a flaccid muscle is stretched, it responds by contracting. This contraction occurs only in the stretched muscle(s) and is (physiologically) accompanied by relaxation of the antagonist(s). There is no contralateral response, and contraction is rapidly initiated and concluded. It is abolished by dorsal root section. The basis for this stretch, or myotatic, reflex (Fig. 7-7) is that the muscle spindle responds to tension by increasing firing rate, stimulating the alpha motoneurons of the stretched muscle(s) only. The reflex can readily be elicited without spinal section and is the basis of the deep tendon reflexes and muscle clonus observable in clinical practice. Being monosynaptic, it is not depressed by drugs (such as meprobamates) that affect interneurons and cause reduced flexor response and reflex spasm.

Clasp-Knife Reflex

Although solely dependent on segmental input, the clasp-knife reflex cannot be demonstrated in a flaccid spinal preparation, since it consists of a sudden relaxation of muscle when tension becomes extremely high. Information is therefore from decerebrate preparations (section above the mid-pons) in which all limbs are rigid. If such a limb is forcibly bent beyond a certain degree, rigidity abruptly disappears, and the limb becomes freely movable. A similar reaction occurs in patients with spasticity. The reflex originates in tendon organs (Fig. 7-7) that respond to *high* tension by firing, is multisynaptic (i.e., involves interneurons), and causes inhibition of the stretched muscle and its synergists and facilitation of the antagonists. Occasionally, the corresponding contralateral muscle is also facilitated, so there is more spread within spinal gray matter than occurs with the very precise stretch reflex (but less than with the flexor response).

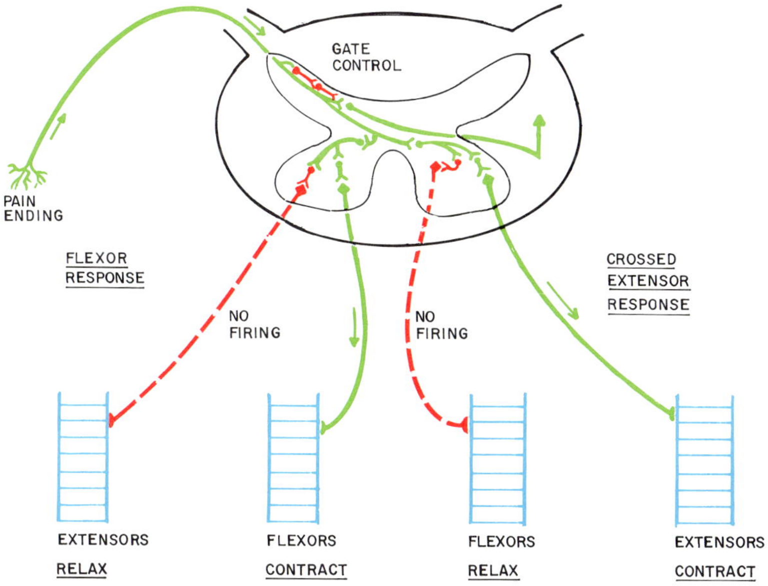

Fig. 7-8. Neural circuits involved in flexor response. Green = activated circuits; red solid = inhibitory circuits; red dashed = inhibited circuits; blue hatched = skeletal muscle.

Flexor Response

If a flaccid limb receives painful stimulation, superficial or deep, generalized flexion of the limb occurs, interpreted teleologically as a *withdrawal response.* It is usually accompanied by extension of the contralateral limb and often, if the cord is intact between hindlimb and forelimb segments, by flexion of the diagonally opposite limb. Although the flexor response is a withdrawal response in all cases (Fig. 7-8), the precise muscle activity depends on the site of stimulation. This phenomenon (local sign) implies topographical representation in segmental sensory and motor gray matter and is usually such as to move the withdrawing limb even farther away from the noxious stimulus. The flexor response, often with crossed extension, is seen in human patients with spasticity and may be so diffuse in spinal gray matter as to amount to a "mass" reflex, which includes incontinence of the bowel and bladder. Stimuli reach the cord through Aδ or C fibers and connect with anterior horn cells only through interneurons. This indirect path accounts for the longer duration of the flexor response (compared with the stretch reflex) and for its marked diffusion into spinal gray matter over several segments on the same and opposite sides.

Other Reflex Responses

Effects of touch and pressure stimuli to the flaccid limb are variable, but often, like pain, they produce a flexor response with crossed extension. The reason is little understood, but even in the intact animal there is a "balance" between pain impulses and those of touch and pressure, and pain may be inhibited by descending influences. In the spinal animal the entire balance at the gate-control area is upset, and deafferentation from suprasegmental influences may lead to neuronal hypersensitivity. A poorly understood reflex that may result from touch or pressure is the *bilateral flexion response,* which clearly differs from flexion with crossed extension. A third response occurs if pressure or touch is applied in the region of the foot pad. This may result in extension of the limb against the stimulating object *(extensor-thrust response),* which shows local sign in that the limb is not merely rigid but is moved to try to remain in contact with the stimulating object. Occasionally, the extensor-thrust response is associated with extension of the diagonally opposite limb and flexion of the other limbs, in which case it is the *positive supporting reaction.* All these responses are multisynaptic, since Aβ fibers conducting touch and pressure make no direct connections with motoneurons. Obviously, some of them are intersegmental rather than segmental, but it is convenient to group them together, as they have features in common and occur in animals with high cervical section (maintained on artificial respiration).

Conclusions Regarding the Organization of the Spinal Cord Gray Matter

Elicitation of the stretch, clasp-knife, and flexor reflexes involves not only contraction of groups of muscles, but also relaxation of their antagonists. This appears to apply to all reflexes and all voluntary

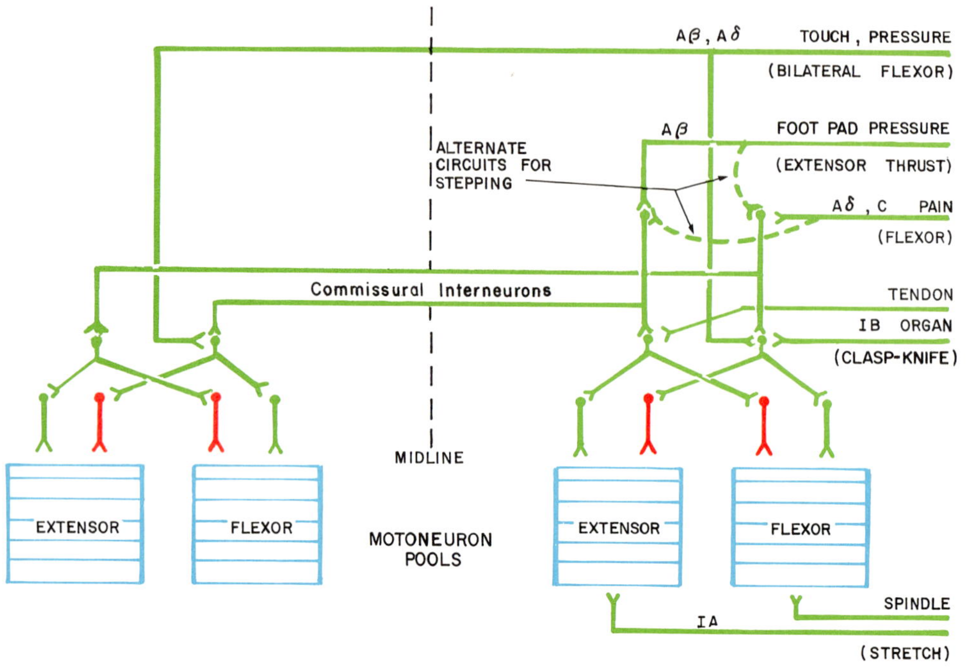

Fig. 7-9. A hypothetical hierarchy of interneurons within the spinal cord, ensuring reciprocal and double reciprocal inhibition, with alternate circuits for stepping movements of spinal origin. How these circuits alternate is not known.

movements, even when carried out under direct "supervision" of the higher centers. It may therefore be assumed that this phenomenon (reciprocal inhibition) is a built-in feature *at the segmental level,* whose purpose is to avoid the impasse of concurrent contraction of opposing muscle groups (with little useful result). Influences acting on motoneurons, with few exceptions, probably do so through two pools of interneurons, one of which might be regarded as "extensor-positive, flexor-negative," and the other as "extensor-negative, flexor-positive." Reciprocal inhibition can be overridden voluntarily, as in isometric exercises, and in the pathological rigidity of basal ganglion disease. At least voluntary overriding appears mediated through pyramidal fibers, making either monosynaptic or unique disynaptic connections with motoneurons, a feature particularly of the primate CNS.

The concept of reciprocal innervation can be extended, since flexion of one limb is often associated with contralateral extension (or vice versa). The term *double reciprocal innervation* is applied to this phenomenon, which might imply a higher pool of interneurons that make connections with one extensor-positive pool and the contralateral extensor-negative pool (with opposite effects on the flexors). Unlike simple reciprocal innervation, double reciprocal inhibition has many exceptions, as in the tonic neck reflexes, bilateral flexion response, and much of the skilled manipulation carried out with the forelimbs, both in primates and subprimates.

On the intersegmental level, reciprocal innervation can be extended still further, since extension of one limb is often associated with extension of the diagonally opposite limb and flexion of the other two. This is *crossed reciprocal innervation* and may imply a third, still higher order of interneurons that extend between segments.

It is apparent (Fig. 7-9) that there is extensive, intrinsic organization within the spinal gray matter, including some topographical representation in posterior and anterior horns and interneuronal connections that have implications both for posture and progressive movement. Thus, most animal progression is associated with rhythmic flexion of the limbs or trunk musculature on one side and then the other, with corresponding contralateral extension. In quadrupeds, diagonally opposite limbs frequently assume similar positions, as in crossed reciprocal innervation, for the purpose of standing and moving. Withdrawal of support by one limb (flexor response) implies transfer of this support to another limb, as in the crossed extensor component of the response.

In this connection, the elicitation of stepping movements in spinal preparations is of great interest. It is occasionally observed that the flexion response, or the extensor-thrust response, gives way to alternating extension and flexion on the two sides, the *stepping response.* Since this occurs in high spinal preparations, it is independent of suprasegmental influences and implies not only the existence of successively higher orders of interneurons, but also a switching mechanism. If pain stimuli are simultane-

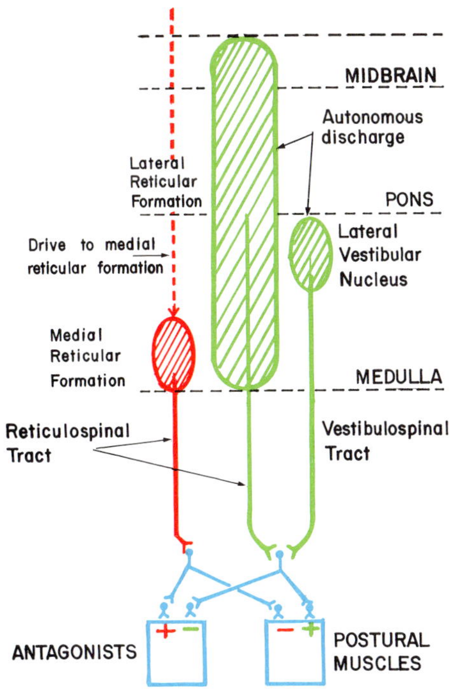

Fig. 7-10. Brain stem centers involved in the maintenance (or inhibition) of postural tonus. Green = facilitatory to postural tonus (autonomous); red = inhibitory to postural tonus (driven from higher centers); blue = postural and antipostural muscle groups; + = facilitation; – = inhibition.

ously applied, say, to both hindlimbs, the elicited flexion-crossed extension responses alternate, again giving a stepping response. There must therefore be some circuitry in the spinal gray matter capable of resolving the dilemma by alternating the expected responses instead of merging or suppressing them – teleologically a much more "intelligent" solution. In rabbits, the contralateral response to flexion is also said to be flexion, and these animals usually hop rather than run.

POSTURAL TONUS AND ITS MODIFICATION

The Origin of Postural Tonus

It is apparent that muscles isolated from descending (suprasegmental) influences have minimal tonus, though they can respond to segmental sensory input. Extensor and flexor tonus are equally low. Since normal animals neither collapse under the influence of gravity nor appear consciously preoccupied with the maintenance of posture, a continuously discharging suprasegmental center presumably is responsible for maintaining unbalanced muscle tonus such that "anti-gravity" muscles maintain the body in an appropriate position. In quadrupeds the anti-gravity muscles are the extensors in all limbs, and it has become commonplace to use the terms *postural tonus* and *extensor tonus* as though they were synonymous. In primates, however, the anti-gravity or postural muscles are the extensors of the lower limbs but the flexors of the upper limbs, since the arms are maintained in a semiflexed position for manipulating the environment.

The level of the "postural center" may be determined by sectioning the brain stem and forebrain and noting the effects on muscle tone. If the brain stem is isolated from the cord (spinal animals), all muscles are flaccid. Section through the mid-pons or mid-mesencephalon is associated with continuous rigidity of postural muscles (all limbs are rigidly extended in subprimates, but hindlimbs are extended and forelimbs flexed in primates, including man), and the animals are not capable of initiating voluntary movement. Section at higher levels (e.g., in the upper midbrain or above the hypothalamus) also results in exaggerated postural tonus, but such animals can perform purposive movements (e.g., walking, running, and chewing) and can therefore override their extensor rigidity.

Such results suggest the existence of a center (or centers) in the lower brain stem (Fig. 7-10) that maintains postural tonus, but whose activity can be modulated by descending influences for the purposes of volitional movement. Experiments show that stimulation of the lateral and rostral parts of the reticular formation in the medulla and pons (and also in the midbrain and subthalamus) facilitates extensor tonus, whereas stimulation of a more localized area, restricted to the medial reticular formation of the medulla, inhibits it. Since mid-pontine section leaves both the lateral and medial parts in communication with the spinal cord (with the lateral obviously dominant), it appears that the medial area requires activation by more rostral centers, whereas the lateral is autonomous and originates continuous (tonic) discharge. Teleologically, this is reasonable, since reduction of postural tonus is needed only intermittently for purposive movements, whereas its maintenance at all other times is desirable. It is believed that both centers act on motoneurons via the reticulospinal tract, probably on the gamma rather than on the alpha motoneurons. In primates, there may be an increasing proportion of alpha motoneuron activity. In either event, reciprocal inhibition is present, and it is assumed that action is exerted through interneurons rather than directly on the motoneurons.

The vestibular nucleus (mainly the lateral division, which is the origin of the vestibulospinal tract) also strongly facilitates postural tonus – again, an autonomous effect.

Modification of Postural Tonus by Tonic Neck and Labyrinthine Reflexes

It has already been seen that postural tonus can be modified for voluntary movement. It can also be modified, though only in fixed patterns, by impulses arising in the proprioceptors of the neck muscles or in the labyrinth, which reflect the position of the head with respect to gravity and the position of the body with respect to the head. The pathways for many of these *postural reflexes* are unknown, but they fall into a group that does not require the midbrain and a group that does.

In animals sectioned at the mid-pontine level, the following reflexes are present:

1. *Tonic neck reflexes.* These originate in proprioceptors of the neck muscles and affect posture in such a way that the front end of the body follows movements of the head. Thus, turning the head upward causes extension of the forelimbs and flexion of the hindlimbs, whereas turning the head to one side causes extension of both limbs on that side and flexion contralaterally.
2. *Tonic labyrinthine reflexes.* The postural changes caused by these reflexes are similar in all four limbs, although their purposes are not understood. In subprimates, there is maximum limb extension when the animal is on its back and maximum flexion when the animal is prone.

The second group of postural reflexes are not present in animals sectioned below the level of the midbrain.

1. *Labyrinthine righting reflexes.* These apparently originate in the otoliths of the labyrinth and result in neck muscle action that restores the head to an upright position. This initial restoration is followed by *body-on-head reflexes,* originating in the proprioceptors of neck muscles, which orientate the body correctly with respect to the head, so that the whole body is in a correct position. (It is possible that the body-on-head righting reflexes do not require the midbrain, but the sequence can only be initiated by orientating the head.)
2. *Labyrinthine linear accelerating reflexes.* In an experimental animal dropped head downward, these reflexes consist of extension of the forelimbs, spreading of the forepaws, and dorsiflexion of the head and may be interpreted as preparation for landing on a surface.
3. *Labyrinthine rotational acceleration reflexes.* The most important of these reflexes is *nystagmus,* by means of which a rotated animal endeavors to keep its eyes fixed on a given point. If rotation is to the left, head and eyes will turn to the right to maintain fixation until the physical limit of such turning is reached; then the eyes will very rapidly straighten to a new fixation point directly ahead of the body. The cycle is repeated, resulting in alternating eye movements that are slow in the direction opposite to the rotation and rapid in the same direction. (In cerebellar disease, nystagmus occurs spontaneously and is designated by the rapid component.) Experimentally, therefore, accelerating rotation to the right causes right nystagmus. During deceleration, nystagmus is again induced, but in the opposite direction, so that deceleration following rotation to the right will cause a left nystagmus. Impulses for these reflexes originate in the semicircular canals.

Evolutionary Changes in Postural Control

Animals with mid-pontine section do not right themselves and will neither stand nor walk spontaneously. Since they usually have extensor rigidity, they can be *placed* in an upright position, and stepping movements can be reflexly elicited, as previously noted. Animals with section above the midbrain can and do right themselves and exhibit spontaneous standing and walking. If section is above the thalamus, all these actions are brisker, better coordinated, more powerful, and appear more rapidly after operation than following midbrain section.

It is now being realized that the results of section at any given level may differ substantially between primates and subprimates. A major change is that primates with midbrain section cannot right themselves, stand, or walk, the thalamus being not merely facilitatory but essential for these activities. Of uncertain meaning is the observation that body-on-head righting in primates is accompanied by a grasp reflex of the upper limbs.

Descending Influences on Postural Tonus

It may be helpful to summarize what are believed to be the main descending pathways modifying postural tonus, presumably to facilitate movement (Fig. 7-11).

1. *Cortically originating fibers of the extrapyramidal system* (COEPS) project directly to the medial reticular area of the medulla and are among the most important activating sources for this area. They are therefore inhibitory to postural tonus.
2. *The midline (vermal) region of the cerebellum* (especially the anterior lobe) projects via the fastigiobulbar and other tracts to the pontomedullary reticular formation. The projection to the medial medullary area appears to predominate and the vermis is therefore inhibitory to postural tonus. The same region projects through the medial part of the lateral ventrolateral thalamic nucleus to cortical areas 4 and 6 and may affect pyramidal discharge.
3. *The intermediate and lateral zones of the cerebellum* project, through the red nucleus and the lateral ventrolateral thalamic nucleus, to areas 4 and 6 of the cortex. They appear to facilitate pyramidal, but not extrapyramidal, fibers and cause a generalized increase of muscle tone, most readily noticed in the more powerful postural muscles. There may also be a direct reduction of flexor tonus, by decreased stimulation of the large-celled red nucleus and consequent reduction of rubrospinal tract activity.
4. *The pyramidal tract* is probably facilitatory to flexor and extensor stretch reflexes, but lack of this facilitation is clinically more obvious in anti-gravity (postural) muscles. Because of the effectively monosynaptic nature of its connections to motoneurons, it could have separate or combined facilitatory effects on opposing muscle groups. It is not clear whether the pyramidal tract effect is autonomous (intrinsic to the cortex) or requires driving by the lateral and intermediate regions of the cerebellum, as in 3.

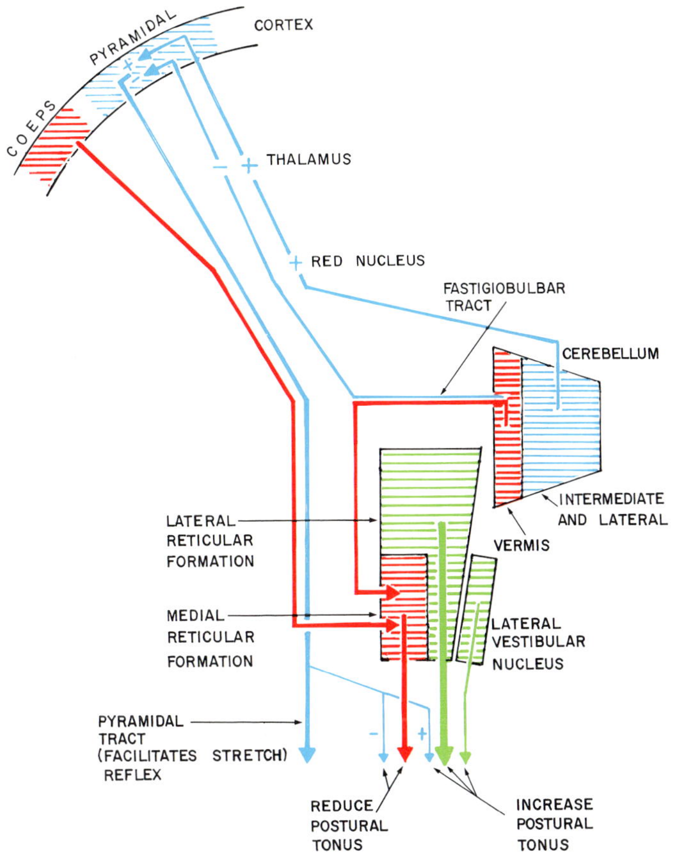

Fig. 7-11. Summary of descending influences on the brain stem postural centers. Red = circuits and areas driving the medial reticular formation (inhibitory to postural tonus); blue = circuits and areas affecting stretch reflexes via the pyramidal tract.

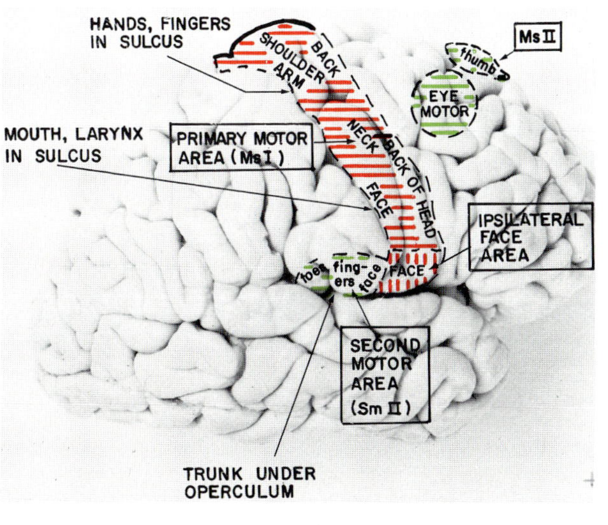

Fig. 7-12. Lateral view of right cerebral hemisphere, showing motor areas. For details, see text.

Thus, postural tonus is largely maintained by the lateral reticular formation and lateral vestibular nucleus, with variable (effectively facilitatory) effects originating in the lateral and intermediate cerebellum and perhaps the pyramidal tracts. Postural tonus is inhibited by the medial reticular area of the medulla; however, this is not autonomous, but requires driving by the midline cerebellum and the COEPS fibers. Since an intact animal exhibits a much less exaggerated postural tonus than a decerebrate animal, there is presumably a tonic inhibitory discharge, probably originating via the COEPS.

CORTICALLY ORIGINATING MOTOR SYSTEMS

Cortical Motor Areas

The concept of a well-defined "motor" strip of cortex, corresponding to the precentral gyrus, has undergone considerable modification. The precentral and postcentral cortex have some degree of overlap in motor and sensory functions, and more anteriorly there no longer seems to be a clear demarcation between the "motor" cortex (area 4) and the "premotor" cortex (area 6), which occupies the free surface of the precentral gyrus and extends on to the middle and superior frontal gyri. Because of radiation of stimuli within the cortex, it is difficult to establish which areas cause a direct motor response and which produce a response only by radiation to other regions. Cortical mapping is facilitated by moderate anesthesia,

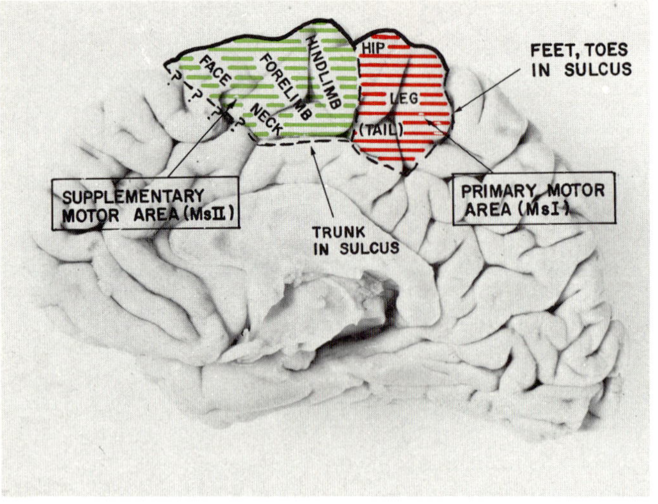

Fig. 7-13. Medial view of right cerebral hemisphere, showing motor areas. For details, see text.

which considerably reduces radiation of stimuli, probably by damping or preventing interneuronal activity. The major regions directly producing motor responses, and in which there appear to be somatotopic (topographical) representation, are the following (Figs. 7-12, 7-13):

1. *Primary motor area* (MsI). This has a major motor and a smaller sensory component and is approximately equivalent to area 4 plus an adjacent strip of area 6. The body is represented upside down, with the back anterior, and representation of hands, feet, face, tongue, and larynx are disproportionately large. Feet and toes (and tail) are represented on the medial surface. Toes, fingers, larynx, and mouth muscles are represented within the central sulcus, and the remainder of the face is represented at the lower free surface of the precentral gyrus as if the neck were sharply hyperextended (i.e., forehead above chin). The anterior margin of MsI is formed (from above downward) by the tail, back of the trunk, arm, hand, back of the neck, scalp, brow, and face. The mouth and larynx part of the motor cortex lies closely behind Broca's speech area, and the arm and hand part closely behind the (less well-defined) writing center of Exner.
2. *Ipsilateral face area.* This is present in the lower anterior precentral gyrus, and therefore is not sharply demarcated from MsI. Stimulation produces ipsilateral facial movements, whereas MsI is almost entirely contralateral.
3. *Second motor area (SmII).* This is also the second sensory area, situated on the undersurface of the parietal operculum, deep to the lower end of the postcentral gyrus. The representation of digits overlaps the free edge of the operculum, and that of the trunk is on the inner surface (with the back at the upper edge of the insula). Stimulation causes diffuse, widespread, complex movements, apparently not mediated by MsI.
4. *Supplementary motor area (MsII).* This lies medially on the superior frontal gyrus, anterior to the paracentral lobule. Leg muscles are represented posteriorly and the head anteriorly; the representation of the back lies adjacent to the cingulate sulcus, and that of the fingers may just overlap onto the upper surface of the hemisphere. Stimulation of this area produces complex bilateral responses but also facilitates MsI.
5. *The eye motor area.* This corresponds approximately to area 8, in the mid-region of the superior and middle frontal gyri. Stimulation causes deviation of the eyes, head, and trunk to the opposite side, with occasional associated autonomic effects, such as

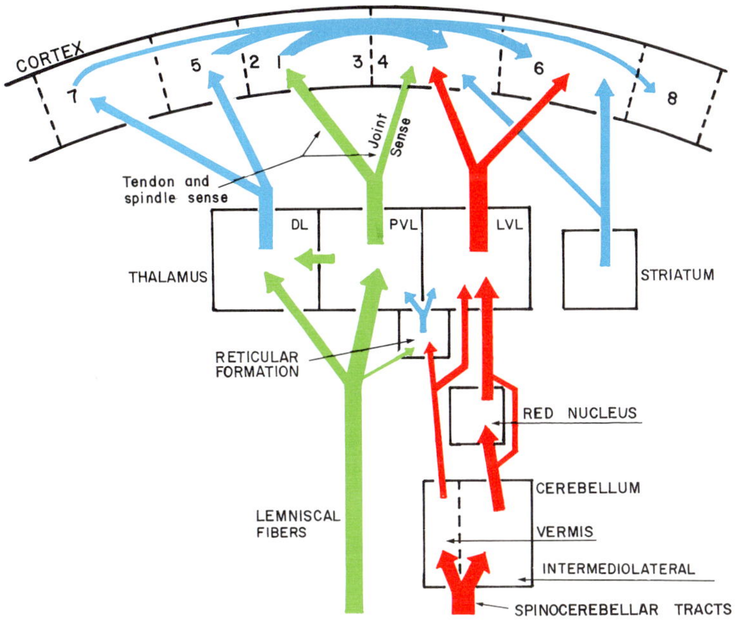

Fig. 7-14. Sensory and related input to MsI (areas 4 and 6) and adjacent regions of the cortex. Green = lemniscal input from medial and spinal lemnisci; red = cerebellar input; blue = other circuits. DL = dorsolateral thalamic nucleus; PVL = posterior ventrolateral (somatosensory) thalamic nucleus; LVL = ventrolateral (cerebellar relay) thalamic nucleus.

lacrimation and alterations of the pupils. The area lies anterior to, but not widely separated from, the eye area of MsI.

Physiologically, it appears likely that the activity of areas other than MsI is normally relayed mainly through MsI. However, ablation of MsI does not entirely prevent the motor effects of stimulating other areas, and in some cases projection fibers have been demonstrated anatomically. The significance of these extra motor areas is not clear, but they are all of high threshold compared to MsI, and tend to cause diffuse truncal and proximal movements (not involving precise distal muscles) such as the assumption of postures.

Organization and Input of Primary Motor Area

Physiological and histological studies indicate a vertical organization in areas MsI and SmI. In MsI the columns (or prisms) are 0.1 to 0.5 mm across, with an individual column, or groups, representing a single muscle. They are so arranged, and the dendritic fields are so large, that larger groupings may also be discerned, representing groups of muscles acting over a joint. Thus, it is functionally correct to state that both muscles and movements are represented in the cortex.

A considerable sensory input, over and above the proprioceptive, is fed into MsI (Fig. 7-14). In addition to muscle spindle and tendon organ input, which apparently reaches MsI and SmI, there are substantial afferents from topographically corresponding areas of SmI and directly (by collateral fibers) from the posterior ventrolateral thalamic nucleus. The lateral ventrolateral nucleus has reciprocal connections with MsI and relays somatotopically from the cerebellum through all deep cerebellar nuclei. There also appears to be significant multimodal input from the thalamic reticular nuclei (auditory, visual, and somatosensory) relayed from the reticular formation to MsI through both the anterior and the lateral ventrolateral thalamic nuclei. This multimodal input is lowest in the alert state and is probably increased in sleep or during anesthesia. There seems to be species variation in the ratio of proprioceptive to other sensory input to MsI, the former being higher in primates.

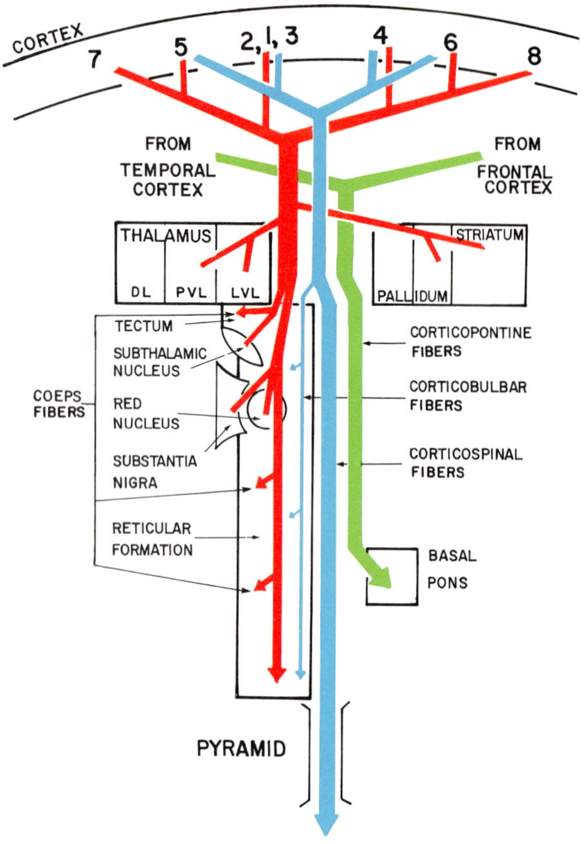

Fig. 7-15. Cortical efferent fibers related to motor function. Blue = pyramidal system; red = COEPS and corticothalamic and corticostriate fibers; green = cortical fibers to the cerebellum (relaying in the basal pons and forming the middle cerebellar peduncles). DL = dorsolateral thalamic nucleus; PVL = posterior ventrolateral (somatosensory) thalamic nucleus; LVL = ventrolateral (cerebellar relay) thalamic nucleus.

Pyramidal and Extrapyramidal Systems

Projection fibers from the motor areas form pyramidal and extrapyramidal groups (Fig. 7-15). Fibers of the *pyramidal* group all originate in the cortex; the corticospinal component passes through the medullary pyramids to reach the cord; corticobulbar tracts or fibers from the corticospinal tract in the brain stem supply brain stem motor nuclei without traversing the pyramids. Nonetheless, they make monosynaptic connections with motoneurons and are functionally "pyramidal." In contrast, *extrapyramidal* fibers may originate in the cortex or in one of numerous subcortical (suprasegmental) centers, relay through the reticular formation, and reach motoneurons multisynaptically. Of these extrapyramidal fibers, those that originate in the cortex are called the COEPS fibers, as previously stated.

It is not possible to differentiate, either by cell type or area, which cortical neurons give rise to pyramidal or to extrapyramidal projection fibers, with the probable exception of the Betz's cells, whose axons are thought to be all pyramidal. However, only 2% of pyramidal tract fibers (mostly those that are 11 to 20μ in diameter) originate in such cells, whereas 90% are small myelinated or nonmyelinated fibers of other origin (from layers III, V, or VI). About 30% of pyramidal fibers originate in area 4, 30% in area 6, and the remaining 40% in areas 3, 1, 2, 5, and 7. The pyramidal tract probably contains no ascending fibers and no descending fibers from the prefrontal, temporal, or occipital regions. Data are not available for the diffuse COEPS fibers, which probably have an even wider cortical origin.

Cortical projection fibers (other than pyramidal) that are probably important in motor function (Fig. 7-15) include at least the following:

1. *Corticostriate and corticopallidal* (the latter run to the lateral pallidum only). They originate mainly in area 6 and make connections with pallidal efferents to the thalamus in the ansa and fasciculus lenticularis.
2. *Corticothalamic,* running to lateral and posterior nuclei of the ventrolateral column of the thalamus.
3. *Corticorubral and corticotectal* (direct) (COEPS).
4. *Corticoreticular,* which project bilaterally without somatotopic distribution. The latency of these fibers is only 2 to 6 milliseconds, suggesting that connections are monosynaptic (COEPS).
5. *Corticopontine,* which, though largely from frontal and temporal areas, includes fibers from the entire cortex, even from areas 4 and 6.

Numerous feedback circuits associated with the COEPS run through the basal ganglia, red nucleus, and cerebellum, reaching the cortex via the relay or reticular nuclei of the thalamus.

Since areas of origin for the pyramidal and COEPS fibers overlap, both travel in the internal capsule, so that human disease associated with hemiplegia (most commonly a result of capsule infarction or hemorrhage) produces a mixture of pyramidal and COEPS symptomatology. *Experimental section of a pyramidal tract* produces several changes in cats and monkeys. The most notable are: a decrease in muscle strength (especially of distal flexors); a decrease in tonus (especially of distal flexors, so that affected limbs hang limply, though they are not actually paralyzed); decreased dexterity with increased use of synergists; preferred use of the unaffected (ipsilateral) limb; and loss of some cutaneous reflexes (abdominal, cremasteric). *Ablation of area 4* results in flaccidity and a Babinski response without fanning of the toes. *Simultaneous removal of areas 4 and 6,* especially if bilateral, causes greater weakness than removal of area 4 alone, with spasticity, hyperreflexia, and fanning of toes in the Babinski response. *Section of the middle two-thirds of the cerebral peduncle, or of the posterolateral white matter in the cord,* causes less weakness than a capsular lesion, with some retention of voluntary and even skilled movement. Many COEPS fibers are presumably spared in such lesions.

On the basis of such experimental work, the clinical features of internal capsular (upper motoneuron)

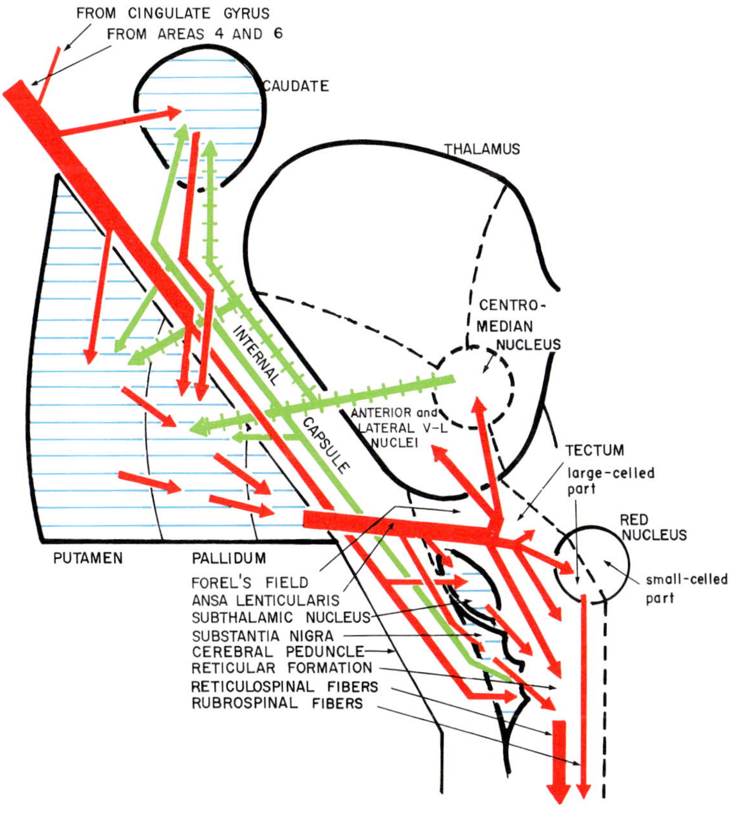

Fig. 7-16. The basal ganglia (blue hatched) and some of their connections. Red = descending (cascading) connections from cortex via the striatum, pallidum, and ansa lenticularis or directly to interpeduncular nuclei; green = feedback circuits from substantia nigra (plain) and centromedian nucleus (cross-marked).

lesions may be analyzed as follows: (1) absence or weakness of voluntary movement, hypotonia (flaccidity), and loss of cutaneous reflexes and Babinski response, due to loss of pyramidal fibers, and (2) spasticity and hyperreflexia (both dependent on exaggerated stretch reflexes), due to damage to COEPS fibers with failure to drive the medial reticular formation. Retention of voluntary or even skilled movements after section of the pyramidal tracts suggests that such movements may be partially mediated through COEPS fibers and thus that absence or weakness of voluntary movement in capsule lesions may be due to damage to both systems simultaneously.

No specific projections can be traced for COEPS fibers beyond the reticular formation, whereas pyramidal fibers are capable of affecting individual muscles or small functional groups in a precise fashion without influencing others at the same segmental level. Although they act partly by activating interneurons, there also seem to be very specific pathways between MsI and anterior horn cells, which are regarded as either monosynaptic or as having a single synapse at the lateral border of the posterior horn (external basilar region, Fig. 7-3). External basilar neurons are unique among interneurons of the cord in that they apparently cannot be fired by segmental sensory afferents, but respond earlier to pyramidal cell (MsI) stimulation than do other interneurons. The effect of the monosynaptic MsI connections is facilitatory, but both flexors and extensors may be involved, so that these pathways cannot be said to have clear-cut inhibitory or facilitatory effects on postural tonus. The later effect of pyramidal stimulation, involving interneurons other than the external basilar interneurons, is probably to facilitate multisynaptic flexor responses rather than monosynaptic stretch responses.

MOTOR FUNCTIONS OF THE BASAL GANGLIA

Structures that may properly be included under the heading "basal ganglia" are not unanimously agreed on. It would appear reasonable that caudate, putamen, pallidum, substantia nigra, and (probably) subthalamic nucleus should be included (Fig. 7-16), whereas the red nucleus appears to belong in part to the reticular formation, but largely to the cerebello-cerebral circuitry. Corticostriate (to caudate and putamen) and corticopallidal fibers (to the lateral division only), together with the reciprocal striato-cortical fibers, are somatotopically organized. Similar point-to-point connections exist in the striatopallidal, pallidosubthalamic, nigrostriatal, nigrothalamic (to

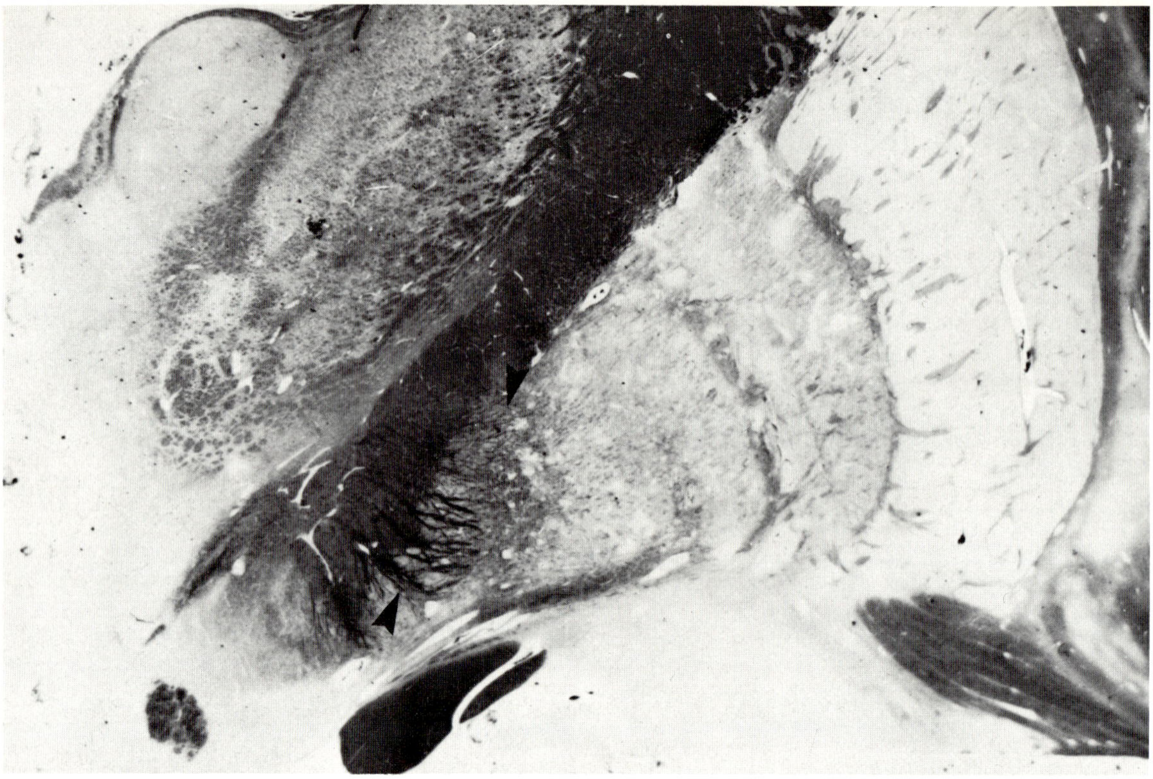

Fig. 7-17. Photograph of transverse section through internal capsule to show the fibers of ansa and fasciculus lenticularis (arrows). (Myelin stain, ×8.)

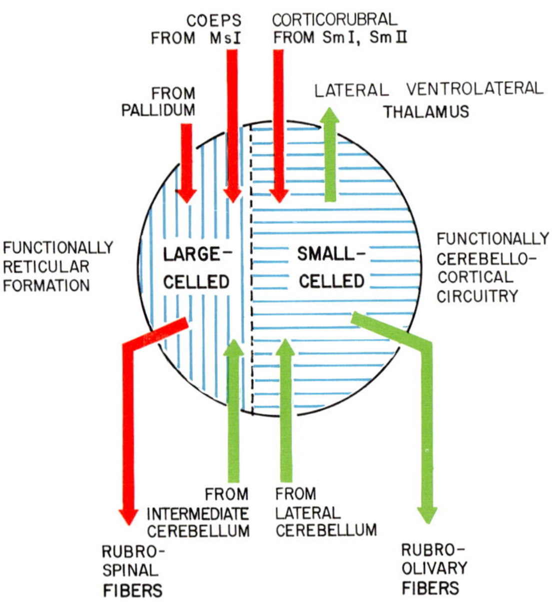

Fig. 7-18. Red nucleus (blue hatched), showing major connections. Green = predominantly cerebellocortical circuits; red = predominantly descending cortical circuits.

lateral nucleus of ventrolateral thalamus), and (probably) pallidothalamic fibers. Presumably, each of these structures therefore has a "body image" (in terms of musculature) inherent in it, and the connections exhibit little convergence or divergence. The major cortical efferents to the basal ganglia pass successively through the putamen (or caudate) and the lateral and medial pallidum, whence a major efferent pathway, the ansa and fasciculus lenticularis, passes under or through the internal capsule to the thalamus (Fig. 7-17).

In spite of extensive investigation, little is known of the functions of the basal ganglia beyond what can be deduced from disease states (see Chap. 24). Experimental stimulation of the basal ganglia often produces no movement or causes movements due to stimulus radiation (excitation spreading to the internal capsule may cause limb flexion; spread to the septal region may cause lip-smacking, swallowing, and salivation). In some experiments, stimulation has caused *adversive* movements, including looking to the opposite side and running in circles away from the stimulated side. Stimulation of the caudate nucleus may inhibit cortically induced movement, due to feedback through the thalamus. In cats, removal of the neocortex does not affect grooming, eating, or sexual behavior, but ablation of the neocortex *and* striate body prevents proper integration of movements into patterns, though the animal remains capable of all appropriate movements in an uncoordinated manner. In primates, lesions of the basal ganglia alone have little clinical effect, but lesions of basal ganglia *and* neocortex cause disturbances somewhat similar to those of basal ganglion disease in man. It appears

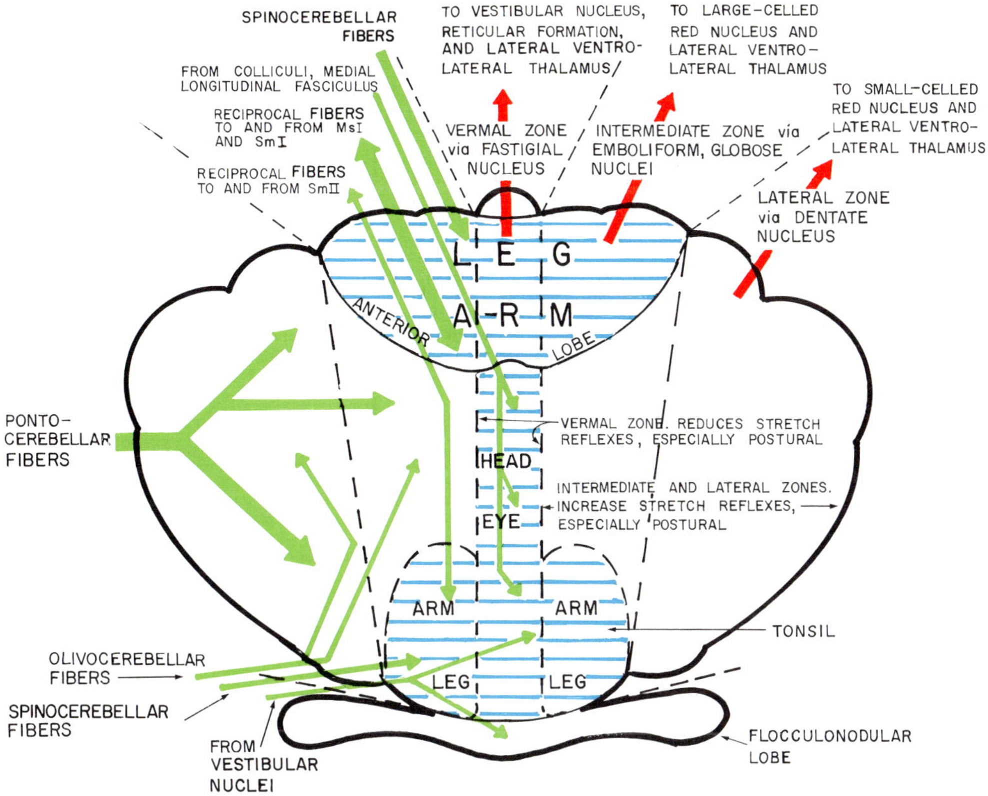

Fig. 7-19. Semischematic representation of cerebellar cortex (imagined as flattened out, upper surface above) showing parasagittal zones and major connections. Blue hatched areas show somatotopic organization. Green = afferent fibers; red = efferent fibers.

that basal ganglia and area 6 of the cortex may act synergistically in modulating (largely inhibiting) the activity of area 4, either by direct cortical connections or by convergence at lower levels, especially at the reticular formation. No consistent pattern of basal ganglion function in the normal animal has yet emerged, in spite of the crippling effects of human lesions in these nuclei.

THE ROLE OF THE RED NUCLEUS

The red nucleus has two functional parts with morphological overlap (Fig. 7-18). Its posterior part is a small, primitive, large-celled area, whose axons form the rubrospinal tract and which may best be regarded as a differentiated part of the brain stem reticular formation. It receives excitatory, monosynaptic COEPS fibers from MsI and from the two "interposed" nuclei (emboliform and globose) of the cerebellum. The more recently developed anterior, small-celled part of the red nucleus does not receive fibers from MsI, but from SmI, SmII, and the contralateral dentate nucleus (the latter connection, at least, is monosynaptic). Efferent fibers pass to the lateral nucleus of the ventrolateral thalamus and to the inferior olives. Since the inferior olive feeds back to the cerebellum, this part of the structure is best regarded as part of the cerebello-cerebral coordinating system.

MOTOR FUNCTION OF THE CEREBELLUM

The cerebellum has no direct connections with lower motoneurons, exerting its influence through the motor systems of the cortex and brain stem. It affects both voluntary activity and postural tonus and receives not only vestibular and proprioceptive input, but also somatosensory, visual, and auditory projections. Anatomically, the major divisions of the cerebellum appear to run laterally (see Chap. 1), but functionally it is best regarded as a series of parasagittal zones (Fig. 7-19). (1) The midline or vermal zone projects to the fastigial and vestibular nuclei and includes the entire flocculonodular lobe, (2) the intermediate or paravermal zone projects to the nucleus interpositus (emboliform and globose nuclei), and (3) the lateral zone projects to the dentate nucleus.

Proprioceptive and somatosensory information is largely projected to the vermal and paravermal zones and is somatotopically organized. Starting superiorly, the body parts are represented in the vermis in this order: leg, arm, head, arm, leg. Visual and auditory representation lie in the posterior (middle) portion of

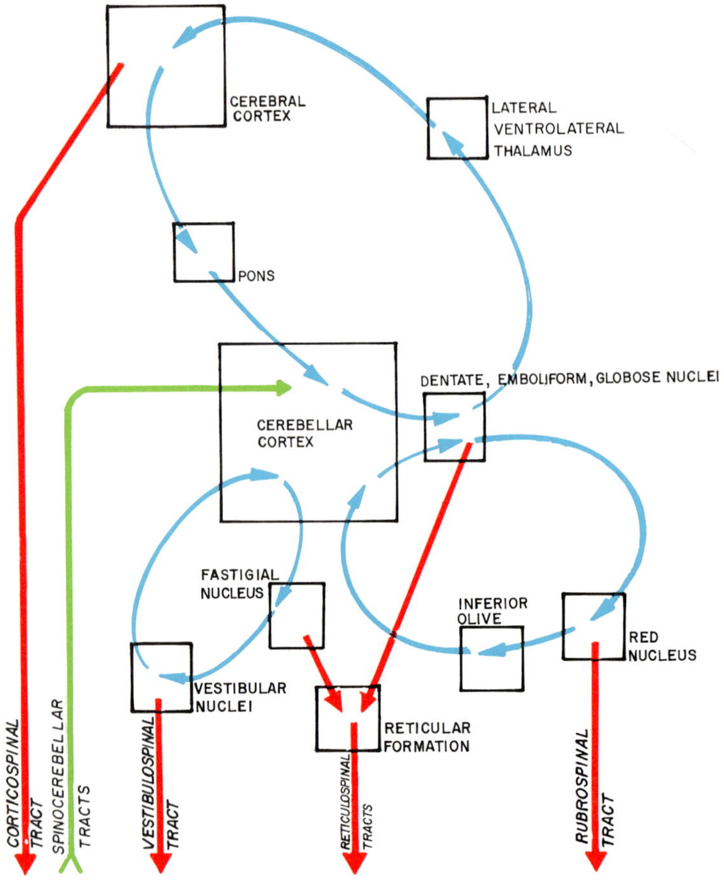

Fig. 7-20. Blue = cerebellar connections, represented as a series of feedback loops; green = spinocerebellar input; red = connections to motor systems.

the vermis, and vestibular input reaches the entire vermis. The rest of the hemispheres (lateral zones) receive input from the pons and inferior olives and do not appear to show somatotopic organization. Somatosensory (in addition to proprioceptive) input is included in the spinocerebellar tracts, and may also be mediated by the spino-olivary and spinoreticular tracts. There are reciprocal somatotopic connections between MsI, SmI, and the upper vermis, SmII and the lower vermis, and cortical areas 18 and 19 and the posterior vermis. Skin stimulation provokes a larger cerebellar response if the cerebral connections are intact, confirming a double sensory input (directly from the ascending tracts and indirectly from the sensory cortex). Much of the cerebellar circuitry is organized as a series of feedback loops (Fig. 7-20).

Equilibration

Equilibration is a function of at least the flocculonodular lobe and probably of the entire vermis. Ablation of the flocculonodular lobe causes loss of balance, in spite of intact postural reflexes and skilled movements. The entire vermis appears to be concerned with standing, which requires vestibular, proprioceptive, and visual input (so that the anatomical input to the vermis corresponds with clinical data). Projection, through the fastigial nucleus, reaches both the reticular formation of the brain stem and the lateral ventrolateral thalamic nucleus and premotor cortex.

Postural Effects

The entire cerebellum appears to be concerned with stretch reflexes and muscle tone, operating through the gamma rather than the alpha motoneurons. Stimulation of the medial anterior lobe inhibits postural muscle stretch reflexes more than those of antagonists, thus effectively inhibiting anti-gravity muscles, apparently through the medial reticular formation. The medial cerebellar projections include fibers from the fastigial nucleus, through the lateral ventrolateral thalamic nucleus, to the cortex. This may be a postural inhibitory pathway additional to that operating through the reticular formation.

Conversely, the intermediate and lateral zones of the cerebellum facilitate stretch reflexes in all muscles, and their absence produces clinical hypotonia. These parts of the cerebellar cortex do not project to the reticular formation, but affect muscle tone through the thalamus and motor cortex. It therefore seems probable that the facilitatory effect of the cerebellum on tonus is exerted through the cortex, possibly by driving the pyramidal neurons. However, unresolved complexities remain in this aspect, as in other aspects, of cerebellar function, since a given area of cerebellar cortex may facilitate or inhibit stretch reflexes and tone, depending on the frequency of electrical stimulation.

Voluntary Movement

Understanding the relationship between the cerebral cortex and cerebellum in the control of voluntary movement probably requires a deep insight into the science of cybernetics and is beyond the scope of this book. Specialized texts may be consulted. The cerebellum, especially its intermediate and lateral zones, is concerned with the rate, range, force, direction, and steadiness of voluntary movements. Since voluntary movement means reducing an initial disparity between the preexisting and the desired positions to zero, continuous feedback is necessary to assess progress. It seems probable that movement is initiated by the cerebral cortex, and that the function of the cerebellum is to detect error and to dampen oscillation. Certainly, cerebellar disease appears to be associated with overdamping at the beginning of a movement (slow start) and underdamping later (intention tremor, slow finish).

Experimentally, lesions of the nucleus interpositus (globose and emboliform nuclei) or dentate nucleus produce ataxia, which is evidence for the involvement of both lateral and intermediate cerebellar zones in control of voluntary movement. The effect of cerebellar ablation might be described as semiquantitative, since partial ablation of the neocerebellum (which excludes the anterior and flocculonodular lobes) causes errors in the force and rate of movements. If ablation includes the dentate nucleus, intention tremor is added, together with errors of range and direction; and if the ablation is bilateral, all signs in man are made considerably worse, including ocular and speech disturbances. The changes resulting from total cerebellar ablation are more severe in primates and include difficulty in balance, as well as hypotonia that is especially obvious, though not necessarily more severe, in the postural or anti-gravity muscles.

BIBLIOGRAPHY

Brodal, A. *Neurological Anatomy in Relation to Clinical Medicine* (2nd ed.). New York, London: Oxford University Press, 1969.

Brooks, V. B., and Stoney, S. D., Jr. Role of pyramidal system in motor control. *Annu. Rev. Physiol.* 33:337-392, 1971.

Eccles, J. C., Ito, M., and Szentágothai, J. *The Cerebellum as a Neuronal Machine.* New York: Springer, 1967.

Elliott, H. C. *Textbook of Neuroanatomy* (2nd ed.). Philadelphia: Lippincott, 1969.

Eyzaguirre, C. *Physiology of the Nervous System.* Chicago: Year Book, 1969.

Gilman, S., Mario, L. A., and Ebel, H. C. Effects of medullary pyramidotomy in the monkey (Pts. I and II). *Brain* 94:495-530, 1971.

Keele, C. A., and Neil, E. (Eds.). *Samson Wright's Applied Physiology* (12th ed.). London: Oxford University Press, 1971.

Nathan, P. W., and Smith, M. C. Effects of two unilateral cordotomies on the motility of the lower limbs. *Brain* 96:471-494, 1973.

O'Brien, J. H., and Conde, H. Functional organisation of the anterior red nucleus. *Brain Res.* 21:345-365, 1970.

Rispal-Padel, L., and Massion, J. Relations between the V-L nucleus and the motor cortex in the cat. *Exp. Brain Res.* 10:331-339, 1970.

Ruch, T. C., Patton, H. D., Woodbury, J. W., and Towe, A. L. *Neurophysiology* (2nd ed.). Philadelphia: Saunders, 1966.

Szabo, J. The efferent projection of the putamen in the monkey. *Exp. Neurol.* 19:463-476, 1967.

Szabo, J. Projections from the body of the caudate nucleus in the rhesus monkey. *Exp. Neurol.* 27:1-15, 1970.

Neuroendocrine Integration

8

Both the central nervous system and a group of endocrine glands controlled by tropic hormones from the pituitary perform homeostatic and adaptive functions in the body, so that harnessing of the two was present at an early evolutionary stage. This integration necessarily involves transduction, from neural impulses to hormones secreted by neural cells. The phenomenon of *neurosecretion* is in some respects similar to neurotransmission (Fig. 8-1). Secretory substances produced by nerve cells travel through the axon to a nerve terminal, where they are stored as large granules, which might be regarded as analogous to the synaptic granules and vesicles in presynaptic knobs. However, the contents of neurosecretory granules, instead of being released into a synaptic cleft or into direct relationship with a muscle or glandular cell, enter small vessels. Thus, neurosecretion differs from neurotransmission in the intervention of a capillary (portal) circulation, as well as in the absence of a specific reuptake mechanism and the lack of a one-to-one relationship between the secreting and target cells.

Neurosecretion occurs in at least three sites in the CNS:

1. In the *neurohypophysis,* where complex neuronal mechanisms converge and cause release of vasopressin (antidiuretic hormone [ADH]) and oxytocin into small vessels of the general circulation.
2. The *median eminence and pituitary stalk,* where equally complex neuronal controls culminate in the release of hypophyseal hypophysiotropic hormones (releasing factors and inhibiting factors) into a special capillary system destined entirely for the adenohypophysis.
3. The *pineal gland,* where neuronal control is conveyed via the peripheral (sympathetic) system and leads to release of melatonin, and probably other methoxyindoles, either into the general circulation or, less probably, into the CSF.

THE NEUROHYPOPHYSIS

Structure

Although situated at the end of the pituitary stalk and in close relation to the adenohypophysis, the neurohypophysis is part of the hypothalamus, specifically of the medial eminence (Fig. 8-2). It is relatively acellular and has considerable vascularity, receiving blood from branches of the inferior hypophyseal artery, itself a direct branch of the internal carotid. These branches form a dense capillary network that drains into the adjacent cavernous sinuses and communicating veins and appears to be largely separate from that of the adenohypophysis. No perikaryons are present (Fig. 8-3), but there are many nerve terminals derived from a prominent nonmyelinated (hypothalamico-hypophyseal) tract passing down the pituitary stalk from cells in the supraoptic and paraventricular nuclei of the anterior hypothalamus. Granular material, stainable by chrome nematoxylin, is present in small amounts in the perikaryons and the tract and in larger amounts in the neurohypophysis itself, apparently in relation to nerve terminals. Electron microscopy shows dense membrane-bound bodies up to 1500 A in diameter, mixed with small vesicles about 400 A in diameter. Similar but smaller bodies are present in the nuclei and tract. The capillaries differ from those of the brain in general in that pores and a small perivascular space are present. Also, the neurohypophysis, like the median eminence, is outside the blood-brain barrier.

Hormones

The stored granular material of the neurohypophysis appears to be a protein-bound peptide. Hormone assays show that its biological activity and degree of stainability are not parallel. The function of the small clear vesicles, which resemble ordinary synaptic vesicles, is unknown, but they appear not to contain peptides. Vasopressin is a peptide containing nine amino acid residues of remarkable phylogenetic constancy: Cys-Tyr-Phe-Glu(NH_2)-Asp(NH_2)-Cys-Pro-Arg-Gly$\cdot NH_2$. Among mammals, only pigs show a different structure (-Lys- replaces -Arg-). The other neurohypophyseal hormone, oxytocin, is also a nonapeptide. It contains Cys-Tyr-Ileu-Glu(NH_2)-Asp(NH_2)-Cys-Pro-Leu-Gly$\cdot NH_2$. A few variations exist in mammals, but in general it closely resembles vasopressin. The amino acid sequences and the ratio between the two peptides are constant for a given species and presumably are genetically determined. Ultracentri-

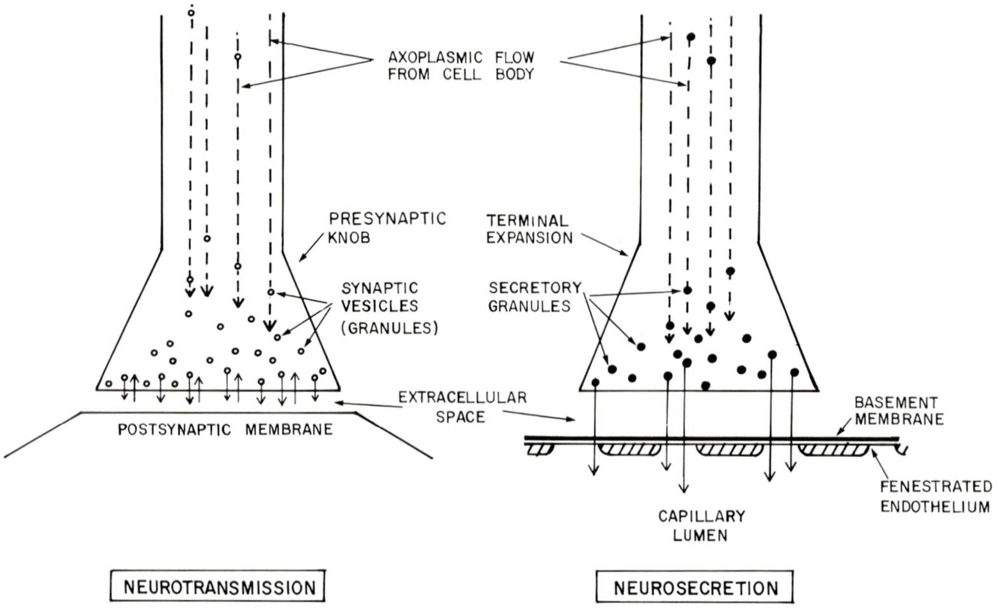

Fig. 8-1. Neurotransmission and neurosecretion contrasted. In the latter, secreted material (e.g., vasopressin, releasing factors) enters capillaries that are not of the cerebral tight-junction type but are fenestrated. There is no reuptake mechanism to the secreting cell, in contrast to its great importance at synapses.

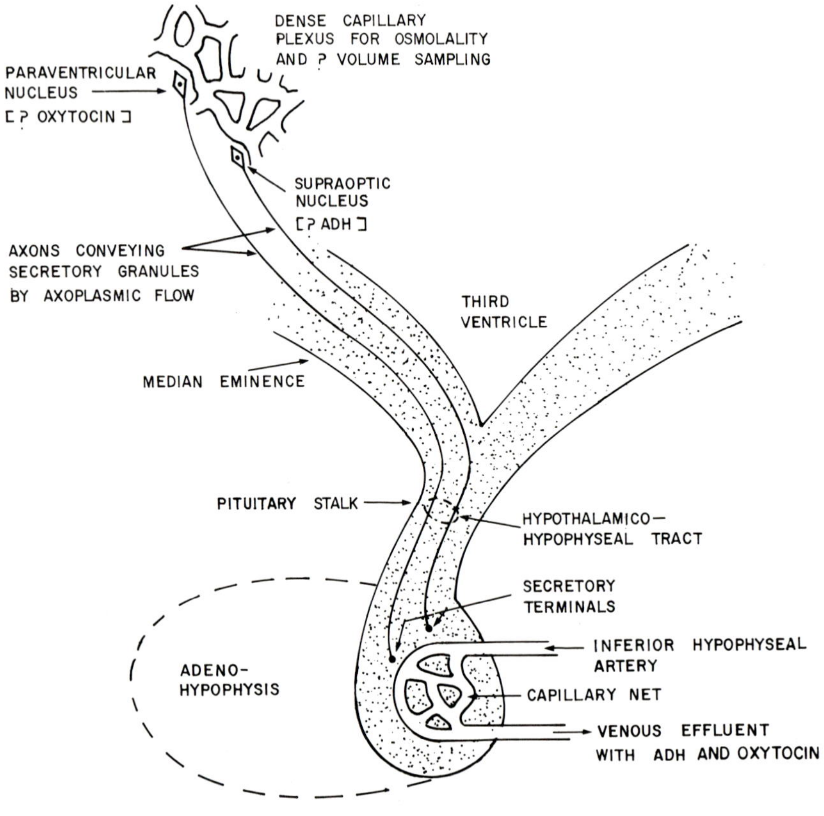

Fig. 8-2. Sagittal section through median eminence and neurohypophysis. Note the hypothalamico-hypophyseal tract (axons of cells in the supraoptic and paraventricular nuclei) and the capillary plexus formed by the inferior hypophyseal artery, a direct branch of the internal carotid vessel. ADH = vasopressin.

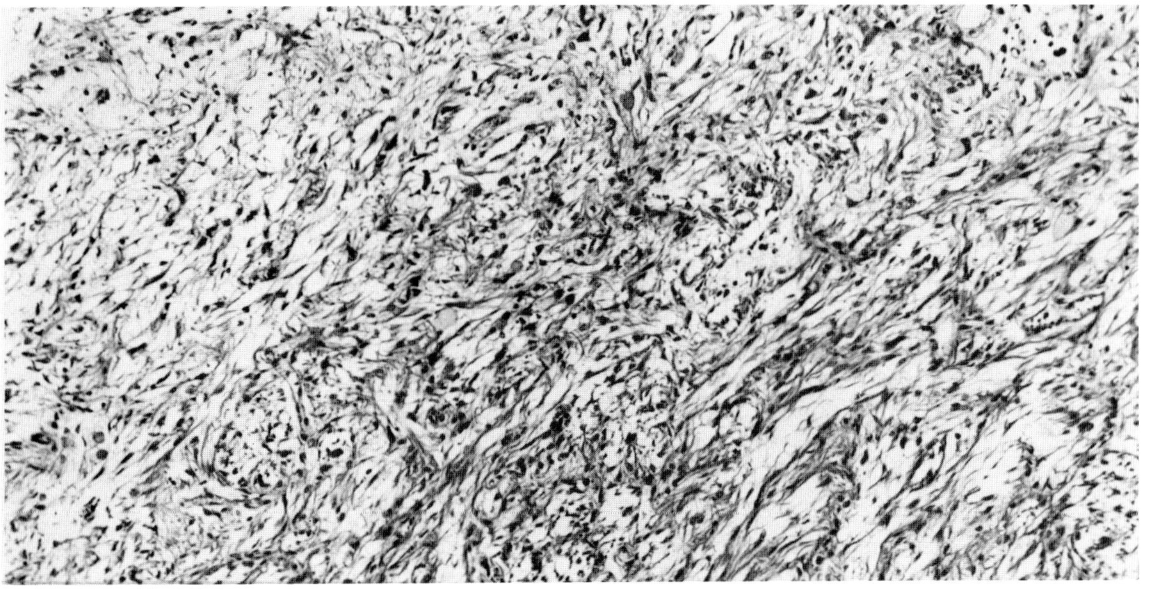

Fig. 8-3. Section of neurohypophysis, showing relative acellularity (nuclei are those of astrocytes and vessels). (H & E, X115; secretory material is not shown by this method.)

fugation confirms the presence of both peptides in secretory granules, but it is not clear whether they occur together or separately. In some mammals there is evidence that vasopressin is formed in the supraoptic nucleus and that oxytocin is formed in the paraventricular nucleus, but this is not confirmed in man. Release of hormones by appropriate stimulation does not reduce neurohypophyseal concentration (although it may reduce stainability), so they must either pass down the hypophyseal stalk or be synthesized within the neurohypophysis at about the same rate as they are released.

Vasopressin

Vasopressin (ADH), which regulates renal water excretion, appears to be the more important of these hormones. Its regulatory function in water excretion implies the existence of osmoreceptors, sensitive to plasma osmolality, and possibly also the existence of volume receptors, sensitive to total plasma volume. Although neither receptor has been located, it seems certain that the osmoreceptors, at least, are in the CNS, possibly in the supraoptic or paraventricular nuclei themselves. Injection of hypertonic solution into the carotid artery stimulates release of ADH (with water retention), whereas hypotonic solutions reduce ADH secretion (with diuresis). However, reduction of total extracellular volume (as by acute hemorrhage) also increases ADH secretion, whereas expansion by transfusing isotonic solutions leads to diuresis. Volume receptors are implied by these observations, since osmolality is normal in the acute stages. If the osmoreceptors are present in the nuclei concerned, neural pathways are probably secondary in physiological osmolality control. However, electrical stimulation of the septal area, and possibly of the amygdala, causes an antidiuretic response, and inappropriate secretion of ADH is associated with some diseases. The location of volume receptors, and therefore of the neural pathways involved, is unknown.

Oxytocin

The role of oxytocin is not always clear. Its only known functions are to increase the rate of sperm passage up the genital canal, to assist in propelling the fetus at birth, and to cause milk injection. Oxytocin is released during lactation and also at coitus, but there is no clear evidence of its release during initiation of labor. There is evidence for concurrent release of both hormones in many situations, but whether this is merely because they are associated in the same granules or because oxytocin has some separate but unrecognized function to perform is not known.

THE ADENOHYPOPHYSIS

Innervation and Blood Supply

The adenohypophysis (pars anterior and pars intermedia, but the latter is not always clearly identifiable in man) appears (Fig. 8-4) to have few afferent nerves, although recent work suggests that fine nerve terminals enter the pars intermedia and make contact with some of its cells.

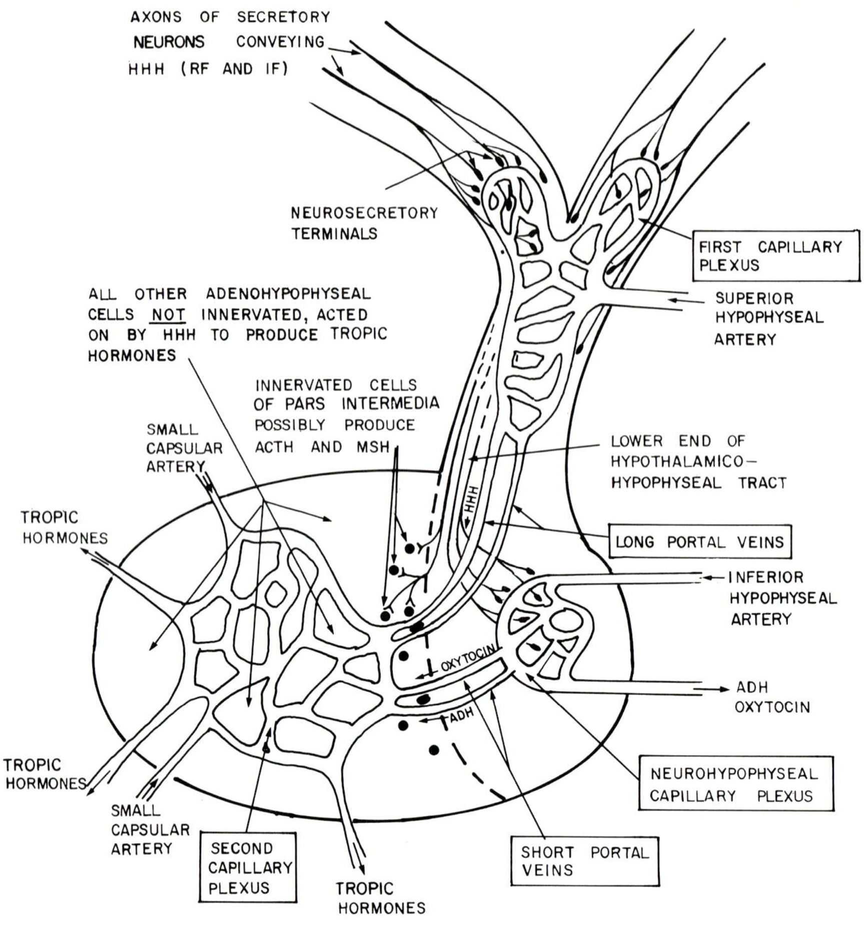

Fig. 8-4. Sagittal section of pituitary and stalk. Note the pituitary portal system, comprising a first plexus supplied by the superior hypophyseal artery, long portal veins, and a second plexus within the adenohypophysis. (The inferior hypophyseal artery also contributes via the neurohypophysis and short portal veins.) A few fibers from the hypothalamico-hypophyseal tract probably reach the adenohypophysis (pars intermedia) and may be involved in ACTH and MSH production. HHH = hypophysiotropic hormone; RF = releasing factor; IF = inhibiting factor; MSH = melanocyte-stimulating hormone; ACTH = adrenocorticotropic hormone.

It has no direct arterial supply except for a few very small vessels that perforate its capsule in the basal region and are capable of sustaining a narrow rim of tissue. The major blood supply is from the *pituitary portal system,* a leash of small veins that originate in a capillary plexus in the central median eminence and pituitary stalk and pass down the stalk (long portal veins) to the adenohypophysis, where they form a second plexus of capillaries and sinusoids among the pituitary cells. The upper plexus is formed by branches of the superior hypophyseal artery, itself springing directly from the internal carotid vessel. A smaller, second component of the portal system (short portal veins) originate in a plexus in the neurohypophysis supplied by the inferior hypophyseal vessel. There is no evidence that there are separate vessel systems for each pituitary hormone, and all the adenohypophyseal vessels anastomose before they unite into several small veins draining into the basal sinuses.

Hormones

At least seven hormones are produced in the adenohypophysis: growth hormone (GH), thyroid-stimulating hormone (TSH) (thyrotropin), follicle-stimulating hormone (FSH), luteinizing hormone (LH), prolactin (PL), adrenocorticotropic hormone (ACTH) (corticotropin) in the pars anterior, and ACTH, together with melanocyte-stimulating hormone (MSH) in the pars intermedia. Several of these hormones have as targets specific organs, some of which in turn produce hormones (e.g., corticosteroids, thyroxine) that may function in a feedback control. However, there is no evidence that feedback hormones are produced in response to PL, GH, or MSH. Indeed, GH may affect all tissues, since, at least in high dosage (but not necessarily physiologically), it antagonizes the actions of insulin, promotes cell uptake of amino

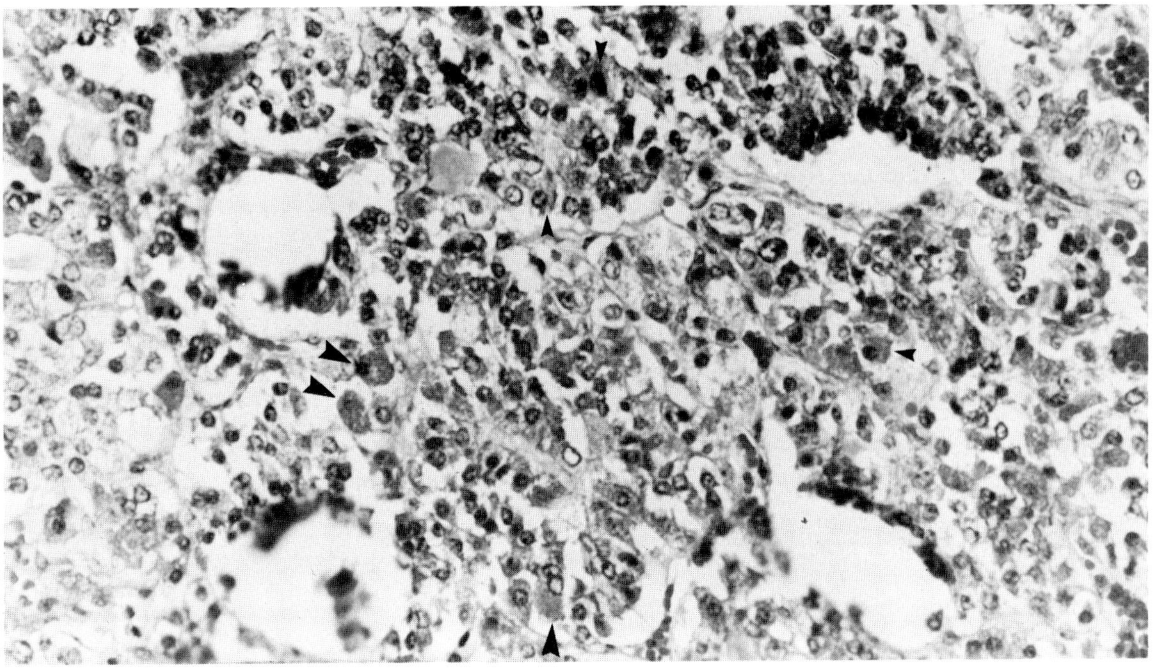

Fig. 8-5. Section of adenohypophysis, showing variation in cellular morphology. At least three cell types may be seen: chromophobes, eosinophils (small arrows), and basophils (large arrows). (Slidder's stain, X 300.)

acids, and causes release of free fatty acids from fat depots. It induces the formation of a substance, *somatomedin* (sulfation factor), in the liver and possibly in other tissues, which stimulates epiphyseal cartilage and causes growth. The importance of MSH in man is largely unknown, but it seems to increase sebaceous secretion. A speculative role in the pathogenesis of paralysis agitans is noted in Chapter 24.

Cell Types in the Adenohypophysis

Three types of cells have long been recognized in the adenohypophysis (Fig. 8-5). These include relatively small, agranular, lightly staining (chromophobe) cells, which appear to form the majority; moderate numbers of larger cells with coarse granules stainable by acid dyes (eosinophils or acidophils); and small numbers of large cells with many or few granules stained by basic dyes such as hematoxylin (basophils). In view of the production of seven hormones, attempts at further subdivision by multiple-stain combinations have been made. Thus, the eosinophils (alpha cells) have been divided into types with large granules, probably releasing PL, and types with medium-sized granules, producing GH. The basophils (beta cells) have been separated into two large angular varieties, one thought to form ACTH and MSH, and the other to form TSH and smaller round cells associated with FSH and LH. The results of such multiple stain methods have not proved to be perfectly reproducible, and more recent investigations have combined the use of isotope-labeled antibodies to pituitary hormones with electron microscopy. Excluding the chromophobes, five cell types have been identified:

GH-producing cells are round or oval and dispersed mainly in the central region. They contain secretion granules 3000 to 3500 A in diameter.

ACTH-producing cells are also found largely in the central region, often surrounded by a cluster of GH-forming cells, and contain granules 2000 A in diameter, found primarily at the periphery of the cell.

TSH-producing cells occur in irregular clusters distinct from the GH and ACTH groups. Their 1500-A granules tend to be peripheral in the cytoplasm and may be uniformly dense or show a dense core.

PL-producing cells are scattered in the central and dorsolateral areas and are irregular in shape, with very coarse granules 8000 A in diameter.

FSH- and LH-producing cells seem to be concentrated in the anterior and ventral pituitary and to contain either or both hormones as granules 2000 to 2500 A in diameter. Cells producing FSH cannot be distinguished from those producing LH, and it is possible that one cell can form both hormones.

The significance of the differential distributions within the adenohypophysis is unknown. MSH-forming cells have not been described. Indeed, the cells of origin of ACTH and MSH are the least certain of any, and it is possible that they are produced by the same or closely similar types. Both are of low molecular weight and are at least partly formed in the pars intermedia, probably by innervated cells. Thus, they may occupy an intermediate position between the directly secreted ADH and oxytocin and those adenohypophyseal hormones whose producing cells are not innervated.

Recently, it has been suggested that there is no permanent specialization of adenohypophyseal cells, any of which may change the hormone they produce without having first to revert to chromophobe status, but this remains to be evaluated.

HYPOTHALAMIC-HYPOPHYSIOTROPIC HORMONES (RELEASING AND INHIBITING FACTORS)

The location of the pituitary and its attachment to the hypothalamus, together with the well-known effects of psychic and environmental factors (stress, coitus, suckling, profound emotion) on pituitary function, long ago suggested a CNS influence on the pituitary mediated through the hypothalamus. The failure to demonstrate any major nerve supply to the adenohypophysis, and the discovery of the pituitary portal system of vessels, indicated that humoral factors might be involved. Confirmation that some neurons were capable of secretion directly into vessels, as in the neurohypophysis, led to speculation that other hypothalamic neurons might be secretory, their hormones being liberated into the first capillary plexus of the portal system and thence conveyed to the pituitary cells. Since seven pituitary hormones are known, and there might be both a releasing and an inhibiting factor for each, a total of 14 such factors were hypothesized. The existence of such factors in no way precludes the possibility that the isolated pituitary might have an intrinsic "basal" secretion rate for each hormone, which would then be modulated by the hypothalamic factors. In fact, the isolated pituitary appears to produce significant amounts only of PL and possibly MSH, suggesting that releasing factors are important for at least the other five hormones and preponderate over inhibiting factors under most physiological conditions. The converse might apply to PL and MSH.

If these speculations are correct, a "chain of command" much like the following can be postulated for each pituitary hormone:

1. Influences from the CNS in general, perhaps especially the limbic and reticular formations, converge on the hypothalamus and modulate the activity of neurosecretory cells by means of the usual neurotransmitters.
2. Neurosecretory cells elaborate and release the appropriate releasing factor (RF) or inhibiting factor (IF) into the pituitary portal system.
3. These factors modulate the production or release of pituitary tropic hormone by the appropriate cell type via the adenyl cyclase—cyclic adenosine monophosphate (cAMP) system.
4. Pituitary tropic hormone is released into the general circulation and acts on its selected target(s), in some instances causing release of a third hormone (corticosteroids, thyroxine).

The isolation, characterization, and synthesis of a few of the releasing and inhibiting factors, with circumstantial evidence for others, have confirmed that this concept is valid. However, there may well be fewer than the postulated 14 factors, with overlapping of activity.

Characterized or Partially Characterized Factors

Thyrotropin-Releasing Factor

Thyrotropin-releasing factor (TRF) has been synthesized. It is a tripeptide (pyro)Glu-His-Pro$\cdot NH_2$, of remarkably constant structure in many mammalian species. Synthetic analogues of lower or, rarely, higher potency have been made. It causes release of TSH and PL, but the effects are separable, since suckling or exogenous estrogen only raises PL, and exogenous thyroxin only lowers TSH. It does not appear that TRF is the normal physiological stimulus for PL production. Surprisingly, hypothyroidism or hyperthyroidism have parallel effects on serum TSH and PL levels.

Luteinizing Hormone Releasing Factor

Luteinizing hormone releasing factor (LRF) has also been isolated and synthesized. It is the decapeptide (pyro)Glu-His-Trp-Ser-Tyr-Gly-Leu-Arg-Pro-Gly$\cdot NH_2$. Synthetic LRFs and LRF antagonists have been made. Other naturally occurring LRFs may exist. Luteinizing hormone releasing factor functions also as a follicle stimulating hormone releasing factor (FRF); it is not known whether or not there is a separate natural FRF. As already noted, pituitary cells producing the two hormones separately have not yet been identified. The factor isolated is often designated LRF/FRF, but at least in some species, a separate crude hypothalamic extract has FRF activity. Since LH and FSH are not naturally produced in parallel, one must suppose either separate releasing factors or possibly separate inhibiting factors (LIF and FIF), which could independently modulate the action of LRF/FRF. Synthetic inhibiting factors with such specificities are known, but so far there is no evidence for naturally occurring factors of this kind.

Growth Hormone Inhibiting Factor

Growth hormone inhibiting factor (GIF) (somatostatin) has been isolated. It is a tetradecapeptide H-Ala-Gly-Cys-Lys-Asp$\cdot NH_2$-Phe-Phe-Trp-Lys-Thr-Phe-Thr-Ser-Cys$\cdot$OH, with the two cystyl residues linked by a disulfide bridge. It is reported to inhibit the formation not only of GH, but also of TSH and sometimes of PL. It may also have a direct action on more peripheral tissues such as the pancreas.

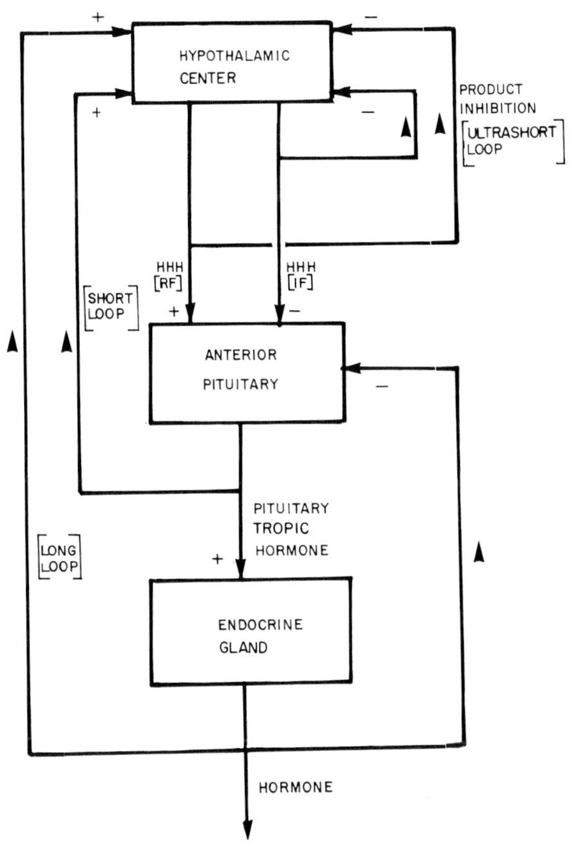

Fig. 8-6. Feedback mechanisms involved in modulation of adenohypophyseal hormone production (arrows pointing upward). Note the possibilities for either inhibition (−) or stimulation (+) at hypothalamic and adenohypophyseal levels, allowing flexible and graded responses.

Other Releasing and Inhibiting Factors

Suggested structures for growth hormone releasing factor (GRF, a possible decapeptide) and melanocyte stimulating hormone inhibiting factor (MIF) remain to be confirmed. Although corticotropin-releasing factor (CRF) was one of the first to be suspected to exist on physiological grounds, it has so far eluded capture and has even occasionally been equated with vasopressin. Certainly, vasopressin does release ACTH, but it is concentrated in the neurohypophysis, rather than in the median eminence as is CRF. Its releasing activity may be associated with the innervation of some ACTH- and MSH-producing cells in the pars intermedia. There is little or no evidence at present for releasing or inhibiting factors other than those that have been mentioned.

Feedback Mechanisms

The concept of a negative feedback at the level of the adenohypophyseal cell (e.g., high blood levels of thyroxine inhibiting the formation of TSH) has been held for some time, but the discovery of releasing and inhibiting factors has led to further elaborations (Fig. 8-6). In the case of a target organ that produces a hormone, feedback could operate at various levels:

1. *Long-loop feedback:* target organ hormone effects on production of hypothalamic hormones.
2. *Short-loop feedback:* pituitary hormone effects on production of hypothalamic hormones.
3. *Ultrashort-loop feedback:* hypothalamic hormone effects on their own production (product inhibition).
4. *"Classic" feedback:* from target organ hormone to pituitary cell.

Where there is probably no target organ hormone (as is the case with GH and PL), long-loop and classic feedback would not be available, and control would depend on the short-loop and ultrashort-loop feedback. Feedback has generally been regarded as negative. This is logical enough in respect to the effect of a target organ hormone, appropriate blood levels of which are the end result of the whole system. However, since both releasing and inhibiting factors are involved, and feedback other than from the target organ hormones occurs, as in short-loop and ultrashort-loop feedback, the possibility of positive feedback must also be considered. There is some evidence that while estrogen and thyroxine have negative feedback effects at the pituitary cell, they exert positive feedback at the hypothalamus, increasing the release of LRF/FRF and TRF respectively. The effect on the pituitary cell appears to be a blockade of releasing factor action, so that a delicately poised system results. It might be assumed that pituitary tropic hormones could have positive feedback to the hypothalamus, since raised levels of such hormones (produced by deficient target organ hormones) would otherwise be antagonized by a reduction of releasing factor secretion.

This is an active field of investigation, and while at present little is known of detailed feedback mechanisms, especially for hormones such as GH and PL, it seems likely that information will be available in the near future, with obvious implications for the treatment of human endocrine disorders.

Sites of Production of Hypothalamic-Hypophysiotropic Hormones (Releasing and Inhibiting Factors)

It is well established that many neurons in the supraoptic and paraventricular nuclei are secretory and that their axons pass down the pituitary stalk to the neurohypophysis and there store or release vasopressin and oxytocin, as appropriate. Electron microscopists have differentiated between the typical

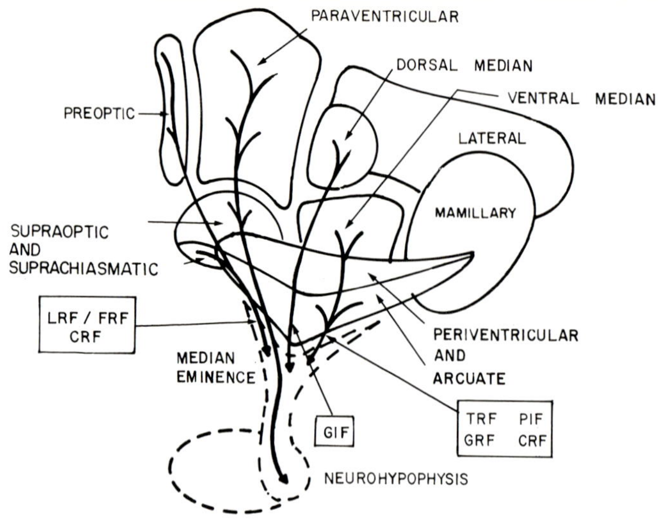

Fig. 8-7. Areas within the hypothalamus that may be concerned in controlling production of pituitary tropic hormones, according to current speculation. Note the anterior group, probably related to LRF/FRF and CRF, and the middle group, related to TRF, GRF, CRF, and PIF (for abbreviations, see text). No function of the posterior areas in hormonal control is established.

(nonsecretory) neurons and those that secrete, the latter having the characteristics of more active metabolic and synthetic activity, including the following:

1. Increased cell, nuclear, and nucleolar size, with folding of the nuclear envelope, suggesting more active transfer of material.
2. Increased rough endoplasmic reticulum containing amorphous material, located especially at the periphery of the cell.
3. A prominent perinuclear Golgi's complex and increased mitochondria and other organelles.
4. The frequent presence (depending on physiological status at the time) of large secretory granules, often with a dense core, 1300 to 1800 A across. Many such cells are found in the supraoptic (SO) and paraventricular (PV) nuclei.

Attempts to locate neurosecretory cells in other parts of the hypothalamus have not been unequivocally successful. Where they are present, they appear to be a much less permanent feature than in the SO and PV areas. They seem to respond to a physiological stimulus and then revert to a resting state, in which they cannot be distinguished from typical nonsecretory forms. In the rabbit, coitus or castration induces neurosecretory changes in about 10% of neurons of the preoptic (PO) and medial supraoptic (suprachiasmatic, SC) regions, associated with increased circulating LH. A few such neurosecretory cells have also been noted in the medial part of the periventricular nuclei (arcuate nuclei, Arc). A further approach to the problem of localization has been the study of uptake of isotope-labeled estrogen by the CNS. This occurs largely in the periventricular (arcuate), preoptic, and ventromedial nuclei, as well as in the corticobasal amygdala, suggesting that such hypothalamic and limbic centers may be involved in the control of LRF/FRF.

Most of the information available, however, has come from meticulous studies involving the destruction, isolation, or stimulation of defined parts of the hypothalamus — studies complicated by the necessity to leave intact the median eminence and stalk, which serve as a final pathway common to discharge of all releasing and inhibiting factors. Such studies indicate that there are two main neurosecretory centers (Fig. 8-7) in addition to that for the neurohypophysis. One is the preoptic-suprachiasmatic (PO-SC) region, and the other includes the ventromedial and arcuate nuclei (VM-Arc). The PO-SC area produces LRF and FRF, and, not surprisingly, since physiologically and chemically they appear to be the same, there is considerable overlap between them. Nonetheless, it has been claimed that some areas, such as PO, produce only LRF, whereas in the region of the adjacent PV nucleus, only FRF is provoked by stimulation. The identity, or lack of identity, of LRF and FRF and a possible multiplicity of factors with similar activity remain confusing. The more posterior VM-Arc region appears to be associated with the formation of TRF, growth hormone releasing factor (GRF), and prolactin inhibiting factor (PIF), though the area for the former may also extend to the SC nuclei, and the area for the latter to the dorsomedial nuclei. Corticotropin releasing factor is apparently associated with an extensive area covering much of both regions. Growth hormone inhibiting factor (somatostatin) may be associated with the dorsomedial nuclei.

To associate a region in the hypothalamus with a factor, whether releasing or inhibiting, is obviously technically difficult. Even then, the meaning of the

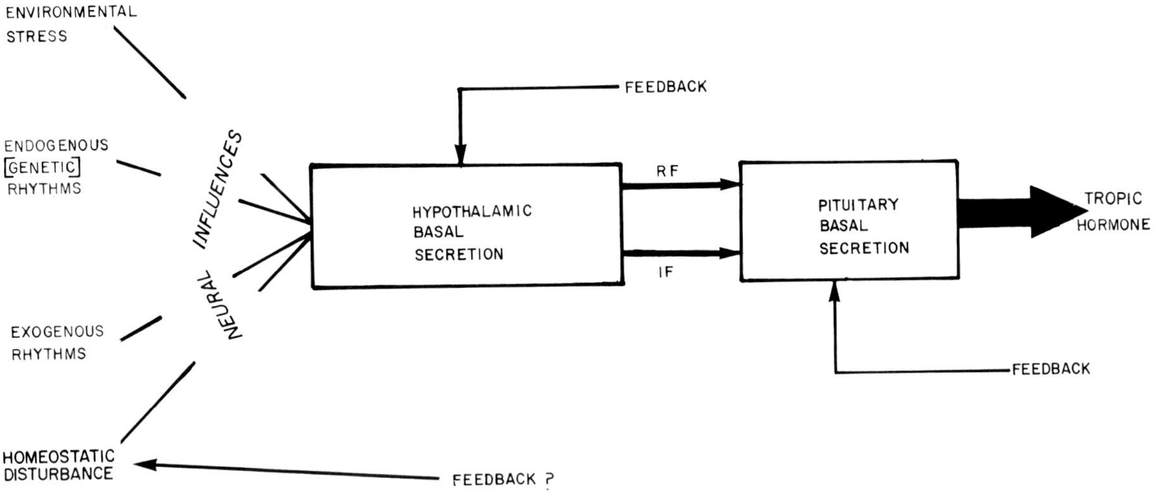

Fig. 8-8. Interplay of factors in modulating secretion of pituitary tropic hormones. RF = releasing factor; IF = inhibiting factor.

association remains to be elucidated. Since the median eminence is relatively acellular and consists largely of axons, glia, and vessels (like the pituitary stalk with which it may be regarded as forming a functional unit), it is unlikely that it is more than a transportation and storage area. It is assumed that the axons are those originating in the areas previously described (PO-SC and VM-Arc, possibly also dorsomedial), though this is not proved in all cases. It is also assumed that the same areas contain the neurosecretory cells (mixed with ordinary neurons) in spite of the inadequacy of electron-microscopic proof. It is less clear whether these "secretory" areas are the point of convergence of feedback and neural controls, or whether integration of humoral and neural influences occurs at a higher level (in or outside the hypothalamus), which in turn controls the secretory areas.

In any event, the level of production of pituitary hormones (Fig. 8-8) depends on at least four factors:

1. The basic level of secretion of the unstimulated (e.g., isolated) pituitary gland, which may vary from zero (always requiring releasing factor to secrete) to high (sometimes requiring inhibiting factor for the maintenance of physiological levels).
2. The basic level of secretion of the unstimulated neurosecretory area (much harder to determine, but not necessarily zero). Thus, there is evidence that after deafferentation, the hypothalamus continues to form CRF and possibly other factors.
3. The effects of the various feedback chains, which may have net inhibitory or releasing results (see p. 159).
4. The effects of neural input to the hypothalamus, which are extremely complex and include the imposition of diurnal rhythms as well as responses to environmental situations.

In the foregoing it has been generally accepted that the effects of releasing and inhibiting factors are exclusively on the adenohypophysis and mediated exclusively via the pituitary portal system. The former assumption is based on the extreme dilution of the hypothalamic factors by the time they reach the general circulation, rather than on any rigorous demonstration that they do not, in fact, affect peripheral structures; and, as has been noted, GIF, at least, can be shown experimentally to have peripheral effects. Transplanted pituitary tissue, however, does not appear sufficiently stimulated by the general circulation to function normally, and it remains probable that the major effects of hypothalamic factors are exerted on the adenohypophysis, although newer assay methods can detect such factors in blood and even in urine. The second assumption, that releasing and inhibiting factors act only via the pituitary portal blood, has been challenged by studies of peculiarities of the ependyma in the infundibular recess, as well as by the detection of such factors in the CSF, in which they might be carried from the third ventricle to the adenohypophysis at the base of the brain via the foramina of Magendie and Luschka. For details of this intriguing work the bibliography refers the reader to more specialized texts and articles.

It seems fair to say that at present there is no evidence that in man such transfer of hypothalamic factors, though it undoubtedly occurs to a minor extent, has clinical significance. If it were to be proved significant, a possible new dimension would be added to the association between noncommunicating hydrocephalus and pituitary-hypothalamic dysfunction, which is presently attributed to distortion and pressure.

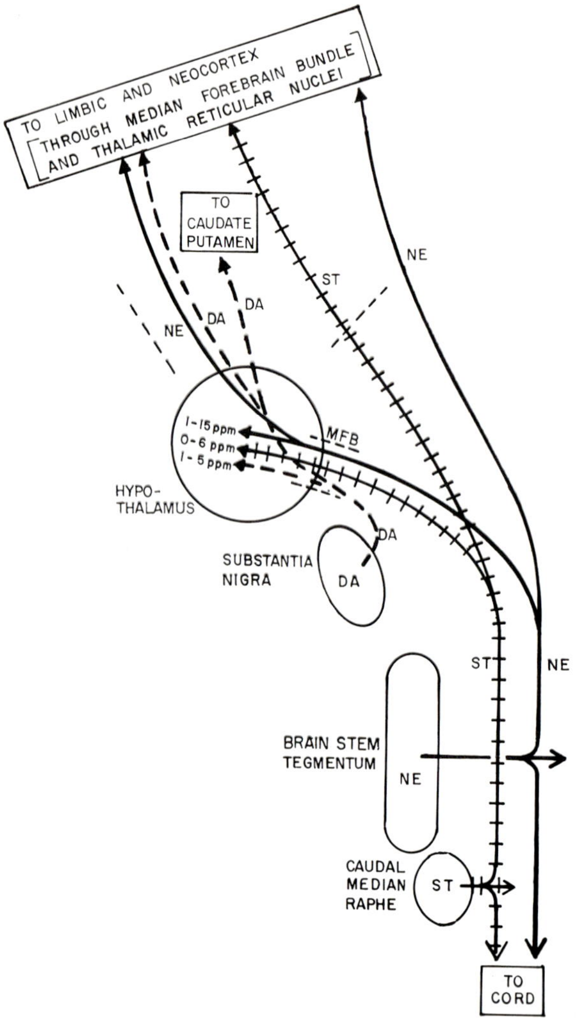

Fig. 8-9. Innervation of the hypothalamus by adrenergic, dopaminergic, and serotonergic fibers originating in the brain stem. Most of these fibers enter the hypothalamus in the median forebrain bundle. Concentrations in the hypothalamus are expressed in parts per million by weight (ppm) and are among the highest in the brain. DA = dopamine; NE = norepinephrine; ST = serotonin; MFB = median forebrain bundle.

NEURAL CONTROL OF HYPOTHALAMIC SECRETORY FUNCTION

The secretion of releasing and inhibiting factors is affected by many stimuli, some of which may operate by humoral mechanisms (e.g., hypoglycemia) and are homeostatic in nature. Others operate wholly or in part through the CNS. These vary from acute physiological stimuli (coitus in rodents) to nonspecific factors such as stress and the diurnal variations observed in hormone levels. The relationship between the factors released and the releasing stimulus is not always apparent. Thus, insulin-induced hypoglycemia releases not only ACTH and GH (presumably by increasing CRF and GRF), but also PL (presumably by reducing PIF or by production of the unknown prolactin releasing factor [PRF]). Also, there is species variation. Most animals respond to stress by increased levels of GH and TSH, but in the stressed rat, both fall. The significance of the diurnal rhythms, in which GH, ACTH, and PL (in both sexes) all rise during sleep, is certainly not immediately apparent. It is difficult to avoid the conclusion that many of the actions of pituitary hormones remain unknown, particularly that of PL.

Whatever the known and unknown purposes served, there is dense innervation of the whole hypothalamus (Fig. 8-9), including many of those intrinsic neurons that seem to be nonsecretory, and levels of many neurotransmitters, including norepinephrine, dopamine, and serotonin, are among the highest in the brain. A dense network of norepinephrine terminals originates from cells of the pons and medulla. Among other functions (Fig. 8-10), this network appears to enhance formation of PIF and reduce PL levels, thereby deinhibiting a dopaminergic system (intrinsic to the hypothalamus) with cell bodies in the arcuate nucleus and terminals in the PO-SC area and allowing increased formation of LRF/FRF. This dopaminergic system is inhibited by estrogen (including oral contraceptives) and testosterone, which produce lowered LRF/FRF levels. Serotonin terminals originate from cells in the caudal midbrain, and concentration of the transmitter in the hypothalamus is sharply reduced by severing these ascending fibers. Serotonergic fibers appear to be inhibitory to LRF/FRF formation. Serotonin metabolism in the hypothalamus is enhanced by exogenous corticosteroids and reduced by adrenalectomy, so it may play a part in the adrenal feedback mechanism. Dopaminergic fibers from elsewhere in the CNS do not reach the hypothalamus in great numbers, but there is a short intrinsic tract (Fig. 8-10), and dopamine concentration, especially in the arcuate region, is high. Incubation of hypothalamic and pituitary tissues (but not pituitary tissue alone) with dopamine increases the release of LH and FSH.

The effects of transmitter amines on the control of estrogen levels have been most convenient for experimental study, but transmitters undoubtedly have equally important roles in the control of adrenal steroids, thyroxine, prolactin, and other hormones.

These systems are mainly ascending, but there is also extensive descending innervation of the hypothalamus from the limbic system, much of it entering from the anterior aspect. Severing these connections eliminates the diurnal rhythmicity of hormone secretion and also prevents the LH response to coitus in rodents, apparently by severing connections with the amygdala. The effects of environmental stress are probably mediated by the limbic system.

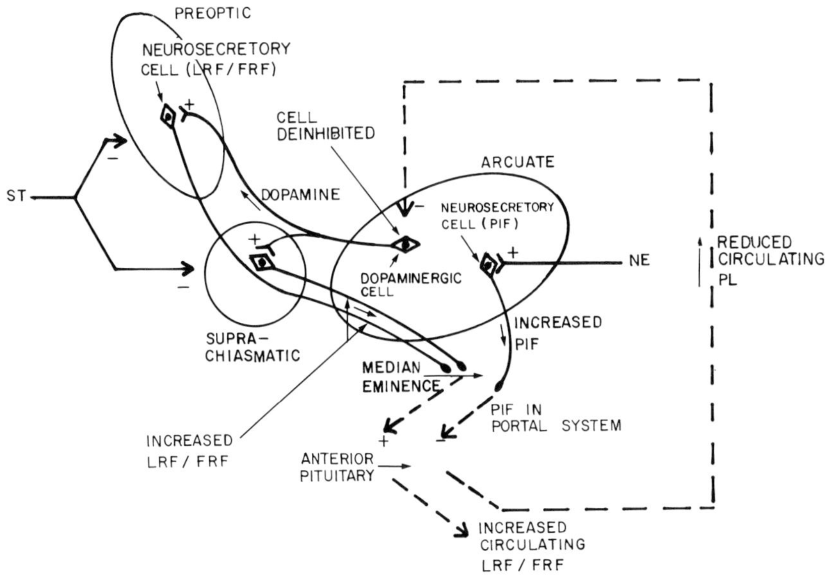

Fig. 8-10. Example of the effects of hypothalamic innervation (modulation of LRF/FRF release – see text). Other, doubtless more fundamental, effects remain for future elucidation. NE = adrenergic terminal; ST = serotonergic terminal; PIF = prolactin inhibiting factor; PL = prolactin.

THE PINEAL GLAND

The pineal of the mammal differs from that of the amphibian in several ways. It no longer has morphologically recognizable photoreceptive cells, but contains a new parenchymal cell, *the pinealocyte,* with an electron-microscopic appearance suggesting secretory function. It has lost all direct neural connections with the CNS, its only innervation being from postganglionic sympathetic neurons in the superior cervical ganglia. It is the only mammalian organ to retain 5-hydroxyindole-O-methyltransferase (5-HIOMT), which synthesizes melatonin and other methoxyindoles and is widespread in amphibian tissues. In summary, the mammalian pineal is no longer a photoneural but a neuroendocrine transducer, responding to norepinephrine secreted by the sympathetic postganglionic nerve terminals.

Structure

The pineal (Fig. 8-11) develops from the neurectoderm of the third ventricle and pia of the tela choroidea, the latter forming the capsule and septa. The septa carry blood vessels and small nerve bundles to penetrate the gland. The neurectoderm forms two types of cells, one apparently an astrocyte, containing a few microtubules and typical glial fibrils, 50 to 60 A in diameter; the processes of these cells end as expansions, frequently containing glycogen, on the true pineal cells, other glial cells, and around the perivascular spaces. The second cell type (pinealocyte) shows numerous microtubules running randomly within the cell body and its extensive branching processes. The nucleus tends to be vesicular. The cytoplasm contains clumps of basophilic material, which is dissolved by ribonuclease, and cell organelles, including a moderate amount of granular endoplasmic reticulum and polyribosomes. The blood supply is from small branches of the medial choroidal arteries. Concurrently, the adrenal cortex and the infant pineal undergo a series of morphological transformations beginning at birth (irrespective of the gestational age) and completed within the first year. The significance of these changes is unknown.

Pineal Metabolism

The pinealocyte synthesizes serotonin, melatonin, and other methoxyindoles from tryptophan (Fig. 8-12) and appears to be stimulated by norepinephrine. Serotonin is synthesized by successive actions of the enzymes tryptophan hydroxylase (confined to serotonin-forming tissues) and L-amino acid decarboxylase (widely distributed). In the pineal, as in other tissues, serotonin is converted to 5-hydroxyindoleacetaldehyde, which is unstable and may then be oxidized to 5-hydroxyindoleacetic acid (5-HIAA) or reduced to 5-hydroxytryptophol. In the pineal only, 5-HIAA or 5-hydroxytryptophan may be methylated by 5-hydroxyindole-O-methyltransferase (5-HIOMT) to form methoxyindoles, but, more important, serotonin itself can be converted to melatonin, N-acetylation being followed by 5-HIOMT methylation. In

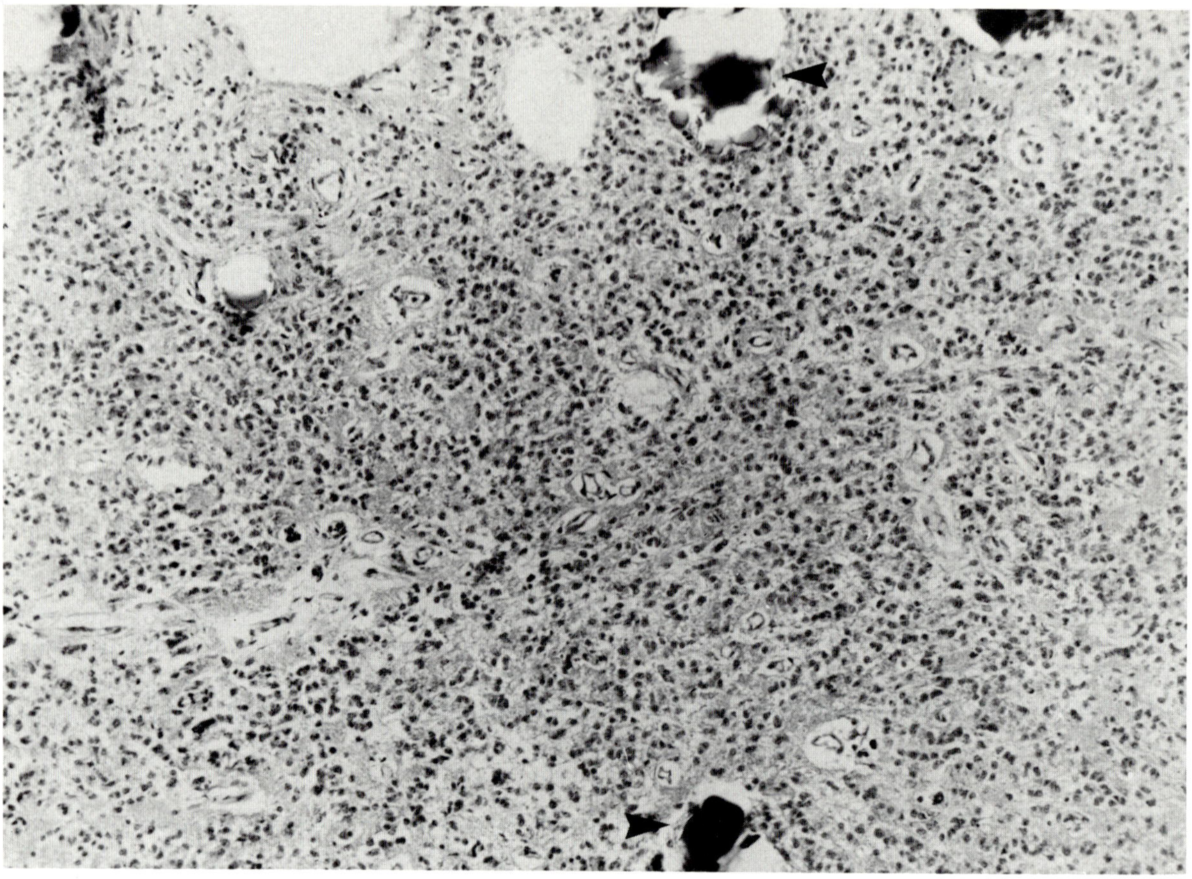

Fig. 8-11. Section of pineal gland (adult). The neurons and astrocytes are scarcely distinguishable with routine stains. Small mineralized granules are seen (arrows) and increase in frequency with advancing age. Thus, the pineal can often be seen radiologically and used in assessing distortions of intracranial contents. (H & E, X115.)

mammals, as far as is known, melatonin is only formed in the pineal. Since it may be found in minute amounts in peripheral tissues and neurons, it is presumed to be secreted by the pineal gland, either into the blood or the CSF. Injected into the blood, it enters all tissues, including the brain, and is chiefly cleared and metabolized by the liver (sulfation or glucuronidation). Injected into the CSF, it is concentrated in some areas, especially in the midbrain and median eminence, where it may be detected for several hours and is then metabolized to an unidentified compound, also stored in the brain. It is therefore probable that some or all pineal melatonin is secreted directly into the bloodstream.

The foregoing summary of pineal metabolism, though based on animal experimentation, may be assumed to be valid in man, since metabolic pathways show considerable phylogenetic constancy. The following comments on pineal physiology, however, cannot be so confidently extrapolated from mammals (largely rodents) to man, since the functional relationships discussed are much less constant. However, the interest and potential significance of human pineal function justifies a brief consideration of its possible roles as an endocrine organ and in "timekeeping" mechanisms.

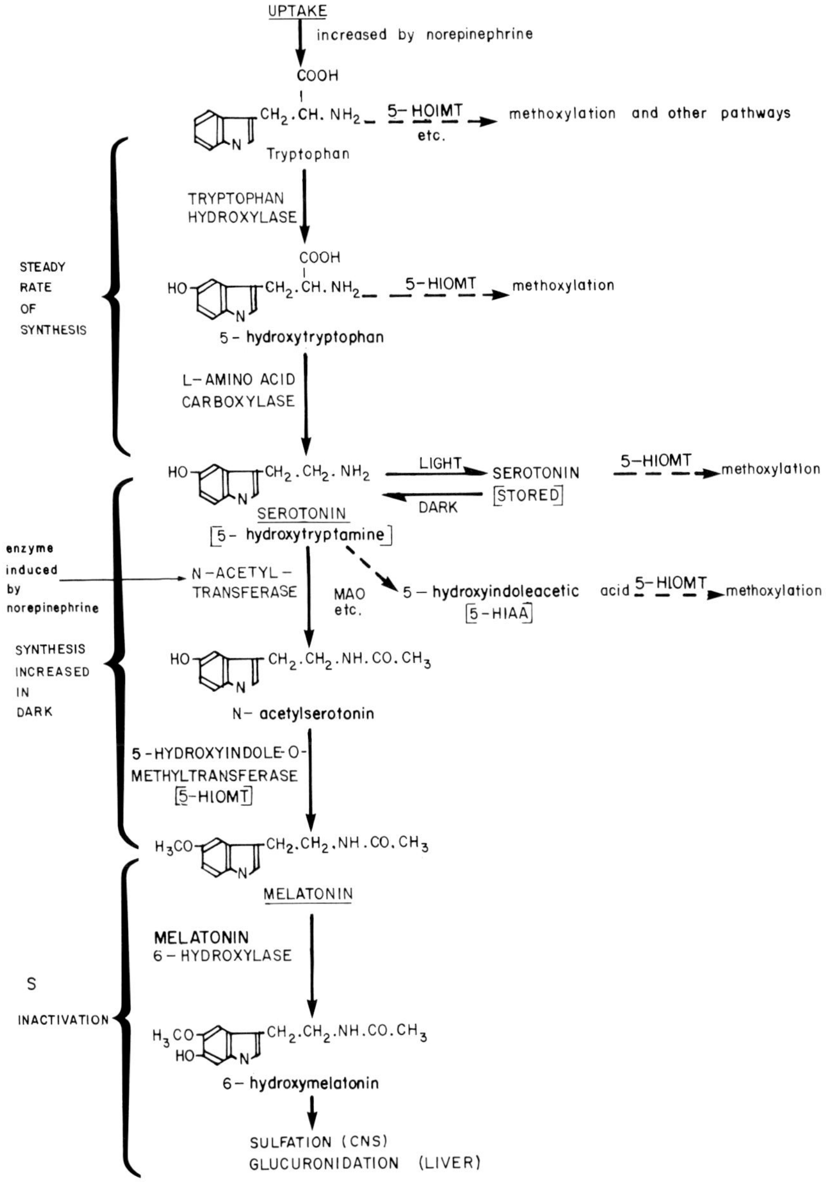

Fig. 8-12. Tryptophan metabolism in the pineal. Serotonin is largely stored during periods of light exposure and partly converted to melatonin during darkness. Note the production of other methoxylated compounds, some of which are probably of equal or greater importance compared with melatonin.

Diurnal Rhythms in Pineal Metabolism

The pineal content of serotonin shows marked daily variation. Normally, it is highest during daylight and lowest at night. Reversing the light-dark cycle changes the serotonin rhythm so that it again becomes highest during periods of light, even if this involves complete phase reversal. Neither constant light, constant darkness, nor blinding abolishes the rhythm, which persists with a regular periodicity of approximately 24 hours. The cycle is totally abolished by various lesions of the CNS or autonomic system, including removal of the superior cervical ganglion and section of the median forebrain bundle. It is therefore not intrinsic to the pineal gland, but rather to some CNS center, possibly the hypothalamus. Control reaches the pineal by a peculiarly roundabout route (Fig. 8-13): from the hypothalamus via the

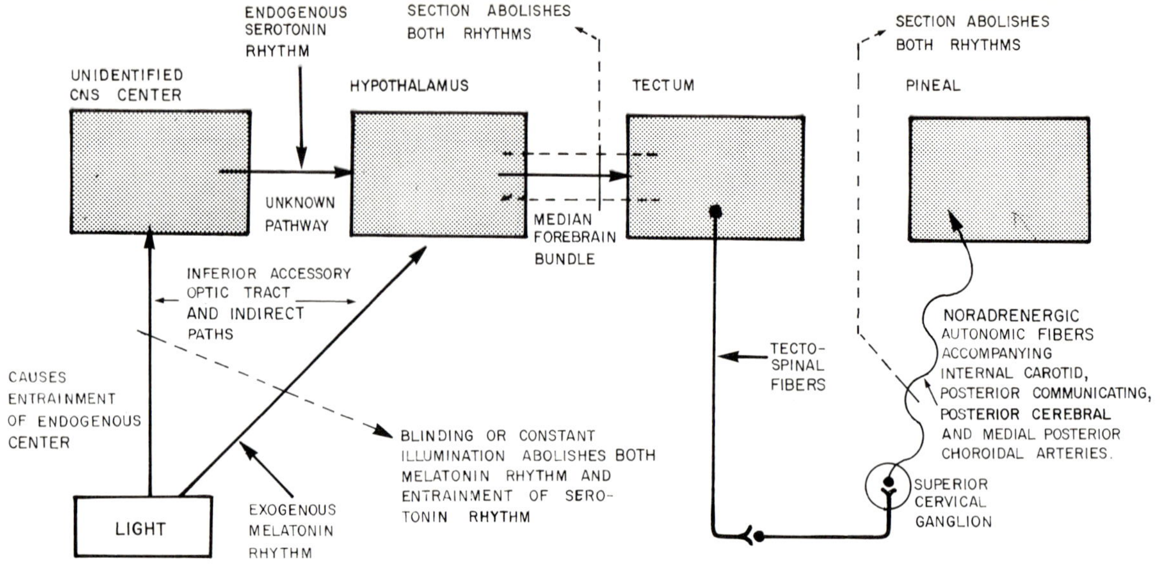

Fig. 8-13. Pathway for pineal innervation. Note the effects of destroying the pathway at various levels. Abolition of a light-dark cycle dissociates the serotonin rhythm (endogenous) from the melatonin rhythm (exogenous).

median forebrain bundle to the tectum; from the tectum by descending autonomic fibers to the upper thoracic cord; thence to the superior cervical ganglia; and by postganglionic fibers that accompany branches of the intracranial vessels and reach the apex of the pineal from the medial posterior choroidal arteries. Since there is an *intrinsic* rhythm of approximately 24 hours, but which is normally brought into phase *(entrained)* with external light, there must be a pathway for light to impinge on the originating (hypothalamic or other) center. Although there are adequate connections between the optic tracts, tegmentum, and hypothalamus, there is said also to be (at least in rats) an *inferior accessory optic tract* directly entering the hypothalamus.

The pineal also demonstrates a rhythm in melatonin production that is inverse to that of serotonin, melatonin levels being highest at night and lowest during the day. As with serotonin, melatonin formation can be entrained by reversing or otherwise changing external lighting conditions. The rhythm is entirely *exogenous* (originates outside the body), since if photic changes are prevented from reaching the CNS, either by blinding, constant light, or constant darkness, melatonin levels cease to fluctuate. By contrast, the serotonin rhythm is *endogenous,* since it persists in the absence of photic stimulation.

There is no daily variation in the activities of tryptophan hydroxylase, L-amino acid decarboxylase, or monoamine oxidase (MAO) (enzymes that produce and inactivate serotonin), but any serotonin formed during the day is bound or stored — about 50% in nerve endings and 50% in pineal cells — and cannot be inactivated by MAO. In the absence of light serotonin is released and either inactivated or converted to melatonin. In melatonin synthesis the rate-limiting enzyme appears to be 5-HIOMT, which is inhibited by light; thus, synthesis of melatonin and other methoxyindoles is higher during darkness. In vitro, melatonin synthesis (i.e., 5-HIOMT activity) is increased by norepinephrine and cyclic AMP, so possibly it is pineal release of norepinephrine that mediates the effects of light.

The Pineal as an Endocrine Gland

In female rats, removal of the pineal causes ovarian hypertrophy, precocious puberty, constant estrus, enlargement of the adenohypophysis, and increased pituitary basophils. Taken together, these effects suggest increased synthesis and release of FSH and LH. All these effects are reversed by the injection of pineal extract, but not by purified melatonin.

In the female it is difficult to dissociate the effects of FSH and LH, but in males it is considered that FSH maintains the testes, whereas LH maintains the prostate and seminal vesicles. Removal of the pineal increases all weights, suggesting increased liberation of FSH and LH. Since pituitary concentrations of these hormones are also raised, the effect must be on gonadotropin synthesis as well as release. Purified melatonin produces atrophy of the prostate and seminal vesicles but not of the testes, suggesting that it inhibits LH only. Serotonin or 5-methoxytryptophol reduces FSH levels and causes testicular atrophy. The results of administering pineal products into the CSF, or directly into the median eminence, also indicate that serotonin and 5-methoxytryptophan inhibit FSH, and melatonin and 5-hydroxytryptophan inhibit LH. Since methoxylated products inhibit gonadotropic hormone production, such production would be expected to be higher during the day, and this has been proved true. There is preliminary evidence that removal of the superior cervical ganglion prevents the nighttime fall in FSH and LH production.

Under natural conditions, the longer nights in winter, with colder weather unsuitable for reproduction, would cause pineal inhibition of FSH and LH synthesis and release. It may be supposed that during hibernation gonadotropin production is virtually shut off, whereas in summer the pineal probably has little or no effect. Experimentally, the pineal effect cannot be extended beyond 20 to 25 weeks, approximately corresponding to the normal winter period, though it is unknown whether fade-out depends on pineal exhaustion or acquired target-organ insensitivity. Antigonadotropic effects of the pineal have been subject to much debate and confusion, for which there are several possible explanations:

1. Many experimental animals are essentially nocturnal, and laboratory lighting conditions are unnatural, with excess light and undue inhibition of pineal activity.
2. Replacement therapy after pinealectomy requires crude pineal extracts, not purified melatonin.
3. It is not yet known which methoxyindoles cross the blood-brain barrier, and intravenous administration therefore produces uncertain results.
4. Pineal effects appear to be limited in time, as previously indicated, and the postoperative or postinjection interval before testing for endocrine alterations therefore affects the result.

The possibility that the pineal has other hormonal actions remains to be investigated. At present, suggestion that it might form "antihormones" that antagonize the action of each pituitary hormone appears unproved. However, pinealectomy leads to increased RNA to DNA ratios, with an absolute RNA increase, in both the adrenal and thyroid, and raised plasma cortisone, TSH, and ACTH have been reported. The possibility that pinealectomy affects the thyroid and adrenal indirectly, by altering estrogen levels, is eliminated by comparing animals that have had oophorectomy with those that have had both pinealectomy and oophorectomy. Melatonin subsequently decreases the RNA to DNA ratio, but because of a rise in DNA rather than a fall in RNA, implying a direct effect on the glands rather than pituitary mediation. Presumably, some other component of pineal extract acts directly on the hypothalamic-pituitary axis.

Administration of pineal extract has been reported as suppressing electrically induced seizures for several hours. It has also been reported that pinealectomy lowers the seizure threshold of the rabbit hippocampal formation, causes seizure-like electrical discharges in other species, delays the lethal effect of pentobarbital, and raises CNS serotonin and gamma-aminobutyric acid by activation of L-amino acid decarboxylase. The use of melatonin in the symptomatic treatment of epilepsy and paralysis agitans has been suggested, and in some species it has been reported to act synergistically with barbiturates in the induction of sleep (perhaps by activation of sleep-inducing serotonin pathways). Clearly, much in this field remains to be investigated.

BIOLOGICAL RHYTHMS

Life at all levels shows biological rhythmic activity, with cycles varying from milliseconds to at least a year. The best understood of these are those approximating 24 hours, which are therefore called "circa-dian." Biological rhythms may originate within the organism (*endogenous* or free-running). These appear to be easily brought into phase (*entrained*) with external rhythms such as the light cycle. Entrainment may involve a slight alteration in cycle length, but circadian rhythms apparently cannot be entrained to any external period of less than 18 to 19 hours. Other types of biological rhythm are entirely dependent on environmental stimuli, and if these cease, the rhythm ceases. Such (*exogenous*) cycles are automatically in phase with the external stimulus and do not require entrainment. It may be difficult to distinguish an exogenous from an endogenous entrained rhythm, the only effective method being to isolate the organism from any conceivable entraining influences (*Zeitgebers*) and see if it persists. Pineal metabolism offers good examples of an entrained endogenous rhythm (serotonin) and an exogenous rhythm (melatonin). It is the temporary dissociation of light-entrained biological rhythms and the light-dark cycle that cause the psychological problems associated with air travel involving changes in time zones.

The mechanism underlying endogenous rhythms is unknown. It must ultimately be based on a series of chemical reactions, most probably occurring somewhere within the CNS, which then "fires off" appropriate responses in other parts of the body. It has been suggested that one function of melatonin is to act as a time signal for other organs, with its release under the control of the (unknown) CNS center. The chemical reactions that produce the rhythms, whatever they may be, seem remarkably immune to the action of drugs and even show a much lower degree of temperature dependence than other chemical and biological activities. Macromolecular synthesis (RNA or protein) has been proposed, and there is evidence that actinomycin D or puromycin may interfere with rhythm generation. In some species the length of the cycle can be modified by changing the ratio of heavy to ordinary water, but the significance of this is totally obscure. Light is by far the most powerful entraining influence, but possible roles for temperature and other factors are not excluded.

The most prominent diurnal rhythm in man is sleeping and waking, which is an entrained cycle apparently originating in the reticular formation. It appears that there is a rostral center in the midbrain and upper pons with activating or arousal activity, and a caudal center in the lower pons and medulla with EEG-synchronizing or sleep-inducing activity. Both are tonically active, but the large sensory input keeps the arousal cycle dominant during the day.

Generally reduced activity of the reticular formation during sleep is reflected in lower blood pressure, reduced heart rate, and raised P_{CO_2} (but constant P_{O_2}) with a pH rise of 0.03. This adult cycle is superimposed on an infantile pattern that has a period of approximately 2 hours, and this pattern is still manifest in the adult as periods of rapid eye movement (REM) sleep.

Other diurnal rhythms include the following:

1. Pulse rate, blood pressure, temperature, and urinary output are maximal during the day.
2. Blood volume, hematocrit, serum Na^+, and serum K^+ are lowest in the early morning.
3. Eosinophil and lymphocyte counts are highest in the morning, monocyte counts are highest about noon, and neutrophil counts are highest in the afternoon.
4. 17-OH-steroids and cortisol are highest at about 6 A.M. and lowest between 8 P.M. and midnight, with urine values running in parallel but 6 to 8 hours later (out of phase). These two rhythms do not seem to be related to the sleep cycle and strongly resist entrainment in night workers. Within the overall 24-hour rhythm, plasma corticosteroids also show bursts of alternating high and low levels, with an irregular periodicity of 1 to 3 hours.
5. At least in experimental animals, there is diurnal variability in susceptibility to toxic agents and response to therapeutic drugs.

These rhythms have obvious implications for clinical medicine. Thus, for example, it is essential to compare plasma levels obtained at about the same time of day to eliminate variations due to biological rhythm (but note that high levels [bursts] of corticosteroids may invalidate comparisons of single samples). Another implication, at present largely unexplored, is that the time of administration may affect the response to drugs or the susceptibility to toxic agents such as anesthetics and narcotics.

BIBLIOGRAPHY

Bajusz, E. (Ed.) *Physiology and Pathology of Adaptation Mechanisms.* Oxford: Pergamon, 1969.

Bernardis, L. L. Localisation of neuroendocrine functions within the hypothalamus. *Can. J. Neurol. Sci.* 1:29-39, 1974.

Blackwell, R. E., and Guillemin, R. Hypothalamic control of adenohypophyseal secretions. *Annu. Rev. Physiol.* 35:357-390, 1973.

Clattenburg, R. E. Ultrastructure of hypothalamic neurones and of the median eminence. *Can. J. Neurol. Sci.* 1:40-58, 1974.

DeFronzo, R. A., and Roth, W. D. Evidence for the existence of a pineal-adrenal and a pineal-thyroid axis. *Acta Endocrinol.* 70:31-42, 1970.

Hastings, J. W. The biology of circadian rhythms from man to micro-organisms. *N. Engl. J. Med.* 282:435-441, 1970.

Hershman, J. M., and Pittman, J. A. Control of thyrotropin secretion in man. *N. Engl. J. Med.* 285:997-1006, 1971.

Hofer, H. O. The Phenomenon of Neurosecretion. In G. H. Bourne (Ed.), *The Structure and Function of Nervous Tissue.* New York: Academic, 1968. Vol. 1, pp. 461-517.

Kenny, G. C. T. The Epiphysis Cerebri. In G. H. Bourne (Ed.), *The Structure and Function of Nervous Tissue.* New York: Academic, 1972. Vol. 6, pp. 253-272.

Kerenyi, N. A., and von Westarp, C. Postnatal transformation of the pineal gland: Effect of constant darkness. *Endocrinology* 88:1077-1079, 1971.

Krieger, D. T. Pathophysiology of Central Nervous System Regulation of Anterior Pituitary Function. In G. E. Gaull (Ed.), *Biology of Brain Dysfunction.* New York: Plenum, 1973. Vol. 2, pp. 351-407.

Martin, J. B. Neural regulation of growth hormone secretion. *N. Engl. J. Med.* 288:1384-1393, 1973.

Martini, L., and Meites, J. *Neurochemical Aspects of Hypothalamic Function.* New York: Academic, 1970.

Reiter, R. J. Comparative physiology: Pineal gland. *Annu. Rev. Physiol.* 35:305-328, 1973.

Schally, A. V., Kastin, A. J., and Arimura, A. The hypothalamus and reproduction. *Am. J. Obstet. Gynecol.* 114:423-442, 1972.

Segre, E. J., and Lloyd, C. W. Neuroendocrine Mechanisms. In J. Minckler (Ed.), *Pathology of the Nervous System.* New York: McGraw-Hill, 1968. Vol. 1, pp. 334-341.

Wolstenholme, G. E. W., and Knight, J. (Eds.) *The Pineal Gland* (Ciba Foundation Symposium). Edinburgh and London: Churchill/Livingstone, 1971.

Some Facets of Neuropharmacology

9

A high proportion of the drugs used in general medicine have actions on the central or peripheral nervous systems, often depending on the freedom with which they cross the blood-brain barrier. However, this chapter is confined to drugs used primarily because of their significant actions on the nervous system — in many cases, effects on both the peripheral and the central nervous system.

Synapses in the peripheral nervous system (PNS) have long served as a model for attempting to understand similar events in the CNS, where the synapse is the most sensitive area to many influences, including drugs. Thus, in deep general anesthesia, axons will respond to stimulation with a propagated action potential at a time when virtually all synaptic activity has ceased. The findings of recent pharmacological and physiological studies, when combined, provide a large body of knowledge about synaptic events. As an example, the only good evidence for the existence of different types of postsynaptic receptors has come from pharmacological studies.

Drugs effective at a synapse with a known neurotransmitter may be used in various ways (Fig. 9-1). They may be needed to mimic or potentiate transmitter activity, as do synthetic drugs acting directly on the postsynaptic membrane, with effects similar to those of the physiological transmitter, or drugs that inhibit inactivating enzymes or prevent reuptake and so prolong activity of endogenous transmitters. Alternatively, drugs may be used to antagonize the transmitter, either at the postsynaptic level (which apparently applies to the clinically effective acetylcholine antagonists and catecholamine antagonists in the PNS) or (in the CNS) by a multitude of presynaptic mechanisms, including inhibition of synthesis and changes in amine reuptake or storage (see Chap. 3 for neurotransmitter metabolism).

A large and historically much older group of drugs acting on the CNS has not so far been associated with any definite site of action or a specific neurotransmitter. This group includes anesthetics, hypnotics, sedatives, tranquilizers, analgesics, and stimulants. Although many of these drugs have been used for centuries, the rationale for their use is much less firm than for those just discussed, and they may be characterized as having unknown (or no) neurotransmitter specificity, though this may later be disproved. As always occurs when the mechanism of a drug's action is unknown, theories have been propounded to explain their activity, and these will be briefly reviewed here.

Certain groups of drugs are associated with specific clinical conditions, and since their actions are often multiple, they are better discussed in association with these conditions (see Chap. 18 for antiepileptic drugs and Chap. 26 for antipsychotic and psychotomimetic drugs).

DRUGS ACTIVE AT CHOLINERGIC SYNAPSES

In the PNS, acetylcholine appears to be the effective transmitter for (1) preganglionic fibers in both sympathetic and parasympathetic divisions, (2) all postganglionic fibers of the parasympathetic and a few of the sympathetic division (including sweat glands), and (3) somatic motor fibers at the neuromuscular junction. As previously noted, acetylcholine is an important neurotransmitter in the CNS, especially for ascending reticular activating system terminals in the cortex. It may possibly be the transmitter for lateral and medial geniculate cells terminating in the visual and auditory cortex and perhaps for other fiber systems. Little is known of postsynaptic receptors for acetylcholine (or indeed for any other transmitter), but it is a long-standing observation that atropine blocks transmission mediated by acetylcholine only in some situations (Fig. 9-2), especially at the postganglionic terminals of parasympathetic and a few sympathetic fibers. Since the same synapses are activated by the alkaloid muscarine, their receptors are termed *muscarinic.* Atropine fails to block transmission at the preganglionic terminals and neuromuscular junction, both of which are stimulated by low concentrations of nicotine; receptors at these sites are termed *nicotinic.* Nicotinic receptors can be further divided, since those at skeletal muscles are blocked by different substances (e.g., the curare group) from those at the preganglionic terminals. Those of the adrenal medulla are blocked by quarternary ammonium compounds such as hexamethonium. Thus, in the PNS, there are at least three types of postsynaptic (acetylcholine) receptors. It is uncertain how many there are in the CNS, but there is evidence for both muscarinic and nicotinic (type unspecified) receptors. Adequate testing would involve direct injection of blocking agents into the CNS, since some fail to cross the blood-brain barrier.

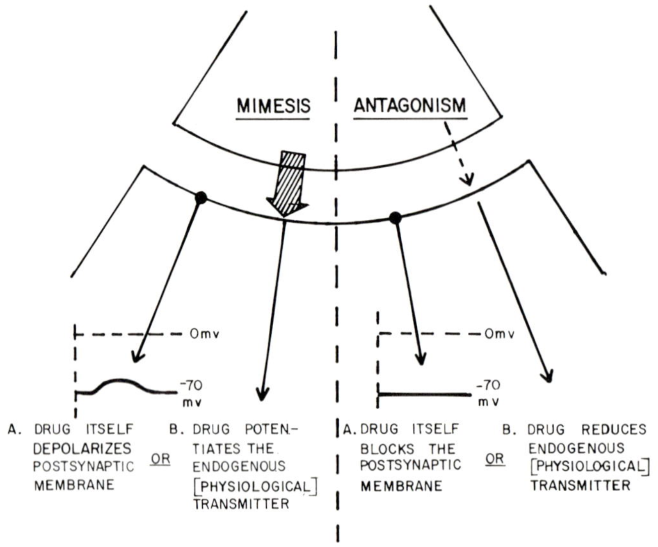

Fig. 9-1. General mechanisms of action of pharmacological agents at synapses, indicating the effect of an action potential on the postsynaptic membrane potential in the presence of mimetic and antagonistic drugs.

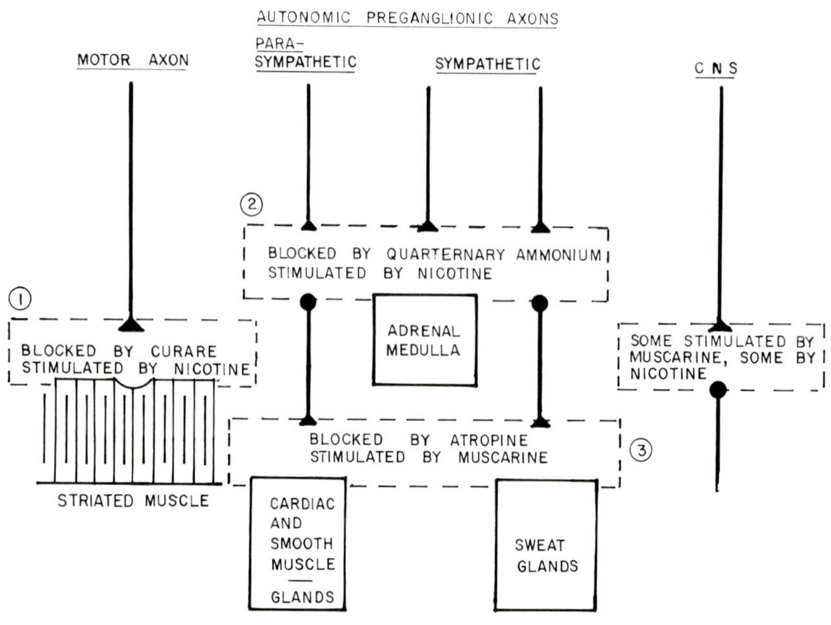

Fig. 9-2. Effects of drugs at cholinergic synapses in the central and peripheral nervous systems. These effects indicate at least three postsynaptic receptors: nicotinic muscular (1), nicotinic ganglionic (2), and muscarinic postganglionic (3). The types in the CNS are not yet clarified.

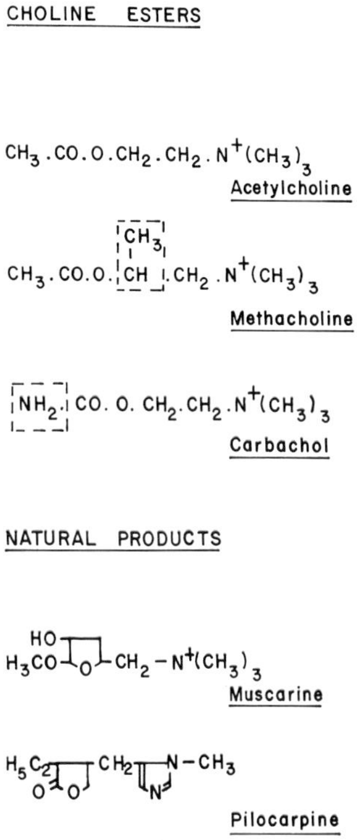

Fig. 9-3. Drugs mimicking the action of acetylcholine.

Drugs Mimicking or Enhancing Acetylcholine Action

Drugs Mimicking Acetylcholine Action

Drugs that mimic the action of acetylcholine (Fig. 9-3), presumably by a direct effect on the postsynaptic receptor, fall into two groups.

Other Cholinesters. These include such drugs as methacholine and carbachol. Because of different chemical constitution, these drugs vary in their resistance to acetylcholinesterase and pseudocholinesterase, but are generally long-acting. Essentially, they have muscarinic (i.e., postganglionic parasympathetic and occasionally sympathetic) actions and are blocked by atropine. However, carbachol, a particularly potent drug, also has nicotinic actions. Its clinical use is restricted to the treatment of glaucoma.

Muscarinic Drugs. These drugs, including muscarine and pilocarpine, both natural products, are active at the same sites as methacholine. They have no significant nicotinic effects and are effectively blocked by atropine. (However, recent evidence suggests that some ganglionic synapses may also be muscarinic and stimulated by pilocarpine.)

Drugs Enhancing the Action of Acetylcholine

Drugs that potentiate the action of acetylcholine (Fig. 9-4) do so by inhibiting acetylcholinesterase, thus prolonging action of the endogenous transmitter on the postsynaptic membrane. With some drugs the inhibition is readily reversible, but in others, inhibition is reversed only with great difficulty, and such drugs (organophosphorus compounds) are potentially dangerous. Therapeutically useful members of the reversible group include the natural product physostigmine (eserine), neostigmine, and edrophonium. Physostigmine, a tertiary amine, has an affinity for acetylcholinesterase 10^4 times than that of acetylcholine itself, but gradually dissociates from the enzyme and is destroyed. It is used in the treatment of glaucoma and as a meiotic. In toxic dosage it may produce a cholinergic crisis. Neostigmine is a quarternary ammonium compound and, in addition to inhibiting acetylcholinesterase, has a direct acetylcholine-like action at some nicotinic synapses, including the neuromuscular junction. Its effects are abolished by atropine, excepting only muscle fasciculation. Edrophonium (Tensilon), another quarternary amine, also has both esterase-inhibiting and direct acetylcholine-like actions, but these are rapid and transient. Physostigmine crosses biological membranes and is absorbed orally better than the others, so that lower dosage is needed.

The virtually irreversible group of acetylcholinesterase inhibitors are environmental toxins used as pesticides and for chemical warfare – the organophosphorus compounds. They include di-isopropyl fluorophosphate (DFP), tetraethyl pyrophosphate, and parathion. Their combination with cholinesterases lasts for weeks or months, and although preferentially affecting pseudocholinesterase, higher doses affect acetylcholinesterase as well. In the absence of treatment, normal levels of acetylcholinesterase in nervous tissue are not regained for up to three months, and the clinical picture includes muscarinic and nicotinic manifestations. The CNS features include restlessness, insomnia, tremor, confusion, ataxia, convulsions, respiratory depression, and circulatory collapse. Hydroxylamines are capable of regenerating the enzyme, and a synthetic drug, pralidoxime, provides reasonably effective treatment, given with atropine. One organophosphorus compound, DFP, has been applied locally in the treatment of glaucoma.

Drugs Antagonizing the Action of Acetylcholine

All clinically effective acetylcholine antagonists appear to act on the postsynaptic (receptor) membrane, and as previously noted, it is on the basis of such actions that three acetylcholine receptors have been postulated. Collectively, this group are known as *cholinergic blocking drugs.*

Atropine and Scopolamine

The prototypal cholinergic-blocking drugs are atropine and scopolamine (Fig. 9-5), both of which

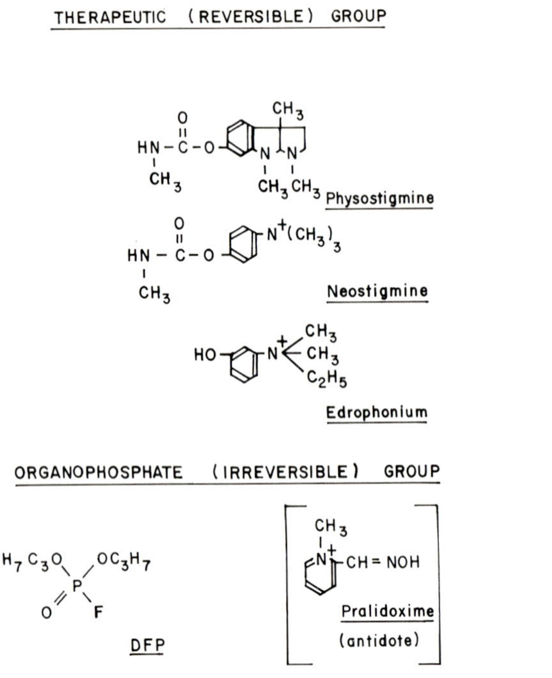

Fig. 9-4. Drugs potentiating the action of endogenous acetylcholine (acetylcholinesterase inhibitors).

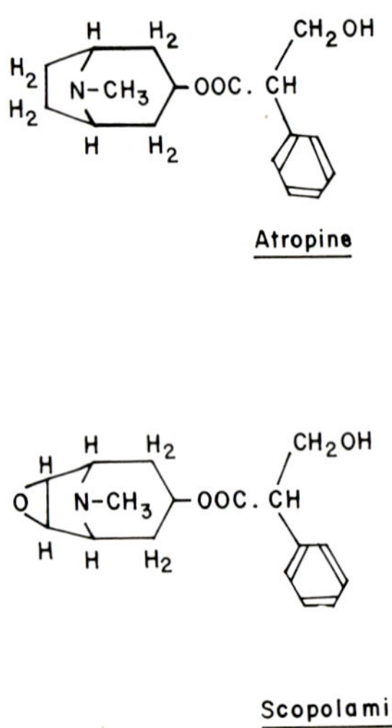

Fig. 9-5. Drugs blocking the action of acetylcholine at muscarinic receptors (postganglionic and CNS).

are complex esters of bases with tropic acid. They compete with acetylcholine for the muscarinic receptors, especially in smooth muscle, cardiac muscle, and glands, and are usually more effective against parenteral cholinergic drugs than against acetylcholine. They block cardiac parasympathetic effects and have some, but less, effect on the gut and the urinary tract; only massive doses have any effect on ganglionic or neuromuscular transmission. Both drugs cause vasodilatation (of unknown mechanism) in the skin, dilatation of the pupil, paralysis of accommodation, and increased intraocular tension. (Adrenergic drugs also cause pupillodilatation, but without paralysis of accommodation. Atropine paralyzes the circular muscle of the pupil, whereas adrenergic drugs stimulate radial muscle.) They (especially scopolamine) cause sedation in low dosage, but increasing concentrations are stimulatory to the CNS, causing delirium and coma. Thus, atropine toxicity is manifested by excitement and mania, hot, dry skin, dilated pupils, and tachycardia. Pilocarpine, perhaps because it fails to cross the blood-brain barrier, improves only the peripheral manifestations. In organophosphorus poisoning, large dosages of atropine may reduce central respiratory depression. Synthetic substituents of atropine are chiefly used for peptic ulcer therapy, many of them having quarternary instead of tertiary nitrogen, which reduces lipid solubility and CNS penetration and adds some helpful ganglionic blocking action. Atropine and scopolamine are of value in the treatment of some cases of parkinsonism (see Chap. 24).

Ganglionic Blocking Agents

Ganglionic blocking agents, which compete at nicotinic receptors, are of limited clinical value and are used mainly to reduce systemic blood pressure. Since the ganglionic transmitter is acetylcholine for both sympathetic and parasympathetic divisions, ganglionic blockade is often accompanied by parasympathetic paralysis (dilatation of the pupils, paralysis of accommodation, dry mouth, constipation, and atony of the bladder). These agents do not penetrate the CNS and indeed remain largely extracellular in all parts of the body; effects they may have on the brain are due to induced hemodynamic changes.

Neuromuscular Blocking Agents

Clinically useful neuromuscular blocking agents (Fig. 9-6) acting at the receptor site include d-tubocurarine and succinylcholine. They are characterized by two quarternary nitrogen atoms (14 A apart) and so are virtually excluded from the CNS. Their effects are potentiated by organophosphorus compounds, general anesthetics, quinine, quinidine, and, less predictably, by many antibiotics. There appear to be two mechanisms of action. One group, including *d*-tubocurarine, gallamine, and benzoquinonium, competes for the receptor site without causing membrane depolarization. The second group, including succinylcholine and decamethonium,

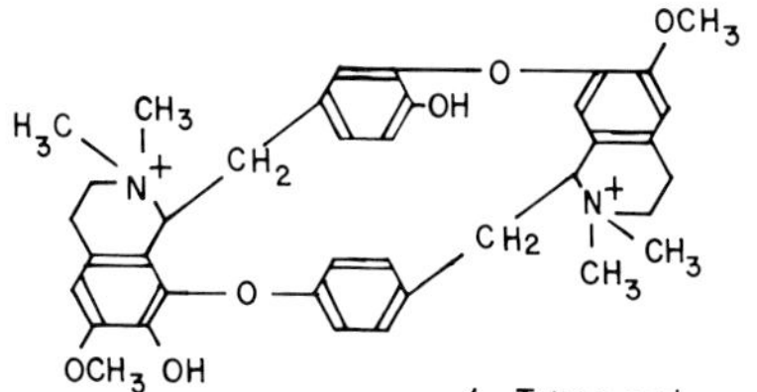

d – Tubocurarine

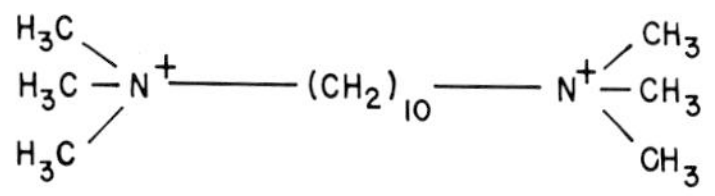

Decamethonium

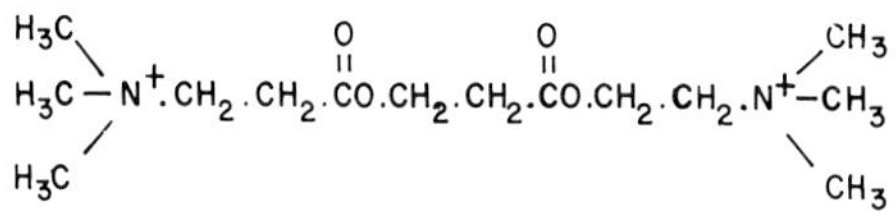

Succinylcholine

Fig. 9-6. Drugs blocking the action of acetylcholine nicotinic receptors of the neuromuscular junction.

causes depolarization followed by repolarization, the membrane remaining insensitive to acetylcholine. Agents of the first group are opposed by neostigmine, edrophonium, and K^+ but potentiated by ether (and also by myasthenia gravis, such drugs being dangerous in this condition), whereas those of the second group are opposed by ether and by *d*-tubocurarine, while edrophonium, anticholinesterases, and K^+ have no effect.

Drugs acting at the neuromuscular junction must be distinguished from those causing muscle relaxation by affecting interneurons of the cord. The latter group are related to tranquilizers, and include mephenesin, methocarbamol, and zoxazolamine. They are different in structure from the blocking agents and readily cross the blood-brain barrier.

DRUGS ACTIVE AT CATECHOLAMINERGIC SITES

Of the three catecholamines, norepinephrine and dopamine are found in high concentrations in the CNS; there is far less epinephrine, which probably has no role in CNS transmission. Norepinephrine and epinephrine are transmitters in the PNS, whereas dopamine apparently has little function (except perhaps as a ganglionic transmitter and an intermediary metabolite). Peripheral postsynaptic receptors are termed *adrenergic* irrespective of their specificity for epinephrine or norepinephrine. Blocking agents for adrenergic synapses have been synthesized and have shown two receptors, alpha and beta, blockaded by different agents. The alpha-beta differentiation does not correspond to sensitivity to epinephrine or norepinephrine, since either may react with both types of receptor. The alpha receptors appear to mediate vasoconstriction, pupilloconstriction (mydriasis), intestinal relaxation with contraction of gut sphincters, contraction of the sphincters and trigone in the bladder, and splenic and pilomotor contraction. The beta receptors mediate effects on the heart (including tachycardia, shortening of the refractory period, increase in conduction rate, and increased contractility), vasodilatation in skeletal muscle, relaxation of bronchial muscle, decreased motility of the stomach, gut, and bladder, pupillodilatation, and glycogenolysis. Sweating is mediated through cholinergic endings.

It is customary to regard norepinephrine as having largely homeostatic functions and epinephrine as an emergency, "fight-or-flight" transmitter, though the adrenal medullary catecholamines are about 20% norepinephrine. Epinephrine increases glycogenolysis, causing release of glycogen from the liver and lactic acid from muscle, increases the release of free fatty acids from adipose tissue, and raises plasma K^+. As in the CNS, monoamine oxidase (MAO) and catechol-O-methyltransferase (COMT) are active in the conversion of norepinephrine and epinephrine to vanillylmandelic acid (VMA), which is a more important peripheral metabolite than MHPG (3-methoxy-4-hydroxyphenylglycol). Pheochromocytomas contain much more norepinephrine than epinephrine. Pharmacological agents for the diagnosis of this tumor either release catecholamines and raise blood pressure (e.g., histamine, methacholine, or tetraethylammonium) or antagonize catecholamines and markedly lower blood pressure (e.g., phentolamine [Regitine]).

Drugs Mimicking Catecholamine Activity

The sympathetic amines (Fig. 9-7) mimic some of the actions of norepinephrine or epinephrine and are antagonized by adrenergic blocking agents. There are two groups: *direct-acting,* such as phenylephrine, which act at receptor sites and are independent of endogenous catecholamines, and the *indirect-acting,* which release stored catecholamine and therefore are of no value if it is absent or reduced, as may occur in chronic denervation or pretreatment with reserpine (see p. 175). This group includes tyramine, amphetamine, and phenylethylamine. A few drugs, of which ephedrine is the best known, exhibit both actions. Theoretically, potentiation of the action of endogenous catecholamines should result from inhibiting their breakdown (analogous to the use of acetylcholinesterase inhibitors), but this does not work in practice. Although a number of inhibitors of MAO are known, they usually do not increase adrenergic activity, perhaps because catecholamines can also be inactivated by COMT (for which no clinically effective inhibitors are

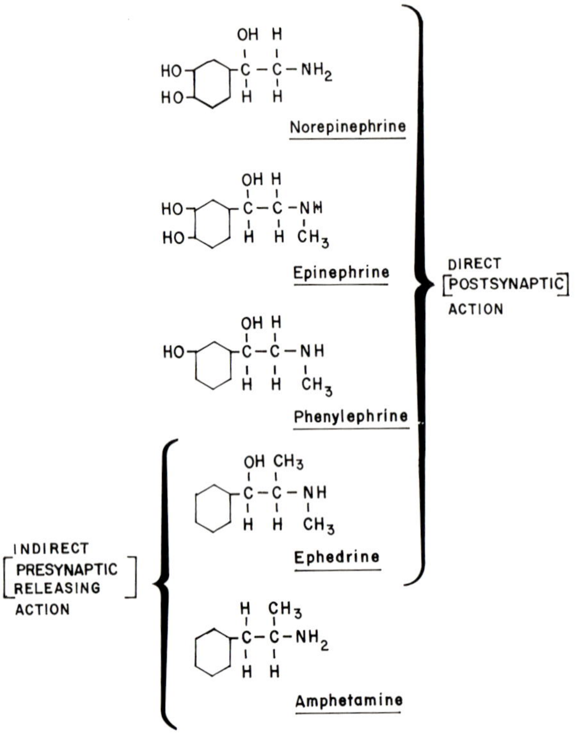

Fig. 9-7. Drugs mimicking the action of catecholamines.

available), and are protected from MAO by rapid, effective reuptake across the presynaptic and granule membranes.

The sympathetic amines are mainly used as vasoconstrictor drugs (alpha receptors) or bronchodilators (beta receptors), though some are CNS stimulants whose mechanism of action appears complex. Ephedrine, which is well absorbed orally, is a versatile drug, acting as a vasoconstrictor, bronchodilator, and CNS stimulant. In excess, it may cause anxiety and wakefulness. It probably acts peripherally by causing release of endogenous catecholamines, but its CNS effects are not altered by reserpine and may be postsynaptic. Most other sympathetic amines cross the blood-brain barrier poorly and have little CNS activity. By synthesis of substituted derivatives, it has been possible to isolate bronchodilator and vasoconstrictor effects partially, and some structure-activity relationships have come to light. Thus, the benzene ring does not appear essential for activity, but if it is present, hydroxylation reduces absorption from the gut and increases susceptibility to COMT. With no substituents on the nitrogen atom, the compound tends to react more with alpha receptors; heavily substituted compounds tend to react with beta receptors. Substitution on the alpha carbon atom prolongs the action of the drug, presumably by protection against enzymes. A –OH group on the beta carbon atom seems to promote storage in synaptic granules.

Drugs Antagonizing or Preventing Catecholamine Activity

Alpha Adrenergic-Blocking Agents

The alpha adrenergic-blocking drugs (Fig. 9-8) prevent vasoconstriction (and other smooth muscle contraction) induced by catecholamines. This method of reducing sympathetic tone must be distinguished from the use of ganglionic blocking agents, which affect the synapse between preganglionic and postganglionic fibers, and of agents such as reserpine, which deplete stores of catecholamines and therefore act presynaptically. Arteriolar smooth muscle has both alpha and beta receptors, but epinephrine and norepinephrine both act more powerfully on the alpha receptors, producing vasoconstriction. If the alpha receptors are blocked, then epinephrine (but not norepinephrine) causes vasodilatation through the beta receptors; in turn, this action may be prevented by beta-blocking agents. Unfortunately, alpha-blocking agents are disappointing in the treatment of chronic hypertension. However, phentolamine is used in the diagnosis of pheochromocytoma and in preventing hypertensive crises during the removal of these tumors. Some of the ergot alkaloids (e.g., ergotamine) are alpha-blocking agents, but cannot be used clinically as such because of side effects, including direct stimulation of smooth muscle and serotonin antagonism. These agents do not appear to affect the CNS, probably because they do not cross the blood-brain barrier.

Beta Adrenergic-Blocking Agents

Beta adrenergic-blocking agents (Fig. 9-8) include propranolol and related drugs, which block the intestinal, bronchial, and, to a lesser extent, the cardiac effects of sympathetic stimulation. They reduce heart rate, myocardial contractility, cardiac output, and the effects of exercise on the heart; the blood pressure may be reduced or unaltered. On the assumption that there may be two separate types of beta receptors, one peculiar to the heart, new beta-blocking drugs are being sought. Beta-blocking agents do not appear to have CNS effects.

Synthetic Analogues

Catecholamines may be depleted by the use of synthetic analogues. Thus, *a*-methyltyrosine (Fig. 9-9) competes with the natural substrate (tyrosine) for the (rate-limiting) enzyme tyrosine hydroxylase; *a*-methyldopa is formed, and competes with dihydroxyphenylalanine for L-amino acid decarboxylase, effectively reducing the synthesis of norepinephrine (and also of serotonin). The subsequent reduction of norepinephrine is prolonged (compared to the depletion of serotonin), perhaps because a-methyldopa is decarboxylated to a-methylnorepinephrine and taken up by storage granules to act as a *false transmitter.* Other substances bearing a –OH radical on

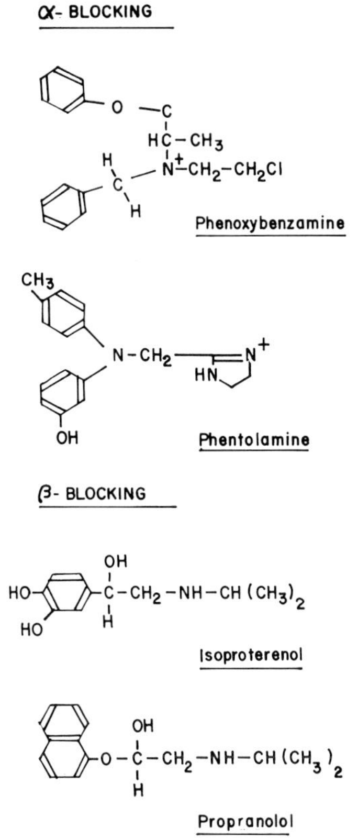

Fig. 9-8. Drugs blocking the action of catecholamines.

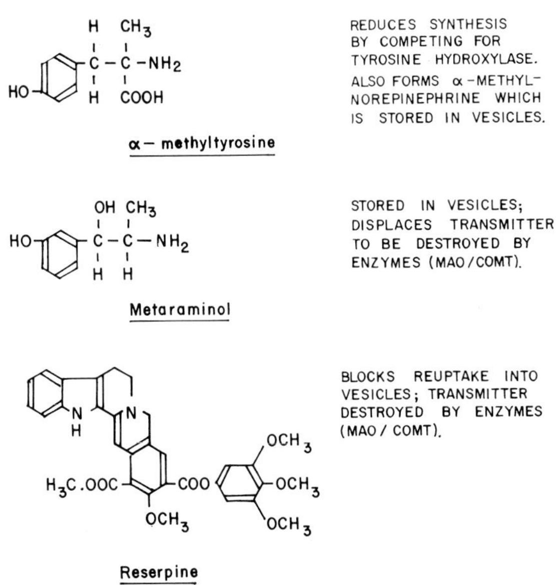

Fig. 9-9. Drugs interfering with storage of catecholamines in synaptic granules or vesicles. If the drugs themselves are stored, they act as false transmitters on release into the synaptic cleft.

the beta carbon atom may be also taken up by storage granules and act as false transmitters, since when released from storage into the synaptic cleft, they do not produce appropriate effects at the postsynaptic membrane, and therefore dilute the activity of physiological transmitters or even compete for receptor sites.

Reserpine

An important group of drugs reducing catecholamine activity are those that either displace transmitters from the storage granules or prevent uptake into granules. Free transmitters trapped in presynaptic cytoplasm are immediately inactivated by MAO, effectively reducing catecholamine concentration. The most important of these drugs is reserpine (Fig. 9-9), which was originally used as an antihypertensive agent, but has been found to be an effective tranquilizer. It depletes levels of norepinephrine, dopamine, and serotonin, affecting both the CNS and PNS, and can be given orally, as it readily crosses the blood-brain barrier. Reserpine has the additional action of inhibiting reuptake from the synaptic cleft; at which point also catecholamine is rapidly inactivated. As has been noted, pretreatment with reserpine abolishes the activity of sympathetic amines that act by increasing the release of endogenous catecholamines.

Other Agents

Guanethimide, a drug somewhat similar to reserpine, causes depletion of stored norepinephrine and may also prevent its release into the synaptic cleft. Oral guanethimide is ineffective, as it does not cross the blood-brain barrier. As previously mentioned, one of the actions of *amphetamine* is to release catecholamines from granules, leading ultimately to their depletion. *Tyramine* and *metaraminol* (Fig. 9-9) displace catecholamines from granules, and the latter enters the granules and acts as a false transmitter. *Cocaine, the tricyclic antidepressants,* and *antihistaminic drugs* block reuptake of catecholamines from the synaptic cleft and increase their inactivation by MAO and COMT.

The effects of drugs on the passage of catecholamines across granule or presynaptic membranes are summarized in Figure 9-10.

DRUGS ACTIVE AT SEROTONERGIC SYNAPSES

So far as is known, serotonin is not a transmitter in the PNS, but plays a significant role in the activities of the reticular formation and perhaps other regions of the CNS. There do not appear to be any clinically effective drugs that mimic or potentiate the action of serotonin. Although MAO inhibitors may double the brain serotonin levels within about an hour, no observable changes have been attributed to the serotonin increase.

Serotonin levels in the brain are depleted by reserpine, the mechanism apparently being the same as for catecholamines, involving release from storage

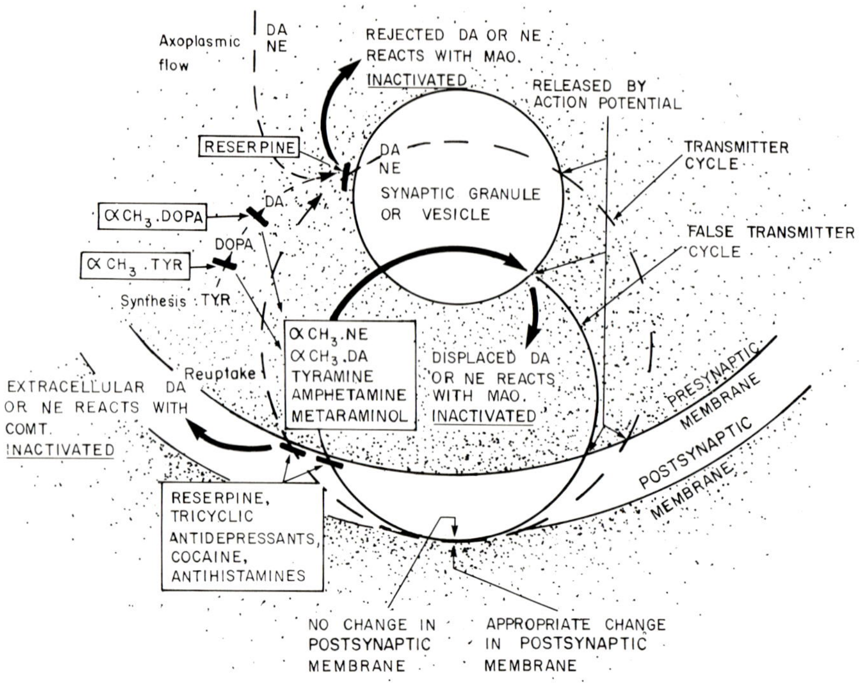

Fig. 9-10. Summary of the effects of drugs on catecholamine reuptake and storage. The dashed circle represents the release-reuptake cycle of normal endogenous catecholamines; the thick bars show the sites of drug blockage. The inner circle represents the effect of abnormal catecholamines taken up by granules and displacing the endogenous transmitter. Transmitter is destroyed by enzymes (MAO and COMT) if reuptake or storage is delayed or prevented. TYR = tyrosine; DA = dopamine; NE = norepinephrine.

sites and subsequent destruction by MAO. Experimentally, synthesis of serotonin may be blocked by p-chlorophenylalanine, which competes for the (rate-limiting) enzyme tryptophan hydroxylase. Since p-chlorophenylalanine is not a tranquilizer, it has been assumed that the tranquilizing effect of reserpine depends on depletion of catecholamines rather than serotonin. Lysergic acid diethylamide (LSD) inhibits the activity of serotonin both on smooth muscle and in the CNS (see Chap. 26).

CENTRAL NERVOUS SYSTEM DEPRESSANTS

The sequence sedation-hypnosis-anesthesia-coma may be regarded as a continuous spectrum and some groups of drugs, e.g., the barbiturate series, may be used as sedatives, hypnotics, or anesthetics. With the exception of the volatile anesthetics, all CNS depressants are, to a variable degree, addictive, as are the minor tranquilizers. The most versatile of the CNS depressants are the barbiturates, of which large numbers have been synthesized, varying considerably in their lipid solubility, ionization at body pH, and rapidity of metabolism. Since the ratio between anesthetic and lethal dosages is approximately 1 to 2, barbiturates are not suitable for the induction of anesthesia unless they are ultra-short-acting. In general, speed of action and drug potency are both positively correlated with high lipid solubility.

Site of Action

The site of action of depressant drugs in the CNS is not known. They affect the reticular formation, causing a reduction in blood pressure, temperature, and respiratory response to increased P_{CO_2}. Fatalities are commonly associated with depression of the respiratory center. However, other brain centers are also affected, as some depressants are anticonvulsive (e.g., in eclampsia, tetanus, and cocaine or strychnine poisoning) and some, including phenobarbital, are antiepileptic. Depressants may abolish electrical excitability in the motor cortex of the monkey. It is generally accepted that synaptic transmission is more susceptible than axonal conduction to CNS depressants, although in vitro it is possible to "anesthetize" axons and abolish action potentials with high drug concentrations.

Metabolic Action

In anesthesia, cerebral oxygen utilization is reduced by 30 to 45%, associated with reduced frequency and amplitude of the EEG. In spite of this, lactate and inorganic phosphate concentrations fall, and glycogen, adenosine triphosphate, and creatine phosphate levels rise. Clearly, with the usual anesthetic concentrations, energy-utilizing processes are depressed before energy production. Toxic doses, however, inhibit cellular respiration, so that these changes are reversed, and there is reduction of energy reserves, as in hypoxia or cyanide poisoning (see Chap. 13). The action of depressant drugs on the CNS is only one facet of their general biological activity. They also cause decreased cell division, motility, bioluminescence, and other effects in all forms of life.

It may be concluded that the receptor sites for depressant agents are not confined to neural tissues. Since anesthesia and depression are by definition reversible, the agent must be readily dissociated from the receptor site. A survey of known depressant agents, ranging from inert gases to complex molecules such as those of the barbiturates and benzodiazepones, makes it highly unlikely that any chemical reaction is involved.

Physicochemical Action

If depression is assumed to have a physicochemical basis, it might well occur at interfaces such as plasma and organelle membranes, which are currently considered to be largely lipoprotein. In view of the observation that anesthetic potency is frequently associated with lipid solubility, early theories of anesthetic activity were that such agents combined with, or were dissolved in, the lipid constituent of membranes, thereby disrupting their structure and possibly blocking the functional pores associated with ionic permeability. Correlation of lipid solubility (oil-water partition) with anesthetic potency is only found for organic molecules containing four carbon atoms or less; the larger ones, in spite of high lipid solubility, show rapidly decreasing anesthetic potency. Studies of the absorption of anesthetic agents by the water of hydration of protein crystals have offered a generally better correlation, in that larger molecules would be excluded from spaces within such crystals. A somewhat different approach is to consider that anesthetic agents may stabilize a layer or layers of water molecules at the surface of cell membranes, forming crystal-like structures (clathrates) and thereby altering the membrane properties.

At present, there appears to be insufficient evidence to rule these various models of anesthetic activity either in or out. It appears possible that all contain an element of truth. Thus, although clathrates on their own are unstable at physiological temperature and pressure, it is conceivable that they might be stabilized by terminal $-NH_2$ groups of protein and thus alter the configuration of the membrane. This in no way excludes the possibility of anesthetic agents' penetrating the lipid portion of the membrane and causing still more disorganization.

Study of the effects of depressant agents on axonal conduction suggests that they do not depolarize the resting membrane, but profoundly affect the increase in Na^+ permeability associated with propagation of the action potential and perhaps also interfere with the activity of the Na^+ pump. If the Na^+ permeability of soma and dendrites were greater than that of axons, as is indicated by the lower resting potential and the rapid depolarization occurring in hypoxia, then it is likely that impaired pumping mechanisms would be detrimental to function, possibly accounting for the finding that anesthetics exert a depressant effect on the soma and dendrites earlier than they do on the axon.

In the formulation of molecular theories of CNS depressant activity, certain general assumptions have been made about molecular fit:

1. Receptor sites have a shape that is inverse to that of the depressant drug.
2. Shapes may be similar in configuration but vary in size.
3. Different receptor sites may be scattered over plasma and organelle membranes.
4. The closer the fit between the drug and the receptor site, the stronger the binding.
5. A drug molecule may simultaneously bind at two, or possibly even more, receptor sites.

One concept of membrane pores views the membrane as an array of macromolecular cylinders packed radially, each approximately 20 A in diameter, leaving pores bounded by three cylinders with a radius of approximately 4 A. (Na^+ and K^+ ions may have either one or two "shells" of hydration — usually one — with diameters of 3.7 and 4.1 A respectively.) Drugs with CNS activity often have a radius equal to or slightly less than 4 A and frequently include groups with sulfur or nitrogen atoms, either of which increases their binding activity. There is some evidence that drugs of relatively small size, which do not accurately fit pores, act as CNS depressants, whereas drugs with larger molecules, more accurate fit, and more active binding tend to act as stimulants.

However, there are many complicating factors. Drug effects depend on concentration. For example, low concentrations of ether cause excitation and high concentrations cause depression; low to moderate concentrations of chlorpromazine cause depression, but high concentrations cause excitation. There are also problems of interpretation, since drugs dissociate behavioral from EEG changes, so that assessment of the EEG is not a satisfactory criterion of drug activity. Furthermore, drugs that are excitatory to only part of the CNS may appear inhibitory in gross behavioral terms.

If drugs with a definite specific synaptic action are excluded, it becomes apparent that the theoretical basis of neuropharmacology is somewhat tenuous. Nonetheless, the subject is of such central importance to clinical medicine that it seems justifiable to discuss it, even if few data are available and most of the discussion must concern theory.

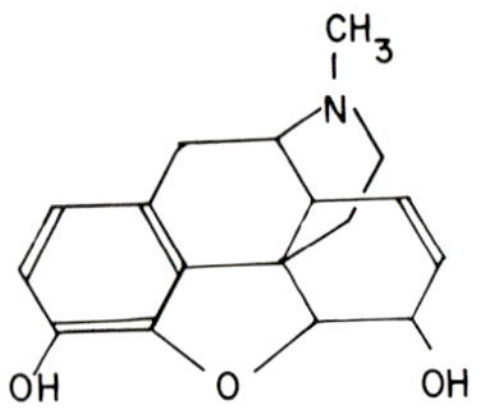

Morphine

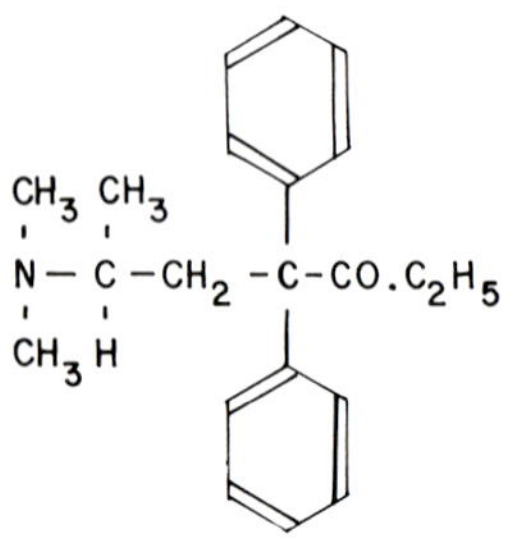

Methadone

Fig. 9-11. Two centrally acting analgesics.

CENTRALLY ACTING (NARCOTIC) ANALGESICS

At least in the form of opium, narcotic analgesics are almost as old as history. The opiate group now includes not only the naturally occurring opium alkaloids (morphine and codeine) but also a large number of synthetic derivatives, synthetic drugs with a similar action, and drugs developed as narcotic antagonists that are effective as analgesics. Little is known of the molecular mechanisms by which narcotic analgesics are effective, and even the topographical sites at which they act (presumably including the midbrain and ascending reticular activating system) are speculative. In varying doses, they are effective against severe chronic pain, apparently reducing both the perception of pain and reaction to it (percept and affect). The use of any of these drugs is accompanied by the phenomena of tolerance (doses must be increased to achieve a satisfactory effect, with a corresponding reduction in side effects) and physical addiction (molecular modification in the CNS, such that withdrawal of the drug leads to profound functional disturbances). With few exceptions, these drugs seem to have part of their structure in common, and this is presumably the major binding part of the molecule, γ-phenyl-N-methylpiperidine.

The dried juice of the opium poppy *(Papaver somniferum)* contains two groups of alkaloids: *phenanthrenes,* which include morphine and codeine (approximately 10% and 0.5% by weight respectively), and *benzylisoquinolines,* of which only papaverine is of clinical significance. Morphine (Fig. 9-11) has phenolic and alcoholic —OH groups, either or both of which are substituted in synthetic derivatives, which may be more or less powerful than the parent morphine or occasionally act as morphine antagonists (e.g., as nalorphine). Morphine is one of the most effective analgesics available, particularly since it is also active against visceral pain. It may produce drowsiness and euphoria or, in other cases, anxiety and nausea. It is a powerful respiratory depressant and causes pupilloconstriction. Occasional side effects include vomiting, constipation, bronchoconstriction, central vasomotor depression, and increased tone of the bladder sphincters. Tolerance to both analgesic and respiratory depressant actions develops rapidly and lasts at least one to two weeks after withdrawal of the drug. Its mechanism is unknown. Codeine is an important, but milder analgesic and seems to have a specific depressant effect on the cough center.

Methadone (Fig. 9-11) is similar in effect to morphine, although lacking its characteristic chemical structure. It is longer-acting, effective orally, and produces less severe tolerance and addiction. It has therefore been used to mitigate the crises of morphine withdrawal.

CENTRAL NERVOUS SYSTEM STIMULANTS

Central nervous system stimulants (Fig. 9-12) are also termed *analeptics* because of their arousal effects. Unlike the depressants, many stimulants have clear preferential sites of action within the CNS. Some are convulsants, such as pentylenetetrazol, picrotoxin, nikethamide, and bemegride, which act preferentially at the brain stem level, and strychnine, which acts on the spinal cord. Many others, including caffeine, amphetamine, ephedrine, cocaine, atropine, pipradol, and methylphenidate, act on the cortex. Some drugs acting on the cortex are psychomotor stimulants rather than convulsants. All stimulants lower the threshold of excitability in the CNS, regionally or diffusely. They may produce cerebral dysrhythmia, and their effects are often associated with increased synaptic transmission. The molecular mechanisms are usually unknown.

Convulsants

It is thought that *strychnine* acts at the Renshaw cell to prevent feedback inhibition of the alpha motoneurons (tetanus toxin may act similarly). *Picrotoxin* is thought to decrease Cl^- permeability, and since increased Cl^- permeability is probably the basis of inhibition, this provides a possible rationale for its convulsant action. Some of the lesser-known convulsants, such as semicarbazide and its derivatives, appear to block enzyme actions that require pyridoxal (including many decarboxylases), and convulsions induced by these agents are aborted by pyridoxal administration. Inhibition of such pyridoxal-dependent enzymes may lower brain

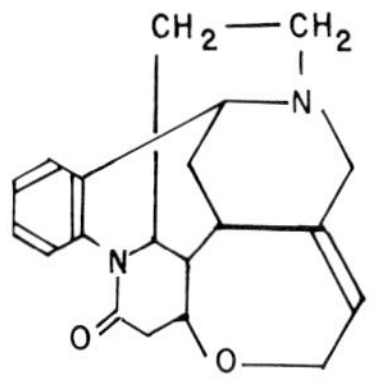

Strychnine

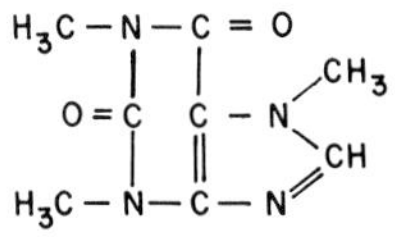

Caffeine

Fig. 9-12. Two centrally acting stimulants.

(particularly cortical) levels of γ-aminobutyric acid, a possible inhibitory modulator of CNS activity (see Chap. 3).

Psychomotor Stimulants

Psychomotor drugs include *caffeine* (a cup of coffee contains 100 to 150 mg of caffeine), which stimulates cortical and medullary centers by unknown mechanisms. *Amphetamines* are also extensively used as psychomotor stimulants; amphetamine itself is a sympathomimetic drug and a MAO inhibitor (combining with the enzyme and inactivating it). Administration of amphetamine is associated with increased production of methylated norepinephrine derivatives, suggesting that there is also impaired reuptake and consequent inactivation by COMT. Although often considered an addictive drug, amphetamine does not cause withdrawal symptoms.

BIBLIOGRAPHY

Baldessarini, R. J. Biogenic amines and behavior. *Annu. Rev. Med.* 23:343-354, 1972.

Goth, A. *Medical Pharmacology* (6th ed.). St. Louis: Mosby, 1972.

Grey, T. C., and Nunn, J. F. (Eds.) *General Anaesthesia* (3rd ed.). London: Butterworth, 1971. Vol. 1.

Hebb, C., and Morris, D. Identification of Acetylcholine and Its Metabolism in Nervous Tissue. In G. H. Bourne (Ed.), *The Structure and Function of Nervous Tissue.* New York: Academic, 1969. Vol. 3, pp. 25-60.

Iversen, L. I. Catecholamine uptake processes. *Br. Med. Bull.* 92:130-135, 1973.

Jenkinson, D. H. Classification and properties of peripheral adrenergic receptors. *Br. Med. Bull.* 92:142-147, 1973.

Page, I. H. Serotonin and the Brain. In G. H. Bourne (Ed.), *The Structure and Function of Nervous Tissue.* New York: Academic, 1969. Vol. 3, pp. 289-307.

Smith, A. D. Mechanisms involved in release of noradrenaline from sympathetic nerves. *Br. Med. Bull.* 92:123-129, 1973.

Disorders of the Central Nervous System

II

General Pathological Reactions of Central Nervous System Cells

10

The central nervous system, composed of multiple areas with different structures, has perhaps more ways of reacting to disease than any other organ. However, the individual brain cell, like a cell anywhere, has a limited repertoire of reactions. Thus, for some types of degeneration or necrosis of neurons or glial cells there is a wide variety of causative factors, often metabolic or vascular. These form the subject matter for this chapter, to avoid reiteration later. On the other hand, certain neuronal or glial changes are virtually pathognomonic of one disease or a closely related group of diseases. Such changes are therefore described in the chapter devoted to the disease or diseases to which they are related.

INTERPRETATION OF NEURONAL MORPHOLOGY

The interpretation of the morphology of neurons in routinely prepared material is complicated by many factors. Some of these can be eliminated in experimental work in small animals, but in the day-to-day practice of medicine, they have to be accepted, lived with, and recognized. In the absence of disease, variations in the appearance of neurons may be due to:

1. Real topographical variation in cell type (e.g., the difference between anterior horn cells and the cells of the thoracic nucleus of Clarke).
2. Local homeostatic conditions immediately preceding death, particularly in patients with acid-base, electrolyte, or water imbalance.
3. The age of the patient.
4. Changes induced by autolysis (before or after death), fixation, dehydration, cutting, embedding, and staining.

The concept of differences in neuronal appearance with varying functional states has been advanced, but there seems to be little definite evidence to bear this out. Electron-microscopic correlates for many of these conditions have not been adequately described. Although autopsy material can be used for electron-microscopic investigation, the resulting artifactual changes are equally, or perhaps even more, formidable than in examination by light microscopy.

Neuronal Artifacts

A particularly common neuronal artifact is the small, contracted, diffusely overstained cell, often surrounded by a perineuronal cleft. Common in both biopsy and autopsy material, it can be produced by minor physical trauma to the tissue or during preparation for microscopic examination. These shrunken or "spiky" cells resemble a type of neuronal shrinkage considered by many a true pathological change, illustrating the difficulties of interpretation. A converse artifact also occurs, with neurons appearing swollen, rounded, and pale-staining, often with an indistinct cell border; the nucleus may be large and pale, or pyknotic. The artifactual nature of this change, which also resembles changes considered truly pathological, can sometimes be inferred from looseness and fragmentation of adjacent tissues. A particularly common but restricted neuronal artifact involves the internal granular layer of the cerebellum, in which cells appear poorly stained and clumped (this may often be predicted grossly from a peculiar "fish-flesh" appearance of the cerebellar cortex).

Accompanying Gliosis

Obviously, most problems arise in the interpretation of acute or subacute neuronal changes without glial alterations. The interpretation of swelling, shrinkage, or changes in staining reactions of neurons, without accompanying vascular or glial changes, must be very cautious. Undoubtedly, the most reliable sign of neuronal disease is disappearance of the neuron, but even this may be difficult to detect unless an appreciable number (perhaps 30% or more) are absent. In these more chronic conditions there is often an associated glial reaction, enabling some confidence in a diagnosis of pathological change. Even here, a note of caution must be sounded, since the presence of considerable numbers of glial fibrils, though often indicative of disease, is normal in some areas, including the brain stem median raphe, the inferior olivary nuclei, and subependymal and subpial areas. In the brain stem, this gliosis may be especially dense, and determination of pathological changes must often rest on unequivocal neuronal or axonal alterations or on spread of the gliosis to other areas.

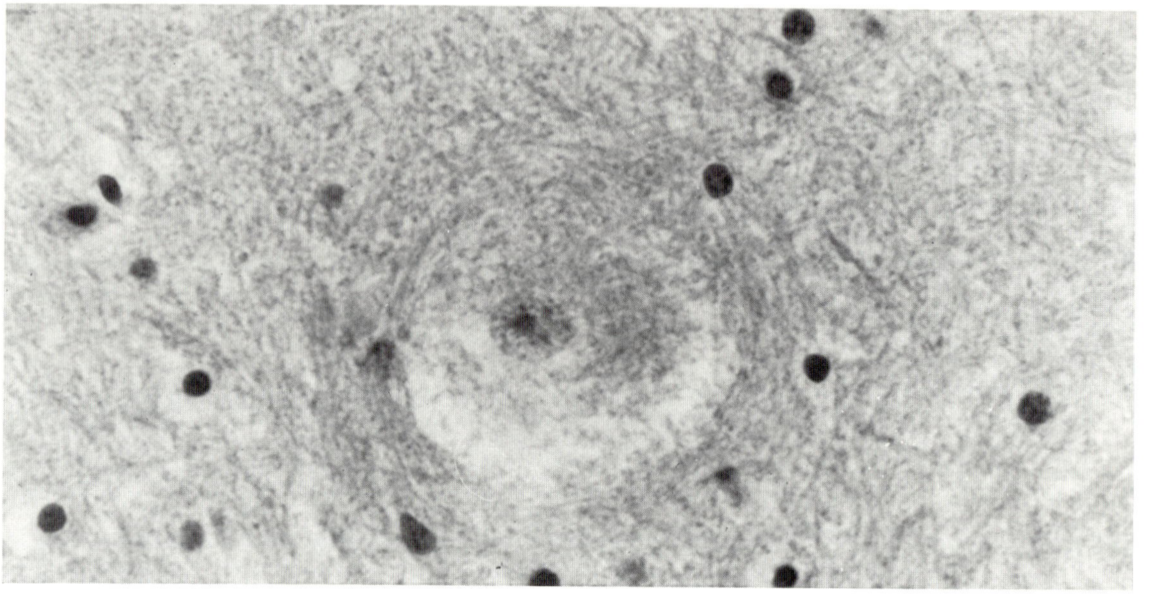

Fig. 10-1. Neuronal swelling (dentate nucleus, severe hyperpyrexia). (H & E, X750.)

Stains

Most neuropathological diagnoses can be made on sections stained routinely, as with hematoxylin and eosin, but special stains are essential to visualize neuronal and glial processes and assist in seeing myelin. The stains most often used are:

1. Basic dyes, such as cresyl violet (Nissl's method) or gallocyanin, which react with ribonucleic acid and therefore stain the granular endoplasmic reticulum (including Nissl bodies) and nucleolus.
2. Stains involving deposition of metallic silver (e.g., methods of Glees, Holmes, Bodian), which are valuable for the demonstration of axons.
3. Stains reacting with compound lipids, such as modified hematoxylin solutions (Weil's, Weigert's, Heidenhain's) or dyes like Luxol-fast blue, which are used for the demonstration of myelin or its breakdown products.
4. Stains for the demonstration of glial fibrils, such as Holzer's and the phosphotungstic acid–hematoxylin techniques.

Many other methods are available for the demonstration of dendrites and processes of glial cells, and histochemical and enzyme histochemical techniques may be used. Frequently, combinations of stains, such as Luxol-gallocyanin or Luxol-Holmes, assist in the orientation of structures and so enable more information to be obtained. However, it must be stressed that, although special stains are of value in confirming impressions gained from sections stained with hematoxylin and eosin and for photographic or other demonstration, and have been indispensable tools in obtaining what knowledge we have of CNS structure, most service neuropathological study is carried out using a routine stain. Special stains should be ordered only as appropriate on selected sections.

GENERAL REACTIONS OF NEURONS

Out of the large number of nonspecific swellings, shrinkages, and discolorations of neurons that have been considered pathological, a relatively small group have survived to be considered (fairly) reliable in routinely prepared material.

Reactions to Generalized Metabolic Deficiencies, Altered Homeostasis, and Endogenous or Exogenous Toxins

A formerly complex and overly eponymous classification has narrowed down to neuronal changes involving swelling and those involving shrinkage. Depending on severity, either change may indicate degeneration (i.e., reversible) or necrosis (i.e., irreversible). Degenerated neurons may become necrotic or recover, as in tissues elsewhere.

Swelling

Neuronal swelling is first manifested by a swollen, pale perikaryon and swollen dendrites, with basophilic or amphophilic cytoplasmic staining, as though RNA were diffuse rather than aggregated in Nissl bodies. The nucleus is also large and pale with an apparently normal nucleolus (Fig. 10-1). Such changes are sometimes associated with infections or hyperthermia and are often seen throughout the CNS; they are frequently reversible. Progression of damage is shown by irregular basophilic rings or granules (not

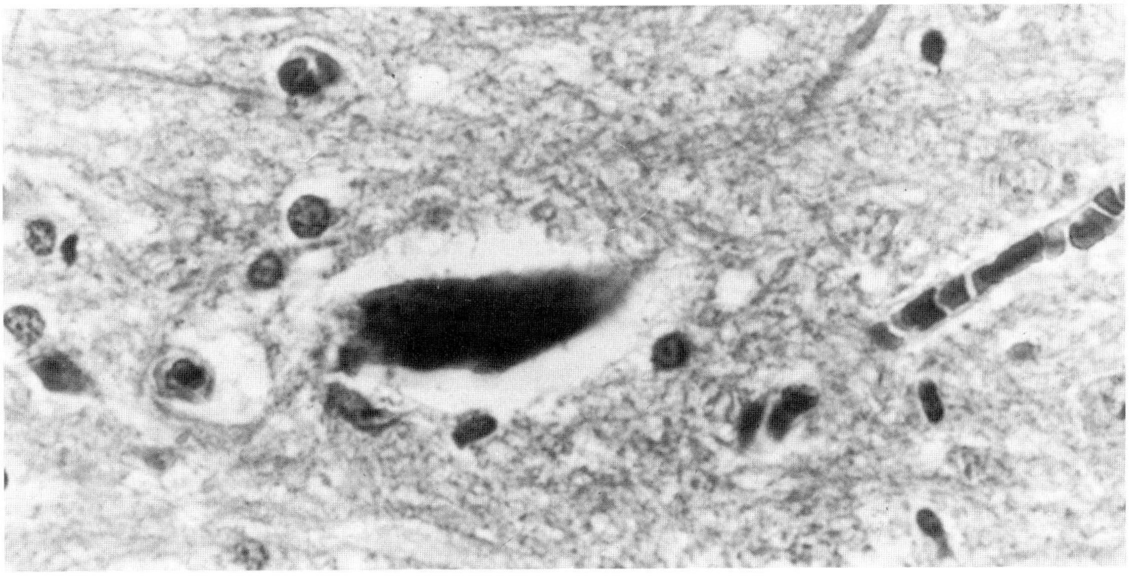

Fig. 10-2. Neuronal shrinkage (trauma to brain stem). (H & E, × 750.)

Nissl bodies) in and around the more swollen cell body. Finally, cytoplasm may vacuolate and disappear, leaving only the basophilic bodies adjacent to a shrunken dark nucleus with an eccentric nucleolus. Such cells may show an increased number of adjacent oligodendroglia (satellitosis) or activated microglial cells (neuronophagia). These changes are described in severe hyperthermia, toxic psychoses, lead poisoning, and focal encephalitis and are essentially irreversible (neuronal necrosis).

Shrinkage

In neuronal shrinkage, the cell margin becomes concave and well defined, the dendrites often tortuous, and the cytoplasm hyperchromic and basophilic. The nucleus is dark and shrunken, with an indistinct nucleolus (Fig. 10-2). With more severe change, the whole neuron becomes a uniform mass of dark, slightly granular material, within which the nucleus cannot always be distinguished. This is presumably irreversible. Such changes may be found in severe heat stroke, prolonged intermittent hypoxia, and at the margins of traumatic cortical hemorrhages. They mainly affect pyramidal and Purkinje's cells, and affected cells are often interspersed with apparently normal neurons. (The difficulty of distinguishing early stages of neuronal shrinkage from spiky artifacts is apparent.)

A special form of neuronal shrinkage associated with ischemia is generally thought to be a reliable pathological change, although it has recently been suggested that it, too, may be imitated by artifact. In *ischemic change,* neurons become shrunken and angular, Nissl bodies are lost and, unlike any of the preceding changes, the cytoplasm becomes eosinophilic (Figs. 10-3, 10-4). A perineuronal space, probably an artifact, is present. The nucleus is shrunken and so dark that the nucleolus may not be distinguishable. The surface of the cell may show minute basophilic dots, perhaps representing degenerating presynaptic knobs. These cells are seen within and adjacent to infarctions and appear to develop within 6 to 12 hours. Possibly related is *homogenizing change,* seen in less severe prolonged ischemia and some severe fevers, possibly associated with hypoxemia. The cell body is pale and eosinophilic and may show either a somewhat refractile or foamy granular cytoplasm. The nucleus loses its membrane and becomes mere clumps of basophilic granules around a more or less eosinophilic nucleolus. Electron microscopy shows the earliest changes to be microvacuolation of the cell body and dendrites, due to swelling of mitochondria and endoplasmic reticulum, and separation of the two layers of the nuclear envelope. This is accompanied and followed by progressive electron density of the nucleus and cytoplasm and by vacuolar shrinkage. The shrunken neuron shows areas of greater and lesser density of unknown significance and appears to be invaded (and possibly removed) by astrocytic processes.

Simple Atrophy

Simple atrophy involves the neuron with all its processes and is seen in the abiotrophies, which are conditions in which neurons degenerate and disappear prematurely (see Chap. 24), in trans-synaptic atrophy, and (rarely) in retrograde trans-synaptic atrophy. Trans-synaptic atrophy occurs in structures that derive virtually their entire input from a single source (e.g., the lateral geniculate body or inferior

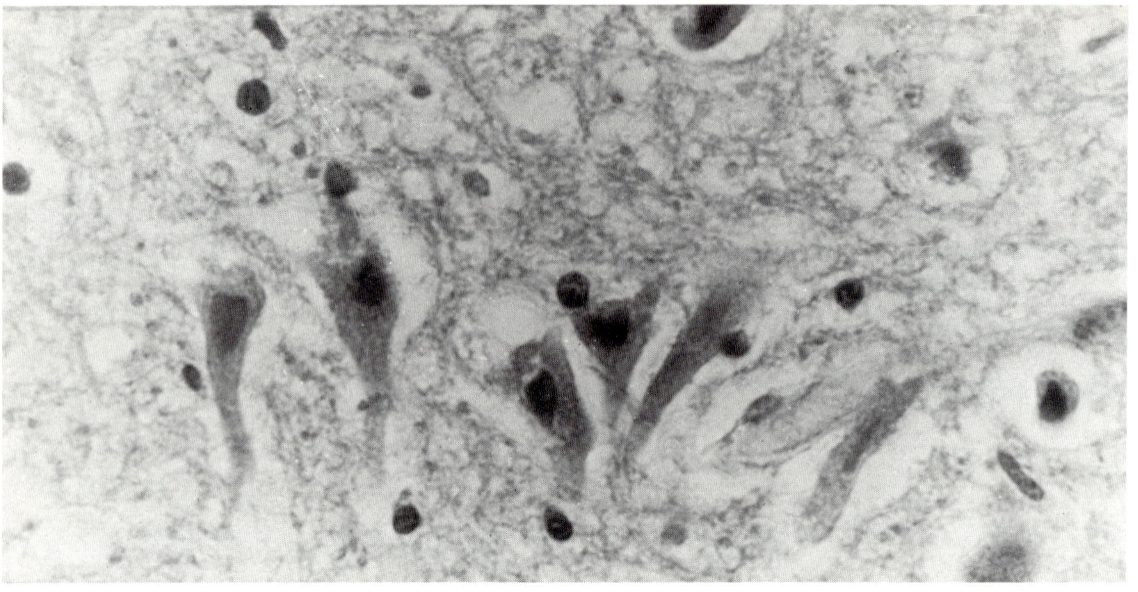

Fig. 10-3. Ischemic neuron (hippocampus). (H & E, ×750.)

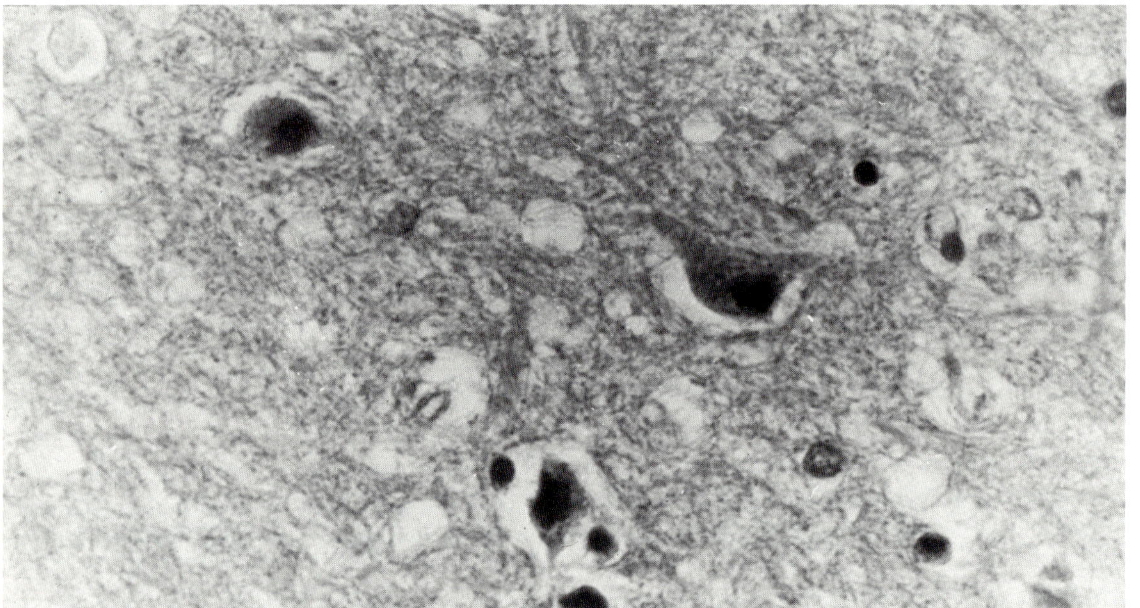

Fig. 10-4. Ischemic neuron (thalamus). (H & E, ×750.)

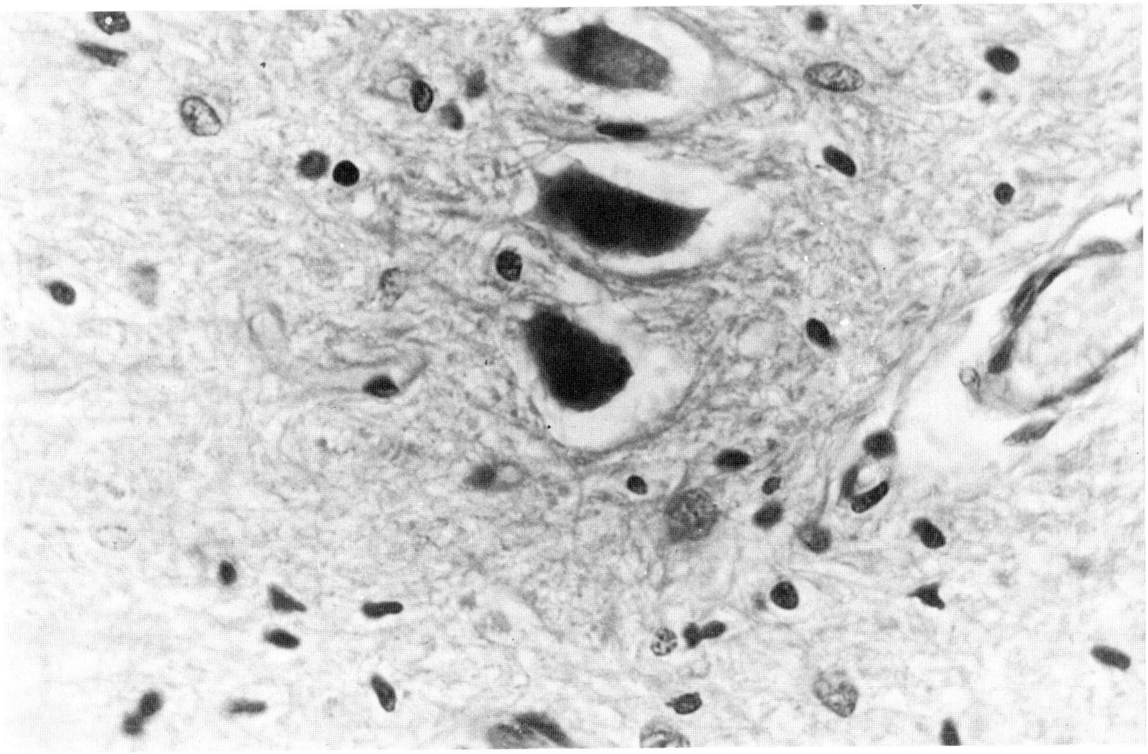

Fig. 10-5. Neuron showing simple atrophy (dentate nucleus, trans-synaptic atrophy). (H & E, ×750.)

olivary nucleus). When this source is destroyed, the neurons are in a state of virtual deafferentation and may atrophy and disappear. Retrograde trans-synaptic atrophy is said to occur in structures whose entire output is to a single destination, which has been destroyed. They are left in the CNS as "culs-de-sac," but as they receive normal input, such degeneration occurs less often. It has been reported in the inferior olives following destruction of cerebellar cortical cells, e.g., by heat stroke. Simple atrophy is also the reaction of neurons whose axons have been severed or irreversibly damaged, if these axons are entirely within the CNS. This is called *Gudden's atrophy* and may be seen in the lateral geniculate body after damage to the optic radiation, in the medial thalamic columns after prefrontal leukotomy, or in the inferior olives after lesions of the cerebellar white matter.

In simple atrophy (Fig. 10-5) the cells become shrunken and concave, with loss of Nissl bodies, but may show variable diffuse hyperchromia. The nucleus is dark and shrunken. There is often thickening and beading of neurofibrils (visible on silver staining). In Gudden's atrophy the residual axon may become tortuous and visible on routine stains. Ultimately, the cells become smaller and paler and disappear, with little glial reaction except for mild diffuse fibrillary gliosis.

Central Chromatolysis (Axonal Reaction)

As noted, neurons lying entirely within the CNS react to axonal loss by simple atrophy. In cells with processes outside the CNS (anterior horn cells, brain stem motor nuclei, dorsal root and corresponding

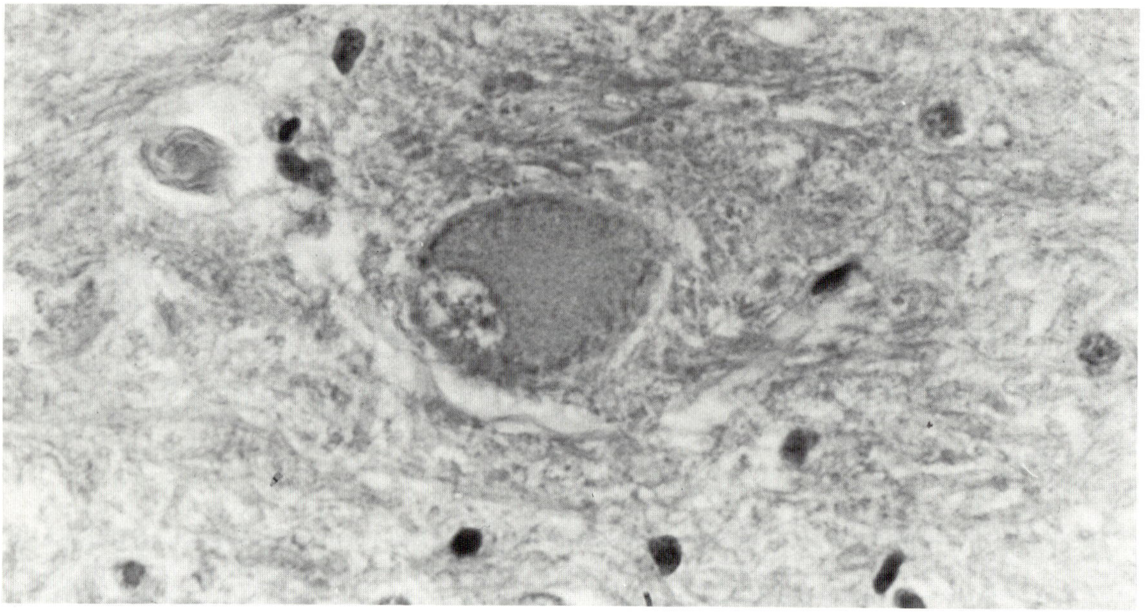

Fig. 10-6. Neuron showing central chromatolysis (medulla, post-traumatic). (H & E, X750.)

cranial nerve ganglia) there appears to be some regeneration of axons, and the cell body shows a reaction characterized by swelling, disappearance of Nissl bodies from all but the edge of the cytoplasm, and often swelling and eccentricity of the nucleus (Fig. 10-6). These changes begin about 48 to 72 hours after acute axonal section, peak after two to three weeks, and regress over the succeeding two to three months. Regression is accompanied by reappearance of Nissl bodies, first in the perinuclear zone, and there may be a stage during which the cell is hyperchromic. Occasionally, cells entirely within the CNS that have lost their axons show transient chromatolysis before passing into Gudden's atrophy. Electron microscopy shows apparent loss of ribosomes and reduced granular endoplasmic reticulum, with increased neurofilaments. Granular endoplasmic reticulum is presumably regenerated from the persistent agranular membranes.

Although this lesion is characteristic of axonal damage and unlikely to represent artifact, it can be misdiagnosed. In the thoracic nucleus of Clarke, the normal neurons are round, with peripheral Nissl bodies and an often eccentric nucleus, and they mimic central chromatolysis. A similar change may be found in nutritional diseases (e.g., in cortical pyramidal cells in pellagra) and in poliomyelitis or subacute sclerosing panencephalitis – conditions usually associated with direct damage to the cell body (though axonal damage cannot be excluded).

Binucleate Neurons

Although neuroblasts and immature neurons continue to differentiate, and even to migrate, for some months after birth, it is improbable that division of neuronal precursors can take place later than term. Occasional neurons are found with two (or, rarely, more) nuclei in patients with traumatic lesions, postencephalitic paralysis agitans, congenital or acquired syphilis, and other conditions, especially in some childhood diseases, including tuberous sclerosis and macrencephaly.

Neuronal Uptake of Blood Pigments

In the vicinity of areas of hemorrhage, even within a few hours after it occurs, neurons that appear otherwise normal (on light microscopy) take up blood pigment that appears as minute rods, granules, or crystals within the cytoplasm. This may occur before pigmentation is seen in glial or mesenchymal cells. Often, because of vascular insufficiency and edema, these neurons also show ischemic change and are presumably necrotic. The ultimate fate of neurons that take up pigment without exhibiting degenerative change at the time is uncertain, but occasional areas

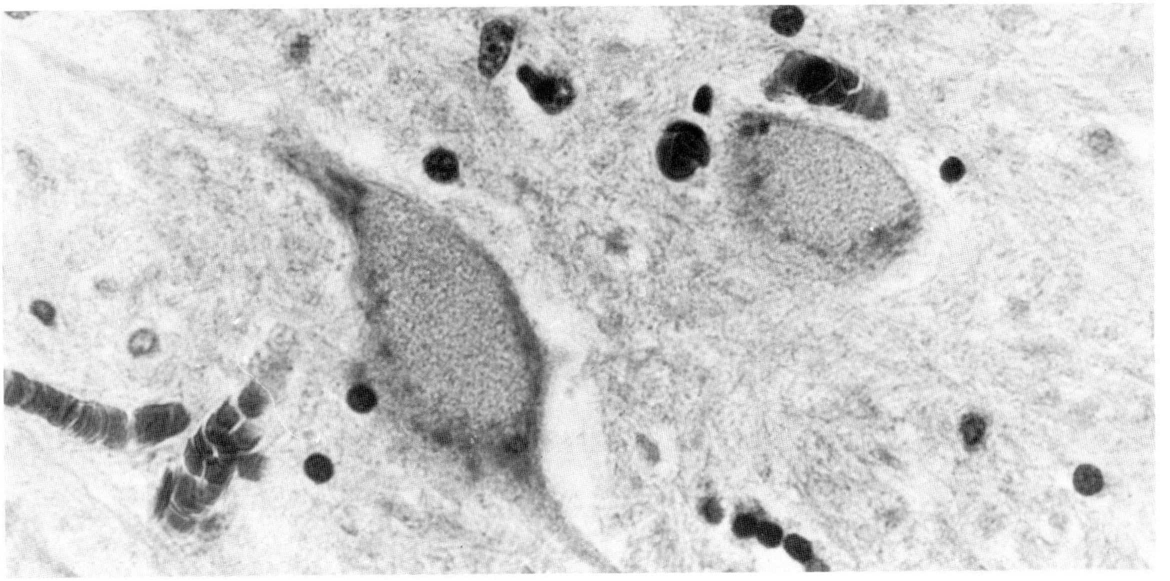

Fig. 10-7. Neuron containing lipofuscin (medulla, 77-year-old patient). (H & E, ×750.)

of fine, dustlike basophilic granules are found incidentally at autopsy that reproduce the shape of neurons, with or without linear aggregates resembling dendrites. The basophilic dust contains iron, and the process is *ferrugination.* Whether or not it represents the end result of neuronal hematin uptake is speculative.

Lipofuscinosis of Neurons

Neurons in the CNS readily accumulate a pigment that resembles lipofuscin ("wear-and-tear" pigment) in other parts of the body. Lipofuscinosis of neurons (Fig. 10-7) cannot be regarded as entirely an aging change (see Chap. 20), since it is found in young age groups in certain regions of the brain and may accompany simple atrophy of neurons. It is common in middle age in the inferior olivary, dentate, and lateral geniculate nuclei, with moderate accumulations in cortical pyramidal cells and motoneurons. It is unusual in Purkinje's cells. Clumps of pigment granules are yellowish-brown in sections stained with hemotoxylin and eosin, are acid-fast, and seem to contain glycolipid. Although probably originating in lysosomes, developed lipofuscin granules are not clearly associated with hydrolytic enzymes such as acid phosphatase.

GENERAL REACTIONS OF ASTROCYTES

Astrocytes are widely distributed in the CNS and may be divided into the fibrous type, occurring largely in white matter and containing glial fibrils, and the protoplasmic type, occurring largely in gray matter, with much lower, but not negligible, fibrillary content. Astrocytes are less sensitive to most noxae than are either neurons or oligodendroglial cells and are largely responsible for such limited reparative powers as the CNS possesses. They may show hyperplasia, hypertrophy, and fibrillary gliosis – all reactive changes – the prime stimulus being destruction of CNS tissue irrespective of cause (e.g., infarction, trauma, abscess, neoplasm). Even minor or incomplete destruction may cause a fine, diffuse fibrillary gliosis, as in neuronal loss of the simple atrophic type, relatively slight degrees of cerebral edema or ischemia, and infectious conditions such as syphilis and some viral diseases. In assessing the significance of areas of gliosis, it must be remembered that in certain situations it is normal. In reactive change, the distinction between a protoplasmic and fibrous astrocyte may be lost, since either is capable of forming fibrillary networks. In extremely adverse conditions, astrocytes, like other cells, undergo degeneration and necrosis. This occurs in areas of complete tissue destruction, such as infarcts, massive hemorrhages, and abscesses, and also in severe chronic edema. Although astrocytes are lost in the center of mass lesions, reactive (reparative) changes occur at the periphery, where damage is less intense.

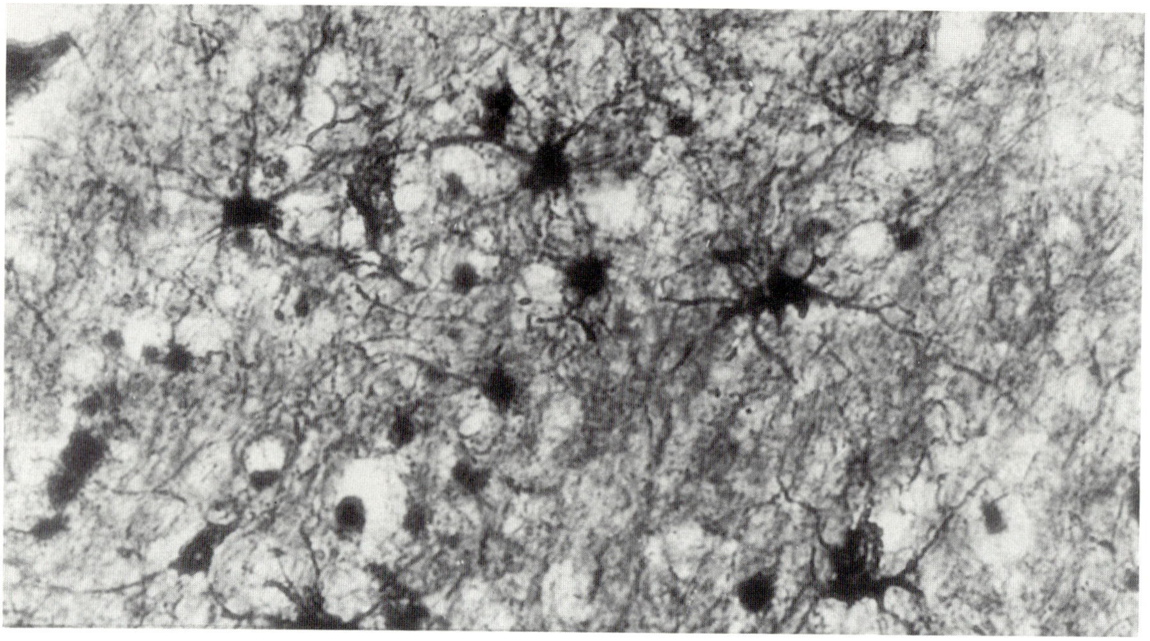

Fig. 10-8. Astrocytes showing degenerative changes (cerebral edema). (Cajal method, ×750.)

Astrocytic Degeneration and Necrosis

In normal CNS sections stained with hematoxylin and eosin, astrocytic cytoplasm is not visible, the nucleus appearing bare in the neuropil. In early degeneration the cell body swells and becomes visible as an homogeneous eosinophilic mass with a central or eccentric nucleus. Subsequently, the astrocytic processes break off as irregular chains of granular debris (not visible with hematoxylin and eosin), and occasionally a few lipid granules appear in the swollen cell body. The nucleus becomes irregular, shrunken, and hyperchromic; and finally, the nucleus and cytoplasm disintegrate and disappear. As well as in mass lesions and edema (Fig. 10-8), regressive astrocytic changes may be seen in acute toxic states (including toxic delirium in uremic and diabetic coma), syphilis of the CNS, and status epilepticus. The electron-microscopic correlates of these changes have not been described.

Reactive Changes in Astrocytes

Astrocytic reaction also starts with hypertrophy of the cell body, but is not accompanied by degeneration of processes. Cytoplasm is uniform, eosinophilic, and somewhat hyaline in appearance (Fig. 10-9), and, if rounded, the cell is termed a *gemistocyte.* Nuclei become larger, darker, and sometimes irregular, often exhibiting a small nucleolus not seen in the resting state. They divide amitotically, and the cells may remain multinucleate or divide (hyperplasia), each daughter cell retaining a portion of the foot process. Although small lipid granules may appear in degenerating astrocytes, there is no evidence that these cells are phagocytic.

Formation of new glial fibrils within the cytoplasm of the cell almost invariably accompanies hyperplasia and hypertrophy (Fig. 10-10). Fibrils are 60 to 80 A wide and do not show periodicity (unlike collagen). Production begins as a network near the nucleus, the fibrils then being formed into parallel bundles (visible on light microscopy), partly by orientation within folds of the nuclear membrane. Production extends within the cell body and processes, and, in tissue culture, astrocytes form a network of intracellular fibrils that may appear continuous from cell to cell. Chemically, glial fibrils differ from collagen by lacking high levels of proline, hydroxyproline, glycine, and cystine, and they more closely resemble the KMEF proteins (keratin, myosin, epidermin, and fibrinogen), showing elasticity and often contractility. (In tissue culture, stimulation of astrocytes leads to slow mechanical contraction of their processes.) Active astrocytes show increased bioenergetic and hydrolytic activity. Although old glial scars are markedly deficient in nuclei, it is not yet proved that the fibers are extracellular.

Fibrillary gliosis in the CNS is not on the same scale as collagen fibrosis in other tissues. Large areas of CNS loss are replaced by fluid-filled cavities rather than by extensive fibrillary gliosis. Cavities may be multiple and irregular, their walls made up of tangentially and irregularly oriented glial fibrils with relatively few astrocytic nuclei. This is termed *cystic gliosis.*

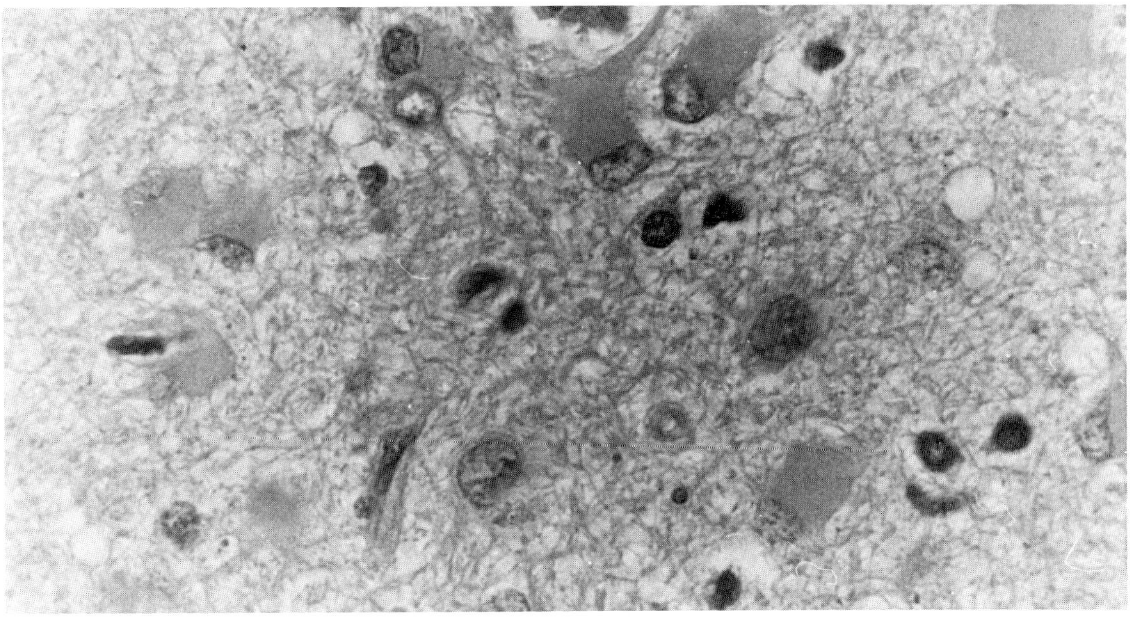

Fig. 10-9. Astrocytes showing reactive hypertrophy of cytoplasm, forming gemistocytes. (H & E, ×750.)

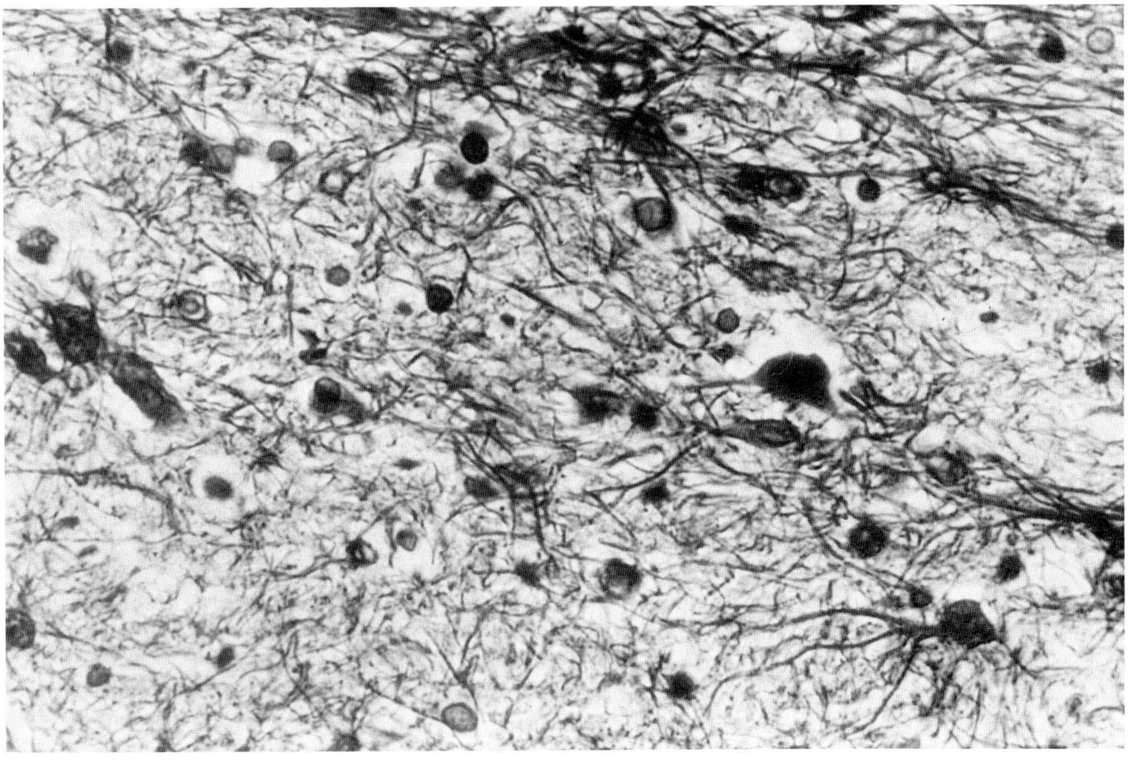

Fig. 10-10. Astrocytes showing new formation of glial fibrils. Electron microscopy has shown that these remain intracellular, but cell cytoplasm is not readily visible, and they often seem to be extracellular. (Holzer's method, ×750.)

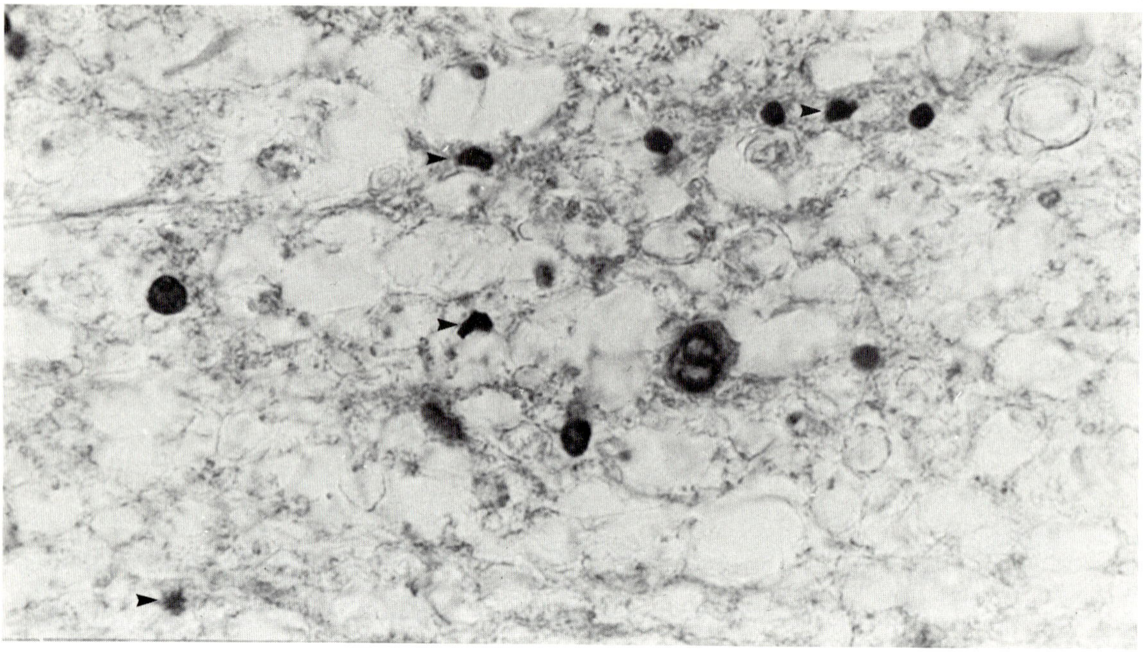

Fig. 10-11. Oligodendroglia showing nuclear pyknosis (arrows) at the margin of a small white-matter infarct. A large, reactive astrocytic nucleus and refractile outlines of swollen myelin sheaths are also seen. (H & E, ×750.)

GENERAL REACTIONS OF OLIGODENDROGLIAL CELLS

Oligodendroglia are widespread, occurring in the vicinity of neurons, where they form *satellite cells,* and in oriented rows among myelinated fiber tracts; the latter are called *interfascicular oligodendroglia.* Little is known of their potentiality for reactive (i.e., reparative) change. Oligodendroglia apparently appear in increased numbers near neurons (satellitosis) in some functional or disease states, suggesting powers of motility, and there is evidence of some myelin regeneration in the CNS, though not on the scale seen peripherally.

Oligodendroglia are relatively sensitive to noxae. Their susceptibility to oxygen deficit in the CNS is second only to that of neurons, though they seem poor in tricarboxylic acid cycle enzymes, implying that they use largely the hexose monophosphate (not energy-producing) and glycolytic pathways. Nonetheless, areas of ischemia that have not progressed to total tissue necrosis frequently show not only characteristic ischemic change in neurons, but also regressive changes in oligodendroglia (Fig. 10-11). Swollen cytoplasm appears as a perinuclear halo or as a narrow, uniformly eosinophilic rim around the nucleus (oligodendroglial cytoplasm is normally not visible on routine stains). The nucleus becomes small, dark, and irregular and may ultimately fragment (karyorrhexis).

The best-known light-microscopic change in oligodendroglia is *acute hydropic swelling* (Fig. 10-12), which is due to rapid enlargement of cytoplasm with accumulation of unstainable material, forming a perinuclear halo; the nucleus may show shrinkage, irregularity, and hyperchromia. Although associated especially with cerebral edema, minor to moderate degrees of this change occur as a postmortem artifact, so that it requires cautious interpretation. Electron microscopy shows the cell bodies and processes of the oligodendroglial cells to be enlarged and extremely electron-lucent.

GENERAL REACTIONS OF EPENDYMAL CELLS

Neither regressive nor reactive changes of the ependymal cells are commonly described. However, many conditions, including marked ventricular dilatation, childhood diseases such as tuberous sclerosis, and chronic infections, result in proliferation of the subependymal astroglial cells. These form nodules that may break through, or even envelop, nests of ependymal cells that appear otherwise normal, a condition called *subependymal gliosis.*

GENERAL REACTIONS OF MICROGLIAL CELLS

Microglia are mesenchymal cells, not glial cells, though they are often a prominent component of CNS reaction to disease. They may undergo hyperplasia or hypertrophy and may become actively ameboid phagocytic cells.

Microglial hypertrophy may be seen in the cortex in subacute inflammatory conditions, especially in

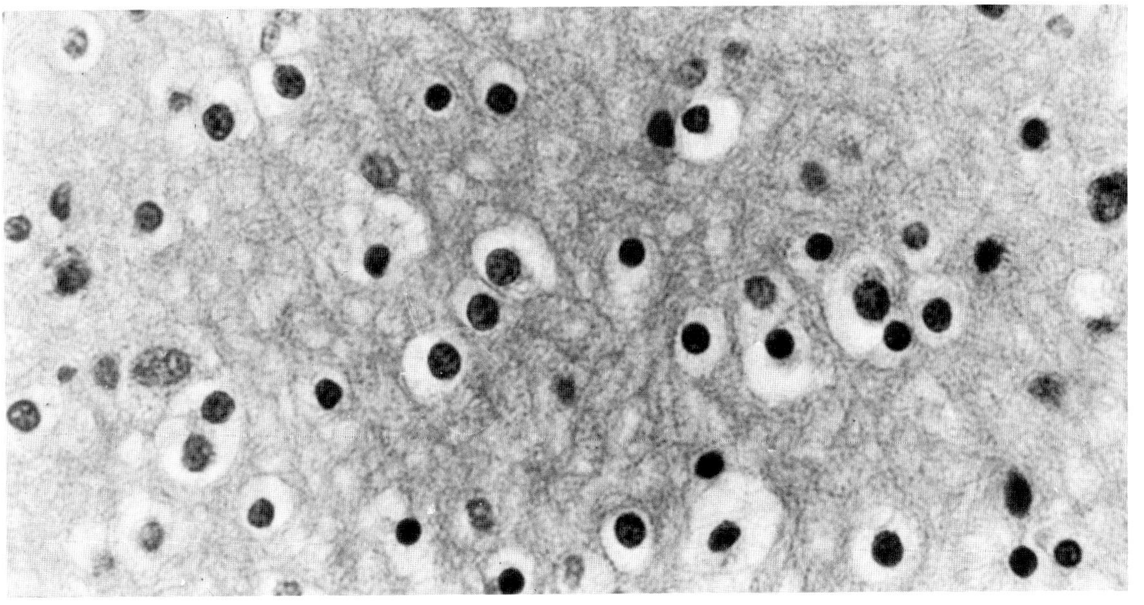

Fig. 10-12. Oligodendroglia showing hydropic swelling (edema). (H & E, ×750.)

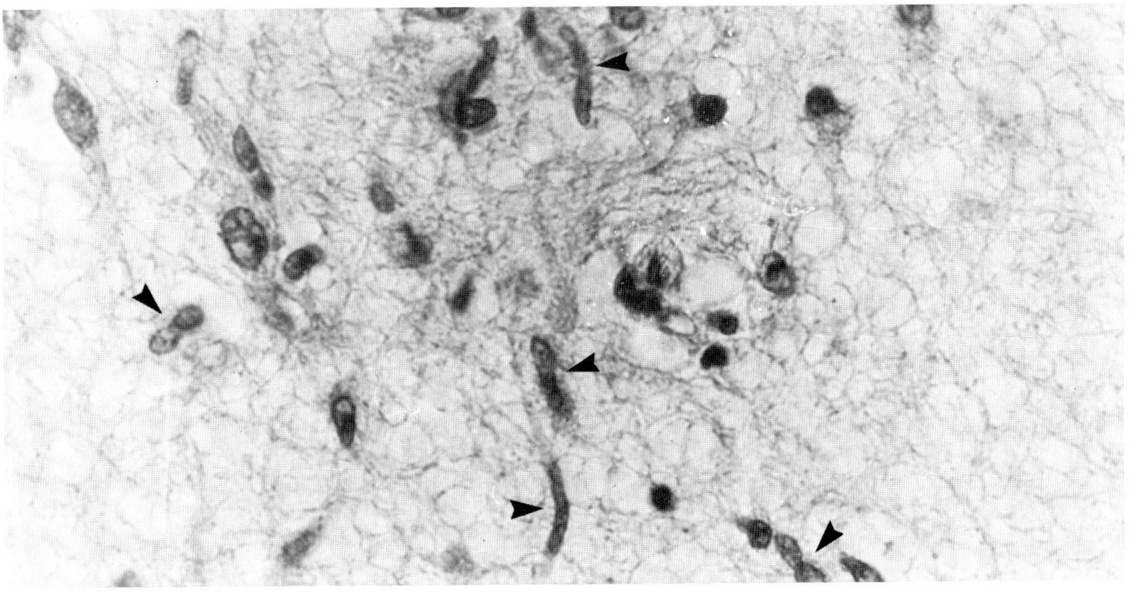

Fig. 10-13. Microglial cells showing reactive changes (arrows), adjacent to area of inflammation. (H & E, ×750.)

tertiary syphilis. The nucleus increases in size, is frequently spindle-shaped or even lobulated, and is orientated perpendicular to the surface. The cell retains its processes, often elongated and widened, and frequently contains stainable iron. In acute, subacute, or chronic encephalomyelitis, *microglial hyperplasia* (proliferation) may appear as "knots," "stars," or more diffuse areas of increased cellularity, especially in the gray matter and reticular formation (Fig. 10-13). In the rickettsial diseases, these hyperplastic cells may be perivascular, and adventitial macrophages may also be proliferating.

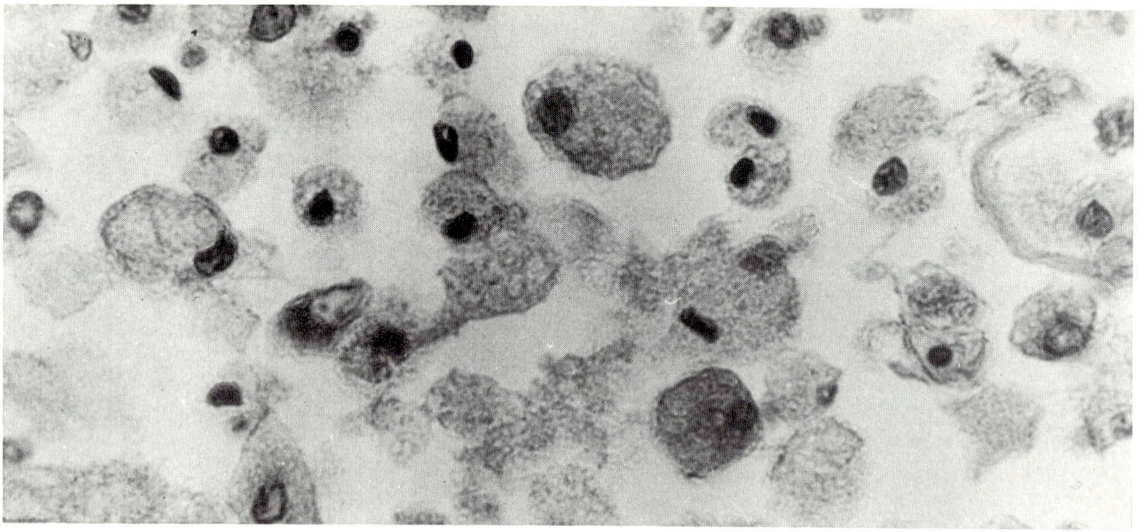

Fig. 10-14. Microglial cells fully converted to active, motile, phagocytic forms known as gitter cells or, in the older literature, compound granular corpuscles. (H & E, X 750.)

The cell may enlarge still further and become relatively globular, retracting its processes and undergoing nuclear division. It is then a characteristic macrophage (Fig. 10-14) and, especially in areas of myelin breakdown, is distended with vacuolar and granular debris and is termed a *gitter cell.* In acute neuronal death, *neuronophagia* may occur, neuronal remnants being surrounded by phagocytic microglial cells.

BIBLIOGRAPHY

Adams, R. D., and Sidman, R. L. *Introduction to Neuropathology.* New York: McGraw-Hill, 1968.

Blackwood, W., McMenemey, W. H., Meyer, A., and Russell, D. S. (Eds.). *Greenfield's Neuropathology* (2nd ed.). London: Arnold, 1963.

Brown, A. W., and Brierley, J. B. Anoxic-ischaemic cell change in rat brain. *J. Neurol. Sci.* 16:59-84, 1972.

Cammermeyer, J. Non-Specific Changes in the Central Nervous System in Normal and Experimental Material. In G. H. Bourne (Ed.), *The Structure and Function of Nervous Tissue.* New York: Academic, 1969. Vol. 6, pp. 131-251.

Luse, S. Astroglia. In J. Minckler (Ed.), *Pathology of the Nervous System.* New York: McGraw-Hill, 1968. Vol. 1, pp. 538-553.

Luse, S. Microglia. In J. Minckler (Ed.), *Pathology of the Nervous System.* New York: McGraw-Hill, 1968. Vol. 1, pp. 531-538.

Luse, S. The Neuron. In J. Minckler (Ed.), *Pathology of the Nervous System.* New York: McGraw-Hill, 1968. Vol. 1, pp. 553-585.

Central Nervous System Dysfunction in Some Common Homeostatic Disorders

11

In view of the large number of homeostatic disorders, it is necessary to confine this chapter to some that are commonly encountered in practice and often associated with CNS dysfunction. This dysfunction is generally reversible if the homeostatic disorder is remedied and may be considered as a metabolic encephalopathy. Disorders such as water, electrolyte, and acid-base imbalance rarely occur in pure form, so that CNS symptomatology is complicated and varied from case to case. However, some significant disorders are often identifiable. These include salt and water imbalance, acid-base imbalance, disorders of other electrolytes, diabetes mellitus, uremia, and liver failure.

The existence of physiological barriers between blood on the one hand and cerebrospinal fluid (CSF) and brain on the other implies an additional line of homeostatic defense for the CNS (see Chap. 4). Knowledge of the mechanisms and function of these barriers is incomplete, and since much investigation has been physiological rather than pathophysiological, more is known of barrier permeability to exogenous substances, such as analogues of thiourea, than even to simple metabolites like $NaHCO_3$ or water. Nonetheless, some generalizations may be made concerning barrier function:

1. The only substances concerned in homeostasis to which the barriers are freely permeable are oxygen, carbon dioxide, and water.
2. The net permeability of the barrier to ions is strictly limited, and ion distribution in the normal CSF — and presumably in brain extracellular fluid (ECF) — implies that ionic passage is at least in part due to active or facilitated transport. The effects of the DC potential may be an additional factor. Some ions, notably Ca^{++}, Mg^{++}, K^+, and HCO_3^-, can be maintained both above and below corresponding plasma levels, implying active transport in both directions.
3. In acutely developing imbalance, initial CSF changes can only be due to rapid diffusion of water or carbon dioxide, although later achievement of abnormal steady-state levels may involve altered transport or even passive diffusion of ions.
4. The known barrier functions are applicable only to normal or near-normal levels of metabolites, and the barrier reaction to gross alterations of metabolite concentration or to abnormal metabolites, such as may occur in renal and hepatic failure, is speculative.
5. Where metabolites are utilized or produced by CNS cells (e.g., O_2, glucose, CO_2, NH_3), or where, under normal conditions, the permeability of the two barriers is thought to be different (as for K^+), assumption of equal concentration in CSF and ECF may not be valid.

SALT-WATER BALANCE

Disorders of salt and water intake, output, or both produce physiological responses by changes in osmolality and total plasma volume; these two parameters may vary independently. In the production of encephalopathy, plasma volume per se is not a factor, and CNS dysfunction is induced by changes in osmolality gradients across the barrier system (taken to include both blood-brain and blood-CSF barriers unless otherwise stated). Except in diabetes mellitus and uremia, osmolality in plasma, CSF, and brain ECF is largely determined by the concentration of NaCl. Important factors for consideration are therefore the rates at which water, Na^+, and Cl^- can cross the barrier system. It is generally assumed, and borne out both by experimental and clinical experience, that the barrier is freely permeable to water in both directions.

Sodium and Chloride Transfer

Little is known of the quantitative aspects of Na^+ transfer (Fig. 11-1), though it is likely that active transfer into CSF and ECF is a factor in the secretion of these fluids. It depends on Na-K—activated adenosinetriphosphatase (ATPase), and CSF secretion is markedly reduced by ouabain. In normal CSF, Na^+ concentration is equal to, or slightly less than, concentration in plasma, since the rapid transfer of water makes it difficult to maintain a significant difference. Experimentally, if plasma Na^+ concentration is reduced but osmolality is normal (as in infusion of glucose) changes in CSF reflect those in plasma, Na^+ and Cl^- concentrations being reduced and glucose concentration increased. If the choroid plexus is bathed in fluid of low NaCl and high glucose concentration with normal osmolality, and the plasma is normal, the rate of CSF secretion increases as though

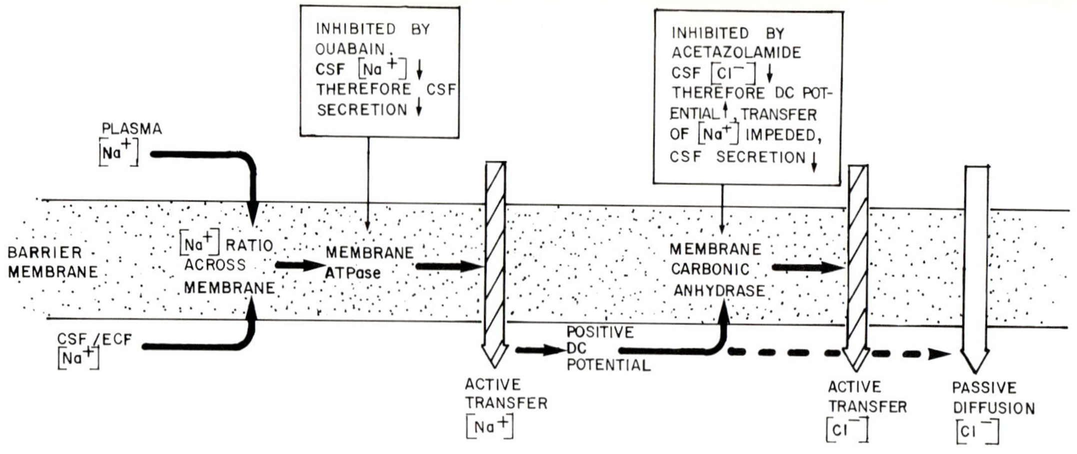

Fig. 11-1. Na^+ and Cl^- transfer across the blood-brain and blood-CSF barriers (cross-hatched arrows = active transfer).

stimulated by low Na^+ or Cl^- concentrations on the CSF side. If the bathing fluid is low in NaCl and of reduced osmolality, production of CSF continues against the adverse osmotic gradient. The rate of Na^+ transfer seems dependent on Na^+ concentration but not on osmolality gradient. Cerebrospinal fluid concentration for Na^+ or Cl^-, plotted against plasma concentration, yields a straight line (constant CSF to plasma ratio) unless plasma concentrations are high, in which case the ratio tends to rise, especially for Cl^-, with a disproportionate increase in CSF values. The disparity between Na^+ and Cl^- in high concentrations may perhaps be explicable by the necessity to maintain constant levels of the other major anion, HCO_3^-, in CSF and ECF.

The mechanism of Cl^- transfer is equally uncertain. The barrier DC potential (3 to 14 mv, CSF positive), perhaps generated by Na^+ transport, may assist chloride transfer. Instead or as well, carbonic anhydrase (confined to the choroid epithelium and glial cells) may play a significant part in barrier transport of Cl^- ions. Its inhibition reduces or abolishes the Cl^- excess that characterizes CSF (compared with plasma) in all species. Thus, the relative importance of passive diffusion and active transport for entry of Cl^- into the CNS is unknown. It appears unlikely that rates of Cl^- transfer can be much out of step with those for Na^+, which, judged by radioisotope measurements, has a half-life of 3 to 6 hours in the human CNS.

In summary, with minor exceptions, transfer of Na^+ and Cl^-, however regulated, maintains a constant ratio between CSF, ECF, and plasma and so corrects transfer of water that may have occurred during the acute stage of salt-water imbalance and may have led to altered intracranial pressure.

Plasma Hypo-Osmolality (Hyponatremia)

Clinical Aspects

The normal osmolality of serum ranges around 290 to 305 mOsm per liter, corresponding to serum Na^+ values of 135 to 145 mEq per liter. Signs of cerebral dysfunction normally appear if the osmolality falls below about 260 to 265, or the blood Na^+ falls below 130.

Early signs of cerebral dysfunction include lethargy, inattention, slight confusion, nausea, and vomiting. In more severe cases there may be convulsions, aphasia, hemiplegia, stupor, or coma, often mimicking the signs of a subdural hematoma. Hypo-osmolality is more often associated with increased water intake, reduced water loss, or both, rather than with a primary deficiency of NaCl. Causes include the following:

1. *Water intoxication,* due to administration of glucose solutions without saline (especially in the presence of morphine or barbiturates), retention of enemas, anuria, psychogenic polydipsia, or the water diuresis test for adrenocortical insufficiency or hypopituitarism.
2. *Excess vasopressin (antidiuretic hormone [ADH]) or ADH-like material,* as in overadministration of ADH, inappropriate secretion of ADH in cerebral injury or disease, lung disease, congestive heart failure, cirrhosis, following surgery or formation of ADH (or similar peptide) by carcinomas, especially oat cell carcinoma of the lung and pancreatic tumors.
3. *Primary loss of sodium without corresponding water loss,* as in adrenocortical insufficiency, renal salt-losing syndrome, and heat prostration.

Pathogenesis

Much experimental work is being done on the effects of hypo-osmolality on the CNS, and results vary considerably with the duration of the experiments, most of which have involved concurrent administration of vasopressin and water, usually in the form of glucose solution. In the most short-term experiments (2 to 3 hours) the only change is increase in water

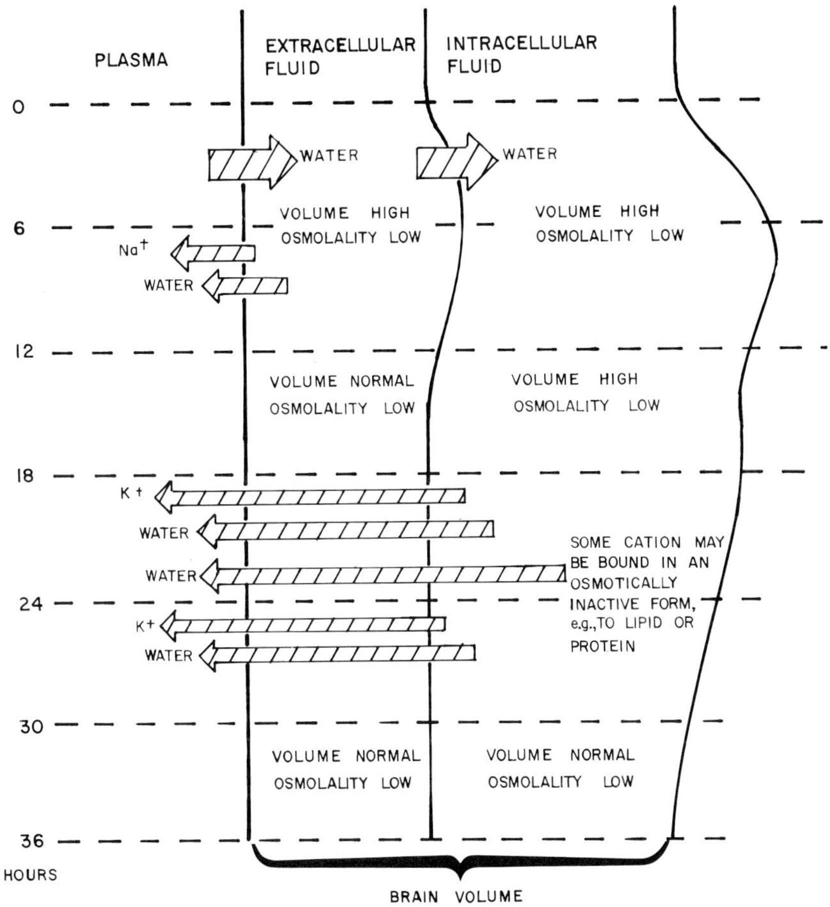

Fig. 11-2. Transfers of water and cation to and from the CNS in serum hypo-osmolality (acute and compensatory phases). The width of each compartment represents its volume at given time after inducing hypo-osmolality.

content of the brain, associated with swelling. Electron microscopy shows swelling of astrocytic processes and widening of extracellular space, mainly in the white matter — changes similar to those in cerebral edema.

Longer-term experiments have involved water-loading for periods of up to three days, with a two-day recovery period, comparing the levels of water and electrolyte content of plasma, muscle, and brain at intervals during this period. After a brief initial period, ECF volume is unchanged in all three tissues, but ECF ion concentrations vary with those of plasma. Swelling is therefore intracellular but averages 20 to 30% in muscle, differing dramatically from about 3% in brain; this difference is associated with cation responses of the tissues.

In muscle there is some early reduction in Na^+ on a dry-weight basis (i.e., an *absolute* reduction), presumably from the ECF's reducing its osmolality to that of the (abnormal) plasma and restoring its normal volume. However, throughout the experiment, the absolute content of K^+ remains unchanged, and excess water must remain in the cells. Similarly (Fig. 11-2), in the CNS, water entry into ECF begins almost immediately, followed within a few hours by losses of Na^+, Cl^-, and water, such that both ions regain their normal ratio to the plasma concentrations, and ECF volume returns to normal (intracellular sodium does not appear to be involved in this loss).

A change that is apparently unique to the CNS and enables it to maintain or regain normal volume starts at about 18 to 24 hours: There is progressive loss of K^+ on a dry-weight basis (presumably from the intracellular fluid), accompanied by loss of water, such that total intracellular cation (approximately Na^+ plus K^+) remains linearly related to total plasma cation (mainly Na^+). The totals are not equal, since it appears that much intracellular cation is osmotically inactive (perhaps bound to protein, lipid, and so on).

The mechanism of cellular K^+ loss, which appears to be peculiar to the CNS, is unknown. It may be a response to low ECF Na^+ levels rather than to low osmolality, so that in addition to restoring normal intracellular fluid volume and intracranial pressure,

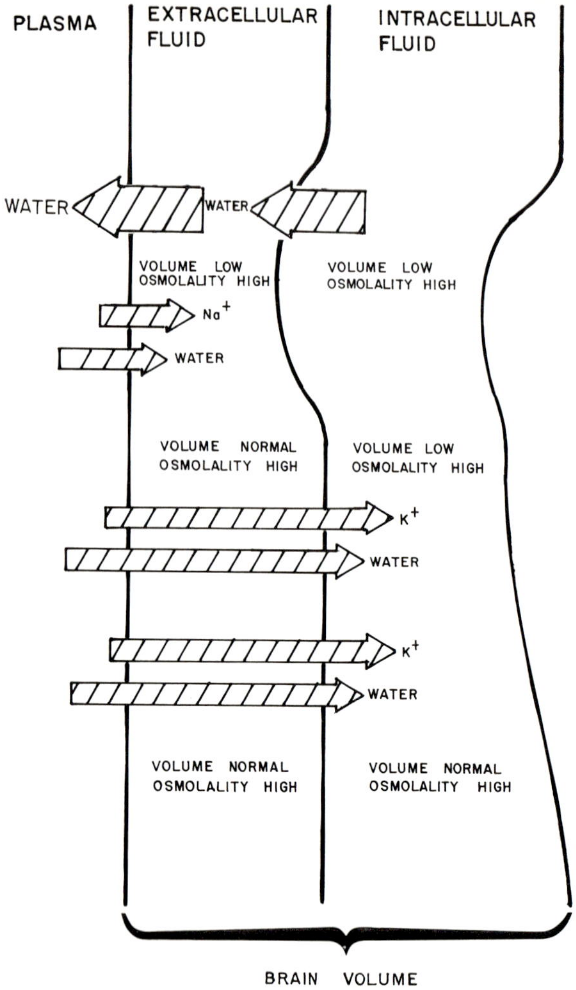

Fig. 11-3. Transfers of water and cation from and to the CNS in serum hyperosmolality (acute and compensatory phases). The width of each compartment represents its volume, but the time scale is not accurately determined, and the changes are indicated in approximate descending sequence.

K^+ loss also tends to restore membrane potential. Whether or not other methods of varying cell osmolality exist in mammals, such as reversible aggregation of amino acids into peptide chains, is unknown.

Thus, except temporarily in precipitous changes of plasma osmolality, there is no significant cerebral edema or swelling, which is in accord with the lack of clinical evidence for increased intracranial tension. Presumably, CNS dysfunction in hypo-osmolality is associated with altered ionic concentrations, but few studies of this relationship have been made.

Plasma Hyperosmolality (Hypernatremia)

Clinical Aspects

Except in untreated diabetic and uremic patients, hyperosmolality is essentially synonymous with hypernatremia, the plasma Na^+ being greater than 160 mEq per liter (osmolality in excess of 325 mOsm per liter). In infancy, the clinical features are irritability, restlessness, hypertonia, twitching, seizures, and nystagmus, occasionally progressing to stupor, coma, and death. The EEG shows high-amplitude, slow-wave activity, with occasional spikes, and permanent sequelae, such as mental retardation and seizures, have been recorded. Similar features are seen in adults, but so many of these patients have had head injuries or cranial surgery that it may be difficult to isolate the hypernatremic features. The causes of hypernatremia include:

1. *Dehydration without corresponding loss of sodium,* as in infantile diarrhea and vomiting, excessive saline in patients with renal disease, diabetes insipidus in unconscious patients, inadequate water intake in unconscious patients (especially with excessive sweating and hyperventilation), or in head injury or brain surgery even without adequate causes for dehydration (impaired secretion of ADH).
2. *Sodium retention,* as in Cushing's disease and hyperaldosteronism.

Pathogenesis

The mechanisms of CNS adaptation to hyperosmolality are less well understood than the clinical aspects (Fig. 11-3). An acute decrease in brain water, accompanied by increased concentrations of Na^+, K^+, and Cl^-, is followed by absolute gains (in terms of dry weight) of at least Na^+ and Cl^- and, probably to a lesser degree, of K^+, presumably as the water content returns to normal. It is assumed, therefore, that after an initial period of brain shrinkage due to rapid extraction of water by the plasma, electrolyte uptake follows, to restore both the extracellular and intracellular fluid volumes to approximately normal levels. However, changes in brain K^+ are less dramatic than in hypo-osmolality, and further biochemical and electron-microscopic observations are required.

Both clinically and experimentally, rapid rehydration of chronically dehydrated subjects frequently causes seizures following a brief period of dramatic clinical improvement. Experimental work indicates that these seizures are due to brain swelling, since plasma restored to normal osmolality is hypo-osmolar relative to the CNS compensated for hyperosmolality, and acute transfer of water into the brain temporarily increases cerebral volume (a situation analogous to water intoxication, but with higher osmolality both inside and outside the brain).

It should be noted that severe degrees of hypernatremia associated with dehydration may indirectly cause cerebral damage by vascular complications such as hypovolemic shock and vascular thrombosis (especially of the superior sagittal sinus). Such complications are more frequent in infants.

Salt-Water Imbalance Secondary to Cerebral Dysfunction

As has been noted, primary cerebral disease, head injury, and neurosurgery are among the *causes* of serum hypo-osmolality and hyperosmolality, apparently because of alterations in release of ADH, which are usually temporary.

Increased ADH Secretion

The more usual change is increased release of ADH (*inappropriate secretion of ADH* [IADH]), which probably occurs in about 25% of neurosurgical cases, half of these severe enough to require fluid restriction. Many of these severe cases are due to subdural hematoma; however, the symptomatology associated with IADH may itself mimic subdural hematoma. The accepted features of IADH include low serum Na^+ (less than 135 mEq per liter), low serum osmolality (less than 280 mOsm per liter), high urine Na^+ (greater than 25 mEq per liter), and urine osmolality greater than that of the plasma — all in the absence of detectable renal or adrenal disease and without peripheral edema or dehydration. The condition responds poorly to hypertonic saline. It may also occur in association with anesthesia, pain, surgery, brain disease or injury, and cerebral edema (in the latter case, a vicious circle is produced). When associated with acute head injury, IADH produces the syndrome formerly termed *cerebral salt-wasting.*

Decreased ADH Secretion

More rarely associated with generalized cerebral disease or head injury is impaired secretion of ADH, leading to diabetes insipidus with polyuria and polydipsia. Such patients show moderate hyperosmolality and hypernatremia, since the primary defect is increased renal loss of water. Antidiuretic hormone (the level determined by radioimmunoassay) may be absent or low relative to the osmolality (i.e., some patients respond to dehydration by increased ADH production, but not at an adequate rate). Whereas IADH may be asymptomatic and is usually temporary, diabetes insipidus is more often permanent, especially if associated with injuries in the region of the third ventricle and a decreased or absent sensation of thirst.

There may be a separate group of patients also presenting with raised plasma osmolality and Na^+ levels but absence of thirst. Although rehydration somewhat reduces plasma osmolality in these patients, it does not return it to normal. They remain susceptible to overhydration and water intoxication, and there appears to be a permanent resetting of the osmoreceptors to high sodium levels. These observations indicate that, at least in man, the thirst center is separate from centers controlling ADH release, and injury or pathological processes can uncouple the two.

ACID-BASE IMBALANCE

The major system controlling the pH of CSF (and presumably brain ECF) in the absence of protein or hemoglobin is the bicarbonate-carbon dioxide buffer mechanism. As stated in the Henderson-Hasselbalch equation,

$$pH = pK' + \log \frac{[HCO_3^-]}{[H_2CO_3]}$$

where pK′ is the apparent dissociation constant of H_2CO_3. Concentration of H_2CO_3 is directly related to the P_{CO_2} by the CO_2 solubility coefficient (S); both pK′ and S are higher in CSF than in plasma, but the former is only slightly higher. There is thus an equilibrium:

$$CO_2 + H_2O \leftrightarrow H_2CO_3 \leftrightarrow H^+ + HCO_3^-$$

This is shifted to the left (i.e., toward evolution of CO_2) by the addition of acid and to the right (toward solution of CO_2) by the addition of alkali. The P_{CO_2} of CSF (not necessarily of ECF) is equal to that of jugular venous blood and 1.23 times higher than that of arterial blood. Since CSF bicarbonate is normally lower than plasma bicarbonate, the pH of CSF is slightly lower (7.29) than that of jugular venous blood (7.31).

Since carbon dioxide is one of the few substances readily diffusible across the barrier system, homeostasis in CSF and ECF must depend on control of bicarbonate levels (Fig. 11-4). With an average plasma HCO_3^- concentration of 26.8 mEq per liter, the normal CSF value is 23.3, a disparity not completely accounted for by the barrier DC potential. Mechanisms of bicarbonate transfer are incompletely understood, and the proportions due to passive diffusion, DC potential, and active transport are unknown. Acute changes in plasma bicarbonate do not produce any significant effect in CSF levels in less than 1 hour. Inhibition of carbonic anhydrase reduces secretion of CSF by about 40%, and one possible mechanism is failure to form bicarbonate ions from carbon dioxide, so that less bicarbonate enters the CSF, the (positive) DC potential increases, and sodium transfer and the osmotically induced flow of water therefore also decrease. (Currently, there seem to be no data on the effects of carbonic anhydrase inhibition on DC potential.) Whatever the mechanism of bicarbonate transfer, changes in plasma bicarbonate will be reflected only slowly in the CSF, since the barrier is relatively impermeable to it; changes in plasma carbon dioxide will produce almost immediate alterations in CSF P_{CO_2}.

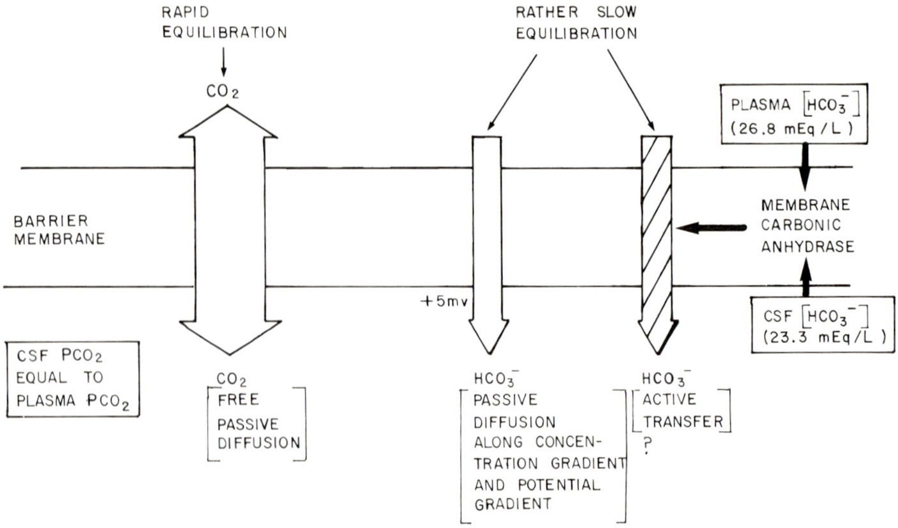

Fig. 11-4. CO_2 and HCO_3^- transfer across the blood-brain and blood-CSF barriers (cross-hatched arrow = suggested active transfer).

Changes in acid-base balance in the plasma are usually characterized as acidosis, in which the pH is reduced, or alkalosis, in which the pH is increased. Each of these is commonly divided into a *respiratory* type, in which the primary change is in P_{CO_2} because of altered ventilation, and a *metabolic* type, in which the primary change is in the amount of fixed anion causing inverse changes in bicarbonate levels, or in the concentration of bicarbonate itself. (Thus, the metabolic acidosis of diabetes is associated with accumulation of keto acids and, to maintain electrical neutrality, a loss of bicarbonate. In metabolic alkalosis due to overadministration of sodium bicarbonate, plasma levels of bicarbonate are raised.)

In all four conditions, the trend is to restore the proper *ratio* of bicarbonate to carbon dioxide and regain an acceptable pH. Although the ratio may be restored, the absolute values of bicarbonate and carbon dioxide may be increased or decreased. Alterations of either P_{CO_2} or HCO_3^- concentration may affect rates of H_2CO_3 dissociation to HCO_3^-, which is catalyzed by carbonic anhydrase in the barrier system. Thus, either raised P_{CO_2} or lowered HCO_3^- concentration might increase dissociation and so produce compensatory changes. Since CSF acidosis is also associated with an increase in the positive DC barrier potential (due to H^+), increased HCO_3^- may diffuse into the CSF.

Respiratory Acidosis

Respiratory acidosis (Fig. 11-5) may be experimentally induced by breathing abnormally high concentrations of carbon dioxide or by hypoventilation. Accumulation of carbon dioxide in the blood is almost immediately reflected by increased P_{CO_2} in the CSF, causing CSF acidosis. Arterial and central chemoreceptors are stimulated and cause an attempted increase in ventilation. However, either ventilation is impaired or the inspired air is rich in carbon dioxide, and these mechanisms are ineffective in reducing arterial P_{CO_2}. After some hours, the plasma bicarbonate begins to rise, followed by increased levels in the CSF, but the compensatory change in bicarbonate concentration is more adequate in the plasma for several days, and CSF acidosis remains relatively poorly compensated. Even so, increased cerebral blood flow (see Chap. 13) reduces the P_{CO_2} difference between CSF and plasma, so that the pH decrease in CSF is usually a little less than in plasma. In chronic, steady-state respiratory acidosis, such as that occurring in many parenchymal lung diseases, there is more adequate

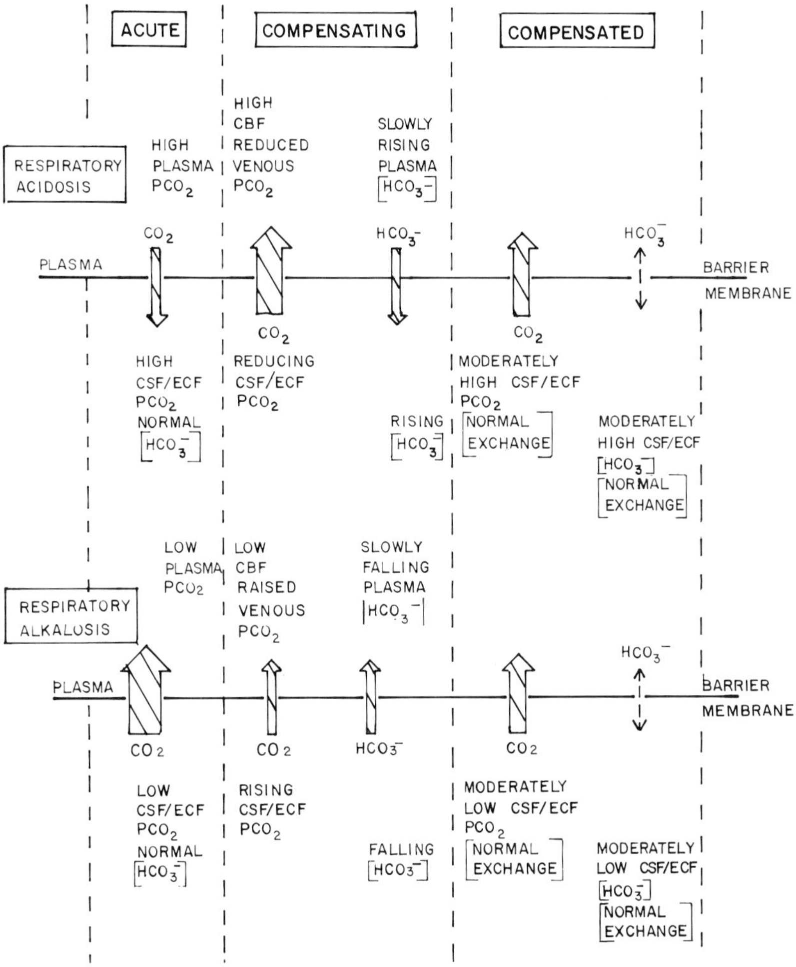

Fig. 11-5. CO_2 and HCO_3^- transfer across the blood-CSF barrier in respiratory acidosis and alkalosis. Changes in cerebral blood flow (CBF), as well as in plasma concentrations, are involved in compensation, which restores normal pH in the CSF.

compensation, with high levels of carbon dioxide and bicarbonate in both fluids, but normal pH ranges.

The association of long-standing hypoxemia and hypercapnia, seen in chronic lung disease, produces CNS acidosis and may be associated with increased blood-brain barrier permeability, leading to cerebral edema.

Respiratory Alkalosis

Acute respiratory alkalosis (Fig. 11-5) may be induced by hyperventilation under experimental conditions, or may be due to low atmospheric Po_2 at high altitudes. Plasma Pco_2 falls, followed by a fall in the CSF level. The kidney compensates by excretion of bicarbonate to reduce the plasma level. A corresponding, somewhat delayed fall in CSF bicarbonate is less marked, so that compensation is again more adequate in the plasma. Cerebral blood flow is reduced, and the difference between CSF and plasma Pco_2 rises. Again, the rise in pH is less in CSF than in plasma. In long-standing respiratory alkalosis, such as that occurring in people living at high altitudes, carbon dioxide and bicarbonate in both fluids stabilize at lower than normal levels, with the maintenance of relatively normal pH.

Metabolic Acid-Base Imbalance

Metabolic acidosis (Fig. 11-6), which is due to the accumulation of anions at a rate faster than they can be removed, is perhaps most common in diabetic ketosis and occurs to some extent in uremia. In acute stages, paradoxical pH changes may be seen in the

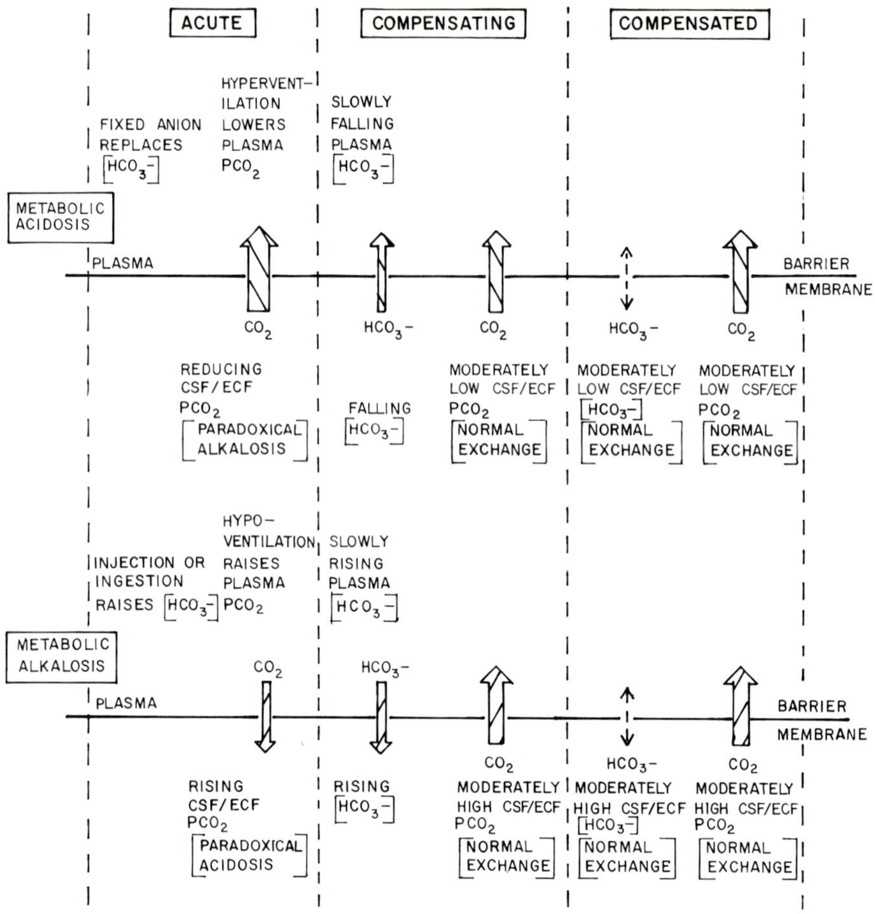

Fig. 11-6. CO_2 and HCO_3^- transfer across the blood-CSF barrier in metabolic acidosis and alkalosis. There is little change in cerebral blood flow.

CSF, emphasizing the importance of using this fluid rather than plasma to estimate the acid-base balance of the CNS. Thus, if NH_4Cl is injected, accumulation of Cl^- rapidly lowers plasma bicarbonate, causing hyperventilation and a compensatory reduction of PCO_2. Since carbon dioxide readily diffuses across the barrier system, CSF PCO_2 rapidly falls, the CSF bicarbonate levels remain normal, and the CSF is alkalotic (temporarily) in spite of the peripheral acidosis. Conversely, injection of $NaHCO_3$ causes a reduction in ventilation, with increased plasma PCO_2; CSF PCO_2 rises in the presence of normal bicarbonate, and CSF shows acidosis in the presence of peripheral alkalosis. These changes are acute only, subsequently compensated by appropriate movements of bicarbonate (out of the CSF in metabolic acidosis and into the CSF in metabolic alkalosis), largely restoring normal pH values. Under clinical conditions (e.g., diabetic ketosis) these metabolic changes develop gradually, and the early paradoxical changes in CSF pH either are less marked than in the experimental situations, or may not be observed at all.

It is apparent that in both respiratory and metabolic acid-base imbalance, CSF bicarbonate changes are in the same direction as in plasma. If PCO_2 is plotted against bicarbonate concentration of CSF in normal subjects or most patients with acid-base imbalance, the values generally fall between lines indicating pH 7.298 and 7.326, suggesting a considerable degree of homeostatic effectiveness. If the distribution ratio of bicarbonate between plasma and CSF is plotted against arterial pH, the relationship suggests passive changes in bicarbonate concentrations superimposed on the normal steady-state differential. There is therefore no proved role for alteration of active bicarbonate transport in acid-base imbalance. In the metabolic disorders, about 40% of the change in plasma bicarbonate is reflected in the CSF, compared with about 70% in respiratory imbalance.

Cerebrospinal Fluid and Control of Respiration

Respiration is affected by (1) chemoreceptors in the aorta and carotid vessels (peripheral receptors), which are stimulated by increased carbon dioxide or reduced oxygen, and (2) chemoreceptors in the medulla (central receptors), situated at or near the

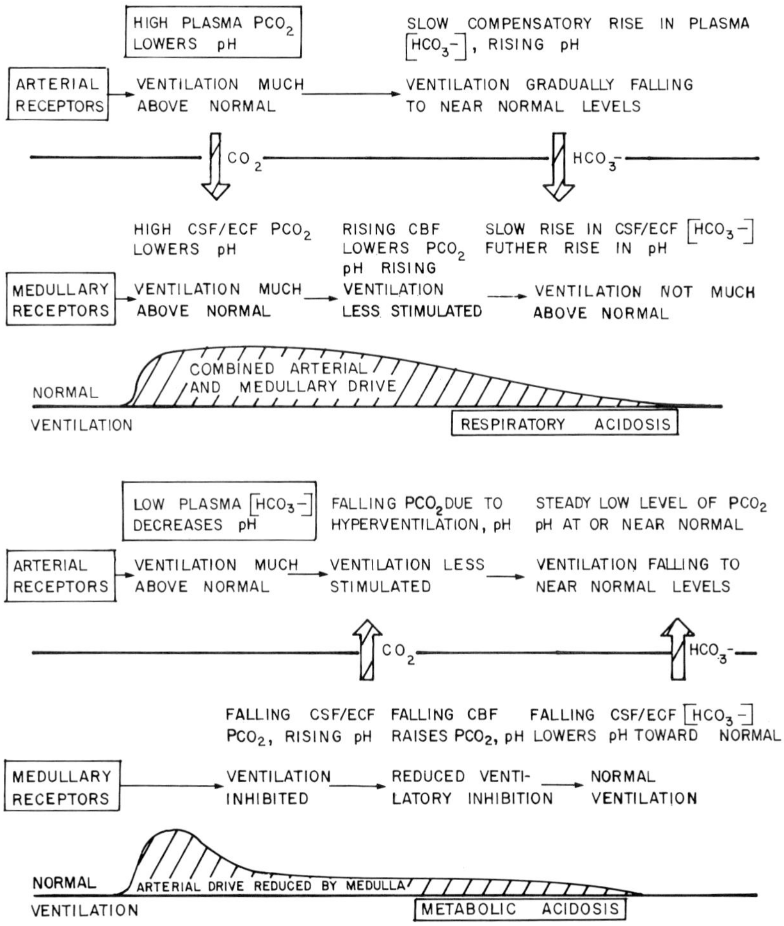

Fig. 11-7. Effects of peripheral (arterial) and medullary receptors on ventilation in respiratory and metabolic acidosis. Because of "paradoxical" alkalosis of CSF early in metabolic acidosis, the effective hyperventilation is considerably reduced.

CSF interface, which respond to altered PCO_2 in the blood or CSF; per unit of pH change, these receptors seem to be from 1.5 to 3.5 times more sensitive than the peripheral receptors.

In the CNS it appears to be H^+ concentration, rather than carbon dioxide or bicarbonate, that is the final effective stimulus of ventilation (and of vasodilatation and control of cerebral blood flow). Receptor localization is complicated by rapid diffusion in the brain ECF, so that application of fluid of predetermined composition immediately produces concentration gradients with the preexisting ECF. Responding chemosensitive cells could lie anywhere along these gradients. The chemosensitive areas in the medulla are commonly depicted on the surface, but it has not yet been proved that they are located there. Where there are paradoxical changes in CSF pH as previously described, peripheral and central receptors may antagonize rather than cooperate, so that during the development and compensation of acid-base imbalance, the chains of events (Fig. 11-7) described in the following paragraphs may be postulated (bearing in mind the carbon dioxide and bicarbonate changes that have been mentioned).

Acute Metabolic Acidosis

In the *acute* phase of metabolic acidosis (such as that following the injection of ammonium chloride), peripheral receptors are stimulated, producing increased ventilation and lowering plasma PCO_2. Low plasma PCO_2 reduces peripheral acidosis and reduces CSF PCO_2, making the CSF alkaline; therefore, it inhibits central receptors and depresses ventilation. Effects on respiration at this stage are thus antagonistic. *Later,* the pH of CSF tends toward normal, due to transfer of bicarbonate from CSF to plasma, and central receptors are deinhibited. Once this stage is reached, arterial pH is more abnormal than CSF pH, so that the peripheral receptors determine ventilation. If chronic metabolic acidosis is *acutely* compensated (as by dialysis in uremic acidosis) CSF bicarbonate remains low, but the plasma level rises, so that CSF is acid relative to plasma, and central receptors will cause persistent hyperventilation until bicarbonate is transferred into the CSF.

Acute Metabolic Alkalosis

In acute metabolic alkalosis (e.g., ingestion of sodium bicarbonate), the situation is opposite to that in metabolic acidosis. *Acutely,* peripheral receptors are inhibited, respiration is reduced, and the plasma P_{CO_2} is raised. This reduces peripheral alkalosis, but makes the CSF acid, stimulating central receptors and increasing ventilation. Again, the effects of the two sets of receptors are antagonistic. *Later,* CSF pH tends toward normal because of transfer of bicarbonate into the CSF, and central receptors cease to be stimulated. Again, arterial pH is more abnormal than CSF pH and henceforward determines the rate of ventilation.

Respiratory Acidosis

Acutely, in respiratory acidosis, peripheral receptors are stimulated, increasing ventilation and reducing plasma P_{CO_2}. Since the initial increase in P_{CO_2} level also involves CSF, central receptors are also stimulated, and both work together in increasing ventilation. *Later,* the CSF pH is restored by bicarbonate transfer, and the central drive is reduced. The pH of the plasma is largely restored by renal bicarbonate retention, and arterial drive is also reduced. Ventilation now becomes relatively normal, but adapted to higher "settings" of P_{CO_2} and bicarbonate.

Respiratory Alkalosis

Acutely, in respiratory alkalosis, P_{CO_2} is low in plasma and CSF, both receptors are inhibited, ventilation is reduced, and P_{CO_2} rises toward normal. *Later,* CSF pH is restored by transfer of bicarbonate from CSF to plasma, and plasma pH by renal bicarbonate loss, so that both drives are reduced. Ventilation is again relatively normal, but adapted to lower "settings" of P_{CO_2} and bicarbonate. In steady-state respiratory alkalosis, such as that occurring in hypoxic hyperventilation, where low P_{CO_2} prevents a decrease in ventilation, carbon dioxide is lost from all body fluids, but the cerebral blood flow rises, to return to normal levels. Alkalosis temporarily persists in the CSF in spite of loss of bicarbonate until additional mechanisms become operative, including a possible active transfer of H^+ from plasma to CSF, or an increase in CSF lactate.

Effect of Brain Lesions on Cerebrospinal Fluid Acid-Base Balance

A recent study of CSF from patients with varying degrees of brain damage, including patients in coma (all breathing spontaneously) showed normal P_{CO_2} in all grades, but significant decreases in pH and bicarbonate levels in coma only. Surprisingly, both arterial and venous P_{CO_2} and the arteriovenous difference were reduced in comatose patients, so that the normal values in CSF were still 6 to 8 mm Hg higher than the venous levels, compared with an insignificant difference in control subjects.

The association of reduced CSF bicarbonate with normal (relatively increased) carbon dioxide implies a breakdown of homeostatic mechanisms in comatose patients. The fall in bicarbonate may indicate accumulation of pyruvate or other fixed acids in the CSF, and failure of carbon dioxide elimination may be due to reduced perfusion of injured brain areas, with or without edema.

OTHER ELECTROLYTE ABNORMALITIES

Other electrolytes (cations) known to be significant in CNS function include K^+, Ca^{++}, and Mg^{++}, which are considered briefly in this section. All are maintained constantly in CSF whatever their concentrations in plasma (within wide limits), generally at significantly different levels.

Potassium CSF 2.9 mEq/L, plasma 4 to 4.6 mEq/L
Calcium CSF 2.3 mEq/L, plasma 4.7 mEq/L
Magnesium CSF 2.2 mEq/L, plasma 1.6 mEq/L

(Figures for Ca^{++} are for the ionized form and ignore protein or other binding.) K^+ and Ca^{++} are maintained at levels significantly lower in CSF than in the plasma, whereas Mg^{++} levels are significantly higher. Ca^{++} and Mg^{++} levels in ECF are probably similar, but K^+ may be lower, since there is a decrease in K^+ concentration as CSF circulates from the ventricles over the surface of the hemispheres. Indeed, the K^+ levels in the subarachnoid fluid are more uniform than those in the ventricles, suggesting that control exerted by the blood-brain barrier on K^+ transfer is even more precise than for the blood-CSF barrier. Variations in brain K^+ are even smaller (although most of it is intracellular, so that small variations in ECF concentration would not be detectable). Thus (with all figures expressed in milliequivalents per liter or per kilogram wet weight.):

	plasma K^+	muscle K^+	CSF K^+	brain K^+
Control	4.15±0.27	110±2.7	2.83±0.8	95.4±1.3
Low plasma K^+	1.58±0.09	72.2±2.6	2.72±0.06	94.5±1.3
High plasma K^+	7.09±0.59	109.8±0.9	3.02±0.12	94.9±0.9

Since CSF K^+ can be maintained above or below plasma levels as circumstances dictate, there may be separate mechanisms for "transport in" and "transport out" of the CNS. The transport-in mechanism should maintain constant K^+ transfer at plasma levels that are low or normal, and it is apparent from the figures that this is approximately the case. Transport out should be minimal at low or normal CSF K^+ levels, but rise sharply when this is exceeded; it may be related to Na^+-K^+ exchange. It is presumed that these mechanisms are present in both barrier systems. (CSF K^+ is altered in respiratory acidosis and alkalosis inversely to the pH, but the mechanism is unknown; metabolic acid-base imbalance has little effect.)

Although the kinetics of Ca^{++} and Mg^{++} exchange have been analyzed less extensively than those K^+ exchange, it is possible that similar dual transfer mechanisms exist for these ions. It is considered that the transport-in mechanism for K^+ and Ca^{++} is a carrier that is largely "saturated" at well below physiological plasma concentrations. Thus, the carrier sites are always occupied at the plasma interface, and a constant amount of ion is transferred. Experimentally, very low plasma concentrations do reduce K^+ and Ca^{++} transport. While CSF concentrations of Ca^{++} and Mg^{++} differ significantly from those in plasma, the degree of independence is not clear. It has been suggested by some investigators that CSF Ca^{++} is virtually independent of plasma level, but others have found some variation. The situation is similar in regard to Mg^{++}, and since both are held reasonably constant, the Ca^{++} to Mg^{++} ratio is also constant at about 1.64 in milligrams per 100 ml.

It is not possible by direct experiment to modify ion concentrations in the brain ECF effectively, but the influence of altered CSF ion concentrations has been noted: Arterial pressure is raised by a reduction in Ca^{++} or Mg^{++}, or by an increase in K^+, along with respiratory stimulation and increased muscular tone. Raised Mg^{++} and Ca^{++} (but not lowered K^+) have opposite effects. Changes are mediated through the brain stem, probably by superficial structures, such as the respiratory center. However, these changes in CSF ion levels are experimentally produced by direct introduction of fluid into the ventricular cavities and bear no relation to the CNS effects of altered plasma levels of K^+, Ca^{++}, or Mg^{++}, which, as has been noted, are not accompanied by major changes in CSF or ECF. Indeed, the effects of altered plasma levels on the CNS appear completely inexplicable. Probably, many of the neuromuscular sequelae of ion imbalance are really direct effects on the peripheral nervous or muscular systems.

Alterations in Plasma Potassium

Normal plasma potassium ranges from 4.0 to 4.6 mEq per liter.

Hyperkalemia

Hyperkalemia is found in pure form in familial periodic paralysis or when excess K^+ salts are administered. As part of a complex electrolyte disturbance, it occurs in acute renal failure, terminal chronic renal failure, dehydration, untreated diabetic coma complicated by acidosis, hyponatremia, some cases of severe head injury, and endocrine abnormalities. Neurological manifestations of hyperkalemia, including muscular involvement, are usually apparent at levels of 7.5 to 8.5 mEq per liter. Acute changes include paresthesias, weakness, and difficulty in walking. Chronic changes include flaccid, areflexic paralysis (often of sudden onset), hypotonia, and paresthesias, with impairment of position and vibration sense.

Hypokalemia

Hypokalemia is more common than hyperkalemia, but is usually less serious, since it does not have disastrous cardiac effects. In pure form it occurs in hypokalemic periodic paralysis, but it is also a feature of K^+-losing nephritis, abuse of diuretic drugs, excessive losses from the gastrointestinal tract, deficient intake (as in prolonged vomiting and the administration of K^+-free parenteral fluids), and recovery from diabetic coma. Some endocrine conditions are also accompanied by low plasma K^+. Clinical features include muscular weakness (less profound than in hyperkalemia and usually sparing cranial nerves). Occasionally, lethargy may progress to delirium, stupor, and coma, but since this is not seen in hypokalemic periodic paralysis, it is probably due to associated metabolic abnormalities rather than to K^+ deficiency per se.

Abnormalities of Serum Calcium

The normal total serum calcium is 9.0 to 10.3 mg per 100 ml.

Hypercalcemia

Hypercalcemia occurs in patients with hyperparathyroidism or with tumors producing parathyroid hormone-like substance, in excessive administration of vitamin D, or Ca^+, or both, sensitivity to vitamin D, metastatic bone disease, and, occasionally, endocrine disorders. It usually becomes apparent when serum calcium exceeds 16 or 17 mg per 100 ml, with profound muscular weakness, hypotonia, occasional increases in deep tendon reflexes, and sometimes dysphagia. Central nervous system features that may occur in hypercalcemia include variable personality changes, lethargy, drowsiness, confusion, impairment of intellect, delirium, hallucinations, coma, and (rarely) death. There may be an increase in CSF protein (which does not necessarily indicate metastatic tumor) and permanent sequelae such as intellectual impairment are noted occasionally. The mechanism of production of CNS symptoms is completely obscure, since, as previously noted, CSF (and presumably ECF) Ca^{++} levels are maintained within narrow limits.

Hypocalcemia

Hypocalcemia usually causes symptoms if serum calcium is less than 6 to 7 mg per 100 ml. Causes include inadvertent removal of the parathyroids during thyroidectomy, malabsorption, low intake of calcium, vitamin D, or both, or elevated serum phosphate, as in chronic renal disease and excessive feeding of cow's milk to infants. In addition to tetany (which also can be produced by reducing CSF Ca^{++}), hypocalcemia may cause seizures (usually of the grand mal type, but occasionally atypical and bizarre), psychotic changes, intellectual impairment, disorders of movement suggesting basal ganglion disease, and increased intracranial tension with papilledema (which may be mistakenly diagnosed as intracranial neoplasm). Again, the mechanism of CNS changes is unknown.

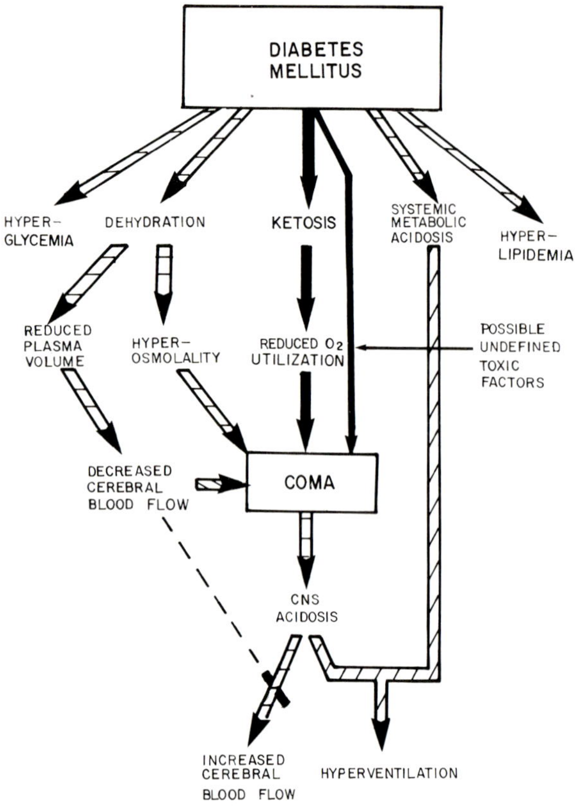

Fig. 11-8. Some of the factors in the production of diabetic (hyperglycemic, ketotic) coma.

Abnormalities of Plasma Magnesium

Normal range of plasma magnesium is 1 to 7 mEq per liter. Except under experimental conditions, it is not clear whether a pure increase or decrease of magnesium level unassociated with other important electrolyte abnormalities can occur. Hypomagnesemia may be associated with a variety of gastrointestinal, renal, and hepatic diseases and produces tetany and CNS dysfunction virtually indistinguishable from that produced by hypocalcemia. The only proof that such effects are due to magnesium deficiency is the response to intramuscular injections of magnesium sulfate, which may be dramatic. Again, since CSF homeostasis for magnesium appears to be good, the relationship between changed plasma levels and CNS symptomatology is unknown.

There is no doubt that both Ca^{++} and Mg^{++} exert effects on the peripheral as well as on the central nervous system. Both ions have a similar effect on axonal conduction, since they reduce permeability to Na^{+} and K^{+} and therefore stabilize the membrane and reduce action potential. However, they have antagonistic actions at the presynaptic membrane, since Ca^{++} promotes the release of acetylcholine and norepinephrine, whereas Mg^{++} antagonizes both. It seems probable that these ions have similar effects on impulse propagation and synaptic conduction within the CNS as they do peripherally, although it is not understood how variations in brain ECF occur across the barrier.

CENTRAL NERVOUS SYSTEM DYSFUNCTION IN DIABETES MELLITUS

Both diabetic (hyperglycemic, ketotic) coma and insulin (hypoglycemic) coma are associated with brain dysfunction and may have permanent sequelae. In addition, overzealous treatment of either carries its own risks. The association of diabetes with hypertension, atherosclerosis, and infection raises additional neurological problems.

Diabetic (Hyperglycemic, Ketotic) Coma

Patients in diabetic (hyperglycemic, ketotic) coma (Fig. 11-8) often have poor skin turgor, low ocular tension, and poor peripheral pulses and may show an increase in the rate and amplitude of respiration. Although such patients are often stuporous rather than comatose, the pupillary reaction to light may be lost early. The characteristic biochemical abnormalities are demonstrable in blood and urine.

As the clinical description indicates, these patients are often both dehydrated and markedly acidotic. Whereas in the alert patient acidosis is well compensated in the CSF and the drive to hyperventilation is reduced, in coma the CSF pH falls, and peripheral and central drives to hyperventilation become additive. Unless dehydration is extreme, the cerebral blood flow of patients in diabetic coma is normal or even slightly increased, but there is about a 50% reduction in oxygen utilization with decreased arteriovenous oxygen difference.

The pathogenesis of diabetic coma is not known with certainty, but is probably multiple. Acidosis is frequently blamed, but the degree of CNS dysfunction is out of proportion to the reduction of CSF pH as compared with other acidotic patients. It has been suggested that acidosis increases barrier permeability and causes cerebral edema, but, in fact, edema is rarely present. It appears most likely that coma is associated with some toxic agents (perhaps keto acids) that prevent the utilization of oxygen, even though it is usually freely available. Hyperosmolality, metabolic acidosis, and reduced blood flow due to dehydration may be additional causes of coma, of varying importance and frequency. Focal neurological dysfunction is not seen unless there is a combination of vascular disease and dehydration, and in such cases autopsy may disclose focal infarction, hyperemia, and cerebral edema. It should be emphasized that many patients in diabetic coma do not die of cerebral dysfunction, but rather of the systemic effects of atherosclerosis, dehydration, hypokalemia, lowered resistance to infection, and other factors.

Cerebrovascular Changes in Diabetes

Diabetes mellitus is associated with hyperlipidemia and increased incidence of atherosclerosis and hypertension. Occlusion of major vessels, such as the coronary or femoral arteries, is increased in all diabetic age groups as compared with nondiabetic controls. However, this does not seem to apply to cerebrovascular accidents. Recent surveys show no statistical difference in occlusion of major cerebral vessels between diabetic and nondiabetic hypertensive patients. Rather, the characteristic diabetic change consists of multiple small areas of cystic gliosis, often of differing ages when seen at autopsy, associated with a generalized reduction in brain weight. Both small infarcts and weight reduction are more marked in the cerebellum and brain stem than in the hemispheres. Particularly characteristic are small linear areas of infarction in the base of the pons, presumably due to blockage of paramedian perforating branches of the basilar artery. The reason for this peculiar susceptibility is unknown.

It is generally observed that intracerebral hemorrhage is decreased in incidence in diabetic, as compared with nondiabetic, hypertensive patients. The cause of this is obscure. However, since hemorrhage in hypertension frequently occurs from small arteries, it is possible that structural changes induced by diabetes, including intimal and medial fibrosis, reduce the liability to rupture.

Central Nervous System Complications of Treatment for Diabetes

Uncompensated diabetes is a serious condition, and treatment tends to be intensive. Iatrogenic CNS dysfunction may be produced in two ways: either by undue reduction in blood glucose to hypoglycemic levels, or by such a rapid reduction in plasma osmolality that the brain becomes relatively hyperosmolar and acutely edematous, a situation analogous to water intoxication.

Insulin-Induced Hypoglycemia

The risk of converting hyperglycemic coma directly to hypoglycemic coma by enthusiastic administration of insulin has long been recognized. The patient in hypoglycemic coma sweats profusely, shows pupillodilatation, and is frequently hyperreflexic, with Babinski responses. Blood sugar is low, but the presence of sugar or even ketone bodies in the urine does not exclude the diagnosis, as they may have been in the bladder since before treatment. In hypoglycemic coma, cerebral blood flow is normal, but cerebral oxygen utilization progressively declines with the available glucose. At blood sugar levels of 20 to 30 mg per 100 ml, oxygen utilization is reduced by 25%, and at 10 to 12 mg per 100 ml, oxygen utilization is only 50% of normal, and the arteriovenous oxygen difference is significantly reduced.

Biochemical investigations in insulin coma have proved difficult, largely because of the great lability of high-energy phosphate compounds, which disappear within 30 to 60 seconds of the cessation of circulation. It has usually been thought that in hypoglycemic coma the brain has reduced or absent adenosine triphosphate (ATP), creatine phosphate (CrP), free and bound glucose, and lactate, with an increase in adenosine diphosphate and monophosphate (ADP, AMP) and inorganic phosphate (Pi), changes being much the same in all areas of the brain. (The term *bound glucose* includes glycogen and possibly some ganglioside hexose and, since it may be reduced by 60 to 80% in acute hypoglycemia, is presumably a readily available substrate.) Recent studies raise the possibility that loss of ATP and CrP is an artifact due to insufficiently rapid freezing, and that in small laboratory animals such as mice, ATP and CrP are well preserved in acute hypoglycemia in spite of precipitous falls of free and bound glucose. Expected falls of ATP and CrP have been found in acute hypoxia. If confirmed, such studies would indicate that hypoglycemic coma not only is a deficiency of energy substrate, but also is a depression of CNS function analogous to that seen in anesthesia.

If blood sugar levels of 10 mg per 100 ml or lower are maintained for a significant period of time, patients remain in irreversible coma until death and at autopsy show widespread neuronal degeneration and necrosis. There may be laminar or total necrosis of the cortex (the visual area is usually spared), with frequent involvement of the hippocampus and basal ganglia (excluding the pallidum). Occasionally, areas of white-matter necrosis are seen.

Insulin-Induced Cerebral Edema

A more recently recognized complication of the treatment of diabetes is sudden development of cerebral edema following rapid reduction of blood sugar by heroic doses of insulin. Autopsy in these patients, who tend to be young and without other complications, confirms severe cerebral edema, the mechanism of which is not clear. Glucose itself can be readily cleared across the barrier system, and it is unlikely that retention of glucose per se is the sole cause of CNS hyperosmolality, although it may be a contributing factor. It has been shown that high intracellular glucose concentrations induce the formation of sorbitol (Fig. 11-9), which can only escape from cells slowly and might therefore remain osmotically active during the treatment of diabetic coma. Other so-called idiogenic solutes may also accumulate in the brain during hyperglycemia in order to maintain osmotic balance and similarly may not be cleared at adequate speed if plasma glucose is rapidly reduced. Their nature is unclear, and it has been thought that they may be dissociated Na^+ and K^+ normally bound to protein or lipid in the cytoplasm (to the extent of about 40% of the total intracellular cation). It is difficult to believe that such cations could not be reassociated at a sufficient rate to obviate hyperosmolality.

It is said that cerebral edema is more likely to develop when experimental hyperglycemia is reduced by insulin rather than by peritoneal dialysis,

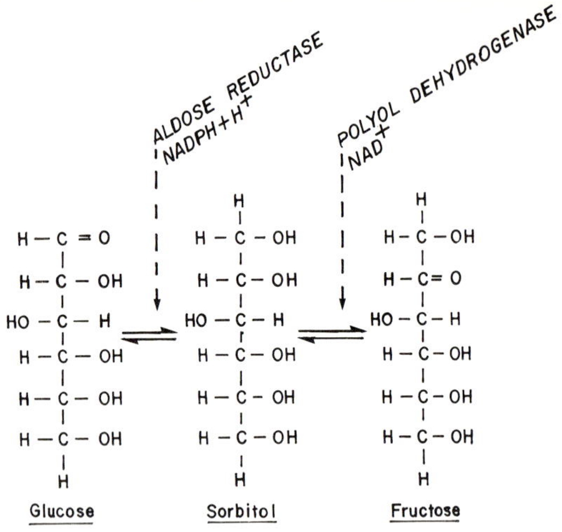

Fig. 11-9. Interconversion of glucose, sorbitol, and fructose. The reaction proceeds slowly in either direction, and sorbitol and fructose pass the cell membrane only with difficulty.

leading to the interesting speculation that insulin may promote cellular absorption of K^+ in the CNS, as in other tissues, and contribute to hyperosmolality at a particularly unfortunate time. Whatever the explanation, the brains of these patients show characteristic gross features of cerebral edema and increased water content. Similar symptoms are seen in experimental animals (and, rarely, in infants) when hypernatremia is acutely corrected by water-loading, presumably on an analogous basis of osmotic imbalance across the barrier system.

CENTRAL NERVOUS SYSTEM DYSFUNCTION IN RENAL DISEASE

A wide range of CNS signs and symptoms are associated with chronic renal disease and uremia. Most of these patients are hypertensive; therefore the majority of the morphological changes seen in the CNS are associated with vascular abnormalities. Renal failure is also associated with multiple disorders of homeostasis, including sodium-water imbalance, acid-base imbalance, and abnormal calcium, magnesium, and phosphorus metabolism, any of which may lead to cerebral dysfunction. In addition, there is retention of urea and other products of protein metabolism, offering the possibility of a metabolic encephalopathy that is specific for renal failure.

Uremic Coma

The spectrum of reversible (and therefore presumably metabolic) CNS impairment in uremia ranges from mild inattention to coma and may include symptoms of basal ganglion dysfunction (abnormal involuntary movements, tremors, rigidity, and asterixis), increased neuromuscular irritability, headache, vomiting, and reduced seizure threshold. Cerebral blood flow is normal in the patients with normal blood pressure, but reduced in the hypertensive group. Irrespective of blood flow, cerebral utilization of oxygen and glucose is low. Concentrations of glucose, ATP, and CrP in the brain are normal or even increased, suggesting metabolic depression (rather than deficiency of energy substrates).

Since these manifestations of uremia are readily reversible by dialysis, it may be assumed that low-molecular-weight compounds are responsible, but no single substance, or even group of substances, has so far been implicated. Experimental infusion of large amounts of urea (as in attempts to treat cerebral edema) do not cause the symptoms of uremia. Brain water content is normal or even slightly reduced, and the absence of edema is consistent with the findings at autopsy. Nonetheless, brain uptake of labeled inulin and sucrose, the CSF to plasma ratio of bromide, and CSF concentrations of urea, uric acid, creatinine, phosphate, and Cl^- are raised. All these changes can be reversed by dialysis, but indicate functional alterations in the barrier system that may be important in the genesis of uremic coma, since they may permit access of substances to the CNS that normally are excluded.

The nature of such substance (or substances) is unclear. Some attention has been directed to low-molecular-weight phenolic acids derived from protein catabolism, which have been shown in vitro to inhibit enzymes concerned with respiration, anaerobic glycolysis, transamination, glutamic acid decarboxylation, and brain nucleotidase activity. More recently, attention has been directed to guanidine compounds, some of which are normal products of protein metabolism (Fig. 11-10). Guanidinoacetic acid is an intermediate in the formation of creatine and creatinine and is itself nontoxic, but guanidine and methylguanidine inhibit oxygen consumption and the activity of several respiratory enzymes. In particular, methylguanidine inhibits the activity of brain Na^+-K^+-ATPase at a concentration only 10% of that present in uremic serum. Guanidinosuccinic acid, the levels of which are raised both in blood and urine, is known to depress transketolase activity by interfering with thiamine metabolism. It may be, therefore, that the peripheral neuropathies of uremia and thiamine deficiency are similar. (Symmetrical pontine myelinolysis is occasionally seen in uremia and is also considered a manifestation of improper thiamine utilization.) Although the guanidine compounds are readily dialyzable, their relationship to the clinical and biochemical features of uremia remains speculative. An additional possible factor in cerebral metabolic changes is the raised level of Pi in plasma, CSF, and (presumably) ECF, perhaps causing feedback inhibition of the conversion of ATP to ADP.

Many uremic patients are glucose-intolerant, and although severe hyperglycemia and ketosis are uncommon, cellular metabolism is altered, and glucose

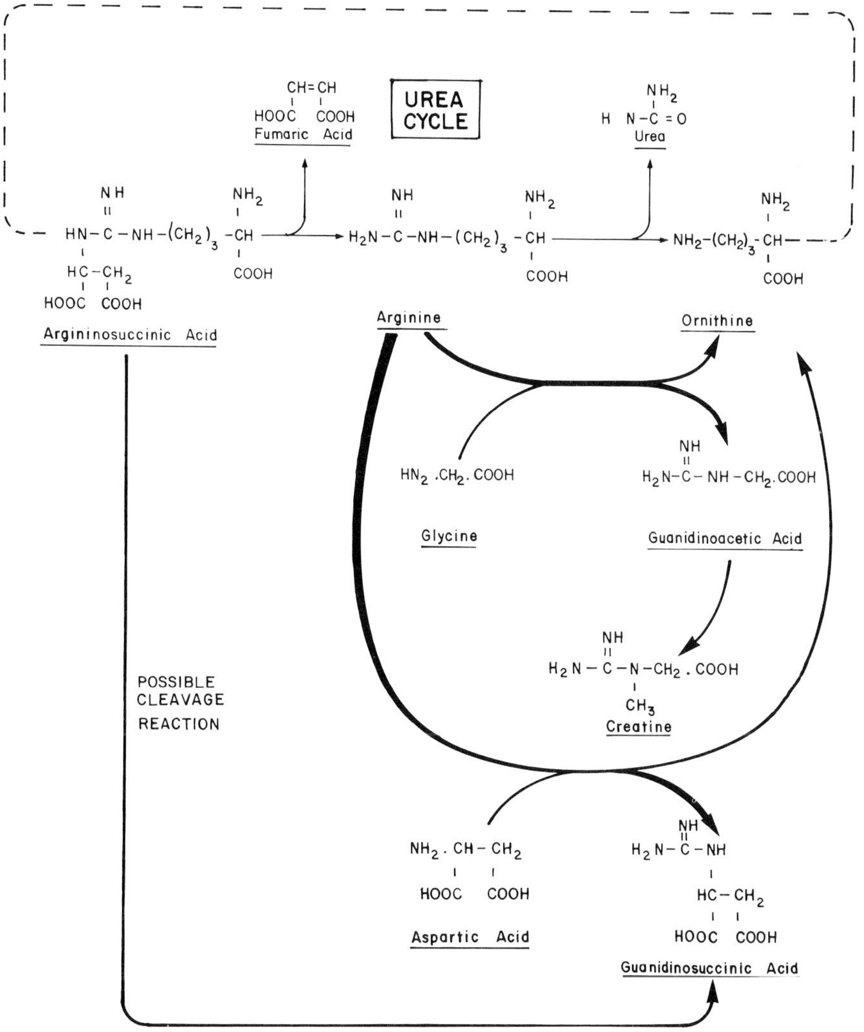

Fig. 11-10. Production of guanidino compounds. Accumulation may be toxic to the CNS in severe uremia.

utilization through the citric acid cycle is reduced (the hexose monophosphate shunt is said to be increased). There is uncoupling of oxidative phosphorylation and decreased synthesis of acetylcoenzyme A, with raised pyruvate levels in the blood. The problem appears to be not lack of insulin, which indeed has a prolonged half-life in uremia but, rather, a target organ insensitivity. Urea concentrations in the CNS are not of necessity associated with changes in NH_4^+ levels, since it appears that not all the necessary enzymes for the urea cycle are present, and the conversion of NH_4^+ to urea therefore occurs elsewhere in the body.

In summary, it may be stated that uremia produces marked but readily reversible changes in CNS function and barrier permeability. The responsible substance is not urea itself, and there may well be several such substances, including abnormal or abnormally accumulated products of protein breakdown, removable by dialysis. Electrolyte alterations, especially of calcium, magnesium, and phosphate, as well as altered utilization of carbohydrate, may contribute to the clinical picture.

Morphological Central Nervous System Changes in Renal Disease

Vascular changes, probably associated with hypertension and accelerated atherosclerosis, are commonly seen in the brains of patients with chronic renal failure. In acute cases these may be limited to congestion, perivascular petechiae, and fresh thrombi in vessels, frequently associated with small perivascular ischemic foci. In more chronic cases in which both arterioles and venules are thickened, with splitting of the internal elastic lamina and degeneration of medial and endothelial cells (or, occasionally, complete necrosis of vessel walls), large or small, single or multiple, intracerebral hemorrhages are often present. Electron-microscopically, endothelial cells may show swelling or shrinkage, with partial separation from the basement membrane, although the intercellular junctions usually remain intact.

Viewed against the background of these vascular changes, and bearing in mind the many possibilities for artifacts in neurons, a catalogue of the morphological associations of uremia in the brain does not look very convincing or specific. These have included:

1. Focal or widespread neuronal changes, characterized by swelling or shrinkage and either acute or chronic.
2. Acute necrosis of the internal granular layer of the cerebellum (which is neither constant nor specific).
3. Areas of focal, pseudolaminar, or other necrosis, sometimes associated with hemorrhage.
4. Focal or perivascular demyelination, with occasional symmetrical demyelination of the pons or even strikingly complete demyelination of the hemispheres, with or without areas of cystic gliosis.
5. Perivascular or generalized regressive changes in astrocytes and oligodendroglia.
6. Glial nodules of mixed cell type, or diffuse astrocytic proliferation.
7. Chronic fibrosis of meninges.
8. Fibrosis and focal infarction of choroid plexus.

Since uremic patients, like others with profound metabolic disturbance, have increased susceptibility to infection, microabscesses, septic emboli, cerebral abscesses, and meningitis may be found in association with chronic renal failure.

Other Cerebral Complications of Renal Disease

Enhanced Drug Sensitivity

A number of cases of enhanced drug sensitivity associated with renal failure are on record. Possible explanations are either that the kidney is failing to excrete drugs normally, or that increased permeability of the barrier system is allowing abnormal access to the CNS (as certainly appears to be the case with penicillin). If not recognized, such drug sensitivity can be dangerous, since the metabolic depression due to uremia, and the action of tranquilizers or sedatives, may be synergistic, and administration of the offending drugs for irritability or seizures may further compromise brain function.

Complications of Peritoneal Dialysis

The treatment of uremia is also not without perils. Peritoneal dialysis is associated with two complications, both unfortunately characterized by drowsiness, headache, confusion, increased blood pressure, and finally coma. One is the development of *cerebral edema* during dialysis. This is presumed to have an osmotic cause, similar to the edema that was mentioned previously as complicating the rapid reduction of blood sugar in diabetes (this mechanism has been experimentally confirmed). The other complication, which is associated with anticoagulation rather than with dialysis per se, is the development of *subdural hematoma.* It is necessary to be aware of both in order to make the appropriate diagnosis.

Neoplasia following Renal Transplantation

Renal transplantation, associated with immunosuppression, carries the usual hazards of infection, often by relatively nonpathogenic organisms, including fungi. In addition, there are reports of neoplasms (especially of the reticuloendothelial system) developing after organ transplantation with immunosuppression. A recent series included 28 epithelial and 24 mesenchymal tumors among 5170 organ recipients. About half the 24 mesenchymal tumors appeared to be primary in the CNS (microglioma, microgliomatosis, unidentified lymphoma) and occurred between six months and four years of transplantation. Rapid development of focal CNS signs in nonfebrile patients with transplants suggests neoplasm rather than infection. So far, there appears to be no evidence for an increase in other primary brain tumors.

Electrolyte and Acid-Base Imbalance

The role of salt-water and acid-base imbalance in producing cerebral symptoms in uremic patients must again be stressed. Some of these patients have severe renal salt loss, and plasma hypo-osmolality and cerebral edema related to water intoxication develop.

CENTRAL NERVOUS SYSTEM DYSFUNCTION IN LIVER FAILURE

Characteristic changes in CNS function are seen in association with extensive liver disease. These include a hepatic encephalopathy, which is characterized by fluctuating psychiatric disorders, increased sleep, and abnormal movements, including corticospinal, extrapyramidal, and cerebellar disturbances, of which the most characteristic is flapping tremor, or asterixis. Occasionally — and particularly if liver failure is of rapid onset, as in acute hepatic necrosis — there may be delirium, convulsions, coma, and decerebrate rigidity (the latter is unusual in that it is clinically reversible with appropriate therapy). Much more rarely, liver disease is associated with focal CNS changes, including irreversible paraplegia.

Biochemical Features of Hepatic Encephalopathy

Except for the rare focal lesions, the features of CNS dysfunction that have been noted are reversible with suitable treatment (including hemodialysis) and are presumed to be on a metabolic basis. Liver disease might cause cerebral dysfunction either by failing to add to the blood some factor essential for cell nutrition, or by failing to remove some substance that is toxic to the CNS. Either of these mechanisms may be associated with hepatic parenchymal damage or with shunting of blood directly from portal to systemic circulations (portocaval shunt).

Liver Tropic Factor

Evidence that the liver contributes some factor essential for cell nutrition is tenuous. It has been noted that during hepatic disease the brain becomes increasingly sensitive to otherwise innocuous levels of hypoxia, electrolyte abnormalities, drugs, and other noxae (a factor that may account for the inconstant associations between brain dysfunction and blood or CSF concentrations of suspected toxic materials). Normal metabolism ceases in brain perfusion preparations after a few hours unless the liver is included in the system, and this effect appears to be at least partly due to lack of cytidine and uridine. Additional tentative evidence for some (undefined) hepatic tropic factor lies in the occasional development of myelin degeneration (e.g., in cerebrospinal tracts), following portocaval shunt.

Possible Toxic Agents

Because of the involvement of the liver in so many facets of metabolism, there has been no shortage of candidates for the role of toxic factor. These have included methionine or other amino acids, products of abnormal tryptophan metabolism, short-chain free fatty acids, and ammonia.

Methionine will precipitate coma in susceptible patients (i.e., with long-standing liver disease), but there is a concurrent rise in blood and CSF ammonia levels. If methionine is administered intravenously instead of orally, or if oral antibiotics are given concurrently, plasma methionine levels rise but ammonia levels do not, since there is no degradation in the gut, and no coma is produced.

Abnormal tryptophan metabolites could be produced by degradation in the gut, although experimentally they have to be given to much higher than clinical levels to affect brain function. Although serotonin levels in the brain may be reduced, intravenous 5-hydroxytryptophan improves the EEG without significantly altering the clinical condition. Small numbers of patients in liver coma have received norepinephrine, epinephrine, and serotonin, with little effect either on the EEG or consciousness (possibly because these factors fail to cross the blood-brain barrier). A few who received levodopa showed a rapid and striking improvement in consciousness and EEG activity, but these changes only lasted 1 to 12 hours. It has been speculated that dopaminergic transmission might be defective in hepatic coma, perhaps because excess S-adenosylmethionine (secondary to raised blood amino acid levels) promotes further conversion to norepinephrine.

Blood levels of *short-chain free fatty acids* are high in hepatic coma and about twice as high in hepatic disease patients with encephalopathy as in those without it. Experimental administration of such acids leads to reversible coma, which also occurs in isovaleric acidemia, a rare error of metabolism causing increased circulating levels of a 4-carbon free fatty acid. The coma of fatty acid administration is associated with depression of the reticular formation and EEG changes similar to those seen in hepatic coma. In tissue preparations, free fatty acids inhibit oxidative phosphorylation and reduce the concentration of ATP. However, there appear to be few studies on barrier permeability in hepatic encephalopathy, and it is not known whether or not intracerebral accumulation of such acids occurs.

Ammonia as a Toxic Agent

Currently, the prime candidate for the production of hepatic encephalopathy is ammonia. It is known that levels of NH_4^+ in the CSF (and presumably ECF) fairly closely reflect those in the blood, there being rapid transfer across the barrier system. In some cases of liver disease, blood and CSF NH_4^+ is extremely high, though in others it appears to be normal. Administration of ammonia to experimental animals or patients with liver disease appears to have little effect. This may be due to the acute nature of the experiments; time induces progressive liver sensitivity to many toxic factors, as has been mentioned. In favor of a direct role for ammonia are the usually high circulating levels and the mitigation of neurological features by reducing such levels (e.g., administration of antibiotics, low protein diet).

Several inborn errors of metabolism are associated with raised ammonia levels, which usually are episodic. The deficient enzymes are most often those of the urea cycle. These diseases include argininosuccinic aciduria, citrullinuria, arginase deficiency, congenital lysine intolerance, and the very rare deficiencies of carbamoyl phosphate synthetase or ornithine transcarbamylase (the latter two absent even from the normal CNS). The neurological features of these diseases during periods of high blood ammonia closely resemble those of hepatic encephalopathy, and the few patients that have been adequately studied at autopsy have usually shown the characteristic change in astrocytes that will be described subsequently.

Since the brain cannot form urea, it presumably relies on two methods for ammonia disposal: first, loss of ammonia to the circulating blood (for urea synthesis elsewhere); and second, as a reserve mechanism, the combination of ammonia with *a*-ketoglutaric acid to form glutamic acid, which can in turn combine with further ammonia to form glutamine (Fig. 11-11). Rapid protein turnover in the normal brain presumably implies considerable ammonia production, and neuronal activity induced by shock or convulsive agents causes a significant rise in blood ammonia. (It is thought that high neuronal activity, mobilizing keto acids for the citric acid cycle, converts glutamic to *a*-ketoglutaric acid with liberation of ammonia, which would then have to be disposed of to the blood.)

In liver failure, glutamine is markedly raised in the brain (but not in other organs). Detoxication of

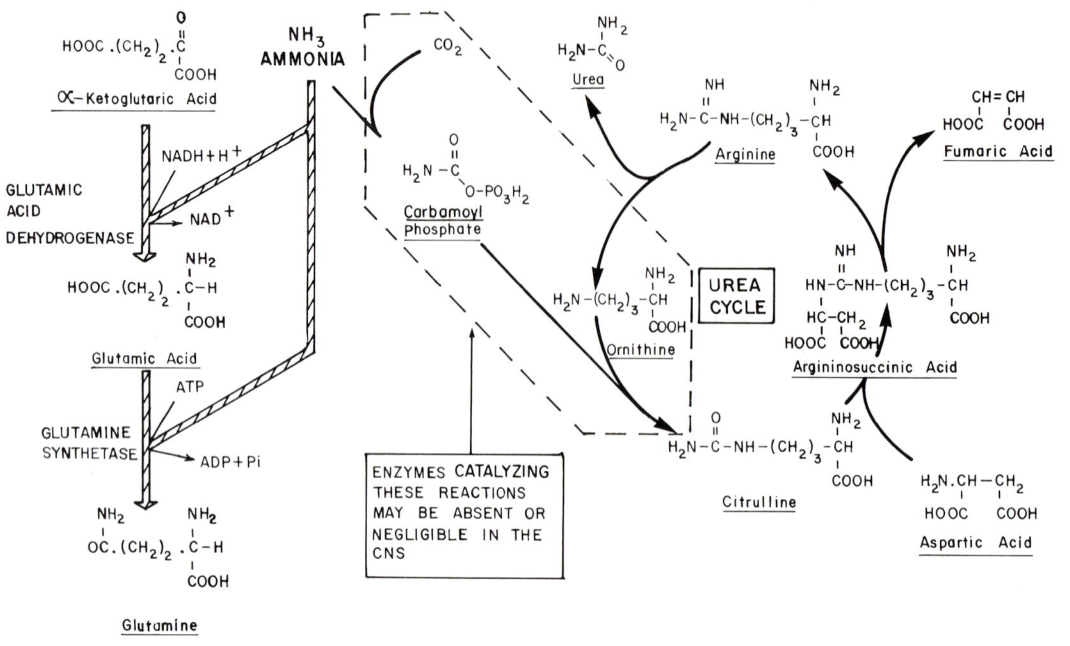

Fig. 11-11. Ammonia metabolism in the CNS. High ammonia concentrations may be a major toxic factor in hepatic encephalopathy.

ammonia by formation of glutamine is bioenergetically expensive. Synthesis of glutamic acid requires glutamate dehydrogenase and nicotinamide adenine dinucleotide (NADH), reducing the supply of NADH for ATP formation and shunting *a*-ketoglutarate out of the tricarboxylic acid cycle. The further synthesis of glutamine requires glutamine synthetase and ATP, thus reducing preformed high-energy phosphate reserves. Therefore, increased brain ammonia may compromise energy metabolism by immobilizing citric acid cycle intermediates and reducing both the supply and the formation of ATP. The possibility that ammonia may be toxic through other mechanisms, such as depletion of acetylcholine or a direct effect on plasma membranes, cannot be excluded.

Brain Metabolism in Hepatic Encephalopathy

Patients with severe hepatic encephalopathy or coma show normal or slightly reduced cerebral blood flow, but a marked decrease in oxygen utilization (30 to 40% in coma), suggesting metabolic depression. Brain concentrations of ATP and CrP are moderately reduced – more so in the brain stem than elsewhere. (Brain stem involvement would explain many of the clinical features, including asterixis, decerebrate and decorticate rigidity, hyperventilation, and coma.) Progressive reduction in ATP levels might also explain the progressive CNS sensitivity to various noxious agents.

Summary of Possible Biochemical Mechanisms

It is noteworthy that if portocaval shunt is carried out in the presence of good liver function, hepatic encephalopathy is rare, suggesting that it results from a failure to detoxify a product absorbed from the gut. On the other hand, in patients with portocaval shunt, rarer CNS changes, such as demyelinative disease, are occasionally seen, suggesting the possibility of some essential "growth factor" derived from the liver. Present evidence suggests that the substance that is not adequately detoxified is ammonia (although other toxic materials are undoubtedly also present), and that the material necessarily contributed by liver cells as a growth factor is uridine, cytidine, or a derivative of one of these.

Morphology of Hepatic Encephalopathy

Relatively constant astrocytic changes are associated with hepatic encephalopathy or coma. These were first observed in an inborn error of copper metabolism (Wilson's disease), in which there is pathological change in the liver and basal ganglia. In Wilson's disease, astrocytes exhibit two changes: in one, there is a large hyperchromatic nucleus and numerous pale, greenish-brown granules in the associated cytoplasm (Alzheimer type I cells); and in the other, a pale, vacuolated, often twisted nucleus, but with very little associated cytoplasm, is visible on light microscopy (Alzheimer type II cells) (Fig. 11-12). Recent investigations suggest a possible relationship between the two types, but type I cells are largely confined to Wilson's disease, and it is only type II that are seen in hepatic encephalopathy.

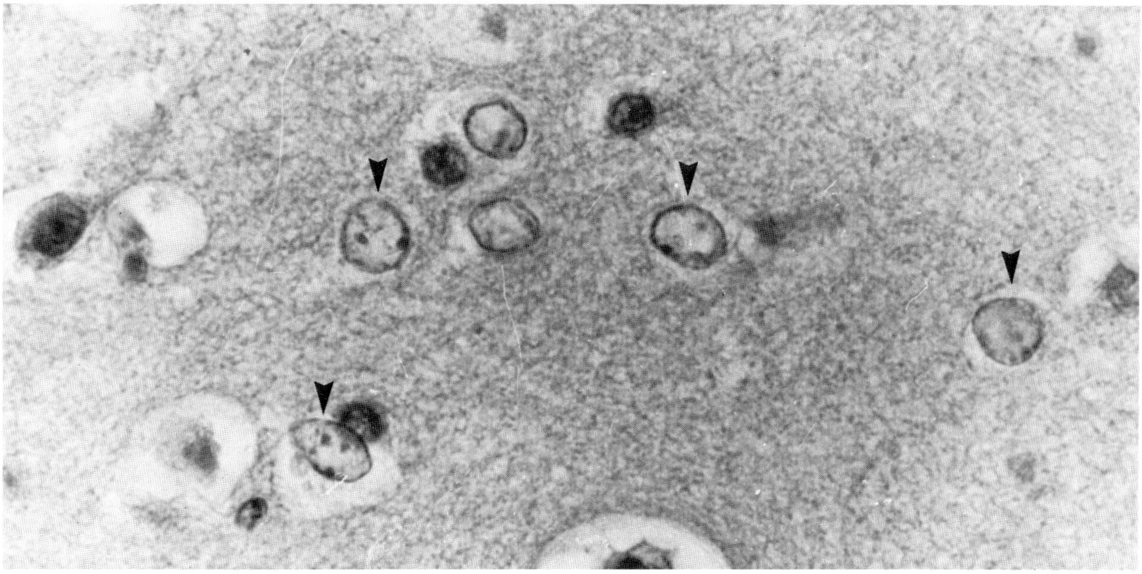

Fig. 11-12. Alzheimer type II astrocytes (arrows). (H & E, X750.)

The production of type II cells has been studied experimentally in rats, which tolerate remarkably high blood ammonia without going into coma. Since the ammonium ion has the same charge and about the same radius as the hydrated potassium ion, it is possible that excess NH_4^+ interferes with the transport of K^+ across the neuronal cell membrane, with disturbance of membrane potential. If this is so, it may be of considerable importance to have a homeostatic mechanism for ammonia in the brain (conversion to glutamic acid and glutamine). The competent compartment of the CNS has not been identified, but may well be the astrocyte (no such mechanism exists in other tissues). Speculating further, such a role for astrocytes might be related to their postulated role of maintaining a constant K^+ concentration in the ECF, and if they take up NH_4^+ in place of K^+, their membrane potential and K^+ absorptive capacity could be altered. Reduced serum K^+ readily precipitates coma in patients with chronic liver disease, and the coma is rapidly relieved by administration of KCl.

Electron microscopy shows a biphasic astrocytic reaction, early swelling being followed by a reaction that includes fibril formation. At first, the entire cell swells and becomes increasingly lucent, losing glial filaments and glycogen granules while other organelles remain unchanged. Irregular, empty, membrane-bound vesicles, up to 2μ across (which are probably localized dilatations of the endoplasmic reticulum) appear, and an unusual feature is folding of the plasmalemma, especially of the end-feet. Swelling varies in intensity from area to area, and in the rat is best seen in the dentate and caudate nucleus. In the second (reactive) phase the nucleolus becomes prominent and the nuclear and plasma membranes increasingly folded. Distended vesicles and increased electron lucency disappear; endoplasmic reticulum, ribosomes, and mitochondria increase, and there is not merely reappearance but a great increase in glial filaments. Astrocytes in the rat cortex do not develop the later (reactive) changes.

Although changes in glial filaments and prominent vacuoles occur in several conditions (including edema and Creutzfeldt-Jakob syndrome), foldings of the plasmalemma and nuclear envelope appear to be specific and might facilitate fluid exchange. The whole sequence could be interpreted as an alteration in fluid balance of the astrocyte, followed by reparative changes. However, no definitive proof has so far been obtained that detoxication of ammonia is carried out in the astrocytes.

More Unusual CNS Changes in Liver Disease

Liver disease appears to be one of the less common but well-established causes of cerebral edema. Although electron-microscopic investigations have not been reported, brains show the usual gross features of edema, including an increase in weight. Edema is particularly associated with acute massive necrosis of the liver, following periods of coma lasting between 24 hours and 10 to 14 days. Although the number of cases is small, the complication appears more often in the younger age group (average age 20 to 25). There appear to have been few studies on barrier permeability or cerebral water content in hepatic encephalopathy, and it is purely speculative to point to similarities in the astrocytic changes that occur in hepatic encephalopathy and in cerebral edema (see Chap. 12).

The introduction of portocaval shunt seems to have been followed by a few new CNS changes that might be generally classified as encephalomyelopathies. One is a symmetrical, incomplete demyelination of the lateral corticospinal tracts, accompanied by mild perivascular lymphocytic infiltration and swelling and distortion of axons. The patients have spastic paraplegia with hyperreflexia and bilateral Babinski responses. It has been reported that Betz's cells are lost from the precentral gyrus; if confirmed, this might be the primary lesion causing corticospinal tract degeneration. Rare cases with cortical involvement have been described, characterized by neuronal loss and Alzheimer type II cells. They have occurred in middle-aged patients with prominent shunting, as well as in younger patients with little shunting but severe parenchymal disease.

BIBLIOGRAPHY

Aronson, S. M. Intracranial vascular lesions in patients with diabetes mellitus. *J. Neuropathol. Exp. Neurol.* 32:183-196, 1973.

Becker, R. M., and Daniel, R. K. Increased antidiuretic hormone production after trauma to craniofacial complex. *J. Trauma* 13:112-115, 1973.

Davson, H. The Blood-Brain Barrier. In G. H. Bourne (Ed.), *The Structure and Function of Nervous Tissue.* New York: Academic, 1972. Vol. 4, pp. 321-445.

Dila, C. L., and Pappius, H. M. Cerebral water and electrolytes: An experimental model of inappropriate secretion of antidiuretic hormone. *Arch. Neurol.* 26:85-90, 1972.

Elliott, F. A. *Clinical Neurology* (2nd ed.). Philadelphia: Saunders, 1971.

Fernandez, J. P., McGinn, J. T., and Hoffman, R. S. Cerebral edema from blood-brain glucose differences complicating peritoneal dialysis. *N. Y. State J. Med.* 68:677-680, 1968.

Fox, J. L., Falik, J. L., and Shalhoub, R. J. Neurosurgical hyponatremia: The role of inappropriate antidiuresis. *J. Neurosurg.* 34:506-514, 1971.

Fulop, M., Tannenbaum, H., and Dreyer, N. Ketotic hyperosmolar coma. *Lancet* 2:635-639, 1973.

Gabbay, K. H. The sorbitol pathway and the complications of diabetes. *N. Engl. J. Med.* 288: 831-836, 1973.

Gordon, E., and Rossand, M. Further studies on cerebrospinal fluid acid-base balance status in patients with brain lesions. *Acta Anaesthesiol. Scand.* 14:97-109, 1970.

Greenhouse, A. H. The Neuropathology of Renal Disease. In J. Minckler (Ed.), *Pathology of the Nervous System.* New York: McGraw-Hill, 1968. Vol. 1, pp. 1029-1042.

Harreveld, van A., Collewijn, H., and Malhotra, S. K. Water, electrolytes and extra-cellular space in hydrated and dehydrated brains. *Am. J. Physiol.* 210:251-256, 1966.

Hogan, G. R., Dodge, P. R., Gill, S. R., Master, S., and Sotos, J. F. Pathogenesis of seizures occurring during restoration of plasma tonicity to normal in animals previously chronically hypernatremic. *Pediatrics* 43:54-64, 1969.

Hogan, G. R., Dodge, P. R., Gill, S. R., Scholl, M. L., and Master, S. Electrophysiologic response of the rabbit brain to chronic hypernatremic dehydration and rehydration. *Pediatrics* 50:769-777, 1972.

Holliday, M. A., Kalayci, M. N., and Harrah, J. Factors that limit brain-volume changes in response to acute and sustained hyper- and hyponatremia. *J. Clin. Invest.* 47:1916-1928, 1968.

Katzman, R., and Pappius, H. M. *Brain Electrolytes and Fluid Metabolism.* Baltimore: Williams & Wilkins, 1973.

Miller, M., and Moses, A. M. Urinary antidiuretic hormone in polyuric disorders and in inappropriate ADH secretion. *Ann. Intern. Med.* 77: 715-721, 1972.

Minkoff, L., Gaertner, G., Darab, M., Mercier, C., and Levin, M. L. Inhibition of brain sodium-potassium ATPase in uremic rats. *J. Lab. Clin. Med.* 80:71-78, 1972.

Norenberg, M. D., and Lapham, L. W. The astrocyte response in experimental portal-systemic encephalopathy. *J. Neuropathol. Exp. Neurol.* 33:422-435, 1974.

Plum, F., and Price, R. W. Acid-base balance of cisternal and lumbar cerebrospinal fluid in hospital patients. *N. Engl. J. Med.* 289:1346-1351, 1973.

Stein, M. F., Cimino, J. E., and Brescia, M. J. Subdural hematoma during dialysis. *N. Y. State J. Med.* 70:2022-2024, 1970.

Walker, C. O., and Schenker, S. Pathogenesis of hepatic encephalopathy with special reference to the role of ammonia. *Am. J. Clin. Nutr.* 23: 619-632, 1970.

Wilson, D. M. Metabolic abnormalities in uremia. *Med. Clin. North Am.* 55:1381-1396, 1971.

Zamora, A. J., Cavanagh, J. B., and Kyu, M. H. Ultrastructural responses of the astrocytes to porto-caval anastomosis in the rat. *J. Neurol. Sci.* 18:25-45, 1973.

Cerebral Edema

12

The brain is edematous when its parenchymal percentage water content is above normal. It is important to distinguish the term *cerebral edema* from others less specific (such as *brain swelling*) that merely imply that the weight of the brain is increased: this might be due to cerebral edema, increased cerebral blood volume, focal lesions such as tumor or abscess, or any combinations of these conditions. It is incorrect to use the terms *cerebral edema* and *brain swelling* interchangeably, and it does not assist in the elucidation of changes in, for example, head injury, where there may be both cerebral edema and increased cerebral blood volume.

Normal Water Content of Brain

The normal water content of the brain varies between the gray and white matter and also within different areas of hemispheric white matter. Commonly accepted ranges of water content are as follows:

Cortex and other large gray masses	81 to 87%
Deep white matter	67 to 74%
Corpus callosum	73 to 76%
Subcortical (arcuate) white matter	77 to 79%

The susceptibility of different regions of the brain to edema is inversely related to the water content, being greatest in the deep white matter and least in the cortex.

PATHOGENESIS

Increased brain water is ultimately derived from plasma and implies a net influx of water across the barrier systems. As noted in Chapter 4, it is probable that the formation of cerebrospinal fluid (CSF) and brain extracellular fluid (ECF) is an active secretory process rather than transudation. Nonetheless, the barriers are much more freely permeable to water than to solutes even of very low molecular weight. Increased water influx into the brain must therefore imply one or more of the following:

1. *Increased secretory activity* at the choroid plexuses and across the brain capillaries.
2. *Increased hydrostatic pressure* within the brain capillaries.
3. *Reduced osmotic differential* between plasma and brain ECF, either because the osmolality of plasma is decreased, or the osmolality of ECF is increased, or both. (Examples of cerebral edema due either to decreased plasma osmolality or to increased brain ECF osmolality were considered in Chap. 11.)
4. *Damage to the barrier system,* enabling plasma protein leakage into the brain ECF (and therefore increasing brain osmolality).

At present, there is no evidence that any form of cerebral edema is due to increased secretory activity across the barrier system (although a relatively unusual form of hydrocephalus associated with choroid plexus papilloma may be caused by this).

The Role of Hydrostatic Pressure in Small Vessels

The effective hydrostatic pressure (Fig. 12-1) across brain capillary endothelium is relatively low because of the complete encasement of the CNS by bone and a slight positive pressure in the CSF. Indeed, this hydrostatic pressure is barely equal to, and may at times be less than, the effective osmotic pressure due to plasma proteins, reinforcing the supposition of active secretion of extracellular fluid (ECF) in the brain. However, reabsorption of ECF into the capillary venules is a passive process, and brain water content is therefore readily upset by a significant alteration of balance between capillary hydrostatic pressure and the osmotic differential across the barrier. The osmotic differential is altered in damage to the barrier system such that there is macromolecular leakage (mainly plasma albumin) into the CNS. As will appear in the subsequent discussion, it seems probable that both barrier damage of this type and increased hydrostatic pressure are of considerable significance in the development of clinical cerebral edema.

The Role of Barrier Damage

Attention has been given, both in clinical and experimental edema, to assessing damage to the barrier system (mainly the blood-brain barrier, since this is so much larger in area than the blood-CSF barrier). One obvious indication of barrier damage would be permeability to molecules that normally

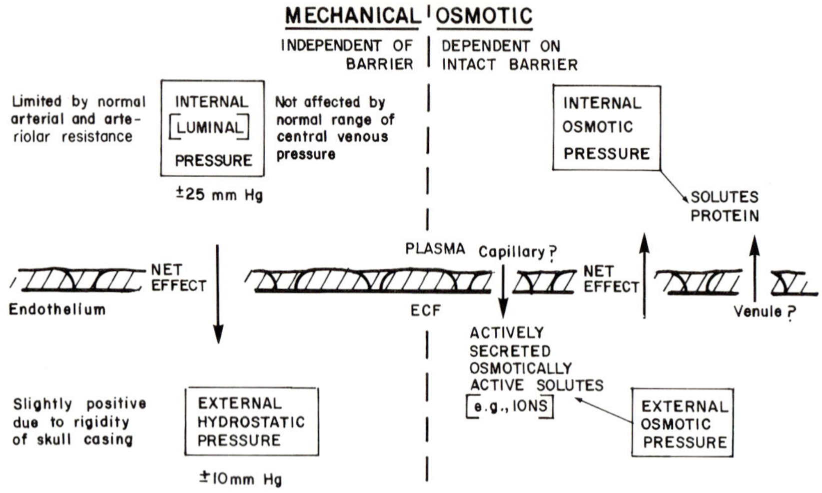

Fig. 12-1. Factors influencing the flux of water across the blood-brain barrier in the normal CNS. Outflow from the plasma depends both on a slight excess hydrostatic pressure in capillaries and active secretion of osmotically active solutes into the ECF. Inflow to the plasma depends on the low internal pressure of venules and the osmotic effect of plasma protein.

are incapable of traversing the barrier — notably, proteins. In many types of cerebral edema, extraction of brain protein shows that it has a high content of albumin, which is normally absent from brain parenchyma.

It is possible to attach fluorescent or colored dyes (such as trypan blue or fluorescein) to proteins and to visualize their escape across the barrier. A further method of assessing barrier damage is to measure the rate of brain uptake of materials that normally penetrate only slowly. In many cases of cerebral edema, uptake of radioisotope-labeled Na^+, K^+, and PO_4^{---} and of nonpolar molecules like urea is markedly increased . There is also a greater accumulation of Br^- and I^-, though it is not entirely clear whether this is due to increased rate of entry or to decrease of the normal active transport back to the plasma. In any event, all these changes suggest damage to the barrier system.

There are degrees of barrier damage, and increases in uptake of radioisotope-labeled ions are a more sensitive indicator of damage than exudation of plasma protein (labeled or otherwise) into the brain extracellular space. To this extent, an accepted classification of cerebral edema into "vasogenic" and "cytotoxic" varieties may not be strictly valid. The distinction is largely based on the permeability of the barrier system to proteins (suitably labeled) and therefore is really effecting a separation into severely damaged and less severely damaged barrier systems, rather than into damaged and normal systems. Even in cytotoxic edema, in which protein does not escape, fluid must derive from the plasma and, unless the toxic materials act by breaking down large molecules and increasing CNS osmolality, for which there is no evidence, it is difficult to envisage any mechanism by which they might produce edema that does not involve an alteration in function of the blood-brain barrier.

CONDITIONS ASSOCIATED WITH CEREBRAL EDEMA

Clinically, cerebral edema is of immense significance because it is common, difficult to reverse, and often fatal. It is a frequent concomitant of ischemia or hypoxia, head injury, focal brain lesions such as an infarct, hemorrhage, abscess, and neoplasm, many types of neurosurgery, and other conditions, including homeostatic disorders (any attempts at their correction), radiation, and the recovery phase of hypothermia.

Experimentally, cerebral edema has been most studied either by the production of "freeze" lesions of the cortex (which cause massive edema of the underlying white matter) or by the production of ischemia (by several methods). Many other experimental procedures, including the implantation of intracranial balloons, implantation of irritant chemicals or tumor cells, thermal injury, stab wounds, and various toxic substances, have also been employed. Considering the wide gamut of clinical and experimental situations producing edema, the overall uniformity of structural and chemical changes is

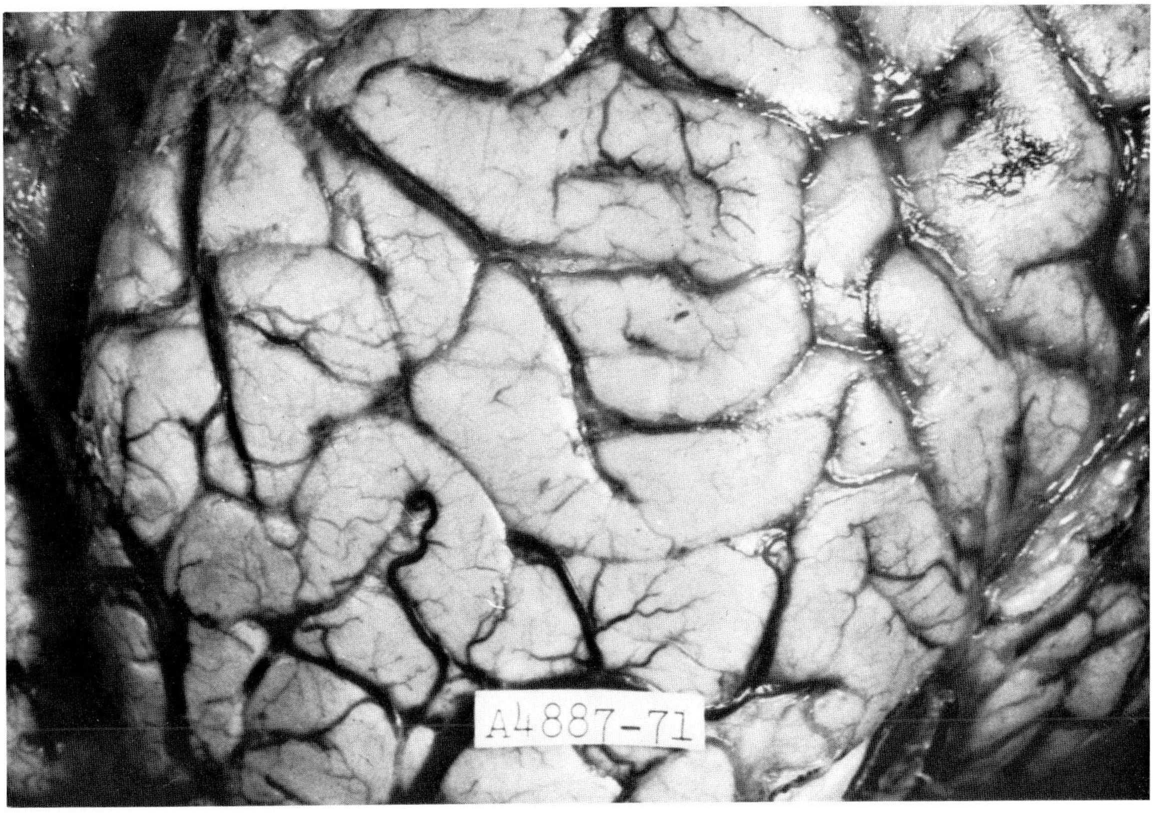

Fig. 12-2. Gyral flattening in diffuse cerebral edema. The normal rounded gyri and perceptible enlargements of subarachnoid space at the outer parts of sulci are not seen.

remarkable. A few exceptional forms that have come to light appear at present to be of little clinical relevance.

MORPHOLOGICAL CHANGES

Total intracranial volume, like normal brain weight, has a range of biological variation. Generally, the brain occupies 85 to 92% of this volume, the remainder being filled by intracranial blood (approximately 100 to 150 ml) and CSF. Approximately 60 to 70 ml of CSF are present in the cranial cavity (about half the total volume); more than half of this is in the subarachnoid space. The total intracranial contents (brain plus blood plus CSF) are enclosed by a rigid, essentially nonexpansible casing, the only significant deficiency being at the foramen magnum. The intracranial space is incompletely divided into three compartments by rigid mesenchymal (dural) septa, the falx and the tentorium. It follows that:

1. Expansion of the brain can only take place at the expense of reduction in the intracranial volumes of CSF, blood, or both.
2. Generalized edema of the brain (mainly of the white matter of the hemispheres) will cause some displacement of the forebrain downward through the tentorial notch (uncal herniation) and of the hindbrain down through the foramen magnum (tonsillar herniation).
3. Localized edema of one hemisphere (as around a neoplasm or infarct, for example) causes the same

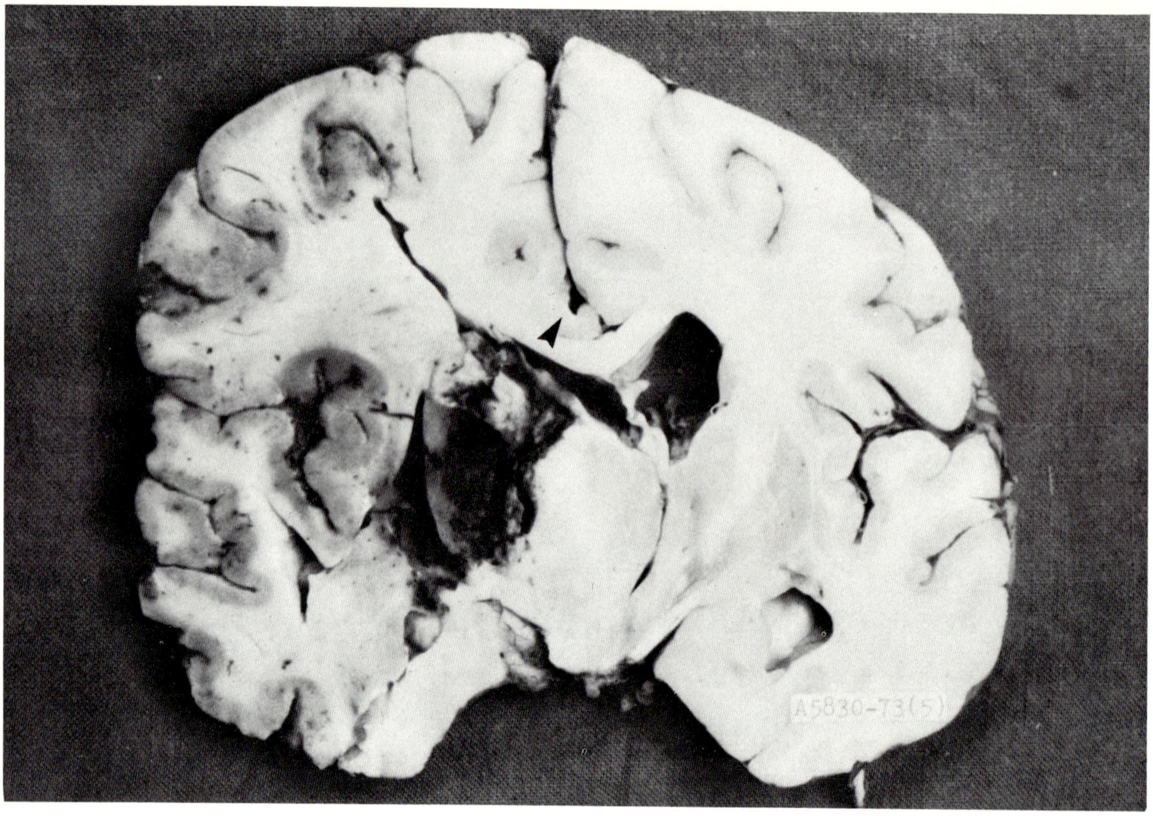

Fig. 12-3. Cingulate herniation. The lower part of the cingulate gyrus is forced across the midline below the free edge of the falx (arrow). Notice also the severe lateral displacement of the third ventricle and surrounding structures. (Infarction due to thrombosis of the right internal carotid artery, with severe right-to-left midline shift.)

changes (usually more marked on the side of the lesion) and also causes a midline shift of the forebrain below the margin of the falx.

It is the *distortion* caused by brain expansion within rigidly confined spaces, together with the effects of raised intracranial pressure on the cerebral blood flow, that are responsible for the very poor prognosis of cerebral edema, compared to edema of any other organ.

Changes in Gross Appearance

Enlargement of the brain due to any cause (including cerebral edema) is manifested by distortion that may be recognized at operation or autopsy. Some caution is needed in interpreting minor degrees of brain expansion at autopsy, since during the interval between death and postmortem examination, the brain may absorb CSF and swell as much as 2 to 4% of its in vivo volume, which leads to a minor degree of uncal and tentorial herniation or "notching." A discussion of the major gross changes in brain enlargement follows.

Gyral Flattening

A section through the normal brain shows rounded gyri separated by approximately triangular areas of subarachnoid space (containing CSF). In areas of severe swelling, section shows rectangular gyri with almost complete obliteration of the subarachnoid

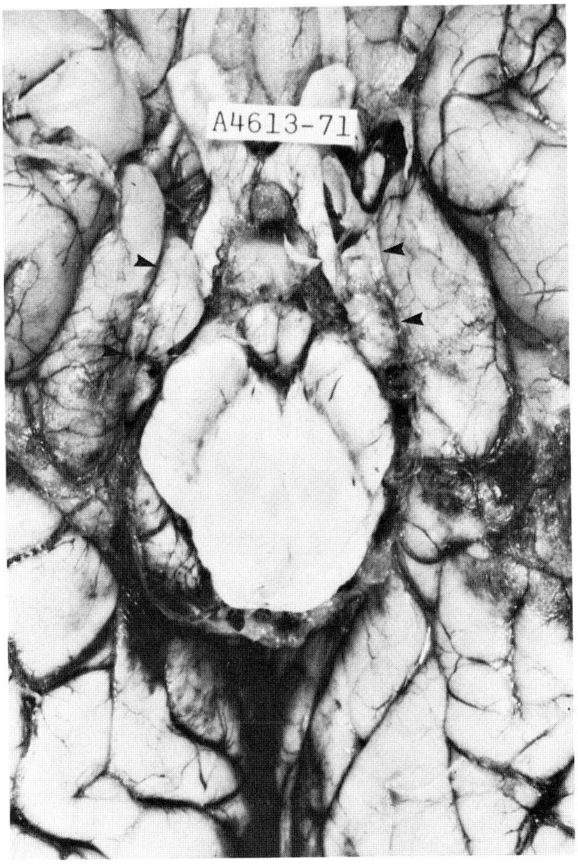

Fig. 12-4. Uncal herniation in diffuse cerebral edema. The medial parts of the uncus on each side are forced downward and medially, causing side-to-side compression of the midbrain and mamillary bodies. The grooves in each uncus (arrows) are caused by the free edge of the tentorium.

space. On the surface, the gyri appear to form a continuous flat sheet (Fig. 12-2), with sulci represented only by narrow lines. During surgery, these areas bulge through the craniotomy site, adding considerably to the technical difficulties of the operation.

Cingulate Herniation

Cingulate herniation is characteristic of unilateral hemisphere enlargement due to a tumor, infarct, hemorrhage, or abscess, usually with associated edema. Since the lower margin of the falx is 1 cm or more above the corpus callosum, the cingulate gyrus on the swollen side is forced across the midline (Fig. 12-3) below the falx, the change being usually most marked anteriorly. This is only one component of a general midline shift seen when the brain is sectioned in the frontal plane. In severe unilateral enlargement, the third ventricle is also forced across to the opposite side, causing considerable distortion of the thalamus and frequently associated with vertical, slitlike thalamic hemorrhages or infarcts.

Uncal Herniation

If either or both cerebral hemispheres expand, the largest deficiency through which brain tissue can be pressed is the tentorial notch on either side of the midbrain. Usually, the uncus, lateral and slightly anterior to the midbrain, is involved (Fig. 12-4), but if the tentorial notch happens to be wide, herniation may extend posteriorly (parallel to the midbrain), involving the parahippocampal gyrus. In diffuse edema the uncal herniation is symmetrical, but in the case of a unilateral mass or lesion, it is more marked on the side of the lesion (Fig. 12-5). The areas of herniation show a sharp indented notch corresponding to the free edge of the tentorium and may become hemorrhagic or even necrotic. Uncal and parahippocampal herniation are external manifestations of a general downward pressure on the central areas of the hemispheres, which can be seen as lateral compression of the thalamus and hypothalamus between the depressed temporal lobes (Fig. 12-6), with caudal midbrain displacement.

Several severe complications can result from uncal herniation, which is often associated with narrowing of the midbrain. With a unilateral mass lesion, the midbrain may be displaced to the opposite side, where the pressure of the tentorial edge indents the cerebral peduncle (Kernohan's notch) and may produce paradoxical ipsilateral motor signs. Uncal herniation causes pressure on veins draining from the midbrain into the great cerebral vein of Galen, producing irregular hemorrhages (Fig. 12-7) of the midbrain and upper pons (Duret's lesions). More rarely, areas of infarction are present in the midbrain, presumably from distortion of perforating arteries, such as those penetrating the posterior perforated substance or arising from superior cerebellar and posterior cerebral vessels. The latter vessels may themselves be compressed on one or both sides, with the most characteristic area of hemorrhagic cortical infarction involving the visual (calcarine) cortex on

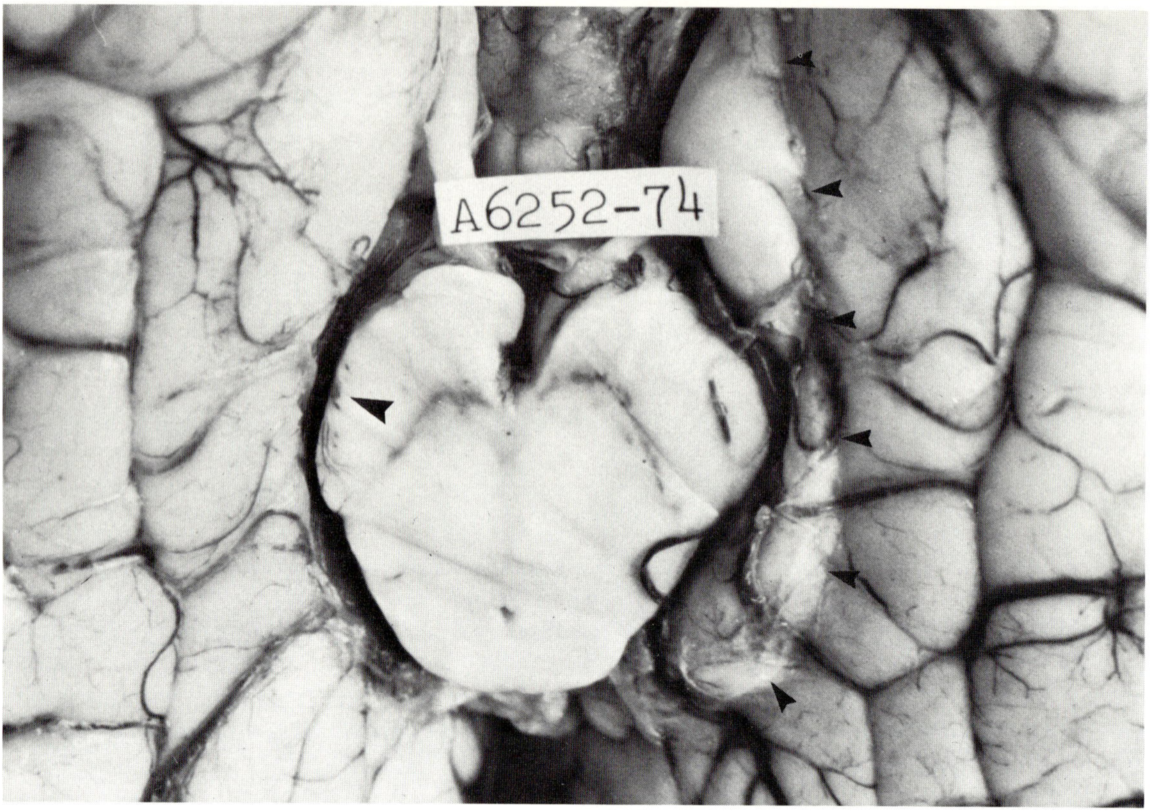

Fig. 12-5. Unilateral uncal herniation in left subdural hematoma. The left uncus and parahippocampal gyrus (small arrows) are herniated, and the midbrain has been forced to the right, with flattening of the right cerebral peduncle against the tentorial edge, Kernohan's notch. This flattening has caused a small area of hemorrhagic infarction (large arrow) in the right peduncle.

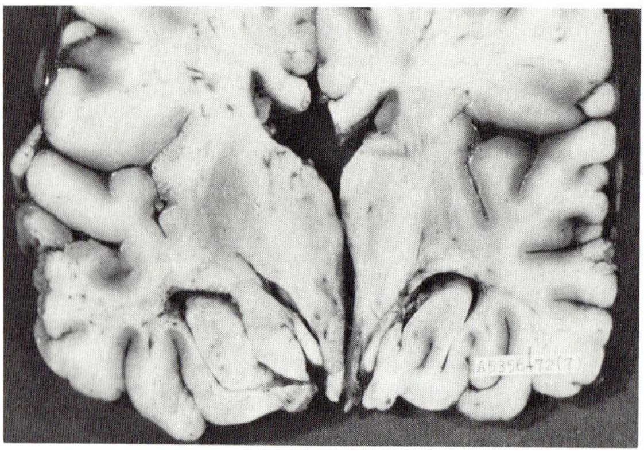

Fig. 12-6. Lateral compression and caudal displacement of the thalamus and adjacent structures, associated with cerebral edema.

one or both sides and sometimes the cuneus; the inferior temporal branches of the posterior cerebral artery are usually spared. Infarction of the superior cerebellum is uncommon. The third cranial nerve may be compressed and distorted, leading to a divergent strabismus. Uncal herniation may occur with none of these complications and rarely produces all of them, but they remain serious potential hazards.

Orbital Herniation

Less often described but often prominent, especially with frontal lesions, is depression of the posterior margin of the orbital cortex (Fig. 12-8) into the middle fossa posterior to the greater wing of the sphenoid. The sylvian fissure is depressed as much as 5 to 8 mm, and the ridge in the orbital cortex is readily mistaken for it in a swollen brain.

Tonsillar Herniation

The tonsils are parts of the posterior cerebellar hemispheres, normally facing each other in the midline rather than downward. If severe pressure is transmitted from the forebrain, or especially if there is a mass in the posterior fossa, the tonsils are herniated downward through the foramen magnum (Fig. 12-9), and this is associated with downward displacement of the posterior inferior cerebellar artery, which can be detected angiographically. The process is usually relatively slow, and symptoms due to compression of the medulla are unusual. Tonsillar herniation should be distinguished from *cerebellar coning,* in

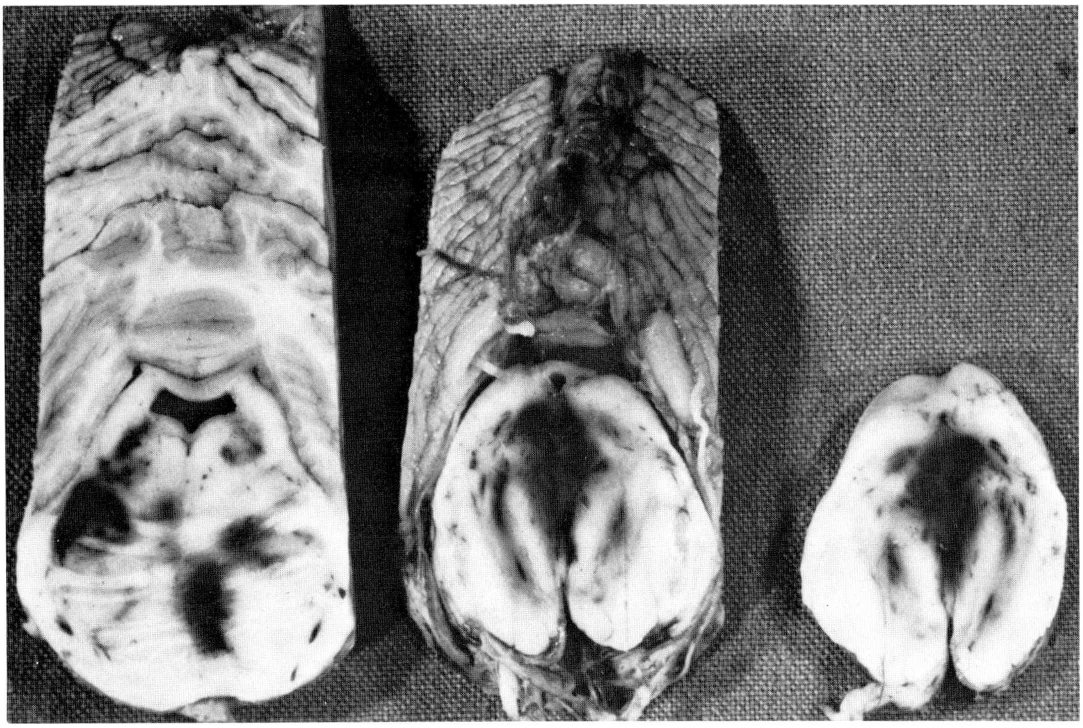

Fig. 12-7. Duret's lesions of the brain stem.

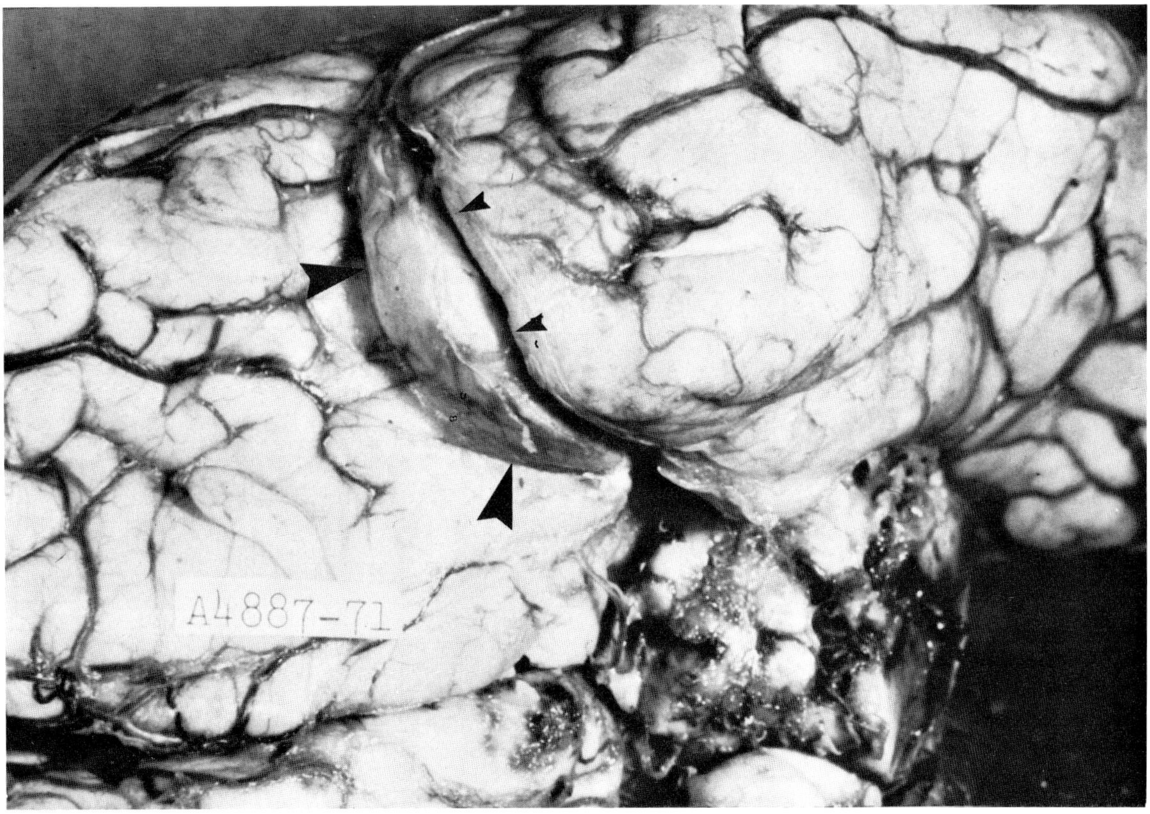

Fig. 12-8. Orbital herniation into the middle fossa (large arrows). The small arrows indicate the depressed sylvian fissure.

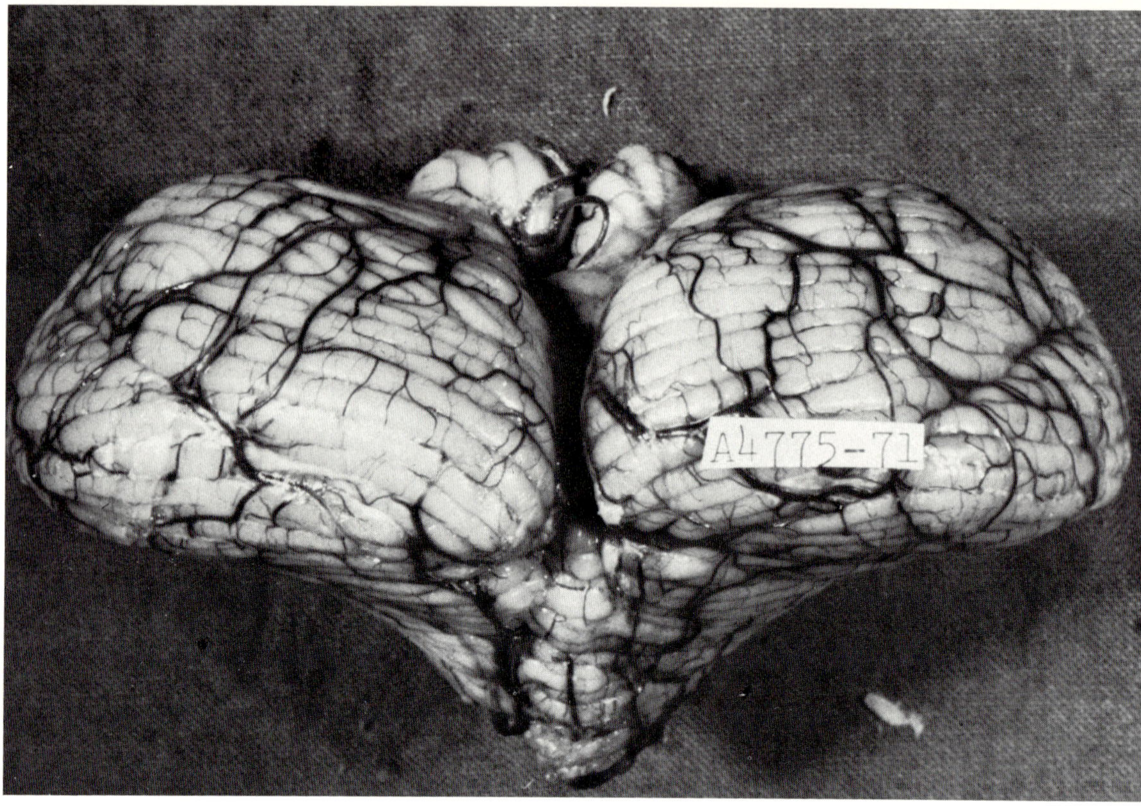

Fig. 12-9. Bilateral tonsillar herniation, viewed from behind after removal of the medulla. The tonsils may be seen projecting beyond the hemispheres (top of photograph; superior cerebellar surface below).

which the tonsils are acutely displaced downward because of a sharp drop in intraspinal pressure (removal of undue quantities of CSF), associated with high intracranial pressure. In cerebellar coning, since movement is rapid, death may occur, presumably from ischemia involving the medullary reticular formation and its vital centers.

Appearance of Cut Surface

In focal edema surrounding a mass lesion, white matter becomes swollen, moist, and often slightly yellow. These changes least affect the corpus callosum, internal capsule, and subcortical white matter; they usually involve the entire hemisphere, but do not significantly cross to the contralateral side. *In diffuse cerebral edema there is usually no visible change in the cerebral white matter.* This is because the maximum possible water increase is about 10%, since the brain already occupies some 90% of the cranial cavity. Assuming half the brain to be white matter, this would involve an extra 0.2 g of water per gram of white matter, or a "dilution" of dry weight from 30 to 25%. In localized edema, as much as 2.5 g of water per gram of white matter may be added, reducing the dry weight from 30% to approximately 8%.

Light-Microscopic Appearances

In *acute focal cerebral edema,* white matter appears poorly stained, whatever method is used. Under high power it is frequently possible to see separation of individual myelin sheaths. The tissue often contains small, irregular "lakes," which are empty or contain amorphous material (Fig. 12-10), presumably plasma protein. Much of the precipitated material separating normal tissue elements is weakly PAS-positive, due to glycoproteins from plasma and increased synthesis of glycogen by astrocytes. By routine staining, astrocytes appear normal, but special techniques show that their processes are irregularly swollen and often fragmented (Fig. 12-11), and that this change may occur within 12 to 18 hours of the onset of edema. The cytoplasm of oligodendroglial cells may form a pale halo around small, dark nuclei (a confusing appearance, as it has no electron-microscopic correlates).

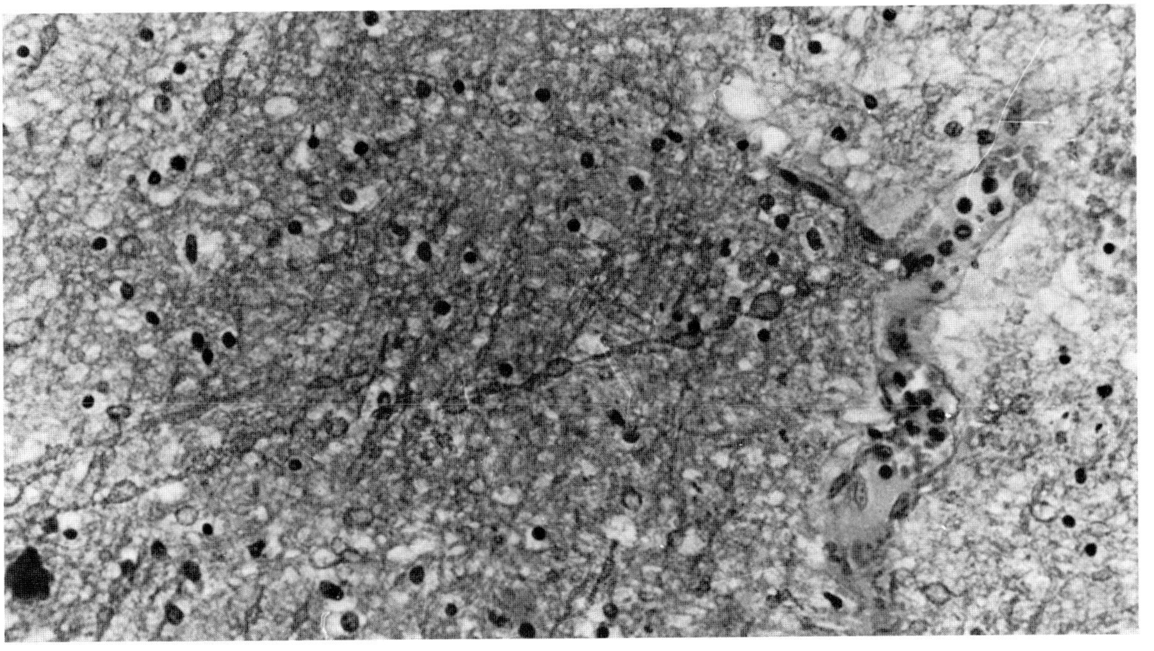

Fig. 12-10. Acute focal edema of white matter, showing transudation of fluid around a vessel, some vascular stasis, spongiosis, and beading of myelin sheaths (adjacent to intracerebral hemorrhage). (Myelin-PAS, ×300.)

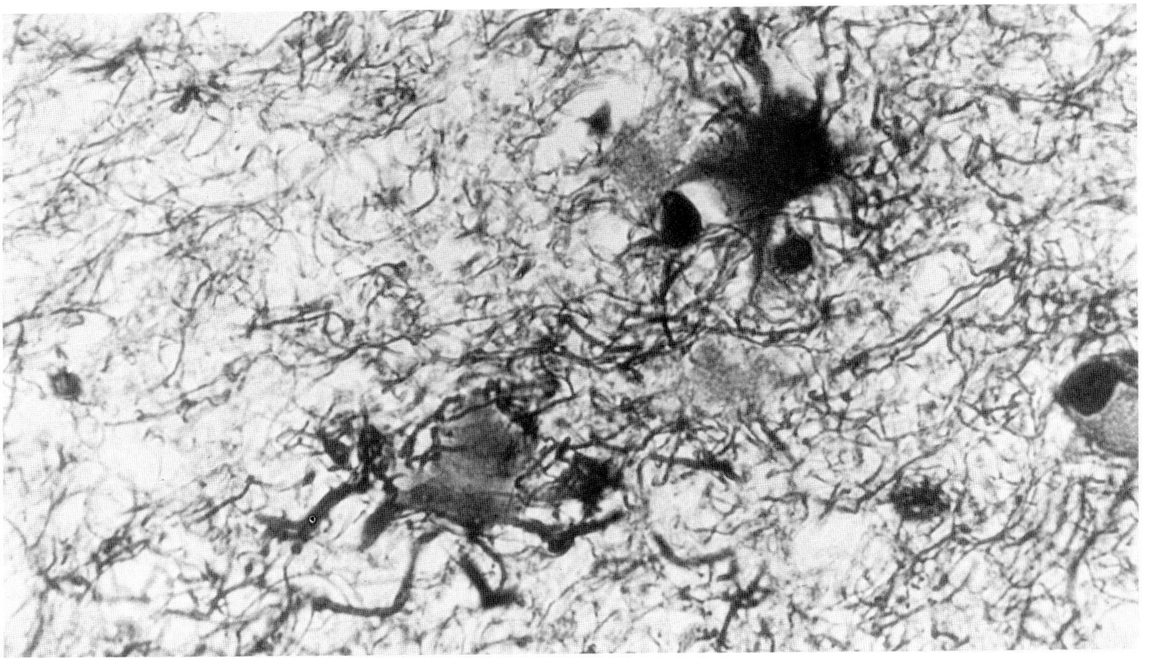

Fig. 12-11. Edema of white matter, the astrocytes showing stunting, irregularity, and fragmentation of processes. Note the loss of oligodendroglial cells and general rarefaction. (Holzer's stain, ×750.)

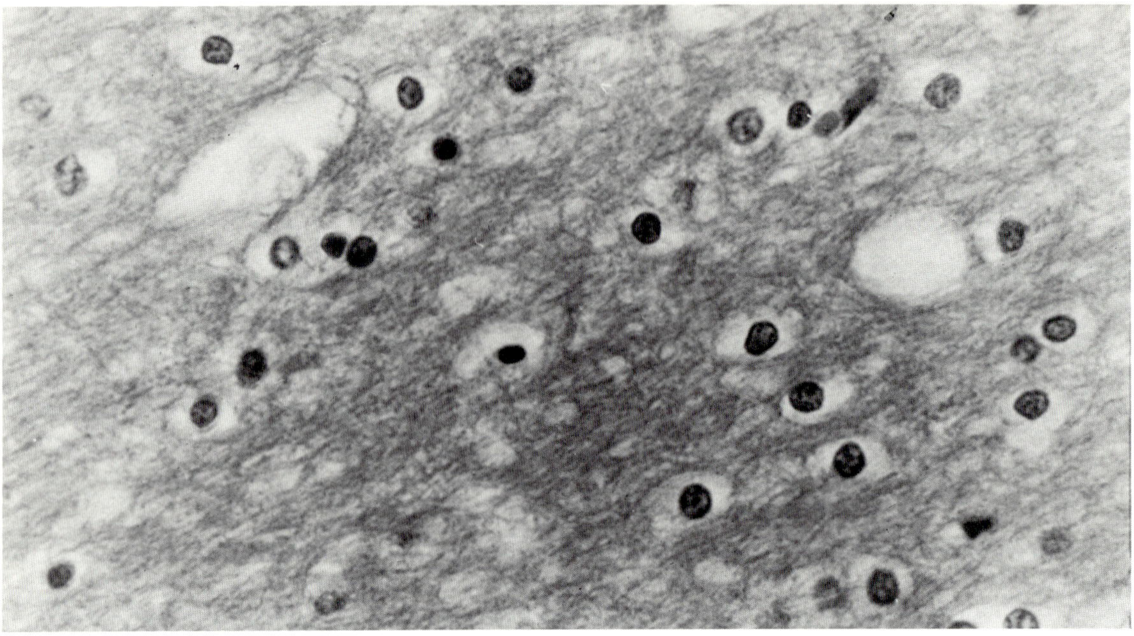

Fig. 12-12. Acute diffuse white-matter edema, showing only minimal spongiosis (but moderate hydropic swelling of oligodendroglia), from a case of head injury. (H & E, ×750.)

In *acute diffuse edema* (Fig. 12-12), pallor and separation of myelinated axons are difficult to see, but staining for astrocytes usually demonstrates the swelling and fragmentation seen in the focal variety.

In *chronic edema* (Fig. 12-13) (as in some cases of hypertension), myelin destruction occurs at a slow rate, although few if any phagocytic cells are visible, and there are only minor accumulations of perivascular neutral fat (myelin breakdown product). Astrocytic nuclei become swollen, and there is progressive irregular swelling, fragmentation, and loss of astrocytic processes. Axons are well preserved. Eventually, myelin may virtually disappear from areas of long-standing edema, and there is a fine, diffuse fibrillary gliosis, with some axonal loss. Oligodendroglial cells are decreased corresponding to myelin loss, and astrocytes do not recover their normal morphological features, retaining short, blunted processes. Small vessels are thick and hyalinized, but the other tissue elements appear "rarefied" on routine stains.

In gray matter, the changes of pure edema are not visible under the light microscope. Gray matter lesions associated with edema may include vacuolation, perivascular hemorrhages, and necrosis.

Electron-Microscopic Appearances

Because of difficulties in tissue preservation, the electron-microscopic appearance of the brain in experimental cerebral edema is much better known than in human edema. However, observations that have accrued from human material fully support accounts of electron-microscopic changes derived from experimental studies. A typical and well-studied experimental method is freezing of the cortex, which causes a focal area of cortical necrosis and massive edema of the underlying white matter. The changes

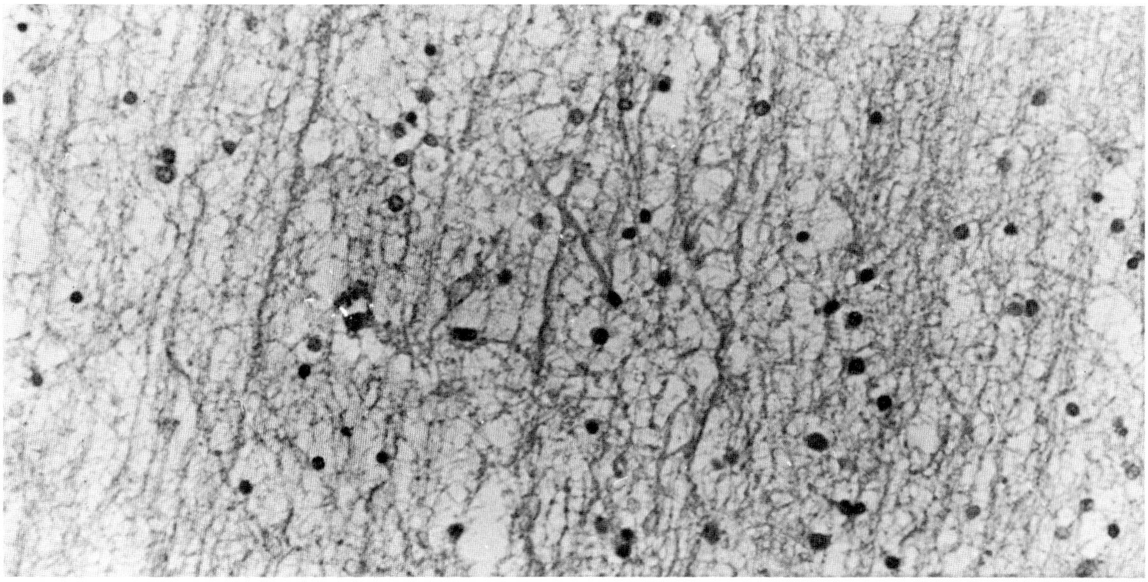

Fig. 12-13. Chronic edema of the white matter, with diffuse rarefaction, no astrocytic hyperplasia, but preservation of axons and general structure. (H & E, × 300.)

induced probably correspond closely to those surrounding mass lesions in the human brain.

It is not clear why edema should be so prominent in white matter and so difficult to detect in gray matter. It seems possible that the normal extracellular space is wider in white matter, that close intercellular junctions (such as synapses) limit possible distension of the extracellular space in gray matter, and also that cell bodies and processes in gray matter, notably the apical dendrites, rapidly absorb ECF (within seconds) as a result of asphyxia following death.

Focal Edema

The major changes seen in edematous white matter (Fig. 12-14) are a marked *increase in the extracellular space,* which may appear empty or may contain small amounts of precipitated amorphous material (usually free of cell organelles), and extreme *distension of astrocytic processes,* especially perivascular foot processes. These show a watery, electron-lucent cytoplasm and may contain irregular membrane-bound vesicles as large as 2μ in diameter. Although it has been suggested that the apparent extracellular space arises from rupture of astrocytic processes, this appears an unnecessary supposition in view of experimental work showing the spread of plasma-like fluid from a focus of cortical or white matter damage, the presence of excess albumin in many cases of cerebral edema, and the usual absence of organelles from the material occupying extracellular spaces. Astrocytic mitochondria are swollen, and the endoplasmic reticulum frequently appears vesicular (probably giving rise to the membrane-bound vesicles). Increased glycogen granules are seen in astrocytic cytoplasm. These changes in astrocytes presumably correspond to the swelling and fragmentation of processes seen with light microscopy.

Changes in myelin sheaths are usually absent or minimal, but there may be a minor degree of splitting

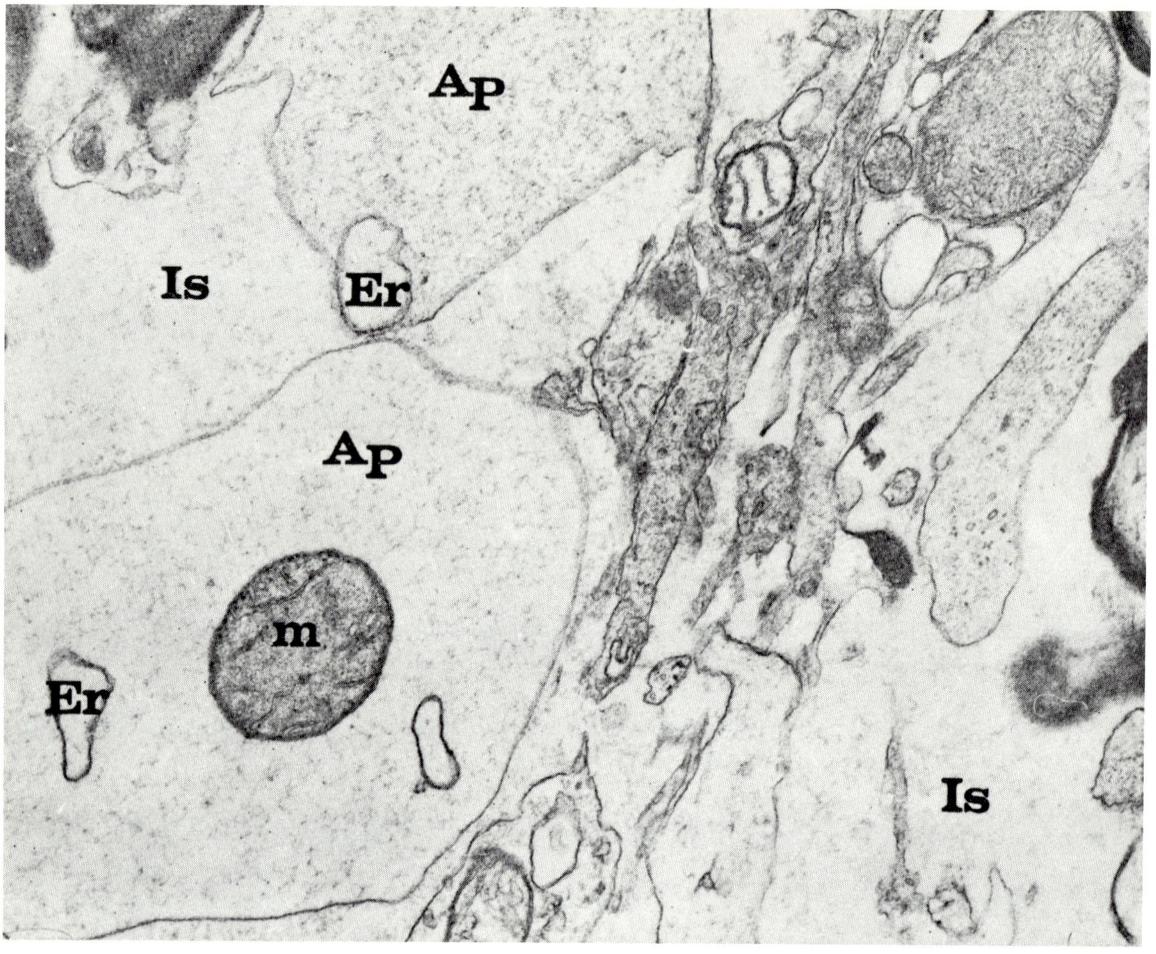

Fig. 12-14. Electron-microscopic appearance of white matter in acute experimental (cold-induced) edema. Astrocytic processes (Ap) are distended and electron-lucent and contain a swollen mitochondrion (m) and vacuolated endoplasmic reticulum (Er). There is a wide extracellular space (Is) containing pale, amorphous material. (X 7000.) (From J. C. Lee and L. Bakay, Ultrasonic changes in the edematous central nervous system, Archives of Neurology *14:37, 1966. Copyright 1966, American Medical Association.)*

at the intra-period line corresponding to a re-creation of the extracellular space. Within two to three days, an increase in intracellular glial fibrils is seen, and, depending on the time of persistence of the edema, fibrillary gliosis may progress as noted in the light-microscopic appearance. Axons do not show significant alteration, and there are no clear descriptions of altered oligodendroglia.

Resolution of white matter edema appears to be achieved largely by transfer of fluid from the extracellular to the intracellular phase, from which presumably it must eventually be returned to the plasma. Where plasma protein, largely albumin and alpha globulin, is extravasated, it is taken up either by damaged astrocytes directly through the cell membrane or by pinocytosis in healthy surviving cells. In either case, it appears to undergo chemical alteration. Little or no change is seen in the structure of capillaries in edematous white matter.

Studies of experimental edema associated with focal lesions suggest that the blood-brain barrier changes are confined to the immediate vicinity of the lesion, and that excess ECF spreads through the white matter in the extracellular space, the vesicular changes in astrocytes being secondary. By the use of markers, such as trypan blue, radioiodine-labeled serum albumin, or low-molecular-weight proteins such as horseradish peroxidase (molecular weight 43,000), it is possible to demonstrate spread of these materials from the damaged focus; this reaches a maximum extent at about three days and then usually regresses. Experiments with radioactive tracers such as ^{24}Na and ^{32}P show that in the necrotic focus these equilibrate almost immediately with plasma, as might be expected from the complete destruction of the barrier system. In normal brain they equilibrate very slowly, and in edematous white matter, they equilibrate at intermediate rates

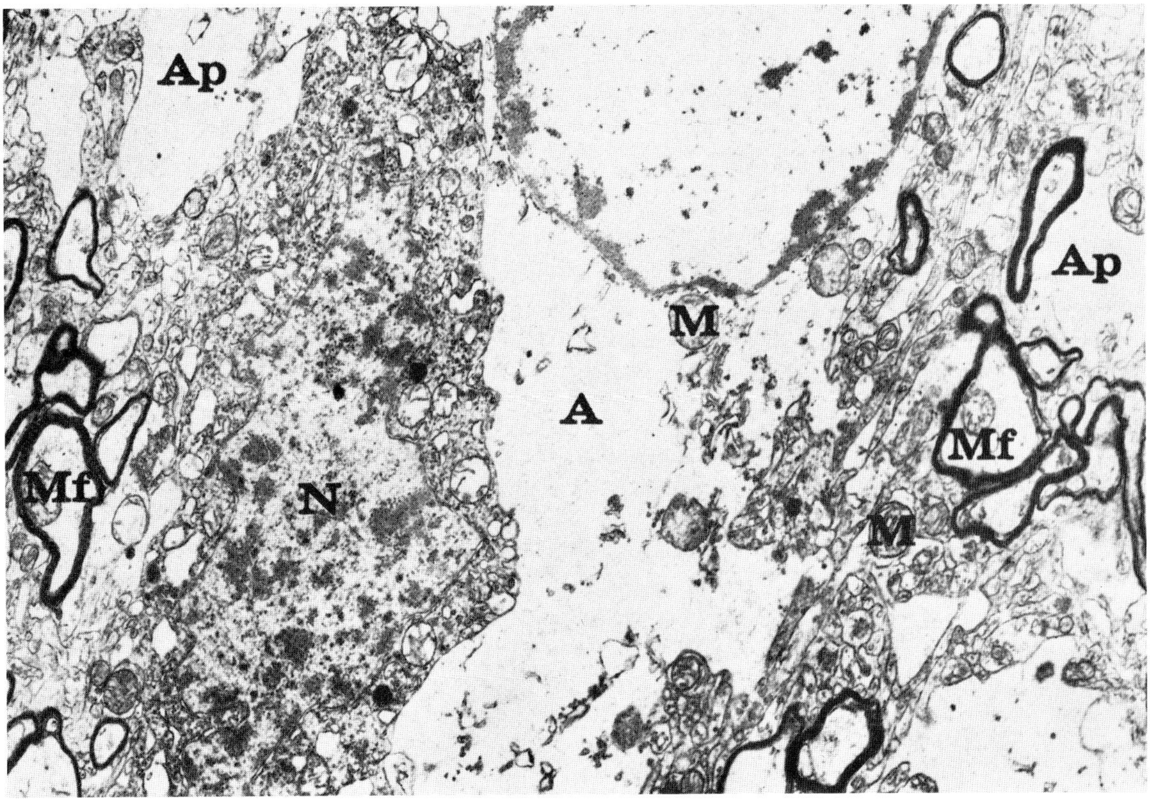

Fig. 12-15. Electron-microscopic appearance of gray matter (cortex) adjacent to a cold-induced injury, showing edema. Astrocytic processes (Ap), contained mitochondria (M), and endoplasmic reticulum. (X 6000.) A = astrocyte; N = nucleus of neuron; Mf = myelinated fibers. (From J. C. Lee and L. Bakay, Ultrasonic changes in the edematous central nervous system, Archives of Neurology 14:40, 1966. Copyright 1966, American Medical Association.)

that are more rapid adjacent to the necrotic focus and slower toward the margin of the edema, again suggesting spread through the extracellular space rather than alterations of the blood-brain barrier in the white matter itself. Such experimental work suggests that, irrespective of molecular weight, materials spread through the distended extracellular space at a uniform rate, representing bulk flow rather than diffusion and presumably due either to a pressure gradient from the necrotic focus or to rhythmic movements of glial cells.

In gray matter (Fig. 12-15) the changes of edema are largely confined to the astrocytes, where they closely resemble those already described. The processes become swollen and watery and contain electron-lucent vesicles, swollen mitochondria, and glycogen granules, the major difference being reduced or absent glial fiber formation. However, there does appear to be a minimal but definite increase in the extracellular space of edematous gray matter. No changes are seen in neurons. Minor changes have been reported in the vessels of gray matter, including some increase in pinocytotic vesicles and slight widening of the capillary basement membrane.

Diffuse Edema

The experimental production of diffuse cerebral edema has proved more difficult than the production of the focal variety. Methods such as trauma, general vascular occlusion, and water intoxication have been used. What relation these may bear to naturally occurring diffuse edema, which may be associated with ischemia, cranial trauma, hypertension, recovery from hypothermia, and other conditions, is not entirely clear. There appears some evidence that the permeability of the barrier system is less severely altered in diffuse than in focal cerebral edema, and that while there is little or no extravasation of protein, there are changes in radioisotope turnover (^{24}Na and ^{41}K). Correspondingly, the increase in endothelial pinocytosis in the gray matter is not seen in these conditions. The changes throughout the brain consist essentially of astrocytic swelling, as previously described, but without any significant enlargement of the extracellular space in the white matter. Presumably, the astrocytes can absorb the extravasated fluid as fast as it is produced.

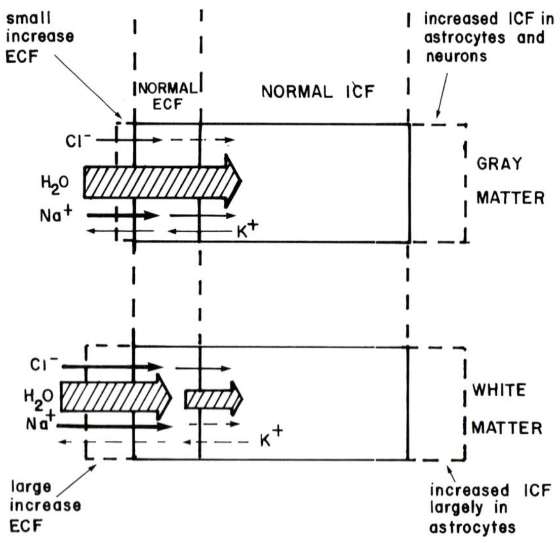

Fig. 12-16. Changes in acute edema in volume of intracellular (ICF) and extracellular (ECF) fluids and corresponding ion fluxes. The solid-line boxes represent normal volumes, and the dashed extensions are an approximate indication of the volume increase in edema. Plasma is assumed to be on the left. The fluxes of water and ions from plasma through ECF to ICF, or vice versa, are indicated very approximately by the thickness of the arrows.

BIOCHEMICAL CHANGES

The increased water content of edematous white matter is presumably accompanied by alterations in electrolyte distribution, notably, Na^+, K^+, and Cl^-. In addition, there are significant changes in energy utilization and bioenergetic patterns, probably accompanied (at least in gray matter) by alterations in other metabolic activities and in concentration of biogenic amines.

Alterations in Water and Electrolyte Content

Although a certain amount of work has been done with human material obtained at operation, most investigation in this field has been carried out on experimental animals. The intrinsic difficulties of such investigations are compounded by the ingenuity of investigators in expressing their results in many different units, making it hard to compare the results of different workers.

In white matter, the normal water content is about 70 to 72%. This figure is appreciably increased in cerebral edema, typically by 4 to 8%, with a corresponding fall in the percentage of dry weight. Much investigation has been carried out on the Na^+ and K^+ content of edematous brain. It is important to draw a distinction between the *concentration* of these ions, expressed in terms of wet weight, and the *absolute content*, expressed in terms of dry weight (total dry weight is presumed to be approximately constant). Studies on experimental animals and on human material (Fig. 12-16) show that the increase in water is accompanied by a significant absolute increase in Na^+ and a somewhat smaller decrease in K^+. Corresponding estimations of the extracellular space (for methods, see Chap. 4) show a significant increase, on the order of 20 to 25%. It is calculated that much of the extra water and Na^+ is in this extracellular space, yielding a concentration of approximately 135 to 140 mEq per kilogram H_2O, roughly corresponding to plasma ultrafiltrate. The absolute decrease in K^+ occurs somewhat later and may reflect both impaired metabolism, resulting in K^+ leakage from cells, and uptake of ECF with exchange of K^+ for Na^+ within the cell to maintain osmolality. Fewer data for the Cl^- content of edematous white matter are available, but it appears to be increased to a greater extent than Na^+. Presumably, some of it is initially intracellular as well as extracellular.

These studies indicate that in edematous gray matter (Fig. 12-16), there is considerably less uptake of water than in edematous white matter. However, the Na^+ uptake is similar to that in white matter, partially balanced by a high loss of K^+. If all the Na^+ remained in the extracellular space, there would be a Na^+ concentration of 280 mEq per liter – at least twice that in plasma. It must therefore be assumed that a considerable part of this excess Na^+ is intracellular and has exchanged with corresponding amounts of K^+, probably as a result of secondary interference with cell metabolism due to edema, or of direct damage from the primary edema-inducing lesion. The Cl^- uptake in the cortex is lower than that in white matter, and estimations of the extracellular space indicate very little increase.

In many experimental situations it is difficult to make other than an arbitrary demarcation between the zone of primary tissue necrosis (e.g., cold-induced) and the surrounding narrow gray zone that may truly exhibit cerebral edema. In the necrotic area itself, the Na^+ and K^+ concentrations are approximately equivalent to those in plasma, indicating the absence of any significant barrier, and Na^+ and K^+ exchanges with plasma are extremely rapid. In edematous gray matter, on the other hand, changes are similar in direction to those occurring in the white matter, and uptake of Cl^- into cells appears to be dependent on increased K^+ concentration in the ECF. If isethionate ion is substituted for Cl^- in the extracellular space, no neuronal or dendritic swelling occurs.

Changes in Energy Metabolism

Edematous brain shows reduced oxygen uptake, which appears to be associated with reduced levels of creatine phosphate, adenosine triphosphate, glucose, and glycogen. However, it shows increased levels of adenosine diphosphate, adenosine monophosphate, inorganic phosphate, and (at least in gray matter) lactate and pyruvate. Most reports indicate increased activity of oxidative enzymes, with the possible exception of lactic dehydrogenase, which has been reported reduced in the edematous brain and increased in CSF. These changes appear to be essentially confined to astrocytes and are not observed in oligodendroglial cells. An increase in anaerobic glycolysis may be associated with decreased efficiency of the tricarboxylic acid cycle, because of the uncoupling of oxidation and phosporylation observed in experimental situations. The cause of this uncoupling is not clear, though accumulation of free fatty acids from the hydrolysis of phospholipids, especially ethanolamine plasmalogen and phosphatidylethanolamine, may be responsible. There appear to be sequential increases in RNA and protein synthesis, presumably associated with the formation of glial filaments and possibly of PAS-positive glycoprotein. These changes start at about 24 hours, peak at three days, and then gradually diminish.

A consideration of the electron-microscopic and biochemical changes in edematous white matter makes it clear that astrocytes are principally affected, and that after an initial period of swelling, they enter a reactive phase. (There seem to be similarities in their behavior in edema and in hepatic encephalopathy [see Chap. 11], though water content of the brain is apparently not increased in the latter condition.)

EDEMA IN HYPOXIA AND ISCHEMIA

Effects of Changes in PO_2, PCO_2, and pH

The clinical association of hypoxemic episodes or hypotension and the development of edema is well known and frequently catastrophic. It is therefore surprising that the blood-brain barrier, at least as judged by the usual methods, appears to be relatively resistant to decreases in oxygen tension. This resistance has usually been assessed by relatively coarse indicators of permeability change, such as dyes linked to protein, and it appears probable that while moderate degrees of hypoxia produce sufficient damage to cause water gain and increased turnover of Na^+ and K^+, severe degrees are necessary to cause permeability to protein. The barrier system is said to persist for at least 12 hours after death, as tested by trypan blue. However, when more permeable dyes such as Astraviolet are used, it becomes permeable within 30 to 60 minutes. Presumably, if it were possible to estimate Na^+ and K^+ turnover, this time would be very appreciably shortened. The apparent failure of hypoxemia to cause barrier damage may therefore reflect insufficiently sophisticated techniques. It could also be due to the more extensive extracranial communications with cerebral vessels in experimental animals compared with those in man, with consequent reduction of stasis and maintenance of a minimal PO_2 (see Chap. 13).

It is difficult to dissociate a reduction in PO_2 from an increase in PCO_2 and accumulation of metabolites such as lactate. Hypercapnia causes a rapid, but transient, increase in the permeability of both blood-brain and blood-CSF barriers to albumin and other substances, even including such nonpolar materials as urea. This generalized permeability increase is apparently not due to altered pH or vasodilatation. In the blood-brain barrier, it is most marked in the brain stem and upper cervical cord. Possible permeability effects of other acid metabolites such as lactate have not been subjected to rigorous testing. Lactate is much less diffusible than carbon dioxide, and its accumulation might lead to structural alterations in protein. A combination of hypoxia and hypercapnia is one experimental method used for the production of edema, said to be confined to the gray matter and characterized by astrocytic swelling, without dilatation of the extracellular space. It is probable that such experiments are complicated by the effects of hypoxemia on the myocardium, leading to increased central venous pressure and stasis of cerebral circulation.

Effects of Reduced Cerebral Blood Flow

Probably the most clinically relevant work has been the production of edema by occlusion of one or more vessels in experimental animals. Collateral circulation from extracranial vessels is often much better developed in such animals than in man, but multiple ligations produce reasonably consistent results. Irreversible cerebral edema develops in some of the experimental animals, and it seems that those in which this does not occur have been protected by one (or both) of two factors: an *effective preexisting collateral circulation* or an *immediate high systemic blood pressure response* to the occlusion. Clearly, both will assist in maintaining circulation in the nominally occluded areas. The animals in which cerebral edema fails to develop show less fall in PO_2 during the period of occlusion than do the others. It is reasonable to assume that these animals also have lower PCO_2, lactate, and other acid metabolites, and that sludging of erythrocytes does not develop. The contrary may be assumed for animals with inadequate immediate pressor response, insufficient collateral circulation, or both. Presumably, one or more of these factors makes the difference between slight and severe barrier damage.

There was loss of autoregulation in both groups, so that restoration of circulation resulted in a luxury perfusion syndrome (see Chap. 14). The group without edema showed a temporary increase in cerebral oxygen utilization, associated with restoration of a normal EEG. The edema group showed a massive increase in oxygen utilization, which persisted for several hours, unassociated with any restoration of electrical activity, but which then fell below normal as edema developed. The group without edema showed a moderate increase in intracranial pressure, presumably associated with increased cerebral blood volume as well as minimal edema. The edema group showed a severe progressive increase associated both with increased blood volume and progressive cerebral edema. The persistence of a high rate of oxygen utilization in this group, with failure to restore neuronal electrical activity, suggests an uncoupling of oxidative phosphorylation, for which the reason is

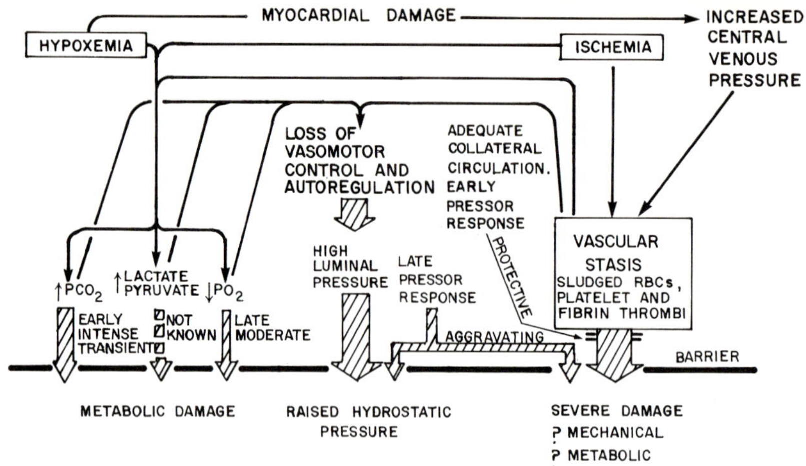

Fig. 12-17. Summary of the possible factors in the pathogenesis of cerebral edema associated with hypoxemia and ischemia. The width of the cross-hatched arrows piercing the barrier indicates the relative importance of these factors according to current knowledge. Note the preventive effect (preventing or reducing stasis) of adequate collateral circulation, or an early pressor response, or both.

unknown. The drug 2, 4-dinitrophenol, which also uncouples oxidative phosphorylation, is capable of producing cerebral edema alone, or enhancing the edema produced by vascular occlusion.

Effects of Embolism

A role for mechanical endothelial damage in the production of edema is suggested by the effects of embolism. Whereas occlusion of vessels for periods up to 12 hours fails to induce protein leakage, solid emboli will do so in 5 to 8 hours. Multiple micro-emboli, as in fat or air embolism, cause almost immediate protein exudation and perivascular hemorrhage. It is probable that sludging in occluded vessels has a similar deleterious effect, especially as it is known to be associated with a patchy failure of restoration of circulation after occlusion has been released (the no-reflow phenomenon).

Effects of Increased Intravascular Pressure

The effects of an adequate immediate pressor response in minimizing edema *during* occlusion are in sharp contrast to the effects of a similar response *after* occlusion is released. In the latter case, cerebral edema develops more rapidly and more extensively, presumably largely due to increased intraluminal pressure in the absence of normal autoregulation.

Distribution of Extravasated Protein

Even where severe barrier damage permits extravasation of protein tracers, their distribution varies with the degree of damage. They may be confined to the region of the basement membrane or may accumulate as perivascular globules, which are probably located in pericytes. Alternatively, they may appear to be concentrated in neurons (presumably, severely damaged by ischemia) in the vicinity of vessels or, more rarely, to be taken up by cells that seem to be astrocytes. Presumably, in all such cases, the protein leakage is minimal and either confined to the immediate vicinity of the vessel or, entering the extracellular space, is promptly taken up by damaged cells. A more characteristic pattern of protein extravasation is a reticular infiltration of the neuropil outlining unstained cellular elements. This presumably corresponds to the massive spread throughout the extracellular spaces seen electron-microscopically.

Conclusions

In summary (Fig. 12-17), current evidence suggests that hypoxemia itself has relatively little effect on barrier permeability unless it is so prolonged and severe that it probably is associated with increased CVP due to myocardial damage (see Chap. 13). Hypercapnia, and possibly other acid metabolites, causes a transient increase in permeability. The major factor in barrier damage and edema in hypoxemia or ischemia is probably vascular stasis, associated with precipitation of fibrin, platelet, or erythrocyte thrombi that cause mechanical damage to the vessel wall. Stasis is aggravated by hypoxemic myocardial damage, poor pressor response, inadequate collateral circulation and vascular occlusion, among other conditions.

CEREBRAL EDEMA IN HEAD INJURY

Swelling of the brain after head injury, even in the absence of significant focal lesions, is a common and serious occurrence for which there appear to be two causes: first, increased cerebral blood volume; second, the development of cerebral edema. *Increased*

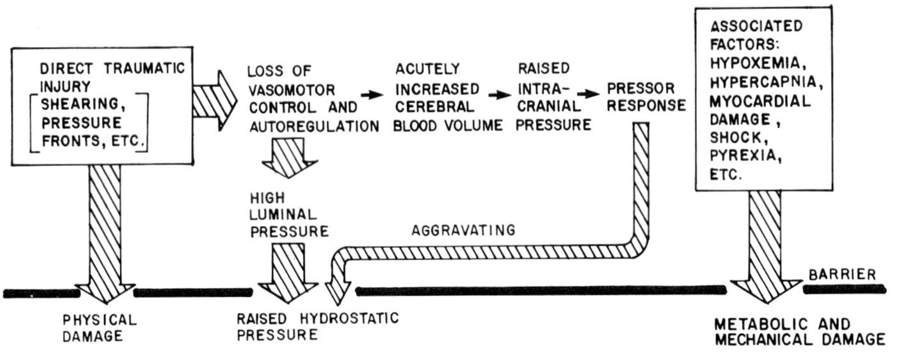

Fig. 12-18. Summary of the possible factors in the pathogenesis of cerebral edema in head injury. The width of the cross-hatched arrows piercing the barrier indicates the relative importance of these factors according to current knowledge. (For metabolic and mechanical damage, see Figure 12-17.) Note the significance of associated factors ("second injury") see Chap. 16).

cerebral blood volume virtually always occurs in head injury because of loss of autoregulation (see Chap. 16). However, the amount of swelling inducible by increased blood volume is limited by the ability of vessels to dilate. *Cerebral edema,* on the other hand, is a frequent but not invariable result of head injury. Once initiated, it often progresses to cause a fatal increase in intracranial tension. The mechanisms leading to cerebral edema in patients with head injuries are therefore of considerable importance (Fig. 12-18).

Direct exposure, handling, or even very minor injury of the brain and its superficial vessels, such as occurs during neurosurgical procedures, may be adequate to induce cerebral edema. In the experimental work on vascular occlusion previously discussed, extravasation of dye (after release of occlusion) occasionally occurred in the area of cortex that had been exposed and perhaps handled at operation. Apparently, manipulation of the brain and cerebral vessels, however gentle, alters barrier permeability. Similar effects might confidently be expected in diffuse head injury, in which there is often contusion and shearing of the brain internally as well as in relation to the skull. Since head injury is also accompanied by loss of autoregulation and consequently by increased pressure in diffusion vessels, mechanical barrier damage and increased luminal pressure may summate in causing edema. The combination of increased cerebral blood volume and early edema raises intracranial pressure and initiates a systemic pressor response that further aggravates the increased luminal pressure, establishing a vicious cycle (see Chap. 13). The vessels seen to dilate in the direct mechanical response are venules and veins, whereas vasospasm is occasionally seen in small arteries.

Head injury is frequently complicated by general changes in homeostasis that the healthy brain can withstand but the injured cannot. Such apparently irrelevant factors may become synergistic and serious. They include respiratory difficulty associated with acidosis and increased P_{CO_2} (which, as already noted, leads to a transient increase in barrier permeability). If acidosis is prolonged, the high permeability may become irreversible. Anemia due to hemorrhage is also dangerous, since it not only reduces the oxygen-carrying capacity of the blood but also reduces plasma osmolality and increases fluid loss into the brain, since plasma volume is initially made up by retention of salt and water and withdrawal of low-protein extracellular fluid from other tissues. Many injured patients are in shock, with reduced skin circulation and often with increased muscle tonus; high body temperature thereby increases the metabolic demands of the brain. Clearly, in addition to appropriate treatment of the CNS injury (see Chap. 16), an important part of treatment of the patient with a head injury is supportive, with correction of hyperpyrexia, acidosis, anemia, hypo-osmolality, and respiratory difficulty ("second injury").

EDEMA IN SYSTEMIC HYPERTENSION

The relation between increased blood pressure and cerebral edema is intricate. Not only may hypertension lead directly to cerebral edema, but also, by increasing intracranial pressure and raising cerebral vascular resistance, edema may in turn lead to hypertension. It is thus easy for a vicious cycle of deterioration to occur, leading finally to the complete cessation of cerebral circulation. This is the cause of "respirator brain" (necrobiosis of the brain), frequently seen in head-injured patients maintained over a considerable period by artificial respiration and other intensive care measures. Such patients have circulating blood that is entirely normal in respect to osmolality, acid-base and electrolyte balance, and oxygenation, but which does not reach the brain at all, because the cerebral circulation is cut off by raised intracranial pressure.

The experimental effects of the systemic pressor response occurring during occlusion of cerebral vessels (beneficial) or following removal of the occlusion (disastrous) have been already noted. Irrespective of primary CNS disease, acute rises in systolic blood pressure may occur clinically, as in malignant hypertension, eclampsia, and pheochromocytoma. This situation has been studied experimentally by inducing acute hypertensive crises with adrenergic drugs. If the (abrupt) increase in systolic pressure is less than 80 mm Hg, no changes are usually seen in the CNS. However, if it exceeds 90 mm Hg, changes almost invariably occur; dye tracers indicate focal barrier damage occurring mainly in the cortex. Moderate protein extravasation occurs from vessels, the protein either being taken up by cells in the vicinity or remaining near the basement membrane and vascular pericytes, indicating a moderate degree of barrier damage, but considerable local damage to cells. Only occasionally do such acute episodes of hypertension produce spreading cerebral edema in the underlying white matter, characterized by protein-containing fluid in the extracellular space and presumably indicating a greater degree of barrier damage.

These sudden episodes of hypertension are usually associated with increased cerebral vascular resistance and decreased blood flow (as compared with the situation in which autoregulation has been abolished). The increased resistance is probably due to focal constrictions of small arteries and arterioles that presumably lead to local ischemia and mechanical damage to the endothelium. It appears likely that the mechanical trauma is the cause of increased permeability and perivascular hemorrhages. Induction of chronic hypertension in experimental animals also causes focal extravasation of protein and tracers in the cortex, and constrictions of small pial arteries have been observed under direct vision.

One of the complications of chronic hypertension in man — albeit not very common — is diffuse demyelination and gliosis involving the white matter of both cerebral hemispheres and resembling the changes seen in chronic edema. Determinations of white matter water content in the hemispheres of hypertensive patients, even in the absence of demyelination or gliosis, have generally shown it to be increased by 3 to 5%. It appears that persistently raised systolic blood pressure may cause not only acute exacerbations with focal hemorrhage and edema in the cortex, similar to that seen with acutely induced hypertension, but also long-term increase in the water content of hemispheric white matter, ultimately leading to diffuse gliosis and demyelination in a few patients.

EDEMA IN OTHER CLINICAL SITUATIONS

Focal Brain Lesions

Almost all types of focal brain lesions, including neoplasms, abscesses, infarcts, and hemorrhages, are associated with edema in the surrounding white matter, usually confined to one hemisphere and failing to cross the corpus callosum. Cerebral edema is particularly severe in association with highly anaplastic astrocytomas, hemorrhages, acute abscesses, or cerebritis, but less so around well-differentiated or metastatic tumors or in association with chronic cerebral abscesses. In all cases, it appears to be due to an increase in barrier permeability to such a degree that there is extravasation of protein and protein-bound dyes, and electron microscopy shows an increase in the extracellular space of white matter, swelling of astrocytic processes, and concomitant alterations in cell organelles. This is a typical example of the "vasogenic" type of edema, similar to that induced by experimental lesions such as cortical freezing or implantation of polysaccharides or tumor. Its pathogenesis is uncertain, but perhaps includes stretching, distortion, spasm, or other mechanical damage to vessels.

Cerebral Edema Following Hypothermia

While body temperature is low, the integrity of the barrier system appears to be normal. However, an occasional complication of rewarming is the rapid development of cerebral edema, usually generalized, presumably because of interference with barrier function. Relatively few investigations have been made into the electron-microscopic or biochemical characteristics of posthypothermic edema. One study on animals killed 3 to 4 hours after rewarming showed an increased brain content of water and Na^+, a moderate reduction in K^+, and some increase in Ca^{++} and Mg^{++}, with a reduced Ca^{++} to Mg^{++} ratio. It is not known whether this type of edema is associated with enlargement of the extracellular space or extravasation of protein, though presumably Na^+ and K^+ turnover across the barrier are increased.

Radiation

Radiation produces a relatively early increase in barrier permeability, associated with extravasation of protein and protein-attached tracers and, presumably, with enlargement of the extracellular space. This type of edema would appear to be similar to that found in association with focal lesions and may be severe and even lethal.

Osmolar Edema

As has already been noted under disorders of homeostasis, edema of the brain may be associated with a reduction in plasma osmolality or with relative increases in brain osmolality during acute treatment of uremia or diabetic coma. These types of edema are not associated with extravasation of protein or enlargement of the extracellular space. They involve changes in *active* Na^+ and K^+ turnover, but the barrier function is normal. Subsequent changes are homeostatic, tending to restore normal intracranial volume.

Edema Associated with Toxins

Only a few cases have been reported of cerebral edema in man associated with the deliberate or acci-

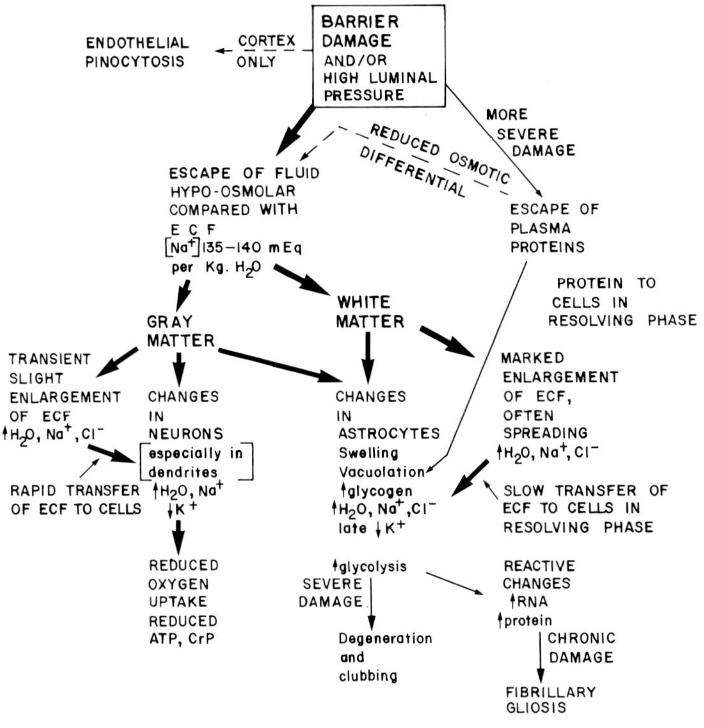

Fig. 12-19. Summary of the pathogenetic mechanisms in cerebral edema. This diagram may be regarded a sequel to the mechanisms shown in Figures 12-17 and 12-18. ATP = adenosine triphosphate; CrP = creatine phosphate.

dental administration of toxic agents. Experimentally, various substances impair the efficiency of the barrier system. One of these, tetraethyl tin (TET), requires mention since it has been the subject of a considerable body of literature on experimental cerebral edema. Administered to rats, TET causes progressive neurological dysfunction, which is reversible if drug administration is discontinued. The morphological changes in the CNS approximately parallel clinical neurological dysfunction in severity, and there is a considerable increase in cerebral water and electrolyte content. As in other types of edema, the absolute content (relative to total dry weight) of Na^+ is increased, the content of K^+ is decreased, and the Na^+ to K^+ ratio rises, indicating exchange of cation within the cells. There is no extravasation of plasma protein, and the edema fluid resembles plasma ultrafiltrate, indicating only minor impairment of the barrier system. Exchange of radioisotopes of Na^+, K^+, and PO_4^{---} is increased. The almost unique feature of TET edema is that, in addition to astrocytic swelling and vacuolation, there is marked accumulation of fluid within the myelin sheaths, where it appears to be accommodated by splitting along the intra-period lines (in what was originally extracellular space). Such splitting might indicate generalized plasmalemma toxicity and be an indication of generalized membrane toxicity in this example of cytotoxic edema.

Although investigations of this experimental model have been of considerable theoretical value, they do not appear directly applicable to any type of human edema so far recognized. Very minor splitting of the myelin sheaths may accompany so-called vasogenic edema and is sometimes seen in inborn errors of metabolism, including maple syrup urine disease, frequently to be followed by demyelination. However, the extent of the myelin splitting in these conditions is in no way comparable to that induced by TET.

SUMMARY OF PATHOGENETIC MECHANISMS IN CEREBRAL EDEMA

Clearly, cerebral edema is a reaction pattern of the CNS and is not a disease per se. However, it is a dangerous complication of the most common types of brain lesion, including infarction, other focal lesions, and head injury. By causing progressively increased intracranial tension, it may initiate clinical deterioration that can only occasionally be successfully reversed (see Chap. 13).

The immediate mechanism of most clinically significant cerebral edema (Fig. 12-19) is damage to the blood-brain barrier (and possibly to the blood-CSF barrier), permitting increased passage of water and electrolytes, mainly Na^+ and Cl^-. Mechanisms of such damage are discussed earlier in this chapter. This is frequently accompanied by sufficient damage to brain cells to cause loss of intracellular K^+, which is presumably exchanged for extracellular Na^+. If damage to the barrier system is more severe, exudation of fluid is greater, and it includes plasma protein, especially albumin and alpha globulin, which accumulates in the extracellular space almost entirely of the white matter. This may be because the normal space is larger in white matter and also because elements of gray matter are held together by junctions, especially synapses, that are difficult to disrupt. Differentiation between vasogenic edema (characterized by extravasation of protein and enlargement of extracellular space), and cytotoxic edema, which lacks these features, may be only partially valid, since the difference may be one of severity of barrier damage, with perhaps an additional element of more generalized plasma-membrane injury in the cytotoxic form. Probably the only type of cerebral edema that can occur in the presence of an entirely intact barrier system is that in which there is an increase in brain osmolality relative to the plasma, as in some homeostatic disorders (see Chap. 11).

The essential cell reacting to cerebral edema is the astrocyte, which in the early stages shows swelling, sometimes fragmentation of processes, dilatation of endoplasmic reticulum, and swelling of mitochondria. Within one to three days the astrocyte passes from the stage of acute swelling to a reactive phase, accompanied by glial fiber formation and increases in RNA and protein synthesis. Edematous tissue shows decreased oxygen utilization yet a general increase in enzyme activity and lactate formation, presumably reflecting the superior ability of the astrocyte, among CNS cells, to survive by anaerobic glycolysis.

BIBLIOGRAPHY

Adachi, M., and Feigin, I. Cerebral edema and the water content of normal white matter. *J. Neurol. Neurosurg. Psychiatry* 29:446-450, 1966.

Adachi, M., Rosenblum, W. L., and Feigin, I. Hypertensive disease and cerebral edema. *J. Neurol. Neurosurg. Psychiatry* 29:451-455, 1966.

Bakay, L. The Movement of Electrolytes and Albumin in Different Types of Cerebral Edema. In E. D. P. de Robertis and R. Carrea (Eds.), *Progress in Brain Research.* Amsterdam: Elsevier, 1965. Vol. 15 *(Biology of Neuroglia)*, pp. 155-183.

Brightman, M. W., Klatzo, I., Olsson, Y., and Reese, T. S. The blood-brain barrier to proteins under normal and pathological conditions. *J. Neurol. Sci.* 10:215-239, 1970.

Bryar, G. E., Goldstein, N. P., Svien, H. J., Sayre, G. P., and Jones, J. D. Experimental cerebral edema: Vital staining with Evans blue during the developmental and regressive phases. *J. Neurosurg.* 30:391-398, 1969.

Davson, H. *Physiology of the Cerebrospinal Fluid.* London: Churchill, 1970.

Feigin, I. Intracranial Tension and Cerebral Edema. In J. Minckler (Ed.), *Pathology of the Nervous System.* New York: McGraw-Hill, 1968. Vol. 1, pp. 424-433.

Feigin, I., Budzilowich, G., Weinberg, S., and Ogata, J. Degeneration of white matter in hypoxia, acidosis and edema. *J. Neuropathol. Exp. Neurol.* 32:125-143, 1973.

Fujita, S., Ueda, T., and Yagi, M. Detection of experimental and clinical brain edema, using an electrical impedance method. *J. Neurosurg.* 37:156-163, 1972.

Gardner, W. J. The plasma protein barriers. *J. Neurol. Sci.* 15:1-12, 1972.

Hirano, A. The Fine Structure of the Brain in Edema. In G. H. Bourne (Ed.), *The Structure and Function of Nervous Tissue.* New York: Academic, 1968. Vol. 2, pp. 69-135.

Katzman, R., and Pappius, H. M. *Brain Electrolytes and Fluid Metabolism.* Baltimore: Williams & Wilkins, 1973.

Klatzo, I. Neuropathologic aspects of brain edema. *J. Neuropathol. Exp. Neurol.* 26:1-14, 1967.

Lee, J. C., and Bakay, L. Ultrastructural changes in the edematous central nervous system. II. Cold-induced edema. *Arch. Neurol.* 14:36-49, 1966.

Olsson, Y., Crowell, R. M., and Klatzo, I. The blood-brain barrier to protein tracers in focal cerebral ischemia and infarction caused by occlusion of the middle cerebral artery. *Acta Neuropathol.* 18:89-102, 1971.

Rasmussen, L. E., and Klatzo, I. Protein and enzyme changes in cold injury edema. *Acta Neuropathol.* 13:12-28, 1969.

Reulen, H. J., Medzihradsky, F., Enzenbach, R., Marguth, F., and Brendel, W. Electrolytes, energy and fluid metabolism in human cerebral edema. *Arch. Neurol.* 21:517-525, 1969.

Sato, Y., Yamaguchi, M., Mullan, S., Evans, J. P., and Ishii, S. Brain edema. A study of biochemical and structural alterations. *Arch. Neurol.* 21:413-424, 1969.

Scheinberg, L. C., Herzog, I., Taylor, J. M., and Katzman, R. Cerebral edema in brain tumors: Ultrastructural and biochemical studies. *Ann. N.Y. Acad. Sci.* 159:509-532, 1969.

Schutta, H. S., Karrell, N. F., and Langfitt, T. W. Brain swelling produced by injury and aggravated by arterial hypertension. *Brain* 91:281-294, 1968.

Siesjö, B. K., and Sørensen, S. C. (Eds.) *Ion Homeostasis of the Brain.* New York: Academic, 1971.

Terauma, T., Meyer, B., Sakamoto, K., Hashi, K., Marc, P., Sterman-Marinchesu, S., and Shinmary, S. Hemodynamic and metabolic concomitants of brain swelling and cerebral edema due to experimental cerebral infarction. *J. Neurosurg.* 36:728-744, 1972.

Disorders of Energy Supply: Hypoxemia, Hypoglycemia, and Ischemia

13

Although there are considerable regional variations in cerebral metabolism, including neurotransmitter synthesis, it is probable that energy-yielding reactions are qualitatively, but not quantitatively, similar in all areas. Certain regions, such as the brain stem, can maintain function for a little longer in the absence of oxygen than others, such as the cortex. Like most organs, the brain has to obtain its supply of oxygen and substrate from the blood, to which it returns catabolic products.

NORMAL OXYGEN AND GLUCOSE SUPPLIES

Role of the Blood-Brain Barrier

So far as is known, oxygen and carbon dioxide are freely diffusible, requiring no energy for transport. Except for water, this seems to be applicable to only a few trace metabolites, possibly including the 2-C and 3-C intermediaries of glucose metabolism. Lactate and pyruvate, the intermediaries in highest plasma concentration, appear to cross freely in both directions, probably by diffusion, though active extrusion of lactate has been suggested. A source of energy significant for most other tissues, which can be used by them to spare glucose, is free fatty acid. It appears that free fatty acid is virtually excluded from the CNS by the blood-brain barrier (Fig. 13-1), leaving glucose and, to a minor extent, amino acids as the only potential substrates for energy-yielding metabolism when nutrition is normal.

Glucose Transfer

Glucose is transferred into the CNS across the blood-cerebrospinal fluid (CSF) barrier (and presumably the blood-brain barrier) by a facilitated transfer system that is completely saturated at plasma glucose concentration of 18 to 20 mg per 100 ml. This transfer is energy-dependent, probably unaffected by insulin, but requires liver factors, possibly cytidine or uridine. Glucose uptake is competitively inhibited by galactose and 3-methylglucose, but not by some other monosaccharides, suggesting several hexose carriers. Uptake apparently depends on the presence of aldose 1-epimerase, which produces a preferentially absorbed form (possibly the 3-aldehyde) and could be a rate-limiting factor in glucose metabolism. Thus, brain hexokinase could phosphorylate glucose 20 to 30 times as fast as it is absorbed, and cerebral metabolic pathways have a much greater capacity than is normally used. Increased cerebral activity or electric stimulation can increase glucose transfer by perhaps 8 to 10 times above the steady-state value. Barbiturates apparently also increase uptake as well as decrease utilization (increasing concentration of brain glucose). The brain appears unable to utilize glucose in the CSF, at least in experimental situations, at levels as high as 600 mg per 100 ml.

Amino Acid Transfer

While there is considerable exchange of amino acids across the blood-brain barrier, it is uncertain that there is significant *net* uptake except during active growth. The half-life of protein in the brain is 6 to 15 days, compared with 2 to 4 days for the liver and 10 to 24 days for muscle. Amino acid concentrations in CSF are negligible, except for glutamic acid and glutamine. There appear to be several carrier systems for amino acids, as in the renal tubules (see Chap. 20). It seems likely that there is net uptake only of glutamic acid, other amino acids either being synthesized in situ by transamination or acquired by exchange across the blood-brain barrier (as is the case for the essential amino acids). Little is known of the control either of facilitated transfer in or of active transfer out, but they probably correspond to the changing needs within the CNS.

Oxygen and Substrate (Glucose) Requirements

That the only substrate available to the brain is glucose is borne out by arteriovenous differences (Fig. 13-2). The difference for oxygen is 6.6 ml per 100 ml, and for carbon dioxide, 6.7 ml per 100 ml, giving a respiratory quotient of 1.0, indicating net metabolism of carbohydrate only. The difference for glucose is 10 mg per 100 ml, of which about 8.5 mg are required for observed normal carbon dioxide production, the remaining 1.5 mg corresponding to an observed arteriovenous difference of 1.2 mg per 100 ml for lactate. In all other respects, cerebral arterial and venous blood are closely similar. The loss of pyruvate is small, and absorption of amino

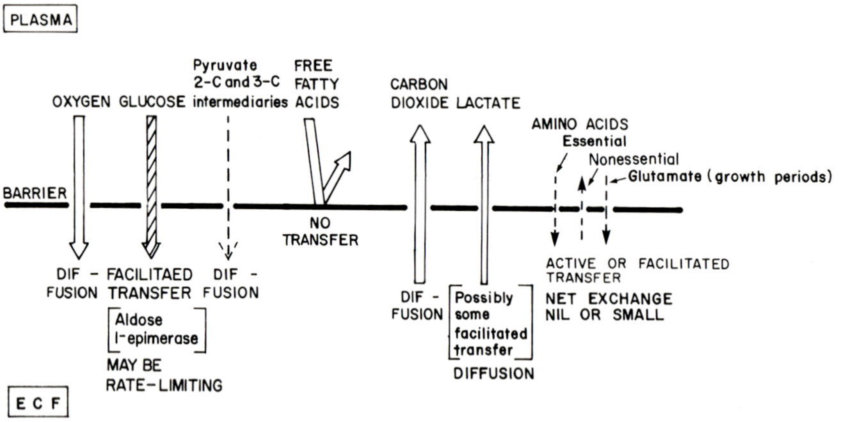

Fig. 13-1. Summary of passage of energy substrates across the blood-brain barrier.

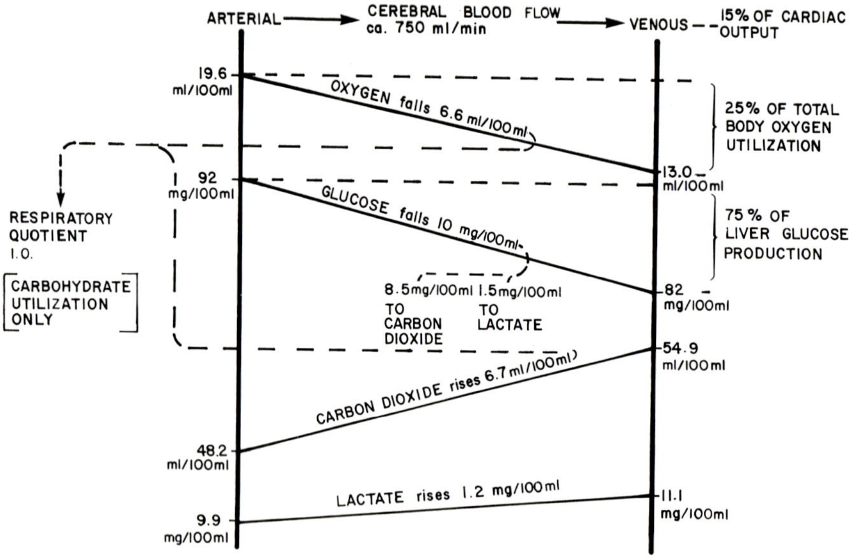

Fig. 13-2. Arteriovenous differences for the brain, indicating that glucose is virtually the only energy substrate, about 85% being converted to CO_2 and 15% to lactate.

acids falls within the limits of experimental error. Corresponding to the increased venous carbon dioxide and lactate is a reduction of the pH from 7.42 to 7.35 and a corresponding slight fall in bicarbonate.

The human brain, about 2.5% of body weight, receives 12.5 to 15.0% of the cardiac output and utilizes 25% of total oxygen consumption and about 75% of glucose liberated from the liver. This very high energy requirement is presumably needed for operation of the ionic pump to maintain neuronal membrane potentials, for facilitated and active transfer of metabolic substrates and products, and for synthesis of RNA, protein, and lipid – all of these being in a state of active turnover.

In spite of the large and continuous obligatory requirements for energy, the CNS is characterized by high dependency on the aerobic metabolism of glucose. Yet it shows a lack of oxygen stores and low reserves of glucose and glycogen; concentration of free glucose is negligible, and concentration of glycogen is only about 0.1% by weight. Glycogen is present in the cytoplasm of astrocytes and neurons and differs slightly from that in the liver by being more highly branched. It has been suggested that up to 85% is in bound form and not readily available, but cerebral glycogen stores can be readily and rapidly depleted. Assuming normal use of about 12 millimols (mM) per minute of adenosine triphosphate (ATP), the steady-state reserve is about 3 mM as ATP and 5 mM as creatine phosphate (CrP), allowing less than 1 minute of normal metabolism. In the absence

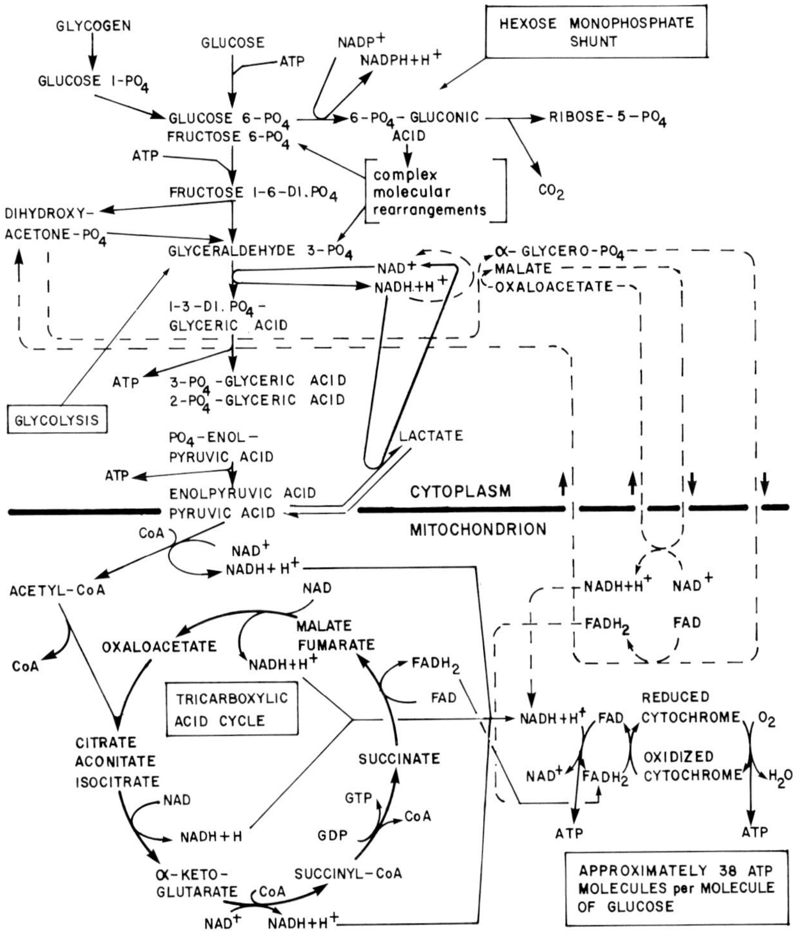

Fig. 13-3. Glucose metabolism in the CNS, showing glycolysis, the tricarboxylic acid cycle, and the hexose monophosphate shunt. Note the shuttle mechanisms (dashed lines) for oxidation of cytoplasmic NADH when little lactate is being formed (i.e., under normal conditions of adequate oxygenation).

of oxygen, the only available endogenous substrates are glucose and glycogen, estimated to yield a further 15 mM, giving a total supply of about 2 1/2 minutes.

METABOLIC PATHWAYS

Glucose Metabolism

The "energy currency" in the CNS, as elsewhere, is ATP, produced from glucose by metabolic processes essentially similar to those in other tissues (Fig. 13-3).

Glycolysis

Glycolysis (Embden-Meyerhof pathway) is an incomplete oxidation that breaks glucose down to pyruvate, with net production of two molecules of ATP and two of pyruvate per molecule of glucose. This pathway neither utilizes oxygen nor produces carbon dioxide, oxidation being by NAD^+, two molecules of which are reduced to $NADH + H^+$. Since the cytoplasmic concentration is extremely low, glycolysis rapidly depletes the supply. To enable the reaction to continue, reduced nicotinamide adenine dinucleatide (NADH) must be reoxidized. In the temporary absence of oxygen this is accomplished by conversion of pyruvate to lactate, the latter being then partially accumulated for future oxidation and partially disposed of to the circulation. Under normal circumstances only about 15% of pyruvate is converted to lactate, an insufficient proportion to oxidize cytoplasmic NADH. Since the nucleotide cannot cross the mitochondrial membrane, it is reoxidized by shuttle mechanisms, reacting either with oxaloacetic acid or with dihydroxyacetone phosphate, respectively producing malic acid or α-glycerophosphate, both of which can diffuse into the mitochondria to be oxidized by mitochondrial nucleotides. Malate reacts with NAD^+ and α-glycerophosphate with flavine adenine nucleotide (FAD). The oxaloacetate-malate shunt appears the most important in the CNS and involves active transport of malate, α-ketoglutarate, glutamic acid, and aspartic acid.

Tricarboxylic Acid Cycle

The tricarboxylic acid cycle (Krebs cycle) (Fig. 13-3) utilizes as substrate about 85% of the pyruvate produced by glycolysis; pyruvate is capable of diffusing into the mitochondria. Two molecules of pyruvate (one molecule of glucose) produce six molecules of carbon dioxide and water. About 50% of the energy of the glucose molecule is trapped as ATP. For each pair of pyruvate molecules entering the tricarboxylic acid cycle, there are formed a further eight molecules of (NADH), two of reduced flavine adenine dinucleotide ($FADH_2$), and two of guanosine triphosphate (GTP), which is equivalent in energy to ATP. NADH reacts with FAD, producing NAD^+ and $FADH_2$, the latter in turn being oxidized by components of the cytochrome system, which react with molecular oxygen to form water. During this process of electron transfer (oxidation), adenosine diphosphate (ADP) is converted to ATP (oxidative phosphorylation), three moles being produced per mole of NADH and two per mole of $FADH_2$. Counting the four net substrate phosphorylations, ten NADH and two $FADH_2$ from both glycolysis and the tricarboxylic acid cycle, a total of 38 molecules of ATP are produced per glucose molecule.

Neither the mechanism of oxidative phosphorylation, nor that by which ATP leaves the mitochondria, is understood. Under abnormal conditions the oxidative exchanges may be completed without production of ATP, so that oxidation and phosphorylation are uncoupled. The whole sequence of coupled oxidation and phosphorylation depends upon spatial configuration within the mitochondrion, and uncoupling may be associated with swelling or other morphological changes. A proportion of the tricarboxylic acid cycle in the CNS is diverted through the γ-aminobutyric acid (GABA) shunt, which is bioenergetically less advantageous (see p. 239).

Hexose Monophosphate Shunt

As in other tissues, a small proportion of glucose (about 1%) passes via the hexose monophosphate shunt (pentose pathway) (Fig. 13-3). This is a complicated series of reactions in which one of six participating molecules of glucose is broken down to carbon dioxide, the others forming intermediary products, most of which rejoin the glycolytic pathway. Apart from ribose, the important product of this reaction is nicotinamide-adenine dinucleotide phosphate (NADPH), necessary for lipid and other syntheses. No oxygen is used. It is presumably essential that no more NADPH is formed than is necessary, since the only method of direct reoxidation involves reaction with NAD^+ and use of a molecule of ATP.

Other Considerations

It is apparent that the catabolism of glucose in the adult CNS is similar to that in other tissues; in addition, a little is used for the synthesis of glycogen. Glycolysis cannot be reversed in the CNS, since some of the necessary enzymes (glucose 6-phosphatase and fructose 1, 6-diphosphatase) are absent. As noted, glucose catabolic pathways are working considerably below their maximum capacity, partly due to limitation of the rate of glucose uptake and partly to inhibitory controls (see p. 240). The reserve of the glycolytic pathway is greater than that of the tricarboxylic acid cycle, so that under conditions of extremely high demand, an increased proportion of pyruvate must converted to lactate. The steady-state proportion of lactate drops abruptly from fetal levels at or about the time of birth, in association with an altered isoenzyme pattern for lactate dehydrogenase (LDH) (the H form increasing from 10 to 40%), which favors conversion to pyruvate.

Distribution of Oxidative Enzymes

The CNS distribution of oxidative enzymes shows a regular pattern from species to species. White matter activity is mainly in the oligodendroglia, with enzymes of the glycolytic and hexose monophosphate pathways prominent. If it were confirmed that oxidative activity of axons is inversely related to numbers of oligodendroglial cells, a possible symbiosis between glia and axons would be implied. Resting astrocytes show variable activity, but reactive forms, including those present in edema, demonstrate a considerable increase in activity. Neurons show considerable levels of enzymes of the tricarboxylic acid cycle, but less of glycolytic or shunt enzymes. Nuclei do not show oxidative activity. The enzyme distribution between gray and white matter and between neurons and glial cells is broadly correlated with the sensitivity of such areas and cells to hypoxemia.

Tricarboxylic and Amino Acids in the Central Nervous System

Interconversion of Tricarboxylic and Amino Acids

Although the ultimate source of energy in the CNS is exogenous glucose, there is considerable and rapid exchange between acid cycle intermediates (α-keto acids) and the mitochondrial pool of alpha amino acids. A major mechanism is transamination, such as the reversible formation of alanine from pyruvate, glutamic acid from α-ketoglutarate, and aspartic acid from oxaloacetate. Glutamic acid takes part in further reactions, including the formation of glutamine and GABA. This rapid shunting of glucose metabolites through lateral pathways explains why, following administration of ^{14}C-labeled glucose (Fig. 13-4), only about 30% of the labeled carbon is immediately recoverable as $^{14}CO_2$, the rest being converted to $^{14}CO_2$ over a period of many hours. In tissue slices, administration of labeled glucose results (after one hour) in 60 to 70% of the activity being present as lactate, 20% as carbon dioxide, about 9% as glutamate, glutamine, or GABA, 2% as aspartate, and 1% as alanine. Although the level for lactate in vitro is high because of the experimental conditions

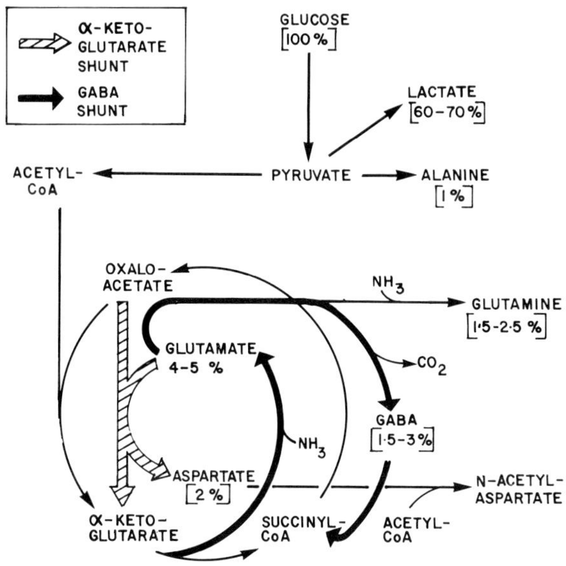

Fig. 13-4. The distribution of ^{14}C in tissue brain slices one hour after the addition of ^{14}C-glucose. The high percentage appearing as lactate is an artifact of the technique used, since glycolytic inhibition appears not to be operating. About 20% of the isotope was recovered as ^{14}C-CO_2 from various reactions.

and lack of glycolytic inhibition, such results illustrate the rapid incorporation of ^{14}C from glucose into the amino acid pool.

Roles of Aspartic and Glutamic Acids

Two amino acids are present in the CNS in uniquely high concentrations, namely, glutamic and N-acetylaspartic acids, both related to tricarboxylic acid cycle intermediates (α-ketoglutaric and oxaloacetic acids).

The formation of N-acetylaspartic acid is by transamination of glutamic and oxaloacetic acids (α-ketoglutarate also being formed), followed by acetylation by acetylcoenzyme A (acetyl-CoA). Its function is not certain, but it may be a "fixed" intracellular anion or a reserve source of acetate for entry into the citric acid cycle in times of pyruvate deficiency.

Glutamic acid may be of dietary origin or formed by transamination reactions from other alpha amino acids (though far more often it is the donor, not the recipient, of the alpha amino group). Some is formed by reaction of NH_4^+ with α-ketoglutaric acid, supplies of which are depleted. This depletion is enhanced if equilibrium is disturbed by the further reaction of glutamic acid with NH_4^+ to form glutamine.

If glutamic acid from the cellular pool forms GABA, which then reacts with α-ketoglutaric acid to form glutamic acid and succinic semialdehyde, only one molecule of α-ketoglutarate is lost. If the glutamic acid itself is formed from α-ketoglutarate, two molecules are lost (for each molecule of GABA formed). The ultimate formation of succinic acid makes the formation and breakdown of GABA an alternative to part of the tricarboxylic acid cycle *(the GABA shunt).* A suggestion that it may replace much of the main cycle is not presently confirmed; it is more generally accepted that 10% of succinate is formed via GABA shunt.

It has been suggested that one role of glutamate may be as an energy source in the temporary absence of pyruvate, since the reaction in which aspartate is formed from glutamate also generates α-ketoglutarate from oxaloacetate, enabling a part of the tricarboxylic acid cycle to proceed *(the α-ketoglutarate shunt).*

It is apparent that some metabolic processes (Fig. 13-4), including aspartate formation, synthesis and breakdown of GABA, and NH_4^+ fixation, involve permanent loss of cycle intermediates (oxaloacetate and α-ketoglutarate). Fortunately, the supply can be replenished by fixation of carbon dioxide onto pyruvic or phosphoenolpyruvic acids, with the formation of malate or oxaloacetate. Thus, the administration of $^{14}CO_2$ or NaH$^{14}CO_3$ results in rapid labeling of malate, oxaloacetate, α-ketoglutarate, aspartate, glutamate, and glutamine.

Energy Balance

Determination of concentrations of intermediate or high-energy compounds is technically difficult, as from the moment circulation ceases, the concentrations of ATP and creatine phosphate (CrP) drop 50 to 90% in 30 seconds, and lactate values rise two to three times. The best results have been obtained in very small experimental animals (rats and mice), which can be almost instantly frozen in liquid nitrogen. Fortunately, interspecies variation in metabolic processes of such phylogenetic constancy may be assumed minimal, and the results are likely to be applicable to man. Such determinations are of great importance, since they must be central to the speed with which irreversible brain damage occurs in complete or partial hypoxia, hypoglycemia, or ischemia, and these conditions represent the primary disease agent, or a frequent and often overwhelming secondary complication, in the majority of common neurological diseases (e.g., cerebrovascular disease, intracranial hemorrhage, head injury, cerebral edema of whatever cause).

Cerebral utilization of oxygen is not by itself a reliable indicator of brain energy balance, since it may merely reflect altered requirements (increased in fever, decreased in anesthesia or hypothermia), with no implication that reserves of ATP are altered. It is even possible, where mitochondria are damaged, that oxidation and phosphorylation might be uncoupled, since increased oxygen utilization may be accompanied by reduced ATP formation. Increases in the concentration of lactate, inorganic phosphate (Pi), and AMP, or in the ratios of NADH to NAD^+ and lactate to pyruvate, or decreases in CrP, appear to be early indicators of reduced intracellular PO_2, followed a little later by reduced ATP and increased ADP. None of these can be measured clinically, since changes in plasma or even in CSF lactate and pyruvate do not necessarily reflect those in the cells. Attempts to estimate NADH by fluorescence in the exposed cortex, if technically and theoretically refined, might be applicable in restricted circumstances.

On a purely theoretical basis, but applicable at least to small animal studies, it has been suggested that energy balance may be expressed as an *energy charge potential* (ECP) in terms of the adenosine nucleotides, such that

$$ECP = \frac{ATP + 0.5ADP}{ATP + ADP + AMP}$$

(ADP = adenosine diphosphate). Since the AMP value is usually very low, any rise may be a sensitive index of energy deficiency. Even this index is liable to error, since in ischemia, AMP may be deaminated to inosine monophosphate (IMP), thus reducing ATP + ADP + AMP and allowing a normal ECP, with reduced ATP. Although a fall in intracellular pH appears to have little *direct* effect on ECP, it does alter some other indices of energy balance. Activities of LDH and creatine phosphokinase are so altered that the lactate to pyruvate ratio rises from 15 to 50, and the concentration of CrP falls by 50%, at a time when ATP, ADP, and AMP levels are normal.

Control of Energy-Yielding Pathways

Neither glycolysis nor the tricarboxylic acid cycle normally proceeds at peak capacity in the brain, apparently largely due to feedback control exerted on critical enzymes when PO_2 is adequate and in part due to limited glucose uptake. Major controls appear to depend on the ratio of ATP to ADP $\times$ Pi, ATP being inhibiting and ADP and Pi being activators. This ratio affects glycolysis directly and the tricarboxylic acid cycle both directly and indirectly (high ATP levels reduce oxidative phosphorylation).

The major control points in the glycolytic pathway (see Fig. 13-3) appear to be the following:

1. *Phosphofructokinase* catalyzes the formation of fructose 1,6-diphosphate from fructose 6-phosphate, is inhibited by its product, and by ATP, CrP, and citrate. The latter serves to correlate the glycolytic and tricarboxylic acid paths. The enzyme is deinhibited by Pi, NH_4^+, ADP, and both 5′ and 3′:5′ AMP. It is inhibited by a fall in pH and deinhibited by a rise in pH, presumably a homeostatic mechanism for intracellular pH.
2. *Hexokinase* catalyzes the formation of glucose 6-phosphate from glucose, is normally restricted by supply of glucose, and is also subject to feedback inhibition from glucose 6-phosphate. It is inhibited by ATP and deinhibited by ADP and Pi.
3. *Pyruvate decarboxylase,* involved in the conversion of pyruvate to acetyl-CoA, is inhibited by the latter (direct feedback inhibition).

Control of the tricarboxylic acid cycle also seems to depend on the concentrations of ATP and citrate (acting as inhibitors) and of Pi, ADP, and AMP (acting as deinhibitors). Control may be largely through the supply of pyruvate, but there seem to be direct effects on two enzymes: isocitric dehydrogenase and succinic dehydrogenase. Synthesis of glycogen is increased by ATP and glucose 6-phosphate, whereas breakdown is accelerated by ADP, AMP, and Pi.

ABNORMAL OXYGEN OR GLUCOSE SUPPLIES

Oxygen deficiency in the CNS may occur with an adequate cerebral blood flow (hypoxemia) or with a reduced blood flow (ischemia). In either case, tissue PO_2 is low (hypoxidosis), though other factors differ. *In pure hypoxemia* with adequate blood flow, there is a normal supply of glucose, and carbon dioxide and lactate are removed. *In pure ischemia* there is a deficient supply of both oxygen and glucose and an accumulation of acid metabolites.

Severe hypoxemia, however, commonly leads to patchy local tissue ischemia, apparently because vasodilatation slows the blood flow, leading to sludging of erythrocytes and other formed elements in the blood. Since considerably more vasodilatation can be induced by high blood carbon dioxide levels without development of local ischemia and therefore presumably without sludging, some additional factor is presumably involved. This is probably the effect of hypoxemia on the myocardium, with a fall in cardiac output and an increase in central venous pressure.

Thus, *clinically significant hypoxemia in man is not clearly separable from ischemia,* and much of the irreversible CNS damage formerly attributed to lack of oxygen may really be due to concomitant myocardial damage. Jugular venous oxygen is a mixed effluent from gray and white matter, and while a venous PO_2 of 35 mm Hg appears high in comparison to that of the myocardium, it can be calculated that the venous blood from gray matter has a PO_2 of only about 17 mm Hg (compared with 50 mm Hg for white matter). Thus the levels for gray matter and the myocardium closely correspond. Either tissue has a limited ability to extract further oxygen and hence approximately equal sensitivity to an oxygen deficit.

Hypoxemia and Anoxemia

Hypoxemia or anoxemia may result from a lowered partial pressure of oxygen in inspired air (decompression, improper anesthesia, altitude, experimental situations); inadequate respiratory exchange (brain stem damage, respiratory muscle paralysis, airway obstruction, cardiopulmonary disease such as diffusion defects or perfusion without ventilation); or a decrease in available hemoglobin (carbon monoxide poisoning, anemia). If accompanied by hyperventilation, hypoxemia is complicated by respiratory alkalosis, decreased cerebral blood flow, and a shift of the oxygen dissociation curve to the left, with impeded release of oxygen to the tissues. If accompanied by anemia, the reduced blood viscosity increases cerebral blood flow. As noted, the hypoxic susceptibility of the myocardium is about equal to that of the CNS, so that the changes in severe hypoxemia may be in part due to circulatory impairment. As will be seen later (Chaps. 15 and 16), normal vascular mechanisms for compensating cerebral blood flow may be lost in conditions also associated with hypoxemia. Inadequate brain perfusion is then compounded.

Anoxemia

Total anoxemia is an experimental rather than a recoverable clinical situation. Neurogenic apnea and an isoelectric EEG appear in mice within 60 seconds, by which time NAD^+ is fully reduced to NADH. CrP is not fully depleted for 3 minutes, at which time ATP is still present in appreciable amounts (energy charge potential 0.56, control 0.91). Lactate continues to accumulate for about 4 minutes, after which it is presumed that glycolysis is inhibited by a fall in intracellular pH. Mortality after inhalation of nitrogen or asphyxia lasting 4 minutes is 50%, probably largely due to myocardial failure. If recovery occurs, normal ATP levels are achieved in 2 minutes, but CrP rises much later, and the abnormally high lactate to pyruvate ratio falls later still. These delays are probably the effects of acidosis on creatine phosphokinase and LDH.

Hypoxemia

Partial oxygen deficiency (hypoxemia) is a common clinical situation. Experimentally, down to an arterial PO_2 of 50 mm Hg (10% inspired oxygen) there is no change in cerebral blood flow, venous PO_2 or lactate, or oxygen utilization. As PO_2 falls from 50 to 30 mm Hg (10.0 to 6.5% inspired oxygen), there is a sequential increase in cerebral blood flow (of about 50%), a fall in venous PO_2 with a rise in lactate, followed by the onset of coma associated with a fall of oxygen utilization. At this point the venous PO_2 has reached its lowest possible level of 16 to 17 mm Hg. Biochemically, the increase in lactate is accompanied by reduced CrP levels, probably because acidosis inhibits creatine phosphokinase. Yet, in spite of coma, even after 30 minutes at an arterial PO_2 of 27 to 28 mm Hg, levels of ATP, ADP, and AMP are normal, and citrate is normal or slightly raised. The profound increase in glycolysis in the presence of normal levels of ATP and citrate and profound acidosis (lactate may be 8 to 10 mEq per kilogram H_2O) is unexplained, but a role for adenyl cyclase and cyclic AMP is possible.

Of particular interest are the effects of still lower values of arterial PO_2. At 15 mm Hg, about half the animals die of myocardial failure, but in the others there is a massive lactate increase (20 to 25 mEq per kilogram H_2O), but normal ATP, ADP, and AMP. At 10 mm Hg, with maintained perfusion, ATP, ADP, and AMP are still normal. Though these data are from small laboratory animals such as rats and mice, they probably also hold true in the human brain.

Such results reinforce the role of cerebral perfusion defects in causing irreversible brain damage and also indicate that coma and EEG changes are not due to lack of ATP (unless on a very localized scale, so far not detectable), but depend on some other unidentified mechanism. At a venous PO_2 of 16 mm Hg, it is calculated that the lowest tissue PO_2 is 4 mm Hg, whereas oxidative phosphorylation can occur at about 1 mm Hg. (The calculation for the lowest tissue value is based on a model of oxygen diffusing through cylinders of tissue around capillaries and may be oversimplified.)

Ischemia

Total brain ischemia as a potentially treatable entity is of course confined to regional involvement, as in occlusive vascular disease (see Chap. 14). *Partial ischemia* is a decrease in blood flow that is usually associated with a reduction in effective perfusion pressure — either a fall in blood pressure due to loss of blood, shock, or heart disease, or raised intracranial pressure from whatever cause. Ischemia is a complication of hypoxemia when the latter is severe enough to affect the myocardium adversely. Whereas in the presence of adequate blood pressure it may be assumed that oxygen deficit in hypoxemia is generally equal in all areas, it appears certain that in reduction of perfusion pressure, the delivery of blood is patchy, so ischemia of moderate severity is a localized phenomenon. The boundary-zone lesions associated with hypotension are the best known examples of this type of ischemia, but it may also prove to be the explanation for selective vulnerability in the CNS (see p. 247).

The biochemical changes of ischemia are qualitatively similar to those in hypoxemia, but are considerably more severe for a given level of arterial PO_2. There is earlier and more severe loss of ATP, and a reduction of total adenosine nucleotides due to partial deamination of AMP to IMP (associated with a rise in NH_4^+). Lactate accumulates to high levels and, together with the released carbon dioxide, may reduce intracellular pH to 6.0.

The maximum period of total ischemia compatible with recovery is widely variable in different areas: from 30 minutes or more in the brain stem down to 5 to 7 minutes in the hemispheres. The latter period corresponds to the time needed for development of "no-reflow" changes in small vessels, implying that even if normal perfusion pressure is restored, no blood will flow through such areas. The morphological changes of no reflow include particulate obstructions, varying from fibrin threads and platelet thrombi to aggregates of sludged erythrocytes, as well as changes in the vessels (swelling and increased pinocytosis in endothelial cells) and surrounding astrocytes (swelling of foot processes), which lead in effect to narrowing of the lumen. No reflow is reduced by measures such as preadministration of hypertonic solutions or inhalation of high carbon dioxide mixtures (either of which might be expected to increase vascular lumens) or by prerinsing vessels with saline or otherwise reducing blood content. Such measures also lengthen the period of total ischemia from which recovery is possible.

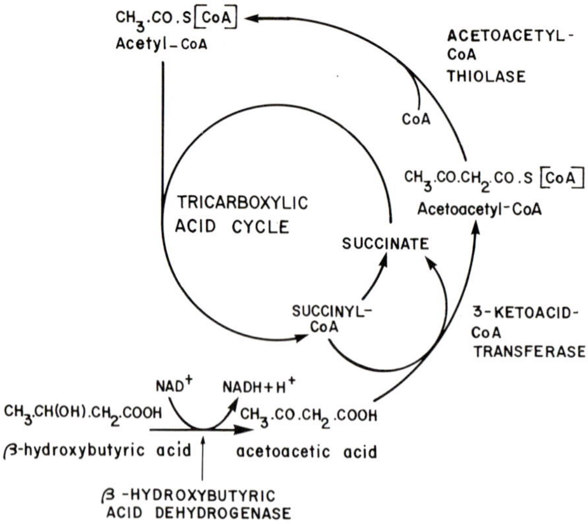

Fig. 13-5. The entry of ketone bodies into the tricarboxylic acid cycle.

A comparison of the changes seen in, and the results of, pure hypoxemia and ischemia make it increasingly doubtful whether reduction of tissue Po_2 per se is, in clinical situations, the major cause of irreversible brain damage. While certainly causing abrupt abrogation of function, it does not seem to be associated with complete loss of energy supplies at levels that the whole organism could otherwise survive. Rather, it would seem that local or general circulatory failure is the important change. The pathogenesis of the former (small-vessel changes) is unclear, though they are of the same nature as seen in vasogenic cerebral edema. "Pure" hypoxemia is not a prominent cause of edema (see Chap. 12).

Hypoglycemia

Hypoglycemia is usually due to hyperinsulinism — either exogenous, as in the treatment of diabetic coma or schizophrenia, or endogenous, as in insulinoma or functional hyperinsulinism (including the idiopathic spontaneous hypoglycemia of infants). Less often, hypoglycemia occurs in pituitary or adrenocortical failure, massive hepatic necrosis, or metabolic diseases such as glycogenosis, galactosemia, or maple syrup urine disease. Since glucose is the only exogenous substrate for normal brain metabolism, severe CNS symptomatology may occur in hypoglycemia.

With blood sugar levels down to 20 to 22 mg per 100 ml, oxygen utilization remains constant, with a small increase in cerebral blood flow and a rise in arteriovenous glucose difference. At 19 mg per 100 ml, oxygen utilization falls to 2.6 ml per 100 g per minute (normal 3.3), and glucose utilization to 2.3 mg per 100 g per minute (normal 4.4). With a progressive fall in blood glucose to 8 mg per 100 ml, oxygen utilization drops to 1.9, glucose utilization to 0.8, and EEG changes followed by coma occur. There is still only a slight increase in cerebral blood flow. This is in contrast to other tissues such as muscle, in which reduced glucose utilization is not accompanied by a fall in oxygen utilization, other substrates such as free fatty acids being used. The brain can utilize acetoacetic and β-hydroxybutyric acids (see below), but in acute hypoglycemia, blood levels of these substances are low. Coma may occur with blood glucose levels of 20 mg per 100 ml, and in such cases it has been suggested that part of the erythrocyte glucose is bound, and plasma levels are lower than the whole blood level would indicate.

In small-animal experiments, hypoglycemia causes depletion of CNS glucose, glycogen, pyruvate, glutamic acid, GABA, glutamine, and alanine, with increased aspartic acid. ATP and CrP are reduced, but less so than in hypoxemia. Depletion of glutamic acid and alanine could be due to conversion to α-ketoglutarate and pyruvate respectively; increased aspartic acid could be due to utilization of the N-acetyl group of N-acetylaspartic acid. Retention of considerable levels of ATP and CrP is presumably in part due to relatively normal intracellular pH, as there is no increased lactate formation. However, there may also be failure of utilization, the biochemical basis of which is unknown.

Experimentally, the brain survives for a limited time by catabolism of endogenous substrate if a glucose-free perfusate at up to three times normal flow rate is used. During this period, the EEG, reflexes, and response to metrazol are normal, and the respiratory quotient drops to values as low as 0.56. Free amino acids, especially glutamic acid, GABA, and glutathione, appear in the perfusate. Of greater clinical interest is the ability to utilize ketone bodies (β-hydroxybutyric and acetoacetic acids) in acute chronic starvation, even though blood glucose levels are not dramatically reduced. In tissue slices, these substances increase respiration even in the presence of adequate glucose. This adaptive charge is not accompanied by altered enzyme levels. The substances appear (Fig. 13-5) to be converted to acetoacetyl-CoA and then acetyl-CoA and so enter the tricarboxylic acid cycle.

Effects of pH on Glucose Metabolism

Changes in pH have a direct effect on glycolysis and the tricarboxylic acid cycle. Acidosis decreases glycolysis and increases glutamic acid utilization, with a net slight decrease in tricarboxylic acid cycle activity; oxygen utilization is slightly reduced, glucose utilization much more so. Alkalosis slightly increases glycolysis and tricarboxylic acid cycle activity, with corresponding slight elevations of oxygen and glucose utilization. These changes may be homeostatic with respect to intracellular pH, but are overridden in hypoxemia and ischemia, perhaps by cyclic AMP, a potent stimulant for glycolysis.

Effects of Hyperbaric Oxygen

Increased tissue Po_2, as in exposure to hyperbaric oxygen, may be toxic to all tissues, including the CNS. It appears to reduce succinic dehydrogenase activity and the oxidation of NADH by FAD, thereby reducing the supply of NAD^+ for the tricarboxylic acid cycle, and lowering ATP. Lysosomal enzymes, including ribonuclease and cathepsins, appear to be activated. Early experimental work on small animals has included attempts to improve survival by the use of energy substrates that are FAD-linked (succinate and α-glycerophosphate) and by administration of reducing agents such as cysteine. Moderately encouraging initial results have been obtained.

REGULATION OF CEREBRAL BLOOD FLOW

Total Blood Flow in Normal Brain

The simplest method for estimating overall cerebral blood flow involves inhalation of an inert nonmetabolizable gas that does not affect respiration, such as nitrous oxide or one of the inert gases. Gas is lost from the cerebral circulation to the CNS, causing an arteriovenous difference. The less the cerebral blood flow, the larger and more persistent will be the arteriovenous difference. It is possible to compute cerebral blood flow by four observations of arteriovenous difference, taken within 10 minutes of the beginning of inhalation. Regional flow rates are determined by inhalation of radioactive gases and direct counting over selected areas.

Under normal conditions the cerebral blood flow is about 55 ml per 100 g brain per minute, for a total of about 750 ml per minute. Of this, about 200 to 225 ml passes through the basilar artery. The remainder passes through the carotid arteries, frequently slightly more on the left than the right. With an arteriovenous oxygen difference of approximately 6 ml per 100 ml, this corresponds to the normal cerebral metabolic rate of 3.3 ml oxygen per 100 g per minute. When a subject is lying or sleeping, the cerebral blood flow rises to about 65 ml per 100 g per minute (presumably because of the increased mean arterial pressure at the carotid syphon), but the arteriovenous oxygen difference decreases and oxygen utilization is unchanged.

In young children, brain metabolism is much more active, with oxygen utilization of 5.1 ml per 100 g per minute and a cerebral blood flow of 100 ml per 100 g per minute or more. Beyond the age of 60, cerebral blood flow may remain at adult levels or may decline, with an increased arteriovenous oxygen difference, perhaps in proportion to cerebral atherosclerosis. Thus, in many elderly persons, oxygen utilization remains normal. In others it may fall, accompanying a decrease in cerebral blood flow, arteriovenous oxygen difference, or both. Although there is a tendency for the lowest levels of oxygen utilization to accompany impaired mentation, it is not possible to separate patients with senile dementia from normal persons on the basis of any of the preceding parameters.

Innervation of Cerebral Vessels

Major vessels and branches in the subarachnoid space are richly supplied with autonomic nerve fibers, apparently of three systems:

1. *Sympathetic (adrenergic) fibers* form a dense branching network between the adventitia and media, showing numerous nodular enlargements. These fibers are almost entirely derived from the superior cervical ganglia, and reach the posterior cerebral arteries along the posterior communicating, rather than the basilar, vessels. Nerve fibers do not enter brain parenchyma except in the region of septal nuclei and accompanying a few midline vessels penetrating the medulla.

2. *Parasympathetic (cholinergic) fibers* are of uncertain origin, but may leave the CNS through the third, seventh, ninth, or tenth cranial nerves. They supply preponderantly the carotid rather than the vertebral-basilar system. This network also is situated between the media and adventitia and appears to parallel the adrenergic system almost exactly, with penetration of the brain only in the same two regions.

3. The fibers of the *third system* are well myelinated and are principally seen on the anterior half of the circle of Willis and its major branches, apparently reaching these vessels from the third cranial nerve. They are probably sensory and are fewer in number than the autonomic motor fibers.

Normal Regional Blood Flow and Metabolic Rates

From subarachnoid vessels, perforating branches without autonomic innervation enter the underlying brain and form a dense capillary plexus, especially in the gray matter. The capillary bed in the cerebral cortex may occupy up to 3% of the volume. In general, capillarization is approximately proportional to neuronal density. The adult cortex is said to contain about 1.4 meters of capillaries per cubic millimeter, a figure that is considerably exceeded in skeletal muscle (6 meters) and myocardium (11 meters). Most of the cortical capillaries aggregate to form small venules that drain directly to the surface, so that there is a considerable segregation of gray and white matter flow.

The average flow rate of 0.55 ml per gram per minute is not uniformly distributed. Flow rates in white matter vary from 0.14 to 0.25 ml per gram per minute, with an average of 0.23. Flow rates in gray matter vary from 0.65 to 1.8 ml per gram per minute (in the superior colliculus), with the rate in the cortex in the range of 0.77 to 1.38. The reticular formation appears to have just about the average flow rate, at 0.59 ml per gram per minute. Much of the estimation of regional cerebral blood flow has been carried out on species other than man, but where it has been possible to check by the use of radioisotopes, the flow rates appear to be applicable to the human brain.

The partial segregation of gray and white matter flow has serious implications for the adequacy of cerebral blood supply. Superficially, the blood supply appears to be generous, since brain weight is only

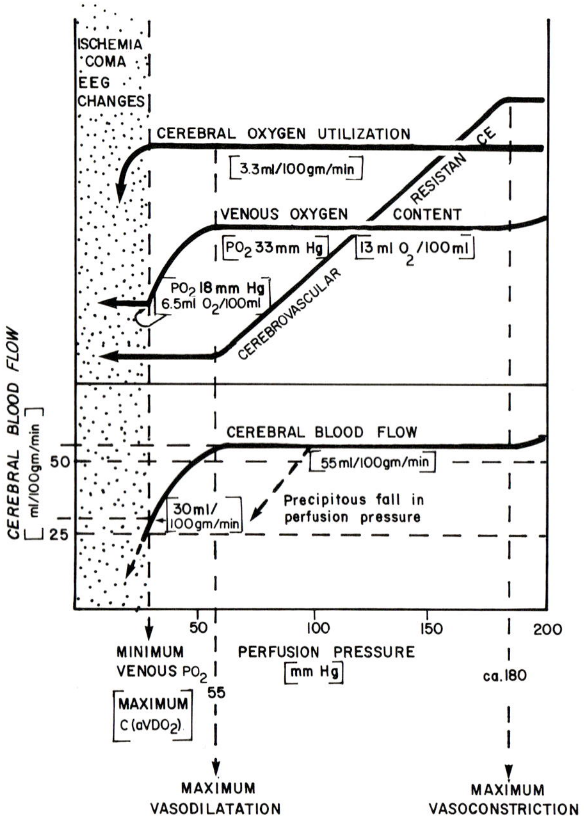

Fig. 13-6. The effect of altered perfusion pressure on total cerebral blood flow and other parameters. Note the parallel falls in blood flow and venous Po_2 (increased O_2 extraction) between perfusion pressures of about 50 and 30 mm Hg, with constant C(aVDO$_2$). Below this level, venous Po_2 cannot be decreased, oxygen utilization falls, and clinical symptoms develop. C(aVDO$_2$) = cerebral arteriovenous oxygen difference.

about 2.5% of total body weight, and the brain receives 12.5% of the cardiac output. However, a comparison of greater functional significance is the venous PO_2 for various organs. Mixed venous blood at the heart has a PO_2 of about 40 mm Hg, compared with a venous blood PO_2 of 62 for the kidney, 45 for the liver and gut, 35 for the brain and resting muscle, 18 for the myocardium, and 16 for exercised muscle (temporary only). The brain appears to have a greater oxygen reserve than the myocardium.

However, if allowance is made for the metabolic differences between gray and white matter (as reflected in blood supply and oxidative enzyme capacity) and for their relative bulk, it may be calculated that the PO_2 for gray-matter venous blood is 17 to 18 mm Hg (approximately the same as for the myocardium or moderately exercised skeletal muscle), whereas that for white matter is about 50 mm Hg. Preliminary experimental work on animals supports these figures for cortical venous blood. Since it is difficult to decrease venous PO_2 below about 16 mm Hg in any tissue, it is apparent that there is very little scope for increasing the arteriovenous oxygen difference in gray matter, and that the most effective compensation for hypoxemia is increased cerebral blood flow. These factors account for the narrow range (arterial PO_2 50 to 30 mm Hg) between the beginning of vasodilatation and the maximum decrease in venous PO_2 and for the early occurrence of personality and EEG changes in hypoxemia.

Response to Altered Perfusion Pressure (Autoregulation)

The effective perfusion pressure (PP) in the CNS is mean arterial pressure minus intracranial pressure (MAP – ICP). Although under normal conditions ICP is approximately equal to jugular venous pressure, this is frequently not true when ICP is raised, a better approximation being obtained by measuring superior sagittal sinus pressure. Within wide limits of perfusion pressure, from 50 to about 200 mm Hg or even higher, the cerebral vasculature is able to compensate for changes by altering vascular resistance (i.e., by dilatation or constriction), thereby maintaining a constant cerebral blood flow (Fig. 13-6). This is true autoregulation and is distinct from vasomotor reactivity to altered plasma carbon dioxide and oxygen levels; the two may be clinically dissociated and probably have different mechanisms.

Fall in Perfusion Pressure

The effectiveness of autoregulation (vasodilatation) as PP falls is to some extent dependent on the rate of fall. Rapid reduction in PP (e.g., a massive hemorrhage) is followed by at least a temporary reduction of cerebral blood flow, even if the pressure falls only to 70 to 80 mm Hg. A steady fall, such as might occur in persistent subacute hemorrhage or increasing ICP, does not reduce cerebral blood flow until the PP drops to the critical level of about 50 mm Hg, which presumably corresponds with the maximum (structurally possible) vasodilatation. Continuing perfusion below this level reduces cerebral blood flow and causes an increased arteriovenous oxygen difference. The classic Cushing's phenomenon appears, presumably due to brain stem ischemia; this consists of systemic hypertension, bradycardia, and respiratory irregularity. The critical cerebral blood flow level for maintenance of consciousness is approximately 30 ml per 100 g per minute; below this level there is a slowing of capillary circulation with the possibility of erythrocyte sludging, formation of microemboli, and failure of some capillary beds to open when adequate PP is reestablished (the no-reflow phenomenon).

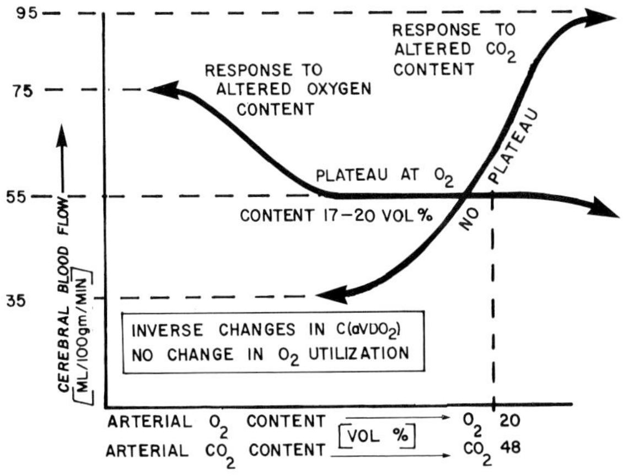

Fig. 13-7. The effects of altered arterial O_2 and CO_2 content on cerebral blood flow. Note the sensitive (steep) response to altered CO_2 content and the much less sensitive (flatter) and less marked O_2 responses. However, the response to low arterial O_2 overrides that to low CO_2 (e.g., in hypoxemic hyperventilation).

Rise in Perfusion Pressure

An upper limit for autoregulation (vasoconstriction) in response to increased perfusion pressure is less clearly established, but cerebral blood flow generally rises at systemic blood pressure of 200 mm Hg. In a few normal persons and hypertensive patients, a PP of only 160 mm Hg leads to increased cerebral blood flow with a reduced arteriovenous oxygen difference. It is probable that if PP levels raising cerebral blood flow were maintained for long periods, blood-brain barrier damage would lead to edema. In persons with chronic hypertension there appears to be upward revision of the lower limit for autoregulation. In one study, a control group tolerated slow reduction of perfusion pressure to 50 to 60 mm Hg without a fall in cerebral blood flow, but an equivalent hypertensive group showed evidence of decreased flow at pressures of 100 to 110 mm Hg. A recognized effect of chronic severe hypertension, at least experimentally, is vasospasm, but it is unknown whether this is a pathological variant of autoregulatory vasoconstriction or has some entirely different genesis.

Preconditions for Effective Autoregulation

Effective autoregulation presupposes that the vessel walls are healthy and that the vessels start in approximately mid-position. Vessels that are already maximally dilated by increased PCO_2 cannot respond to a fall in PP by further dilatation, so that autoregulation appears to be abolished. Severely atherosclerotic vessels cannot dilate or contract, so that even moderate variations in PP cannot be compensated. Also, as noted previously, autoregulation may be impaired by an upward revision of steady-state pressure in patients with chronic hypertension.

Response to Altered Oxygen or Carbon Dioxide Concentration (Vasomotor Control)

The direct effect of oxygen on cerebral blood flow appears to be much less finely adjusted than that of carbon dioxide, but since oxygen deficiency is virtually always associated with carbon dioxide excess, this may not be physiologically disadvantageous.

Effects of Altered PO_2

If arterial PO_2 is reduced, compensatory vasodilatation does not occur until it falls below 50 mm Hg, and the maximum increase in cerebral blood flow inducible by an oxygen deficit (Fig. 13-7) is about 50% (up to 75 to 80 ml per 100 g per minute), a far smaller increase than can be achieved by hypercapnia. In experimental or voluntary hyperventilation, PCO_2 is reduced, and initial vasoconstriction occurs; this effect is overridden by the dilatation of vasoconstriction-induced cerebral oxygen deficit at a venous PO_2 of 18 to 19 mm Hg (cerebral blood flow 60% of normal).

Recent studies indicate that increased arterial PO_2 has a vasoconstrictor effect; inhalation of 100% oxygen at atmospheric pressure reduces cerebral blood flow by 13%, and at 3 atmospheres by 25%. Different effects are exerted on the carotid and vertebral flows; only the former is markedly decreased. Since experimental evidence suggests that a reduction in PCO_2 also constricts only the carotid vessels, there may be differences in vasomotor control of blood supply to the brain stem and to the forebrain.

Effects of Altered PCO_2

Much is known of responses to altered PCO_2, since this can be readily changed independently of PO_2, whereas the converse is more difficult. Hyperventilation (reduced arterial PCO_2) causes sufficient vasoconstriction to reduce cerebral blood flow to about 34 ml per 100 g per minute, leaving oxygen utilization unchanged (increased arteriovenous oxygen difference). Inhalation of 5 to 7% carbon dioxide in air almost doubles cerebral blood flow (to 95 to 100 ml per 100 g per minute), again without a change in metabolic rate (decreased oxygen difference). The vasodilatation that accompanies raised PCO_2 in plasma (reduced vascular resistance) reduces flow through a partially occluded vessel because of dilatation of healthy collaterals. Metabolic acid-base imbalance has less marked, less constant effects on cerebral blood flow. In diabetic acidosis, cerebral blood flow is approximately normal, although oxygen utilization (and therefore the arteriovenous oxygen difference) is reduced.

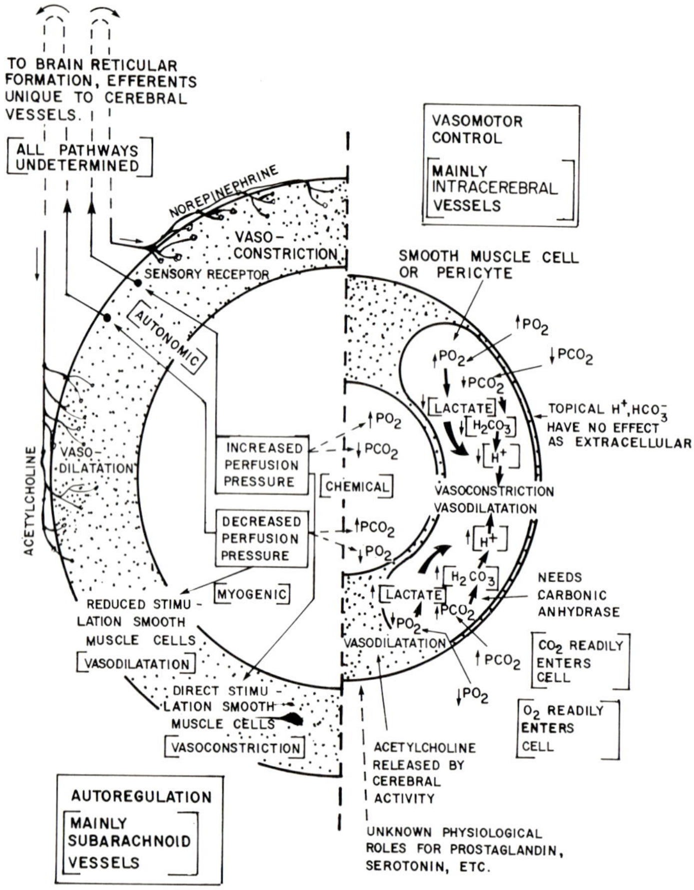

Fig. 13-8. Mechanisms of autoregulation (left) and chemical vasomotor control (right), according to current thinking. The stippled area represents a vessel wall, containing on the right a greatly disproportionate smooth muscle cell or pericyte (unstippled).

Mechanisms of Autoregulation and Vasomotor Control

It is increasingly difficult to maintain a unitary concept for autoregulation and vasomotor control. In many patients with strokes, autoregulation (response to changes in perfusion pressure) is diminished or abolished, whereas vasomotor control (response to carbon dioxide) remains intact. In disorders of the central autonomic system, such as the Shy-Drager syndrome (idiopathic orthostatic hypotension), a similar dissociation is noted, and it may be reproduced experimentally by alpha-adrenergic blocking agents (phenoxybenzamine, thymoxamine) which abolish responses to altered perfusion pressure, but leave carbon dioxide responses intact. In patients with stroke, this dissociation seems more common when lesions involve the brain stem or diencephalon than with cortical lesions, suggesting central autonomic involvement.

Autoregulation in Relation to Autonomic Innervation

Observations such as those above, and the copious autonomic innervation of subarachnoid vessels, suggest that the autonomic nervous system may play a prominent role in autoregulatory responses (Fig. 13-8), though direct evidence for this role is lacking. Experimentally, while sympathetic stimulation causes cerebrovascular constriction, it causes even more constriction in other vessels and therefore a tendency for cerebral blood flow to increase, apparently contrary to the desired effect. Most studies of parasympathetic stimulation have shown no effect on cerebral blood flow, although a recent study involving stimulation of the facial nerve within the cranium did demonstrate a slight ipsilateral increase in blood flow (vasodilatation).

Presumably, if the autonomic system is involved in autoregulation, there must be separate pathways within the central and peripheral nervous systems by which the cerebral vasculature alone can be caused to contract. These pathways would be different from those that mediate Cushing's phenomenon, in which general vasoconstriction, more intense in extracerebral vessels, shunts blood into the cranial cavity. This phenomenon is apparently dependent on a brain stem center that is believed to be directly sensitive to reduced PO_2.

Although reduction of arterial P_{CO_2} (producing vasoconstriction) is said to deplete neurotransmitters in subarachnoid vessels, it appears likely that this is a secondary effect, and that the autonomic system is not responsible for vasomotor control.

Vasomotor Control in Relation to H^+ Concentration

Vasomotor control appears (Fig. 13-8) to be a direct vascular response to altered P_{O_2} or P_{CO_2}, P_{CO_2} being very much more effective. While one effect of reduced arterial P_{O_2} is autonomic, via a brain stem center that is probably in the midbrain (Cushing's phenomenon), there is clear evidence that reduced P_{O_2} directly causes vasodilatation and some evidence that increased P_{O_2} decreases at least the carotid part of the brain circulation.

The effects of altered arterial P_{CO_2}, on the other hand, make it appear to be one of the most sensitive agents in vasomotor control, very likely acting on the small penetrating arteries, arterioles, and capillaries rather than on subarachnoid vessels. Thus, it has been demonstrated that (presumably regional) activity in the brain, such as that induced by mental arithmetic (frontal cortex) or visual stimuli (occipital cortex), causes regional variations in cortical blood flow, which are not associated with measurable alterations in total cerebral blood flow. The effects of metabolic acidosis or alkalosis at a constant P_{CO_2} are very small.

Since it is difficult to dissociate P_{CO_2} and pH, there has been speculation as to whether it is CO_2 or H^+ concentration that is ultimately responsible for vasomotor control, and whether extracellular or intracellular concentrations are important. Since the relationship between CO_2 and H^+ is based on the conversion of CO_2 to H_2CO_3, a reaction catalyzed by carbonic anhydrase, recent experimental work with a carbonic anhydrase inhibitor (acetazolamide) is of interest. Cerebral blood flow was assessed indirectly by measurement of cortical temperature and P_{O_2}, and acetazolamide apparently abolished the vasomotor effects of altered arterial P_{CO_2}. This work would imply that either H^+ or HCO_3^- concentration, but not P_{CO_2}, is the ultimately responsible agent, and since local applications of bicarbonate or weak acids to the cortex fail to produce vasomotor changes, an intracellular site of action is suggested.

It is therefore probable that though alterations in P_{CO_2} are the *effective* cause of vasomotor control (since only CO_2, not H^+ or HCO_3^-, can freely enter cells), the intracellular P_{CO_2} *operates through changes in concentration of H^+ or HCO_3^-*. Experimental evidence indicates that CO_2 entering the cell causes a much larger change in H^+ than in HCO_3^-, so the former is probably the ultimately responsible agent.

Acetazolamide has no effect on the vasomotor response to P_{O_2}, and there is no direct evidence as to how this effect is mediated. It would seem economical to postulate that intracellular P_{O_2} is inversely related to lactate concentration and this in turn affects intracellular pH, so that the final mechanism is the same as for P_{CO_2} changes, but is delayed until there is a significant switch from aerobic to anaerobic metabolism.

Other Theories of Autoregulation and Vasomotor Control

While the above theory of vasomotor control is in a sense myogenic, insofar as it is the intracellular pH of smooth muscle cells that is presumed to be effective, the *myogenic theory of autoregulation* suggests that reactions to altered perfusion pressure are due to a direct mechanical effect on arterial smooth muscle, rather than being mediated through the autonomic nervous system. The theory postulates that asynchronous, spontaneous, rhythmic contraction is a general property of smooth muscle cells and is responsible for vascular tone. This spontaneous activity is increased if the intraluminal pressure (perfusion pressure) rises, leading to vasoconstriction, with the contrary effect if intraluminal pressure falls. At present, evidence in favor of this hypothesis seems inconclusive.

Another possibility is that the effects of altered perfusion pressure (autoregulation) are mediated by alteration in P_{CO_2} or pH, so that there is no distinction between the mechanisms of autoregulation and vasomotor control. The balance of evidence appears to favor separate mechanisms, as outlined above.

It is possible that other chemical factors are involved in controlling the caliber of cerebral vessels, especially perhaps the regional vessels. Active cortex liberates considerable amounts of acetylcholine and shows vasodilatation. If atropine is added, vasodilatation is reduced and delayed, whereas it is enhanced by eserine or cholinomimetic drugs. Suggested roles for serotonin and for the prostaglandins are at present speculative. The relationship, if any, between normal autoregulation and (pathological) vasospasm (see Chap. 15) remains obscure.

MORPHOLOGY OF BRAIN DAMAGE

Hypoxemia, hypoglycemia, and ischemia are all characterized by a subnormal supply of metabolic substrates with or without accumulation of waste products, and the histological changes in each are generally similar. The topographical distribution of these changes depends both on vessel distribution and a poorly understood phenomenon known as *selective vulnerability.*

Selective Vulnerability

The predisposition of certain regions in the brain to damage by noxae to which all regions are equally exposed (selective vulnerability) has led to several explanatory hypotheses:

The *vascular hypothesis* suggests that the reserve of vascular supply to various areas of the brain may be widely different. Expressed in other terms, some areas might be using almost all the oxygen and substrate normally supplied, whereas others are extracting relatively less. This is certainly true of gray and white matter, but the vascular hypothesis extends to differences between gray areas. In such circumstances, a reduction in Po_2 or blood supply would clearly damage most severely those areas already using virtually their entire normal oxygen input, whereas other areas would have a considerable reserve. In view of the previous discussion of the role of ischemia in hypoxemic damage, it may be that the vulnerable component in these areas is not the neural parenchyma itself, but the vessels, and the vulnerability is not to hypoxia per se, but to vascular stasis.

The *theory of pathoclisis* suggests that there are metabolic peculiarities in different areas that affect their susceptibility to oxygen deficiency and possibly to glucose deficiency. While such metabolic differences are certainly recognized, as in different parts of the pyramidal layer of the hippocampus, they cannot be conclusively associated with selective vulnerability in ischemia or hypoxemia.

Brain swelling (presumably due to edema) may be associated with compression of vessels such as the anterior choroidal, posterior cerebral, and superior cerebellar arteries. Some areas exhibiting selective vulnerability, such as the hippocampus, parieto-occipital cortex, and dentate nucleus, are in the peripheral territories of such vessels and are therefore most affected by decreased flow or oxygen deficiency. While compression of these vessels may be associated with uncal herniation, this is not specific for ischemia or hypoxemia, and the theory fails to account for other areas of selective vulnerability.

According to a fourth theory, large cells may be more susceptible to oxygen deficiency or metabolite accumulation than smaller cells, simply because their central areas are at a considerable distance from the nearest capillary. Such a concept might account for the susceptibility of Purkinje's cells and large pyramidal cells of the cortex.

These theories are not mutually exclusive, and no unifying concept of selective vulnerability currently exists. It is probable that stasis due to associated myocardial insufficiency may play a role in hypoxemia and hypotension, but probably a lesser role in hypoglycemia, since the myocardium can utilize fatty acids for oxidation.

General Relationship of Microscopic Changes to Degree of Oxygen or Substrate Deficiency

The histological changes in damaged regions depend on the severity and duration of ischemia, hypoxemia, or hypoglycemia, as well as on the differing metabolic requirements of CNS cells. Neurons have a very limited ability to survive by anaerobic glycolysis, probably surviving longest in the brain stem and hypothalamus. Oligodendroglial cells are intermediate in their resistance to substrate or oxygen deficiency, whereas astrocytes and the mesenchymal framework of the brain (vascular tissue) are much more resistant.

Therefore, the least degree of tissue destruction is manifested as *selective necrosis of neurons.* Necrotic neurons exhibit many specific and semispecific changes, including ischemic necrosis (not often seen in hypoglycemia) and shrinkage or swelling, often followed by cell necrosis and disappearance (see Chap. 10). There is usually a mild to moderate astrocytic reaction, characterized by astrocytic hypertrophy and hyperplasia and later by fine, diffuse fibrillary gliosis. Loss of neurons entails loss of their axons and myelin, but this proceeds at a relatively slow pace, apparent in the acute phase as spongiosis of white matter with slight axonal and myelin fragmentation (changes that are often barely apparent, since fibers from undamaged sources remain intact). If the patient survives, the white matter shows mild pallor, often accompanied by fine, diffuse fibrillary gliosis.

In more severe damage, the neuronal changes are accompanied by *swelling, pyknosis, and rhexis of oligodendroglial cells.* This leads to demyelination, the white matter showing acute myelin breakdown (see Chap. 21), followed by fibrillary gliosis and even minor cystic change. The axons of surviving neurons may persist for months or years in this demyelinated, gliosed tissue.

If substrate or oxygen deprivation is very severe or prolonged, there is *total tissue necrosis,* involving the astrocytes and mesenchymal framework as well, and the changes seen then resemble those of infarction (see Chap. 14), except in their topographical distribution. Cells, cellular processes, and vessels disappear in the central area, to be replaced by irregular cystic spaces, often containing granular debris. In the long term there is replacement by multilocular cavities, surrounded by a zone of fibrillary gliosis.

Hypoxemic Damage

In pure hypoxemia, such as that occurring at high altitudes, there is a remarkably rapid onset of clinical symptoms, including listlessness, apathy, drowsiness, and markedly deficient judgment — so rapid that appropriate corrective action, even if possible, is frequently not taken. Within a few seconds, these manifestations may be followed by coma, convulsions, and cessation of electrical activity (within 20 seconds in the cortex and 30 to 90 seconds in the medulla). Some patients who survive show an unexplained secondary failure: After the appearance of mild or even severe symptoms, they may temporarily recover for some hours or days and then again relapse.

The pathological changes are not uniformly distributed, and areas of selective vulnerability include the cerebral cortex (especially the deeper layers 3 and 4), the pallidum, and the hippocampus (particularly sector H_1 and H_{3-5}, see Fig. 13-9). Commonly involved but less pathognomonic are the striatum, thalamus, and Purkinje's cells, the latter especially when deep within cerebellar folia. The hypothalamus, brain stem, and spinal cord are generally well preserved. Involvement of the cortex may include one or more adjacent layers or the entire thickness. If the former, the end result if the patient survives is a thin layer of cystic gliosis involving only the destroyed laminae (laminar necrosis); if the latter, cystic gliosis involves the entire cortex (Fig. 13-10) or variable layers from region to region (pseudolaminar necrosis).

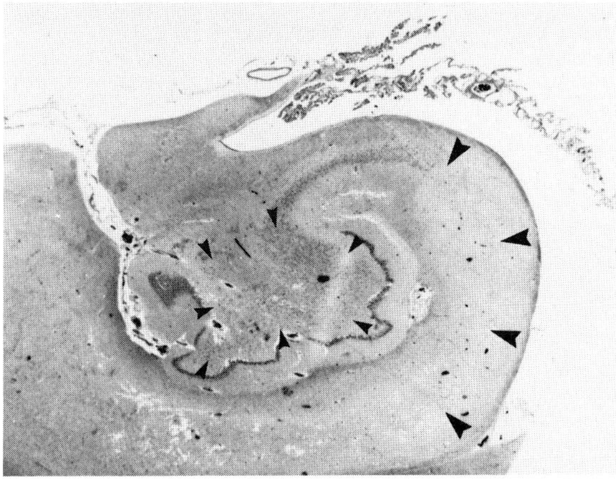

Fig. 13-9. Section of hippocampus at the level of the lateral geniculate body (more anteriorly, it is difficult to interpret the more complex structure). There is ischemic neuronal loss from sectors H_1 (large arrows) and much of sectors $H_{3\text{-}5}$ (small arrows). Surviving neurons are seen in the intervening compact sector H_2, and some are seen in H_3.

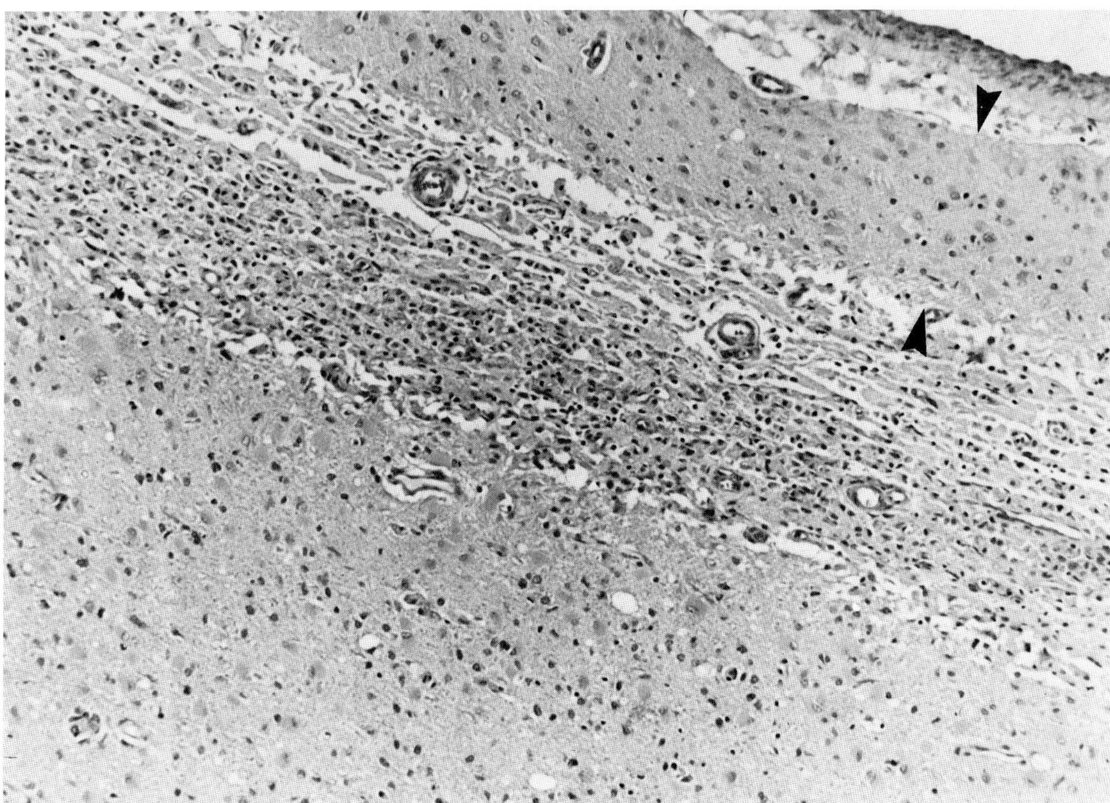

Figure 13-10. Cortex, showing subacute hypoxemic necrosis (pseudolaminar, full-thickness except molecular layer). Hyperplastic (gemistocytic) astrocytes may be seen in the molecular layer (arrows) and the superficial white matter below the cortex. (H & E, × 115.)

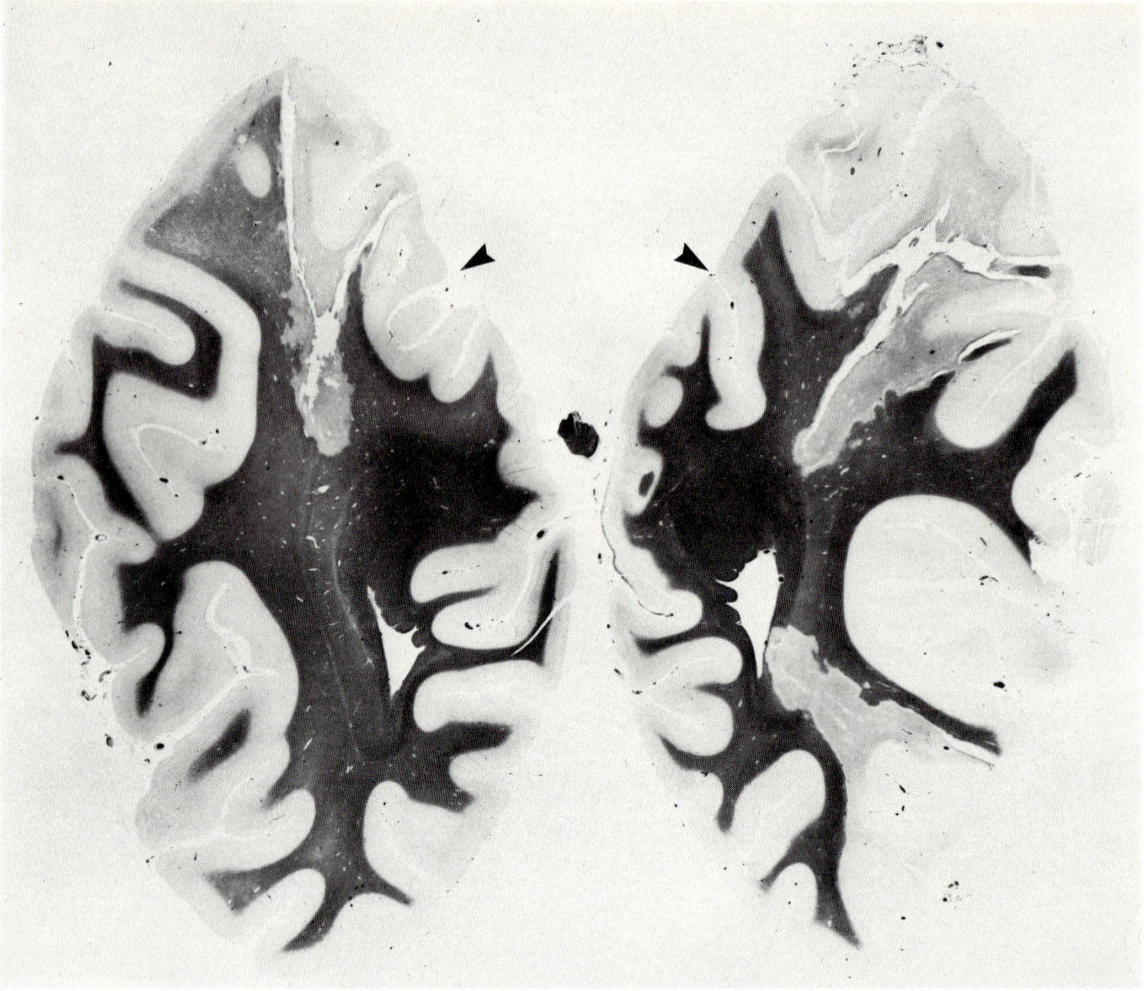

Fig. 13-11. Transverse (frontal) section of hemispheres, showing boundary zones between the middle cerebral and adjacent arterial territories. The existence of such zones in hemispheric white matter as well as in the cortex is clearly demonstrated. The hemispheres have become slightly rotated in processing, and arrows mark the medial surfaces, which should be parallel and close together. No boundary-zone lesion is present inferiorly on the left. (Occipito-parietal sections.)

In *carbon monoxide poisoning* the brain shows a characteristic bright pink coloration and compensatory vasodilatation, and petechiae are often seen in the white matter and corpus callosum. The pallidum may appear to be anemic. Patients who survive frequently show laminar or pseudolaminar necrosis in the cortex, cystic gliosis of the pallidum, and usually involvement of the substantia nigra (reticular part), the hippocampus (in the sectors previously indicated), and Purkinje's cells. Occasionally, destruction in the white matter is seen in the absence of typical gray matter changes and is characterized by demyelination, with only moderate axonal damage, perhaps related to the development of cerebral edema.

The distribution of lesions in *cyanide poisoning* is similar, except that white matter may be more often and more severely affected, perhaps indicating a direct effect of cyanide on myelin metabolism.

Ischemic Damage

Where the perfusion pressure is inadequate because of a reduction in systolic pressure, a somewhat different distribution of damage may be found. Characteristic cerebral lesions due to systemic hypotension are full-thickness or laminar cortical necrosis, especially marked in the boundary zones between the supply territories of major cerebral vessels (Fig. 13-11). These "watershed" areas include the superior aspect of the superior frontal gyrus and the superior parietal lobule, part of the lateral occipital surface, and the medial surface in the region of the parieto-occipital fissure. The changes are frequently more severe deep in the sulci than on the surface. In patients who sur-

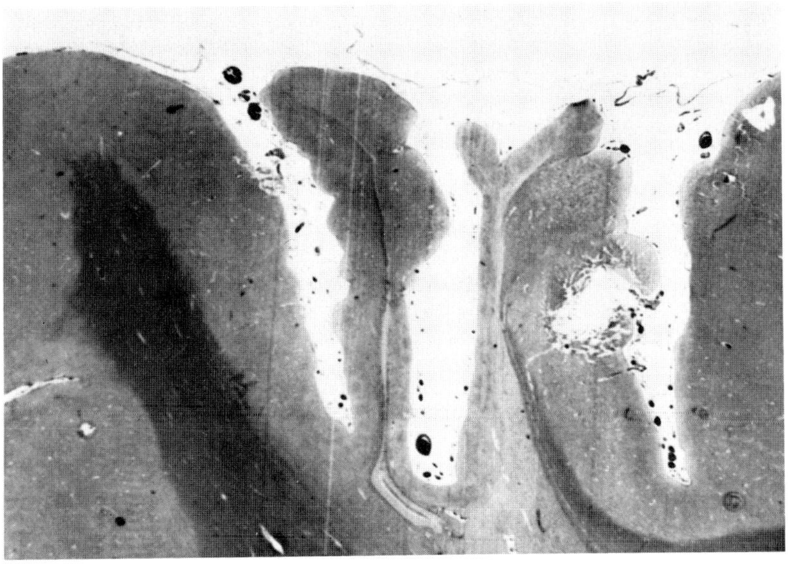

Fig. 13-12. Transverse section from region of superior frontal gyrus, showing old boundary-zone lesion with sclerotic microgyri (ulegyria). (Myelin, ×5.)

vive, sclerotic microgyria may develop (Fig. 13-12). Some gyri, because of their survival on the surface relative to ischemia in the sulci, appear mushroom-shaped on transverse section. Other areas of gray matter may also be involved in systemic hypotension, including the basal ganglia and thalamus, sectors H_1 and $H_{3\text{-}5}$ of the hippocampus, and the cerebellar cortex. Occasionally, in the absence of gray matter lesions, severe cystic gliosis of the white matter is seen in survivors, frequently maximal in the region of the lateral ventricle and extending into the superior and middle frontal gyri and along the lateral surface of the occipital horn. The mechanism of this localization is not clear, although these lesions are sometimes regarded as boundary-zone effects in the white matter.

It should be noted again that, irrespective of the cause, whether hypoxemia, hypoglycemia, or ischemia, the microscopic changes are virtually identical, except for the usual lack of neuronal ischemic necrosis in hypoglycemia. Only lesion distribution, together with the clinical history (which is more reliable), may give etiological hints in long-term survivors. Even the areas of selective vulnerability overlap considerably.

Hypoglycemic Damage

Changes induced by hypoglycemia appear to be concentrated in the cortex, where there may be laminar or pseudolaminar necrosis, principally involving the deeper layers. The caudate and putamen are usually severely affected, especially the small neurons, as well as the hippocampus. The cerebellar cortex and cerebral white matter are less often damaged, and neuronal loss in the thalamus is absent or confined to the lateral areas.

EFFECT OF INCREASED INTRACRANIAL PRESSURE ON BLOOD FLOW

A rise in intracranial pressure per se, if it could be diffusely distributed throughout the CNS so that no pressure gradients were created, would not cause clinical symptoms, because increased hydrostatic pressure does not adversely affect neuronal function. However, a truly uniform increase in intracranial pressure throughout the craniospinal axis cannot be achieved (except perhaps experimentally).

In clinical situations involving raised intracranial pressure there are two major problems. The first is nonuniform expansion of the brain (even cerebral edema mainly affects the hemispheres), resulting in *displacements of the neuraxis* within the craniospinal cavity (see Chap. 12). The second is *interference with adequate blood supply.* Under normal conditions, when intracranial pressure (ICP) is low, perfusion pressure (PP) in the cerebral vessels may be taken as the mean arterial pressure (MAP) at the base of the skull. However, since the vessel walls are not rigid tubes, any increase in ICP must be subtracted from the MAP in calculating the effective perfusion pressure. If raised ICP significantly lowers PP, two compensatory mechanisms are activated. As noted above, autonomic mechanisms exist that can to some extent compensate for reduced perfusion pressure due to raised ICP by increasing the MAP (Cushing's phenomenon). Autoregulation is also an important line of defense, not only against reduced blood pressure, but also against increased ICP, any decrease in

PP causing active vasodilatation of cerebral vessels (principally those in the subarachnoid space).

The major contents of the cranial cavity are brain, blood, and CSF. Increased ICP may be caused by an increase in volume of any one or more of these, but principally of the brain. Such an increase may be due to cerebral edema or to a focal lesion such as tumor, abscess, or hematoma. Neoplasms of other intracranial tissues, such as the meninges or pituitary, or developmental tumors may also raise ICP. A significant increase in cerebral blood volume may occur in impaired autoregulation (vasoparalysis), which may be a significant factor in head injury. Increased CSF volume (hydrocephalus) will be considered separately (see Chap. 19).

Under normal conditions the brain constitutes at least 85% of the cranial volume, the blood up to 10%, and the cerebrospinal fluid about 5%. In the earliest stages of development of cerebral edema or growth of a focal lesion, CSF can be partially expelled from the cranial cavity without causing symptoms. Probably 30 to 40 ml (50%) can be so expelled, but the ventricular system and the large subarachnoid cisterns cannot be completely obliterated without producing unacceptable distortions. Compression of the interpeduncular system would involve massive distortion at the base of the brain and midbrain, and obliteration of the cisterna magna would prevent egress of CSF into the subarachnoid space.

The Development of Increased Intracranial Pressure

In the early stages of increased ICP, autoregulation remains intact. The condition at that time is reversible if expansion of the causative lesion can be arrested. The following stages of progression may be discerned.

1. In response to reduced perfusion pressure, autoregulation causes a controlled vasodilatation. Arterial resistance falls, capillary and venous resistance are unchanged, and cerebral blood flow is maintained at normal levels. The vasodilatation itself contributes slightly to further raising of ICP, but the mechanism is effective, and cerebral blood flow remains normal until PP drops to about 40 to 50 mm Hg, at which stage no further vasodilatation is possible.

2. A further fall in PP causes a drop in cerebral blood flow, and Cushing's phenomenon is invoked causing systemic hypertension. The resulting increase in MAP approximately keeps pace with the increasing ICP, so that PP is kept constant at or slightly above 40 mm Hg. At this stage, arterial resistance is low, capillary resistance is slightly low because of vasomotor dilatation, and venous resistance is normal or slightly increased because of the compressive effect of ICP on the dural sinuses. Capillary dilatation and raised venous pressure cause a slight reduction in flow rate, and the lowered arterial and slightly raised venous resistance cause increased capillary pressure. This combination of capillary changes may be of serious prognostic import (see below).

Experimental work indicates that there is some variation in the PP at which Cushing's phenomenon appears. If increased ICP is associated with distortion in the tentorial area (e.g., uncal herniation), as it usually is in clinical situations, Cushing's phenomenon tends to occur early (with a relatively high PP). It is probable that the area receptive to reduced PO_2 is in the midbrain which discharges through the medullary reticular formation and peripheral sympathetic nervous system. The phenomenon is abolished by removal of the sympathetic ganglia.

Up to this stage, autoregulation and vasomotor control are intact; cerebral blood flow is maintained at marginal levels by increasing MAP in parallel with ICP, but there is increased intracapillary pressure and relatively slow capillary flow. The rise in ICP is still reversible, *but the prognosis may at this point be drastically changed for the worse by one or both of two eventualities, namely,* complete loss of autoregulation *(vasoparalysis) or the* development of cerebral edema, *to which the capillary changes noted in the preceding paragraph predispose.*

3. The third (irreversible) stage of progression features the concurrent development of vasoparalysis and edema.

Vasoparalysis must be distinguished from maximal vasodilatation, from which it differs in greater distension of the vessels, total lack of response to increased PP, and absent vessel tone. As a result of this loss of tone, arteries may now be compressed by ICP, and conversely increases in MAP are transmitted to surrounding tissues, further augmenting ICP. There is no longer any distinct segregation of pressures inside and outside the vessels. Cerebral blood volume, as well as cerebral blood flow, is now proportional to PP, so that progressive increases in MAP cause an increase in blood volume and are directly transmitted to the ICP as pressure waves. At this stage, arterial resistance is high, since it is influenced by ICP; venous resistance is high for the same reason; and capillary resistance is normal or slightly low. There is marked slowing of capillary flow in spite of high intraluminal pressure. Vasomotor control is also lost and the vessels show no constriction response to reduced PCO_2.

The terminal event is often the development of a train of flat pressure waves with an amplitude of 50 to 100 mm Hg, lasting 5 to 20 minutes, apparently triggered by small increases in MAP, which raise cerebral blood volume and are acutely reflected in the ICP. Pressure waves tend to continue until ICP is equal to MAP, at which time cerebral circulation ceases. The cause of vasoparalysis in increased ICP, fundamental as it often is to the death of such patients, is unknown.

As already noted, capillaries are dilated with relatively slow flow and also have increased luminal pressure. Both circumstances contribute to damage to the endothelium and blood-brain barrier and initiate vasogenic edema. Locally increased PCO_2 and reduced pH cannot be ruled out as initiating factors in the development of edema, but stasis, with formation of fibrin, platelet, and erythrocyte aggregates, is a more likely cause (see Chap. 12). The resulting swelling of endothelial cells and astrocytic processes causes such a sharp increase in capillary resistance that this suddenly becomes the main component of the total cerebrovascular resistance.

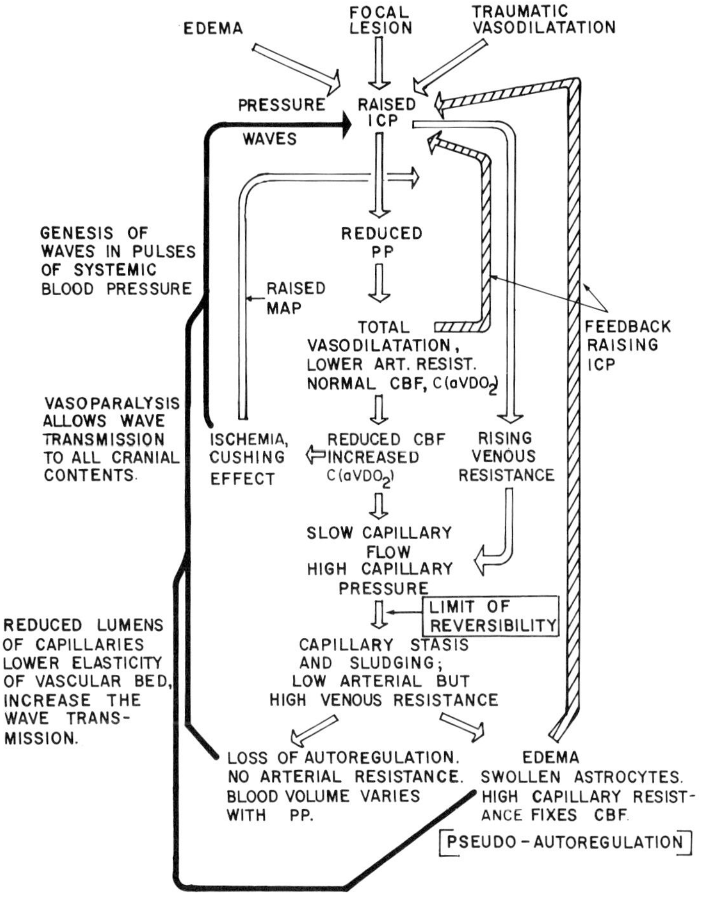

Fig. 13-13. Diagrammatic summary of events that may follow increased intracranial pressure (open arrows). Cross-hatched arrows show positive (deleterious) feedback mechanisms. Solid arrows indicate genesis of pressure waves. Note the limit of reversibility. ICP = intracranial pressure; MAP = mean arterial pressure; PP = perfusion pressure; C(aVDO$_2$) = arteriovenous oxygen difference; CBF = cerebral blood flow.

Once edema has developed, the cerebral blood flow is at a fixed low level, independent of PP (pseudo-autoregulation).

When, as is usual, cerebral edema and vasoparalysis both develop with severely increased ICP, there is progressive fall and fixation of cerebral blood flow, and shift of cerebrovascular resistance from arteries to capillaries and veins. Autoregulation and vasomotor control are lost. Loss of the elasticity of the capillary reservoir because of edema means that each surge in arterial pressure causes an even sharper pressure wave than if edema were absent. Consideration of the chain of events in increased ICP (Fig. 13-13) makes it clear that each deterioration contributes to the next, and that rising ICP is a deteriorating vicious circle, for which therapy is difficult and prognosis, except in the early stages, is gloomy.

BIBLIOGRAPHY

Albers, R. W., Siegel, G. J., Katzman, R., and Agranoff, B. W. *Basic Neurochemistry.* Boston: Little, Brown, 1972.

Corbett, J. L., Eidelman, B. H., and Debarge, O. Modification of cerebral vasoconstriction with hyperventilation in normal man by thymoxamine. *Lancet* 2:461-463, 1972.

Eidelman, B. H., Corbett, J. L., Debarge, O., and Frankel, H. Absence of cerebral vasoconstriction with hyperventilation in tetraplegic man. *Lancet* 2:457-460, 1972.

Englund, G. Neuropathology of Cardiorespiratory Diseases. In J. Minckler (Ed.), *Pathology of the Nervous System.* New York: McGraw-Hill, 1968. Vol. 1, pp. 997-1005.

Ferendelli, J. A., and Chang, M-M. Brain metabolism during hypoglycemia. *Arch. Neurol.* 28:173-177, 1973.

Harper, A. M., Deshmukh, V. D., Rowan, J. O., and Jennett, W. B. The influence of sympathetic nervous activity on cerebral blood flow. *Arch. Neurol.* 27:1-6, 1972.
Hekmatpanah, J. Cerebral blood-flow dynamics in hypotension and cardiac arrest. *Neurology* 23: 174-180, 1973.
Hicks, S. P. Vascular Pathophysiology and Acute and Chronic Oxygen Deprivation. In J. Minckler (Ed.), *Pathology of the Nervous System.* New York: McGraw-Hill, 1968. Vol. 1, pp. 341-350.
Hoff, J. T., Sengupta, D., Harper, M., and Jennett, B. Effect of α-adrenergic blockade on response of cerebral circulation to hypocapnia in the baboon. *Lancet* 2:1337-1339, 1972.
Ingvar, D. H., and Lassen, N. A. Cerebral blood-flow and cerebral metabolism. *Triangle* 9:234-243, 1970.
Kanai, N., Hayakama, T., and Mogami, H. Blood-flow changes in carotid and vertebral arteries by hyperbaric oxygenation. *Neurology* 23:159-163, 1973.
Kjeldsborg, C. R. Respirator Brain. In J. Minckler (Ed.), *Pathology of the Nervous System.* New York: McGraw-Hill, 1972. Vol. 3, pp. 2952-2961.
Lindenberg, R. Systemic Oxygen Deficiencies. In J. Minckler (Ed.), *Pathology of the Nervous System.* New York: McGraw-Hill, 1971. Vol. 2, pp. 1583-1617.
Lowell, H. M., and Bloor, B. M. The effect of increased intracranial pressure on cerebrovascular hemodynamics. *J. Neurosurg.* 34:760-769, 1971.
Mahler, H. R., and Cordes, E. H. *Biological Chemistry* (2nd ed.). New York: Harper & Row, 1971.
Meyer, J. S., Shimazu, K., Okamoto, S., Koto, A., Ohuchi, T., Sari, A., and Ericsson, A. D. Effects of α-adrenergic blockade on autoregulation and chemical vasomotor control of cerebral blood flow in stroke. *Stroke* 4:187-200, 1973.
Miller, J. D., Stanek, A. E., and Langfitt, T. W. Cerebral blood flow regulation during experimental brain compression. *J. Neurosurg.* 39:186-196, 1973.
Patel, K. K., Hartmann, J. F., and Cohen, M. M. Effect of pH on metabolism and ultrastructure of guinea-pig cerebral cortex slices. *Stroke* 4:221-231, 1973.
Quastel, J. H. Carbohydrate Metabolism in the Nervous System. In G. H. Bourne (Ed.), *The Structure and Function of Nervous Tissue.* New York: Academic, 1969. Vol. 3, pp. 61-107.
Sacks, W. Disorders of Glucose Metabolism in Brain Dysfunction. In G. E. Gaull (Ed.), *Biology of Brain Dysfunction.* New York: Plenum, 1973. Vol. 1, pp. 143-189.
Schwartz, P. Localization and Extension of Cerebrospinal Disease. In J. Minckler (Ed.), *Pathology of the Nervous System.* New York: McGraw-Hill, 1968. Vol. 1, pp. 380-392.
Shinohara, Y. Mechanism of chemical control and vasomotor activity. *Neurology* 23:186-195, 1973.
Siesjö, B. K., and Plum, F. Pathophysiology of Anoxic Brain Damage. In G. E. Gaull (Ed.), *Biology of Brain Dysfunction.* New York: Plenum, 1973. Vol. 1, pp. 319-372.
Sokoloff, L. Metabolism of ketone bodies by the brain. *Annu. Rev. Med.* 23:271-280, 1972.
Steegmann, A. T. The Neuropathology of Cardiac Arrest. In J. Minckler (Ed.), *Pathology of the Nervous System.* New York: McGraw-Hill, 1968. Vol. 1, pp. 1005-1029.
Strandgaard, S., Olesen, J., Skinhøj, E., and Lassen, N. A. Autoregulation of brain circulation in severe arterial hypertension. *Br. Med. J.* 1:507-510, 1973.
Symon, L., Held, K., and Dorsch, N. W. C. A study of regional autoregulation in the cerebral circulation to increased perfusion pressure in normocapnia and hypercapnia. *Stroke* 4:139-147, 1973.
Waltz, A. G. Disorders of the Cerebral Circulation. In G. E. Gaull (Ed.), *Biology of Brain Dysfunction.* New York: Plenum, 1973. Vol. 2, pp. 75-113.
White, A., Handler, P., and Smith, E. L. *Principles of Biochemistry* (5th ed.). New York: McGraw-Hill, 1973.
Woodhall, B., Kramer, R. S., Currie, W. D., and Sanders, A. P. Brain energetics and neurosurgery. *J. Neurosurg.* 34:3-14, 1971.

Cerebrovascular Disease

14

The previous chapter dealt with changes in the central nervous system due to reduction in perfusion pressure or to deficient oxygenation or glucose content of the blood. Any such lesions that progress to total tissue necrosis may be regarded as infarction, such as those occurring in the pallidum or deeper layers of the cortex in hypoxemia or in the boundary zones in systemic hypotension. The present chapter deals with *regional* CNS infarction due to vascular disease, or occlusion, or both, in which the distribution bears an obvious relationship to the vessel involved.

Since the majority of these vascular accidents involve the internal carotid, middle cerebral, or basilar arteries, they frequently produce hemiplegia or other massive pareses, loss or abnormalities of speech, and disturbances in the level of consciousness. In popular parlance, such lesions, of acute or subacute onset, are called *strokes*. Occlusive cerebrovascular disease with infarction is by far the most common cause of strokes, the other major cause being intracranial hemorrhage.

From the point of view of diagnosis, treatment, and autopsy examination of the brain, it is important to realize that, first, it is not necessary for a vessel to be completely occluded to produce extensive cerebral infarction. Second, the vascular lesion causing infarction may be located in the internal carotid or vertebral vessels in the neck and may therefore be missed on routine autopsy examination of the brain. Such extracranial vascular lesions account for an appreciable number of cerebral infarcts. (Extraspinal vascular disease is the most common cause of infarction in the spinal cord.) Third, vascular disease, usually atherosclerosis, is common and often asymptomatic, and therefore autopsy may disclose severe stenosis of major vessels at the base of the brain without clinical or morphological evidence of infarction.

It is therefore obvious that stenosis is a necessary but not sufficient factor leading to cerebral infarction. Others probably include abnormal systemic blood pressure, duration of vascular narrowing, and the adequacy of collateral circulation, which is partly a function of individual variability and partly of the time available for its development. The overwhelming majority of cerebral infarcts are associated with atherosclerosis of extracranial or intracranial vessels, and since atherosclerosis is a generalized disease there is often an association between cerebrovascular and coronary insufficiency. Reduced cardiac efficiency by reducing systolic pressure, may often be a factor in the production of strokes.

VASCULAR DISEASES ASSOCIATED WITH CENTRAL NERVOUS SYSTEM INFARCTION

Atherosclerosis

Atherosclerosis is a disease of large arteries, from the aorta down to those about 2 mm in external diameter. Atherosclerosis is clinically most important when it affects the coronary and cerebral vessels and causes severe reduction of blood flow. As noted previously, venous PO_2 in the myocardium and cerebral gray matter is approximately 18 mm Hg, representing almost maximal oxygen extraction. These tissues are therefore peculiarly susceptible to a reduction in blood flow, and in many patients with cerebrovascular atherosclerosis, potential or actual coronary insufficiency is a complicating factor.

Although changes leading to atherosclerosis are said to begin shortly after birth, grossly visible lesions in the carotid or vertebrobasilar systems are rare before the second or third decade, when flat yellow spots or streaks may be seen in the intima, earlier in the carotid than in the vertebrobasilar system. These spots or streaks are made more obvious by a fat stain such as scharlach R. Foam cells and free neutral lipid are present in the intima, but there is little connective-tissue change. Intracranial vessels do not often show significant involvement until after the age of 30, after which atherosclerotic lesions rapidly increase, usually becoming more severe in males than females. By the age of 50, lesions are usually widespread in the neck vessels and major vasculature at the base of the brain, including the first few centimeters of the middle and posterior cerebral arteries. These lesions are elevated and show marked intimal fibrosis, extracellular and intracellular fat at the base and edges, varying degrees of degeneration and necrosis, deposition of cholesterol, calcification, and occasional lymphocytic infiltration. This subintimal reaction is the major factor narrowing the lumen of diseased vessels. After the age of 50 there is an increasing tendency for plaques to form in smaller

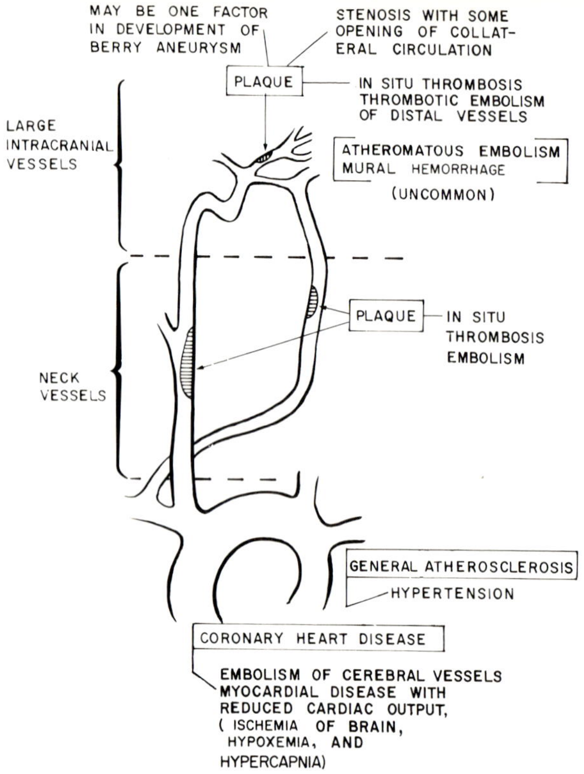

Fig. 14-1. Relationships between atherosclerosis and occlusive cerebrovascular disease.

vessels, including the anterior cerebral and posterior inferior cerebellar arteries.

Atherosclerotic plaques may be concentric or eccentric and even without complications can produce an 80 to 90% reduction in the lumen (stenosis). However, they are liable to the same complications as in other parts of the body (Fig. 14-1), the most frequent and serious being in situ thrombosis on the plaque, presumably associated with loss of endothelium and increased fluid turbulence. Less often, the contents of the plaque may be released into the circulation, leaving an atheromatous ulcer and causing embolism in the direction of blood flow (atheromatous embolism). More commonly, portions of thrombus from the plaque may detach and cause embolism more distally (thrombotic embolism). Relatively infrequently, the microscopic hemorrhages often present in old plaques may become grossly enlarged, dissecting within the wall of the vessel and occluding the lumen (intramural hemorrhage). In the intracranial vessels, the major causes of atherosclerotic strokes appear to be in situ thrombosis or severe stenosis associated with other circulatory factors such as a fall in blood pressure. Strokes due to involvement of the neck vessels are commonly due to in situ thrombosis and may also be associated with atheromatous or thrombotic embolism. Strokes associated with atheroma of the coronary vessels may be due to thrombotic emboli arising in the heart as a result of myocardial infarction or auricular fibrillation.

Rheumatic Fever

The cardiac and vascular lesions of rheumatic fever may cause occlusion of relatively large cerebral vessels, the former by thrombotic embolism and the latter by in situ thrombosis in apparently normal vessels, even as large as the middle cerebral artery. Other rheumatic vascular changes are rarely associated with thrombosis. Aschoff bodies occasionally occur in the adventitia of large vessels such as the vertebral artery, and small arteries may show necrotizing panarteritis or proliferative endarteritis, thrombosis being rare in either case. Vascular lumens may be occluded by the inflammatory or proliferative change, but the subarachnoid and perforating arteries involved are so small that even the normal collateral circulation is adequate to prevent infarction.

Thromboangiitis Obliterans

Thromboangiitis obliterans (Buerger's disease), if it exists as a nosological entity (see textbooks of general pathology), involves small subarachnoid arteries by endothelial proliferation and thrombosis, so that ultimately vessel segments appear white and shrunken. Depending on the length of the segments involved and on the collateral circulation, infarction varies from microscopic foci to parts of complete gyri. More rarely, the internal carotid artery or vessels at the base of the brain may be involved – again with thrombosis and cerebral infarction. (It seems not improbable that cases of large-vessel involvement may be early atherosclerosis, whereas small-vessel involvement may be atypical rheumatic fever.)

Temporal Arteritis

Temporal (giant cell) arteritis is a diffuse disease, usually involving subarachnoid rather than intracerebral vessels. Some cases are associated with the clinical syndrome of temporal arteritis. In addition to the chronic inflammatory and giant cell reaction, necrotizing changes with vascular thrombosis may occur, with areas of infarction varying from microscopic to involvement of whole segments of gyri. Only rarely are vessels such as the anterior or middle cerebral arteries involved, causing classic strokes.

Periarteritis Nodosa

Periarteritis nodosa involves the CNS in some 10% of cases, though it rarely *presents* as a CNS disease. In this condition, necrosis and acute or chronic inflammation are frequently associated with thrombosis, the disease involving subarachnoid and perforating arteries and larger arterioles in short segments. Acute and chronic lesions may coexist. Weakening of

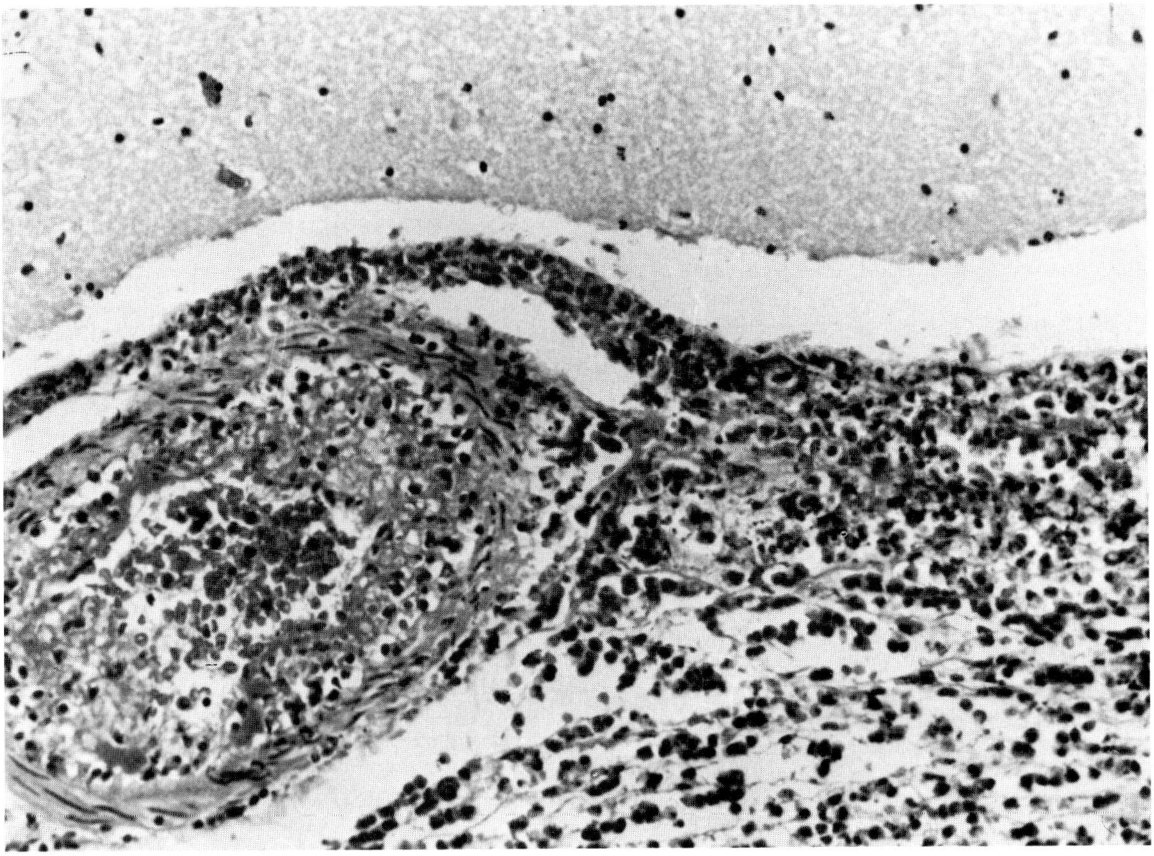

Fig. 14-2. Inflammation of the wall of a small subarachnoid artery in purulent leptomeningitis. The vessel is not thrombosed. (H & E, X300.)

vessel walls may be accompanied by subarachnoid or intracerebral hemorrhage, but only rarely are the large vessels involved with extensive infarction. More typically, the lesions are distributed as in thromboangiitis obliterans or temporal arteritis, or take the form of hemorrhage.

Pulseless Disease, Disseminated Lupus Erythematosus, and Thrombotic Microangiopathy

Pulseless disease (Takayashu's disease), characteristically involving the large elastic or muscular arteries, is only an occasional cause of cerebral infarction. *Disseminated lupus erythematosus* occasionally involves the CNS, but usually affects vessels less than 100μ in diameter. The meninges may appear thick and fibrosed, with small thrombosed vessels, and either granular cortical atrophy or somewhat larger lesions arranged around the sulci may be seen. Massive infarction does not occur. *Thrombotic microangiopathy* may produce diffuse CNS symptomatology, including hemiplegia, convulsions, and coma. It is a disease of precapillary arterioles, causing endothelial hyperplasia and thrombosis, with widespread parenchymal damage and petechial hemorrhage, but not infarction.

Summary of Arterial Diseases Causing Cerebral Infarction

It is apparent that virtually the only vascular disease leading to stroke is atherosclerosis. Rarely, large vessels may be occluded in rheumatic fever, pulseless disease, temporal arteritis, and thromboangiitis obliterans. Most of these diseases, however, involve smaller vessels and produce ischemic lesions varying from multiple focal (often with a granular superficial appearance to the cortex and adherent leptomeninges) to segments of gyri. Similar small-vessel inflammation (Fig. 14-2), often with thrombosis and small infarcts, may complicate bacterial meningitis.

Thrombosis of Intracranial Veins and Sinuses

Although involvement of venous channels in systemic vascular disease is rare, intracranial venous or sinus thrombosis is not unusual as a complication of local infections such as meningitis, otitis, mastoiditis, or infections in the central region of the face. In addition, "spontaneous" thrombosis of sinuses in the absence of any obvious predisposing lesion occurs.

Associated factors include malnutrition, dehydration, high fever, right ventricular failure, head injury, cerebral infarction or hemorrhage, polycythemia, abortion, puerperium, and the use of oral estrogens as a contraceptive measure. Increased blood coagulation (as with oral contraceptives) or viscosity (as in polycythemia or dehydration), venous stasis (as in right ventricular failure), mechanical injury (as in head trauma), vasospasm (as in trauma and subarachnoid hemorrhage), and local or general infection are undoubtedly predisposing conditions, but all, of course, frequently occur without sinus or venous thrombosis, and the exact relationship is unclear. In thromboses following labor or abortion, retrograde sinus embolism from thrombosed pelvic veins has been postulated, apparently without any clear evidence. A large proportion of sinus thromboses not associated with local sepsis occur in debilitated children (under the age of 30 months, with most under 12 months), many of them showing severe nutritional disturbances, dehydration, and hyperpyrexia. A few similar marasmic cases occur in old age with similar associations.

The number of cases in children has decreased dramatically with the advent of adequate fluid therapy and antibiotics. In the infectious group, the superior sagittal sinus is most often involved if there is diffuse bacterial meningitis; involvement of the lateral sinus is associated with otitis, mastoiditis, or cellulitis of the scalp; in cases of bacteremia, there may be multiple sinus involvement. In the noninfectious cases, including marasmic examples in infancy and old age, the superior sagittal or lateral sinuses are most frequently affected.

Because of the extensive venous collateralization on the surface of the hemispheres, the effects of sinus thrombosis depend very much on additional involvement of cortical veins. Thus, if only a part of the superior sagittal sinus is involved, no other vascular changes may be present. If the entire sinus is involved, there may be superior frontal congestion and hemorrhage, particularly if thrombosis extends into the lateral sinuses. However, if the draining veins show thrombosis, severe hemorrhagic infarction of the dorsal hemispheres is likely to occur.

Cavernous sinus thrombosis (with or without meningitis) may occur in association with facial infections, but does not lead to cerebral infarction. Sometimes it is associated with pituitary infarction or with paresis of the external ocular muscles, since the third, fourth, and sixth cranial nerves pass through it.

Cardiac Disease

Both cardiac disease per se and cardiac surgery are associated with significant numbers of cerebrovascular occlusive episodes. In *congenital heart disease* these may take the form of emboli that arise in systemic veins or the right atrium and pass through a patent foramen ovale or arise within the heart itself, or result from surgical procedures. In situ thrombosis in cerebral vessels is associated especially with cyanotic congenital heart disease, probably because polycythemia causes increased viscosity and stagnation of blood flow, with endothelial damage. The major dural sinuses, internal carotid or middle cerebral arteries, or smaller penetrating vessels may be affected. Similar changes may occur in *acquired heart disease,* either in cases where emboli arise from the heart (bland or infected), or when there is diminished cardiac output with increased central venous pressure, which frequently contributes to infarction.

Serious brain lesions associated with open heart surgery are not rare, although less than 1% are fatal. Various types of embolism (Fig. 14-3) may occur (air, fat, antifoam, thrombotic, calcified material, or heart muscle emboli), or episodes of hypotension or hypoxemia in combination with severe cerebrovascular stenosis may lead to infarction. The inherent risks of hypotension, hypoxemia, altered acid-base and electrolyte balance, and surgically induced thrombocythemia are also present. The use of large quantities of stored blood may lead to hypoglycemia, and hypothermia occasionally causes cerebral edema.

CEREBROVASCULAR ANATOMY

The clinical significance of occlusion or severe stenosis of a vessel can neither be deduced nor understood if the distribution of that vessel is unknown. Thus, the distribution of named cerebral arteries and the venous and sinus drainage of the CNS will be discussed briefly.

Although large arteries such as the anterior, middle, and posterior cerebral arteries, and, to a lesser extent, the cerebellar arteries, are fairly constant, smaller vessels show considerable variability and reciprocity. A small right posterior inferior cerebellar vessel may be compensated by an increase in size of the corresponding vessel on the left, by an increase in distribution of the superior cerebellar artery on the right, or both. Similarly, there is often reciprocity between the sizes of the anterior choroidal and posterior communicating arteries, which run reasonably closely together at the base of the brain. Only general patterns can be outlined for cortical branches or perforating vessels, but the overall areas supplied, at least by the anterior, middle, and posterior cerebral arteries and the vertebrobasilar system, are fairly constant, and these are the vessels most commonly involved in occlusive or stenotic lesions leading to clinical stroke.

Collateralization

There has been, and is, considerable disagreement as to the adequacy of collateralization of cerebral vessels (Fig. 14-4). For the main vessels supplying the cerebral hemispheres there are two levels of anastomosis.

The first is formed by the circle of Willis (Fig. 14-5), in which the two anterior cerebral vessels are joined by an anterior communicating artery, and the internal carotid and posterior cerebral arteries of each side are joined by a posterior communicating artery. This would be a very satisfactory arrangement if the circle of Willis were immune from atherosclerosis and always made up of vessels of useful caliber. In fact, one or both of the posterior communicating

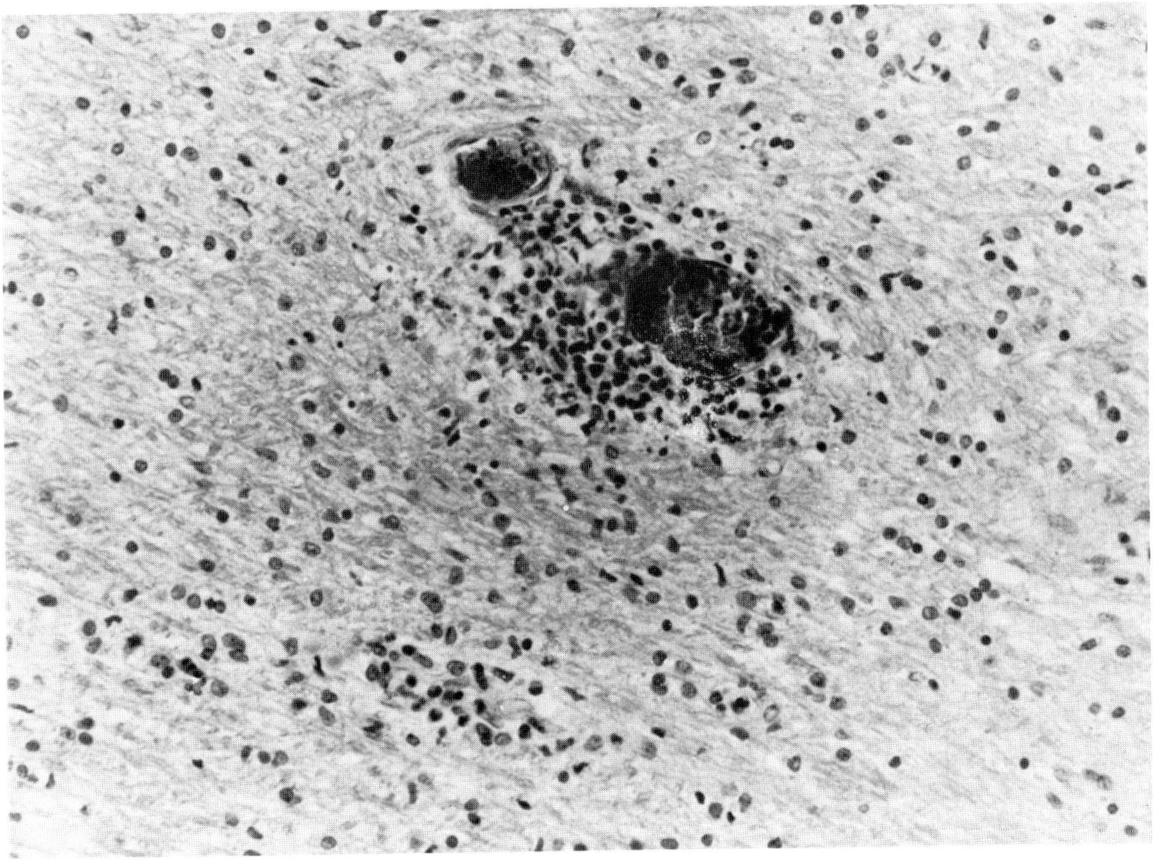

Fig. 14-3. Embolism associated with open heart surgery (three days postoperatively). Amorphous debris occupies a small vessel lumen, and there is a neutrophilic exudate. (H & E, ×300.)

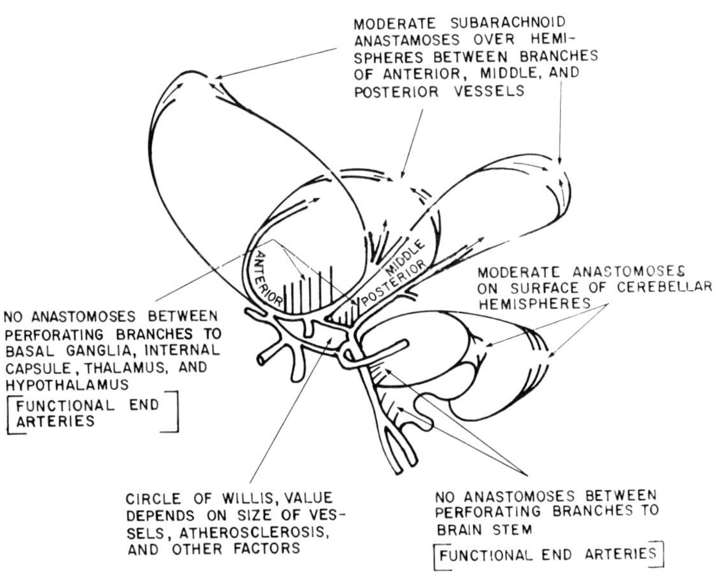

Fig. 14-4. Two levels of collateralization of vessels supplying cerebral hemispheres: first, at the circle of Willis, joining major supply vessels at the base of the brain; second, in the subarachnoid space, where territories of supply (of anterior, middle, and posterior cerebral arteries) meet – the boundary zones.

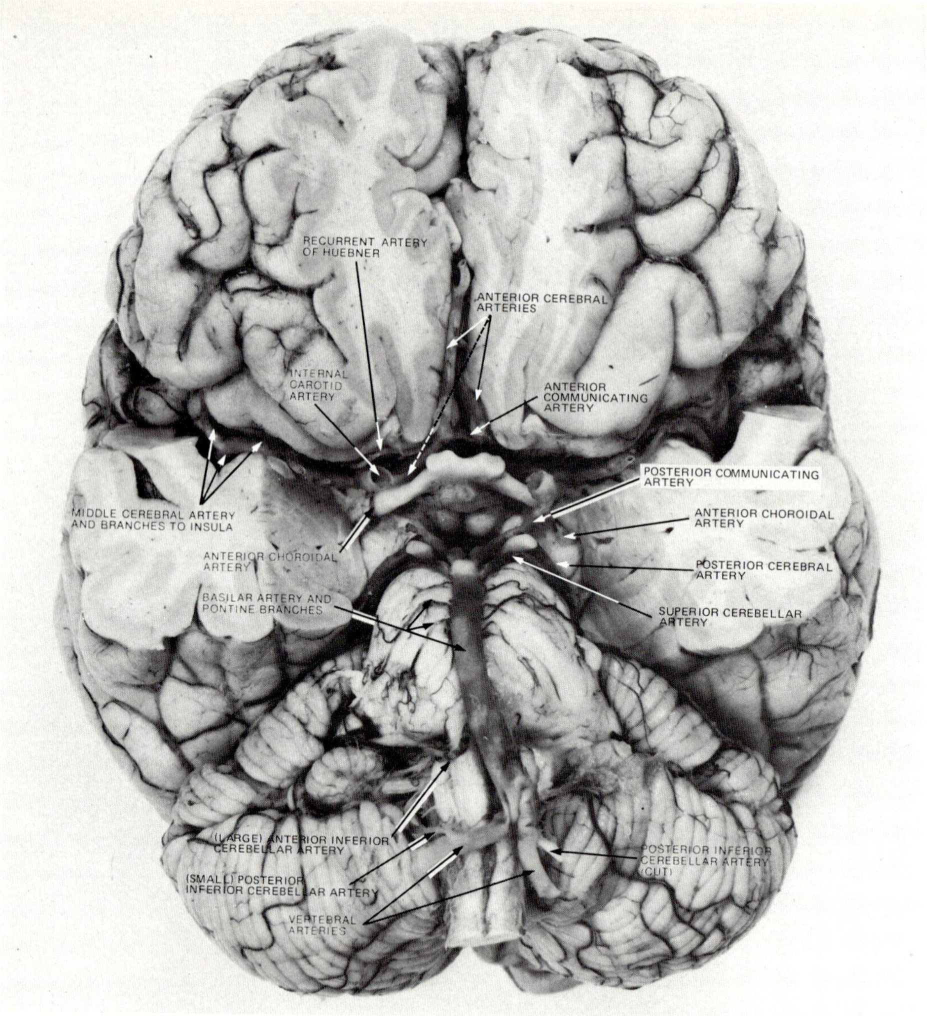

Fig. 14-5. The circle of Willis and main arteries at the base of the brain.

vessels is often very small, and the vessels forming the circle are usually affected by atherosclerosis at an early stage of the disease. Not uncommonly, the posterior cerebral artery on one or even both sides originates from the internal carotid (persistent fetal configuration), so that the posterior communicating vessel on that side is large, but the segment connecting the basilar artery with the junction of posterior communicating and posterior cerebral vessels is small. Occasionally, both anterior cerebral arteries are supplied from one internal carotid, the root of the contralateral anterior cerebral (between the internal carotid and anterior communicating vessels) being hypoplastic. The most reliable part of the circle of Willis is the anterior communicating vessel. For this reason, where there is occlusion of one internal carotid artery, it is uncommon to see infarction in the territory of the ipsilateral anterior cerebral vessel, whereas the middle cerebral territory is almost always infarcted. Thus, the circle of Willis is better in conception than in design.

The second level of collateralization consists of small branches in the subarachnoid space that pass from one vascular territory to the adjacent territory, bridging the boundary-zone or "watershed" area. These are most frequent between the middle and anterior vessels, the posterior territory being somewhat isolated. Cortical branches of any major artery tend to be nonanastomosing, so that if a branch is occluded proximally, it can only fill from across the boundary zone, not from adjacent cortical branches of its own parent vessel. The penetrating (intracerebral) arteries, though they have scanty capillary anastomoses, are functional end-arteries. If they are blocked, infarction occurs in their area of supply.

Almost invariably, neither the circle of Willis nor the subarachnoid collaterals are capable of compensating for occlusion of middle cerebral (or internal carotid) arteries. Sudden occlusion in young people (e.g., embolic), in whom the subarachnoid collateral circulation is poorly developed, causes an area of infarction corresponding to the anatomical area supplied by the vessel. In older patients with moderate atherosclerosis and better-developed collaterals, particularly if the infarction is of relatively slow onset and associated with preceding stenosis, the collateral supply may be sufficient to reduce the area infarcted considerably, although never to zero. In these circumstances, it is surprising that anastomoses between the intracranial and extracranial circulations, so prominent in subprimates, have become progressively less effective in man. It appears unlikely, in their reduced state in humans, that they make a significant contribution to cerebral blood flow except, infrequently, through the ophthalmic artery (retrograde flow) in patients with slowly progressive internal carotid stenosis.

Surprisingly, the preceding remarks apply only to the relatively *well*-supplied cerebral cortex and its underlying white matter. Other areas, supplied largely by median or paramedian penetrating vessels (the basal ganglia, thalamus, internal capsule, hypothalamus, and entire brain stem) are at much greater risk, since each perforating vessel is a functional end-artery with a few capillary anastomoses only; if it is blocked, there is no collateral circulation. The cerebellum appears to be in an intermediate position, since it has an effective collateral circulation at the subarachnoid level. Again, this merely reduces areas of infarction and does not prevent them.

Branches of the Internal Carotid Artery Prior to Its Bifurcation

The internal carotid originates at the level of the upper border of the thyroid cartilage and runs upward deep to the sternomastoid muscle and close to the jugular vein and the vagus. Rarely, a persistent hypoglossal artery connects it to the vertebral artery, but usually there are no extracranial branches. The internal carotid passes medially through the petrous temporal bone to the medial wall of the cavernous sinus, supplying small caroticotympanic vessels to the middle ear. In the cavernous sinus it passes forward, first slightly downward and then upward, to emerge through the dura near the anterior clinoid process. The cavernous carotid supplies a meningohypophyseal branch to the basal dura and the neurohypophysis, capsular branches in the floor of the sella with extensive bilateral anastomoses, and a branch supplying the parts of the third, fourth, fifth, and sixth cranial nerves within the sinus and the trigeminal ganglion. Embryological communications (which normally disappear) are the trigeminal and hypoglossal (otic) arteries, which connect the cavernous carotid to the upper part of the basilar artery.

In the subarachnoid space the carotid artery passes upward, posteriorly and laterally, to end beneath the anterior perforated substance by dividing into the anterior and middle cerebral vessels. In addition to supplying small branches to the optic nerve, optic chiasm, and hypothalamus, it produces four named branches:

1. The *superior hypophyseal* artery passes to the pituitary stalk and anastomoses with its fellow of the opposite side, producing the proximal plexus of capillaries for the pituitary portal system.
2. The *ophthalmic artery* enters the orbit through the optic canal and divides into the central artery of the retina (an end-artery), small muscular vessels, and the lacrimal, supraorbital, anterior and posterior ethmoidal, dorsonasal, and frontal arteries. These supply the contents of the orbit and adjacent skin regions and form numerous anastomoses with branches of the external carotid artery.
3. The *posterior communicating artery* (Fig. 14-5) is the embryological stem of the posterior cerebral vessel, supply of the latter being taken over by the basilar artery only at a later stage. Often, it persists as the main posterior cerebral supply, or it may be hypoplastic. It supplies branches to the posterior optic chiasm and tract, posterior hypothalamus and adjacent cerebral peduncle, and the anterior part of the thalamus (including the anterior nucleus and the anterior ventrolateral nucleus). The largest is the premamillary artery.
4. The *anterior choroidal artery* (Fig. 14-5) is the last branch of the internal carotid in about 75% of cases, but occasionally arises from the middle cerebral or posterior communicating vessel. It passes posteriorly above the uncus and enters the choroid plexus near the lateral geniculate body; but before reaching the latter, it supplies small branches to the optic tract, medial pallidum and adjacent internal capsule, uncus and adjacent amygdala (and occasionally to the anterior hippocampus), and parts of the ventrolateral midbrain. Branches arising at the level of the lateral geniculate body supply its lateral half, a small inferior part of the posterior limb of the internal capsule, and the choroid plexus of the inferior horn, with numerous anastomoses with the posterior choroidal vessels.

The Anterior Cerebral Artery and Its Branches

The anterior cerebral artery passes forward and medially toward the midline immediately below the anterior perforated substance, above the optic tract and chiasm. At the medial margin of the hemisphere, it is connected with its fellow by the anterior communicating artery (Fig. 14-5). This proximal portion provides minute branches to the optic nerve and chiasm, and 5 to 10 medial striate arteries arise from its superior surface to pass laterally and backward (i.e., retracing the path of the parent vessel), enter the anterior perforated substance, and supply the anterior inferior parts of the caudate and putamen and intervening internal capsule, pillars of the fornix, medial anterior commissure, anterior hypothalamus, and septum pellucidum. One of these striate arteries, the recurrent artery of Huebner (Fig. 14-5), may appear significantly larger than the others. Viewed from the lateral aspect, the medial striate arteries form the anterior third of a fan-shaped series supplying the caudate and putamen, the posterior two-thirds being derived from the middle cerebral vessel. All are end-arteries, with only capillary anastomoses. The anterior communicating artery is

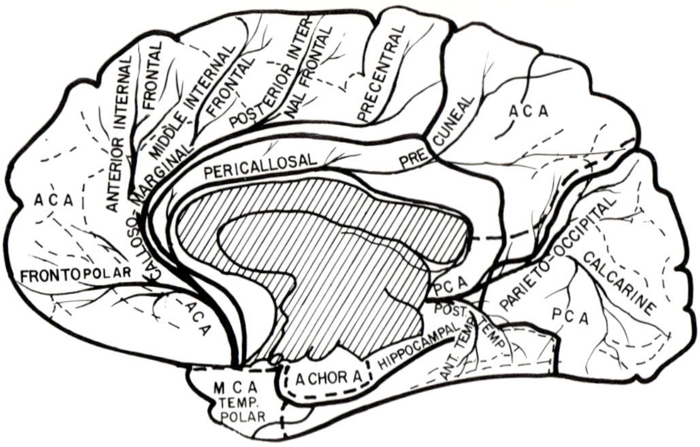

Fig. 14-6. Medial aspect of right cerebral hemisphere, showing arterial territories (heavy dashed lines) and major supply vessels. ACA, MCA, and PCA = anterior, middle, and posterior cerebral arteries respectively. A Chor. A = anterior choroidal artery; Temp. polar = temporal polar branch of MCA; Ant. Temp. and Post. Temp. = anterior and posterior temporal branches respectively of PCA.

short (1 to 3 mm) and may supply small branches to the region of the anterior hypothalamus and corpus callosum.

Immediately distal to the anterior communicating vessel, the anterior cerebral artery supplies local branches to the adjacent structures (Fig. 14-9) (septum pellucidum, fornix, corpus callosum) and then cortical branches (orbital and frontopolar) to the medial orbital surface, olfactory bulb and tract (Fig. 14-7), frontal pole, and anterior superior frontal gyrus. (For locations of structures see figures, Chap. 1.) In front of the genu the vessel divides into callosomarginal and pericallosal branches (Fig. 14-6), passing respectively above and below the cingulate gyrus and supplying the medial surface of the hemisphere and a 1- to 3-cm band of its superior surface, as far back as the parieto-occipital fissure. A small terminal branch of the pericallosal trunk may pass round the splenium and forward in the tela choroidea of the third ventricle, as far as the foramen of Monro.

The Middle Cerebral Artery and Its Branches

The middle cerebral artery passes laterally from its origin across the anterior perforated substance (Fig. 14-5), enters the sylvian fissure, and divides into two or more main cortical branches that pass posteriorly and upward on the surface of the insula. The proximal portion, as far as the main bifurcation, averages 1.6 to 2 cm in length; seven to ten striate arteries arise from this segment and enter the perforated substance as a medial and lateral group. The three to six small vessels of the medial striate series are in line with those from the anterior cerebral artery; they penetrate the medial third of the perforated substance and terminate largely in the lateral pallidum. The three to six lateral striate vessels are larger and occasionally arise from the bifurcation or even from cortical branches within the sylvian fissure. They turn backward toward the midline deep to the middle cerebral vessel, penetrate the lateral two-thirds of the perforated substance, and follow sweeping curves to supply most of the putamen, caudate nucleus, and intervening internal capsule (Figs. 14-9, 14-10). The largest may be sufficiently distinct to be termed the lenticulostriate artery. Although there are capillary anastomoses, these vessels function as end-arteries. The only other occasional branch of the proximal middle cerebral artery supplies the temporal pole (Fig. 14-7).

The large cortical branches of the middle cerebral artery arise in somewhat inconstant fashion deep in the sylvian fissure and emerge over the upper and lower opercula to supply the entire lateral and superior aspects of the hemisphere (Fig. 14-8), apart from a narrow superior strip supplied by the anterior artery in front and the posterior behind. In addition to supplying the cortex, these vessels supply the underlying white matter, the claustrum, and the lateral part of the amygdala.

Posterior Cerebral Arteries and Their Branches

The posterior cerebral artery originates by bifurcation of the basilar artery at the upper border of the pons (Fig. 14-5) and passes round the midbrain to reach the cortical surface at the lower (anterior) end of the parieto-occipital fissure. About 1 cm from its

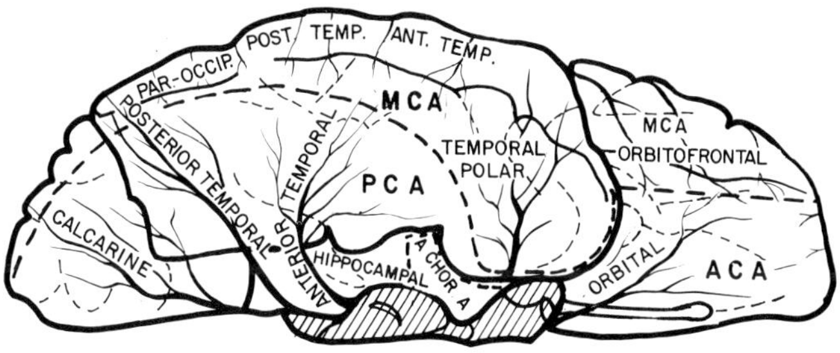

Fig. 14-7. Basal aspect of right cerebral hemisphere, showing arterial territories (heavy dashed lines) and major supply vessels. ACA, MCA, and PCA = anterior, middle, and posterior cerebral arteries respectively. A Chor. A = anterior choroidal artery. Par.-occip., Post. Temp., and Ant. Temp. = parieto-occipital, posterior temporal, and anterior temporal branches respectively of MCA.

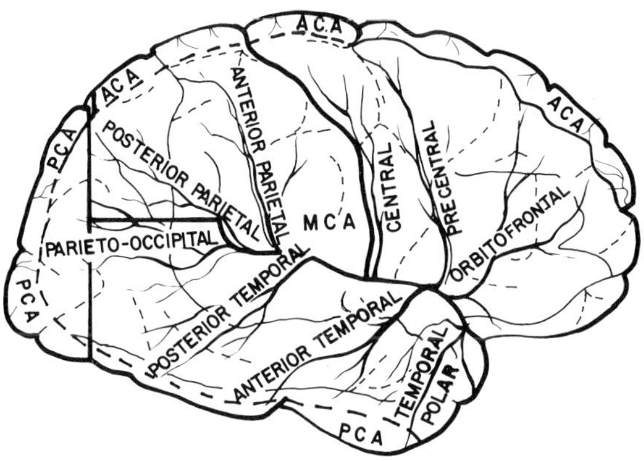

Fig. 14-8. Lateral aspect of right cerebral hemisphere, showing arterial territories (heavy dashed lines) and major supply vessels. ACA, MCA, and PCA = anterior, middle, and posterior cerebral arteries respectively.

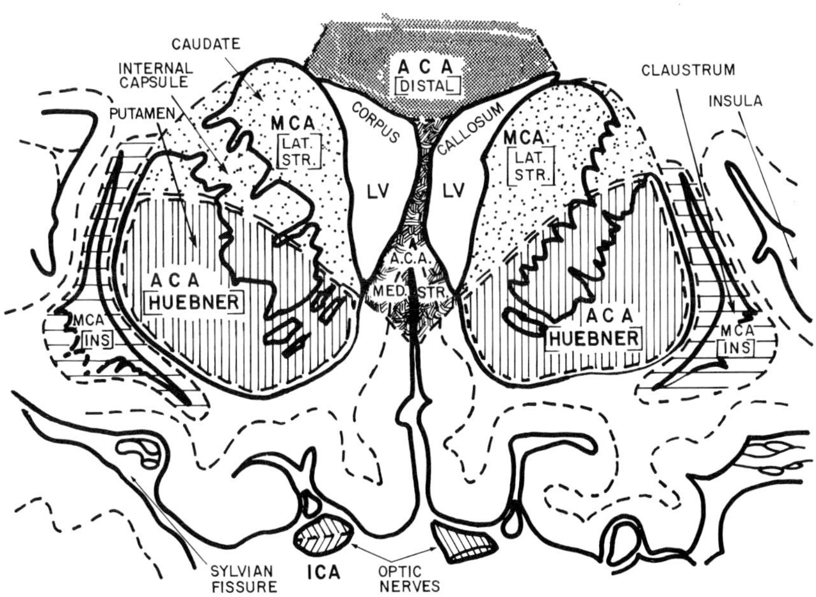

Fig. 14-9. Frontal section of hemispheres just anterior to the third ventricle, showing the blood supply of deep structures. ACA [distal], ACA [med. str.], and ACA [Huebner] = distal callosal, medial striate, and Huebner's recurrent branches respectively of the anterior cerebral artery. MCA [ins] and MCA [lat. str.] = insular and lateral striate branches respectively of middle cerebral artery. LV = lateral ventricle.

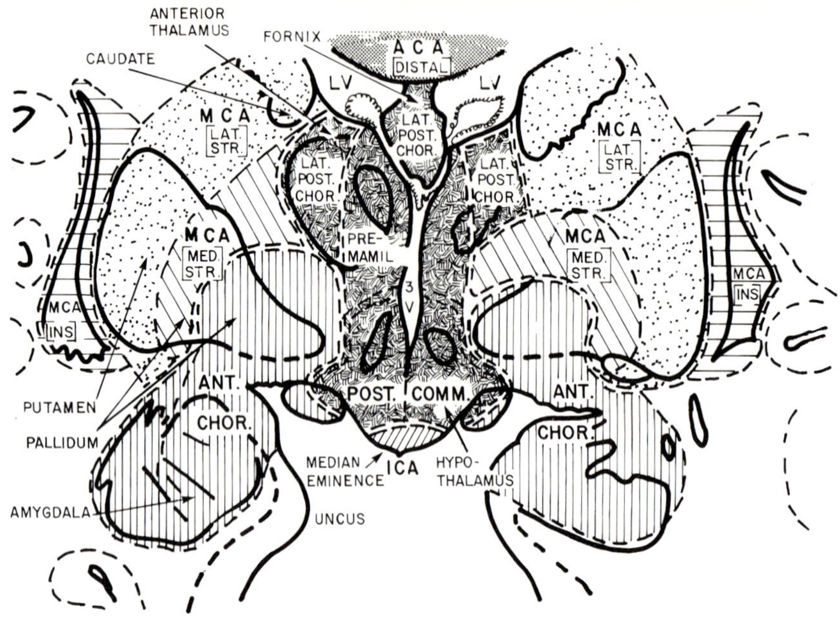

Fig. 14-10. Frontal section of hemispheres through the median eminence, showing the blood supply of deep and basal structures. ACA [distal] = distal callosal branches of anterior cerebral artery. MCA [ins], MCA [med. str.], and MCA [lat. str.] = insular, medial striate, and lateral striate branches respectively of middle cerebral artery. Lat. Post. Chor. = lateral posterior choroidal artery; Premamil. = premamillary artery; Post. Comm. = posterior communicating artery; ICA = internal carotid artery; Ant. Chor. = anterior choroidal artery. LV and 3V = lateral and third ventricles respectively.

origin, it is joined by the posterior communicating vessel (see p. 261).

At or close to its origin, the posterior cerebral artery gives off a large number of small branches (thalamogeniculate and thalamoperforating arteries), which penetrate the posterior perforated substance to supply the posterior hypothalamus and the ventral two-thirds of the middle and posterior thalamus, including the medial geniculate body and the medial part of the lateral geniculate body (Fig. 14-11). As the artery passes round the midbrain, small branches are supplied to the cerebral peduncles and deeper tissues of the ventral mesencephalon, and the medial and lateral posterior choroidal arteries are given off. The small medial choroidal vessels run near the midline in the tela choroidea of the third ventricle and supply the pineal body and a small superior part of the medial thalamic column. The much larger lateral choroidal vessels supply branches to the choroid plexus of the lateral and third ventricles and the dorsal thalamus, including most of the dorsolateral column and pulvinar (Figs. 14-10, 14-11). Other small branches from the posterior cerebral vessel supply the hippocampus (sometimes excluding a small anterior portion) and the splenium of the corpus callosum.

On the lateral aspect of the midbrain, the posterior cerebral artery gives rise to anterior and posterior temporal branches, which supply the cortex and the underlying white matter of the inferior surfaces of the temporal and occipital lobes (Fig. 14-7). The vessel terminates at the junction of the parieto-occipital and calcarine fissures by dividing into similarly named arteries, supplying the medial surface of the parietal and occipital lobes (Fig. 14-6) and a small strip of the superior surfaces adjacent to the midline. The field of supply of the calcarine vessel extends as far as the occipital pole.

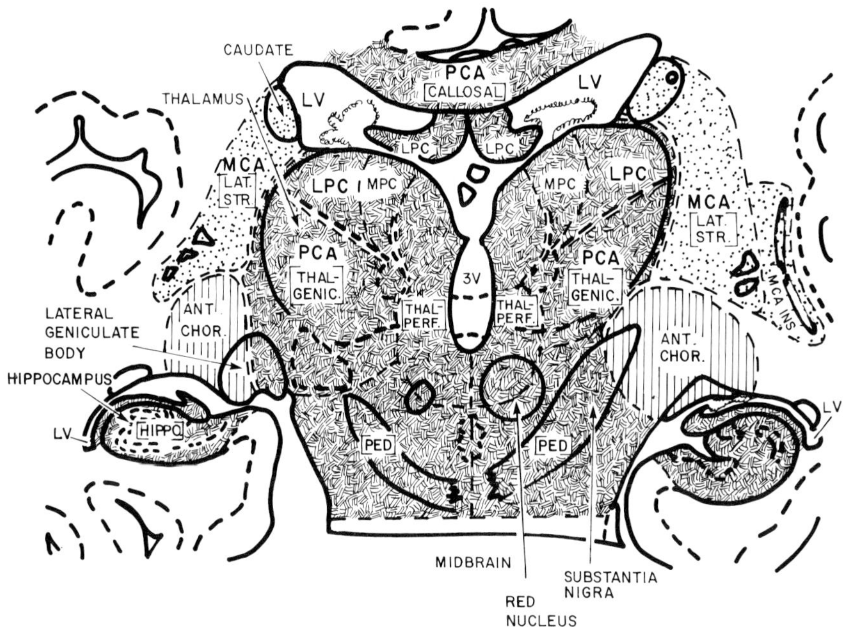

Fig. 14-11. Frontal section of hemispheres through midbrain, showing the blood supply of deep and midbrain structures. MCA [ins] and MCA [lat. str.] = insular and lateral striate branches respectively of middle cerebral artery. PCA [callosal], LPC, MPC, [Thal. Genic.], [Thal. Perf.], and [Ped.] = callosal, lateral posterior choroidal, medial posterior choroidal, thalamogeniculate, thalamoperforating, and peduncular branches respectively of the posterior cerebral and posterior communicating arteries. Ant. Chor. = anterior choroidal artery. LV and 3V = lateral and third ventricles respectively.

The Vertebrobasilar System and Brain Stem Arteries

The *vertebral artery* (the first branch of the subclavian) passes medially and ascends through the transverse foramina of the upper six cervical vertebrae to enter the cranial cavity through the foramen magnum. In its course through the neck it provides segmental branches to the spinal cord and spinal column, and deep muscular branches that anastomose with the external carotid system. There is frequently a perceptible narrowing and a sharp curve as the vessel enters the cranial cavity, which (like the irregular course of the internal carotid vessel) may exert a damping effect on the pulse pressure. The left vertebral artery is frequently larger than the right, and the basilar artery, which is formed by the junction of the vertebral arteries near the lower border of the pons, is often deviated in the opposite direction (i.e., to the right). In extreme sideways movement of the head, the vertebral artery tends to become occluded on the opposite side at the level of the atlantoaxial joint, and this occasionally produces transient ischemia. Within the cranial cavity (Fig. 14-12), the vessel supplies small perforating arteries to the medulla and branches to the basal meninges, the anterior spinal and posterior cerebellar arteries, and sometimes to a posterior spinal vessel.

The *basilar artery,* which is a single structure running in or near the midline from the lower to upper border of the pons, supplies small pontine branches, as well as the anterior inferior and superior cerebellar vessels and a small artery to the cochlea and labyrinth.

The *anterior spinal artery* arises from the medial aspect of the vertebral near its termination and passes medially and caudally to join with its fellow from the opposite side and form a single midline vessel. The anterior spinal vessels themselves, and the small arterial square they form with the distal segments of

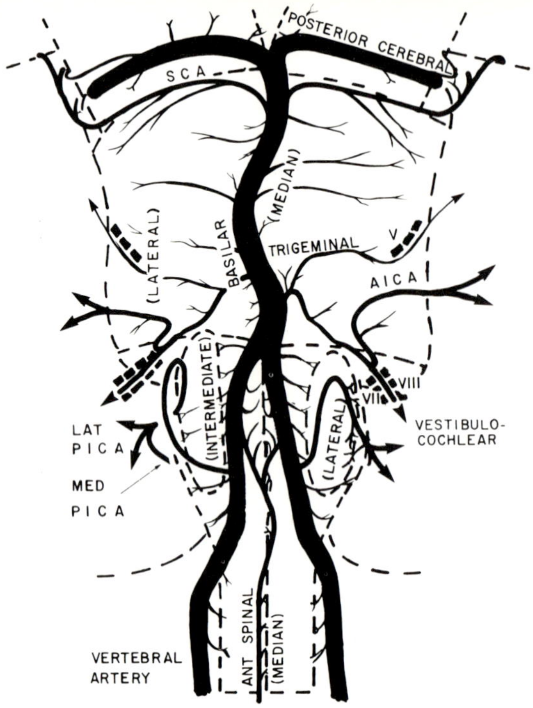

Fig. 14-12. Major arteries of the vertebrobasilar system. AICA = anterior inferior cerebellar artery; lat. PICA and med. PICA = lateral and medial cerebellar branches of the posterior inferior cerebellar artery; SCA = superior cerebellar artery; V, VII, and VIII = roots of fifth, seventh, and eighth cranial nerves respectively.

the vertebral vessels, provide perforating midline arteries to the medulla, the uppermost of which are inclined upward, supplying the tegmentum of the pons as high as the sixth nerve nucleus.

Other medullary branches arise from the vertebral artery: a middle group between the origins of the posterior inferior cerebellar and the anterior spinal vessels, which enters both the medial and lateral medullary sulci; and a lower group below the origin of the posterior inferior cerebellar, which enters the lateral sulcus along the emerging nerve rootlets. (The dorsolateral medulla is supplied by branches of the posterior inferior cerebellar artery.)

Arteries supplying the pons arise largely from the basilar artery, although some vessels entering the medulla are inclined upward, as previously indicated, and others entering the midbrain are inclined downward. Six to ten median pontine vessels enter the pons just lateral to the midline, and about an equal number of lateral arteries enter after branching on the anterolateral and lateral pontine surface. All arteries supplying the medulla, pons, and midbrain are functionally end-arteries. In about one-third of brains the artery to the labyrinth and cochlea originates directly from the basilar vessel and runs with the seventh and eighth nerves to supply vestibular and cochlear structures, with branches to the dura.

Cerebellar Arteries

The *superior cerebellar artery* arises from the basilar artery prior to its bifurcation and runs around the midbrain parallel to the posterior cerebral vessel, supplying small branches to the dorsolateral midbrain, especially the collicular region. It divides into medial and lateral cortical branches, which supply the entire upper surface of the cerebellum and underlying white matter, usually including the dentate nucleus.

The *anterior inferior cerebellar artery,* the smallest of the three cerebellar arteries, originates from the lower part of the basilar artery, and runs horizontally to the internal auditory meatus, in which it often makes a tight loop before running laterally on the anterior margin of the cerebellum. In about two-thirds of brains, the artery to the labyrinth and cochlea originates from this loop. The anterior inferior cerebellar artery supplies the anterior margin of the cerebellum, flocculus, choroid plexus of the lateral recess, and much of the middle cerebellar peduncle and roof nuclei.

The *posterior inferior cerebellar vessel* originates 1 to 2 cm below the union of the two vertebral arteries, passes upward, loops downward, and finally turns medially onto the vermis to form medial and lateral branches. In its course it provides penetrating vessels for the dorsolateral medulla and usually gives origin to the posterior spinal vessel. The medial terminal branches supply the inferior vermis and choroid plexus of the fourth ventricle, and the lateral branches supply the remainder of the posterior and inferior surfaces of the cerebellar hemispheres, including the tonsils. There are rich anastomoses on the surface of the cerebellum (although the penetrating vessels are functional end-arteries), and the sizes of the six cerebellar vessels are often inversely related. The posterior spinal artery usually arises from the posterior inferior cerebellar artery (although sometimes directly from the vertebral artery), divides into ascending and descending branches that supply minute vessels to the dorsolateral medulla, and anastomoses inferiorly with the posterior anastomosing arterial tract.

Arterial Supply to the Spinal Cord

Up to five longitudinal arterial trunks may be recognized in the subarachnoid space overlying the cord (Fig. 14-13). The most prominent is a midline anterior vessel. Less obvious are four posterior vessels, two lying medial and two (smaller and less constant) lying lateral to the dorsal roots. These are referred to as *anterior and posterior spinal arteries,*

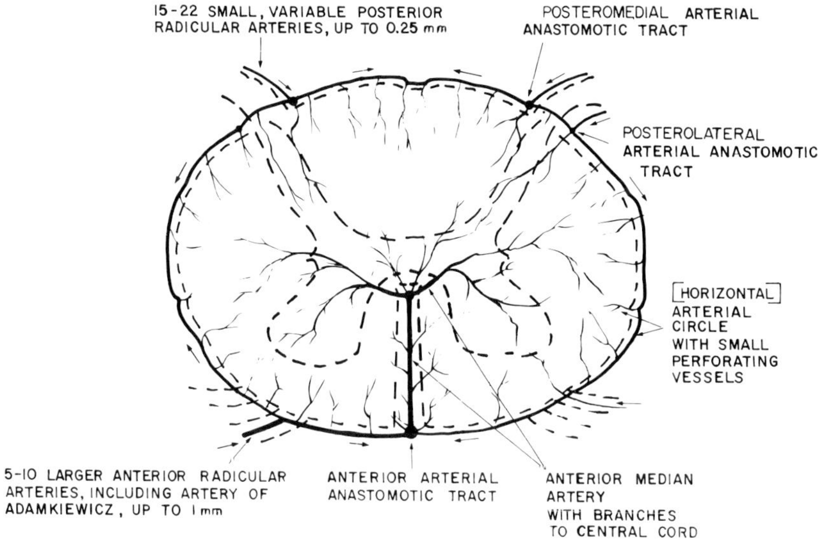

Fig. 14-13. Arterial supply to the spinal cord (transverse section).

or *anterior and posterior arterial anastomotic tracts,* and are continuous superiorly with the corresponding arteries arising at the level of the medulla. All longitudinal vessels are connected by horizontal branches, usually forming at least one complete arterial circle round each spinal segment.

Embryologically, the blood supply to this spinal arterial plexus arises from the radicular arteries that accompany each anterior and posterior nerve root, although there is a small contribution from the spinal arteries of the medulla. The radicular arteries arise from the extracranial vertebral arteries (C-1 to C-6), the ascending cervical branch of the subclavian (C-7 to C-8), the superior intercostal branch of the subclavian (T-1 to T-2), the intercostal vessels (T-3 to T-12), the lumbar vessels (L-1 to L-4), the ileolumbar vessel (L-5), and the medial and lateral sacral arteries (S-1 to S-3). However, the majority of the radicular arteries disappear or become so small that they supply only the root itself.

The adult cord has 5 to 10 anterior radicular vessels, 0.2 to 1.0 (rarely up to 2.0) mm in diameter, and 15 to 22 posterior radicular vessels, 0.2 to 0.25 mm across; the latter are evenly distributed up and down the cord. The distribution of the residual anterior vessels is irregular. In the cervical region there are usually two or three of equal size, the most constant being at C-6. In the upper thoracic region there are only one or two small vessels, whereas the lower thoracic and lumbar cord is supplied by one to three vessels, which usually are prominent. The most prominent usually lies between T-8 and T-12 (artery of Adamkiewicz) or (rarely) as low as L-3. If it is situated between T-8 and T-10, it often supplies the entire lumbosacral enlargement, although there may be a small vessel at L-5 or S-1. If it is situated from T-11 to L-3, there are usually no vessels caudal to it, but there are a few small radicular arteries between T-7 and T-9. There is no evidence for a consistent craniad or caudad flow in the longitudinal trunks. Blood probably flows both up and down from any point at which the trunk is joined by a radicular artery. Inferiorly, the anterior vessel terminates as the artery of the terminal filament (filum terminale).

The intraspinal arteries (Fig. 14-13) include a peripheral group arising all around the cord and passing toward the central gray matter, and a large central group that originates from the horizontal anterior median arteries. The latter originate from the anterior arterial anastomotic tract and run dorsally in the anterior median fissure. Their central branches radiate to the gray commissure, thoracic nucleus of Clarke, anterior and lateral gray matter, and to much of the anterior and lateral white matter. It is apparent that considerable overlap exists between the supply territories of the central and peripheral group. Vertical (intersegmental) anastomoses exist within the cord, but there appears to be little functional anastomosis between the central and peripheral arteries in spite of their territorial overlap. The capillary network in the white matter is uniformly sparse; that of the gray matter is markedly denser, especially in areas corresponding to cell columns.

Venous Drainage from the Brain and Cord

Venous effluent from the cortex and underlying white matter drains superficially to the subarachnoid space and divides chiefly into a larger superior drainage to the superior sagittal sinus and a smaller inferior drainage largely to the transverse sinus (Fig. 14-14). However, there are extensive superficial anastomoses between these two systems.

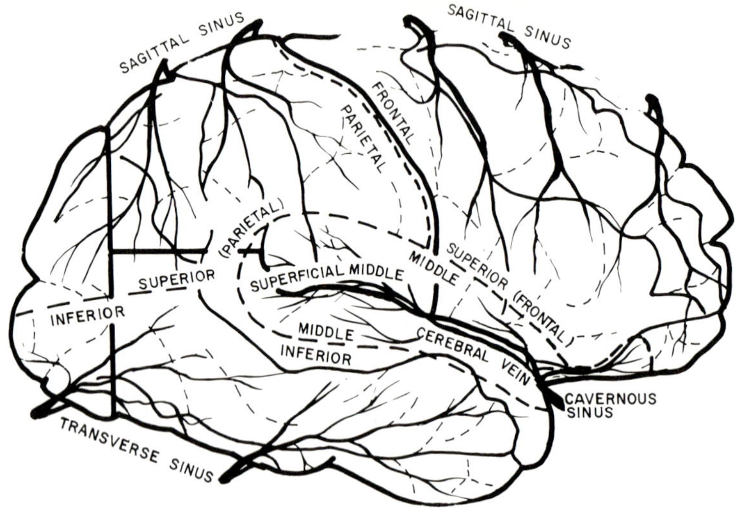

Fig. 14-14. Superficial venous drainage of (lateral) right cerebral hemisphere. Dashed lines approximately separate the superior (frontal), superior (parietal), middle, and inferior fields of drainage.

The superior drainage includes the upper part of the lateral surface and most of the medial surface of the hemispheres and consists of a frontal group of two to three trunks entering the superior sagittal sinus at right angles or posteriorly, and a parietal group of two to three trunks entering the sinus in an anterior direction (that is, against the flow). No vessels run directly from the occipital lobe into the sinus. All the superior draining veins enter the sinus proper and not the lateral lacunae and do so by crossing the subdural space.

The inferior veins drain the lower lateral and inferior surfaces of the temporal and occipital lobes, collecting into one to three trunks, whose terminal segments are frequently embedded in the tentorium before reaching the transverse sinus.

Between the superior and inferior draining veins is a small middle group, consisting of a *superficial middle cerebral vein* that drains the opercular regions into the cavernous or sphenoparietal sinus and a *deep middle cerebral vein* that drains the insular cortex, ultimately into the great cerebral vein of Galen. Occasionally, there are prominent single anastomotic veins from the middle group either to the superior sagittal sinus *(inferior anastomotic vein of Trollard)* or to the transverse sinus (*superior anastomotic vein of Labbé*).

The brain also has a deep internal drainage, with extensive anastomoses in the hemispheric white matter, connecting it to the superficial plexus. Deep veins discharge through the great cerebral vein, which originates below the posterior corpus callosum and joins the inferior sagittal sinus to form the straight sinus. In its course of about 2 cm, the great cerebral vein receives the internal occipital veins from the medial occipital lobes and small branches from the cingulate gyrus, posterior midbrain, and superior cerebellum.

The *great cerebral vein (vein of Galen)* (Fig. 14-15) originates by the confluence of four veins, the basal and internal cerebral of each side. The *basal vein* is formed lateral to the optic chiasm by the junction of the anterior cerebral vein (same course as the anterior cerebral artery) and the deep middle cerebral vein (from the insula). It passes backward above the uncus and round the midbrain to reach the great cerebral vein, receiving numerous small tributaries from structures at the base of the brain and often connected to its fellow of the opposite side by transverse communicating vessels. The *internal cerebral vein* originates just behind the foramen of Monro by the junction of vessels that drain the septal region, basal ganglia, internal capsule, and some of the deep white matter. It passes posteriorly in the tela choroidea, receiving tributaries from the thalamus and the choroid plexus. Beneath the posterior corpus callosum it joins its fellow from the opposite side and the two basal veins to form the great cerebral vein.

Drainage from the superior sagittal and straight sinuses reaches the torcula, where it is diverted into the two transverse sinuses, ultimately reaching the jugular veins. There is an extensive network of dural sinuses in the base of the skull, which have communications with the extracranial venous system through the orbit and the skull, with potential spread of infection into the cranial cavity.

The venous drainage of the spinal cord generally retraces the route of the arterial supply. Whereas arteries are more prominent anteriorly, the veins are more prominent posteriorly, where they form an irregular subarachnoid plexus. This plexus is drained by radicular veins that accompany spinal nerves to join the vertebral plexus.

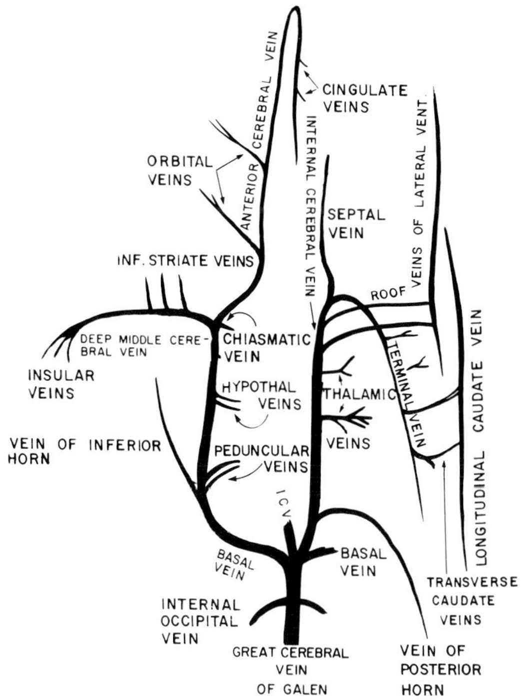

Fig. 14-15. Deep venous drainage of cerebral hemispheres viewed from above. For the sake of clarity, the branches forming the basal vein are omitted on the right, and those forming the internal cerebral vein are omitted on the left. ICV = internal cerebral vein.

PRECIPITATING FACTORS IN CEREBRAL INFARCTION

Atherosclerosis is widespread in males past the age of 40 and women past the age of 55 to 60, but cerebrovascular accidents only account for 16 to 20% of deaths in Western countries. Even severe degrees of stenosis (80 to 90%) may not cause ischemic changes in the territory supplied. Since uncomplicated cerebrovascular atherosclerosis per se does not lead to infarction, there must be other conditions that effectively occlude one or more large vessels, in association with, or in the absence of, atherosclerosis.

At autopsy, 25 to 35% of cerebral infarcts do not appear to be associated with total occlusion of any vessel. This figure might be diminished by more adequate examination of the carotid and vertebral arteries of the neck. However, even in series that have been so studied, there remain 10 to 25% of morphologically inexplicable cases.

It is possible to recognize four major situations that may lead to cerebral infarction, the first two and some cases of the third being associated with vascular disease, almost always atherosclerosis.

1. In situ thrombosis, which is commonly associated with atheroma, but occasionally with other vascular diseases (see p. 256).
2. Severe arterial stenosis (80% or more), complicated by other factors such as hemorrhage, myocardial disease, and the "steal" syndrome.
3. Embolic arterial occlusion (impaction by a thrombus, atherosclerotic plaque material, fat, air, and so on).
4. Venous or sinus obstruction.

In Situ Thrombosis

Thrombosis in major vessels is usually associated with disease of the vessel wall. In an overwhelming majority of such cases atherosclerotic plaques are found either in the cranial cavity or in the carotid or vertebral arteries in the neck. Rarely, thrombosis complicates other vascular diseases. Even more rarely, it may occur as a result of changes in blood coagulability in normal vessels (e.g., sickle cell anemia, polycythemia, or thrombocythemia following surgery). Spontaneous thrombosis in young women is allegedly associated with oral contraceptives, but the validity of this association rests on collecting data from a suitably large control group, and most published studies do not meet this criterion.

Severe Stenosis with Complicating Factors

A significant proportion of cerebral infarcts examined at autopsy during the acute stage do not appear to be associated with total vascular occlusion, although severe atherosclerotic stenosis is often present. In such cases, even a small fall in systemic blood pressure will severely reduce blood flow in the stenosed segment; such hypotension could occur physiologically during sleep or as a result of coronary insufficiency, which is common in the same age group. Particularly in the vertebrobasilar system, reversals in the normal direction of blood flow *(steal syndrome)* may cause ischemia. Such flow change may occur in thrombotic occlusion of the subclavian artery if it and its branches distal to the occlusion are filled by retrograde flow through the ipsilateral vertebral vessel via the numerous muscular anastomoses. Occasionally, other factors that impede blood flow or reduce PO_2, such as attempted strangulation, attempted suffocation, or carbon monoxide poisoning, may be implicated in the pathogenesis of stenotic infarction.

Embolism

Cerebral vascular emboli, as elsewhere, may be solitary or multiple, large or small. If they cause sudden large vessel occlusion, there has been no time for development of collateral circulation, such as may occur in association with stenosis. Embolism associated with stroke is usually thrombotic – from the

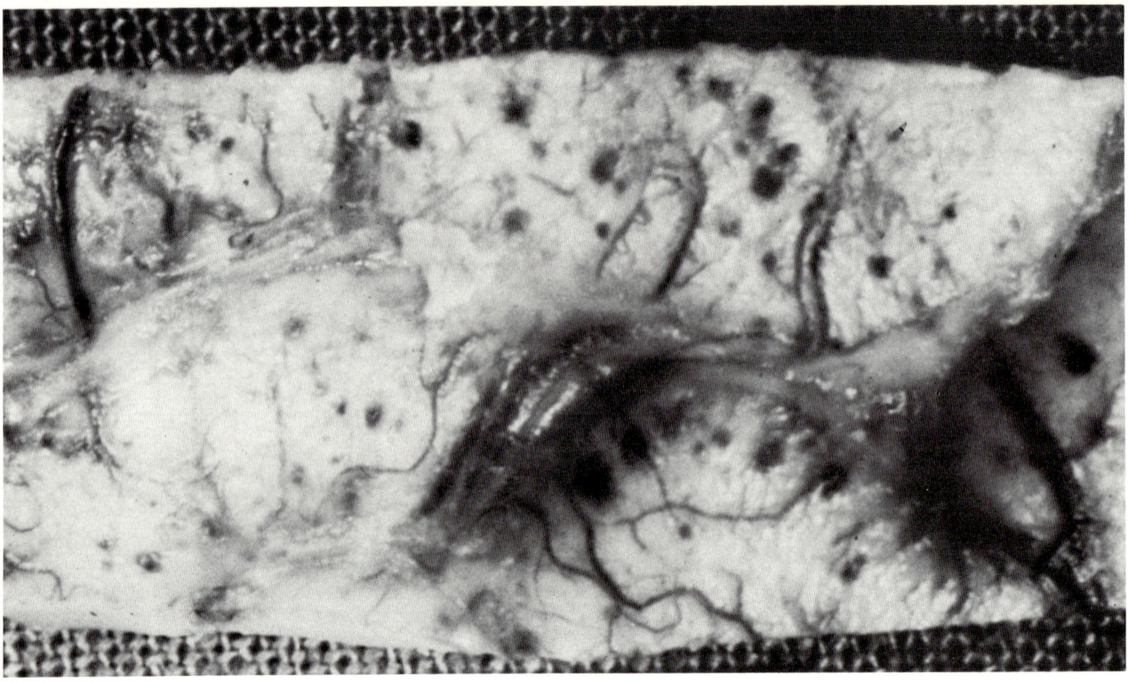

Fig. 14-16. Fat embolism. Close-up of brain surface with meninges, showing numerous petechial hemorrhages.

heart or carotid artery — or associated with dislodged atherosclerotic plaque material from neck vessels. Other types (not usually associated with a massive infarct) include fat or air embolism associated with injury and miscellaneous forms of emboli that may occur in open heart surgery.

Thrombi causing embolism may arise in the left side of the heart in association with coronary insufficiency or occasionally in association with rheumatic fever. In a few cases they arise from large vessels in the neck, although it may be that in situ thrombosis is a more common complication in these vessels. In some patients with a clinical history strongly suggestive of embolism, nothing is found at autopsy, and it has been hypothesized that in these patients, a thrombus lodging in a large vessel may (1) remain in situ, (2) break up into smaller fragments and pass into more distal branches (where it usually escapes detection at autopsy), or (3) be completely lysed by plasma fibrinolysin.

Occasionally, infected emboli from suppuration in the lung, bacterial endocarditis, or pyemia reach the brain. In most cases these are small and multiple and lead to miliary cerebral abscesses rather than to infarction. Lesions include multiple petechial hemorrhages, diffuse suppuration, abscesses, or, occasionally, mycotic aneurysm.

Fat embolism is associated with injury to bone, subcutaneous tissue, or fatty viscera. In this condition, globules of circulating neutral fat block precapillary arterioles or capillaries, especially in the brain, kidneys, or lungs. Symptoms usually do not appear until three to six days after injury and vary from minor headache and fatigue to coma and death, occasionally with such focal signs as hemiplegia. At autopsy, multiple petechial lesions are seen (Fig. 14-16), more often in white than in gray matter, perhaps because white matter capillaries have fewer anastomoses and are therefore more susceptible to ischemia if blocked. As noted in Chapter 12, fat embolism is associated with severe localized damage to the blood-brain barrier, and there is rapid development of perivascular hemorrhage and necrosis, with protein transudation (Fig. 14-17). Early perivascular demyelination occurs, and in patients who survive somewhat longer, small miliary foci of microglial proliferation, occasionally overt gitter cells, are seen.

Air embolism is an occasional complication of abortion, lung injury or lung operations, artificial pneumothorax, and damage to neck vessels and may even complicate neurosurgical procedures if the patient is in a sitting position. The prognosis depends on the amount of air, since death is due to foam formation within the cardiac chambers, resulting in a precipitous drop in cardiac output. If the patient is alive after 10 to 15 minutes, the prognosis is usually good, although permanent ischemic spasticity or blindness has been reported. Positive autopsy findings in the CNS in acute deaths consist only of gas bubbles in the superficial vessels (Fig. 14-18).

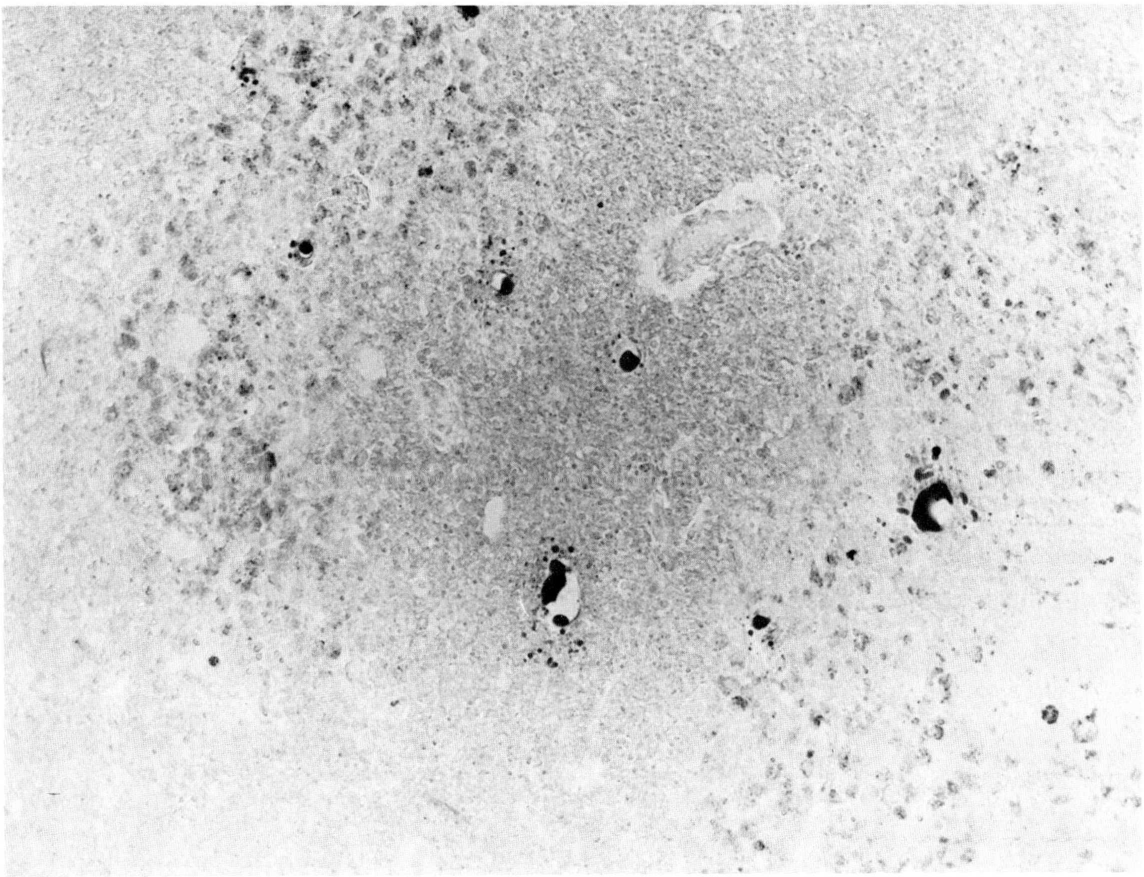

Fig. 14-17. Fat embolism. Vessels contain small globules of neutral fat (dark), and there are focal areas of hemorrhage and necrosis in the white matter, with normal tissue intervening. (Oil Red O, ×115.)

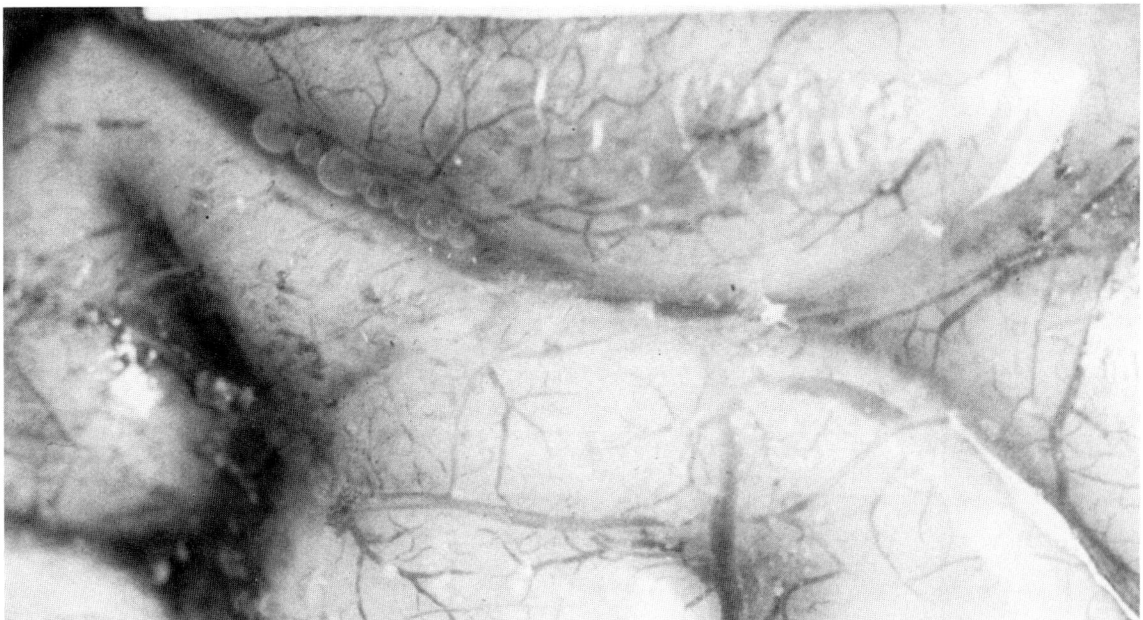

Fig. 14-18. Air embolism following insufflation of fallopian tube. The carotid and vertebral vessels were ligated before cutting to avoid artifact. A line of gas bubbles is clearly visible.

Venous and Sinus Thrombosis

The factors associated with thrombosis of the dural sinuses or cortical veins have already been noted. Central nervous system damage depends on the extent of the thrombus and particularly on the presence or absence of vein involvement. Total thrombosis of the superior sagittal sinus has been reported in experimental animals with no observable CNS damage at all and in human subjects with a minimal degree of subarachnoid and cortical petechial hemorrhage, confined to the upper medial margin of the hemispheres. If it spreads into the transverse sinuses, hemorrhagic infarction is increased; and if it involves superficial veins, the good collateral subarachnoid connections between the superior and inferior venous plexuses are ineffective, since the effluent from each individual emergent vein is blocked at the surface, and severe hemorrhagic infarction results. Thrombosis of the great cerebral vein rarely causes hemorrhagic infarction of the entire deep territory; changes are often confined to a small zone, including the posterior midbrain and thalamus. Other areas presumably drain superficially through anastomic vessels.

TRANSIENT ISCHEMIC ATTACKS

A transient ischemic attack is an episode of focal neurological deficit lasting less than 24 hours and sometimes only a few minutes. In such cases, transient hemiparesis or aphasia may be associated with temporary blindness, but the latter, on its own, does not constitute a transient ischemic attack unless other etiological factors are excluded. Most transient ischemic attacks occur after the age of 40. They are common after 50, being more numerous and more serious in males. An individual patient may have many such attacks, frequently considered as a warning of impending stroke. However, follow-up for two to three years suggests a completed stroke incidence between 18 and 63%.

There is said to be a strong positive association between transient ischemic attacks and abnormal ECGs that are presumed to be a result of coronary insufficiency. Many such attacks may therefore be on the basis of emboli arising in the heart. Others are known to be associated with stenosis of the internal carotid artery, low blood pressure, high blood pressure with hypertensive crises, or blood diseases such as leukemia or polycythemia. Angiographic findings may be normal and known predisposing factors absent; some transient ischemic attacks remain unexplained. Either the carotid or vertebrobasilar systems may be involved, and it is possible that a dislodged thrombus from neck-vessel plaques that are not readily seen radiologically accounts for some cases.

VASCULAR RESPONSES TO INFARCTION

Typical Response to Occlusion

Within the area rendered ischemic there is a dramatic fall in perfusion pressure, together with reduced PO_2 and accumulation of carbon dioxide and lactate, so that autoregulation and vasomotor control cooperate to produce maximal vasodilatation. At the periphery, this leads to the opening up of such collateral circulation as may be available through the subarachnoid vessels. For a varying width at the edge of the occluded territory, this collateral circulation will maintain at least structural, if not functional, integrity, so that changes are potentially reversible. In the center, unless the total occluded area is very small, the collateral circulation is ineffective and ischemia persists, causing irreversible tissue damage and complete loss of vascular tonus (a change from maximal vasodilatation to vasoparalysis). The vasoparalysis is almost always reversible, the smooth muscle cells maintaining their structural integrity. Thus, a central ischemic zone is surrounded by hyperemic brain, and according to the relative sizes of these areas, presumed infarcts sometimes show reduced, sometimes increased, regional blood flow.

If the occlusion is permanent, but the patient survives, the occluding material becomes organized, and distal vessels become atrophic except in the border area where they fill from collaterals. Collateral hyperemia persists for several weeks, but normal flow rates are ultimately restored except in the central infarcted area; its avascularity corresponds to the morphological appearance of cystic gliosis (see Chap. 10).

Responses to Restoration of Blood Flow

There are exceptions to this typical course of events. The occluding material may fragment and pass into smaller vessels, or may be lysed. In this case, normal perfusion pressure is suddenly restored to an area where there is vasoparalysis (Fig. 14-19) and therefore no effective vascular resistance. Flow is then directly proportional to perfusion pressure. However, since metabolism has ceased except in the vessel walls, effluent blood is high in oxygen and low in carbon dioxide and veins contain red arterial-like blood; the condition is termed *luxury perfusion syndrome.* This hyperemia may last for 7 to 14 days, but since vasoparalysis is reversible, the vessels ultimately respond to perfusion pressure and constrict to normal levels. Electrical activity is absent both during and after the hyperperfusion phase. Fragmentation of a thrombus and its passage to more distal vessels may lead to edema and perivascular hemorrhages in more proximal parts of the occluded territory, due to restoration of normal perfusion pressure in vessels with a blood-brain barrier sufficiently damaged to permit both protein and red cell loss. The more distal areas remain protected by the broken fragments lodged in smaller vessels. If the thrombus is lysed completely and rapidly, such changes may involve the entire occluded area.

Effects of Collateral Circulation

Such effects are not seen from opening up of the collateral circulation, since this is a gradual event with no acute rise in perfusion pressure. However,

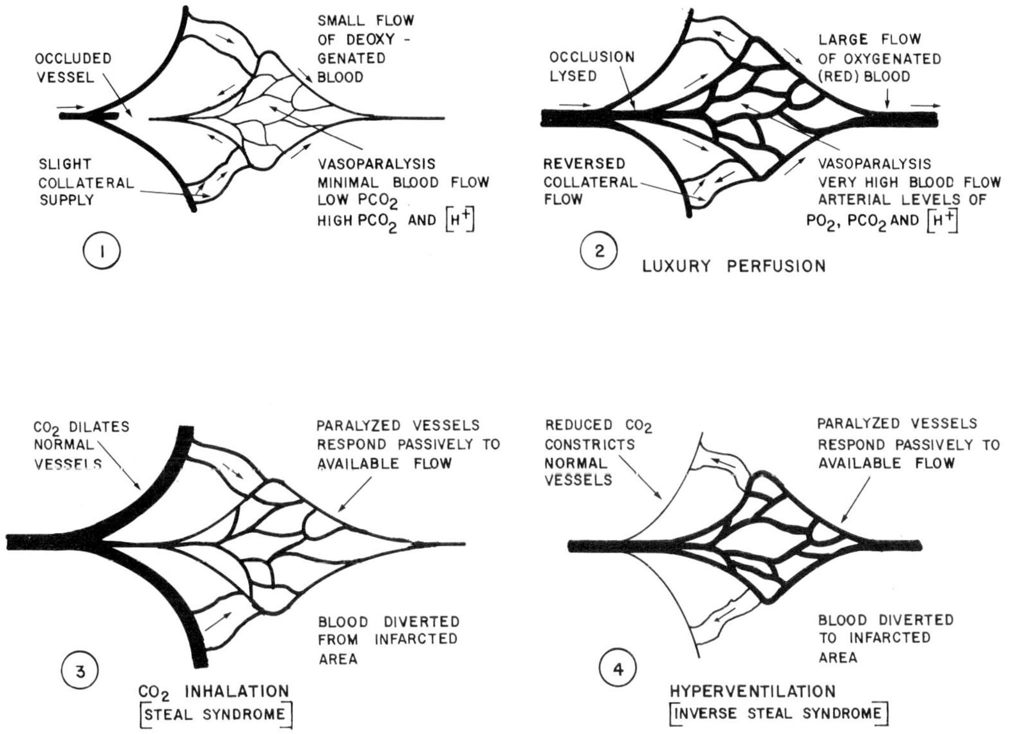

Fig. 14-19. Diagrammatic representation of occlusion of (1) a cerebral vessel and (2) the luxury perfusion syndrome that results if the occlusion lyses or fragments while vasoparalysis persists. Lower diagrams show the paradoxical effects of (3) hypercapnia and (4) hypocapnia on circulation through such an area.

there may be sufficient stasis and barrier damage due to collateral dilatation, especially within the margin of the occluded area, to cause a zone of cerebral edema surrounding an infarct, which spreads through adjacent noninfarcted brain for 24 to 48 hours. It is resolution of this edema, rather than increasing collateral supply to the infarct, that accounts for the partial improvement usually seen in strokes after the acute stage.

The existence of vasoparalysis in ischemic lesions nullifies any value that induced vasodilatation might have as a therapeutic measure (Fig. 14-19), since it dilates vessels only in healthy areas and therefore diverts blood away from the infarct (intracerebral steal syndrome). Vasoconstriction induced by hyperventilation, since it also affects vessels only in the normal brain, will paradoxically divert blood into the lesion (inverse steal syndrome).

Effects on Total Cerebral Blood Flow

In addition to the complicated and variable local vascular changes, there is evidence of a generalized decrease in cerebral blood flow during the acute stages of cerebrovascular accidents, the mechanism of which is completely uncertain. Involvement of the reticular formation is hardly likely in occlusion within the carotid system, unless it is secondary to edema and shift of the brain stem. It might be speculated that the connections of the infarcted areas are themselves less active than normal areas and therefore require less oxygen. Since many patients with cerebral infarction are stuporous or comatose, reduced cerebral oxygen utilization ($CMRO_2$) and carbon dioxide production might cause constriction of vessels as a result of normal vasomotor control.

METABOLIC CHANGES IN INFARCTION

The essential metabolic changes have already been outlined (Chap. 13). They include loss of adenosine triphosphate (ATP) and creatine phosphate (CrP) within 30 to 60 seconds, a dramatic fall in Po_2 to near zero, and accumulation of carbon dioxide, lactate, other acid metabolites, and inorganic phosphate. These changes are accompanied by an almost instantaneous failure of neuronal function and by electrical silence.

Enzyme histochemical studies have confirmed the persistence of necessary enzymes for aerobic and anaerobic metabolism for at least 12 to 24 hours after vascular occlusion. All enzymes investigated, namely, adenosinetriphosphatase (ATPase), succinic dehydrogenase (SDH), lactic dehydrogenase (LDH),

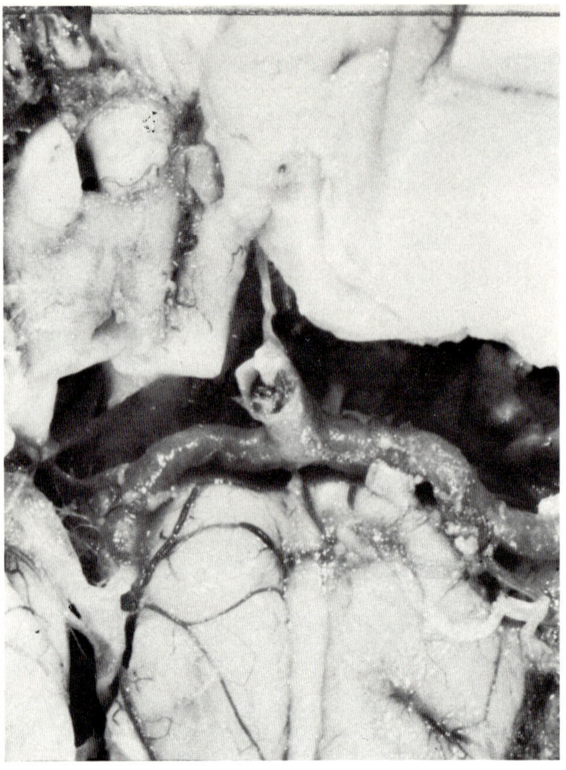

Fig. 14-20. Right internal carotid artery occluded by thrombotic embolus from the same vessel in the neck. Note that the thrombus extends along the anterior cerebral vessel only as far as its junction with the anterior communicating artery.

cytochrome oxidase, and nicotinamide-adenine dinucleotide (NAD^+) diaphorase, disappear at approximately the same rate, contemporaneously with obvious morphological disintegration (see p. 279). Investigation of these changes in animals, even in monkeys, is complicated by a much more efficient collateral circulation than in the human brain, including extracranial anastomoses. However, there seems to be no reason to doubt that the effects of human infarction are qualitatively similar, although perhaps more acute in onset.

More interesting changes in enzyme distribution and activity are observed in the marginal zone, where reactive rather than regressive changes are occurring. Thus, ATPase, SDH, and NAD^+ diaphorase show a moderate to marked increase within 24 to 36 hours; LDH shows a more gradual increase one to eight weeks following infarction. No changes are seen in the levels of cytochrome oxidase. Lysosomal hydrolases are increased in activity. The ATPase reaction is normally most intense in vessels and diffusely distributed in the neuropil; but at the infarct margin, it is increased in vessels (proliferation) and also in astrocytes and at the edge of gitter-cell (microglial or macrophage) cytoplasm. SDH and NAD^+ diaphorase reactions, normally intense in neurons and neuropil and slight in axons and oligodendroglial cells, show early intensification in the marginal zone, associated with globular axonal swelling and increased activity in the (previously unvisualized) astrocytes. LDH activity is also increased in macrophages within a week and in astrocytes within eight weeks.

Thus, there are two types of marginal reaction: an early, temporary one, reflecting the globular accumulation of axoplasm (incoming axons) and manifested by SDH and NAD^+ diaphorase activity; and a longer lasting change, reflecting an increase in general metabolic activity in macrophages and astrocytes, including an apparent significant switch to aerobic metabolism in the latter.

DISTRIBUTION AND SYMPTOMATOLOGY OF INFARCTS

The two major aspects of any CNS reaction are its distribution and its morphological characteristics. In a consideration of the distribution of infarction, the necessity for an adequate knowledge of vascular neuroanatomy becomes apparent.

Infarcts of Cerebral Hemispheres

Since the distribution of the supratentorial vessels is relatively constant, the clinical picture associated with their occlusion is more reliable and uniform. Thus, occlusion of the anterior cerebral vessels leads to lower limb monoplegia, often with cortical sensory disturbance; or if bilateral (as it often is with severe atherosclerosis), it leads to spastic paraplegia. Occlusion of the internal carotid or the middle cerebral vessel (Fig. 14-20) leads to hemiplegia, more marked in the arm than the leg, cortical sensory disturbances (hemianesthesia), aphasia if the dominant hemisphere is involved, and complete or partial hemianopsia (Figs. 14-21 to 14-24). Involvement of the posterior cerebral artery (Fig. 14-25) may lead to homonymous hemianopsia, with sparing of the macular region (because of middle cerebral collaterals), hemiparesis, disturbances of sensation, and alexia if the dominant hemisphere is involved. For detailed accounts, textbooks of clinical neurology should be consulted.

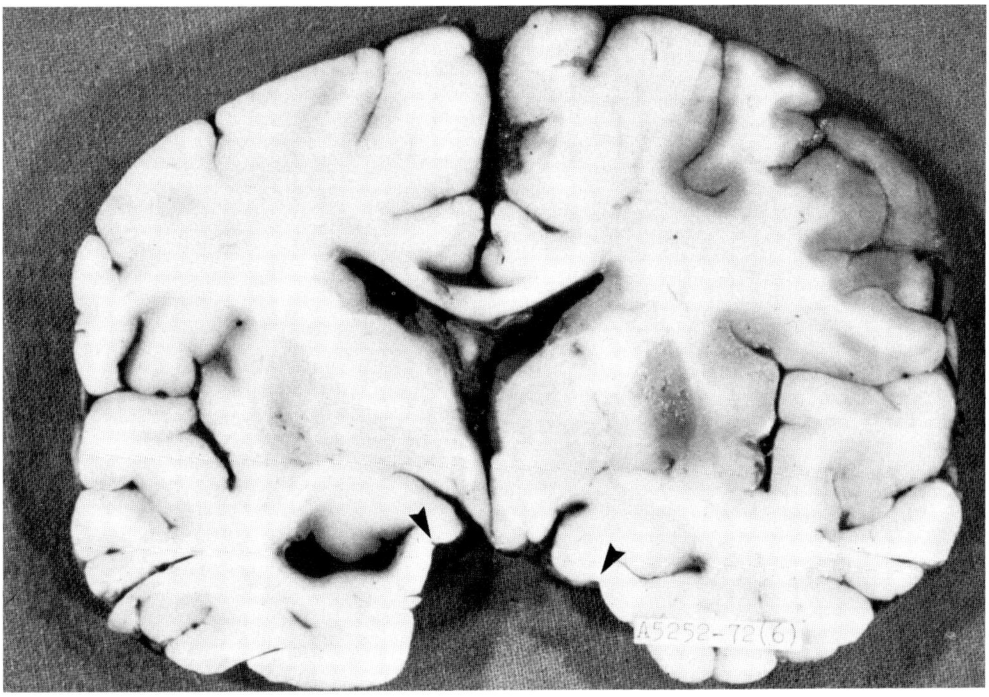

Fig. 14-21. Recent infarction of left middle cerebral arterial territory (right in photograph). Infarcted cortex and basal ganglia are dark and somewhat swollen, and there is an early left-to-right midline shift with bilateral uncal herniation (arrows), due to edema.

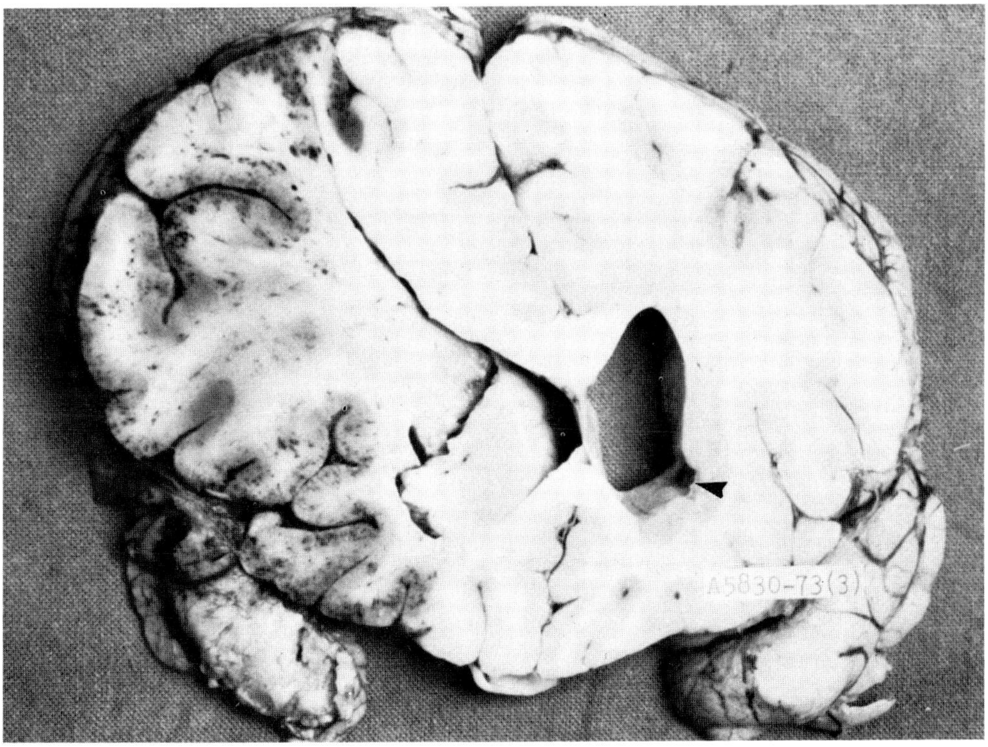

Fig. 14-22. Infarction of right middle cerebral arterial territory (left in the photograph). The infarcted cortex is dark and shows radial hemorrhages, occasionally confluent. Infarcted white matter and basal ganglia are soft and readily separate from adjacent noninfarcted (but edematous) tissue. The lower anterior basal ganglia, supplied by the anterior cerebral artery, survive. A small remote infarct is present in the left caudate nucleus (arrow).

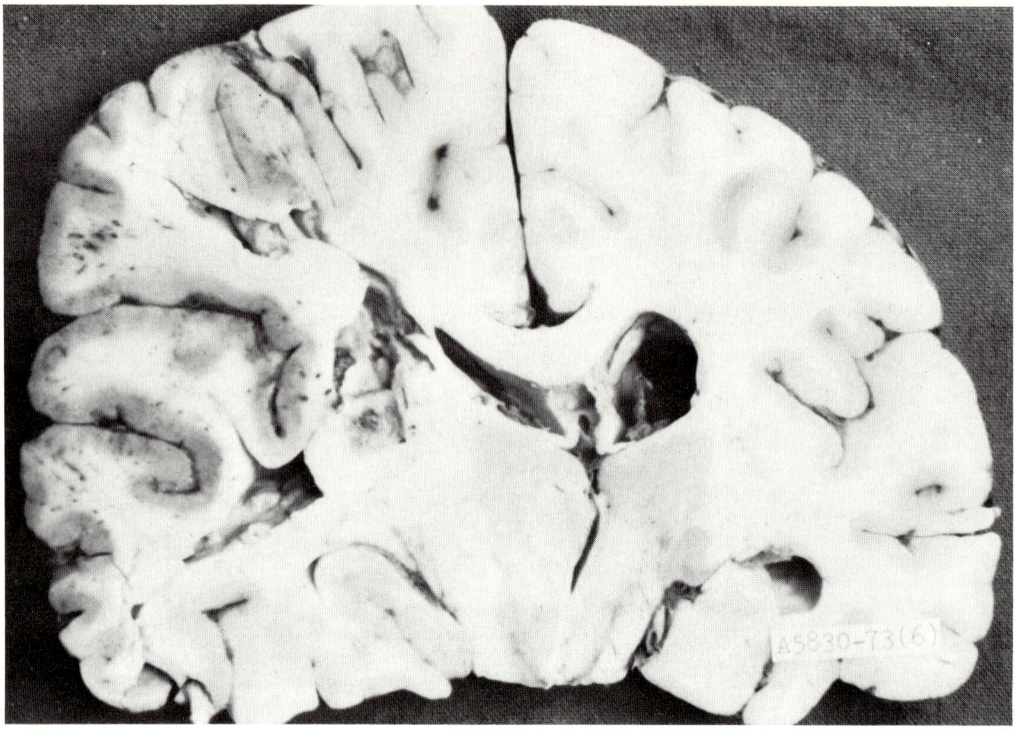

Fig. 14-23. Infarction of right middle cerebral arterial territory (same patient as in Fig. 14-22). This more posterior section shows the preservation of the thalamus and lower internal capsule, as well as of the medial and basal cortex, none of which is supplied by the middle cerebral vessel.

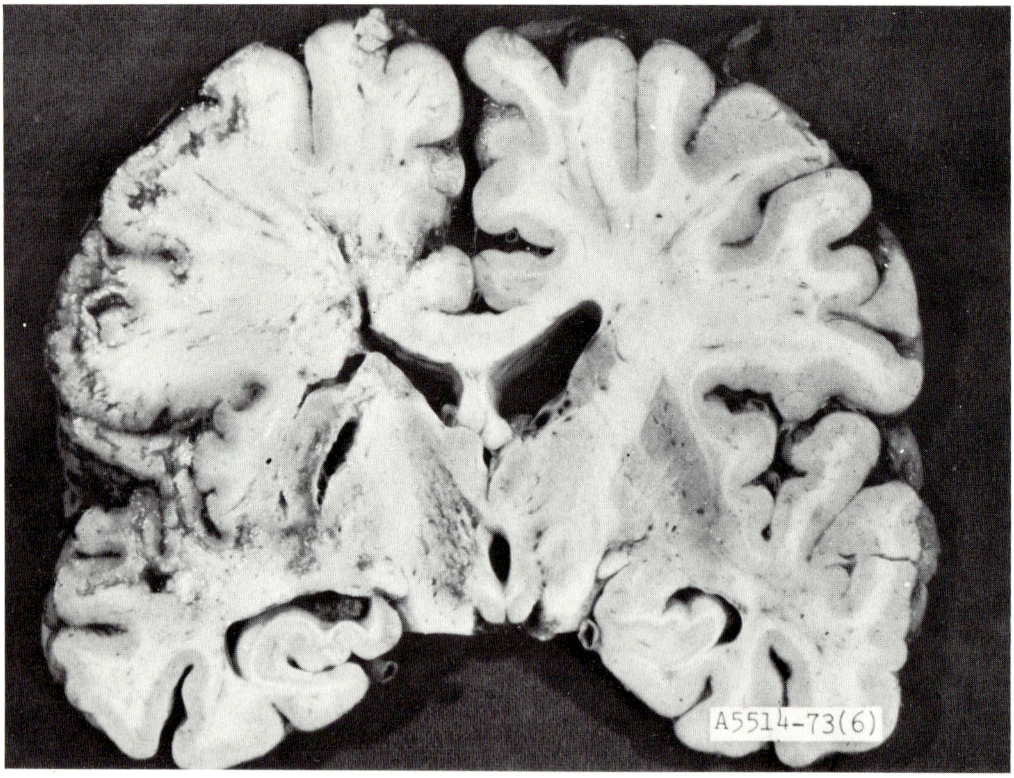

Fig. 14-24. Older infarction of right middle cerebral arterial territory, showing early cystic change and liquefaction in cortical areas, around the lateral angle of the lateral ventricle, and in the basal ganglia. Edema has resolved, and there is no residual midline shift, but infarction of part of the thalamus and subthalamus shows that the posterior cerebral or posterior communicating penetrating branches were compressed or distorted by edema in the acute stage.

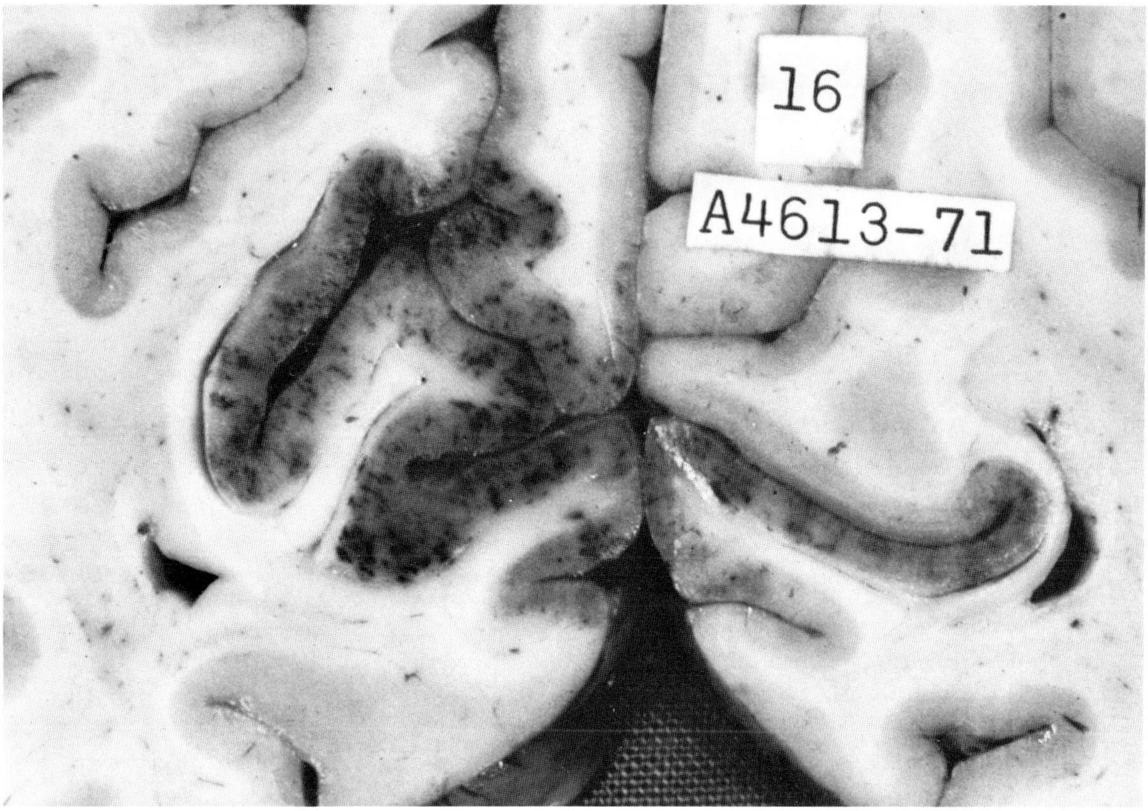

Fig. 14-25. Recent occlusion of both posterior cerebral arteries (by bilateral uncal herniation in a head injury). The calcarine and pericalcarine cortex, having the highest metabolic requirements, shows multiple perivascular hemorrhages.

Infarcts of Cerebellum and Brain Stem

The clinical significance of occlusion of the cerebellar arteries lies more in the small branches they supply to the brain stem than in the loss of blood supply to the cerebellum.

Superior Cerebellar Artery

Occlusion of the superior cerebellar artery by atherosclerosis or embolism is rare, but it may be blocked in basilar thrombosis. It is susceptible to compression by uncal herniation. The features include cerebellar dysfunction on the same side and contralateral sensory loss. They are associated with infarction of the superior cerebellar cortex, dentate nucleus, and superior cerebellar peduncle; of lateral and spinal lemniscus and part of the medial lemniscus; and of the adjacent dorsolateral midbrain and upper pons.

Anterior Inferior Cerebellar Artery

Occlusion of the anterior inferior cerebellar artery is rare, though it is occasionally damaged in operations for the removal of acoustic neurilemomas. The clinical features include cerebellar dysfunction on the same side, loss of the sensations of pain, temperature, and light touch on the same side of the face, facial paralysis, deafness, Horner's syndrome, and incomplete pain and temperature loss on the opposite side of the body. These features are due to involvement of the flocculus and anterior margin of the cerebellar cortex; the caudal part of the middle and the inferior cerebellar peduncles; part of the spinal tract and nucleus of the fifth nerve; the seventh and eighth cranial nerves and cochlear nuclei; some spinocerebellar and spinothalamic fibers; and part of the reticular formation.

Posterior Inferior Cerebellar Artery

The posterior inferior cerebellar artery is the most commonly involved cerebellar vessel in thrombotic and embolic phenomena. Symptoms (lateral medullary syndrome) may include dizziness, difficulty in gait with falling to the affected side, nystagmus, dysphagia, Horner's syndrome on the same side, and loss of pain and temperature sense on the same side of the face and the opposite side of the body. The cerebellar cortex is often spared because of free anastomoses from the opposite vessel and the superior cerebellar artery. Among the structures involved

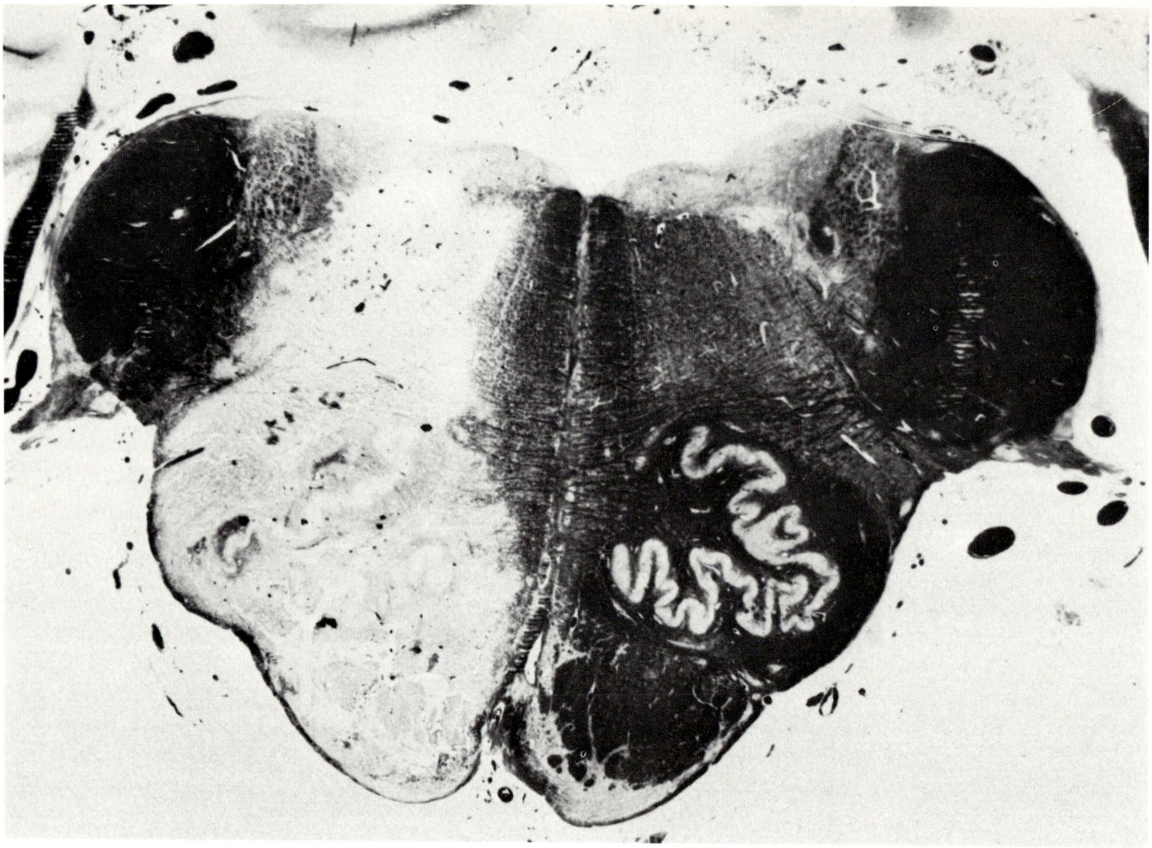

Fig. 14-26. Medullary infarction due to occlusion of the vertebral artery by atheromatous thrombosis. Blockage of the penetrating and posterior inferior cerebellar vessels has produced a combined medial and lateral medullary syndrome (see text).

are the descending tract and nucleus of the fifth nerve; the spinal vestibular nucleus with its fibers to the medial longitudinal fasciculus; the ambiguus nucleus; fibers of the ninth and tenth nerves within the brain stem; autonomic pathways such as the central tegmental tract; lateral spinothalamic and spinocerebellar fibers; olivocerebellar fibers; and the ventral part of the inferior cerebellar peduncle.

Vertebral and Basilar Arteries

Although the small perforating branches directly supplying the brain stem are not usually themselves involved by atherosclerosis or embolism, disease or thrombosis of the vertebral or basilar arteries may cause their occlusion at source, leading to brain stem ischemia; as has been noted, each is functionally an end-artery. The most common syndrome associated with thrombosis of the vertebrobasilar system is the medial medullary syndrome (Fig. 14-26) characterized by contralateral hemiplegia, hemianesthesia, and ipsilateral weakness and atrophy of the tongue. The major structures involved (supplied by paramedian perforating branches of the vertebral arteries) are the pyramid, medial lemniscus, nucleus and emergent fibers of the twelfth cranial nerve, and parts of the inferior olive and reticular formation.

If infarction occurs in the pons (supplied by the paramedian and lateral branches of the basilar vessel), it is usually confined to the basal part (Fig. 14-27). It may be relatively asymptomatic or may involve pyramidal fibers, resulting in hemiplegia. Such lesions seem particularly common in diabetic patients. Sparing of the tegmentum is presumably due to its being supplied largely by ascending and descending branches of the medullary and midbrain vessels.

Infarcts of Spinal Cord

Direct involvement of the intraspinal or superficial spinal arteries is an unusual cause of infarction of the spinal cord. These vessels may occasionally show atherosclerotic, syphilitic, or inflammatory lesions, but embolism appears to be very rare. They may also be locally compressed by disc protrusion, osteoarthritic changes of the epiphyseal or intervertebral joints, or other mass lesions.

More often, cord infarction is associated with vascular changes in more remote vessels, such as atherosclerosis, syphilis, or dissecting aneurysm of

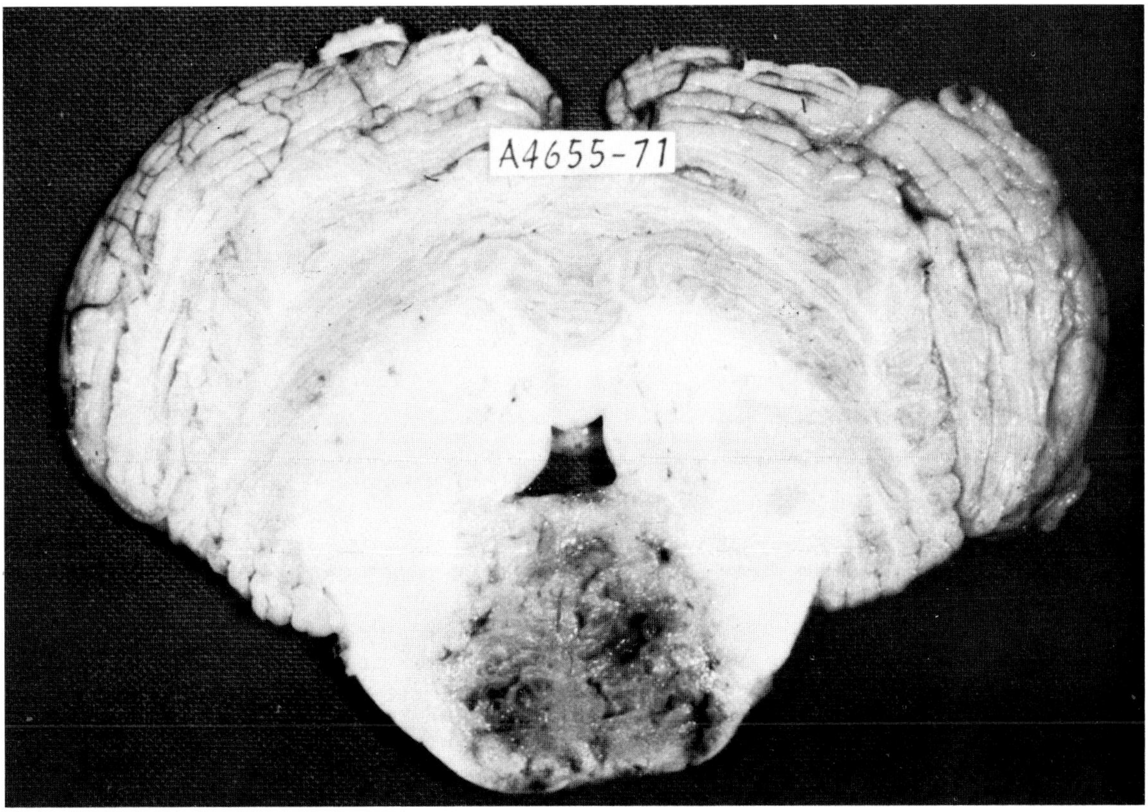

Fig. 14-27. Pontine infarction associated with basilar artery thrombosis (atherosclerotic).

the aorta; changes following aortic surgery; or thrombosis or embolism involving the aorta or iliac vessels. Surgical occlusion lasting over 15 to 20 minutes is particularly dangerous above the level of the renal arteries, since it cuts off supply through the artery of Adamkiewicz and its collateral branches, causing ischemic lesions from about T-8 to T-10 downward. Occlusion above the left subclavian artery may lead to ischemic lesions from the midcervical cord downward, most severe in the lumbosacral region.

Cord infarction varies both in longitudinal and transverse extent. Total transverse infarction (effectively, transection of the cord) is common, especially in the lumbosacral region. Anterior infarction, which spares only the posterior columns and dorsal horns, is also frequently seen. Lesser degrees of anterior softening involving only the central area of the cord are uncommon, and purely posterior infarction is rare. As in the brain, the gray matter is more susceptible than the white, and the ischemic vulnerability of neurons (in decreasing order) appears to be alpha motoneurons, Renshaw cells, gamma motoneurons, and dorsal horn cells. Severe anterior and descending degeneration (see Chap. 21) is seen beyond the segments of infarction.

The symptomatology of spinal cord infarction is variable. There may be complete interruption of long fibers with clinical features similar to transection or transverse myelitis. Other combinations of sensory, upper motoneuron, lower motoneuron, and sphincter disturbances, not always symmetrical, may be seen. If the lesions are restricted, they may be only an incidental autopsy finding.

MORPHOLOGY OF INFARCTS

Gross Changes

Gross changes are usually not apparent within 6 hours of occlusion, but between 6 and 48 hours, infarcted gray matter and infarcted white matter both soften and swell. The gray becomes darker and slightly brownish; the white becomes, if anything, even more pale. After about 48 hours, gray and white matter, but especially the latter, become soft and mushy, with a marked tendency to artifactual fragmentation, clefting, and failure to hold normal shape. Early liquefaction or cavitation can usually be seen between two and three weeks, the spaces being irregular and ragged. After a few months, the final stage of cyst formation is reached, the lesion being converted to unilocular or multilocular cysts, traversed and separated by fibrovascular (mesenchymal) strands and lined by a smooth, pale cream or brown-stained wall. There is some increase in consistency due to fibrillary gliosis and thus cystic gliosis is present.

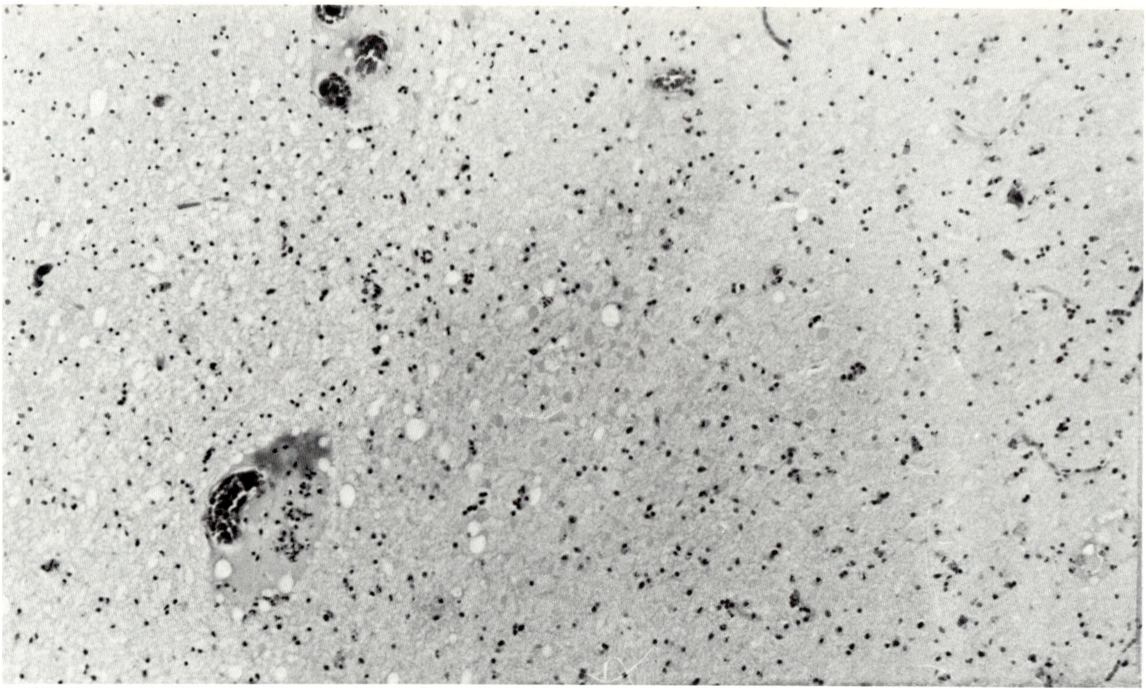

Fig. 14-28. Early infarct (24 to 48 hours). A pool of plasma with a few extravasated red cells surrounds a distended capillary. Neutrophils have escaped into the surrounding brain, oligodendroglial cells are pyknotic, and there is spongiosis and rarefaction. (H & E, ×115.)

Microscopic Changes

Microscopically, the earliest changes are seen in neurons, usually within 6 hours. These include not only ischemic necrosis, but various types of sclerosis and swelling (see Chap. 10). Between 6 and 24 hours, neuronal necrosis progresses, and by about 24 hours (Fig. 14-28), neurons are either pyknotic or disintegrating, oligodendroglial cells show swelling and nuclear pyknosis, and astrocytic processes are fragmented. There is proliferation of endothelial cells, and some vessels (especially veins) are occluded by a thrombus containing leukocytes. Small numbers of neutrophils have left the vessels and are migrating among disintegrating parenchyma. Myelin-staining begins to deteriorate at 8 to 12 hours. Within one to two days, myelin and axons become swollen and beaded, and the infarct is sharply demarcated from surrounding viable, but edematous, tissue. Mitotic activity may be seen at the margin in endothelial and microglial cells.

After about five days (Fig. 14-29), there is virtual disappearance of neural and glial cells from the infarcted area (though vessels are still prominent), and increasing numbers of actively phagocytic (gitter) cells, containing PAS-positive lipid, are present. The edge of the infarct is intensely active, with proliferation of endothelial cells and macrophages and early hypertrophy and hyperplasia of astrocytes. From the fifth to the thirtieth day is a phase of resorption of necrotic tissue, with prominent endothelial, phagocytic, and fibroplastic activity and progressive deposition of collagen and glial fibers. The infarct liquefies during this stage.

The period from four weeks up to three to six months shows a continuation of resorptive changes at a gradually decreasing tempo, gitter cells becoming fewer and endothelial hyperplasia less apparent. Glial fibrils are laid down in the walls of the cavities (Fig. 14-30), following which the astrocytes cease to divide and revert to a resting stage, in which their cytoplasm is again inapparent.

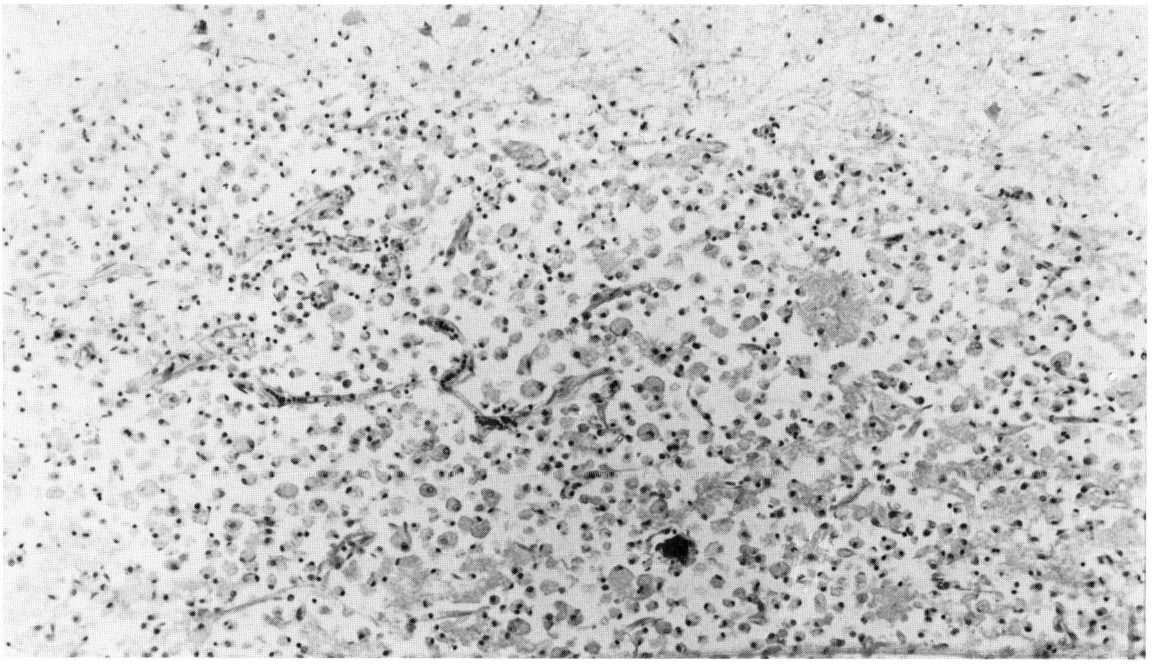

Fig. 14-29. Early infarct (5 to 7 days), showing total disintegration of neuropil, residual vessels, large numbers of gitter cells, and early astroglial hypertrophy at the periphery. (H & E, X115.)

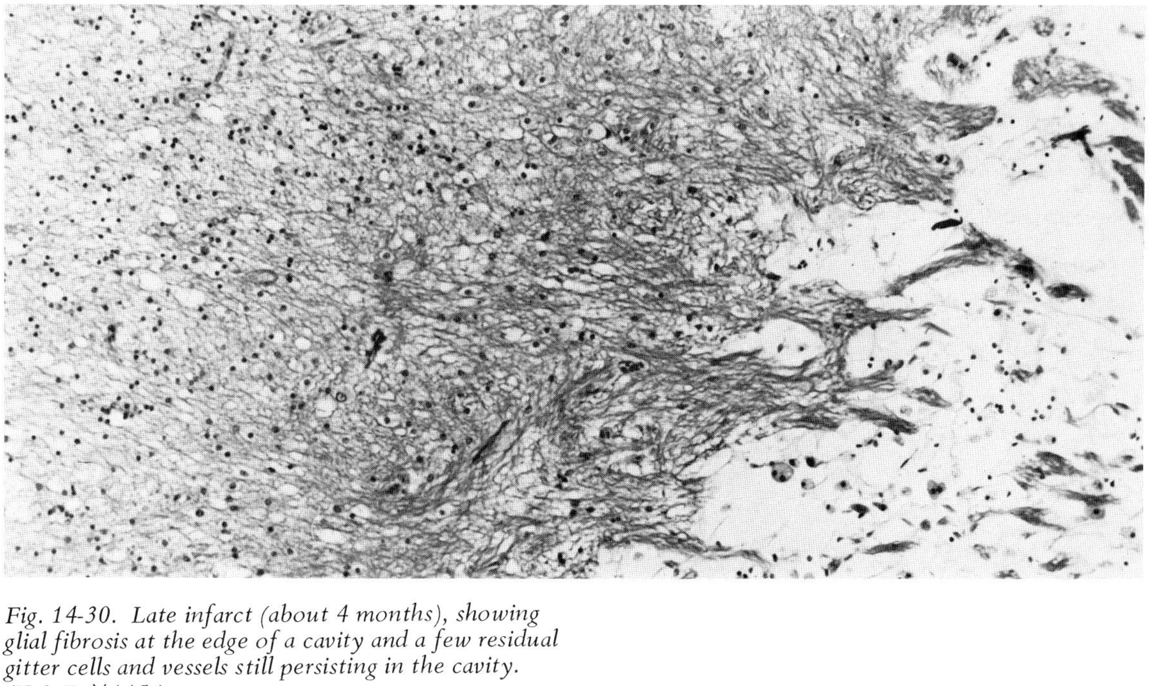

Fig. 14-30. Late infarct (about 4 months), showing glial fibrosis at the edge of a cavity and a few residual gitter cells and vessels still persisting in the cavity. (H & E, X115.)

BIBLIOGRAPHY

Blackwood, W., McMenemey, W. H., Meyer, A., and Russell, D. S. (Eds.) *Greenfield's Neuropathology* (2nd ed.). London: Arnold, 1963.

Castaigne, P., Lhermitte, F., Gauthier, J. C., Escourelle, R., Derouesné, C., der Agopian, P., and Popa, C. Arterial occlusions in the vertebrobasilar system. *Brain* 96:133-154, 1973.

Eklöf, B., and Schwartz, S. I. Effects of subclavian steal and compromised cephalic blood-flow on cerebral circulation. *Surgery* 68:431-441, 1970.

Fazio, C. Vascular Pathology of the Spinal Cord. In J. Minckler (Ed.), *Pathology of the Nervous System.* New York: McGraw-Hill, 1971. Vol. 2, pp. 1548-1567.

Ford, D. H., and Kaplan, H. A. *The Brain Vascular System.* Amsterdam: Elsevier, 1966.

Garcia, J. H., Cox, J. V., and Hudgins, W. R. Ultrastructure of the microvasculature in experimental cerebral infarction. *Acta Neuropathol.* 18:273-285, 1971.

Gillilan, L. A. The arterial and venous blood supplies to the forebrain (including the internal capsule) of primates. *Neurology* 18:653-670, 1968.

Kogure, K., Busto, R., Scheinberg, P., and Reinmuth, O. M. Energy metabolites and water content in rat brain during the early stage of development of cerebral infarction. *Brain* 97:103-114, 1974.

Lazorthes, G., Géraud, J., and Bès, A. The contribution of haemodynamic investigations to the study of cerebral vascular pathology. *Triangle* 9:250-257, 1970.

Stephens, R. B., and Stilwell, D. L. *Arteries and Veins of the Human Brain.* Springfield, Ill.: Thomas, 1969.

Vaughn, J. E., and Skoff, R. P. Neuroglia in Experimentally Altered Nervous System. In G. H. Bourne (Ed.), *The Structure and Function of Nervous Tissue.* New York: Academic, 1972. Vol. 5, pp. 39-72.

Zulch, K. J. Hemorrhage, Thrombosis, Embolism. In J. Minckler (Ed.), *Pathology of the Nervous System.* New York: McGraw-Hill, 1971. Vol. 2, pp. 1499-1536.

Intracranial Hemorrhage

15

In this chapter, the term *intracranial hemorrhage* is restricted to one massive hemorrhage (rarely, two or three) within the cranial cavity that is the primary cause of cerebral damage. This deliberately excludes multiple small petechiae or hemorrhages, such as may complicate many forms of intracranial disease (e.g., fat embolism, head injury, blood dyscrasias, or disseminated infections), but in which the volume of extravasated blood is not a major cause of symptoms.

Massive hemorrhage within the cranial cavity may develop catastrophically, as a complication of systemic hypertension or the rupture of abnormal intracranial vessels. It then constitutes one form of stroke. Alternatively, the onset may be insidious over a period of hours or even days, with a progressive increase in intracranial pressure and usually lateralizing signs, as in extradural or subdural hemorrhages associated with head injury. Cases of acute or subacute onset also occur from hemorrhage into a brain tumor or in association with lymphoma or blood dyscrasia. The clinical picture is thus widely variable, but irrespective of its rate of development, the accumulation of a significant volume of blood within the cranial cavity is a serious, often lethal, condition.

Sites of Hemorrhage

Because of the concentric nature of the cranial contents, five primary locations (Fig. 15-1) for intracranial bleeding are commonly recognized, though it must be emphasized that blood may spread from one to another.

Extradural Hemorrhage

Extradural hemorrhage separates the outer layer of the dura from the skull bones. It may originate from the meningeal vessels (most often the middle meningeal, but occasionally the posterior meningeal vessel) or from venous sinuses. It is virtually always associated with head injury. However, in children, it is not necessarily associated with skull fracture (see Chap. 16).

Subdural Hemorrhage

Subdural hemorrhages are more common than extradural bleeding. They are rarely of purely arterial origin and thus commonly have an insidious onset. A large proportion of subdural hemorrhages are associated with overt trauma, but sometimes in elderly people in whom there is widening of the subarachnoid space (and even more often in patients with dementia and cerebral atrophy), subdural hemorrhages may occur in the absence of any elicitable history of trauma. Even then, it is considered that minor, forgotten blows to the head are the usual precipitating factor (see Chap. 16).

Subarachnoid Hemorrhage

Subarachnoid hemorrhage is a relatively frequent condition, usually of dramatic onset and commonly due to berry aneurysms of major cerebral arteries, arteriovenous malformations, or systemic hypertension. Diffuse, usually minor subarachnoid hemorrhage also occurs in head injury. Blood in the subarachnoid space need not be primary, as some intracerebral hemorrhages rupture into the subarachnoid space, especially from superficially situated lesions such as cortical arteriovenous malformations. Secondary subarachnoid hemorrhage in the posterior fossa and at the base of the brain may mimic the distribution seen with a vertebrobasilar berry aneurysm, but actually be due to escape of intraventricular blood through the foramina of Luschka and Magendie.

Intracerebral Hemorrhage

It is in the intracerebral hemorrhage group that it is necessary to make a clear distinction between a massive extravasation of blood that forms a space-occupying lesion and the multiple petechial hemorrhages associated with embolism (including fat embolism), blood dyscrasias, hemorrhagic infarction, and other conditions. In the latter, areas of hemorrhage are intimately mixed with brain tissue, presenting a mottled appearance. The space-occupying hemorrhage is a massive blood clot, firm and dark after fixation and devoid of cerebral tissue, which has been pushed aside or destroyed. Systemic hypertension is probably the most common cause of intracerebral hemorrhage (Fig. 15-2), but some arise from arteriovenous malformations, focal lesions such as primary and metastatic neoplasms, or clotting defects associated with lymphoma, leukemia, or anticoagulant therapy (Fig. 15-3).

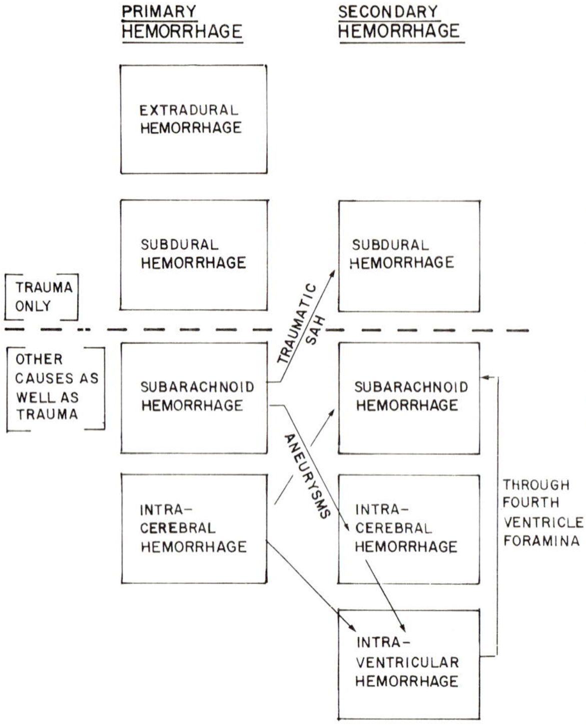

Fig. 15-1. Primary and secondary intracranial hemorrhage in five sites, and common routes of primary to secondary spread. SAH = subarachnoid hemorrhage.

Secondary hemorrhage may occur within the brain, usually associated with rupture of a berry aneurysm. Thus, hemorrhage from aneurysms of the middle cerebral vessels frequently dissects upward and may reach the lateral ventricle, whereas bleeding from anterior communicating aneurysms dissects laterally into the adjacent frontal lobes and posteriorly (through the lamina terminalis) into the third ventricle.

Intraventricular Hemorrhage

Since massive hemorrhage from the choroid plexus does not occur, intraventricular hemorrhage is by definition secondary. Thus, it may complicate hypertensive hemorrhage of the basal ganglia, which frequently dissects into the lateral ventricle, or frontal white matter hemorrhage, which may reach the anterior horn. Or, as already noted, hemorrhage from berry aneurysms may pass through the brain and reach the ventricular system. Since intraventricular hemorrhage frequently reaches the subarachnoid space at the ventral brain stem and base of the brain, it may at times be difficult to determine the original bleeding site.

Relation Between Site and Etiology

Within the brain, bleeding tends to localize by etiology. Thus, the relatively few hemorrhages primarily in the cortex are often associated with arteriovenous malformations. Lesions in the hemispheric white matter are likely to be due to hypertension, hemorrhage into a neoplasm, or clotting defects. Occasionally, massive white matter hemorrhage is seen in head injury, but is an unusual complication (see Chap. 16). Hemorrhages in the basal ganglia are almost always associated with systemic hypertension and usually originate in the lower part of the putamen. Hemorrhage originating in the thalamus is uncommon; again, hypertension and arteriovenous malformation are the most likely causes. Primary brain stem hemorrhages are relatively unusual and are far outnumbered by the secondary bleeding episodes (Duret's lesions) associated with increased intracranial tension (see Chap. 12). Cerebellar hemorrhages are usually due to hypertension.

These are only statistical generalizations, and no etiology can be completely excluded, whatever the site of bleeding.

EFFECTS OF INTRACRANIAL HEMORRHAGE

Hemorrhage in other parts of the body, unless repetitive or so massive as to compromise circulatory efficiency, is of relatively minor significance. In the central nervous system, an acute hemorrhage of 75 to 100 ml of blood is extremely serious and may prove lethal. The effects of course vary with suddenness, size, and location, but may be considered to include tissue destruction, space-occupying effects with raised intracranial pressure, and the induction of cerebral edema, vasospasm, and hydrocephalus.

Tissue Destruction

Intracerebral hemorrhage is usually due to arterial hypertension or arteriovenous malformation. A small lesion can produce surprising tissue destruction, including the self-destruction of vascular malformations. Since the basal ganglia and internal capsule are common sites of intracerebral hemorrhage, varying combinations of hemiplegia, hemianesthesia, and hemianopia may occur. Hemorrhage tends to spread widely in the white matter, but largely by dissection among the components of major fiber tracts, so that if the patient survives, the residual damage from even a large clot may be minor. Primary brain stem hemorrhages may be almost immediately fatal, presumably by involving the reticular formation; the destructive effects of a cerebellar hemorrhage are less severe.

Hemorrhage as a Mass Lesion

Intracerebral hemorrhage is, in most instances, in only one cerebral hemisphere and therefore acts as an asymmetrical mass lesion, causing a contralateral midline shift, ipsilateral or bilateral uncal herniation with brain stem distortion, and often Duret's lesions. Brain stem lesions are normally fatal before they achieve significant size, but cerebellar lesions may

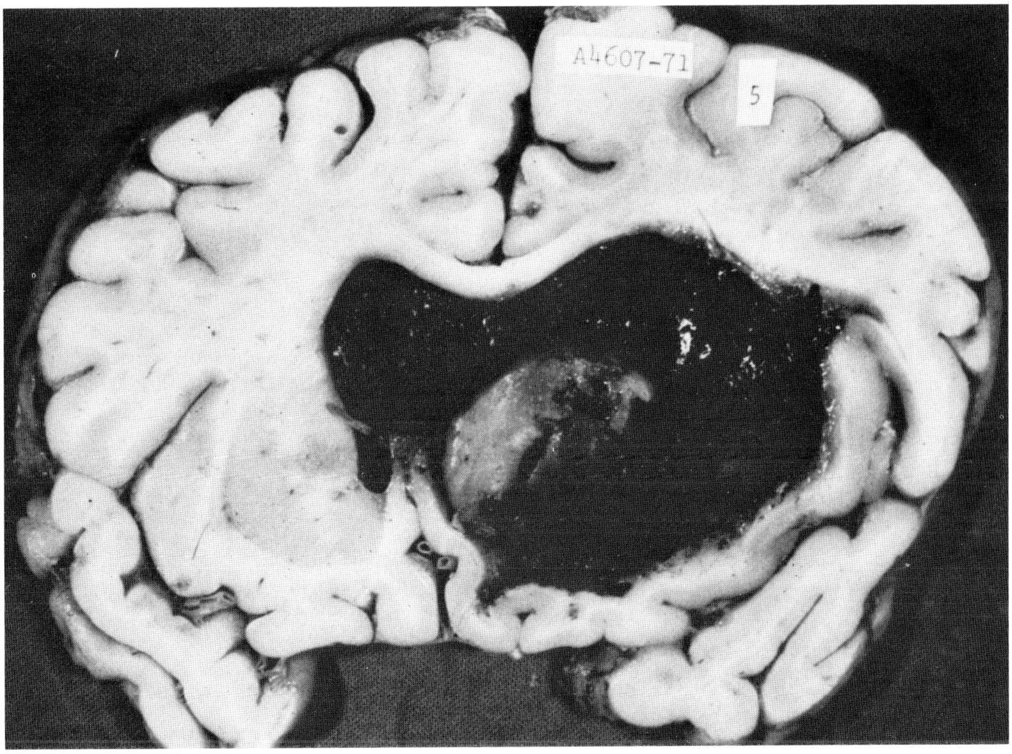

Fig. 15-2. Hypertensive intracerebral hemorrhage (central hemorrhage), probably originating in the basal ganglia and rupturing into the ventricles.

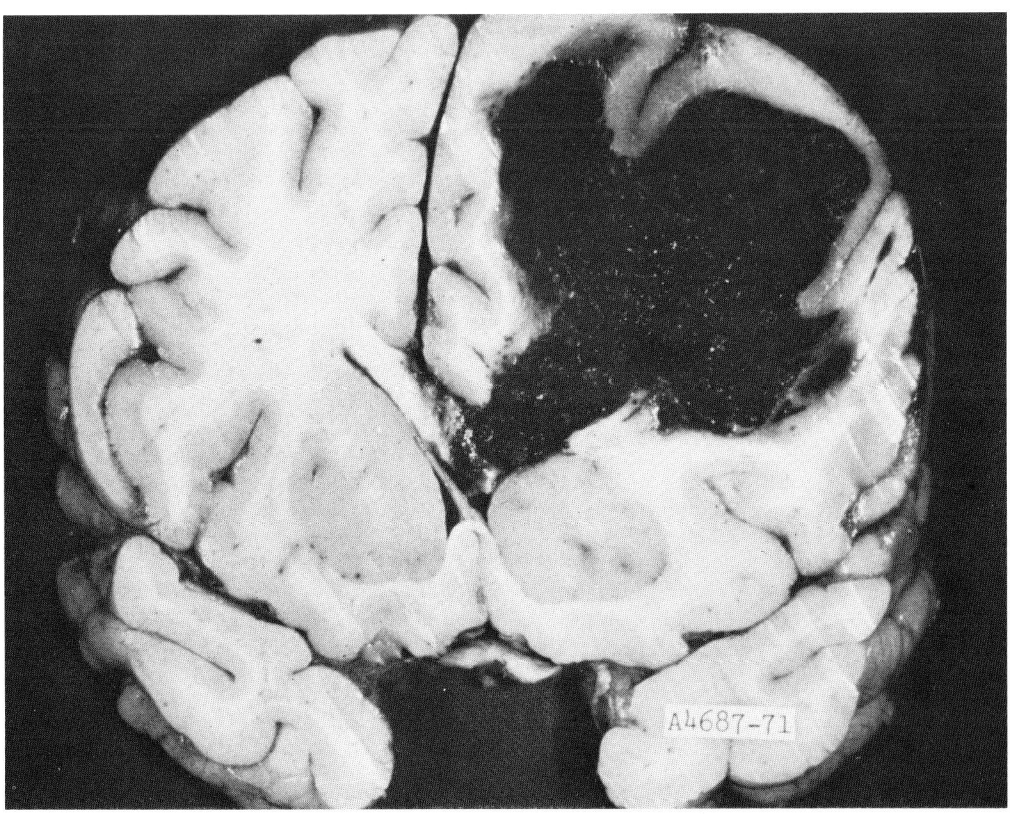

Fig. 15-3. Intracerebral hemorrhage associated with anticoagulant therapy (peripheral hemorrhage), originating in the white matter and rupturing into the ventricles.

rupture into the fourth ventricle and cause pressure distortion and ischemia of the brain stem, along with severe tonsillar herniation.

While subarachnoid hemorrhage, which can distribute itself through the subarachnoid space and displace cerebrospinal fluid (CSF) into the spinal subarachnoid space, may not cause significant brain displacement, it does cause a moderate to severe rise in intracranial pressure. Extradural and subdural hemorrhages are most commonly unilateral and produce severe brain shifts, as noted for a unilateral intracerebral hemorrhage. The occasional bilateral subdural hemorrhage may fail to produce lateralizing signs, but causes a significant rise in intracranial pressure, with marked uncal and tonsillar herniation and the usual sequelae.

Induction of Cerebral Edema

Intracerebral hemorrhage is a potent cause of cerebral edema. A hemorrhage that of itself might be tolerated by the CNS is often found associated with massive swelling and softening of the entire cerebral hemisphere. The increase in intracranial pressure and cerebral displacement due to the hemorrhage itself are frequently greatly accentuated by this edema, but the cause of its rapid appearance and spread is not clear. It seems reasonable to speculate that release of substances such as serotonin, prostaglandins, and vasoactive kinins from platelets and other elements of the hematoma may have a direct effect on vessels in the hemisphere — either increasing their permeability and permitting the escape of excess fluid and protein, or producing local vasospasm with subsequent damage to the endothelium and blood-brain barrier, or by both mechanisms.

Vasospasm

Occurrence in Subarachnoid Hemorrhage

Although spasm of small intracerebral vessels may be associated with cerebral edema, vasospasm has been most studied as it involves the relatively large vessels at the base of the brain, in association with subarachnoid hemorrhage.

Incidence and Duration. The incidence of vasospasm in subarachnoid hemorrhage has been estimated at 10 to 45%. It may frequently be visualized angiographically as a uniform narrowing of vessels, often concentrated in the region of a ruptured aneurysm, and affecting with particular frequency the internal carotid artery in the subarachnoid space.

Spasm may be observed from the first day up to several weeks after an acute hemorrhage, although in some of the longer-persisting cases, angiographic narrowing appears to be less regular. At this stage there may be structural changes in the vessel wall. Such changes include subendothelial granulation tissue with thickening of the intima, usually involving vessels near the site of hemorrhage, and do not usually become marked until the fourth week. They must therefore be regarded as sequelae of the vasospasm (on the basis of an anoxic or mechanical insult to the vessel) and are in no sense the cause of the original vascular narrowing.

Relationship to Total Cerebral Blood Flow. Subarachnoid hemorrhage is usually associated with a bilateral diffuse decrease in cerebral blood flow, but it is not certain that this is directly attributable to generalized vascular spasm, at least as determined by angiography. Indeed, the cause of this global decrease is unclear, but it appears to be an autoregulatory phenomenon. It may be secondary to decreased oxygen utilization; cerebral blood flow may fall to extremely low levels, yet many patients in whom this occurs make full recovery without neurological impairment. The concept of such a generalized metabolic change is supported by diffuse EEG changes, with an excess of slow-wave activity proportional to the fall in cerebral blood flow. It has been suggested that such changes may be an effect of products of hemolysis on the underlying cortex. Such hemolysis would also result in local CSF acidosis, leading to hyperventilation and respiratory alkalosis. Either such alkalosis, or an increase in blood pressure secondary to raised intracranial pressure could produce autoregulatory vasoconstriction and the observed fall in cerebral blood flow. Both the cause and the effects of this general reduction in blood supply require much further investigation. No autopsy findings have been correlated with it.

Relationship to Focal Ischemia and Infarction. At autopsy, a proportion of patients who have had a subarachnoid hemorrhage exhibit areas of infarction corresponding to vessel distribution. Although these autopsy findings have not yet been adequately correlated with spasm that was observed by angiography, a correspondence between such spasm and the neurological features and brain scan findings suggestive of ischemia in surviving patients has been reported. Presumably the intensity and duration of spasm, and availability of collateral circulation, determine whether or not infarction occurs.

Experimental Vasospasm

Occurring not only in subarachnoid hemorrhage, but also in head injury and as a complication of vessel handling in neurosurgical procedures, vasospasm has been the subject of much experimentation. It can be produced with moderate consistency in many species, either by trauma to basal vessels (handling or puncture) or by subarachnoid injection of blood. Injections of saline or dextran either have no effect or cause slight dilatation. Such experimental spasm is usually acute and of short duration, being maximal in 2 to 3 minutes and lasting only 1 to 8 hours. However, if followed by a second injection of blood, spasm becomes more severe and prolonged. This continued presence of blood corresponds more closely to clinical conditions. There is some evidence that clinical vasospasm itself might be biphasic, with an early acute stage in the first hour, followed by chronic and possibly more diffuse contraction at 24 to 72 hours and lasting up to several weeks.

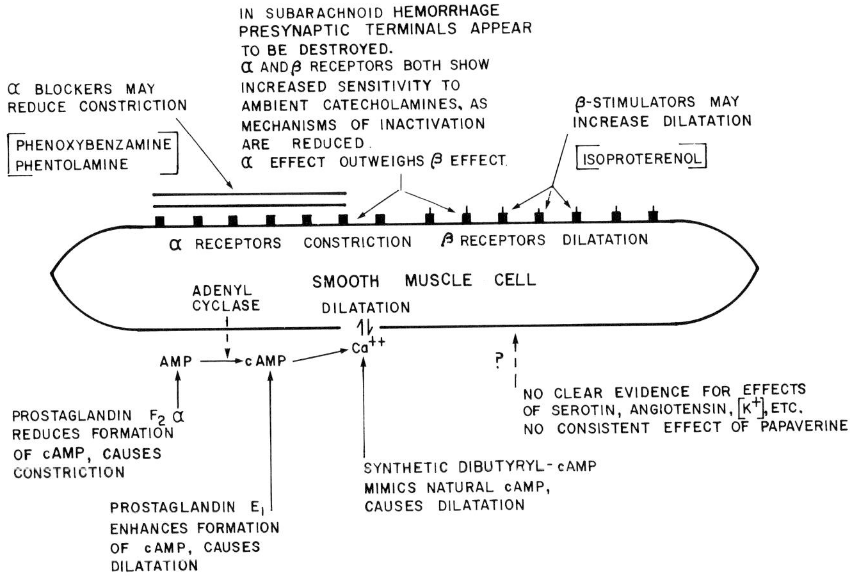

Fig. 15-4. Some of the possible factors involved in the production of vasospasm. The squares represent alpha- and beta-adrenergic receptors on a smooth muscle cell. Note that the effects of prostaglandins appear to be independent of adrenergic (or any other) receptors. cAMP = cyclic AMP (adenosine 3':5'-monophosphate).

Theories of Pathogenesis in Relationship to Therapy

Although mechanical spasm is an occasional surgical hazard, the prolonged spasm associated with subarachnoid hemorrhage, either spontaneous or traumatic, is a more important problem.

Role of Catecholamines. Vasospasm can be elicited after cervical sympathectomy and is therefore not neurally mediated. Catecholamine granules are nonetheless depleted in spastic vessels. If this is due to damage to nerve terminals and so to inability to bind ambient amines, as seems probable, the vessel receptors, both alpha and beta, might be hypersensitive to existing low catecholamine levels, with the alpha (constrictor) effect outweighing the beta (dilator) effect. Correspondingly, alpha-blocking and beta-adrenergic drugs have been tried, each with some experimental and clinical success, to redress the alpha-beta balance in favor of dilatation (Fig. 15-4). Phenoxybenzamine, an alpha blocker, experimentally alleviated blood-induced, but not mechanical spasm, though there was a time lag when it was given parenterally. Phentolamine, another alpha blocker, relieves both types of experimental spasm. Since it relieves mechanical spasm in a vessel where hematogenous spasm has already been reduced by phenoxybenzamine, it presumably has routes of action in addition to alpha blockade. The beta-adrenergic drug isoproterenol has shown promise in clinical trials. However, it must be used with care, as it increases myocardial contractility and can cause arrhythmias. In a small series of cases it appeared to improve the prognosis markedly, but further evidence concerning its effects is still needed.

Role of Serotonin. There are candidates other than ambient catecholamines for spasmogenic agents, possibly liberated from the blood during lysis. *Serotonin* has been proposed, but there is no conclusive evidence that it has spasmogenic action. Further, a serotonin antagonist, methysergide (1-methyl-D-lysergic acid butanolamide), fails to reduce spasm.

Role of Prostaglandins. Prostaglandins both are present in the normal CNS and are liberated from lysis of subarachnoid blood. There has been great recent interest in their possible role, not only in the genesis of spasm, but also in normal autoregulation. They are 20-carbon lipids, with the center of the chain cross-linked to form a 5-carbon ring. Depending on configuration and substituents, they have been classified into series A, B, E, and F. Many are vasoactive, causing dilatation or constriction, but the effects vary somewhat between species. They act via the adenyl cyclase - cyclic adenosine monophosphate (AMP) system to control Ca^{++} release across membranes and are independent of the catecholamine mechanism. (Synthetic dibutyryl-3', 5', cyclic AMP has shown some experimental promise as a spasmolytic agent.) Animal experiments suggest that prostaglandin E_1 alleviates spasm and may even increase cerebral blood flow through normal vessels, whereas prostaglandin F_{2a} causes vasoconstriction and enhances the spasm due to subarachnoid hemorrhage. Both are present in the normal CNS and released to the cerebrospinal fluid by serotonin or electrical stimulation. Their role in normal autoregulation may prove to be more certain than their effect in subarachnoid hemorrhage, but clearly they are potential agents, not only in the genesis of spasm, but also in its therapy. Further work on these potentialities is actively proceeding.

Other Agents. There is little support for significant effects of angiotensin, or raised CSF K^+ concentrations, in the production of vasospasm. There is no theoretical support for the use of papaverine, which is frequently, but not consistently advocated for the treatment of vasospasm. The clinical results are rarely satisfactory. In monkeys, locally applied papaverine alleviates hematogenous spasm for short periods, perhaps for the first phase only of a biphasic spasm. Its dubious value and the absence of any other accepted therapy indicate the urgency of the search for drugs effective against this dangerous condition.

Hydrocephalus

Extravasation of considerable amounts of blood into the subarachnoid space commonly leads to an intense reaction on the part of the meninges. This reaction includes a considerable degree of fibrosis and scarring between the arachnoid and pial layers. Clinically, in a few patients with subarachnoid hemorrhage, hydrocephalus has developed in the acute or chronic stage. However, there has been little investigation into the frequency of ventricular dilatation, perhaps because of the undesirability of air encephalography in such sick patients.

However, angiograms are usually obtained, and it has been shown that the width of the lateral ventricles can be assessed with considerable accuracy by visualization of the thalamostriate vein. In one series of 50 patients, about 40% showed appreciable ventricular widening, although this bore no relationship to the acute symptomatology. In one of the few patients in whom angiography was repeated, there was a regression in ventricular size. It appears that there might often be a temporary hydrocephalus, associated with clots and other debris in the cisterns at the base of the brain, or even with temporary blockage of the villi, whereas only in a few patients does sufficient fibrosis develop (perhaps especially over the hemispheres where the subarachnoid space is narrow) to cause a permanent delay of CSF flow. Temporary ventricular dilatation appears to be associated more commonly with aneurysms of anterior communicating arteries than with aneurysms of the middle cerebral arteries, perhaps because of the frequent leakage of blood into the ventricles from the former lesions.

HYPERTENSIVE BRAIN DISEASE

Systemic hypertension has a number of CNS manifestations, the most important of which is intracranial hemorrhage, usually intracerebral but sometimes primarily subarachnoid. There is a strong statistical correlation between intracranial hemorrhage and known clinical hypertension (or in the absence of a clinical history, between intracranial hemorrhage of otherwise undetermined etiology, increased heart weight, and hypertrophy of the left ventricle). Rare CNS manifestations occurring with hypertension include hypertensive encephalopathy, associated with sudden blood pressure rises in malignant hypertension, and chronic demyelination of the cerebral hemispheres, more marked in the occipital regions (Binswanger's dementia).

Effect on Autoregulatory Capacity

At least in early hypertension, cerebrovascular autoregulation ensures normal cerebral blood flow and oxygenation by vasoconstriction in the face of increased perfusion pressure. In healthy vessels, vasoconstriction is effective up to a mean arterial pressure of 180 mm Hg and, for short periods, probably up to considerably higher pressures. Beyond such levels, increased pressure is transmitted through arterial and arteriolar resistance to the capillaries, with the likelihood of damage to these vessels. Persistent chronic hypertension changes autoregulatory capacity in two ways: First, there appears to be *habituation to the permanently raised pressure levels,* with an increase in both the upper and lower limits for autoregulation. In a normal person, a fall of mean arterial pressure to 45 to 50 mm Hg is necessary to attain maximal vasodilatation. In hypertensive patients, this occurs at 80 to 90 mm Hg, so that a fall of pressure below this level cannot be compensated, and cerebral blood flow drops in parallel with perfusion pressure. The second effect is *acceleration and intensification of degenerative vessel changes* at all levels, from subarachnoid arteries to arterioles, of such a nature that ultimately autoregulatory capacity is virtually abolished. At this stage, cerebral blood flow will be at all times proportional to perfusion pressure. Even the therapeutic reduction of blood pressure to more normal levels may cause severe ischemia in the brain of the hypertensive patient. During treatment it is important to remember that chronic hypertensive patients have modified and impaired autoregulatory capacity.

Effect on Brain Vessels

Subarachnoid Vessels

It is generally accepted that hypertension causes severe and premature atherosclerotic changes in medium-sized and small arteries (e.g., the named arteries of the brain and at least their major cortical branches). It is not uncommon to see atherosclerosis in the form of small plaques, 1 to 2 mm in diameter, extending along the middle cerebral vessels on the insula, the anterior cerebral vessels above the corpus callosum, and the cerebellar vessels, especially the posterior cerebellar artery. These plaques are less common in normotensive persons.

Perforating Vessels over 300μ in Diameter

True atherosclerotic plaques are not usually seen in the perforating vessels, neither in the striate arteries supplying the basal ganglia nor in vessels entering the cerebral and cerebellar hemispheres, thalamus, or brain stem. However, in the larger of these vessels, say those with a diameter exceeding 300μ, arteriosclerotic changes occur that somewhat resemble those of atherosclerosis (Fig. 15-5), though discrete

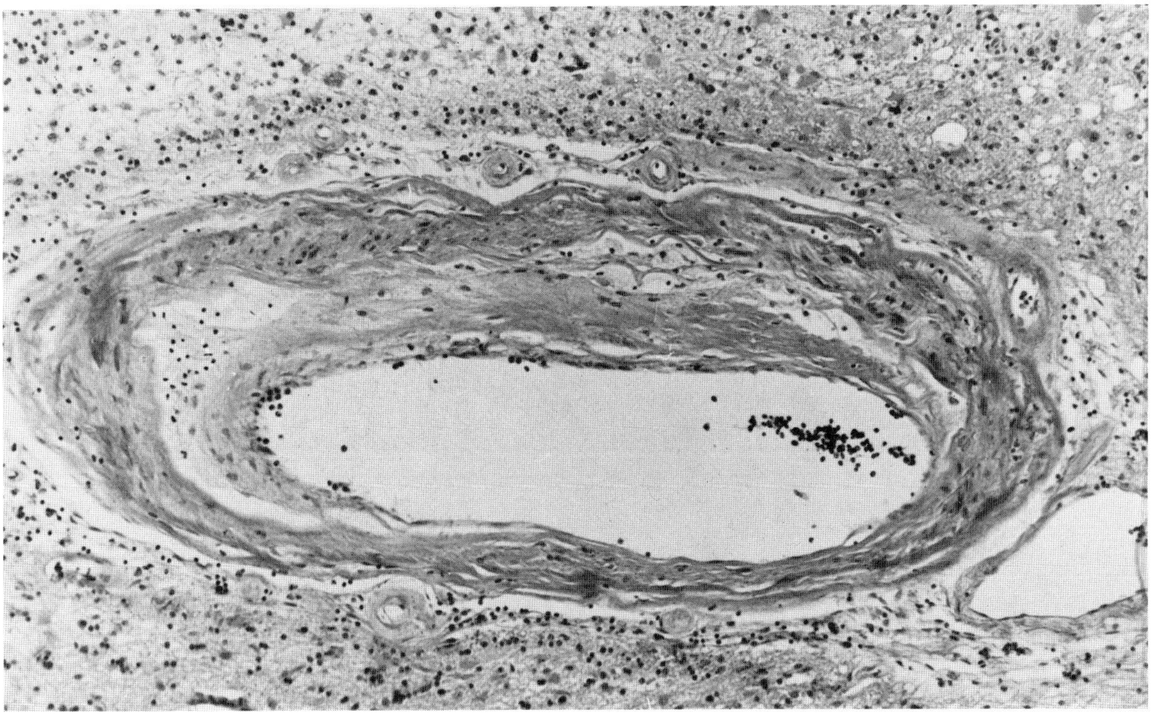

Fig. 15-5. Hypertensive changes in large perforating vessel bearing some resemblance to atherosclerosis. (H & E, ×115.)

plaque formation is not apparent. Changes include splitting and reduplication of the internal elastic lamina, cellular proliferation below the intima, with foam cells and free lipid, and increased collagen in all layers, but no muscular hypertrophy.

Perforating Vessels less than 300μ in Diameter

Morphology. In vessels less than 300μ in diameter, best studied in the basal ganglia but occurring in many other regions, there is hyalinization (transformation of media and intima into hyaline, eosinophilic material, apparently derived from collagen), often associated with local fusiform or saccular dilatations (Figs. 15-6, 15-7). More hyaline material, apparently derived from plasma, is deposited either in the dilatations or actually in the vessel lumen, causing complete occlusion. These dilatations, which may or may not be partially filled with plasma hyalin, apparently correspond to the aneurysms described earlier by Charcot and Bouchard, although it had been suggested that these occur in the slightly larger, arteriosclerotic vessels.

All the affected perforating arteries are very tortuous, and sections traverse them at all angles, producing artifacts. However, the existence of dilatations, whether or not they should be regarded as true aneurysms, appears indisputable. Originally demonstrated by multiple section as small dilatations (400 to 500μ) of the basal ganglion vessels, they have also been shown by microangiography prior to dissection. They are more common in hypertensive patients (but occasionally are seen in normotensive persons), are present at a considerably lower age than in normal persons, and have a characteristic distribution.

Distribution of Lesions. These degenerative changes are more common in the putamen, pallidum,

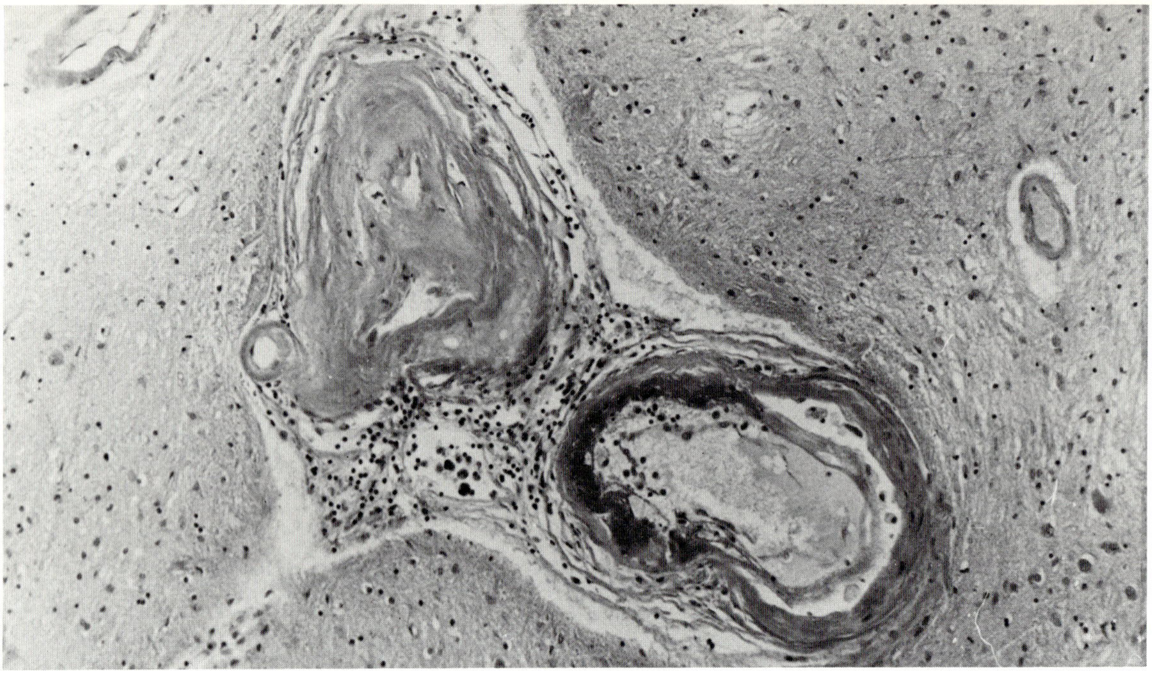

Fig. 15-6. Hypertensive changes in small arteries with mild perivascular lymphocytic cuffing. The upper vessel is hyalinized and virtually occluded, and the lower shows acute hyaline change in a part of the wall (left). (H & E, X115.)

and thalamus than in the caudate or internal capsule. They are common at the junction of the cortex and white matter in all areas except the anterior frontal lobe and are less frequent in the pons and cerebellum, where, however, they tend to be large. Aneurysms are most often present at branching points, and sometimes there are several on one vessel. Their wall thickness is 10 to 200μ, and they are occasionally surrounded by siderophages and reactive astrocytes, suggesting local hemorrhage.

Perforating vessels supplying the basal ganglia have been extensively studied in connection with primary intracerebral hemorrhage. The small medial striate vessels that pass to the lateral pallidum are only 100 to 200μ in diameter and frequently show no dilatations. The larger lateral striate vessels (300 to 400μ) pass unbranched to the level of the anterior commissure, this segment showing arteriosclerotic changes. At about the level of the commissure they form three or four main branches (plus small branches) to the putamen, pass unbranched through the internal capsule, and end in the caudate. Vessels above the anterior commissure are the ones that commonly show hyaline change and fusiform or saccular dilatation. Lengthening and tortuosity in the lower arteriosclerotic segments are almost equally common in the normotensive group. Each branch of a striate artery is, in effect, an end-artery, with relatively few capillary anastomoses to adjacent vessels.

Morphological Changes in Brain Parenchyma

The most characteristic CNS sequel of hypertension is massive intracerebral (or sometimes subarachnoid) hemorrhage. Many European investigators divide intracerebral hemorrhage into a "typical" group, occurring in the basal ganglia (Fig. 15-2), thalamus,

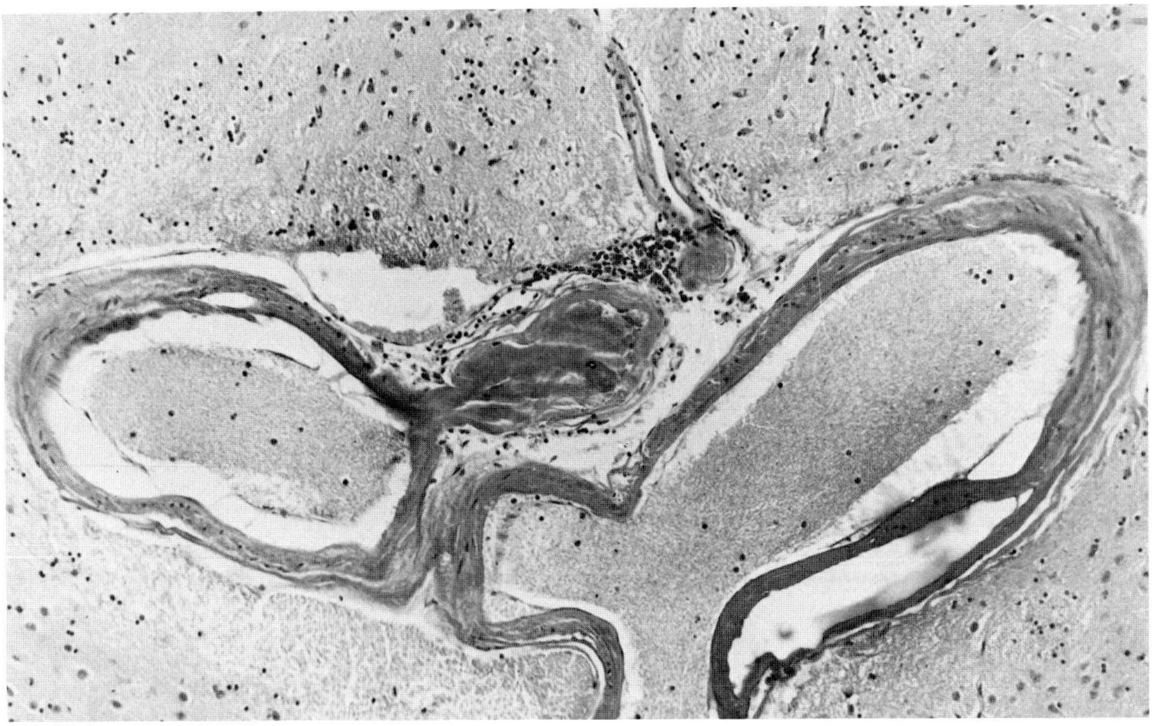

Fig. 15-7. Hypertensive changes in small arteries, including dilatation that suggests early "aneurysm" formation. (H & E, ×115.)

or cerebellum and associated with hypertension, and an "atypical" (peripheral) group, in normotensive persons (Fig. 15-3), and of multiple etiology.

Hypertensive Hemorrhage

The typical hypertensive hemorrhage is frequently centered at the base of the putamen and, if examined before fixation, shows a large central blood clot surrounded by a mixed area of blood and torn tissue. If the clot is washed away, torn ends of small striate arteries may be seen projecting into the lower margin. At the periphery of the lesion, petechiae and edema develop because of vessel compression, and hemorrhage may spread in the frontal, parietal, or temporal white matter up to the cortex or into the lateral (occasionally third) ventricles. The putamen and adjacent gray matter are destroyed. Other such hemorrhages occur in the thalamus, usually with rupture into the lateral or third ventricles, and in the cerebellum, where they probably start near the dentate nucleus and may rupture into the fourth ventricle or subarachnoid space.

Since the vessels involved are small, the causative lesion is destroyed by the hemorrhage, but examination of the contralateral hemisphere demonstrates aneurysmal dilatations in most cases, from which it is assumed hemorrhages arise. Some support for this assumption lies in the frequent discovery of iron-laden macrophages and reactive astrocytes around the aneurysms. If the patient survives (which is much less common with typical hemorrhages than with the more peripheral type), a zone of organizing granulation tissue forms at the periphery, showing early endothelial hyperplasia and neutrophilic exudate, followed by exudation of lymphocytes, proliferation

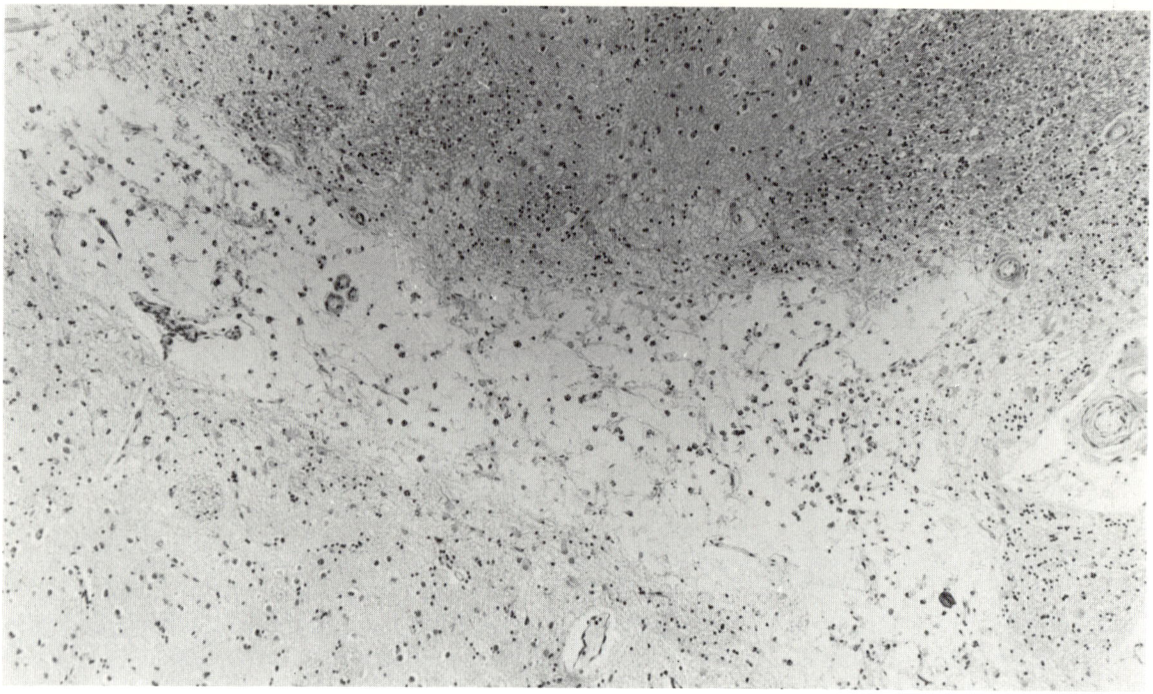

Fig. 15-8. Status lacunaris in basal ganglia of a hypertensive patient. The photograph shows one lacuna, with iron-containing macrophages and an irregular border containing a few reactive astrocytes. (H & E, ×115.)

of gitter cells containing iron and fat, and marked mesenchymal (capillary and fibroblastic) proliferation. Small hemorrhages are usually converted to mesenchymal (rather than glial) scars, whereas larger ones liquefy centrally, due to autolysis, and ultimately form cavities with extensive mesenchymal and glial fibrosis in the walls. The rarity with which such lesions are found at autopsy testifies to the high acute mortality of this type of brain disease.

Minor Lesions Associated with Degeneration of Small Vessels

A frequent incidental finding in the CNS of hypertensive patients who have not bled, or on the contralateral side from a fatal hemorrhage, is the presence of small, cystic, often irregular areas, largely confined to the basal ganglia and thalamus. Such *status lacunaris* (Fig. 15-8) is much more frequent in hypertensive patients than in others. The small cavities are old miliary infarcts and do not contain a vessel. They may show a few gitter cells and a narrow marginal zone of gliosis and fibrosis. They probably result from hyaline occlusion of small vessels. *Status cribrosus* is common in all elderly people irrespective of blood pressure and consists of small cystic foci up to 0.5 to 0.6 cm in diameter (Fig. 15-9), largely in the putamen and less in the thalamus; they surround an artery and vein (and therefore are different from "lacunae"). The etiology of status cribrosus is unknown. Suggestions that it is due to pulsation of tortuous vessels or resorption of inadequately nourished perivascular tissue require substantiation.

Lesions Possibly Associated with Hypertensive Spasm of Perforating Vessels

Occasionally, more widespread changes are seen in the CNS of hypertensive patients, irrespective of massive hemorrhage. These vary from small cortical foci of selective ischemic neuronal necrosis to such large areas of infarction as a complete gyrus. Foci may also be multiple. A vascular thrombus may be seen,

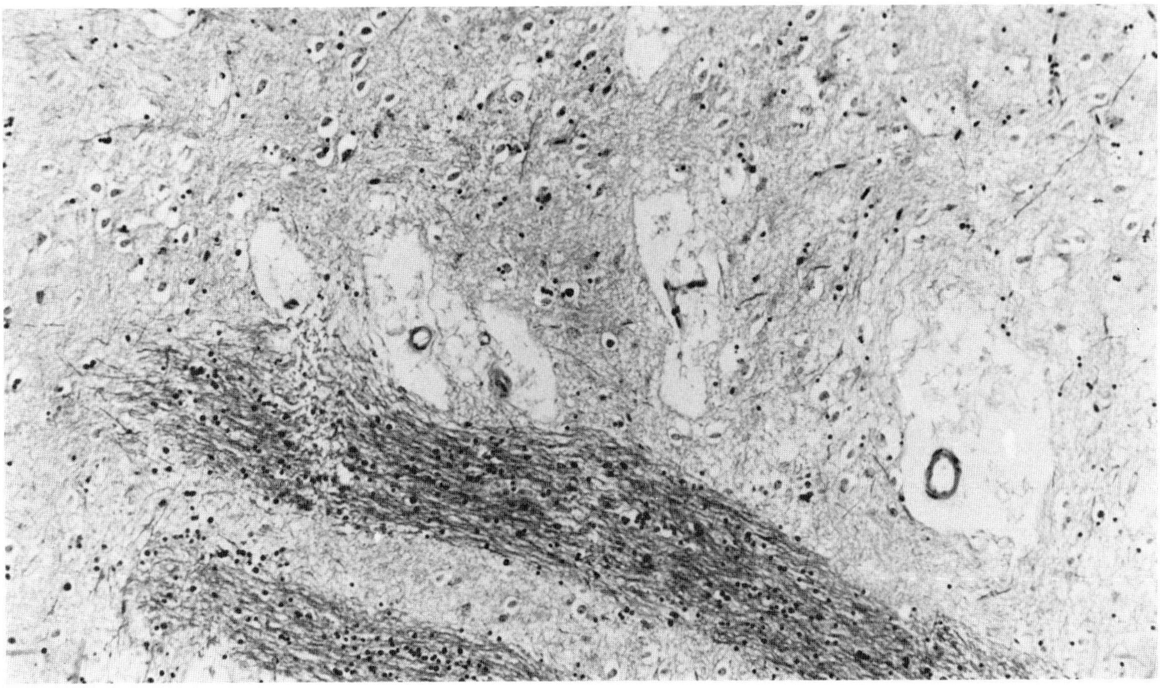

Fig. 15-9. Status cribrosus in basal ganglia of an elderly normotensive person. Small spaces with a well-defined border contain a central vessel. No microglial or astroglial reaction is present. (H & E, X115.)

and it is possible that vasospasm is an etiological factor in producing such lesions. This would imply pathological irritability of vessels superimposed on the already maximal autoregulatory vasoconstriction caused by increased perfusion pressure. Depending on the duration and the size of the vessel involved, vasospasm can lead to transient functional disturbances, selective neuronal loss, or local infarction. Much of the investigative work on hypertensive vasospasm is on animals, but in patients with hypertension the effects of atherosclerosis and accompanying myocardial disease are complicating factors in causing brain disease; some of the CNS lesions may be embolic. Occasionally, old peripheral hemorrhages may be seen, including slit hemorrhages, which lie immediately below and parallel to the cortex.

Vasospasm may be a generalized and significant factor in hypertensive encephalopathic crises, in which there are brain parenchymal changes similar to those just described, together with mild to severe (often focal) edema, multiple petechiae, perivascular plasma exudate, and recent infarcts. It appears that these crises are preceded by acutely rising blood pressure, probably causing the vasospasm (possibly an exaggerated myogenic reflex). If vital areas in the brain stem are affected, such a crisis may cause early death, with little or no morphological change.

Lesions Possibly Associated with Chronic Edema

An uncommon and not readily explicable complication (or at least association) of hypertension is Binswanger's dementia, in which there is demyelination, more marked in the occipital and temporal lobes than in frontal and parietal lobes, and which may involve one or several convolutions or even a complete lobe. It is often associated with severe atrophy of the central white matter and with dilatation of the lateral ventricles, especially their posterior horns. Demyelinated areas may be plaquelike or diffuse and accompanied by marked astroglial proliferation; the vessels show typical hypertensive arteriosclerotic and hyaline changes. The overlying cortex and often the arcuate fibers are intact. The distribu-

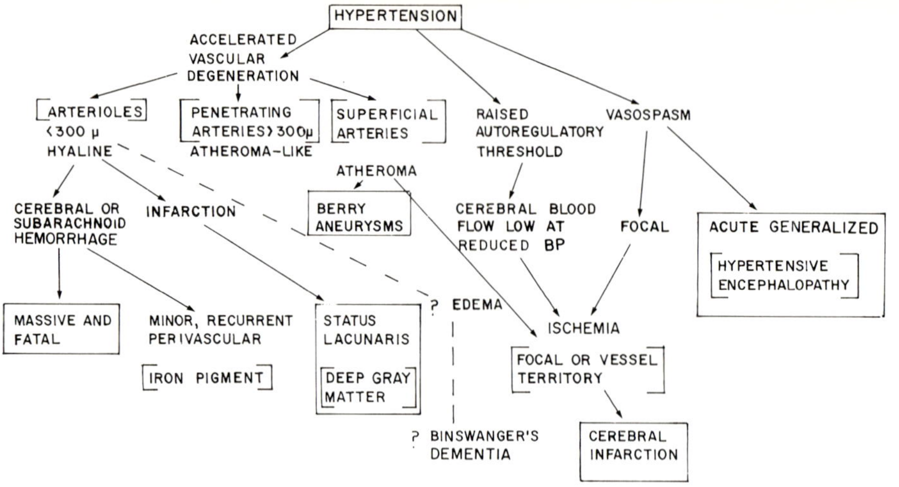

Fig. 15-10. Summary of the pathogenesis of hypertensive brain disease.

tion and morphology are those of chronic edema — again possibly due to diffuse, subacute vessel damage.

The central nervous system complications of systemic hypertension are summarized in Figure 15-10.

SUBARACHNOID HEMORRHAGE

In approximately 10% of cases, acute cerebrovascular disease (stroke) is due to acute subarachnoid hemorrhage, usually associated with berry aneurysm, arteriovenous malformation, or hypertension. Subarachnoid hemorrhage is most common after the age of 40, with a peak incidence at 55 to 60 years of age. There is a lower age peak, at about 30 to 40, associated with arteriovenous malformations. Subarachnoid hemorrhage is slightly more common in women, particularly in association with aneurysms, where the ratio is about 3:2. Taking all groups together, 50 to 55% of subarachnoid hemorrhages appear to be due to berry aneurysms and 5 to 10% to other vascular malformation.

The remainder show neither of these lesions, and it is surmised that in this group the hemorrhages are due to hypertension, since there is a marked association with both severe hypertension and atherosclerosis. Although the pial circulation does not include capillaries, it appears to contain small arteries, 100 to 400μ in diameter. It is conceivable that these arteries might show the same arteriosclerotic and hyaline changes as occur in the penetrating vessels of the brain, though there appear to be few reports on this subject.

The incidence of subarachnoid hemorrhage appears to be somewhat higher than usual during pregnancy, and most such cases are associated with vascular malformations or aneurysms. A small series of 44 pregnant patients with arteriovenous malformations showed peak incidences of hemorrhage from 16 to 20 weeks and from 31 to 35 weeks. Among a series of 77 aneurysms that bled during pregnancy, the incidence of bleeding increased as pregnancy advanced. Surprisingly few episodes of bleeding occur during labor or in the postpartum period, and the cause of the increased hemorrhage during pregnancy is not clear. The rapid rise in cardiac output that occurs in the first trimester and during the second stage of labor does not correlate with bleeding. The hypervolemia of approximately 50% (occurring in all pregnancies) may be an etiological factor.

Although the peak incidences of subarachnoid hemorrhage are in adulthood, such hemorrhages may also occur during childhood. A slightly smaller proportion of these (36%) are associated with aneurysm. A considerably larger proportion (27%) are associated with arteriovenous malformation. The remainder show no lesion, and since hypertension is infrequent in children, the etiology of these hemorrhages remains problematical. The possibility of small aneurysms or malformations that have been completely destroyed in the course of the bleeding episode is speculative but cannot be disregarded, either in children or older age groups.

Cerebral (Berry) Aneurysms

Except for a tiny proportion due to trauma, infection, or rare vascular diseases, aneurysms of cerebral vessels are saccular lesions (Fig. 15-11), usually occurring on major arteries at the base of the brain and of unknown etiology. Rupture of these aneurysms (Fig. 15-12) with subarachnoid hemorrhage causes 2 to 5% of sudden, unexpected adult deaths. There is no association of aneurysms with other diseases, except for a slight increase in association with aortic coarctation and polycystic disease of the kidney (with a common background of hypertension). Familial cases are rare, and there is currently no evidence for a genetic, even polygenic, background.

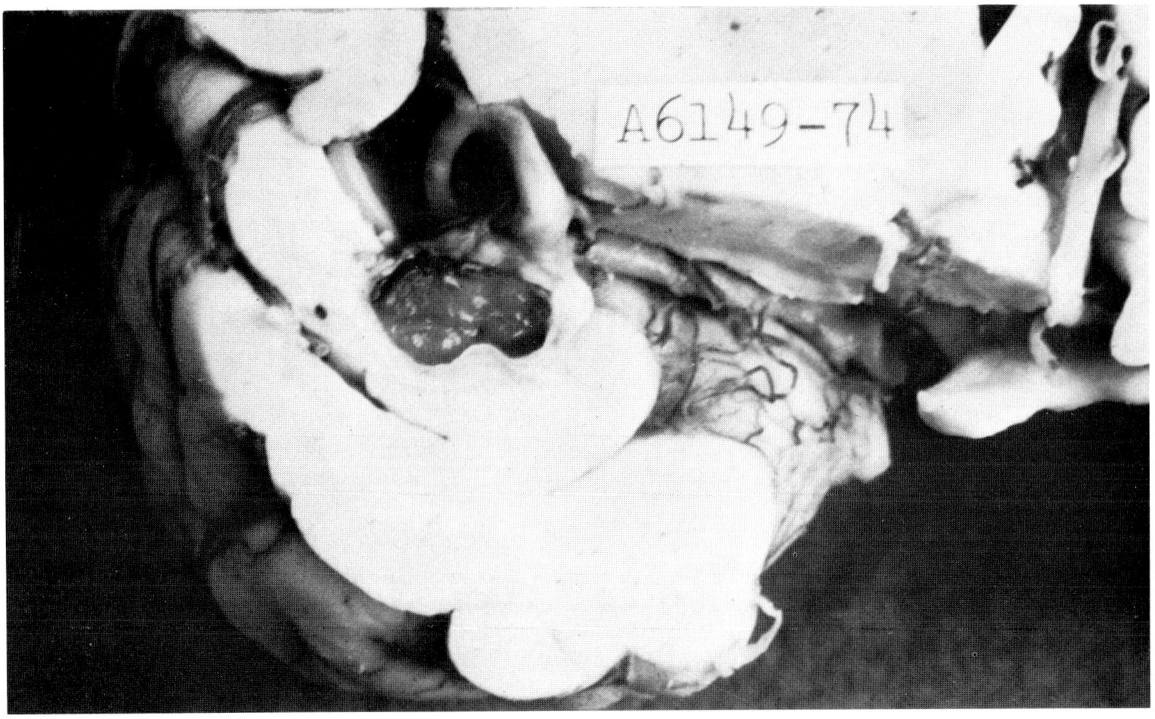

Fig. 15-11. Unruptured berry aneurysm on the (right) middle cerebral vessel. Incidental autopsy discovery.

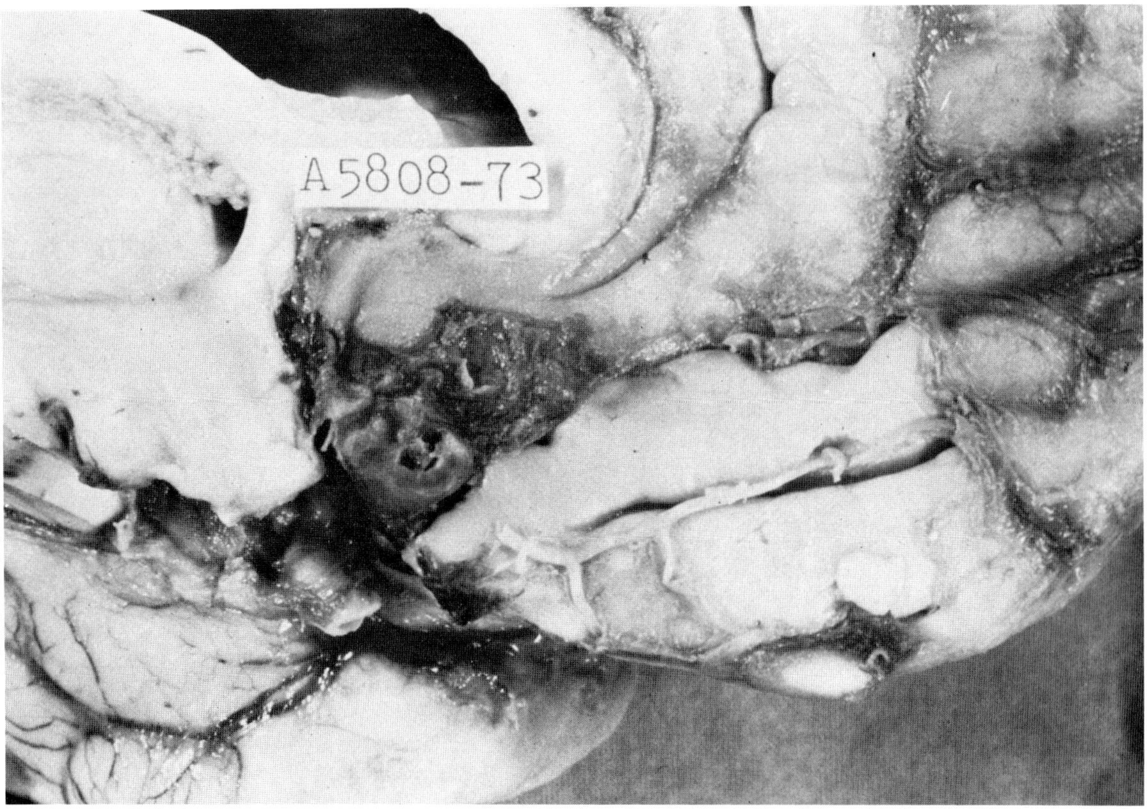

Fig. 15-12. Ruptured berry aneurysm of the anterior communicating artery. The extensive subarachnoid hemorrhage was washed away before fixation to locate the lesion.

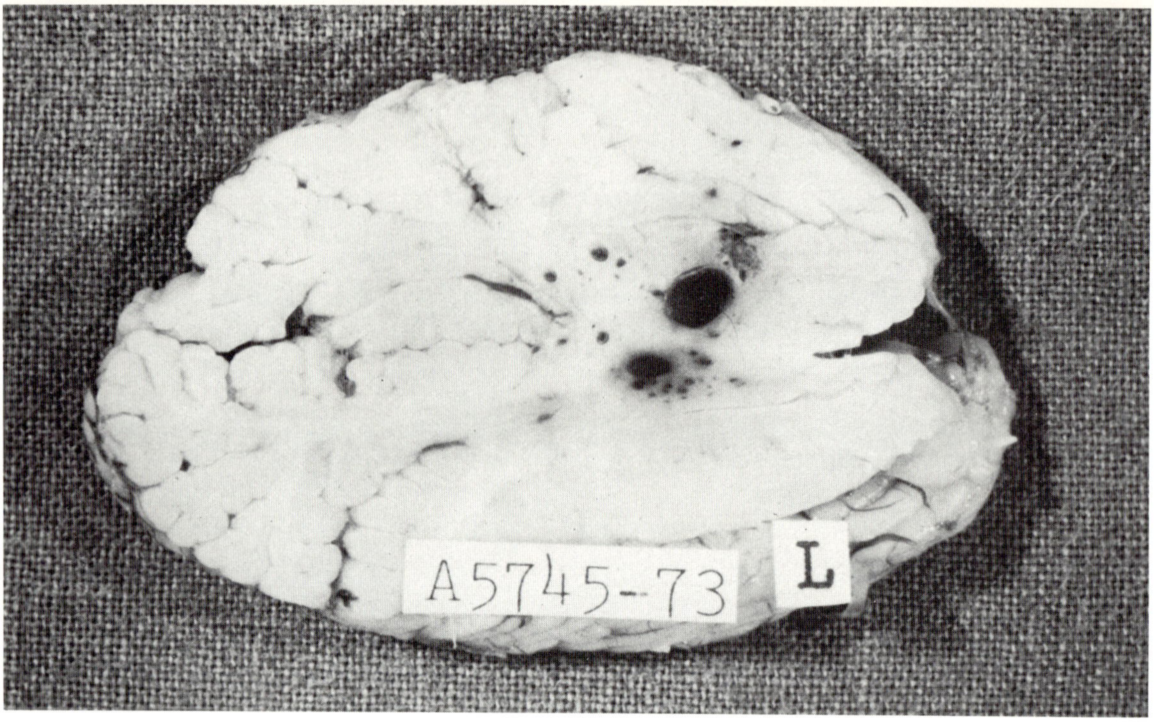

Fig. 15-13. A small, incidentally discovered telangiectasia.

Distribution

About 30% of cerebral aneurysms occur on the anterior communicating artery, 25% on or near the posterior communicating vessels, and 20% on the first inch or so of the middle cerebral vessels. The remainder are distributed either more distally on the anterior cerebral arteries, at the bifurcation of the internal carotids, or in the posterior fossa. It is said that 15 to 20% of aneurysms are multiple, a common association being the anterior communicating artery with one middle cerebral artery. They vary in diameter from 3 to 25 mm and often rupture in the 7- to 15-mm range, generally at the apex.

Morphology

Aneurysms are commonly found at points of bifurcation or in areas corresponding to the origin of fetal vessels that have disappeared during maturation of the cerebrovascular system. The aneurysm wall is composed almost entirely of collagen, with a partial lining of endothelial cells, and is devoid of elastic or muscular tissue. Lymphocytes or even acute inflammatory cells may be seen within the wall, and at the point of rupture, there may be an exudate of neutrophils, eosinophils, and eosinophilic material, presumably plasma protein. At the aneurysmal neck, where it joins the parent vessel or vessels, the media and internal elastic lamina of the latter cease abruptly. Aneurysms are frequently surrounded by dense collagenous tissue, often orange-stained by iron, presumably indicating previous subclinical leakage. The lumen contains varying amounts of laminated antemortem clot and may be completely filled with such material. Where two aneurysms occur on one vessel, it is usually the proximal that ruptures, suggesting that pulsation rather than mean internal pressure is the major predisposing factor.

Etiology and Pathogenesis

The etiology of berry aneurysms is unknown. Only rare examples are seen in infancy and childhood. Their frequent siting at a vascular bifurcation or the point of occlusion of an embryonal vessel suggests weakness of the vessel wall at such points. Studies of normal vessels have shown frequent defects in the media and slight microherniation of the internal elastic lamina. However, in this respect, human vessels are not different from those of subprimates, in which aneurysms seem not to develop. A partial explanation for this discrepancy may be the additional weakening effect of atherosclerosis (rare in animals) on the vascular wall, and often the effect of the mechanical stress of systemic hypertension.

In experimental models it can be shown that the impact of a fluid flow is maximal at the apex of the

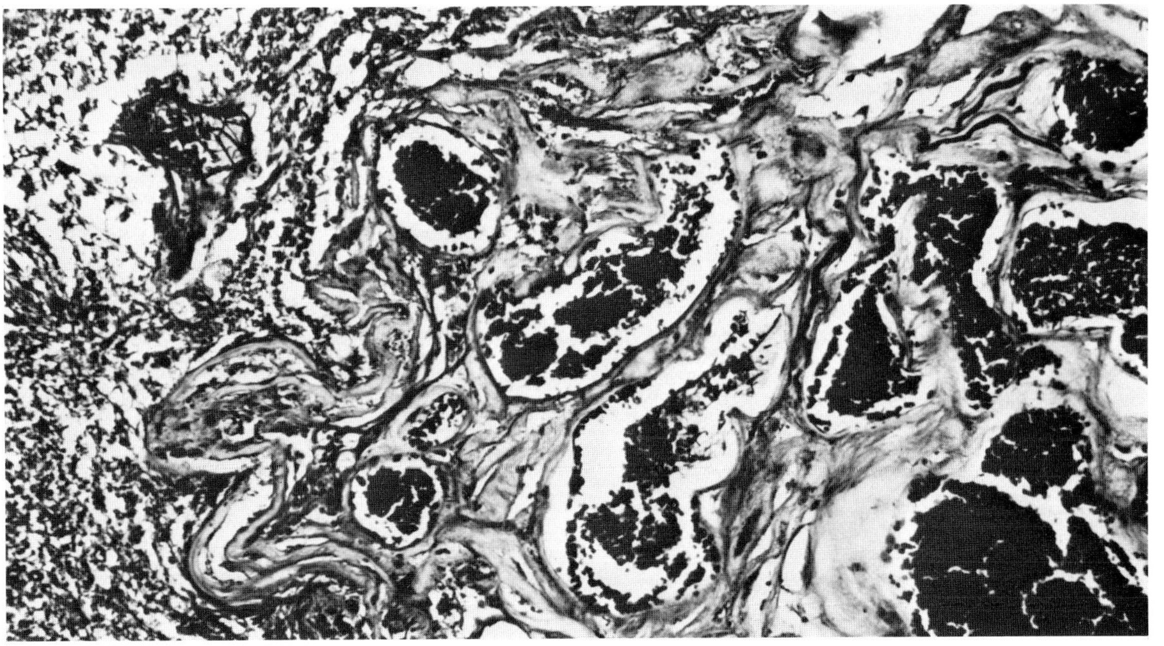

Fig. 15-14. Incidentally discovered cavernous angioma. (Trichrome, X 115.)

point of division of the channel (which corresponds to the situation of aneurysms). Thus, it is possible that these lesions are due to a complex of factors, including a physiological weakness of the vessel wall at the point of bifurcation, aggravated by fluid flow dynamics, hypertension, and the additional destructive effects of atherosclerosis. The factors that precipitate aneurysmal rupture are not clear. Even where histories have been adequate, in only a minority of cases has rupture occurred during undue exertion.

Vascular Malformations

As in other parts of the body, various types of vessel malformation occur within the cranial cavity. Some are associated with familial syndromes, such as ataxia-telangiectasia, Sturge-Weber syndrome, and the von Hippel-Lindau syndrome (see Chap. 19). These represent only a minority of intracranial vascular malformations and are not considered further here. The sporadic lesions include telangiectasias and varices as well as venous, cavernous, and arteriovenous hemangiomas.

Telangiectasias

Telangiectasias are single, small, almost invariably nonsymptomatic lesions, with distended, thin-walled vessels separated by glial tissue (Fig. 15-13). They rarely bleed and are usually incidental discoveries at autopsy, frequently showing calcification.

Varices

Varices are usually single, small lesions, consisting of either one or a small cluster of dilated veins, most often seen in the basal pons. They rarely bleed.

Venous Angiomas

Venous angiomas occur on the surface of the spinal cord, usually posteriorly, and are a rare source of hemorrhage, although they may undergo thrombosis and cause segmental venous infarction.

Cavernous Angiomas

Cavernous angiomas consist of a mass, 1 cm or more in diameter, of distended, sinusoidal, blood-filled spaces (Fig. 15-14), with walls that contain little or no elastin or muscle and without intervening glial tissue. They may cause massive bleeding and be entirely destroyed when this occurs, since they have little mechanical strength. Their existence has been established largely by their incidental discovery at autopsy.

Arteriovenous Angiomas

Arteriovenous angiomas are the most likely to cause serious intracranial (usually subarachnoid) bleeding and are markedly variable in size. They consist of a mass of vessels (Fig. 15-15) of indeterminate structure, somewhat resembling veins, except for the irregularity

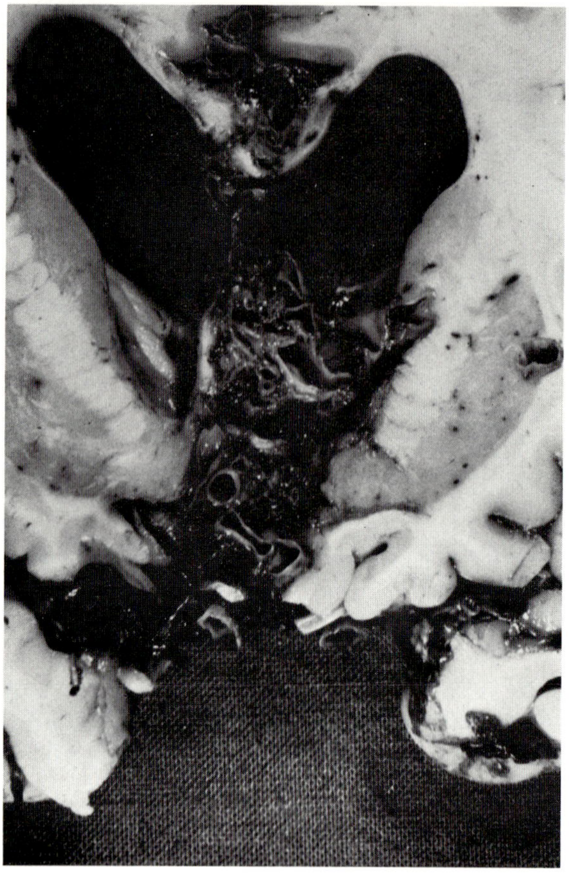

Fig. 15-15. Large arteriovenous malformation at the base of the brain, following the course of, and replacing, the anterior cerebral vessels of both sides.

in wall thickness, with blood supplied by one or more conspicuous, enlarged "feeder" arteries. If less than about 2.5 cm in diameter, they may be extremely difficult to find after a massive intracranial hemorrhage. Smaller lesions may occur in any part of the brain, but larger ones are unusual in the posterior fossa. Most of these angiomas involve the cortex and meninges, although a few present as carotid cavernous fistulas.

BIBLIOGRAPHY

Adachi, M., Rosenblum, W. I., and Feigin, I. Hypertensive disease and cerebral edema. *J. Neurol. Neurosurg. Psychiatry* 29:451-455, 1966.

Aronson, S. M. Vascular Malformations. In J. Minckler (Ed.), *Pathology of the Nervous System.* New York: McGraw-Hill, 1971. Vol. 2, pp. 1884-1897.

Bailey, O. T. Aneurysms. In J. Minckler (Ed.), *Pathology of the Nervous System.* New York: McGraw-Hill, 1971. Vol. 2, pp. 1870-1884.

Cole, F. M., and Yates, P. O. The occurrence and significance of intracerebral microaneurysms. *J. Pathol. Bacteriol.* 93:393-411, 1967.

Denton, I. C., Jr., White, R. P., and Rubinstein, J. T. The effect of prostaglandins E_1, A_1 and $F_{2\alpha}$ on the cerebral circulation of dogs and monkeys. *J. Neurosurg.* 36:34-42, 1972.

Echlin, F. Experimental vasospasm, acute and chronic, due to blood in the subarachnoid space. *J. Neurosurg.* 35:646-656, 1971.

Flamm, E. S., Yaşargil, M. G., and Ransohoff, J., II Alteration of experimental vasospasm by adrenergic blockade. *J. Neurosurg.* 37:294-301, 1972.

Hashi, K., et al. Cerebral hemodynamic and metabolic changes after experimental subarachnoid hemorrhage. *J. Neurol. Sci.* 17:1-14, 1972.

Heilbrun, M. P., Olesen, J., and Lassen, N. A. Regional cerebral blood-flow studies in subarachnoid hemorrhage. *J. Neurosurg.* 37:36-44, 1972.

McCormick, W. F. Vascular Disorders of Nervous Tissue: Anomalies, Malformations and Aneurysms. In G. H. Bourne (Ed.), *The Structure and Function of Nervous Tissue.* New York: Academic, 1969. Vol. 3, pp. 537-596.

Nagai, H., et al. Experimental cerebral vasospasm: I. Factors contributing to early spasm. *J. Neurosurg.* 41:285-292, 1974.

Nakano, J., Chang, A. C. K., and Fisher, R. G. Effects of prostaglandins E_1, E_2, A_1, A_2 and $F_{2\alpha}$ on canine carotid arterial blood-flow, cerebrospinal fluid pressure and intraocular pressure. *J. Neurosurg.* 38:32-39, 1973.

Parkes, J. D., and James, I. M. Electroencephalographic and cerebral blood-flow changes following spontaneous subarachnoid hemorrhage. *Brain* 94:69-76, 1971.

Pelofsky, S., Jacobson, E. D., and Fisher, R. G. Effect of prostaglandin E_1 on experimental vasospasm. *J. Neurosurg.* 36:634-639, 1972.

Pennink, M., White, R. P., Crockarell, J. R., and Robertson, J. T. Role of prostaglandin $F_{2\alpha}$ in the genesis of experimental cerebral vasospasm. *J. Neurosurg.* 37:398-406, 1972.

Petruk, K. C., et al. Cerebral blood-flow following induced subarachnoid hemorrhage in the monkey. *J. Neurosurg.* 37:316-324, 1972.

Simeone, F. A., Trepper, P. J., and Brown, D. J. Cerebral blood-flow evaluation of prolonged experimental vasospasm. *J. Neurosurg.* 37:302-311, 1972.

Skinhøj, E., and Strandgaad, S. Pathogenesis of hypertensive encephalopathy. *Lancet* 1:461-462, 1973.

Smigiel, M. R., Jr., and Sundt, T. M., Jr., Comparative effectiveness of α-blockade and β-stimulation in modifying experimental basilar arterial spasm. *J. Neurosurg.* 41:300-305, 1974.

Weeks, J. R. Prostaglandins. *Annu. Rev. Pharmacol.* 12:317-336, 1972.

Weir, B., et al. Vasospasm in response to repeated subarachnoid hemorrhages in the monkey. *J. Neurosurg.* 33:395-406, 1970.

Yamamoto, Y. L., et al. Experimental vasoconstriction of cerebral arteries by prostaglandins. *J. Neurosurg.* 37:385-397, 1972.

Zülch, K. J. Hemorrhage, Thrombosis, Embolism. In J. Minckler (Ed.), *Pathology of the Nervous System.* New York: McGraw-Hill, 1971. Vol. 2, pp. 1499-1536.

Craniospinal Injury

16

Statistics from Western countries indicate that major head injury is involved in about 11% of accidents that are disabling beyond one day and 15% of accidents causing long-term serious disablement. Of fatal accidents, 33% are associated with head injury as the only or a major component of the fatal lesions. In civilian practice, more than 50% of head injuries are associated with motor vehicle accidents, and the remainder are largely due to falls or blows to the head. Of the injured who die, probably 40 to 50% die before reaching the hospital. Of those that reach the hospital, 40% die within one day and a further 35% within one week.

In considering the causes of the morbidity and mortality associated with craniospinal injury and in deciding on the therapeutic measures to be taken, it is imperative to make a distinction between the *primary lesion* (direct results), which is due to disruption produced by physical force and is present from the moment of injury, and the *second accident* (indirect results), which is due not to disruptive effects on the craniospinal contents but to other changes, such as alteration in cerebrovascular tone and caliber and injuries elsewhere in the body, particularly those involving the cardiopulmonary system that result in alterations of blood pressure, arterial PO_2, or acid-base balance. The importance of this distinction is that while often little can be done for the direct effects, intelligent and painstaking anticipation of possible secondary deterioration may enable countermeasures to be taken that will materially improve the prognosis. A significant but unknown proportion, perhaps as high as 50%, of fatalities and long-term disabilities associated with craniospinal injury is due to the indirect, not the direct, sequelae. It must be emphasized that factors such as reduced PO_2 or acidosis, which may be relatively innocuous to the intact uninjured brain, act synergistically with brain damage to cause profound and even lethal depression of central nervous system function.

Traumatic intracranial hemorrhage may seem to occupy an anomalous position between primary and secondary craniospinal damage, in that the causative lesions (vessel damage) are present immediately, but extravasation of blood may not occur for some time (from minutes to days). Thus, the clinical manifestations of the primary lesion may overlap with those of secondary brain damage. However, since such hemorrhages are a direct and inevitable result of physical damage to vessels inflicted at the time of injury, intracranial hemorrhage is considered here to be a primary lesion, in spite of its later clinical presentation.

Both clinically and experimentally, cranial injury has tended to overshadow lesions inflicted on the spinal cord, although there has recently been a resurgence of interest in cord injury. Meticulous examination of the entire neuraxis in cases of accident has indicated a frequent association of cranial and spinal injuries, particularly involving the cervicomedullary region. In the assessment of head injury, the possibility of cord damage should always be considered and attempts made to localize it. Because many of the pathogenetic mechanisms and morphological manifestations are somewhat different in the brain and spinal cord, they are dealt with separately in the following discussion. This in no sense implies that they are mutually exclusive, and indeed it will become apparent that some of the mechanisms and changes are similar in both.

PATHOGENESIS OF PRIMARY INTRACRANIAL INJURY

By definition, primary intracranial injury is a direct disruptive effect of the absorption of mechanical energy by the head that results in immediate lesions (except for the necessary time for accumulation of extravasated blood, which was mentioned previously). Analysis of the effects of applying physical force – either to the head directly or to the body in such a way as to cause hyperextension of the head on the neck – is extremely difficult, and a considerable amount of experimental work has been carried out in this area. Since the degree of protection afforded by soft-tissue structures, the shape of the skull, and the mass ratio of brain to skull vary from species to species, some divergences and discrepancies are apparent in the results. More impressive, however, are the remarkable similarities obtained in experimental work on species as diverse as the cat, dog, monkey, and baboon and the similarity of many of the lesions observed to those found clinically. These findings encourage the supposition that the results of analysis of such lesions in animals are to a considerable degree applicable to human head injury.

It is important to try to distinguish between concussive and nonconcussive blows in experimental animals, since the analysis of higher mental function in these species is not feasible. The criteria for concussion in animals are:

1. An immediate flaccid paralysis with loss of response to stimuli.
2. Apnea for at least several seconds.
3. Bradycardia associated with dysrhythmias for periods usually measurable in minutes and generally accompanied by lowered systemic blood pressure and an increase in pulse pressure (subconcussive blows tend to increase the heart rate).

Human experience makes it reasonably clear – and it has been confirmed experimentally – that concussion can be produced in the absence of skull fracture or of grossly (and perhaps even microscopically) observable brain lesions. Both concussion and more severe brain lesions can be produced not only by direct impact to the head, but also by body impact that causes hyperextension of the cervical spine.

Theoretical considerations indicate that physical force might produce intracranial lesions in one or more of several ways: local deformation (indentation) of the skull; generalized deformation of the skull; linear acceleration; rotational forces (probably mainly produced by hyperextension of the neck, but perhaps also by pivoting the head on the neck and by lateral head movements); and the creation of pressure fronts originating at the point of impact. In penetrating injury, wounding of the brain by missile or bony fragments and the creation of a pressure wave by passage of foreign bodies must be added. An attempted assessment of the significance of such mechanisms follows.

Local Indentation of the Skull

Even in the absence of fracture, experimental work has shown instantaneous indentation of the skull at the time of striking with a blunt object, with the maximum depression occurring in about 0.5 milliseconds, followed by three or four oscillations and a return to rest within 5 milliseconds. (Indentation and subsequent oscillations might produce alternating positive and negative pressure immediately below the point of impact. Speculatively, either of these could be associated with the production of lesions, either by compression or cavitation, though there is no evidence that they are significant factors.) Depending on the force of the impact, the skull may or may not be fractured. The minimum fracture is a simple linear crack though the center of impact, extending variably toward the base of the skull at each end. More severe impact produces a stellate fracture with radiating cracks; even more force produces a permanently depressed fracture, with the triangular segments of bone breaking off at their bases and remaining below the inner table. Such depressed fracture may be associated with laceration or wounding of the dura, leptomeninges, and brain directly underneath.

In addition to meningeal and brain lacerations associated with depressed fracture, two other effects of local skull deformation may be envisaged. One is the propagation of a pressure wave, which has been experimentally demonstrated; it tends to pass toward the foramen magnum as the only opening of any significant size. The association of such a pressure front with morphological brain damage is unclear, but it may be one factor in producing changes in the cervicomedullary region. These will be taken up in the discussion of the effects of rotational stress. A second possible effect is instantaneous forcing of the entire brain to the opposite side of the skull. Pressure effects produced by such a brain shift would summate algebraically with those produced by linear acceleration or deceleration (Fig. 16-1) and will be discussed in that context.

It appears that the only unequivocal effect of local indentation – and then only when this is severe enough to be associated with fracture – is laceration of the underlying meninges and brain (which is one form of coup injury, to be discussed below).

Generalized Deformation of the Skull

It might be envisaged that a severe blow to the skull would lead to flattening in the direction of impact, with a corresponding widening of diameters at right angles to the impact line. There is little evidence that such an event, if it occurs, is productive of lesions in the brain. Such changes would be maximal in the application of blows to the head supported against a rigid object. Although this is not a usual type of injury, there is documentation that it causes extremely severe skull damage with remarkably little change in the underlying brain; indeed, consciousness may not be lost. It is assumed that the force of the blow is partly absorbed by fracturing of the skull and partly by the supporting object, and that other forces such as linear or rotational acceleration are not involved.

Linear Acceleration

A blow to the head with a blunt object of appreciable mass, in addition to producing local deformation, almost invariably causes sudden acceleration of the skull and contents in the direction of the blow (*linear acceleration*). Much attention has been given to acceleration as a possible causative factor for contusions (bruises) of the surface of the brain. Contusions are usually visible immediately after injury as areas of multiple petechial or larger coalescent hemorrhages in the cortex. They have long been classified as *coup lesions* if occurring adjacent to the point of impact, *contrecoup lesions* if occurring at approximately the opposite end of the brain, and (more recently) as *intermediate coup lesions* if occurring in other areas of the cortex or in the deeper structures, particularly at the tentorial edge and lower border of the falx.

Positive and Negative Pressures Produced by Acceleration

It was originally hypothesized that coup lesions were due to sudden positive pressure generated by accelera-

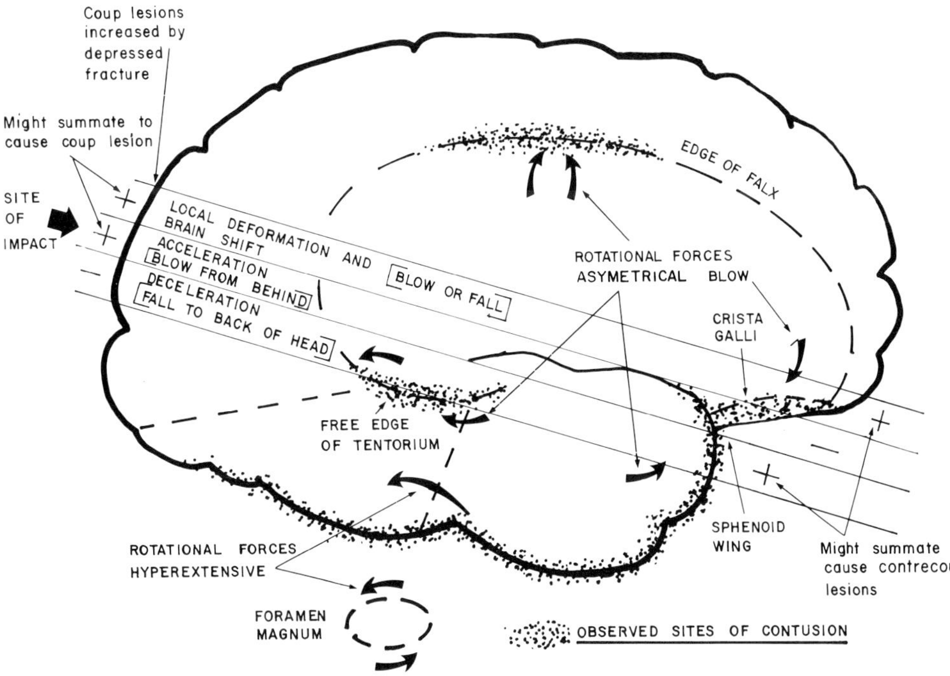

Fig. 16-1. Lateral view of brain (falx and tentorium indicated by dashed lines), showing observed common sites of contusion. The three parallel lines indicate possible summation of positive and negative pressures due to acceleration, deceleration, and whole-brain shift. Arrows indicate theoretical locations of rotational forces in relation to areas of relative brain fixation.

tion of the skull against the inertia of the brain, and that contrecoup lesions were generated at the opposite pole by a negative pressure (cavitation), due to the skull's moving away from the brain before the latter was set in motion. Recently, this concept has been challenged on both observational and theoretical grounds, the latter applying especially to the concept of cavitation due to negative pressure. One feasible result of negative pressure might be release of dissolved gases from blood or cerebrospinal fluid to form small bubbles, yielding lesions orientated on a vascular basis. Such lesions are not seen. Alternatively, negative pressure might produce flash vaporization of dissolved gases, or small vacuum cavities if tissue expansion exceeded its own tensile strength. However, in either case, collapse of such cavities would generate severe stress, laceration, and destruction (implosion). Neither experimentally nor clinically are disruptive lesions seen in contrecoup situations, and even in coup lesions they are only associated with depressed fracture and dural tear. There seem to be no grounds for supposing that negative pressure per se is responsible for any observed lesions in head injury, although the negative pressure may algebraically summate with pressures created by brain shift due to deformation and modify the effect of the lesions.

Summation with Pressures Produced by Local Deformation

That such summation might occur is indicated by reports of the dissimilar distribution of coup and contrecoup lesions in patients who have suffered blows to the unsupported head, compared with those who have struck their head against an immovable object. In the former, coup lesions are more common than contrecoup lesions. This might be explained by the positive pressure of skull acceleration and the positive pressure of skull indentation being additive at the point of impact, whereas at the opposite end of the skull, the negative pressure of skull acceleration is opposed to the instantaneous positive pressure of whole-brain shift due to deformation and partially cancels such positive pressure. Greater deformation is therefore necessary to produce contrecoup lesions (Fig. 16-1). In falls against an immovable object, on the other hand, the head is normally still accelerating, and a negative acceleration pressure at the point of impact will be opposed by the positive pressure due to skull deformation. Opposite the point of impact, the positive pressure of skull acceleration is additive to the positive pressure due to brain shift. Correspondingly, contrecoup lesions tend to be more common and more severe than coup lesions.

Observations Casting Doubt on the Role of Linear Acceleration

Irregularities in the distribution of coup and contrecoup lesions, however, both in clinical and experimental work, cast doubt on the simple acceleration hypothesis. In monkeys subjected to occipital blows, contrecoup lesions in the orbital and temporal regions are common, whereas coup lesions are usually confined to the cerebellum and even then are relatively uncommon. Coup lesions exceed contrecoup lesions only in the presence of occipital skull fracture. With frontal blows, coup lesions do not occur unless there is frontal fracture, and contrecoup lesions are rare. The facial bones with their air sinuses fracture readily and may spare the brain by thus absorbing much of the energy of impact.

Thus, coup lesions are usually small and restricted except in the presence of depressed fracture, and contrecoup lesions are common only with occipital blows. Similar observations have repeatedly been made in clinical practice, where it has also been observed that blows to the side of the head produce ipsilateral and contralateral contusions in approximately equal numbers, these lesions again usually involving temporopolar and orbital areas and sometimes the medial cortex adjacent to the free edge of the falx.

It appears that in the absence of sufficient local deformation to produce subimpact contusions (usually with skull fracture), the site of election for cortical contusions, irrespective of the site of impact, is the orbitotemporal region adjacent to the wing of the sphenoid bone. Similar lesions are commonly seen in relation to the edge of the falx, or at the base of the brain and midbrain in relation to the edge of the tentorium. Such a distribution of contusions is not so far predictable from any model based on linear acceleration forces and is more in keeping with the theoretical effects of rotational stresses.

Rotational Stresses

Rotational stresses are produced either by body blows that move the body relative to the head (hyperextension of the neck) or by head impacts that may also produce hyperextension or lateral or pivoting stresses if they do not pass through the center of gravity of the head.

Relationship to Contusion and Hemorrhage

Theoretical predictions indicate that irrespective of the plane of rotation, maximal stress is set up in the vicinity of the sphenoid wing and corresponds closely to the distribution of orbitotemporal contusions (Fig. 16-1). Shearing stresses would be expected within the brain, the outer parts being constrained to move in conformity with the skull, whereas the inertia of the deeper areas causes them to lag behind.

Transparent skull prostheses have clearly demonstrated that the brain oscillates in a rotary fashion on application of any significant blow. Such oscillations would be the least productive of lesions where the brain was free to move without impact and most damaging where it was tethered by bony or fibrous irregularities, as at the sphenoid wing, crista galli, edge of the falx, and edge of the tentorium. Shearing stresses would be essentially tangential to the surface and would therefore tend to rupture radially arranged structures, notably including penetrating arteries and draining veins. Bridging veins in the region of the superior sagittal sinus and the sylvian fissure (ectopic vessels) would also be liable to tearing.

It currently appears that the rotational model would account for subdural hemorrhage, subarachnoid hemorrhage, the small petechial or confluent hemorrhages seen in the contused cortex and less often in the white matter, and also for the predilection of contusions for areas of irregularity in the skull. A further predictable and experimentally verified result of shearing stresses would be rupture of centrifugally or centripetally directed axons in the hemispheric white matter. Retracted, torn axonal ends have been observed following head injury.

If such a concept reflects the true importance of rotational forces in producing brain injury, this may go some way toward explaining the apparent ineffectiveness of crash helmets in reducing severe head injury in sportsmen and cyclists. These helmets are designed to reduce linear acceleration-deceleration stresses. However, by virtue of their weight, they are likely to increase rather than to decrease rotational stresses, especially hyperextension.

Relationship to Concussion

It further appears probable that rotational forces associated with hyperextension of the neck may be largely responsible for damage to the cervicomedullary region. Experimental application of blows graded in a range from subconcussive to contusional has shown that restriction of the mobility of the neck, as by the application of a plastic collar, approximately doubles the force needed, either to the head or to the body, to produce a condition resembling concussion.

Morphological Changes in Concussion. Although the morphological substrate of concussion has not been clearly defined, observations such as that above have led to close examination of the cervicomedullary region and to claims that subtle morphological and functional changes can be demonstrated earlier in this region than in other parts of the CNS. These include an early and temporary increase in blood-brain barrier permeability to vital dyes, the occasional presence of small perivascular hemorrhages, and changes in neurons, particularly of the lower medullary reticular formation, which resemble central chromatolysis, with loss of central Nissl bodies, swelling, and eccentric displacement of the nucleus. Changes in neurons require at least 24 hours for their development. Axonal rupture and myelin degeneration have been described in the ventrolateral white matter of the upper two cervical segments. How injury causes these changes is not clear, but hyperextension could involve direct contusion of the lower medulla and upper cervical segments against the rim of the foramen magnum and upper cervical vertebrae, causing axonal damage and central chromatolysis (axonal reaction).

Pathogenesis of Concussion. A major role is undoubtedly played by the rotational forces of hyperextension, but a possible contribution by pressure waves generated at the point of impact and leading to shearing stress cannot be excluded. Such waves focus in the area of the foramen magnum in models if the foramen is closed by an elastic but not by a rigid membrane (in the latter case, the point of maximum pressure is a few centimeters anterior to the foramen magnum, nearer the geometric center of the cranial cavity).

In addition to disruption by shearing stresses, a change in the sol-gel configuration of protein (syneresis) has been suggested as one cause of concussion. The concept receives some support from the presence in the brains of professional boxers (who suffer repeated subconcussive and concussive blows) of small plaques of degenerate amyloid-like material and neurofibrils, resembling Alzheimer's disease. Biochemical changes associated with concussion include instantaneous reduction of adenosine triphosphate and creatine phosphate, with accumulation of lactate and inorganic phosphate, suggesting disruption of neuronal function even at the macromolecular level. The EEG of the brain stem reticular formation shows high-amplitude slow waves, and there is temporary desynchronization of the cortical EEG.

There is not universal agreement that concussion is associated with injury only to the reticular formation. In an attempt to correlate retrograde and post-traumatic amnesia with concussion, it has been suggested that the amnesias are due to a "functional" separation of diencephalic structures from the cortex, largely affecting oligosynaptic, myelinated, larger-fiber pathways; whereas concussion, representing a greater degree of shearing stress, disconnects midbrain and cortex by involving small multisynaptic nonmyelinated fibers, such as those of the ascending reticular activating system. These hypotheses need not be mutually exclusive, since the degree of rotational stress disconnecting the midbrain from the cortex may be of the same order as that producing changes in the cervicomedullary region, and it does not appear likely that cortical disconnection per se would account for the cardiorespiratory symptoms that accompany concussion.

Penetrating Injuries

Other than the local injury associated with a depressed fracture, penetrating injuries or perforating (through-and-through) injuries are usually associated with missiles of low mass but high velocity, which penetrate but do not displace the head. They produce direct brain damage as a result of disruption, laceration, or wounding, which may be confined largely to the path of the missile or, particularly near the entry wound, may be cone-shaped, due to fragmentation and dislodgement of pieces of skull.

Passage of a high-velocity missile through a skull filled with materials ranging from clay to gelatine is accompanied by instantaneous, intense, radially transmitted pressure, causing total fragmentation of the skull, with relatively little damage to the clay or gelatin content, though it is temporarily extruded through the entry wound during passage of the missile. Presumably, such pressure fronts may also be reflected toward the foramen magnum. An interesting association has been suggested between high-velocity missile wounds of the brain and the development of meningeal adhesions in the cervicomedullary region, associated with Lhermitte's phenomenon (a peculiar sensation often described as electrical, passing down the arms or legs in association with sudden jarring or hyperflexion of the head; it also occurs following cord irradiation, again, possibly due to the formation of adhesions).

PATHOGENESIS OF SECONDARY BRAIN INJURY

Secondary brain injury is not due to direct physical force causing disruption in the CNS at the gross or microscopic level but instead is mediated either by alterations in the cerebral vasculature (other than rupture) or by changes in other parts of the body, principally involving inefficiency of the cardiorespiratory system. Both mechanisms will only be considered briefly, since much of the relevant material has either already been discussed in previous chapters or will be found in textbooks of general physiology and medicine.

Alterations in Cerebral Vessels and the Blood-Brain Barrier

Induction of Vasoparalysis

Direct observation through a transparent synthetic calvarium indicates that trauma, even at subconcussive levels, produces severe dilatation of the subarachnoid vessels. Further investigation shows that changes extend beyond the subarachnoid vessels and include dilatation of small venules and veins, with slowing of blood flow. Cerebral blood flow following severe injury is proportional to perfusion pressure, confirming the directly observed loss of autoregulation (i.e., vasoparalysis). An increase in pressure and flow is therefore transmitted to the capillaries, and red, oxygenated blood is seen in the veins, indicating a functional shunt. (At present it is not clear whether some arteriovenous bypass exists.) In closed head injuries an increase in cerebral blood volume, occasionally up to four times normal, with a peak approximately 30 minutes following injury, has been observed, also reflecting abolition of autoregulation. Vasoparalysis occurs both in concussional and more severe head injury and precedes changes in arterial blood-gas concentration, therefore being independent of any such changes.

In concussion and even more in severe head injuries, cardiac dysrhythmia with reduced cardiac output and increased central venous pressure often occurs and there is cerebral venous dilatation and partial stasis. There is thus dilatation of the entire cerebral vasculature, and if this causes a twofold or greater increase over the normal cerebral blood volume (120 to 150 ml), an early and significant rise in intracranial pressure occurs. In the early stages this rise is independent of any evidence of blood-brain barrier damage and appears earlier than any possible development of cerebral edema.

Induction of Edema

Even concussive blows (in experimental animals) are associated with temporary permeability of the blood-brain barrier at the cervicomedullary region, extravasation of vital dyes occurring for periods up to an hour. As the force used is increased, this change extends throughout the central nervous system and becomes more enduring, suggesting a functional disruption of the blood-brain barrier, undoubtedly leading to cerebral edema.

Thus, the development of edema, a frequent complication of head injury, may be due to at least two factors (both affecting the integrity of the vessel wall): alteration in the barrier function and paralysis of autoregulation. (It should be noted that an experimentally observed decrease in electrical impedance due to trauma, which develops within a minute, cannot be due to edema and increased extracellular fluid, since it occurs too early. It may represent a further manifestation of functional membrane damage.) If increased central venous pressure significantly increases cerebral circulation time, or arteriovenous shunts reduce circulation to the capillary bed, stasis and hypoxemia may also contribute to the development of edema. (However, as noted in Chapter 12, hypoxemia per se does not appear important in the induction of edema.)

Increased Intracranial Pressure due to Vasoparalysis and Edema

Thus, in many cases of head injury, a significant increase in intracranial pressure often develops within 1 to 3 hours, partly due to increased cerebral blood volume and developing cerebral edema. The potentially lethal spiraling deterioration associated with increased intracranial pressure and compensatory increases in blood pressure, until finally the two become approximately equal and cerebral circulation ceases, was discussed in Chapter 13. This catastrophe can occur in patients in whom there is no mass lesion in the usual sense (e.g., massive depressed fracture or significant intracranial hemorrhage).

Metabolic Effects of Vasoparalysis and Edema

Significant tissue acidosis results from stasis, edema, ischemia due to bypass, or any combination of these conditions, and there are reduced levels of ATP, CrP, and glucose, with accumulation of lactate and inorganic phosphate. One of the earliest morphological features is increased accumulation of glycogen granules within a few hours in the cytoplasm of astrocytes. It has been suggested that there might be failure of neuronal utilization because of physical or metabolic damage, glucose being transferred from neurons to astrocytes. Certainly, autoradiography indicates an increase in glycogen synthesis, but this might be an early reactive change in the astrocytes. The phenomenon is not peculiar to traumatic brain injury, but it is particularly marked in many of these cases, suggesting that both mechanisms might be operative.

Other Vascular Changes

The existence of regional as well as generalized vasoparalysis has been demonstrated (at least in children) by the estimation of regional cerebral blood flow. The normal "washout curve" of xenon shows a fast component due to rapid blood flow in gray matter and a slower component due to the less rapid flow in white matter. In some cases of head injury, a triphasic curve is observed, the abnormal third component being even faster than that for normal gray matter and presumably representing a functional or anatomical shunt mechanism.

An effect paradoxically opposite to paralysis of autoregulation is sometimes observed. As noted previously, vasospasm may occur if arteries sustain mechanical trauma, or in the presence of subarachnoid hemorrhage, and either or both of these may be involved in diffuse head injury. Spasm has been demonstrated angiographically in up to 30% of cases of head injury with variable distribution. It may be diffuse, either involving major basal vessels or extending to larger cortical vessels over the hemispheres; or it may be localized at contusion sites, especially in association with depressed fracture or extradural or subdural hemorrhage. It has occasionally been observed in the vicinity of penetrating injuries. The intracavernous part of the internal carotid artery appears to be the most susceptible area. Vasospasm may persist for a day or two or up to six weeks though, in the more chronic cases, narrowing observed on angiography may be due to vessel-wall damage, sometimes distinguishable as irregularities of contour.

Alterations in the Cardio-Respiratory System

Injury in other parts of the body may have a severe indirect effect on the CNS, which, if combined with direct brain damage, may act synergistically to produce otherwise unexpected death or permanent sequelae.

The vascular system may be involved either by direct cardiac damage or blood loss. Severe hemorrhage acutely reduces circulating blood volume, and although generalized vasoconstriction effectively shunts more blood to the CNS, cerebral blood flow may still be insufficient, perfusion pressure lowered, and, especially if intracranial pressure is raised, ischemic changes may occur. Circulating volume may be made up later from extracellular fluid or administered fluids, but unless much of the replacement is blood or plasma, hemodilution lowers both the osmotic pressure (favoring development of cerebral edema) and the arterial PO_2 (favoring development of hypoxemic lesions). These changes are compounded if injury to the heart results in reduced cardiac output and raised central venous pressure.

Another significant problem in many cases is the development of respiratory acidosis, associated with chest injury, pulmonary hemorrhage, aspiration, or other ventilatory insufficiency. Since there may also be primary depression of respiratory drive due to the CNS injury, spiraling deterioration is readily established, leading to reduced arterial P_{O_2} and increased P_{CO_2}. In the early stages, a compensatory rise in cerebral blood flow occurs if vasomotor reactivity is retained. If vasoparalysis is already established, cerebral blood flow is maximal, depending only on perfusion pressure. In chronic respiratory acidosis in the absence of vasoparalysis, cerebral blood flow may eventually fall to subnormal levels (decompensation). This may in part be due to the effects of acidosis on the heart, leading to tachycardia and reduced cardiac output, and in part to acidosis-induced damage to the blood-brain barrier, causing cerebral edema. In experimental respiratory acidosis there are early and severe EEG changes, reduction and clumping of synaptic vesicles, and a minor degree of astrocytic swelling, occurring in the early phase of increased cerebral blood flow. This probably indicates interference with ATP formation even in the presence of adequate oxygen, glucose, and metabolite removal (metabolic hypoxidosis).

Hyperpyrexia is not uncommon in patients with head injury and may be of CNS origin, associated with infection or due to reduced heat loss from the skin because of shock and vasoconstriction. A degree of hyperpyrexia that is without observable effects on the normal CNS may cause significant impairment in brain-injured patients.

In summary, the second accident, which so often complicates the primary mechanical disruptive effects of head injury, may be due to effects on vessel caliber, including vasoparalysis and vasospasm, altered barrier permeability, or changes in the quality and quantity of perfusion (alterations of pressure, total flow, oxygen and carbon dioxide concentration, and temperature). Many of these factors, if continuously monitored, can probably be kept within normal limits, perhaps making a significant contribution to improving the prognosis of patients with head injuries.

THE MORPHOLOGY OF HEAD INJURY

The descriptions of the morphological sequelae of head injury given in this section are confined to the primary effects. Secondary lesions associated with alterations in cerebral vessels or cardiopulmonary insufficiency have been dealt with in the preceding chapters. It suffices to say that in fatal cases, autopsy may show almost any combination of direct and indirect brain damage.

Large autopsied series of fatal head injuries show a wide range of lesions. If death was immediate, very little change may be seen in the CNS, since there has been inadequate time for morphological alterations to develop. With longer survival, there may be varying combinations of lesions, which can be classified as contusions (bruises), penetrating or lacerating lesions (brain wounds), and hemorrhage of such volume as to constitute a significant space-occupying lesion. This latter occurs in very few even of those patients who come to autopsy, emphasizing that the rise in intracranial pressure accompanying head injury is almost always due to the indirect effects that have been discussed.

Minimal Morphological Changes in Fatal Head Injury

Many patients with head injury suffer what may be regarded for practical purposes as immediate death (within a few seconds or a few minutes) and are dead on admission to the hospital even under the most favorable circumstances. As previously indicated, such patients will not show significant space-occupying hemorrhage or cerebral edema, nor can the subtle changes described in experimental lesions at the cervicomedullary junction be manifested so soon. Even the small perivascular hemorrhages of contusion may not have developed in the short period between injury and death. Patients with depressed skull fracture and laceration of the dura, or with penetrating or perforating wounds, naturally show brain laceration. There are, in fact, only two changes almost invariably found in death due to head injury, even if it is virtually immediate. The first is vasodilatation or vasoparalysis, manifested by a mild to moderate increase in brain weight, and dilated vessels, often best seen grossly in the frontal white matter and basal ganglia (Fig. 16-2). Microscopically, dilatation appears particularly to involve small vessels of the cerebellum and brain stem, especially beneath the ependyma of the fourth ventricle. The second change is minor hemorrhage, not amounting to hematoma formation, best seen as slight, diffuse blood-staining of CSF in the subarachnoid and ventricular spaces.

With further minutes of survival time, contusion hemorrhages may become apparent, and there may even be early hematoma formation, especially if large arteries are damaged by skull fracture or penetrating injury.

Contusions

Contusions have been extensively referred to in the preceding discussion under such terms as *coup, contre-coup,* and *intermediate coup lesions.* In order to make an adequate distinction between contusion and wounding, the term *contusion* is best applied to cortical lesions only in the absence of dural perforation. Contusions are largely associated with rotational stresses following head or body impact and usually present as hemorrhages or occasionally as areas of nonhemorrhagic necrosis. In the immature brain, they may appear as lacerations.

Contusion hemorrhages (the usual form of contusion) are multiple, petechial, or occasionally coalescent, initially perivascular, and present within seconds or minutes of impact, occasionally increasing in size for a few hours. Rarely, they develop into hematomas. They are often in the form of radial streaks in the cortex (Fig. 16-3), accompanied by minor, diffuse blood-staining of adjacent subarachnoid fluid. They are more likely to become coalescent deep in the cortical sulci, where they may form small globular lesions a few millimeters across. The reaction of the brain tissue, as to any other hemorrhage, includes microglial activation at 36 to 40 hours, gitter-cell and astroglial reaction at five to six days, and total resorption in three to twelve weeks, depending on size. Small petechiae give rise to microscopic gliomesen-

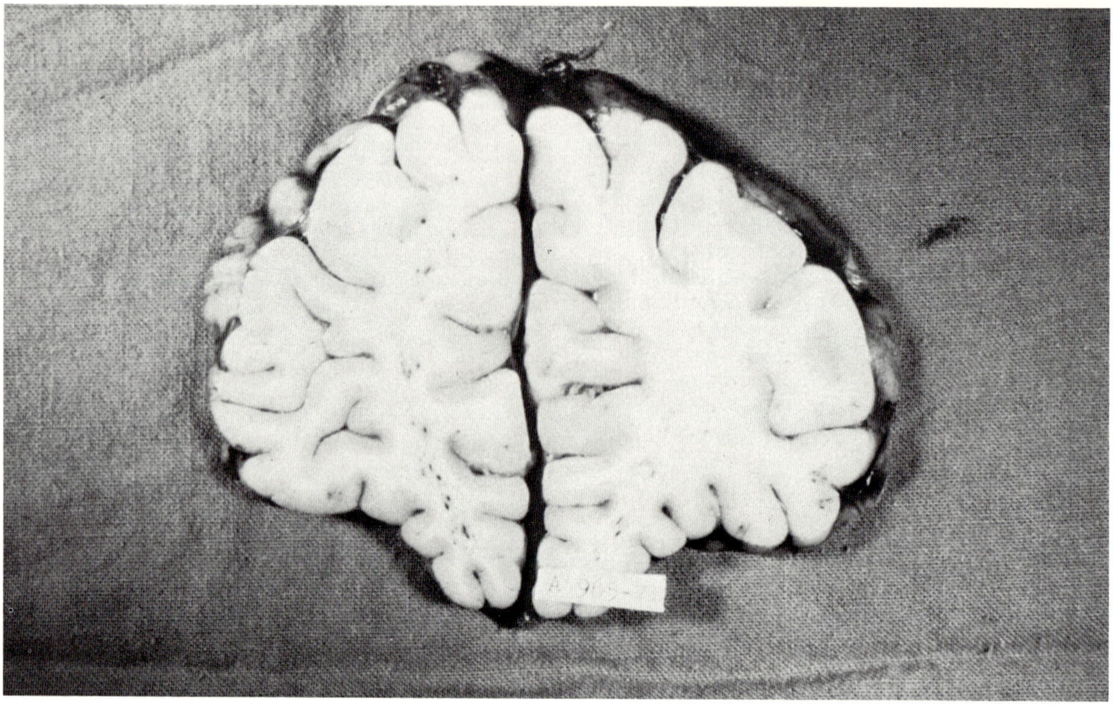

Fig. 16-2. Minimal changes seen in death due to head injury, occurring shortly after injury, include vasodilatation, which, as here, is often most prominent in the frontal white matter.

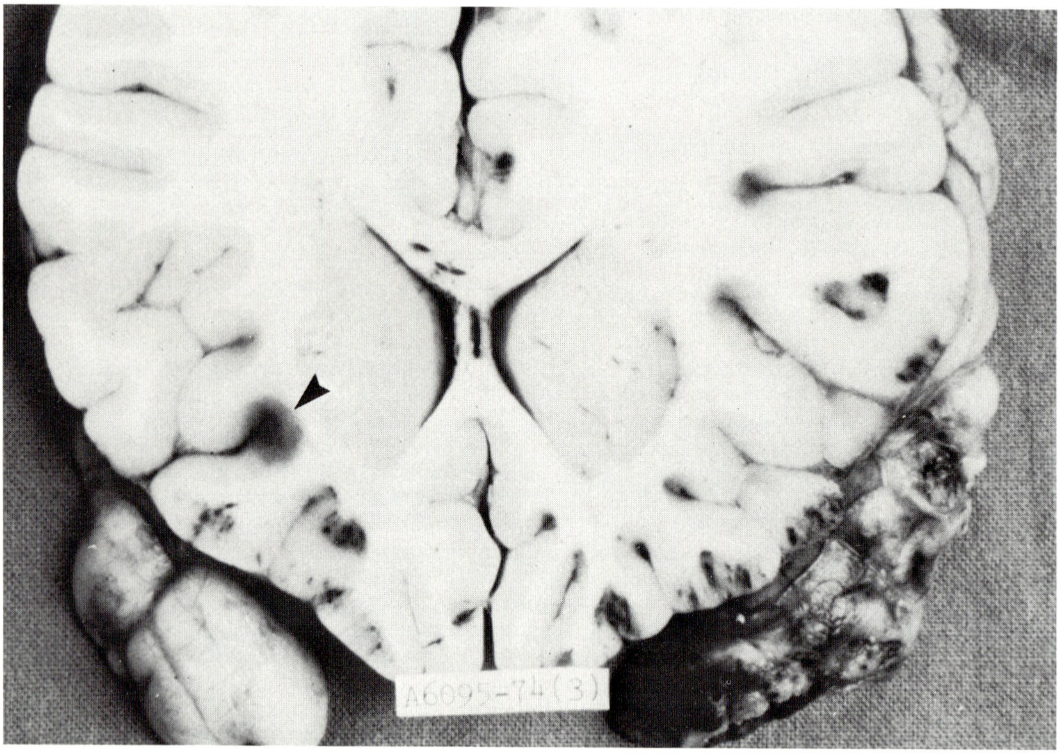

Fig. 16-3. Cortical contusions in the orbitotemporal area, especially on the left. The cortical hemorrhages tend to be radial and linear, and coalescent hemorrhages forming a small hematoma may be seen on the right (arrow). A few small rotational hemorrhages are also present in the corpus callosum, adjacent to the edge of the falx, and elsewhere.

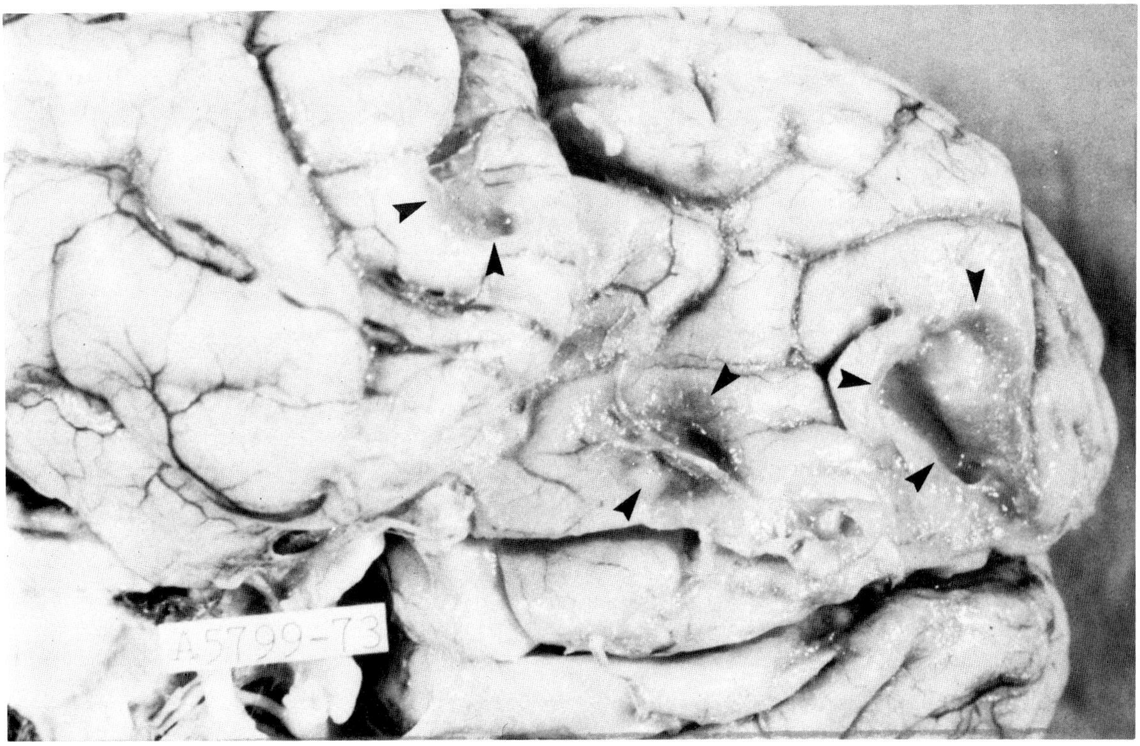

Fig. 16-4. Old areas of contusion necrosis in the right orbitotemporal region (arrows), situated on the gyral crowns and open to the subarachnoid space.

chymal scars; larger hemorrhages form small cystic cavities.

Contusion necrosis is not visible for about 12 hours. Lesions gradually become swollen and soft, reaching maximum size at five to seven days and resolving slowly over the next few months, with the formation of superficial, cystic, slightly discolored cavities in the superficial cortex and white matter (Fig. 16-4). These cavities are directly open to the subarachnoid space, since the molecular layer is involved (unlike infarcts). They are found at the crests of gyri and appear wedge-shaped on transverse section. The intervening sulcal cortex is intact. These features enable distinction of post-traumatic lesions (état vermoulu or plaques jaunes) from small cortical infarcts. Contusion necrosis is unusual except in the orbitotemporal cortex.

In immature brains, clefts in the hemispheric white matter may be the only evidence of injury and can readily be mistaken for artifacts due to postmortem handling. They occur in the same areas that are involved in adults, particularly the orbitotemporal, superior frontal, and (occasionally) occipital regions. Lacerations are rare in adults, but they are occasionally seen in the corpus callosum, septum pellucidum, cerebral peduncles, or at the junction of the pons and medulla.

Intracranial Hematomas

Even in autopsies intracranial hematomas are relatively infrequent. Subdural hemorrhages are found in about 5%, extradural hemorrhages in about 1.5%, and intracerebral hemorrhages in about 0.5% of autopsies following fatal head injuries.

Extradural Hemorrhage

Extradural hemorrhage is usually associated with blunt rather than penetrating injury and occasionally develops in children in the absence of skull fracture. Development of an extradural hematoma clearly implies separation of the outer layer of the dura from the skull, and since the attachment is normally firmer at the base and in the occipital region, extradural hemorrhage is rare in these areas. In infancy, the entire dura seems to be firmly attached, and the incidence of extradural hemorrhage is low.

Hemorrhage may occur either from arteries or veins, but venous pressure cannot extend the traumatic stripping of the dura. Arterial pressure can do so, and most of the life-menacing extradural hemorrhages are arterial, arising usually from the middle meningeal vessels, but occasionally from posterior meningeal vessels. An acutely developing mass of 75 ml or more may endanger life; a smaller amount will do so if there is severe vasodilatation and edema.

Extradural hematomas are organized from the dura, and migration of mesenchymal cells and new vessel formation is usually conspicuous between six to nine days. Vascular channels are relatively few, and secondary hemorrhages are correspondingly infrequent. Small extradural hematomas are con-

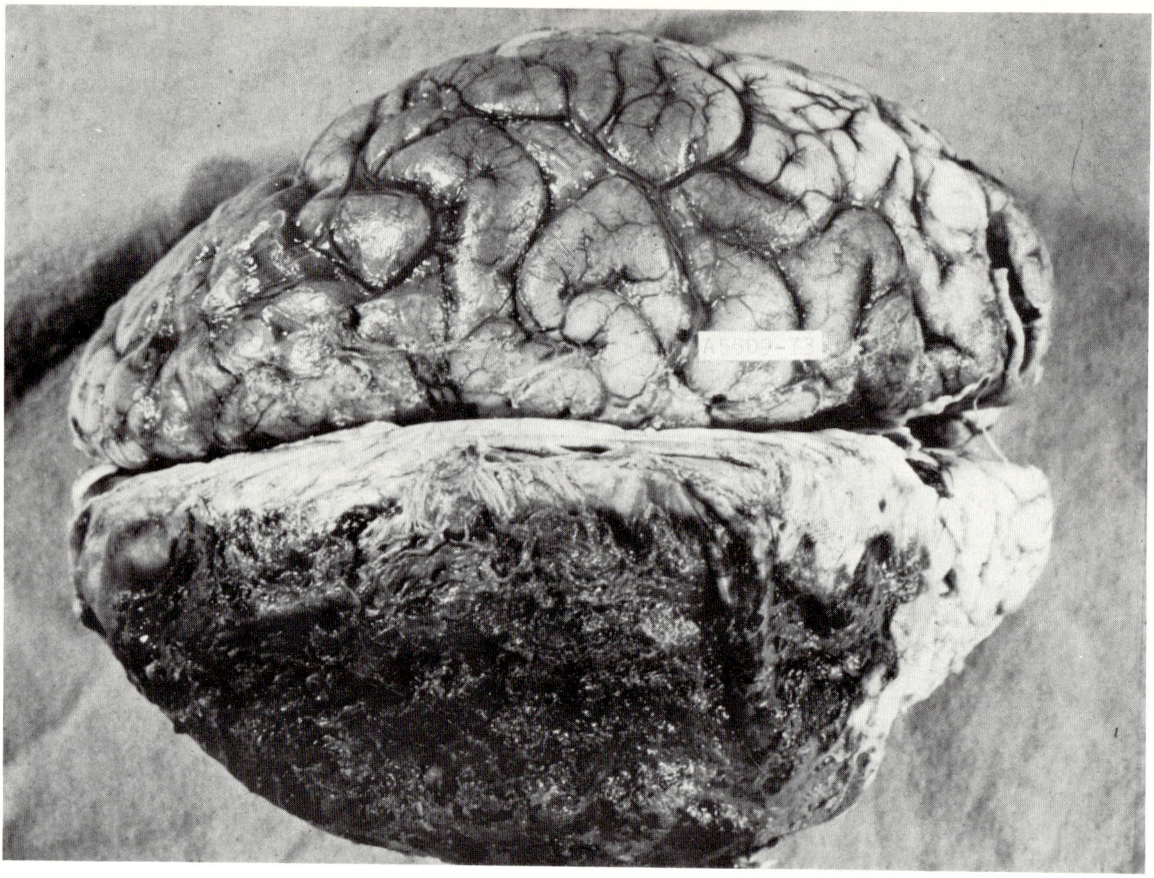

Fig. 16-5. Subdural hematoma. The dura from the upper hemisphere has been turned downward to reveal a massive organizing blood clot on its deep surface. Note that there were no changes in the underlying arachnoid, except some discoloration due to blood pigment, and no dural-arachnoidal adhesions.

verted to collagenous scars, but larger ones form cysts with a collagenous rim and containing thin, variably blood-stained fluid.

Dural tears are associated with a small extradural hematoma essential for their repair, with organization starting from the adventitia of small vessels and the inner lining of the dura. If the blood clot is washed away, as by fistulas passing into the middle ear or the nose, the dura may need surgical repair to forestall retrograde infection of the cranial cavity. If dural tears involve sinuses, severe hemorrhage may result, particularly from the superior sagittal or lateral vessels. Bleeding may be internal, external, or both and is difficult to control because of the rigidity of the sinus walls. Sinus tears are usually associated with fracture in adults, but in infants can occur without them. Lesser damage to the wall of the sinus may cause thrombosis. Fractures at the base, although rarely tearing the cavernous sinuses, may injure the carotid artery, leading to a carotid-cavernous sinus fistula.

Subdural Hemorrhage

Subdural hemorrhage is probably always due to trauma, although the injury may be so slight, especially in elderly people, that no such history is obtained. Probably the commonest sources of subdural bleeding are cortical hemorrhagic contusions associated with tearing of the arachnoid, and tears or lacerations of the dura, especially if sinuses are involved. About 30% of subdural hemorrhages are due to rupture of bridging veins — either those adjacent to the superior sagittal sinus or ectopic vessels that enter the dura from the region of the sylvian fissure and run between its two layers to the superior sagittal or lateral sinus. (The sylvian fissure area often shows quite firm adhesions between arachnoid and the dura, representing persistence of the embryonic condition.) Even the most exacting examination fails to reveal a source for subdural bleeding in about 10% of cases.

Hemorrhage is most common over the upper and lateral aspects of the hemispheres (Fig. 16-5), unilaterally or bilaterally, but may also occur in the temporal regions. It seems to be associated with blows in the anteroposterior rather than in the lateral direction, and

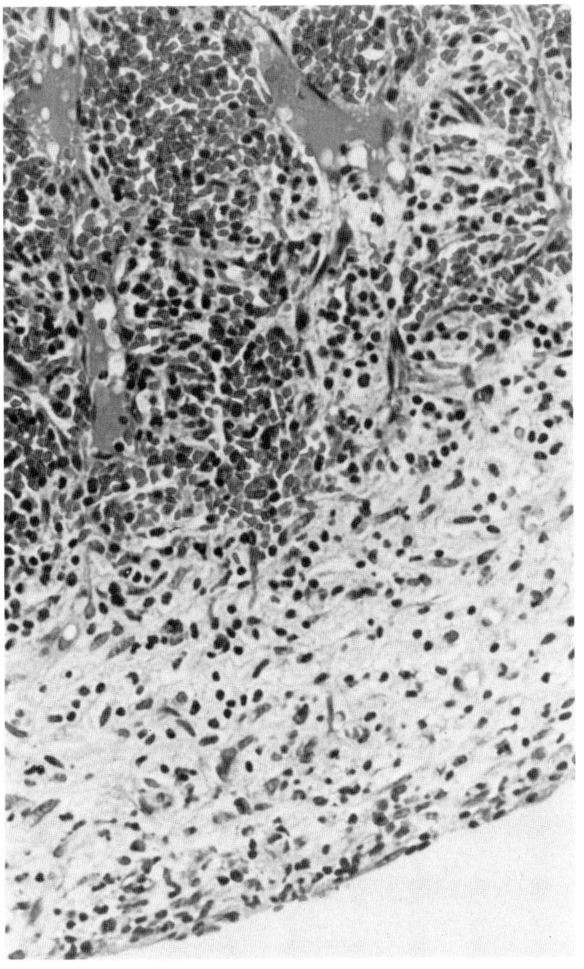

Fig. 16-6. An early stage in the organization of a subdural hematoma. The inner membrane is clearly seen and contains mononuclear cells and vessels. Prominent capillaries are invading the blood clot. (H & E, ×300.)

there is little relation between the side of the blow and the side on which hemorrhage develops. Since subdural hemorrhages are usually mainly venous in origin, development is slower than for extradural hemorrhages, and the possibilities of treatment are therefore greater. Patients with accumulations of 100 to 200 ml of blood may survive, even with considerable deformation of the brain. However, *acute* subdural hematomas may develop following penetrating head injury with cerebral laceration and arterial bleeding. Such hematomas are difficult to treat and carry a rather poor prognosis.

Subdural hematomas are organized entirely from the dura, not from the arachnoid. Cells derived from the inner lining of the dura and its perivascular mesenchyme migrate into the clot directly and also spread over the surface facing the arachnoid (Fig. 16-6). Organization begins at 5 to 7 days and is proceeding rapidly at 10 to 20 days. The formation of the thin inner membrane (facing the arachnoid) and a thicker outer membrane is usually complete in four to eight weeks (Fig. 16-7). The organizing blood clot is very vascular, and secondary hemorrhages are frequent, probably accounting for recurrence of symptoms and expansion of the lesion.

It has been suggested that such expansion might be due to hyperosmolality from the breakdown products of blood, but the osmolality of resolving subdural hematomas is the same as in blood and CSF. The mechanism of resolution in infants appears to be somewhat different, as the blood is very rapidly removed and the clot converted to a clear fluid (subdural effusion), enclosed by delicate membranes. If the membranes are not adequately removed, the effusion may recur after evacuation; but, again, its osmolality is that of blood and CSF.

Subarachnoid Hemorrhage

Subarachnoid hemorrhage is usually diffuse and thin (Fig. 16-8) rather than forming a definite hematoma, although a firm clot is occasionally seen if arteries are torn. Presumably because of dilution by CSF, such hemorrhages do not usually clot. Red cells are lysed within two to seven days and removed partly by bulk flow (see Chap. 4), but largely by leptomeningeal phagocytic cells that are active within two days, reach a peak at two to four weeks, and disappear after two to three months, leaving little or no scar tissue. Residual iron-staining of astrocytes in the molecular layer of the cortex is frequently the only persistent change. However, there is occasional development of permanent communicating hydrocephalus, which appears to be a common temporary phenomenon during the resolution stage. Where permanent, it is presumably associated with fibrosis of the meninges, either in the posterior fossa or over the surface of the brain, or possibly with permanent damage to the arachnoidal granulations (pacchionian bodies) and arachnoid villi, and becomes clinically significant.

Intraventricular Hemorrhage

Intraventricular hemorrhage, to the extent of blood-stained CSF, is virtually inevitable. Major hemorrhage, which is not often seen, arises from veins in the ventricular walls, tears of the septum pellucidum or major cerebral damage.

Intracerebral Hemorrhage

Intracerebral hemorrhage is unusual, at least to the extent of becoming a significant space-occupying lesion. It is probably associated with rotational accelerations, since most occurs in the temporal or frontal lobes, with only occasional bleeding in other regions (Fig. 16-9). The frontal hematomas tend to be associated with a severe occipital blow, and temporal lesions with a lateral blow and showing a slight

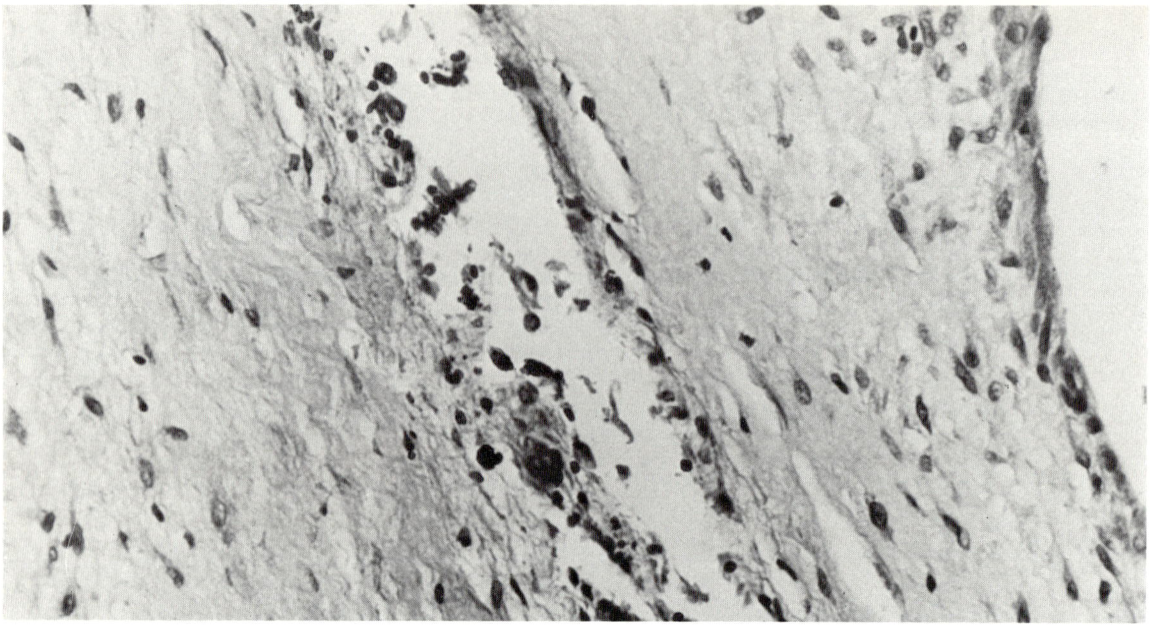

Fig. 16-7. A well-organized subdural hematoma, showing the inner (right) and part of the outer membrane, the former clot being now represented only by a cleft containing macrophages filled with iron pigment. (H & E, X300.)

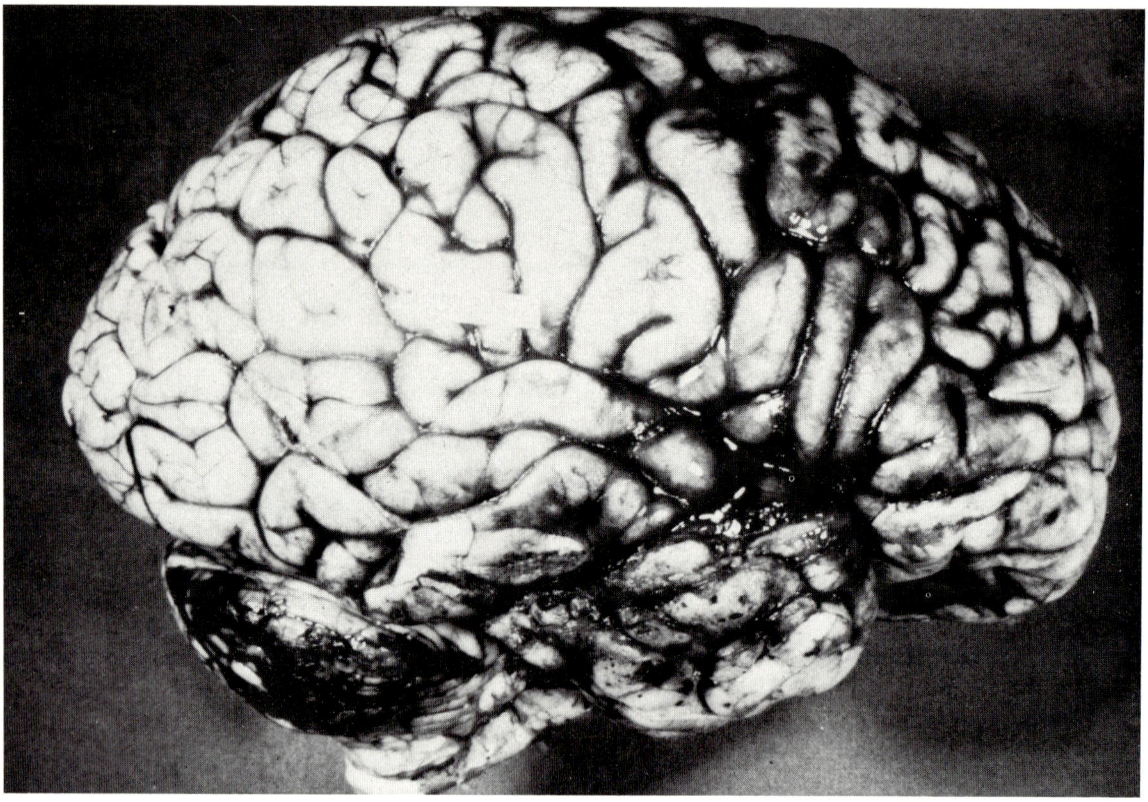

Fig. 16-8. Minor subarachnoid hemorrhage, such as that often seen in patients with head injury. Temporal lobe contusion can also be seen.

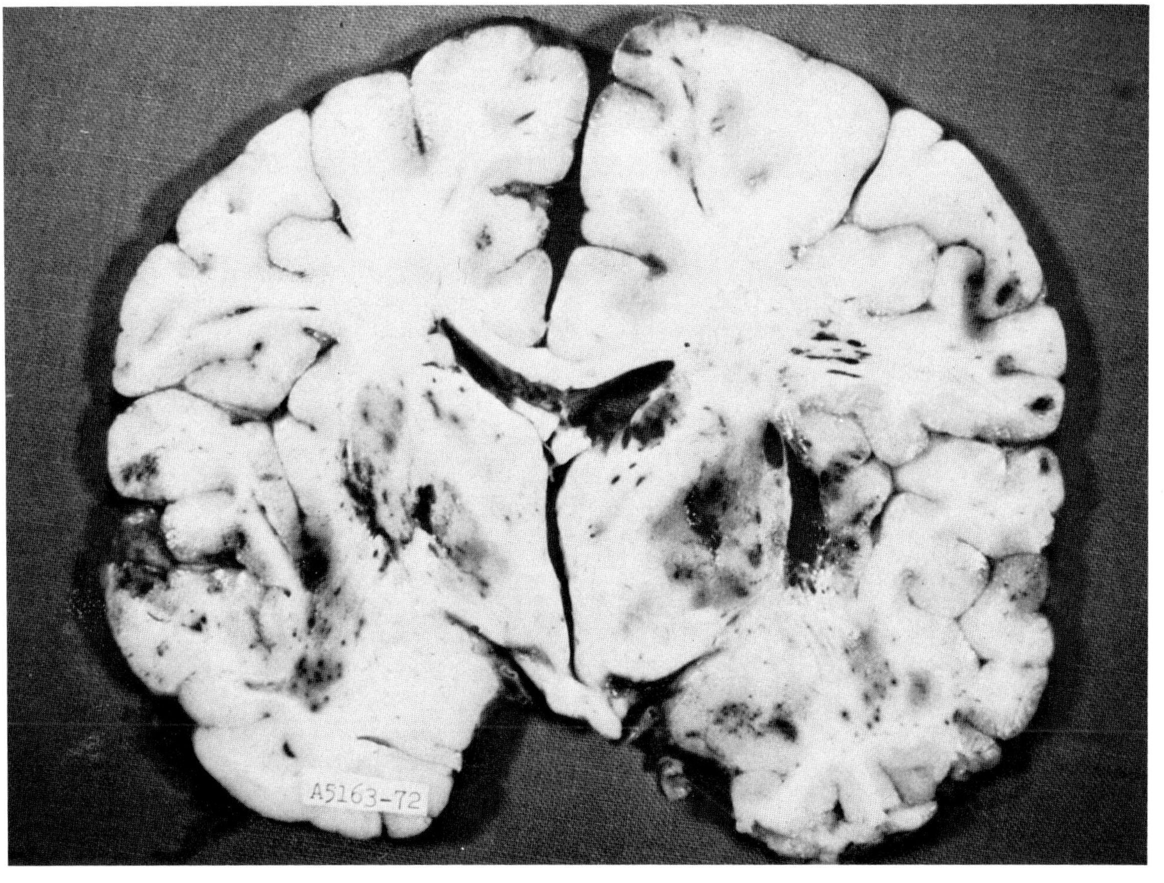

Fig. 16-9. Generalized intracerebral petechiae, perivascular hemorrhages, and small coalescent hemorrhages in head injury, probably due to rotational (shearing) stresses and unusually marked in the deep gray matter. Hemorrhages larger than these (space-occupying) are distinctly unusual.

preponderance on the side of impact. In patients who survive, resolution of these hemorrhages is by lysis, with formation of gliomesenchymal scars or cavities, depending on size.

Brain Wounds

General Characteristics

Brain wounds are due to penetration of the brain and therefore are invariably associated with rupture of the dura. They may be extended by bone fragments detached from the skull, particularly in the orbital cortex, since the bone of the orbital roof tends to form thin, brittle fragments (Fig. 16-10). In injuries from low-velocity objects (blows or falls), the shape of the wound may reflect that of the object, being rounded or irregular (hammer, other blunt object) linear (axe), or narrow and elongated (screwdriver, steel rod). Wounds are associated with tearing and pulping of brain substance, and retained foreign bodies, notably bone fragments, may be present. Hemorrhage is variable and is not a reliable index of survival time, since such severe injury may produce localized vasospasm, and wounded areas may remain ischemic for as long as one hour, and then bleed copiously.

Wounds by small, high-velocity missiles, such as bullets or fragments of shrapnel, are far less frequent in civilian than in military practice. They may be classified as *depressed* if the missile bounces off the external surface of the skull tangentially; *penetrating* if it enters the cranium and remains there; or *perforating* (through-and-through) if it both enters and leaves the cranial cavity. Depressed missile wounds are rare and are associated with severe laceration of bone, meninges, and vessels at the point of impact, variable laceration of the brain, and softening due to vascular damage that may considerably outweigh the primary injury. Penetrating wounds are the most common and are usually due to a single bullet of medium velocity, though they may be complicated by explosive gases and bone fragments or be multiple in shotgun wounds. Occasionally, the bullet may ricochet inside the skull, so that more than one linear tract is found.

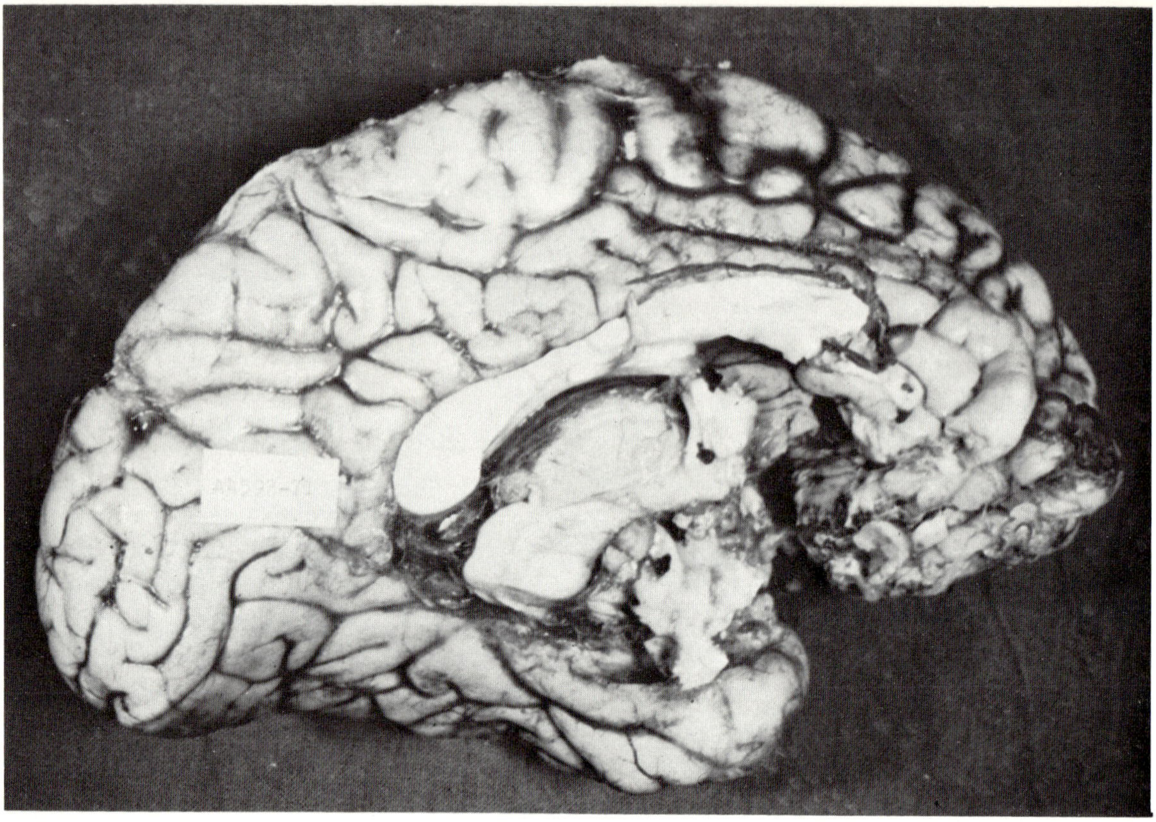

Fig. 16-10. Laceration of the posterior orbital region (left hemisphere) by thin bone plates detached from the orbital roof (frontal blow).

Special Characteristics of Bullet Wounds

Penetrating and perforating bullet tracts within the brain (Fig. 16-11) are slightly wider than the bullet, especially in their mid-portion, and the wall frequently shows a zone of necrosis and laceration adjacent to the cavity, a middle zone of pale ischemic necrosis, and a zone of petechial or confluent hemorrhage adjacent to normal brain. The cause of the zones is not clear, but they are present even in immediately fatal wounds. As has been noted, a missile of medium or high velocity produces very severe centrifugal force, which may be responsible for the zone of ischemic necrosis, and also can produce unexpected fractures of the skull (particularly in the orbital region, where the bone is thin) and contusions at the edge of the tentorium and foramen magnum. Hemorrhage from bullet wounds may be either immediate or delayed for an hour or two and is not usually extensive unless a major vessel is torn. However, raised intracranial pressure may develop in these patients, possibly associated with edema or altered autoregulation.

Post-Traumatic Lesions

The many potential short-term and long-term sequelae of head injury may be briefly listed.

Infection

Infection may occur in open injuries and includes epidural or subdural empyema, leptomeningitis, diffuse encephalitis, single or multiple brain abscesses, and pyocephalus. Localized brain infections especially are often associated with retained fragments of foreign material. Military experience has shown that these fragments, even if metallic, are often contaminated with skin bacteria such as *Staphylococcus epidermidis.*

Hydrocephalus

Hydrocephalus is an uncommon sequela of head injury (some possible mechanisms in its development were discussed in Chapter 15). Occasionally, hemorrhage may block the aqueduct, producing a symmetrical, noncommunicating hydrocephalus. There is little evidence for postulated excess CSF formation in the postconcussional syndrome.

Delayed Hemorrhage

Hemorrhage may develop in almost any part of the brain days to months after injury. It is probably due to partial tearing of a vessel, with ultimate development of an area of vessel rupture or aneurysm (often termed a *false aneurysm*).

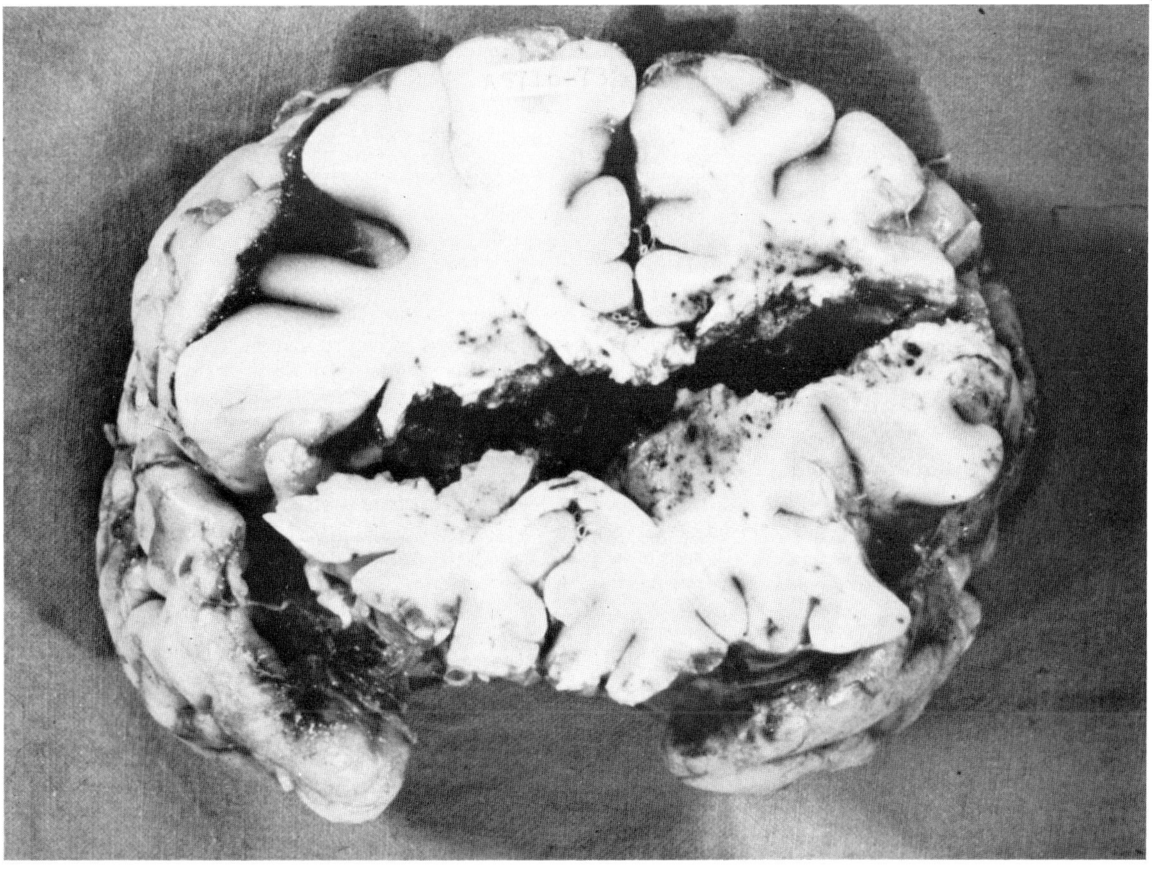

Fig. 16-11. Transverse bullet wound (entry to left of photograph), showing central widening. The zone of ischemic necrosis described in the text is not seen here.

Cranial Nerve Damage

Rotational stresses and subarachnoid hemorrhage occasionally damage cranial nerves, including the olfactory nerve filaments, optic nerve, nerves to the ocular muscles, and, if there is basal fracture, branches of the fifth, seventh, and eighth nerves. Sequelae include anosmia, ocular pareses, facial paresis, deafness, and dizziness. The latter two might also be due to bony damage involving the cochlea and labyrinth.

Protracted Post-Traumatic Encephalopathy

Protracted post-traumatic encephalopathy is a term often applied to patients unconscious from the time of an accident, with evidence of severe brain stem dysfunction, such as oculomotor, postural, and respiratory disorders and extensor spasms, who may survive in such a state for periods of months. These cases are due to secondary damage, hypoxemic or circulatory, most severe in the deep structures and brain stem and attributable to edema, uncal herniation, brain stem displacement, and damage to perforating vessels at the rostral brain stem level.

Psychopathy

Following severe head injury, there appears to be a considerable incidence of psychological deficit, from which children recover better than adults. The morphological substrate is unknown.

Post-Traumatic Epilepsy

Epilepsy is a well-recognized complication of moderate or severe head injury and is discussed further in Chapter 18.

SPINAL CORD INJURY

Mechanisms

Trauma to the spinal cord or cauda equina may occur at any level but is particularly common in the cervical region as an accompaniment to head injury, where it is frequently neglected in routine autopsies. Mechanisms of cord injury include hyperextension or hyperflexion, often with a rotational component, and stretching of the cord or roots is accentuated by disc prolapse or severe spondylolisthesis. More severe cord injuries are associated with fracture dislocation of the spinal column, mostly in the cervical but also in the lower thoracic region. Penetrating wounds, usually posterior, occasionally occur.

Transient Cord Damage

The spinal cord, like the brain, may suffer from concussion, which is temporary and from which patients completely recover. There is immediate but temporary loss of ascending and descending conduction and segmental function in the area of the trauma, with no demonstrable bone fracture or external change in the cord. The few autopsy studies available have shown localized edema, perivascular hemorrhage, occasional small ischemic softenings, neuronal changes resembling central chromatolysis, and some beading and swelling of myelin and (occasionally) axons. Any small ischemic areas presumably form gliomesenchymal scars, but otherwise the condition appears to be one from which patients recover and may be regarded as primary vascular stasis and edema. Of course, in autopsied patients it can only be assumed that permanent, complete restoration of function would have occurred if death had not supervened. In such patients, the changes described may be more severe than usual.

Permanent Cord Damage

More severe injuries cause permanent, partial or complete, functional transection of the cord, which may or may not be associated with physical laceration or actual transection. Interference with ascending and descending pathways and local segmental function is, at least in part, permanent, and death in such patients may be due to intercurrent infection of the lung or bladder or trophic ulcerations of the skin. In patients without physical transection, variable recovery may occur, presumably due to axonal growth. There may be a return of sensation, first of pressure, then of touch, pain, and temperature. Finally, some motor function may return. Recovery is limited by gliosis in the disrupted cord and probably also by failure of regenerating axons to make the appropriate physiological connections.

The tragic morbidity, as much as the mortality, associated with spinal cord injury has led to intensive investigation into the pathogenesis of traumatic cord lesions. The results of these studies will be reviewed, followed by a discussion of their relation to observations on human subjects.

Experimental Spinal Cord Injury

Technique

A standard method of producing experimental cord injury consists of exposing the cord (usually with the dura intact) by laminectomy, applying a graded force, and assessing morphological changes and, more recently, vascular, physiological, and biochemical effects. The findings are then compared with the clinical results in controls subjected to laminectomy only. A force of 300 g-cm usually produces a severe but transient paraplegia, whereas increasing the force to 400 g-cm usually causes irreversible clinical changes. Thus, much of the research has focused on the results of the application of force at these levels, mainly in primates.

Morphological Correlates of Reversible Cord Damage

A force of 300 g-cm (reversible clinical weakness) leads to central edema, hemorrhage, and diapedesis of leukocytes, and there may be a central area of hemorrhagic necrosis with some neuronal loss. Lesions tend to be centered immediately posterior to the central canal and spread to involve adjacent white and gray matter, the latter more severely.

Small confluent hemorrhages and hematomas are associated with early distension and small tears of venules; diapedesis of erythrocytes around postcapillary and muscular venules is present at about 15 minutes, and gross gray-matter hemorrhage appears at 1 hour. The endothelium of both capillaries and venules shows a marked increase in pinocytosis. The cause of vessel tearing is unknown, but perhaps is shearing stress. The reason for endothelial changes may be arterial constriction, since some vessels apparently fail to perfuse. White matter shows occupation of a widened space between axons and their myelin sheaths by clear, non-protein-containing fluid at 15 minutes, some attenuation of myelin at 30 minutes, and variable axonal shrinkage with free myelin figures at 1 to 4 hours, with mild swelling of astrocytic processes.

Thus, investigations suggest that even at this level of force there is probably some irreversible, though clinically inapparent change in both gray and white matter.

Morphological Correlates of Irreversible Cord Damage

A force of 400 g-cm or more (severe or total irreversible paraplegia) causes severe edema and hemorrhage within a few hours, followed by massive hemorrhagic and inflammatory necrosis, with destruction of parenchymal elements and even vessels. Peripheral white matter retains some normal myelinated axons. The lesions are progressive for several hours. Focal hemorrhages in the gray matter rapidly coalesce (minimal changes in the central anterior horns only; maximal changes in all except the tips of the dorsal horns). White-matter hemorrhages do not coalesce, but are associated with massive edema that may lead to necrosis. The changes in vessels are similar to those observed with the force of 300 g-cm, but are considerably more severe.

Areas of retained circulation have been assessed by the dye thioflavine S, which stains endothelium; the contused segments of cord are removed within 10 seconds (one circulation time) of dye injection. In control cords there is general fluorescence, which is more marked in gray than white matter. In contused cord, the patterns in gray and white matter differ. In gray matter, small areas of nonfluorescence (hemorrhage) are visible at 5 minutes, are appreciably larger at 15 minutes, and coalesce to involve much of the gray matter by about 30 minutes. From 1 to 24 hours (the limits of the experiment) contused gray matter shows virtually no fluorescence and histologically is totally hemorrhagic. The white matter, on the other hand, appears normal at 5 minutes, shows slightly reduced fluorescence at 15 minutes, but restoration of normal levels at 30 minutes, except for small nonfluorescent (hemorrhagic) spots. From 1 to 8 hours there is again a decrease in fluorescence (with some edema and extravasation of the dye), followed by an increase almost to control values at 24 hours, except near the white matter hemorrhages and the central gray matter.

Effects on Water Content and Metabolism of Cord

Other experiments have shown that cord contused at a force of 300 g-cm or less (with little hemorrhage) shows increased water content within 5 minutes. This persists for some 15 days and presumably is edema.

Increased lactate is detectable within minutes, persists at least 12 to 18 hours, and is presumably associated, as in the brain, with a change to anaerobic metabolism and reduction in ATP levels. Rapid decreases in cord tissue Po_2 and blood flow have also been reported.

Possible Role of Norepinephrine in Pathogenesis of Vascular Damage

The mechanism of the vascular damage, leading to massive gray and some white matter hemorrhage, is undetermined. Direct physical damage, leading to tears in the venules, seems inadequate to explain total hemorrhagic necrosis. Thrombosis in the earliest stages has not been reported, and arterial spasm with stasis appears the most probable mechanism. Following contusion, irregularity and spasm of cord vessels occurs, particularly affecting the anterior median arteries, which supply much of the gray and adjacent white matter.

Serotonin concentration shows very little change, but there are dramatic rises in norepinephrine, associated with a reduction in dopamine. Even slight injury raises cord norepinephrine. A force of 400 g-cm doubles the level in 25 to 30 minutes and raises it to five times normal in about an hour. Norepinephrine diffuses one to two segments along the cord and begins to drop at 3 to 4 hours, finally reaching subnormal levels. Injection of norepinephrine into the cord, producing concentrations more than double the normal, exactly reproduces the hemorrhagic necrosis observed in trauma, whereas injection of saline has no effect. (This tendency of the cord to liberate norepinephrine readily probably accounts for the ready elicitation of the Cushing phenomenon by minor cord manipulation or pressure.)

Alpha-methyltyrosine, given 15 minutes after cord compression, reduces and in some cases prevents central hemorrhage and converts a normally irreversible process into a reversible one, with restoration of adequate cord function.

It is uncertain whether the increase in norepinephrine levels is due to release from granules, increased synthesis, reduced reuptake or inactivation, or any combination of these processes. Unfortunately, necessary dosages of α-methyltyrosine are toxic to the human kidney, but it is possible that fractional dosage, concurrent forced diuresis, or the substitution of another similar compound may enable human trials to take place.

Tentative Conclusions

In summary, experimental work indicates that, in the absence of physical transection, the effect of injury on the cord is largely vascular. Mechanical rupture is only a minor factor, most damage being secondary to vascular spasm and stasis, possibly due to norepinephrine release. This vascular damage leads to white-matter edema. Although the cord does not have a tight bony casing, the pia arachnoid is sufficiently strong to resist the stretching, and the edema causes additional ischemia.

Morphological Observations in Clinical Cord Damage

The morphological correlates of human spinal cord concussion (see p. 314), presumably corresponding to the experimental impact of a force of 300 g-cm or less, show considerable correspondences with those of the experimental studies just discussed.

More severe spinal cord injury is often characterized by central spindle-shaped hematomyelia, widest at the point of injury, which tends to be confined to gray matter. Since the blood clots within about 30 minutes, evacuation is difficult, but there appears to be relatively little compression of white matter in patients who survive. These changes are most common in the cervical or lumbosacral enlargements. Resolution appears to be complete by four to six months, leaving a central cavity surrounded by a glial scar, often iron-stained. It seems reasonable to regard as analagous experimental central hemorrhagic necrosis and the central hematomyelia observed clinically. The apparent lack of white-matter changes in human material may be due to the impossibility of sampling at appropriate times after injury, so that many stages of the experimental process have not yet been observed in human material.

Complete transection of the cord does not appear to be accompanied by a massive hemorrhagic reaction. Rather, minor hemorrhage is present in the cord and meninges at the transection, followed by localized softening, ascending and descending degeneration, leptomeningeal fibrosis, and often formation of meningeal cysts. The microscopic changes resemble those seen in wounding of the brain, with successive phases of necrosis, resorption, and glial-mesenchymal fibrosis.

Cord injury may also be associated with continuing compression, as in disc prolapse or spondylolisthesis, leading to hyperemia, perivascular hemorrhage, and parenchymal necrosis, sometimes sparing the anterolateral tracts and anterior gray matter. These lesions also show the sequence of necrosis, absorption, and glial-mesenchymal proliferation, and arachnoid cysts may compress the cord or nerve roots. It seems more likely that these changes are due to ischemia than that they are directly attributable to stretching or pressure atrophy.

BIBLIOGRAPHY

Bailey, F. W. Trauma of the Spinal Cord. In J. Minckler (Ed.), *Pathology of the Nervous System.* New York: McGraw-Hill, 1971. Vol. 2, pp. 1765-1774.

Cervós-Navarro, J., Valencak, E., and Liepert, M. Circulatory Disturbances and Ultrastructural Correlates in Hyper- and Hypo-Ventilation. In *Head Injuries* (Proc. Int. Symp. on Head Injuries). Edinburgh and London: Churchill/Livingstone, 1971. Pp. 207-213.

Davis, D., et al. The pathological findings in fatal craniospinal injuries. *J. Neurosurg.* 34:603-613, 1971.

Douglas, J. M., Nahum, A. M., and Roberts, S. B. Impedance changes in deep brain structures following experimental head impact in primates. *J. Trauma* 12:315-326, 1972.

Ducker, T. B., Kindt, G. W., and Kempfe, L. G. Pathological findings in acute experimental cord trauma. *J. Neurosurg.* 35:700-708, 1971.

Evans, J. P. Prevention of the Second Accident – An Important Cause of Morbidity and Death in Head Injury. In *Head Injuries* (Proc. Int. Symp. on Head Injuries). Edinburgh and London: Churchill/Livingstone, 1971. Pp. 36-38.

Fried, L. C., and Goodkin, R. Microangiographic observations of the experimentally traumatized spinal cord. *J. Neurosurg.* 35:709-714, 1971.

Gurdjian, E. S. Mechanisms of Impact Injury of the Head. In *Head Injuries* (Proc. Int. Symp. on Head Injuries). Edinburgh and London: Churchill/Livingstone, 1971. Pp. 17-22.

Jamieson, K. G., and Yelland, J. D. N. Traumatic intracerebral hematoma. *J. Neurosurg.* 37:528-532, 1972.

Kasoff, S. S., Zugesser, L. H., and Shulman, K. Compartmental abnormalities of regional cerebral blood-flow in children with head trauma. *J. Neurosurg.* 36:463-470, 1972.

Klatzo, I. Some Early Reactions of Brain Tissue to Injury. In *Head Injuries* (Proc. Int. Symp. on Head Injuries). Edinburgh and London: Churchill/Livingstone, 1971. Pp. 214-221.

Lecuire, J., Dechaume, J. P., and Deruty, R. Long Term Prognosis of the Prolonged and Serious Traumatic Comas. In *Head Injuries* (Proc. Int. Symp. on Head Injuries). Edinburgh and London: Churchill/Livingstone, 1971. Pp. 141-144.

Lindenberg, R. Trauma of Meninges and Brain. In J. Minckler (Ed.), *Pathology of the Nervous System.* New York: McGraw-Hill, 1971. Vol. 2, pp. 1705-1765.

Loew, F. Pathophysiological Basis for the Management of Head Injuries. In *Head Injuries* (Proc. Int. Symp. on Head Injuries). Edinburgh and London: Churchill/Livingstone, 1971. Pp. 223-228.

Merksey, H., and Woodforde, J. M. Psychiatric sequelae of minor head injury. *Brain* 95:521-528, 1972.

Ommaya, A. K., Grubb, R. L., Jr., and Naumann, R. A. Coup and contre-coup injury: Observations on the mechanics of visible brain injuries in the rhesus monkey. *J. Neurosurg.* 35:503-516, 1971.

Osterholm, J. L., and Mathews, G. J. Altered norepinephrine metabolism following experimental spinal cord injury (Pts. I and II). *J. Neurosurg.* 36:386-401, 1972.

Paul, R. L., Polanco, O., Turney, S. Z., McAslau, T. C., and Cowley, R. A. Intracranial pressure responses to alterations in arterial carbon dioxide in patients with head injuries. *J. Neurosurg.* 36: 714-720, 1972.

Ringkjøb, R. Care at the Roadside – Prevention of Second Accident. In *Head Injuries* (Proc. Int. Symp. on Head Injuries). Edinburgh and London: Churchill/Livingstone, 1971. Pp. 32-36.

Seitelberger, F., and Jellinger, K. Protracted Post-Traumatic Encephalopathy. In *Head Injuries* (Proc. Int. Symp. on Head Injuries). Edinburgh and London: Churchill/Livingstone, 1971. Pp. 240-249.

Weir. B. The osmolality of subdural hematoma fluid. *J. Neurosurg.* 34:528-533, 1971.

Weiss, G. H., and Caveness, W. F. Prognostic factors in the persistence of post-traumatic epilepsy. *J. Neurosurg.* 37:164-169, 1972.

Birth Injury

17

Exactly which central nervous system lesions constitute birth injury is extremely difficult to determine. There is little doubt that in infants who die in the early neonatal period and in whom autopsy discloses significant lesions in the brain or cord but nowhere else, it is reasonable to ascribe death to birth injury. But a second and larger group, of much greater social and economic importance, includes children who exhibit any combination of mental retardation, psychopathic changes, cerebral palsy, and seizures. Brain dysfunction is apparent in infancy but not necessarily from birth, and the brains of these patients on pathological examination show lesions compatible not only with damage originating at or about the time of birth, but also with postnatal conditions including epilepsy, central nervous system infection, and head injury. The problem of attribution of such lesions is further discussed on p. 325.

A tentative definition of *birth injury* might be the following: "Birth injury consists of damage to the brain, spinal cord, nerve roots, or any combination of such damage, irrespective of when it becomes clinically manifest, which is currently thought to be due to abnormalities in the process of separation of infant from mother, whether acquired before (due to placental separation or disease) or during the process of birth." Such a definition – which is anything but succinct – covers both the acute and the presumed chronic sequelae of birth injury and also takes account of the children who die in the early neonatal period and exhibit brain lesions that on histological grounds must be considered to antedate parturition. Such lesions may arise from placental disease or incipient or actual placental separation during the last few weeks of pregnancy.

It should be noted that *injury* in this context is not necessarily analogous with *injury* in the preceding chapter. There, the word *injury* implied lesions directly or indirectly due to physical trauma. Birth injury has many etiological factors. Physical trauma is only one kind of CNS insult in these patients, and probably in most cases is not the most important one.

In contrast to the large amount of physiological and biochemical investigation that has been possible in human subjects in diseases such as cerebrovascular accidents and head injury, the nature of the birth process makes studies on human subjects exceedingly difficult. Investigations into pathogenetic mechanisms in monkeys have been necessarily confined to manipulation of one or two parameters at a time (e.g., arterial PO_2). Thus, the results yield only a partial model of the multiple physiological and pathological changes that may occur during birth. Furthermore, the findings of such studies are not necessarily applicable to other species. Particular caution is required in applying experimental results to the human CNS, which has many features that appear to be unique. Therefore, most of the many theories as to the etiology and pathogenesis of human craniospinal birth injury are based on interpretation of morphological data and have not been experimentally verified. Comparison with adult CNS damage has been a cornerstone, and although this may be valid, it is necessary to take into account the differences in biochemistry and physiology between the neonate and the adult.

In the pages that follow, theories of the etiopathogenesis of birth injury are reviewed, and the acute and (presumed) chronic lesions are described. Birth injury is believed to be a significant cause of mental retardation, epilepsy, cerebral palsy, and psychopathy. Mental retardation and epilepsy are discussed in succeeding chapters, but a brief consideration of cerebral palsy is included here.

ETIOLOGY AND PATHOGENESIS OF CEREBROSPINAL BIRTH INJURY

The fetal head is large in proportion to the body, is relatively rigid and incompressible, and is the presenting part in the majority of deliveries. It is therefore liable to bear the brunt of any difficulties due to disproportion between the fetal head and maternal pelvis or due to lack of changes in the birth canal that permit of its greater dilatation (but do not occur until the last few weeks of pregnancy). Even premature infants, who are usually smaller than normal, are liable to mechanical birth injury by being forced through a birth canal that is not fully prepared for delivery.

Even in a normal delivery, following presentation of the fetal head at the vulva uterine contractions force fetal blood into the head, which is subject only to atmospheric pressure. This phenomenon is well demonstrated by the frequent occurrence of a caput succedaneum, which may consist of edema or a hema-

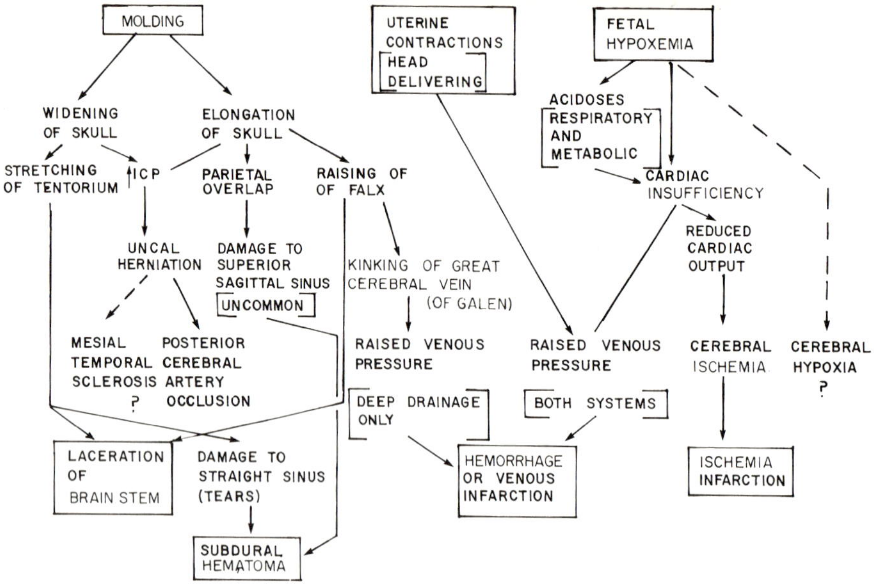

Fig. 17-1. Schematic summary of probable pathogenetic mechanisms in birth injury. ICP = intracranial pressure. For details, see text.

toma of the scalp. Such expulsion of blood from the intrauterine to the extrauterine parts of the fetus, and accompanying obstruction of venous return, must involve not only the scalp, but also the contents of the cranial cavity, and lead to raised intracranial pressure and slowing of cerebral circulation. If uterine contraction is particularly forceful or prolonged, or in the presence of other factors also predisposing to brain damage, these intracranial effects may cause brain injury.

Perhaps more important than either of the preceding events is the risk of hypoxemia, since the pressure generated by uterine contractions exceeds the fetal systolic pressure and inhibits respiratory movements (even if the mouth and nose have been delivered). Fortunately, resistance to hypoxemia of the fetal heart and brain is considerably higher than in the infant or adult, and if delivery proceeds within a reasonable time without significant complications, these periods of temporary oxygen deprivation do not appear to be damaging. In prolonged delivery, especially if due to disproportion, but also if associated with inadequate uterine contractions, hypoxemia is likely to be prolonged and to cause damage to the heart and brain. Risks to the adequate oxygenation of the fetus also occur in maternal distress, diffuse placental disease, significant placental infarction, or premature separation with retroplacental hemorrhage, and occasionally also if the umbilical cord becomes knotted, wrapped around the neck, or prolapsed through the vulva, causing deficient fetal perfusion.

An additional problem may arise in breech deliveries, in which there is difficulty in extracting the aftercoming head. Attempts to do so may be associated with stretching or hyperflexion of the spinal column, with potential damage to the spinal cord, possibly the lower brain stem, and to nerve roots, particularly in the cervical region. The risks of CNS damage in fetal malposition and malpresentation may be a strong indication for cesarean section.

Some of the mechanisms that may cause birth injury are summarized in Figure 17-1 and are discussed in detail in the following sections.

Mechanical Injury to the Fetus

It is accepted that even in normal deliveries there is some molding of the fetal head, with overlapping of the parietal bones due to lateral compression and often also of the frontal over the parietal bones due to anteroposterior compression. The midline parietal overlapping is in the region of the superior sagittal sinus and the bridging veins that join this sinus, and it seems reasonable to assume that if molding is severe, these structures may be damaged. This could include rupture of bridging veins, leading to subdural hematomas on one or both sides, or damage to the sinus itself, leading occasionally to a tear but more often to endothelial damage and subsequent sinus thrombosis.

However, these effects on the superior sagittal sinus and its branches are less common and probably of less significance than damage caused at the junction of the falx and tentorium. Lateral narrowing of the head (parietal overlap) is accompanied as a compensatory measure by occipitofrontal elongation, causing tightening of the falx and central raising (peaking) of the tentorium. Such stress may be associated with tears in the region of the straight sinus or at the junction of the sinus and the great cerebral vein of Galen. On the other hand, occipitofrontal compression leads to compensatory lateral widening of the skull and lateral stretching of the tentorium — again with the possibility of tears involving the straight sinus and the great cerebral vein. Such damage in the region of the straight sinus may lead to hemorrhage between the two layers of tentorium and in the posterior falx, but more commonly to subdural hemorrhage; if the latter involves the posterior fossa, brain stem compression and decompensation may cause death, or there may be laceration or lesser injuries of the brain stem (particularly of the midbrain) or of the cerebellum. Upward herniation of the superior cerebellum through the tentorial notch may cause acute occlusion of the posterior cerebral artery and might, in theory, be a cause of mesial temporal sclerosis and subsequent development of epilepsy (see Chap. 18).

These effects might be regarded as directly due to mechanical stress. An additional hazard associated with tentorial peaking is severe angulation at the junction of the straight sinus and the great cerebral vein of Galen, with localized venous obstruction of the deep drainage area. This will be discussed in the next section.

In some infants, usually associated with presentation of a part other than the head, mechanical injury may result from the manipulations necessary to complete delivery. Traction on the aftercoming head may damage the cervical cord or medulla, since the extensibility of the spinal column in extreme traction (about 2 cm) is appreciably greater than that of the cord (about 0.25 cm). Lacerations of the cord and medulla, or even total separation of the cord from the medulla, may occasionally occur and cause sudden death. With less severe lesions, damage is mainly in the cervical cord, with upper and lower motoneuron lesions involving the leg and arm respectively. Intercostal muscle paralysis may leave only diaphragmatic breathing, which is a precarious state that may lead to respiratory failure and death. There is often associated brachial plexus injury (Erb's palsy or Klumpke's palsy), producing paralysis of an arm, but this relatively minor lesion more often results from direct or indirect traction on the arm in attempts to assist delivery.

Venous Obstruction due to Uterine Contraction with Head Partially Delivered

One of the classic theories of the causation of birth injury, already briefly alluded to, proposes that blood is squeezed out of the body into the head (by intrauterine pressure) after the head has presented. This causes increased cerebral blood volume and dilatation of cerebral vessels. The tissue damage that can be caused is attested to by the often hemorrhagic nature of caput succedaneum of the scalp. The frequent presence of small amounts of blood in the cerebrospinal fluid of clinically normal neonates may well be due to a temporary increase in venous pressure. In some respects, the manifestations might be expected to overlap those of mechanical trauma, which may cause rupture or thrombosis of dural sinuses, tearing of bridging veins, and angulation of the great cerebral vein on the straight sinus, with central venous obstruction. Total suspension of central venous return would be associated with stasis and hypoxemia, damaging the endothelium and predisposing to thrombosis.

A special role for the great cerebral vein in the cerebral circulation has been considered, but remains undetermined. Occasionally, it is distended to become as much as 1.5 to 2.0 cm in diameter and almost spherical, and it has been reported as having a significant autonomic innervation. Since the intracranial pressure during uterine contraction must be uniform, both superficial and deep venous drainages should be equally susceptible to increased pressure and stasis, and hemorrhagic infarction should be equally common, both at the superior margins of the hemispheres and in the deep white matter and basal ganglia. However, hemorrhage or hemorrhagic infarction occurs in the deep structures much more frequently, and some additional factor, possibly angulation or some peculiarity of the great cerebral vein, must be responsible for this. Certainly, the dilatation of the vein lies immediately distal to the postulated point of obstruction. It remains speculative whether or not it has an autonomic as well as an obstructive basis and what purpose the innervation of the vein might normally serve.

An additional explanation for raised intracranial venous pressure in many cases might be hypoxemic cardiac failure, complicating the allocation of lesions to localized intracranial pathogenetic mechanisms. (However, this would not raise intracranial pressure to nearly as high a point as does normal contraction, in which intrauterine pressure may rise to 180 mm Hg, with pressures as high as 250 mm Hg having been recorded.) Perhaps the intermittency of uterine contraction (except in extreme delay of labor) makes these high pressures less damaging than the moderate but prolonged increases caused by congestive cardiac failure.

Hypoxemia

Causative Factors

The fortunate fetus may expect a virtually instantaneous transition from oxygenation via the umbilical cord to oxygenation via the lungs. However, if transplacental oxygenation terminates prematurely, or pulmonary oxygenation begins late, there is a period during which the fetus is subject to hypoxemia of varying degrees.

As noted, *premature cessation or inadequacy of transplacental oxygenation* may be associated with placental disease, infarction, or premature separation, or, less often, knotting, twisting, or prolapse of the cord. During arrested labor with intense uterine contractions, the pressure developed may cause prolonged embarrassment of the placental and cord circulation.

Delay in the onset of pulmonary oxygenation may be neurogenic, due to severe damage to the brain stem already incurred during difficult delivery, or it may be due to inadequate clearing of the airways or to aspiration of amniotic fluid. Postnatal development of lung disease, particularly, hyaline membrane disease (respiratory distress syndrome), may occur so early that hypoxemic effects on the CNS overlap with those of prenatal or intranatal origin.

Indirect Effects on Central Nervous System: Acidosis and Myocardial Damage

Hypoxemia is not an isolated development, but induces many changes besides decreased arterial PO_2. It is associated with hypercapnia or respiratory acidosis, which is also due to inadequate respiratory or placental gas exchange, and also with metabolic acidosis, because of increased anaerobic metabolism and production of lactate. While the neonatal brain has a much greater capacity for glycolysis than the adult brain, presumably because of the different lactic dehydrogenase isoenzyme pattern, this capacity is not limitless. It delays the effects of hypoxemia sufficiently to enable the infant to survive a normal delivery, but not to survive a prolonged, complicated delivery.

Hypoxemia equally severely affects the heart, and brain damage and irreversible myocardial damage may be almost contemporaneous (see Chap. 13). Thus, the direct effects of hypoxemia on the CNS may be considerably compounded by myocardial damage; since the effect of hypoxemia on brain stem nuclei may have a reciprocal deteriorating effect on myocardial function, there is the potential for a vicious circle of deterioration.

Experimental Observations on Pathogenesis of Hypoxemic Lesions

Recent experimental work using newborn monkeys makes it appear that the direct effects of tissue hypoxia (hypoxidosis) on the CNS may not be a major factor in human cerebral birth injury and implicates more strongly the associated metabolic changes and effects on the cardiovascular system.

Total Acute Asphyxia (Anoxemia). In one series of experiments, total acute asphyxia was induced by clamping the umbilical cord and placing a rubber bag over the head for varying periods. The blood pressure rose briefly, due to increased vascular resistance (clamping off the placental circulation), and then fell for about 2 minutes, presumably due to progressive myocardial hypoxidosis. This was followed by a rise in blood pressure lasting a few minutes (and apparently associated with endogenous catecholamine secretion) and then a progressive fall to total cessation of circulation in 13 to 15 minutes.

If asphyxia was terminated in less than 10 minutes by active respiration (when there was still sufficient circulation), there appeared to be no permanent CNS sequelae. However, clinically and morphologically detectable brain damage increased with periods of asphyxia lasting 10 to 18 minutes. With longer periods (e.g., 25 minutes), the monkeys did not survive long enough for morphological changes to develop. Brain damage could be slightly delayed by barbiturate anesthesia, which reduces oxygen utilization, or by infusion of alkali plus glucose, so long as circulation persisted.

Unexpectedly, morphological changes in the CNS, if present (i.e., following about 10 to 18 minutes of asphyxia), were essentially confined to the brain stem and diencephalon and did not involve the cortex, cerebral white matter, or basal ganglia; thus they differed completely from the pattern in human birth injury. The susceptibility of brain stem and diencephalic structures correlated reasonably well with regional oxygen utilization and capillarization. Damage occurred in uniform order, the inferior colliculi being followed in succession by the superior olives, sensory nucleus of the fifth nerve, gracilis and cuneate nuclei, medial and spinal vestibular nuclei, lateral and posterior nuclei of the ventrolateral thalamus, and, finally, most other brain stem and thalamic structures. (Only occasional animals, all thought to have had intrauterine asphyxia *preceding* the experimental procedure, showed cortical and basal ganglion lesions such as are commonly seen in the human.) Since the distribution of lesions was correlated with oxygen utilization, and the effects of myocardial damage on the CNS were minimal in such short-term experiments, these CNS lesions were considered to be truly hypoxemic.

Partial Prolonged Asphyxia (Hypoxemia). Other experiments imposed partial prolonged, rather than total acute, asphyxia. Several techniques were used, including administration of oxytoxin to enhance uterine contractions, constriction of the maternal aorta, partial placental separation, and maternal hypotension induced by halothane. Hypoxia, hypercapnia, and mixed respiratory and metabolic acidosis developed in some of the mothers given halothane, while the fetuses showed bradycardia, reduced blood pressure, and reduced pulse pressure, all of which became increasingly severe as abnormalities of PO_2, PCO_2, and acid-base balance became more pronounced.

Clamping of the maternal aorta (normal pressure 70 mm Hg) led to a progressive fall of pressure below the clamp and to increasing fetal distress. At a maternal aortic pressure of 40 mm Hg (fetal blood, $PO_2 <$ 13 mm Hg), fetal death occurred in 30 to 60 minutes. A fetal blood PO_2 of 15 to 17 mm Hg could be tolerated indefinitely, but the further (relatively small) drop to 13 to 14 mm Hg caused progressive deterioration in PO_2, PCO_2, acid-base balance, and cardiovascular function. The fetal blood pressure showed a considerable decrease in basal level, superimposed on which were periodic episodes of even more severe hypotension, the fetuses finally dying of myocardial failure. If maternal aortic pressure was maintained at 40 to 60 mm Hg (fetal blood PO_2, 13 to 15 mm Hg), a proportion of fetuses survived long enough for morphological brain injury to become apparent. The changes seen in these fetuses closely mimicked the combinations of cortical, cerebral white matter, and basal ganglia changes associated with human birth injury to be discussed. In these cases, in addition to hypoxemia, these were metabolic changes and myocardial failure. The hypoxemic CNS lesions seen in the acute lesions failed to develop.

Conclusions from the Experiments. If such results are applicable to the human fetus, it appears that hypoxemic birth injury is associated with respiratory and metabolic acidosis, brain perfusion being maintained but probably not at adequate levels. In many monkey fetuses following hypotension, the brain showed swelling, probably due to increased cerebral blood volume, and there was a shift of extracellular fluid to the intracellular compartment. Blood flow appeared to be reduced in the hemispheres, with the areas supplied by the posterior cerebral arteries being least affected. The cerebellum showed areas of necrosis, but the brain stem was little affected. Attempts at postmortem vascular perfusion showed the no-reflow phenomenon in many areas, presumably due to stasis and sludging. However, it was not rigorously established whether these areas corresponded to boundary zones and were therefore on a hemodynamic basis, or whether they were related to unequal metabolic requirements in different areas.

Clinicopathological Observations on the Pathogenesis of Hypoxemic Lesions

Distribution of Cerebral Hemorrhage in Relation to Venous Development. Independently of this experimental work, a significant role for stasis induced by myocardial failure and increased central venous pressure has been postulated by observing the distribution of intracerebral hemorrhage in human birth injury. It has been claimed that in premature infants with predominantly deep venous drainage, lesions tend to involve particularly the germinal matrix in the wall of the lateral ventricles. On the other hand, lesions tend to be largely peripheral in full-term or postmature infants, in whom major metabolic activity has shifted from the neuroepithelial cells of the germinal matrix to the developing cerebral cortex and in whom the superficial drainage predominates. However, this correlation of age with lesion distribution is not accepted by all observers.

Possible Role of Arterial Hypotension. There appears to be considerable evidence for a role for the metabolic effects of prolonged hypoxemia in the causation of cerebral birth injury. Furthermore, it seems that many such lesions are related to increased central venous pressure following myocardial damage. There appears to be somewhat less evidence for a direct role for arterial hypotension due to myocardial hypoxemia, although lesions directly due to decreased perfusion pressure probably do form part of the spectrum of birth injury. Many infants who survive for months or years show chronic, gliotic changes, the distribution of which corresponds to the boundary zone between the middle and anterior, or between the anterior and posterior, cerebral vessels. The common finding of severe atrophic changes involving the entire dorsal halves of the hemispheres may be regarded as an extension of such boundary zone lesions.

Nonhemorrhagic white-matter lesions are frequent in birth injury, and while it is difficult to conceive of these lesions as due to venous stasis, it is well known, both from clinical and experimental evidence, that lesions in the subependymal white matter, especially at the lateral angles of the ventricles and lateral aspects of the occipital horns, may follow periods of arterial hypotension in the absence of impaired venous return.

A few birth-injured brains show infarction in the territories of the posterior cerebral artery. It is assumed that, as in adults, such lesions are due to localized compression of the vessels associated with uncal herniation.

Increased Cerebral Blood Volume. Brain swelling is often observed in infants who die with acute birth injury, the most reliable criteria being tonsillar herniation, uncal herniation, or both. Gyral flattening depends on the maturity of the fetus and only correlates randomly with tonsillar or uncal herniation. Brain water content appears to be inversely rather than directly correlated with swelling. Since this is not compatible with cerebral edema, and since the solid content of blood is actually higher than that of neonatal brain, it seems probable that neonatal brain swelling is associated with an increase in cerebral blood volume rather than with edema. This is reasonable in view of the known difficulties of venous return, and brain swelling might also be associated with generalized vasodilatation due to abnormal vasomotor control. However, little information is available on the status of either autoregulation or vasomotor control in the neonate.

Role of Placental Abnormalities. Occasionally, infants dying shortly after birth, apparently of brain injury, show morphological and histological changes that it is difficult to conceive of as having developed in the short period following parturition (e.g., areas of softening, with gitter cells, in infants who die 12 to 24 hours after birth). Since similar lesions may also be seen in older infants at a time compatible with perinatal birth injury, it seems probable that the mechanisms are similar, and that the prenatal lesions are also associated with hypoxemia and its complications, either due to premature involutionary changes or partial premature separation of the placenta. The best-known example of such a lesion is neonatal hypoxic leukoencephalopathy (periventricular encephalomalacia).

MORPHOLOGY OF ACUTE BIRTH INJURY

When brain damage causes death in the neonatal period, the relationship of the lesions to the process of birth is usually unequivocal, although the changes found occasionally appear to have originated prior to parturition, as previously mentioned.

Hemorrhage in the Vicinity of the Dura

Dural tears may involve the tentorium, sometimes crossing the straight sinus and leading to extensive hemorrhage. Much less commonly, they are found in the falx, and occasionally the superior sagittal sinus is torn. Dural sinuses may be dilated, and thrombosis is seen, usually in the superior sagittal vessel. Bridging veins may be torn, leading to subdural hematoma over the hemispheres, but a more common site of hemorrhage is the posterior fossa, where it is usually associated with tears at the junction of falx and tentorium and damage to the great cerebral vein. Intradural hemorrhage between the layers of the falx or tentorium may occur, but extradural hemorrhage is rare in infants (see Chap. 16).

Subarachnoid Hemorrhage

Subarachnoid hemorrhage is most often found in the posterior fossa and at the base of the brain, usually

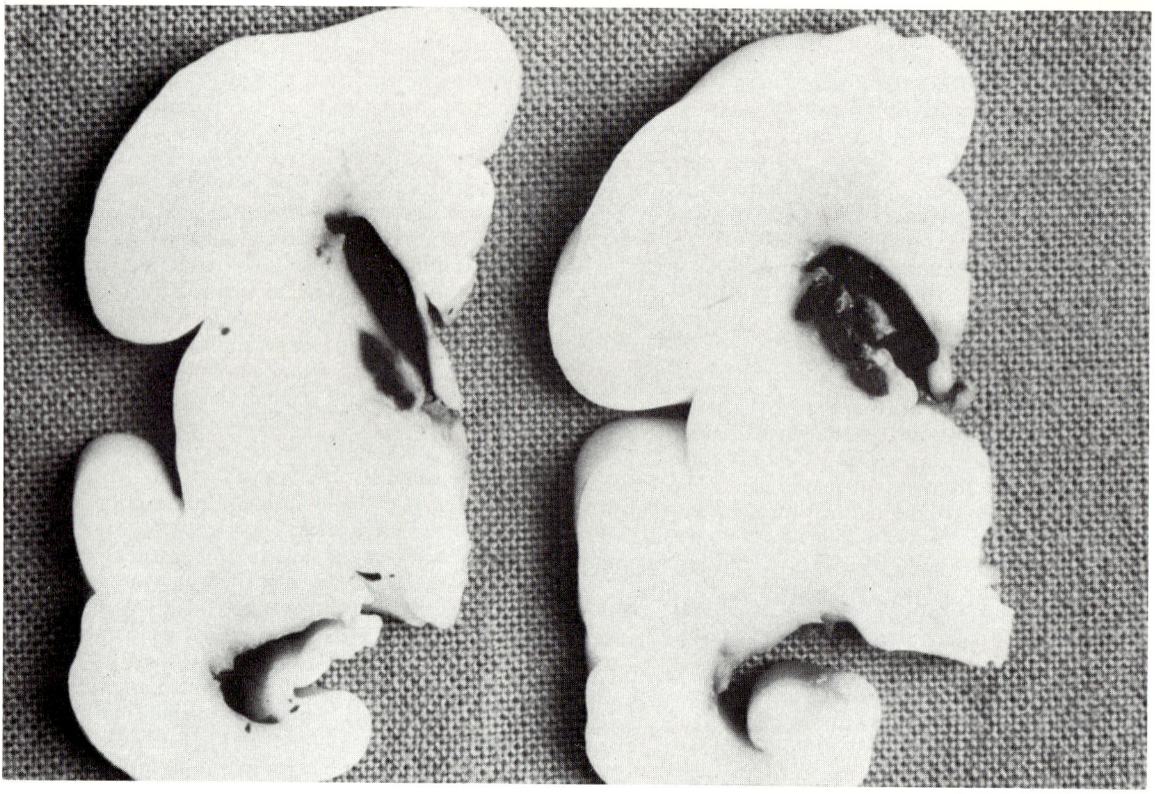

Fig. 17-2. Subependymal (germinal matrix) and intraventricular neonatal hemorrhage.

having escaped from the ventricles. Scattered subarachnoid hemorrhages may be seen over the hemispheres, particularly at the upper margin, in association with severe molding and damage to the superior sagittal sinus and bridging veins.

Intraventricular Hemorrhage

Intraventricular hemorrhage is frequently bilateral, although it may be unilateral or asymmetrical. It appears most often to originate from veins in the walls of the lateral ventricles (Fig. 17-2), notably the terminal and lateral ventricular vessels, which are large and thin-walled and supported only by the loose residual neuroepithelial tissue (germinal matrix) that is conspicuous in full-term infants and even more prominent in prematures. Because of these weaknesses, these vessels are thought to bleed readily as a result of increased venous pressure. Since they are subependymal, they may cause massive intraventricular hemorrhage with casts of clotted blood (Fig. 17-3), but only minimal involvement of brain tissue.

Intracerebral Hemorrhage

Massive intracerebral hemorrhage is relatively unusual, although minor bleeding in the germinal matrix virtually always accompanies ventricular hemorrhage. The lesion in the matrix tissue has been described as hemorrhagic necrosis, but the histological appearance (Fig. 17-4) is merely that of extravasated red blood cells surrounding parenchymal (mainly neuroepithelial) cells; the latter show little morphological change. The veins are distended and often show antemortem thrombus, but the site of rupture is often not seen. In a relatively small proportion of cases, said to be more common with extreme prematurity, the matrix hemorrhage not only ruptures into the ventricles, but also spreads to occupy some, or even a large part, of the hemispheric white matter. The areas affected are largely those supplied by the subependymal tributaries of the great cerebral vein. Not only white matter, but also parts of the basal ganglia and thalamus, may be involved, a common site being the head of the caudate nucleus. The hemorrhagic

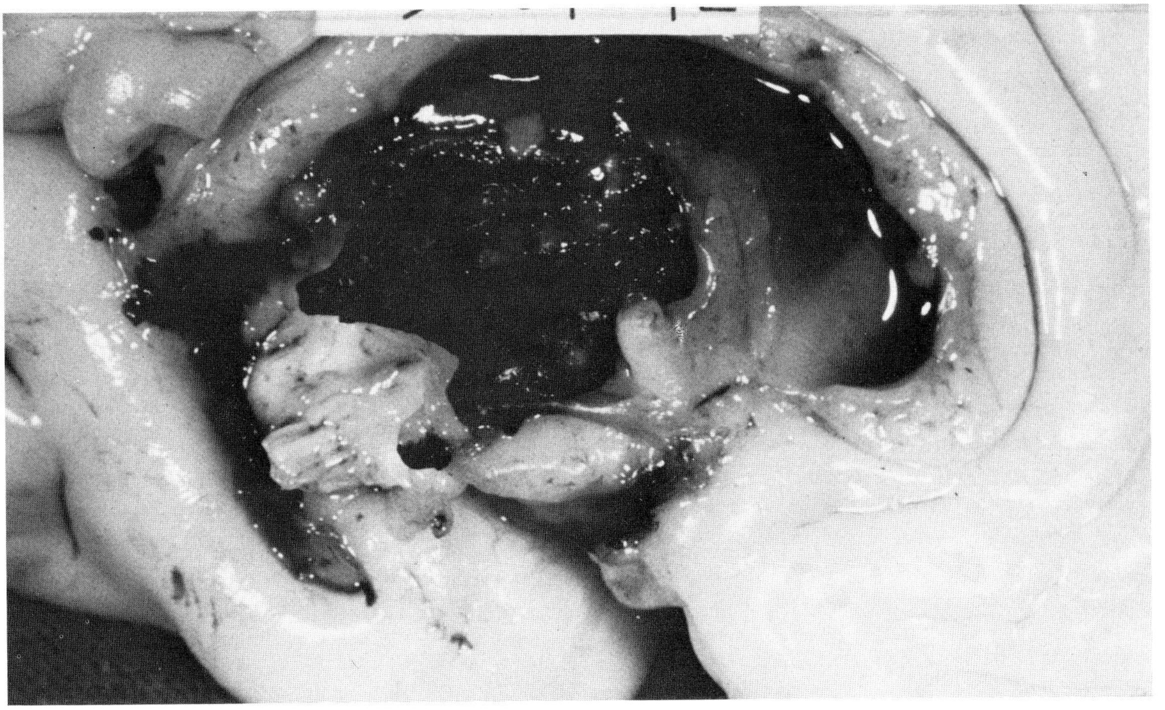

Fig. 17-3. Intraventricular hemorrhage of third ventricle in neonate, showing typical cast.

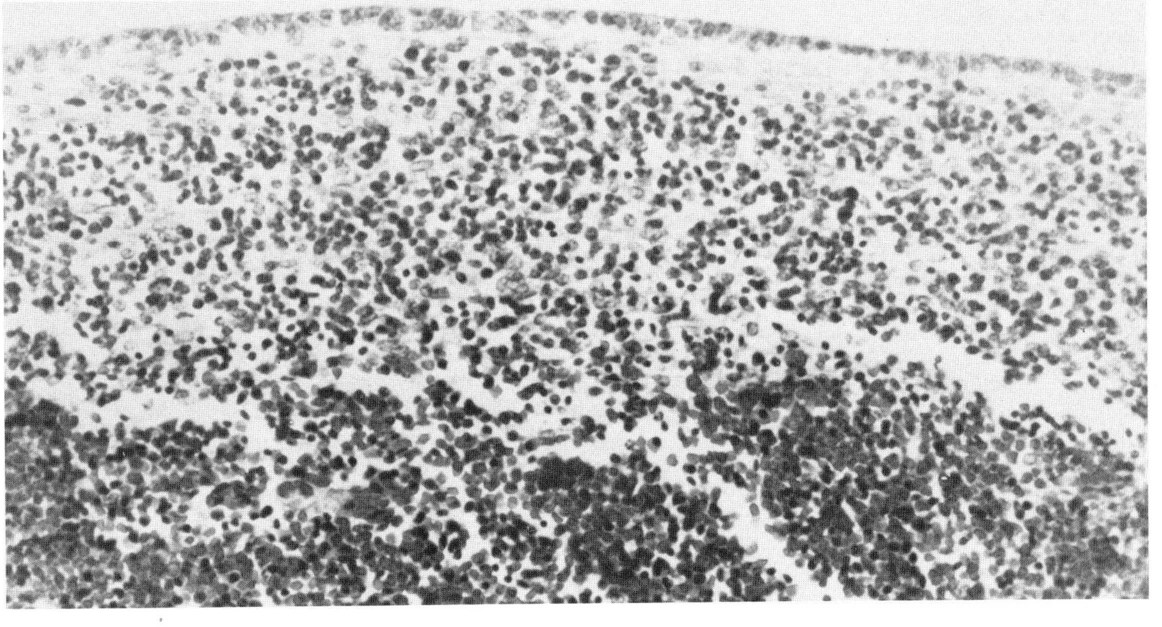

Fig. 17-4. Microscopic appearance of germinal matrix hemorrhage. Intact (not necrotic) neuroepithelial cells remain beneath the ependyma. The lower part of the photomicrograph is occupied by extravasated blood, but the veins from which this presumably originated are not shown. (H & E, X300.)

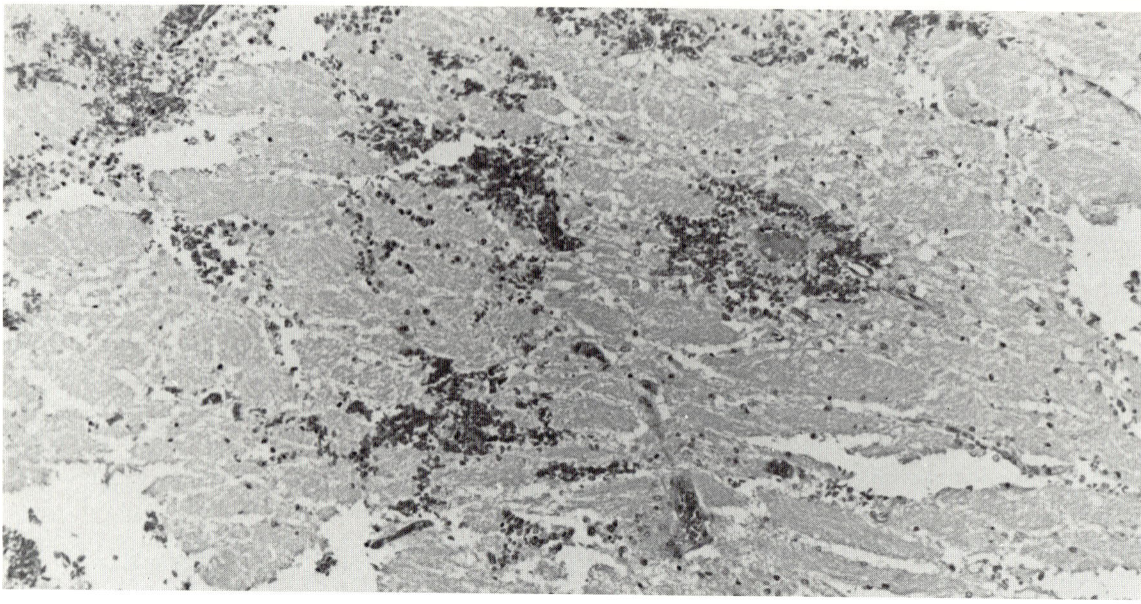

Fig. 17-5. Perivascular (perivenous) hemorrhages in deep white matter. This infant also showed germinal matrix hemorrhage. (H & E, X115.)

lesions are not of the massive disruptive type associated with arterial rupture, but represent a coalescence of perivenous and perivenular diapedetic hemorrhages (Fig. 17-5). Less commonly, and usually in later premature or full-term infants, similar confluent diapedetic hemorrhages may be seen in the cortex and underlying white matter of the superior frontal gyri, probably associated with damage to the superior sagittal sinus and its tributary veins.

Nonhemorrhagic Cortical Necrosis

Acute cortical necrosis is usually nonhemorrhagic and shows a widely variable distribution. The degree of cortical devastation varies from selective ischemic necrosis of neurons through laminar necrosis, most marked in the depths of the sulci, to full-thickness necrosis of entire gyri or even virtually entire lobes. The most common lesions are found in the boundary zones between the anterior and middle, or anterior and posterior, cerebral arteries; lesions in the middle and posterior boundary zone are unusual. It is sometimes difficult to equate areas of damage with vascular territories, as when the entire dorsal half of the hemispheres is scarred. Possibly this is due to an even more severe fall of blood pressure and represents an exceptional extension of boundary-zone lesions. In animals, selective cortical necrosis may involve posterior frontal and posterior parietal regions, leaving the postcentral gyrus relatively intact, presumably on a basis of metabolic peculiarities (topism), but such a pattern is not characteristic of human birth injury.

Nonhemorrhagic Lesions of the White Matter or Basal Ganglia

Nonhemorrhagic lesions of the white matter and basal ganglia tend to be symmetrical and to involve the caudate and putamen, the deeper parts of the cerebral white matter, or both. In the white matter they often take the form of irregular foci a few millimeters in diameter, seen grossly as small, whitish spots that tend to be grouped around the lateral aspects of the lateral ventricles – again, in the subependymal venous drainage areas. They are not often associated with similarly distributed deep cerebral hemorrhage and seem difficult to explain on the basis of venous stasis. However, boundary zones are also present in the white matter, where they extend from the superolateral hemisphere to the lateral ventricles. Lesions involving white matter alone, without ischemic changes in the overlying cortex, can be produced (at least in adult animals) by acute reduction in blood pressure.

Admittedly, such lesions are hard to explain, but the poor vascularity of the white matter, its greater distance from the subarachnoid supply vessels, and a possible asphyxial shunt mechanism diverting blood to the cortex may combine to outweigh its considerably lower metabolic requirements relative to the overlying cortex. It is this type of nonhemorrhagic, periventricular lesion, demonstrably originating before parturition, that has necessitated the extension of the concept of *birth injury* to include lesions acquired before birth as a result of placental disease. Such lesions are not likely to be due to venous stasis; it would seem more probable that they are of hypotensive origin.

Changes in the basal ganglia, as in the cortex, vary from selective ischemic necrosis of neurons to irregular ("geographical") areas of total tissue infarction and tend to be topistic. Thus, the pallidum is rarely involved.

Stretch Injury of the Cerebellum, Brain Stem, or Cervical Cord

The lesions of stretch injury of the cerebellum, brain stem, and cervical cord are frequently missed in a routine autopsy, in which the brain and cord are separated at the level of the lower medulla and the cord may not be examined at all. However, thorough investigations suggest that, especially in association with traction on the cord or undue flexion, severe mechanical deformation, sometimes associated with laceration, may occur in the brain stem, cerebellum, or cervical cord. Such lesions seem to be of purely mechanical origin. Usually, only minor intracerebral and subarachnoid bleeding occurs, though there may be epidural hemorrhage that is most marked posteriorly in the cervical spinal canal. This may be a sensitive indication of damage in this area in the absence of other gross lesions.

THE MORPHOLOGY OF CHRONIC BIRTH INJURY

Cerebral birth injury is not necessarily immediately fatal, and in patients who survive, phases of resorption and gliomesenchymal fibrosis will occur in much the same time sequence as in association with cerebral infarct or traumatic injury (see Chaps. 14 and 16). The end result is therefore a brain with areas of tissue destruction and scarring, and structurally normal areas that function abnormally because of release from either stimulatory or inhibitory influences from damaged centers. Because of the immaturity of the CNS at birth, the difficulty in testing CNS function in the first year of life, and the fact that some CNS functions are not operative until early or late childhood, sequelae of birth injury may not become apparent for months or even years. Thus, any relationship observed is circumstantial and has largely been inferred from histories and from observations at autopsy.

A history of abnormalities during gestation or labor is frequently obtained in children with birth injuries. Depending on the interval between birth and the onset of clinical symptoms, this history becomes progressively less reliable, particularly in large families. The mother herself may not have adequate recollections of the gestation or labor, and hospital records are often fragmentary, both with regard to the course of labor and the neonatal condition of the infant.

The types of brain damage discovered at autopsy in these children can usually be plausibly derived from the changes regarded as characteristic of acute birth injury. Again, there are unfortunately many fallacies. During the period between birth and clinical onset there may have been infections, minor episodes of trauma, and sometimes convulsions, which, in the early stages, were considered "febrile." Since the type of brain damage produced by seizures and trauma overlaps that found following birth injury (hypoxemia, ischemia, and edema being common factors), it often becomes questionable whether the neuropathological changes in a given case are in fact sequelae of birth injury, result entirely from later seizures or trauma, or represent both factors superimposed. On the other hand, trauma from falls may be due to antecedent birth injury that causes abnormalities of gait (ataxia, dyskinesia, or spasticity), and seizures may also frequently indicate preceding brain damage. Thus, by the time an autopsy is performed, there is usually a spectrum of pathological features, from which it is extremely difficult to disentangle the lesions of the original birth injury.

The association of abnormalities of mental and motor development and of convulsive disorders with birth injury, although circumstantial and based on the lines of evidence noted above, is reasonably convincing. Prospective studies involving large populations of infants with adequate records of labor and neonatal status who are followed for many years to determine the incidence and type of CNS disease are in progress to provide additional and more convincing correlations.

Types of Lesions Found at Autopsy

Lesions of the Cerebral Cortex

When relatively localized, lesions of the cerebral cortex occur *either* in the parasagittal frontoparietal region (anterior and middle cerebral artery boundary zone) *or* around the calcarine sulcus and on the inferior surface of the occipital and posterior temporal lobes (posterior cerebral artery occlusion). They vary from (1) somewhat granular cortex with adherent leptomeninges, in which vertical zones of gliomesenchymal fibrosis and neuronal loss are probably centered on perforating arteries, through (2) areas of laminar or pseudolaminar necrosis principally situated deep in the sulci, to (3) areas of sclerotic ulegyria, in which the normal pattern is replaced by irregular, small gyri that on cross section appear normal at the apex, but are sclerotic deep in the sulci (mushroom gyri).

In areas where the cortex is not completely destroyed, myelin staining may show irregular areas of increased myelination (status marmoratus), the origin of which will be discussed subsequently (p. 326). Small vessels overlying the damaged cortex may show intimal fibrosis and calcification of the

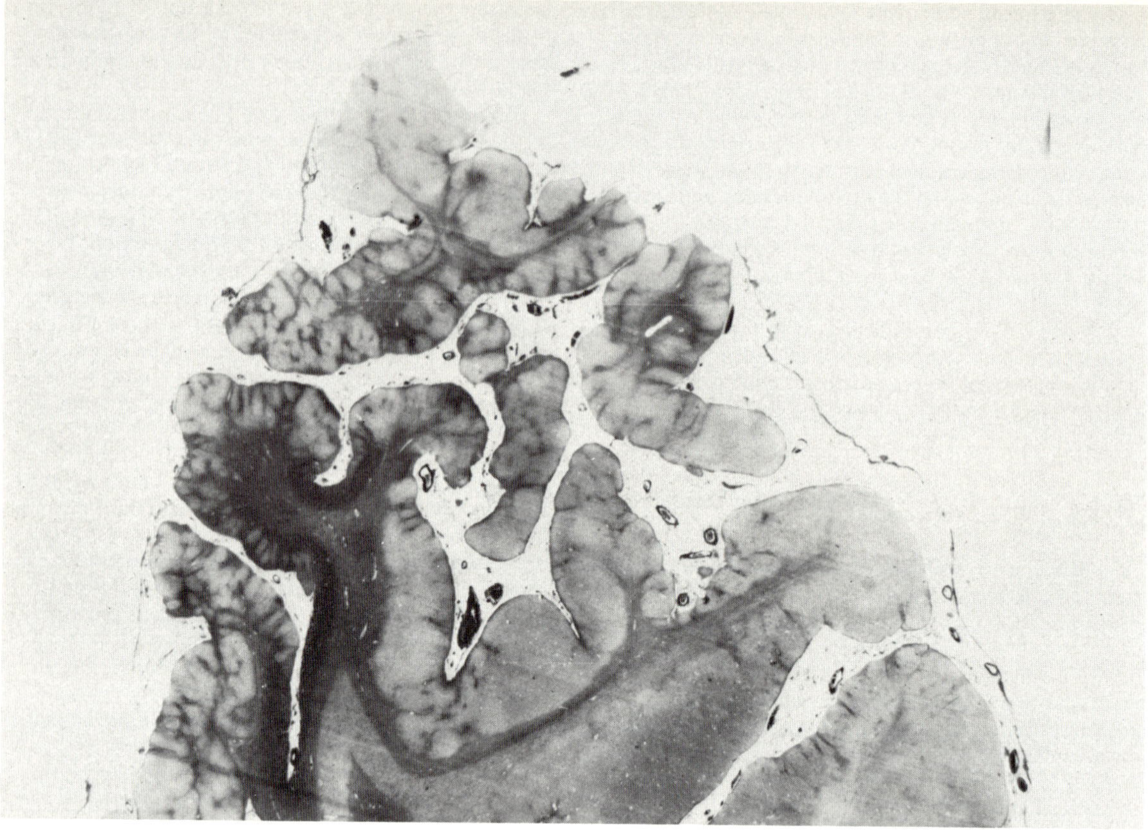

Fig. 17-6. Transverse section of the upper margin of the left cerebral hemisphere (parietal region). The gyri are shrunken and distorted, and areas of cortical gliosis are apparently following the radial orientation of perforating vessels. (Holzer's stain, X 5.)

internal elastic lamina. In widespread lesions, most of the cortex shows shrinkage and ulegyria (Fig. 17-6), only the orbital, temporal and inferior occipital surfaces remaining relatively normal. As has been noted, these distributions probably reflect ischemia as a result of hypoxemic cardiac failure, or compression of the posterior cerebral vessel by the uncus during brain swelling. Occasional areas of ulegyria are found which are not readily explicable on either of the above bases, and their pathogenesis is obscure.

Lesions of the Cerebral and Cerebellar White Matter

Lesions of the cerebral (and, rarely, cerebellar) white matter may or may not involve overlying cortex. They vary from small, multiple areas of cystic gliosis, frequently distributed laterally to the lateral ventricles, to large cavities extending up to or destroying the overlying cortex (porencephalia). Where extensive, they may cause regular or irregular ventricular dilatations. Bordering or overlying cortex may show ulegyria or at least granular changes, and cavities are separated from the subarachnoid space by a gliomeningeal membrane. Brownish-yellow staining of the walls of the periventricular cavities suggests that they have developed from central hemorrhagic white-matter lesions. Siderosis of the larger porencephalic or superficial cavities is less common, and these perhaps have developed from ischemic infarcts.

Lesions of the Central Gray Matter

Lesions of the central gray matter are often associated with white-matter lesions, but may occur in isolation. They are most marked in the caudate nucleus, putamen, and anterior or medial parts of the thalamus. Lesions include multiple small cystic spaces (status lacunaris), diffuse fibrillary gliosis, and varying, often severe, neuronal loss. The amygdala is occasionally involved. A somewhat intriguing finding, most marked in the putamen but also seen in the caudate nucleus, is the presence of irregular hypermyelinated areas (status marmoratus), which also show gliosis and neuronal loss. Status marmoratus occurs only with other manifestations of hypoxemic brain damage, and as noted previously, may also be seen in the cortex. It seems to be due to reactive collateral proliferation of damaged axons, the sprouts becoming heavily myelinated. Status dysmyelinatus may be seen in the pallidum, with loss of neurons and of myelinated pallidal efferent fibers (ansa and fasciculus lenticularis). Minor subependymal damage is manifested as transventricular adhesions between the upper surface of the caudate nucleus and the undersurface of the corpus callosum.

Cerebellar and Brain Stem Lesions

In spite of the presumed frequency and importance of lesions in the brain stem in acute birth injury, few sequelae are found in the chronic cases, presumably because significant brain stem injury is likely to be immediately or rapidly fatal. Isolated lesions of the third, fourth, sixth, and seventh cranial motor nuclei, the inferior olives, and occasionally the superior cerebellar surface and dentate nucleus have been described. Birth injury may represent one cause of isolated nuclear palsies.

Superimposed or Inconstant Lesions

Other types of lesions found in the CNS are those apparently due to convulsions (recent laminar necrosis of the cortex and Purkinje's cell loss) or to retrograde degeneration (neuronal loss and minimal gliosis in the lateral geniculate body or other thalamic nuclei, associated with damage to corresponding areas of cortex). In a proportion of cases there is scarring of the medial temporal lobe, especially of the uncus and amygdala, often attributed to the original birth injury and thought to cause some cases of epilepsy (see Chap. 18).

CEREBRAL PALSY

Cerebral palsy is an administrative rather than a medical term, applied to CNS disorders that are nonprogressive, affect motor function (and, usually to a lesser extent, mental function), and are congenital or apparent within the first two years of life. The incidence is 1 per 200 to 500 live births. Spasticity is much more frequent than dyskinesia, and ataxia is found only occasionally, so that the usual morphological substrate includes parts of the pyramidal and extrapyramidal systems, but not often the cerebellum. About 90% of cases are due to birth injury, but there are others due to postnatal lesions such as trauma or infection. Over 50% of cerebral palsy patients are mentally retarded, and about 30% are epileptic.

Pathological studies in many cases show gross and microscopic changes like those already described for chronic birth injury. Hypoxemia seems to be a common etiological factor, due to such diverse causes as maternal anemia, cardiac or respiratory disease, infection, infarction or detachment of the placenta, knots or compression of the umbilical cord, oversedation or improper anesthesia, delay in delivery, neonatal pneumonitis, and respiratory distress syndrome. A few cases are associated with dural tears and subdural hematomas or with spinal cord or brain stem damage. Cerebral palsy may also be associated with kernicterus (see the next section).

As noted, in a few cases cerebral palsy appears to be independent of birth injury. Some of these cases are associated with intrauterine infections such as cytomegalovirus or toxoplasmosis or with postnatal meningitis. Other cases are due to hydrocephalus, and tend to be predominantly spastic with little athetosis, since the basal ganglia remain intact, although there is severe thinning and atrophy of the motor and premotor cortex. A small group of cerebral palsy patients have other developmental defects. Very occasional antecedents include toxemia of pregnancy, maternal hepatic or renal disease, and postmaturity.

As in chronic birth injury in general, prematurity appears to be a significant contributing factor to the development of cerebral palsy; 25% or more of cerebral palsy patients are prematurely delivered, compared with less than 5% of the general population. Prematurity appears not only to predispose the infant to mechanical damage in the birth canal, but also to increase considerably the mortality and morbidity of associated brain-damaging factors, such as hypoxemia and kernicterus.

KERNICTERUS

Kernicterus is a CNS disease most commonly seen in neonates, especially in premature infants, but is occasionally seen in other conditions such as the Crigler-Najjar syndrome. It is characterized by a high plasma level of unconjugated bilirubin not bound to serum albumin and therefore apparently able to cross the blood-brain barrier. Either conjugation (to glucuronic acid in the liver), which reduces solubility in lipid, or attachment to serum albumin protects the CNS. Kernicterus is associated with the following:

1. Impaired liver conjugation (deficiency of glucuronyltransferase), as seen temporarily in neonates and accentuated by prematurity or occurring in rare inborn errors of metabolism.
2. Increased erythrocyte destruction, especially in Rh or ABO incompatibility of mother and fetus, but also in neonatal sepsis and rare metabolic errors (such as glucose 6-phosphate dehydrogenase deficiency).
3. High plasma bilirubin (20 to 40 mg per 100 ml) in excess of albumin-binding capacity, low serum albumin or dissociation of the albumin-bilirubin complex by acidosis, free fatty acids, salicylates, or sulfonamides or other drugs. Free bilirubin appears to be directly toxic to the CNS and is bound by brain mitochondria, producing swelling and cristal irregularities. Oxidation and phosphorylation are uncoupled, and the formation of adenosine triphosphate is impaired — a type of cytotoxic hypoxia. Hypoxemia and excess unconjugated bilirubin do not seem to act synergistically to cause kernicterus, except insofar as there is metabolic acidosis. Presumably, tissue PO_2 is immaterial once oxidative phosphorylation is uncoupled.

Seen grossly, CNS tissue in kernicterus is characterized by yellow staining of some areas of gray matter, observed in the fresh state (Fig. 17-7) and sometimes seen even better in formalin-fixed material. The cranial nerve nuclei, anterior horns, periaqueductal and subependymal gray matter of the brain stem, dentate and olivary nuclei, subthalamic nucleus, and hippocampus usually show the deepest staining, with variable involvement of the pallidum, cerebellar ver-

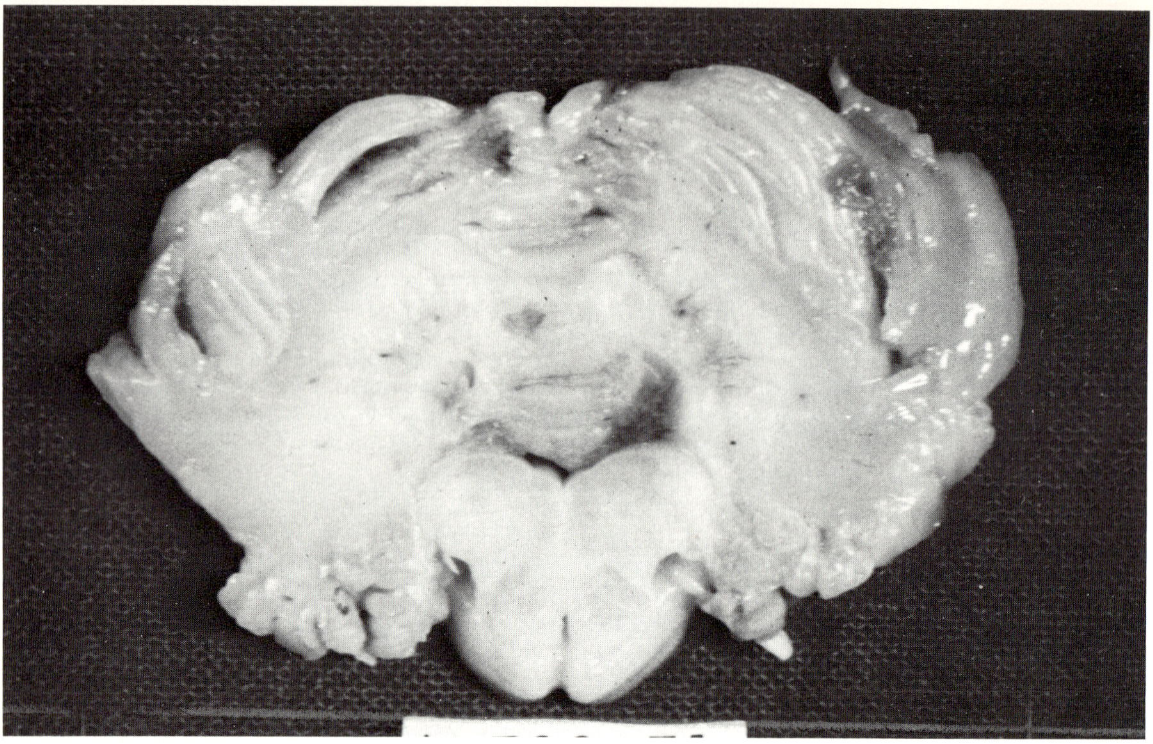

Fig. 17-7. Kernicterus in transverse section of cerebellum and brain stem. Bile-staining of the inferior olives and entire floor of the fourth ventricle may be seen.

mis, flocculus, and, to a lesser extent, the putamen and thalamus. (Bile-staining of other areas, especially the cortex and hemispheric white matter, indicates ischemic or other damage involving the blood-brain barrier and is not related to kernicterus.)

Bile pigment is difficult or impossible to visualize microscopically in kernicterus. The changes seen include sclerosis or ischemic necrosis of neurons, with variable diffuse yellowish staining of neurons, neuropil, and occasionally astrocytes. The intensity of neuronal damage bears little relation to the amount of gross pigmentation, and permanent neuronal loss and gliosis in the survivors is usually limited to the pallidum (one or both divisions), subthalamic nucleus, and hippocampus (sectors H_1 and H_2 and occasionally $H_{3\text{-}5}$). Permanent changes do not occur in the other pigmented areas. There is as yet no explanation for this selective vulnerability, either to acute pigmentation or to residual permenent damage, though the latter at least shows considerable similarity to vulnerability in hypoxemia (see Chap. 13).

Motor dysfunction is not a conspicuous feature of the acute, jaundiced stage. Predominantly, survivors show dyskinesias such as chorea and athetosis, together with deafness and paralysis of upward gaze (Parinaud's oculoglandular syndrome). They may also be retarded and epileptic.

BIBLIOGRAPHY

Cowger, M. L. Bilirubin Encephalopathy. In G. E. Gaull (Ed.), *Biology of Brain Dysfunction.* New York: Plenum, 1973. Vol. 2, pp. 265-293.

Meyers, R. E. Two patterns of perinatal brain damage and their conditions of occurrence. *Am. J. Obstet. Gynecol.* 112:246-276, 1972.

Osterberg, K. Kernicterus. In J. Minckler (Ed.), *Pathology of the Nervous System.* New York: McGraw-Hill, 1971. Vol. 2, pp. 1338-1342.

Schwartz, P. Birth Injuries. In J. Minckler (Ed.), *Pathology of the Nervous System.* New York: McGraw-Hill, 1971. Vol. 2, pp. 1774-1806.

Schwartz, P., and Anderson, G. A. W. Birth Lesions of the Nervous System. In J. Minckler (Ed.), *Pathology of the Nervous System.* New York: McGraw-Hill, 1971. Vol. 2, pp. 2926-2952.

Towbin, A. Central nervous system damage in the human fetus and newborn infant. *Amer. J. Dis. Child.* 119:529-542, 1970.

Towbin, A. Cerebral Palsy. In J. Minckler (Ed.), *Pathology of the Nervous System.* New York: McGraw-Hill, 1971. Vol. 2, pp. 1832-1850.

Epilepsy and Convulsions

18

Epilepsy is characterized by episodic manifestations of central nervous system dysfunction, which may or may not be associated with clinical signs of brain damage. These manifestations represent an extreme degree of synchronization of large groups of neurons, usually in the cerebral cortex, and are often associated with electroencephalographic changes characterized by synchronization and high amplitude, which are present during and sometimes between the clinical episodes. Attacks may be apparently spontaneous or may occur in relation to a sensory input to which, however, they represent an inappropriate, incoordinated, and excessive reaction. They may not involve convulsions, but instead may include disturbances of movement, sensation, behavior, consciousness, or any combination thereof. Epilepsy is not the only cause of episodic disturbances of cerebral function. The differential diagnosis includes disorders of cerebral blood flow, psychiatric disorders, hypoglycemia or other metabolic disturbances, and the effects of drugs.

Epilepsy may be divided into a primary (idiopathic) form, which is thought to be on a constitutional or genetic basis, and a secondary (symptomatic) variety. Secondary epilepsy is associated with focal or general lesions in the CNS (e.g., injury, tumors, encephalopathy, storage disease) or with such systemic factors as anoxia, hypoglycemia, hypocalcemia, eclampsia, and others. It seems probable that there is no sharp dividing line between the primary and secondary forms, but rather that *the development of epileptic symptoms depends on a balance between the intrinsic seizure threshold for the brain, determined genetically, and superimposed lesions producing epilepsy by structural brain damage.* In this view, the only morphological lesions in primary epilepsy are secondary to ischemia, hypoxemia, and similar factors, whereas the likelihood of epilepsy developing after brain damage (such as head injury) varies with the genetic seizure threshold of the individual.

The term *convulsions* is restricted to motor manifestations of hypersynchronous CNS activity. Convulsions are therefore only one possible form of epilepsy. The term is also used on an age-orientated basis (infantile convulsions) and in respect to motor seizures precipitated by drugs or alterations in homeostasis (e.g., strychnine ingestion, hypoglycemia). It seems appropriate to use the term *convulsions* for nonprogressive motor seizures over a limited period, whether due to recognized or unknown factors, and to restrict the term *epilepsy* to recurrent, often progressive, episodes of synchronized CNS activity, frequently but not necessarily motor, and not associated with systemic disease.

An important property of all seizures is that they appear capable of producing permanent modifications in the seizure threshold of the CNS, so that there is increasing predisposition to further episodes. While this property may be of little importance in convulsions of extracranial origin, such as those due to drugs or homeostatic disorders, which are normally self-limiting in time, it is of considerable importance in seizures of cerebral origin, whether primary or secondary epilepsy. It is a strong argument for early and adequate anticonvulsant therapy, which may even be used prophylactically (as after head injury) to prevent or reduce convulsions and decelerate this self-perpetuating tendency. It is less clear whether this tendency to "imprint" other areas of the brain with lowered seizure threshold applies to nonmotor manifestations.

CONVULSIONS OF SYSTEMIC (EXTRACEREBRAL) ORIGIN

Motor seizures of extracerebral origin are not initially associated with morphological brain damage, but with factors capable of producing neuronal hypersynchrony and motor discharge, even in the presence of a seizure threshold normal for the age of the patient.

Convulsions may be caused by innumerable drugs, apart from the recognized convulsants such as strychnine and picrotoxin. These drugs include antibiotics, especially in the presence of renal failure (penicillin, carbomycin, erythromycin, streptomycin, and bacitracin), some antimalarial drugs, anticholinesterases (diisopropyl fluorophosphate and physostigmine), some antihistamines, tricyclic antidepressants (amitryptyline), morphine, ammonium salts, high doses of pyridoxine, environmental poisons such as DDT and lead, and hydrazide derivatives, including isoniazid. Deficiency states may also be associated with convulsions, notably lack of oxygen, glucose (leucine and isovaleric acid lower the blood-sugar level of infants), pyridoxine and other vitamins of the B group, and calcium. Convulsions may also result from accidental or therapeutic electric shock. Convulsions occur as a complication of severe hypertension and eclampsia, and it is postulated that there is alteration of the blood-brain barrier in these conditions, leading to the escape of fluid and acute edema (dyshoric encephalopathy). Convulsions also occur in association with childhood febrile conditions, especially between the ages of 3 and 7; the degree of fever need not be very high (see below). They are also reported in severe hepatic insufficiency, aminoacidopathies, allergies, endocrine diseases, heat stroke, and congenital heart disease.

Neonatal Convulsions (Mixed Cerebral and Extracerebral Origins)

Convulsions developing during the first 30 days of life may be of varying etiology, and their adequate investigation is important prognostically as well as therapeutically – in particular, for assessing the likelihood of continuing childhood epilepsy. The incidence of neonatal convulsions appears to vary between 2 and 8 per 1000 live births.

About 30 to 35% of neonatal convulsions are associated with hypocalcemia (blood calcium of less than 7.0 mg per 100 ml). Hypocalcemic seizures are characterized by facial spasm followed by rhythmic jerking of one or more limbs, often accompanied by apnea and cyanosis. In many cases they seem to be due to the high phosphate content of cow's milk and artificial formulas, as compared with human breast milk. They usually respond well to intravenous calcium and, in the long run, to administration of low-phosphate formula. The prognosis is generally good, and epilepsy develops in few, if any, of these infants.

Another 30 to 35% are associated with antepartem or intrapartem injury to the CNS, are not amenable to any form of therapy other than anticonvulsant drugs, and carry an extremely poor prognosis. Only about 20% of these patients become normal; the rest develop epilepsy, cerebral palsy, mental retardation, or any combination of these.

Of the remaining 30 to 35% of patients, the majority do not show demonstrable etiological factors; convulsions cease spontaneously and the long-term prognosis is good. In a few infants the convulsions are associated with hypoglycemia, and the prognosis is relatively good (i.e., epilepsy develops in only a few). In a few others convulsions are associated with perinatal CNS infection or developmental anomalies, and many of these infants become epileptic.

Convulsions in the approximately one-third of patients in whom there is no demonstrable cause, and in whom prognosis is good, have not been convincingly explained. However, experimental work indicates that there is normally a low seizure threshold in the immature brain, and that this increases with maturation until adult levels of relative seizure resistance are reached. If these findings are applicable to the human infant, one might assume that the unexplained, and indeed some of the "explained," convulsions (such as those associated with only moderate depression of plasma calcium or glucose), may simply represent the effects of trivial insults on immature brains that physiologically have a low seizure threshold. Conceptually, they are cases of temporary, age-limited "primary epilepsy."

Clinically atypical infantile convulsions (salaam attacks and myoclonus epilepsy) will be discussed under secondary epilepsies. However, in some patients, salaam attacks are due to a biochemical lesion (pyridoxal dependency), and with early, adequate treatment permanent epilepsy may be prevented.

Febrile Convulsions

Infants and young children may have generalized convulsions in association with pyrexia, even though low-grade, due to anything from a minor, nonspecific infection to serious exanthematous disease. Febrile convulsions almost invariably first occur under the age of 3 years. A first convulsion occurring later than this should be viewed with suspicion as possible true epilepsy. They usually cease spontaneously by the age of 10 years. They appear to share at least one characteristic with epilepsy, namely, familial incidence, since the siblings of patients with febrile convulsions show three times the incidence of such convulsions when compared with the siblings of a control population. However, unlike the EEG in true epilepsy, the EEG in patients with febrile convulsions is normal between seizures.

Since the criteria for febrile convulsions are poorly standardized, accurate incidence figures are not available, but it is suggested that about 2% of infants and children have one or more, and that of these, about 30% go on to develop nonfebrile convulsions or true epilepsy. It is open to question whether those who so progress do so because all febrile convulsions are at least a forme fruste of primary epilepsy, or because the convulsions have been sufficiently severe to produce hypoxic brain damage and secondary epileptogenic foci. Further studies, including adequate postmortem investigation, are necessary.

As has been noted, experimental work suggests that the seizure threshold of immature brains is lower than that of the adult. Just as this may explain a proportion of neonatal convulsions, it perhaps also may explain febrile convulsions in infants and children. According to this view, it might be suggested that those children with a genetically determined low threshold, to which the further reduction in threshold due to immaturity is added, are the ones who progress from febrile convulsions to true epilepsy. Since this would also be the group in whom anoxic damage is likely to be most severe because convulsions were more marked, it may be difficult to confirm such a hypothesis.

CLASSIFICATION OF EPILEPSY

A pragmatic separation of cases of epilepsy into primary and secondary, the former on a presumed genetic basis with a low seizure threshold and the latter due to CNS damage of many types associated with a normal seizure threshold, was mentioned at the beginning of the chapter, along with the warning

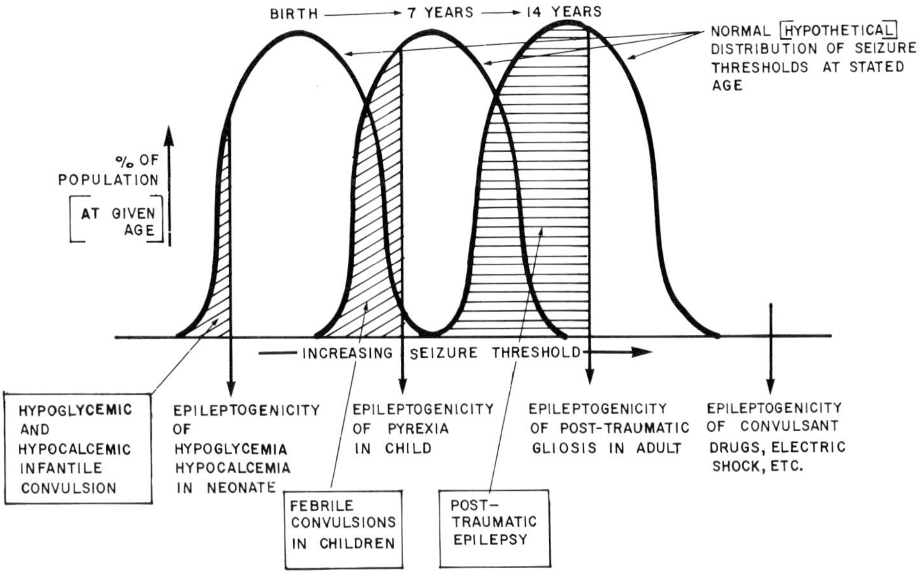

Fig. 18-1. Distribution of seizure threshold (bell-shaped curve) and its increase with age throughout childhood. Convulsions of infancy and childhood, and perhaps symptomatic adult epilepsy, occur in patients with thresholds near the lower limit of normal for their ages. Primary epilepsy presumably represents a genetically determined seizure threshold at or below normal infant levels, which fails to advance normally with age.

that this might be a somewhat artificial distinction. Seizure thresholds represent a continuous spectrum with a normal bell-curve distribution (Fig. 18-1), and are called normal (i.e., high) if seizures can be elicited only by such agents as convulsant drugs or electric shock; *moderate* if seizures are precipitated by such factors as fatigue, teething, fever, and alcohol; and low if seizures apparently occur spontaneously with no recognized precipitating factor. Since the development of an epileptic seizure represents an overwhelming of the seizure threshold by one of many precipitating factors, including structural brain damage, there can be no valid theoretical distinction between primary and secondary types. However, from the pragmatic viewpoints of prognosis and treatment the distinction is useful.

Primary Epilepsy

The primary epilepsies are generalized from their onset and show bilateral, symmetrical, synchronous, high-amplitude EEG activity during the episodes, with variable EEG activity in the interictal stage.

Grand Mal Seizures

Major (grand mal) seizures usually have a prodromal period, characterized by irritability and a feeling of tension, which may last for hours or days. Attacks occur without other warning, with unconsciousness, rigidity, sometimes a cry, apnea, and urination. After a few seconds, tonic spasms of the face, trunk, and limbs occur, progressing through interrupted tonus and clonus to coma and flaccidity. The return of consciousness is gradual, and postictal confusion, headache, and drowsiness are common.

Petit Mal Seizures

Minor (petit mal) seizures may take the form of absence, or lapse, attacks, myoclonic or akinetic seizures, or any combination thereof, and usually last for a few seconds only. Patients subject to petit mal may progress to grand mal, or the two types of attack may alternate in the same patient. *Absences* are characterized by abrupt cessation of activity with the eyes staring or rolling upward, nonresponsiveness to external stimuli, and then a sudden return to whatever activity was going on before the attack. The patient is often unaware that an attack has occurred. Multiple and often frequent (10 up to 100 attacks each day), petit mal seizures are characterized by bilateral, synchronous spike and slow-wave EEG activity (3 cps). Some patients also have *myoclonic seizures,* which are short periods of jerking of one or more limbs, or *akinetic seizures,* in which there is an abrupt loss of postural tone. The association of absences with myoclonic and akinetic seizures is the *petit mal triad.*

Not only is 3-cps EEG activity observed in patients, it is also found in about 50% of siblings between the ages of 4 and 16, suggesting an inherited (genetic) basis, which appears to be autosomally dominant, with age-dependent penetrance. Theta rhythms, which are 4- to 7-cps, bilaterally symmetrical waves, best detected in the parietal area, are also more common in this group of patients and siblings than in control populations. Normally only detectable in children between the ages of 2 and 7, they may be the most suitable for genetic analysis of families, since patients with only myoclonic or akinetic seizures may not show 3-cps spike and wave activity.

Major or minor seizures may also occur in secondary epilepsy. However, in this case, minor seizures are not necessarily associated with their characteristic EEG activity, or they may be focal instead of bilaterally symmetrical.

Secondary Epilepsy

In secondary epilepsy, a CNS focus (occasionally multiple foci) has become epileptogenic following disease or brain injury. At least in the early stages, epileptic discharge may be focal; it may or may not progress to generalized seizures like those of primary epilepsy. Since, as already noted, the occurrence of motor and possibly other types of seizures appears to lower the seizure threshold of the brain, the initial focal stage may become unrecognizable later in the progression of the disease.

Early Focal Manifestations

Depending on the site of the epileptogenic focus, there is often an aura or focal seizure (not present in primary epilepsy) preceding generalization, and the type of focal activity varies with the area of the cortex affected.

Motor and Premotor Cortex Seizures. These originate as focal motor activity (Jacksonian epilepsy), which may be initially clonic or tonic in nature.

Sensory Cortex Seizures. These originate as sensory disturbances, which are usually paresthesias rather than dysesthesias.

Occipital Cortex Seizures. These may originate either as negative seizures, in which there is impairment of vision, or positive seizures, in which visual hallucinations occur. These are usually fragmentary and apparently meaningless, but if the adjacent temporal cortex is also involved, hallucinations may take the form of meaningful scenes.

Frontal Cortex Seizures. These originate as episodes of coma without any describable aura and may therefore be confused with primary grand mal epilepsy. Occasionally, coma is preceded by episodes of altered psychic content. Secondary epilepsy due to frontal lesions appears to show a higher-than-average predisposition to status epilepticus.

Temporal Cortex Seizures. The temporal lobe is the original seizure focus in about one-third of all cases of epilepsy, with several types of aura, usually with psychic content. The auras include unpleasant sensations, ranging from the epigastric region to the throat or mouth; hallucinations of many sensory modalities, including vertigo; disturbances of memory (including déjà vu and jamais vu); dreamy states; affective disorders, such as anxiety, ecstasy, depression, or paranoia; or, occasionally, primary automatisms with overt motor activity, usually of a gustatory or sexual nature.

Spread of Epileptogenic Activity

Any of these focal manifestations may be followed by spread of various types. They may, for example, spread *sequentially* along a gyrus (classic Jacksonian epilepsy), *centrifugally* over the cortex, irrespective of the gyral pattern (as when adversive head-turning occurs in a spread from temporal or anterior frontal foci to the premotor cortex), or *deeply* through the corticothalamic fibers, to involve the reticular activating system, leading to generalized grand mal seizures.

Where there are diffuse cerebral pathological changes, such as those seen in anoxia, lipidosis, encephalitis, and tuberous sclerosis, multifocal epilepsy may occur.

Secondary Epilepsy following Head Injury (All Age Groups)

Of particular importance among the secondary epilepsies are those that follow head injury, especially of the penetrating variety or when accompanied by significant intracranial hemorrhage. Post-traumatic epilepsy may follow an episode of trauma at any age, whereas most of the idiopathic epilepsies begin in childhood. (As many as 17% of patients with idiopathic epilepsy are, however, said to have their first convulsion after the age of 25.)

A study of 820 consecutive patients with penetrating brain injuries showed that 43% still had epileptic seizures five years later. Although this study was carried out over a long period, advances in surgical management (such as early primary debridement) appeared to have brought little improvement. Available evidence suggests that different areas of neocortex, even in the normal person, have a variable epileptogenic potentiality. Correspondingly, it has been observed that epilepsy develops in a much higher proportion (60 to 70%) of patients with injuries involving the medial temporal, premotor, motor, and parietal regions than in patients with injuries involving the anterior frontal, lateral temporal, or occipital regions. Patients with injuries in the upper medial cortex (within 5 cm of the superior sagittal sinus) generally show a much lower incidence of post-traumatic epilepsy.

A majority of patients begin to have seizures during the first week after injury, often Jacksonian or focal in nature; some have their initial seizure between the second and seventh week; and relatively few show their first seizure more than 8 weeks after injury. Seizures beginning after the first week often appear to originate in the temporal lobe. The early Jacksonian group appear to carry a better prognosis. Only 30% of patients who had their initial seizure within seven days of injury became permanently epileptic, whereas of those who had their initial fit from the second week onward, about 80% became epileptic. Patients who had only a single seizure within minutes of injury or who had no seizures at all during the acute or subacute stage rarely had permanent epileptic sequelae. In less severe, nonpenetrating injury the incidence of epilepsy is considerably lower.

Other Causes of Secondary Epilepsy (All Age Groups)

Epilepsy may also complicate other cerebral lesions, most often in adults. Focal inflammatory lesions, such as cerebral abscess or cysticercosis, carry almost as high a risk as head injury. Epilepsy only occasionally complicates cerebrovascular accidents, encephalitis, raised intracranial pressure, or multiple sclerosis (in the latter, usually when the lesions are cortical or immediately subcortical).

Secondary Epilepsy Peculiar to Infants and Children

Infantile Spasms. A distinctive manifestation of secondary epilepsy is the infantile spasm, usually first seen between the third and seventh months of life, associated with momentary movements of nodding and flexion of the body, often with outstretched arms (salaam attacks). There is a characteristic EEG (hypsarrhythmia), which shows high-amplitude, irregular, slow spike and wave forms and absence of a fixed focus. Those due to *diffuse cerebral pathological changes* are frequently associated with mental retardation and may alternate with grand mal seizures. Another group, due to *genetically determined pyridoxal dependency,* respond to therapy with massive pyridoxal dosage and may not progress to true epilepsy. Associated with infantile spasms may be chronic episodes of abnormal posture maintained for seconds or minutes, often with arm flexion and extension of the legs.

Progressive Myoclonus Epilepsy. Another secondary epilepsy of childhood is progressive myoclonus epilepsy, a clinical syndrome with several etiologies. Some cases are familial and others sporadic. Girls are affected more often than boys. Onset, with grand mal seizures, is usually between the ages of 6 and 13 years. The seizures are followed by irregular twitchings of part of a muscle or a muscle group, only occasionally sufficiently strong to cause movement. Later in the course of the disease, complex myoclonus causes movements of the trunk and limbs, often so violent and frequent as to render the patient helpless. Still later, extrapyramidal disturbances and progressive dementia occur, and death follows a state of rigid immobilization, dementia, marasmus, and intercurrent infection.

This characteristic picture may be a manifestation of *late infantile or juvenile ganglioside storage disease* (such cases begin earlier and have a shorter clinical course); may be associated with *nonspecific degenerative CNS changes,* including neuronal loss, especially from the pallidum, substantia nigra, and dentate nucleus; or may show the characteristic intracytoplasmic, PAS-positive, neuronal inclusions of *Lafora's disease,* accompanied by changes in the liver and muscle. In the latter two groups, there appears to be recessive inheritance and frequently a history of parental consanguinity.

ETIOLOGY OF EPILEPSY

The electroencephalographic and clinical features of convulsions and epilepsy make it apparent that they involve massive synchronous discharge from large groups of neurons (hypersynchronization). This is associated with a lowered seizure threshold in those with idiopathic epilepsy and with powerfully epileptogenic foci able to overcome a (presumably) normal threshold in those with secondary epilepsy. Convulsions may be associated with a temporarily low threshold (in infants and children) and with the action of systemic factors that affect energy metabolism and membrane polarization in the brain. In patients with symptomatic (secondary) epilepsy, precipitating factors are clearly present, but genetic lowering of the seizure threshold has not been excluded. An interplay of the two factors may be significant in determining which patients with head injury, for example, will ultimately develop epilepsy.

Primary Epilepsy

Nothing is known of the etiology of the reduced seizure threshold in persons with primary epilepsy, although it is presumed to be a biochemical defect on an inherited basis. The mode of inheritance is not clear, but the familial incidence is undisputed, as is frequent concordance in monozygotic twins. In one study of 14 pairs of such twins, 10 pairs were both epileptic, but in four pairs, only one. Other kinships have been described containing numerous persons with overt epilepsy in three or four consecutive generations. Electroencephalographic studies have been extensively employed in attempted genetic analysis. In one such study it was found that of clinically normal siblings of epileptic children, 8% showed some epileptiform features in the EEG, compared with 0.8% in a control population. This figure is even higher in kinships with petit mal. If normal siblings are tested at the appropriate age, both the 3-cps spike and wave activity and parietal theta rhythms show statistically significant increases over the incidence in control populations.

Thus, there is a clearly enhanced familial incidence with subclinical changes in siblings, and yet no clear dominant or recessive inheritance. Presumably, what is inherited is a level of seizure threshold (i.e., predisposition or resistance to epileptic seizures). This inheritance could be on a multiple-gene (polygenic) basis or could be an autosomal dominant with incomplete penetrance, as perhaps is suggested by the results of EEG studies.

Secondary Epilepsy and Convulsions

Among the secondary epilepsies and convulsions, familial incidence has been demonstrated only in the group of febrile convulsions occurring in young children. The possible relationship to epilepsy has already been discussed. There is at present no clear evidence of increased familial incidence of both febrile convulsions and epilepsy in single kinships.

Since presumably the seizure threshold in a population is a continuous variable, a role for low thresholds in the development of post-traumatic and other secondary epilepsies could be postulated, but to date there is no clear evidence for or against such a role. In secondary epilepsy, abnormalities of the EEG may precede clinical seizures or occur in the absence of seizures. However, it is difficult to be dogmatic about the latter, since the necessary duration of follow-up to exclude development of epilepsy completely is unknown. In patients with diffuse neurological disease, about 2.5% may show an epileptiform EEG without seizures; in approximately 0.5%, seizures eventually develop, especially if the disease is progressive and the patient is under the age of 20. However, all these findings are as compatible with the progressive epileptogenicity of focal lesions as with the preexistence of a low threshold. Continuing studies are needed to elucidate these relationships.

Birth Injury and Epilepsy

The absence of a precipitating factor (epileptogenic focus) in idiopathic or primary epilepsy is not accepted by many, and a relationship between primary epilepsy and birth injury has been widely postulated. The birth injury usually proposed is damage to the region of the uncus occurring during birth or as a result of prenatal, intranatal, or postnatal asphyxia. More recently, a relation between the overriding of bones during skull molding and possible damage to the underlying cortex has also been suggested.

The morphological substrate of epilepsy is discussed later. It suffices to say at this point that there is no type of brain damage unique to epilepsy and no type of brain damage present in all cases of epilepsy; in many well-documented cases, in which competent autopsy examinations were made, no detectable epileptogenic focus was found. Many of the lesions seen in epileptic brains are a result, not a cause, of epileptic seizures.

There is no concrete evidence that birth injury is a cause of *primary epilepsy*. As noted in the preceding chapter, birth injury is, of course, a major cause of brain damage associated with *secondary epilepsy* and other severe CNS dysfunction.

PATHOGENESIS OF EPILEPSY

A consideration of pathogenetic mechanisms has to account for at least the following aspects of epilepsy:

1. The frequent presence of abnormal EEG activity between clinical attacks (interictal phase), representing the background on which seizures are superposed.
2. The factor or factors that precipitate the clinical seizure (preictal phase).
3. The factor or factors that lead to termination of a seizure (ictal and postictal phases).
4. The mechanism whereby a focal hypersynchronized discharge may spread through the CNS.
5. The mechanism whereby epileptic discharge causes a permanent molecular alteration in neuronal populations that increases the likelihood of their producing hypersynchronized discharges (seizures) in the future.
6. The mechanisms leading to morphological brain damage, with possible further enhancement of the epileptic process.

Information on many of these aspects is extremely scanty. Current techniques provide more information about the behavior of individual neurons in epileptic foci than about the manner in which their discharge is originated and spread.

Electrophysiological Changes in Neurons

Changes have been studied experimentally in epileptogenic foci produced by the application of penicillin to the cortex or similar procedures. In such foci, in between periods of abnormal electrical discharge or overt seizures, the neurons cannot be recognized as abnormal by any of the electrophysiological parameters tested; membrane conductance responds to inhibitory and excitatory postsynaptic potentials, and generation of action potential is normal. Changes discussed in the succeeding sections are illustrated in Figure 18-2.

Changes in Neuronal Membrane Potential

During periods of abnormal electrical activity, some neurons exhibit a period of prolonged membrane depolarization associated with the generation of multiple action potentials. This is called the *paroxysmal depolarization shift* (PDS). The PDS resembles an excitatory postsynaptic potential (EPSP) (see Chap. 4), except that it is much longer (several hundredths of a second) and larger (20 to 30 mv) and generates a fast train of action potentials. It has longer latency than, and may appear after, a normal EPSP, separated from it by an interval of normal membrane potential. Since the cell responds normally to excitatory and inhibitory synaptic impulses, it is probable that there is no change in the neuronal membrane, but that the effect, due to an abnormally sustained barrage of excitatory impulses, represents a pathological exaggeration of a normal EPSP. The PDS is presumably a result of interneuronal exitatory feedback (within the focus), which involves the entire soma-dendrite membrane (whereas physiological input tends to be localized according to its site of origin). The PDS is preictal and indeed is separated from the convulsion by a period of hyperpolarization (PHS) resembling an exaggerated inhibitory postsynaptic potential (IPSP). Following the PDS and PHS, a long period of afterdepolarization accompanies the tonic phase of the seizure. Afterhyperpolarization then develops, and persists through the clonic into the postictal phase.

Not all neurons show the PDS or subsequent changes. Some remain hyperpolarized throughout the preictal, ictal, and postictal phases, and this hyperpolarization may be most marked during the convulsive phase. Waves of temporary depolarization may be superposed on the hyperpolarization — again suggesting that neuronal membranes in the focus remain capable of normal responses to physiological stimuli. The hyperpolarization may be considerable (i.e., between −75 and −80 mv); it cannot be due solely to increased Cl^- permeability as is the normal IPSP, but implies a significant increase in K^+ permeability.

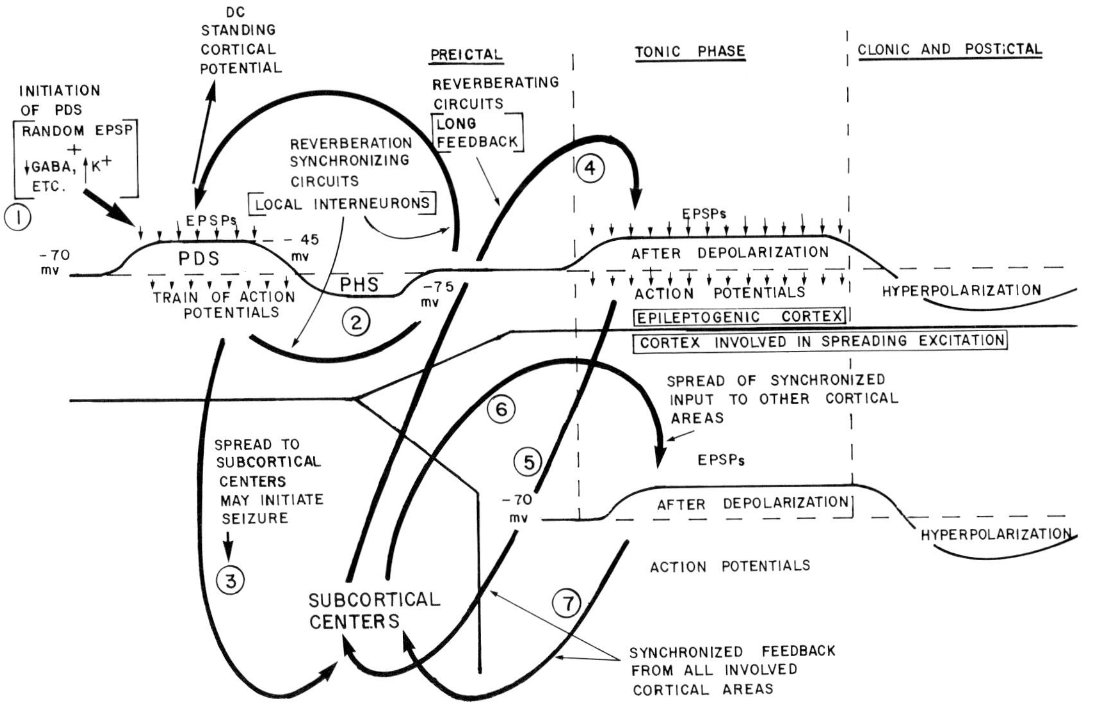

Fig. 18-2. Possible sequence of electrophysiological events (1 to 7) involved in the initiation (1 and 2), focal synchronization (3 to 5), and spread (6 and 7) of an epileptic seizure. For abbreviations and details, see text.

Changes in Cortical Standing Potential

The normal cortical EEG is probably the resultant of postsynaptic potentials (PSPs) generated mainly by pyramidal cells, since these are uniformly orientated. Any PSPs generated by interneurons, which are granular cells with an apparently random arrangement, would tend to be self-canceling. It has been demonstrated that cortical potential gradients are radially orientated. Similarly, the cortical standing potential probably results from pyramidal cell activity. During seizures there is a negative shift in this potential, which becomes positive during the postictal phase, and the size of the shift is proportional to the change in neuronal membrane potential. Since it is recorded from the extracellular fluid (ECF), the negative shift represents a shift of ECF potential toward that of the intracellular fluid and therefore indicates membrane depolarization.

Hypersynchronization

Physiologically, the discharge from cortical neurons may be random or synchronous, the latter implying a subcortical driving mechanism. Not only synchronous cell discharge, but also cells with a uniform discharge frequency even out of phase may still produce a synchronous EEG record. Synchronization of the EEG during convulsive activity therefore represents a greater than normal uniformity in discharge frequency of individual neurons, but not necessarily an increase in synchronization and could of itself originate by short feedback mechanisms within the cortical focus. However, the observed EEG spike *amplitudes* (as high as 5 to 10 mv) must imply increased synchronization in addition to uniform discharge frequency. Such hypersynchronization within the epileptogenic focus might be produced by the fast train of action potentials generated through interneurons early in the PDS, presumably returning through feedback circuits involving subcortical structures. Synchronous depolarization might be entirely due to such synaptic mechanisms, but a possible role for depolarization spread centrifugally, not dependent on neuronal circuits, cannot be excluded. This *field depolarization* might involve generalized modulators of CNS activity (such as glutamate or γ-aminobutyric acid [GABA]), but not synaptic neurotransmitters.

Possible Precipitating Factors in Clinical and Experimental Lesions

In secondary epilepsies there is a focal lesion representing the initial epileptogenic focus that is more or less comparable with the experimentally produced lesion; it varies widely, from gliosis through malformation to tumors. At least two possible mechanisms might account for the readiness with which neurons, both in such clinical foci and in experimental lesions,

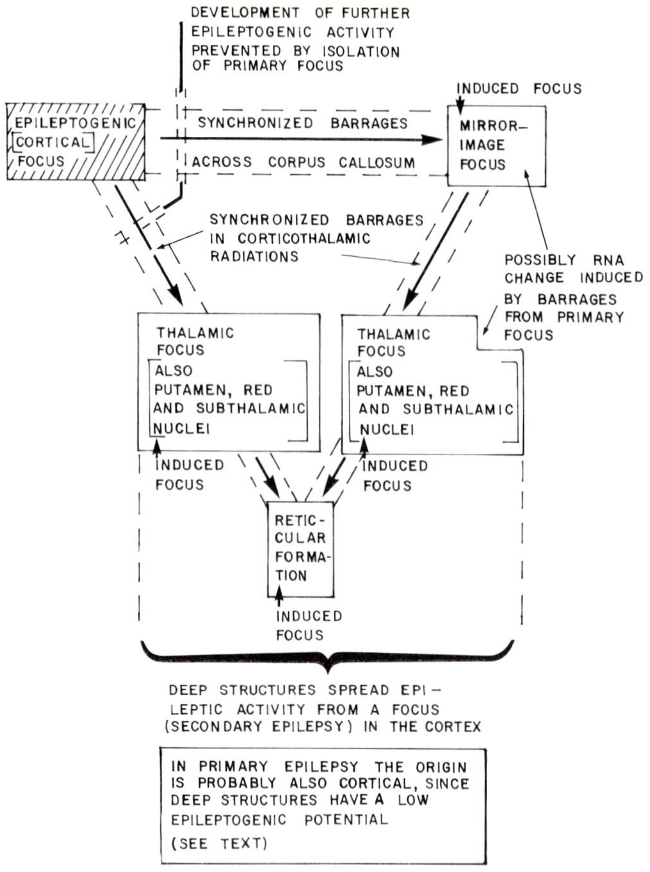

Fig. 18-3. Routes of spread of epileptic discharges. For details, see text.

undergo depolarization. One is *partial deafferentation* and consequent increased sensitivity to neurotransmitters. Another is an *increase in extracellular K^+ concentration,* since in such foci, neurons are not surrounded by normal glial cells or processes, but rather by glial processes packed with fibrils, or even by reticulin or collagen fibers. If, as has been proposed, glial cells have a physiological role in maintaining normal K^+ levels in the ECF, taking up the K^+ lost from active neurons, such absence of normal neuron-glial relationships could cause abnormal prolongation of neuronal depolarization.

The Spread of Epileptic Activity

Formation of Secondary Epileptogenic Foci

Lesions in the motor or premotor cortex of monkeys (produced by application of alumina cream or by freezing) are consistently followed by focal seizures with characteristic EEGs. Later, independent *secondary epileptogenic foci* develop consistently in a similar area of the contralateral cortex (mirror focus) and also bilaterally in the putamen, subthalamic nucleus, red nucleus, and several nuclei of the thalamus (Fig. 18-3). Such foci develop over 3 to 10 months; they usually develop in the ipsilateral deep structures first, then in the mirror focus, and finally in the contralateral deep structures.

The areas in which independently discharging foci develop are the same areas from which electrical activity can be recorded when the primary epileptogenic focus is stimulated. Secondary foci persist after connections with the primary lesion are severed, but are aborted if these connections are severed before or shortly after inducing the primary lesion. The frequency of their development is reduced by anticonvulsant drugs. The higher the degree of CNS organization, the longer it takes for such secondary foci to form. In man, periods of years, rather than months, seem to be necessary.

How the secondary foci develop is completely unclear, but they are presumably related to the arrival of barrages of synchronous, high-frequency impulses from the primary focus and the induction of electrophysiological changes as noted in the primary focus. The possibility that some "epileptogenic agent" accompanies axoplasmic flow cannot be ruled out, but preliminary indications of altered ribonucleic acid (RNA) in the secondary foci suggest possible synaptic facilitation, perhaps akin to that involved in learning. The liability of the CNS to such "imprinting" by persistent epileptic discharge underlines the need for early and adequate anticonvulsant therapy.

Routes of Spread

Observations such as these emphasize the importance of anatomical pathways in the development of generalized bilaterally symmetrical seizures resembling those of primary or idiopathic epilepsy. The most significant of these long-range pathways appears to be the corpus callosum, which connects mainly corresponding areas of the cortex on the two sides, and the reciprocal thalamocortical connections that also connect with the reticular formation of the thalamus and brain stem.

The Reticular Activating System and Primary Epilepsy

Since primary epilepsy is generalized and symmetrical from the start, and immediate loss of consciousness is a feature of both minor and major attacks, it has been suggested that the epileptogenic focus in primary epilepsy lies in deep structures that are involved in consciousness and radiate widely to the cortex. Such criteria pinpoint the reticular formation, and the term *centrencephalic epilepsy* has been coined to express this concept. However, it is not universally accepted. Tumors of the central gray matter and brain stem produce epilepsy only in 3 to 8% of cases, compared with 32% in tumors of the occipital cortex and up to 80% in tumors of the frontal cortex.

The results of studies of electrical or convulsant-drug stimulation of different parts of the CNS support the peculiar susceptibility of the cortex and certain subcortical structures, particularly the frontal cortex, amygdala, and adjacent temporal cortex. Although generalized seizures may be initiated from the cortex in the absence of brain stem lesions, destruction or damage of the brain stem in many cases seems to prevent their occurrence, suggesting that the role of the reticular formation lies in facilitating the spread of activity from a cortical epileptogenic area throughout the CNS.

The synchronizing activities of the ascending reticular activating system are poorly developed in immature animals, but the experimental evidence indicates that seizure threshold in such animals is low. The injection of metrazol into either carotid artery of a patient with primary epilepsy (and no evidence of a focal lesion) immediately leads to a generalized seizure, which is promptly aborted by the intracarotid injection of amobarbital on the same side. Since the carotid artery does not supply the thalamus or brain stem, it would appear that epileptogenic activity is exerted directly on the cortex. Injection of metrazol into the vertebral arteries, which supply the thalamus and reticular formation, does not initiate seizures in such patients. Indeed, it may reduce seizure activity, presumably by activating the alerting component of the ascending reticular activating system (see Chap. 5).

The findings outlined in the preceding paragraphs would suggest that the ascending reticular activating system does not have a role in the initiation of primary epilepsy, but may be a route of spread.

Attempts to Suppress the Spread of Epileptogenic Activity

The deliberate induction of destructive lesions by stereotaxic surgery in such areas as the amygdala, pallidum, lateral thalamus, thalamic fasciculus, and fornix has been reported. In the relatively small number of cases so far on record, and in which there is a wide distribution of induced lesions, there appears to be improvement in some cases, particularly of frontal lobe epilepsy, but the effect on primary epilepsy has not as yet been determined.

The cerebellum appears to have an inhibitory effect on the development of epileptic seizures: Although naturally occurring cerebellar lesions do not appreciably alter the incidence of epilepsy, the deliberate experimental irritation of the cerebellum (by application of cobalt powder or electrical stimulation) increases cerebellar discharge and inhibits epileptic seizures and EEG activity. (The application of cobalt powder to the cerebral cortex, on the other hand, produces epileptogenic foci.)

The Biochemical Correlates of Epilepsy

A large body of clinical and experimental data on the biochemical changes associated with epilepsy is available. Such data include changes in tissue slices incubated in vitro, as well as the biochemical CNS changes in vivo following induction of convulsions by many methods. It is therefore difficult to derive coherent information, but there is a consensus that certain changes are characteristic.

Bioenergetic Changes

Bioenergetic changes are numerous. There is a localized increase in cerebral blood flow; depletion of oxygen, glucose, glycogen, adenosine triphosphate, and creatine phosphate; a fall in pH and rises in inorganic phosphate, lactate, and carbon dioxide. Presumably, the attempt to maintain membrane polarization involves heavy utilization of both anaerobic and aerobic cycles, and adequate supplies of B-group vitamins are essential. While convulsive activity involves regional depletion of high-energy phosphates, experimental work suggests that there may not be a complete switch from aerobic to anaerobic metabolism, provided adequate oxygenation and ventilation are maintained. Thus, the hypoxic changes following numerous epileptic seizures may not be entirely due to excessive metabolic demand (and therefore inevitable), but may in part be due to deficient oxygenation of the blood because

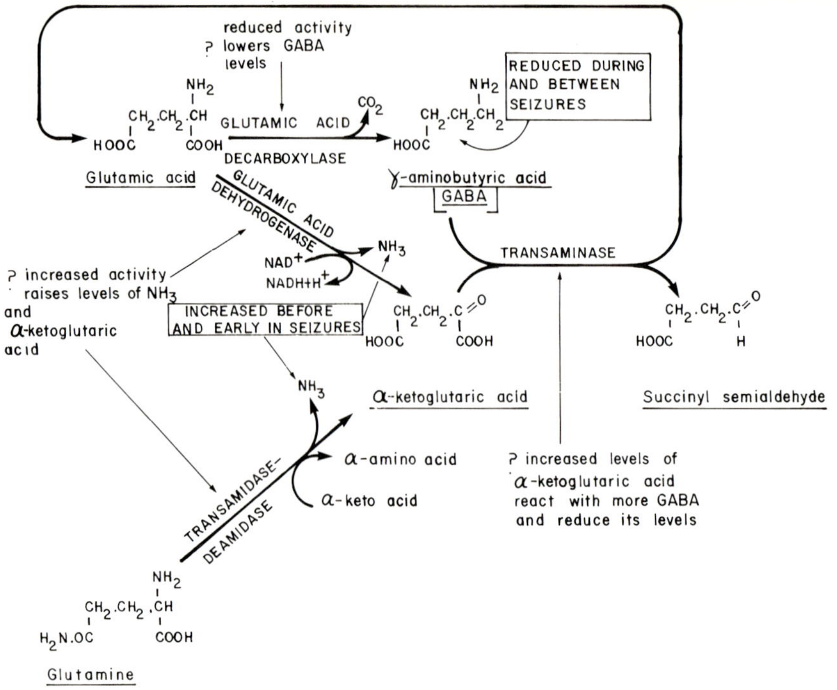

Fig. 18-4. Possible changes in enzyme activity in epileptogenic foci, with resulting decrease in concentration of the inhibitory modulator GABA.

of muscular spasm and excessive bronchial secretion (and therefore in part preventable). Between seizures, carbohydrate metabolism and oxygen utilization are normal, and there are no confirmed alterations in oxidative enzyme activity.

Changes in γ-Aminobutyric Acid and Ammonia

Levels of GABA appear to be low, not only during seizures, but also in the interictal phase, perhaps due to reduced activity of glutamic acid decarboxylase (a pyridoxal-dependent enzyme). Production of ammonia is said to rise before and in the early stages of convulsion, but the significance of this change is unclear, since the major mechanism for producing ammonia in the brain is the conversion of glutamine or glutamic acid to α-ketoglutaric acid, which in turn reacts with GABA to form glutamic acid and succinate. It might be hypothesized that the levels of GABA are reduced not only by the defective synthesis, but also by excessive transamination to succinate (Fig. 18-4). Speculatively, a disturbance of glutamic acid metabolism, leading to reduced levels of GABA, which is considered to be an inhibitory modulator or neurotransmitter, might contribute to depolarization (see Chap. 3).

Changes in Acetylcholine Binding

Under normal conditions, brain acetylcholine is bound in synaptic terminals, and any that is freed outside the cell is rapidly inactivated by acetylcholinesterase. In epileptogenic foci there is said to be an increase in extracellular acetylcholine and a decrease in the bound form, accompanied by increased (perhaps compensatory) levels of acetylcholinesterase. In the terminal stages of a convulsion the proportion of bound acetylcholine rises nearer to normal levels, although it is not known whether this contributes to the cessation of cortical discharge.

Electrolyte Disturbances

Electrolyte disturbances in epileptogenic foci include increased intracellular Na^+ and decreased K^+ concentrations, with converse changes in ECF, presumably associated with a greater permeability of neuronal membranes in depolarization. This may be attributable to free acetylcholine or other neurotransmitters.

Experimentally, extracellular K^+ increases the release of norepinephrine, an action requiring the presence of Ca^{++}; diphenylhydantoin (DPH) reduces such release and has anticonvulsant effects. (Synthetic derivatives of DPH that do not affect norepinephrine release have no effect on convulsive activity.) Apparently, DPH and Ca^{++} act competitively at the cell membrane, probably including the synapses where Ca^{++} is necessary for neurotransmitter release. Correspondingly, DPH is known to prevent intracellular Ca^{++} accumulation in many tissues; it reverses myotonia, decreases cardiac contractility, and reduces inappropriate secretion of vasopressin.

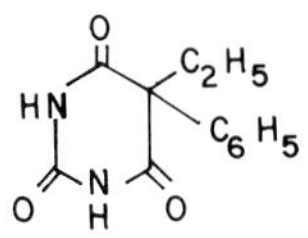

Phenobarbital

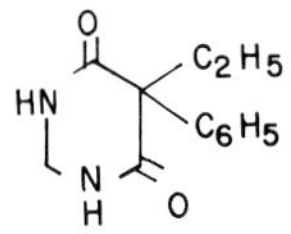

Primidone

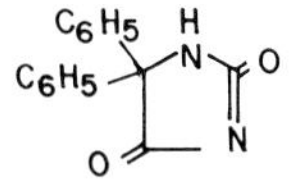

Diphenylhydantoin

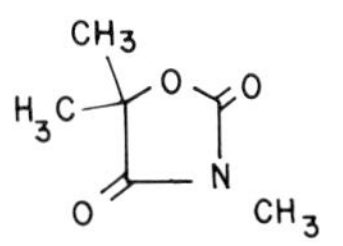

Trimethadione

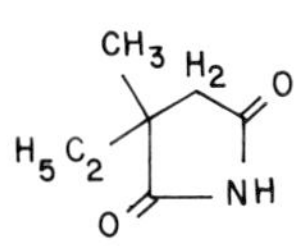

Ethosuximide

Fig. 18-5. Some drugs used in the treatment of epilepsy.

Optimum Ca^{++} concentration is necessary for transmitter release, but high Ca^{++} levels depress CNS function. Raised cerebrospinal fluid Ca^{++} has anticonvulsant activity (contrary to the effect of K^{+}). There is a 20- to 30-minute latency in anticonvulsant activity after CSF Ca^{++} levels are raised; this may reflect the time needed for ECF diffusion, since Ca^{++} binds to plasma membranes that must be progressively saturated before the ions can diffuse further. (Convulsant drug molecules, although larger than Ca^{++} diffuse from CSF to ECF much faster.) Once Ca^{++} is bound to the plasma membrane, its protective effect is prolonged. Increasing K^{+} concentration in the CSF (and therefore presumably in ECF) changes the shape of postsynaptic potentials, and causes a late component in the apical dendritic wave which progressively increases in size and duration, and which may correspond to the PDS in epileptogenic foci. Ca^{++} delays and reduces this change.

Although there is no direct evidence of the mode of action of convulsant drugs such as metrazol on extracellular K^{+} concentration, they have been observed to cause astrocytic swelling. Thus, there is a possible failure of glial function that could cause a secondary increase in ECF K^{+} concentration (and also possibly cause defective transport of glucose, capillary obstruction, and other problems). The K^{+} to Ca^{++} balance in ECF may be a significant determinant of seizure threshold.

Effects of Folates and Folate Derivatives

Anticonvulsant drugs reduce plasma and CSF levels of folic acid and may even cause megaloblastic anemia. Some patients treated with these drugs show apathy and diffuse CNS symptomatology, said to be improved by folate, but only at the expense of more frequent seizures. Experimental administration of sodium folate in high dosage (or small amounts directly into CSF) causes convulsions. Experimentally induced epileptogenic foci and the secondary mirror foci both show increased folate. Chemotherapeutic drugs such as methotrexate and aminopterin (which are folate derivatives) are epileptogenic, probably by concentration at the synaptosomal membrane. Although it appears improbable that folic acid has an etiological role in primary epilepsy, it does antagonize anticonvulsants, especially DPH. However, the mechanism of this antagonism is unknown.

Interference in Pathogenetic Mechanisms by Anticonvulsant Drugs

The drugs used in the treatment of epilepsy fall into the general class of drugs known as depressants (see Chap. 9). However, they differ somewhat from other depressants in that they increase the seizure threshold yet cause little general drowsiness. Screening of anticonvulsant drugs by assessing their effects on electrically or drug-induced convulsions in animals has proved of considerable value, though the ultimate test is their efficacy in clinical use.

Theoretically, anticonvulsants might act directly on the epileptogenic focus or prevent the generalization of seizure activity throughout the brain; since they may prevent convulsions but do not alter the interictal EEG record, the latter appears more likely. It must be stressed that drugs do not abolish any epileptogenic focus, but are palliative in that they prevent or reduce seizures. Because of the imprinting effect of recurrent convulsions and resulting multiplication of epileptogenic centers, such palliation is of vital importance in preventing progression of the disease. They are of equal importance in primary and in secondary epilepsy.

Most of the useful anticonvulsants are based on heterocyclic rings with carbonyl groupings (Fig. 18-5), but their mode of molecular activity is unknown. It seems likely that the ability of the hydantoins to compete with Ca^{++} for membrane-binding may reduce the release of neurotransmitters (see p. 338), but why such action should only be apparent in the circuits concerned with epileptic discharge is unknown.

Most members of this group of drugs have side effects that may be potentially serious. Pharmacology texts should be consulted for the details. The most important groups are:

1. *Barbiturates and similar compounds,* especially phenobarbital and primidone, particularly effective in grand mal and psychomotor seizures.
2. *Hydantoins,* especially DPH, for the same conditions.
3. *Oxazolidones,* such as trimethadione, particularly efficacious in petit mal.
4. *Succinimides,* such as ethosuximide, also for petit mal.
5. *Other drugs,* such as acetazolamide (grand and petit mal), meprobamate (petit mal), and diazepam (petit mal and status epilepticus). The latter two are better known as anti-anxiety drugs (tranquilizers) (see Chap. 26).

Summary of Theories of Pathogenesis

The etiological and pathogenetic factors in epilepsy are still in considerable doubt, but the foregoing discussion, although necessarily diffuse, at least suggests some of the factors and mechanisms involved. These may be summarized as follows:

1. The origin of the discharge is in the cerebral cortex in most, if not all, cases; only in secondary epilepsy, however, does pathological examination usually disclose an epileptogenic focus. In such a focus, the seizure threshold may be lowered by deafferentation hypersensitivity or raised ECF K^+ concentration due to the absence of normal astrocytic cytoplasm. In primary epilepsy the threshold is genetically low. Seizure thresholds are normally low in infancy but rise during childhood.

2. Both experimental and natural foci show reduction of neuronal population and fibrillary gliosis, but no pathognomonic features. At least some such foci have low GABA concentration between, as well as during, seizures, perhaps due to reduced activity of glutamic acid decarboxylase and diversion of glutamic acid metabolism to other pathways.

3. Immediately preceding, during, and after a seizure (preictal, ictal, and postictal phases), neurons in epileptogenic foci show severe depolarization and increased membrane permeability, resulting in a gain of Na^+ and a loss of K^+ by the cell, with opposite changes in ECF concentrations; massively increased aerobic and anaerobic metabolism to rectify these changes; adenosine triphosphate depletion; and increased free acetylcholine (and perhaps increases in other transmitters). Causes of this severe depolarization include GABA deficiency, deafferentation sensitivity, high ECF K^+ concentration (a vicious circle), unidentified genetic mechanisms, and random EPSPs, any of which may act synergistically.

4. Although neuronal membranes retain their capacity to respond to superimposed excitatory and inhibitory postsynaptic potentials at all times (and are therefore presumed to be functionally normal), many of the neurons in a focus show a sequence of polarization changes, all of which are very long in comparison with normal postsynaptic potentials. These include a prolonged depolarization shift (PDS) and a prolonged hyperpolarization shift (PHS) in the preictal phase, with the former generating a long train of rapid action potentials. Such trains, acting through intracortical feedback circuits, may lead to equalization of discharge frequency and hypersynchronization. The tonic phase of the seizure is accompanied by a very prolonged depolarization that is perhaps initiated by feedback from subcortical circuits, such as those passing through the thalamus and reticular formation, and resulting in further trains of synchronized potentials. The clonic and postictal phases are characterized by a long period of hyperpolarization.

5. The cortical focus shows rapid, high-amplitude synchronous discharge during and sometimes between seizures, presumably associated with intracortical feedback synchronization, whether or not this generates a generalized convulsion. There are changes in the transcortical potential in connection with a seizure – it is negative during convulsive activity and positive after – presumably originating in the radially orientated pyramidal cells and reflecting depolarization and hyperpolarization respectively.

6. Local spread may occur along gyri (Jacksonian march) or centrifugally, presumably through association fibers.

7. Generalization occurs through the normal anatomical pathways of the focus, predominantly to the thalamus and reticular formation and to mirror-image cortex via the corpus callosum.

8. Whether local or general, spread causes permanent modification of the "target" areas, lowering their seizure thresholds; in turn, they become epileptogenic foci. The nature of such modification is unknown, but it may involve synaptic facilitation with RNA changes and thus may be analogous to the learning process.

9. Prolonged, severe, or frequent seizures – and especially status epilepticus – may cause such imbalance between energy supplies and requirements as to produce structural (hypoxic or hypoglycemic) damage in the CNS, varying from selective ischemic neuronal necrosis to laminar infarction and possibly accentuated by increased intracranial pressure due to intense vasodilatation and edema caused by local acidosis. The energy imbalance is not solely due to high energy requirements. It is also related to spasm of respiratory muscle and excess bronchial secretions.

MORPHOLOGY OF EPILEPSY

It should be stressed again that there is no one pathological change or group of changes found in all cases of epilepsy; nor is there a unique lesion found only in epilepsy and not in other conditions. The following notes briefly review the findings in idiopathic epilepsy, post-traumatic epilepsy, and the unique Lafora type of progressive myoclonus epilepsy. In any of these conditions, or in any other type of epilepsy, there may be found in the brain lesions that are characteristic of systemic hypoxemia or hypoglycemia (see Chap. 13). These lesions may result

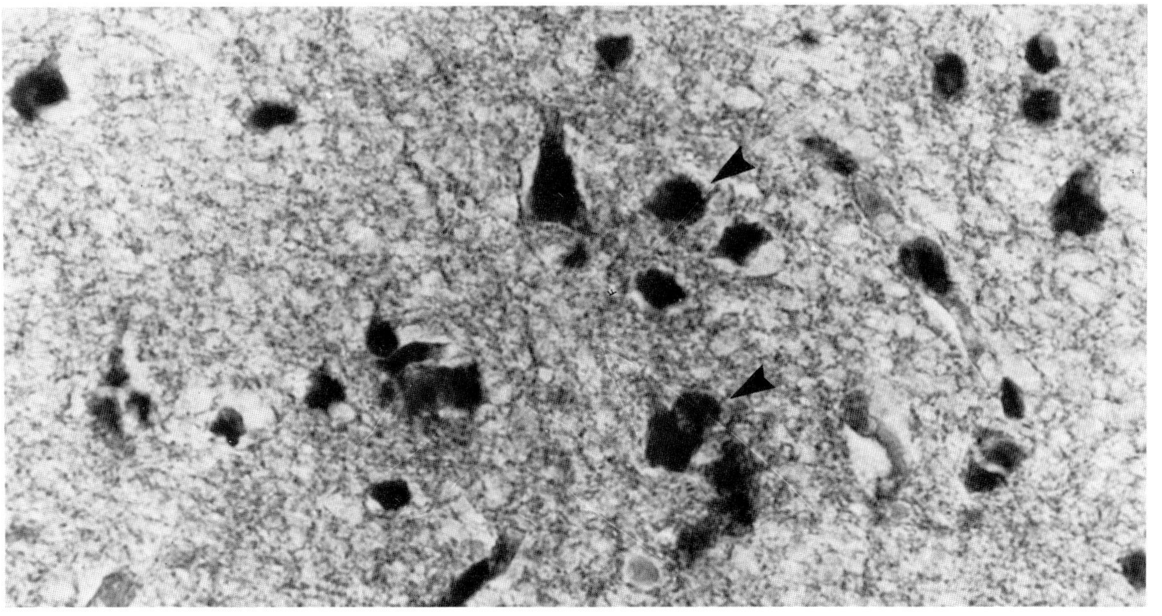

Fig. 18-6. Myoclonus epilepsy, showing two rounded bodies with faint radial striations at the edges (arrows). (PAS, ×750.)

partly from hypoxemia due to apnea and excessive bronchial mucus secretion during seizures and may also reflect a relative deficiency of oxygen and substrate due to the massive neuronal metabolic activity.

Idiopathic Epilepsy

In idiopathic epilepsy the most frequent finding, probably secondary, is selective neuronal loss and dense fibrillary gliosis in the medial part of the temporal lobe, especially the hippocampal gyrus. Within the hippocampus the layer of large pyramidal cells is most often involved, especially the end-plate (H_{3-5}) and the major broad diffuse band (H_1); clearly, this distribution is precisely that associated with hypoxemia and ischemia. Similar changes may involve the entire hippocampus, or there may be remote infarction (cystic gliosis). Neuronal loss and fibrillary gliosis may extend inferiorly and laterally into the adjacent neocortex (through the parahippocampal gyrus) and anteriorly into the uncus and amygdala. Such changes probably reflect the combined effects of hypoxemia and uncal herniation, the latter due to increased cerebral blood volume (and perhaps edema) during and after seizures.

A general term for the preceding temporal lobe lesions is *mesial temporal sclerosis* (*Ammon's horn sclerosis* implies involvement of the anterior part of the hippocampal gyrus only, and is therefore merely one component of mesial temporal sclerosis). The alternative term *incisural sclerosis* has been used on the assumption that such lesions were caused by injury against the edge (incisure) of the tentorium during birth, but there is no conclusive evidence for dating the lesion so early.

Mesial temporal sclerosis is usually unilateral. Bilateral sclerosis tends to be associated with Korsakoff's psychosis (characterized by amnesia, confabulation, and apathy) rather than with epilepsy. The frequency is 35 to 65% in cases with adequate pathological confirmation. Obviously, in a considerable proportion of cases, no temporal lobe lesions are found; further, identical lesions have been described in patients without epilepsy. (Remarkably, the surgical removal of a microscopically normal temporal lobe has been reported as curing or improving the clinical condition.) It remains to be proved that mesial temporal sclerosis in idiopathic epilepsy is not a sequel of multiple epileptic seizures with their resulting hypoxemia, cerebral vasodilatation, and possibly edema. Each of the latter two is capable of causing uncal herniation.

The occurrence of *secondary* temporal lobe epilepsy with subsequent generalization of seizures, as a sequel to mesial temporal sclerosis due to birth injury, as to any other cause, is of course perfectly feasible. However, it is important to distinguish clearly between *secondary epilepsy due to temporal lobe lesions and idiopathic epilepsy causing temporal lobe sclerosis* — a fundamental difference not always clearly realized in the past.

Other lesions are recorded, but less frequently, in idiopathic epilepsy. Abnormal cells in the cortex include tangential, bipolar neurons, termed *Cajal-Retzius cells,* which are immature cells resembling neuroblasts, and irregularly scattered large neurons. The presence and significance of these cells is doubtful in many cases, but often they appear to represent cortical immaturity. Moderate or severe subpial gliosis (*Chaslin's gliosis*) may be found diffusely in the cerebral hemispheres, and areas of laminar or total cortical necrosis may be focal, lobar, or even hemispheric. In addition, subcortical structures may be involved, and there may be diffuse neuronal loss and fibrillary gliosis in the thalamus (especially the lateral nucleus), caudate and putamen, cerebellar cortex, and dentate and inferior olivary nuclei. Clearly, many of these lesions reflect hypoxemia and are secondary to repeated seizures.

Post-Traumatic Epilepsy

Depending on the site of injury, focal or extensive areas of cortical scarring, with fibrillary gliosis and neuronal loss, are found in post-traumatic epilepsy and may be particularly prominent in penetrating wounds. In addition, there may be yellow-stained, irregular gyri, especially in the orbitotemporal region (taches jaunes, état vermoulu), indicating remote cortical contusions (see Chap. 16). It has already been noted that the tendency for post-traumatic epilepsy to develop varies according to the area of cortex that is damaged. Mesial temporal sclerosis is not common in post-traumatic epilepsy, unless the temporal lobe was the site of primary injury, but the other neocortical, subcortical, and brain stem lesions that have been noted may occur if convulsions have been prolonged or severe.

Progressive Myoclonus Epilepsy (Lafora Type)

As previously noted, progressive myoclonus epilepsy of the Lafora type is an inherited disease with characteristic histopathological lesions. It probably represents a rare inborn error of glucose metabolism, with accumulations of glucose polymers (not normal glycogen) in the brain and viscera. Gross findings are confined to mild or moderate generalized atrophy. Microscopy shows moderate to extensive neuronal loss from all areas, notably the thalamus, pallidum, and dentate nuclei, together with widespread, periodic acid—Schiff stain positive, rounded, laminated, intracytoplasmic neuronal inclusions (occasionally apparently free in the neuropil) (Fig. 18-6). Similar abnormal stored material, in the form of irregular granules, occurs in the liver parenchymal cells and myocardium and possibly also in skeletal muscle.

Other cases, which clinically present as progressive myoclonus epilepsy, may prove on histological examination to show nonspecific neuronal loss and gliosis without Lafora's bodies or to be examples of amaurotic familial idiocy.

BIBLIOGRAPHY

Ayala, G. F., Matsumoto, H., and Gumnit, R. J. Excitability changes and inhibitory mechanisms in neocortical neurones during seizures. *J. Neurophysiol.* 33:73-85, 1970.

Doose, H., Gerken, H., Horstmann, T., and Völzke, E. Genetic factors in spike-wave absences. *Epilepsia* 14, 57-75, 1973.

Falconer, M. A. Genetic and related aetiological factors in temporal lobe epilepsy. *Epilepsia* 12:13-31, 1971.

Goddard, G., McIntyre, D., and Leech, C. A permanent change in brain function resulting from daily electrical stimulation. *Exp. Neurol.* 25:295-330, 1969.

Green, J. R., Halpern, L. M., Thomas, E. D., Jr., and Amick-Corkill, J. A. The effect of diphenylhydantoin on the activity of selected enzymes in chronic isolated cerebral cortex of cat. *Epilepsia* 14:223-232, 1973.

Hommes, O. R., and Obbens, E. A. M. T. The epileptogenic action of Na-folate in the rat. *J. Neurol. Sci.* 16:271-281, 1972.

Isaacson, R. L., Schwartz, H., Persoff, N., and Pinson, L. The role of the corpus callosum in the establishment of areas of secondary epileptiform activity. *Epilepsia* 12:133-146, 1971.

Matsumoto, H., Ayala, G. F., and Gumnit, R. J. Neuronal behavior and triggering mechanism in cortical epileptic focus. *J. Neurophysiol.* 32:688-703, 1969.

Nieto, D., and Escobar, A. Epilepsy. In J. Minckler (Ed.), *Pathology of the Nervous System.* New York: McGraw-Hill, 1972. Vol. 3, pp. 2627-2634.

Ottino, C. A., Meglio, M., Rossi, G. F., and Tercoro, E. An experimental study of the structures mediating bilateral synchrony of epileptic discharges of cortical origin. *Epilepsia* 12:299-311, 1971.

Petsche, H., and Brazier, M. A. B. (Eds.). *Synchronization of EEG Activity in Epilepsies.* New York: Springer, 1972.

Pollen, D. A., and Trachtenberg, M. C. Neuroglia: Gliosis and epilepsy. *Science* 167:1252-1253, 1970.

Scholz, W. Cerebral Changes Due to Convulsive Disorders. In J. Minckler (Ed.), *Pathology of the Nervous System.* New York: McGraw-Hill, 1972. Vol. 3, pp. 2635-2654.

Sutherland, J. M., and Tait, H. The epilepsies: Modern treatment and diagnosis. Edinburgh: Livingstone, 1969.

Taylor, D. C., and Ounsted, C. Biological mechanisms influencing the outcome of seizures in response to fever. *Epilepsia* 12:133-146, 1971.

Wilder, B. J., King, R. L., and Schmidt, R. P. Cortical and subcortical secondary epileptogenesis. *Neurology* 19:643-652, 1969.

Williams, D. The thalamus and epilepsy. *Brain* 88: 539-556, 1965.

Woodbury, D. M., and Kemp, J. W. Pharmacology and mechanism of action of diphenylhydantoin. *Psychiatr. Neurol. Neurochir.* 74:91-115, 1971.

Zivin, L., and Marsan, C. A. Incidence and prognostic significance of "epileptiform activity" in the EEG of non-epileptic subjects. *Brain* 91:751-778, 1968.

Malformations and Hydrocephalus

19

An abnormality of shape or of size is difficult to define precisely. Thus, morphological abnormalities may be visible at the naked-eye, light-microscopic, or only at the electron-microscopic level. They may be clearly defined either quantitatively (e.g., supernumerary digits) or functionally (e.g., most congenital heart defects), or they may merge with the physiological range of variation (e.g., genu valgum, pes cavus, or low-set ears). Minor anomalies of no functional significance (such as abnormal dermatoglyphics) are particularly noted in association with chromosomal abnormalities and are missed unless specifically sought. However indefinable, a malformation is nonetheless generally understood as an abnormality of form present from birth, outside the range of biological variation, and often associated with functional inadequacy. Because of the complicated organogenesis of the heart and the CNS, and the importance of their normal function, malformations of these two organs are the most frequently of concern. Many common CNS malformations are isolated, with other parts of the body normal, but they may form part of a multisystem syndrome, often due to chromosomal anomalies.

Perhaps in contradistinction to other organs, a mere diminution in size, not associated with other striking abnormalities, is often referred to as a malformation in the CNS. Reduction in weight by 20 to 30% in most other organs would hardly be regarded as noteworthy, but there are reasonable justifications for making an exception for the brain:

1. A brain weight below normal (micrencephaly) is usually associated with severe dysfunction, including mental retardation, motor disorders, and epilepsy.
2. The same agents that are known to produce CNS malformations of a more striking character have frequently been implicated in the etiology of micrencephaly.
3. There is a relatively constant histological abnormality in these small brains, with failure of neuronal processes, especially dendrites, to develop adequately.
4. In some cases of micrencephaly, and possibly in all if sufficiently detailed examination were carried out, there are abnormalities of gyral pattern that would rank as true malformations. To detect them is time-consuming, requires an intimate knowledge of the normal convolutions at varying ages, and probably presupposes a greater familiarity with the normal range of variation, especially of secondary and tertiary sulci, than is presently available.

The development of a malformation is restricted to the period during which an organ reaches its final form. For most, this period of organogenesis is complete by about the thirteenth week of gestation. Most agents producing malformations (teratogens) therefore operate during the first trimester. However, the human CNS remains incomplete at 13 weeks, its major cellular migrations occurring up to the sixth or seventh month. The final definition of gyral pattern is completed in postnatal life. Teratogenic agents may therefore affect the CNS over a much longer period of time than they affect other organ systems, although the later they act, the less dramatic the malformation produced. Thus, while malformations characterized by failure of the neural tube to close or failure of the hemispheres to separate must originate within the first 8 to 10 weeks, micrencephaly may be due to agents operating as late as the sixth to seventh month.

Known teratogenic agents account for few CNS malformations, most being of unknown etiology. A list of agents producing CNS malformations in laboratory animals is almost endless but must be viewed with skepticism as for any other organ, since a given agent varies widely in its effect from species to species. As in general in teratology, the CNS effects of a teratogenic agent are probably more dependent on the time it acts than on its nature. Intrauterine infections, irradiation, and hypoxia may produce dramatic CNS malformations during the early weeks of gestation or may be responsible for micrencephaly if acting in later months. In terms of etiological agents known or suspected, there is great overlap between this and the succeeding chapter (on mental retardation). Many cases of mental retardation are associated with micrencephaly, and agents causing micrencephaly are also productive of major malformations.

Selected Aspects of Neuroembryology

Adequate studies on early human embryonic stages are few, and available descriptions are complicated by the fact that some authors date by days following conception, others by the length of the fetus, and still others by the number of somites. In round figures, a 1.5-mm fetus is 8 days old and has two somites; a 3-mm fetus is 25 days old and has 20 somites; and a 4.5-mm fetus is 30 days old and has 31 somites. Beyond this stage, it is usual to refer to periods of gestation: a 2-month fetus is 25 to 30 mm and a 3-month fetus about 80 mm in length. In the sequence of major developmental stages of the human CNS that follows, the gestation periods are merely approximate, since there is often no consensus in the literature.

Day 18. The neural plate is formed in the dorsal midline.

Day 21. Fusion of the neural folds starts in the cervical region and extends caudally.

Day 25. The anterior neuropore is closed, and the neural crests and sensory placodes are formed.

Day 26. The posterior neuropore is closed (more caudal regions of the spinal cord are formed by excavation in the midline mesenchyme and do not pass through an open-plate stage).

Day 28. Brain vesicles are clearly delineated, and the permanent 90-degree flexion of the prosencephalon on the mesencephalon is present. The peripheral nervous system shows clear segmentation, with formation of autonomic and dorsal root ganglia. The internal carotid arteries are present, with anterior and posterior branches beginning to differentiate from the perineural plexus (the anterior branch will form the anterior cerebral, middle cerebral, and anterior choroidal vessels at a later stage, and the posterior branch will form the posterior communicating and posterior cerebral arteries and their branches).

Day 35. Telencephalic vesicles and optic rudiments are present. Anterior nerve roots appear in the brain stem and cord. The basilar artery differentiates ventral to the brain stem and joins the posterior cerebral vessels.

Day 42. The rudiments of all cell masses for future diencephalic, telencephalic, and axial structures in the brain and spinal cord can be discerned. The infundibulum comes into contact with Rathke's pouch.

Day 49. Telencephalic vesicles are prominent, and the anterior commissure is present in the lamina terminalis. The pineal recess develops. Thickening of the lips of the upper fourth ventricle indicates the beginning of cerebellar formation. The vertebral arteries join the basilar artery. Vascularization of the brain starts, and choroid plexuses begin to be formed in the ventricles.

Day 56. The optic chiasm, olfactory bulbs, and all cranial nerves are present and well formed. Cerebellar thickenings begin to fuse in the midline to form the vermis. A definitive anterior communicating artery completes the circle of Willis. True CSF secretion starts at this stage (fluid previously in the ventricular system arose from the extracellular space of the CNS and surrounding mesenchyme).

Day 70. The telencephalic vesicles completely hide the diencephalon. The sylvian fissure is just visible, and migrating neurons begin to reach the cortical surface. The vertebral arches of the spinal column are closed.

Day 84. The striate body (future caudate and putamen) becomes fused to the lateral aspect of the thalamus. Growth of the hemispheres produces a C-shaped caudate nucleus, and the amygdala is formed. The aqueduct has assumed its adult form, and the foramina of the fourth ventricle are open. (It has been supposed that this is a necessary preliminary to the formation of a subarachnoid space, which is allegedly dissected out by CSF. However, current evidence suggests the independent formation of a subarachnoid space, even in the absence of CSF.)

Days 91 to 98. The medial aspects of the hemispheres fuse dorsal and posterior to the lamina terminalis, producing a continuity of tissue within which the corpus callosum and hippocampal commissure start to develop. The cerebellar vermis is completely formed, and the flocculonodular node becomes apparent. The cord shows cervical and lumbosacral enlargements, and the central canal is of adult configuration.

Three to Five Months. The intersegmental and long tracts of the cord and brain stem develop, and myelination begins in nerve roots – first in the ventral nerve roots. At about 5 months, the basal ganglia have assumed adult configuration, the central, parieto-occipital, and calcarine fissures are present, and the spinal column has begun to outgrow the spinal cord.

Six Months. The cortex is well stratified. The median longitudinal fasciculus is myelinated. During this period (about 5 to 7 months) myelination of many of the long tracts in the cord starts in the cervical region and spreads caudally. The corticospinal axons appear, but are not myelinated at this time.

Seven Months. The corpus callosum is now complete and has displaced the hippocampal commissure posteriorly. All primary sulci are present, and the septal region has been split by anterior growth of the corpus callosum into the septum pellucidum lying above and the olfactory and parolfactory gyri lying below.

Eight Months to Term. Myelination occurs in the long tracts of the brain stem (vestibulospinal, rubrospinal, and reticulospinal) and in the basal ganglia, thalamus, and white matter of the cerebellum.

Term to Two Years. During this period the morphological growth of the brain is completed, with enlargement of the frontal and temporal lobes, growth of the opercula over the insula, and completion of the secondary and tertiary sulci. Considerable myelination goes on during this period, first involving incoming sensory projection tracts, then motor projection tracts, and finally the association and commissural fibers. (It may be noted as a general rule that myelination usually starts near the cell body and spreads distally, and also that it tends to occur in phylogenetic sequence.)

Teratogenic Agents

Since malformations of the CNS are common in man, a tremendous amount of experimental work has been done to try and elucidate their causes. Because of marked species variability, particularly in responses to chemical teratogens, the applicability of some of this work to man is not clear, but it certainly offers stern warnings. Among drugs that produce widespread malformations in laboratory animals, often involving the CNS, are those used in the chemotherapy of neoplasms and infections, psychotropic drugs, azo dyes, aminobenzine derivatives, substances interfering with metabolism, such as galactose, 2-deoxyglucose, and imipramine, and many other agents, including such common drugs as salicylates. Although there is little evidence that drugs produce CNS malformations in man, it would seem desirable that the administration of drugs to women during pregnancy be curtailed (insofar as possible) as a precautionary measure. The first trimester is not the only vulnerable period, because the development of the CNS continues throughout pregnancy.

Nutritional Deficiencies

Vitamin deficiencies and deficiencies in trace metals such as copper and zinc may cause CNS malformations in animals. Excessive vitamin A may lead to anencephaly. Production of some specific dietary deficiencies requires purified and often synthetic diets, and it is unlikely that they occur even in the most adverse human dietary situations. Severe, generalized malnutrition has been shown to reduce brain weight and retard development of neurons, but does not appear to be associated with malformations, presumably because the total metabolic needs of the fetus in the organogenetic stage are small, and it is capable of satisfying these needs at the expense of the mother. In man, there is evidence, to be discussed subsequently, that dietary restrictions retard CNS development, and there is also an association between CNS malformations and low socioeconomic status. Since the latter involves many adverse factors other than dietary deficiency, the precise nature of this correlation is unknown.

Oxygen Deficiency

Oxygen deficiency in animals has produced anencephaly, cyclopia, and other malformations, but in man the only clear association appears to be a small number of cases in which maternal carbon monoxide poisoning resulted in offspring with necrosis of the basal ganglia and micropolygyria. The human fetus is less sensitive than postnatal man to oxygen deficiency (see Chap. 17), being equipped with fetal hemoglobin, isoenzymes of lactic dehydrogenase adapted to convert pyruvate to lactate, and adequate placental transfer of lactate to the mother.

Infections

A small but significant proportion of human CNS malformations (using that term in its broadest sense) are associated with placental and fetal infections. Among the defects produced by rubella virus are hydrocephalus, micrencephaly, meningomyelocele, and absent corpus callosum. *Toxoplasma* and cytomegalovirus apparently act somewhat later and may produce micrencephaly, hydrocephalus, and necrosis with calcification. Associations of CNS malformations with such agents as mumps virus, influenza virus, infectious hepatitis virus, coxsackie virus B, and others are less positive, and syphilis, although causing extensive inflammatory changes, is not apparently teratogenic.

Hormonal and Immunological Changes

In experimental animals, hormonal changes are frequently teratogenic. In man, the only such association appears to be with maternal diabetes or prediabetes, which shows a statistically significant correlation with micrencephaly, hydrocephalus, and mental retardation. A possible role for antibodies directed against fetal CNS has been substantiated in experimental animals, but in man a projected association between increased maternal antihuman lymphocyte antibody and fetal mental retardation remains to be established.

Chromosomal Abnormalities

Spontaneous abnormalities of karyotype in man are associated with CNS malformations, usually of somewhat minor nature, but often accompanied by mental retardation. Mongolism, or Down's syndrome, (trisomy 21) is the best known, but changes are also seen in other types of autosomal trisomy. Trisomy 13–15 may be associated with a severe malformation (holoprosencephaly). Less dramatic chromosomal changes such as translocation or deletion may also be associated with retardation and often with micrencephaly and other changes. Mutations can be induced by varying methods, including administration of purines and pyrimidines, nitrogen mustard, and colchicine, and by irradiation. Irradiation is firmly established as a teratogen in man.

Epidemiological Observations

Certain factors are clinically recognized as increasing the risk of fetal malformation, although the mechanism of such associations is unknown. A firstborn child has a slightly higher risk of anencephaly and spina bifida, and increasing maternal age increases the likelihood of Down's syndrome. It is probable, but less well documented, that increasing paternal age also raises the incidence of Down's syndrome, suggesting that in both parents, advancing age is associated with an increasing risk of nondisjunction. Many studies have indicated a distinct effect of the season of birth on the incidence of both anencephaly and spina bifida, although the results are sometimes conflicting. Associations have been suggested (with varying degrees of objectivity) between the incidence of malformations and maternal ill-health, trauma, emotional stress, race, and geographical situation, but such associations have not been established.

General Observations

The preceding list of teratogenic factors is not complete, either in respect to agents that have been proved teratogenic in experimental situations or in respect to theories as to what might be teratogenic in the clinical setting. The factors mentioned suffice to indicate the extremely wide range of potentially teratogenic agents in the environment, and the advisability of protecting the mother throughout pregnancy from at least the more tangible of these agents, such as drugs, irradiation, and dietary deficiency. Even so, it is unlikely that such protection will have more than a marginal effect on the incidence of CNS malformations or mental retardation, since a definite etiological agent can be identified only for a very small group. There is no clear distinction between agents producing malformations and those producing mental retardation; the time of action is probably the significant factor.

An agent operating early in pregnancy may cause failure of normal brain development, but if such changes are sufficiently localized, they need not be associated with mental retardation. Absence of the corpus callosum, Chiari type I malformation, and many of the lower grades of spina bifida are compatible with effectively normal intellectual development. The same agent acting later is likely to interfere with active cells proliferating and migrating to form (largely) the cerebral cortex, with the possible consequences of decreased brain weight, abnormal gyri and cortical architecture, and inadequate development of dendrites – all likely to be associated with mental retardation.

TYPES OF MALFORMATIONS

In theory, malformations result from the interplay of three factors (genetic background, teratogenic agent, and the agent's time of action). In fact, the agent for the great majority of human malformations is unknown, as has been emphasized. Attempts to incriminate background levels of radiation so far have been unconvincing.

The incidence of major CNS malformations is approximately 1% of live births, and by far the most common are anencephaly, which is not compatible with prolonged survival, and spina bifida, which may vary from an incidental radiological finding with normal function to part of a more generalized malformation associated with hydrocephalus and infection. Both conditions are more frequent with advancing maternal age and likely to occur in either the first birth, a late birth, or the last births of large sibships.

Classification of CNS malformations is incomplete, since not only the etiology, but often also the pathogenesis is unknown. The two commonest conditions (noted above) involve varying nonclosure of the neural tube (dysraphia), but there is no consensus as to whether this represents a primary failure of closure, or rupture of a neural tube that had already closed. Spina bifida may be associated with another common malformation, the Arnold-Chiari deformity, but the latter may also occur in isolation. It cannot reasonably be regarded as a dysraphic state and is difficult to fit into any classification.

Another group of disorders, rare but striking, involve failure of normal development of the telencephalic vesicles, commonly associated with absence of the olfactory tracts and bulbs and abnormal facial development. This group is referred to as *arhinencephaly* (from the absence of olfactory tracts and bulbs) or *holoprosencephaly* (because of the abnormal prosencephalic development). Some cases of holoprosencephaly are associated with absent corpus callosum, but the latter can also occur as an isolated defect that again defies neat classification.

Teratogenic agents acting after the first trimester are likely to affect the cerebral and cerebellar cortex, inducing, in sequence, defects in cell proliferation, migration, and maturation and leading to micrencephaly, together with agenesis, hypoplasia, polymicrogyria, or other defects of the cerebellum. Mental retardation is almost invariably present.

Since there is, in effect, no classification, the most important malformations will simply be considered seriatim.

The complicated pathway followed by the CSF (see Chap. 4) from the choroid plexuses to the subarachnoid space and venous sinuses implies that many CNS malformations might be associated with obstruction and therefore with accumulation of CSF under pressure (hydrocephalus). Since the clinical features of hydrocephalus, and many aspects of its pathogenesis and diagnosis, are the same irrespective of the site of block, and also since hydrocephalus may develop as a result of infections, trauma, subarachnoid hemorrhage, or other unidentified factors, it is dealt with in a later section in this chapter and merely mentioned in passing here.

Anencephaly

Anencephaly is more common in female than male fetuses and is often associated with hydramnios and prematurity. In all cases there is loss of diencephalic and telencephalic structures and no recognizable brain tissue above the tentorium. Usually, the cerebellum and brain stem are also absent and the fetuses are stillborn; but if these structures are present, the anencephalic infant may survive for a few hours or days.

The face is normal in anencephaly, but the eyes appear to protrude because of the absent cranial vault. The cranial floor is present and relatively normal, but the frontal, squamous temporal, parietal, and squamous occipital bones, if present at all, are only rudimentary. The base of the skull is covered by vascular, irregular tissue that merges at the edge into normal skin. This covering consists largely of vascular meningeal tissue, although islands of glial cells, occasional neurons, and fragments of choroid plexus may be found. The trigeminal ganglia can usually be located, and a little adenohypophyseal tissue is usually present, though often displaced to the roof of the pharynx or within the sphenoid bone. The lack of pituitary development is presumably due to the absence of hypophyseal stimulating hormones and is associated with unusually small adrenals that lack a fetal zone. Major vessels are hypoplastic and do not penetrate the vascular mass, except that if the cerebellum and brain stem are present, the vertebral and basilar arteries are well formed.

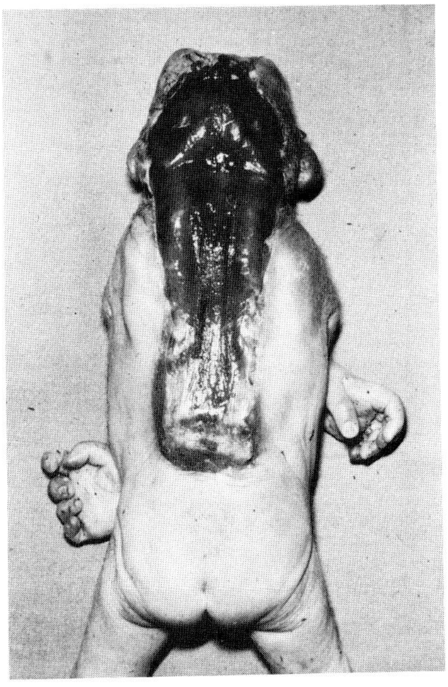

Fig. 19-1. Dorsal view of stillborn anencephalic fetus, showing the absence of skin and exposed vascular tissue on the dorsal and upper head (anencephaly) and a similar middorsal defect of the trunk (rachischisis). The protuberant orbits (above) and ears (laterally) are clearly visible in this rear view.

Some cases of anencephaly are associated with rachischisis, in which the cord is unrecognizable, the neural arches unclosed, and a thin, narrow mid-dorsal strip of vascular tissue extends from the cervical to lumbar region, resembling that on the surface of the skull (Fig. 19-1). Sympathetic and dorsal root ganglia are invariably present, and examination often reveals the proximal fibers of the dorsal root ganglion cells in the midline vascular tissue. Careful dissection often shows the remains of anterior roots, with marked schwannosis.

Etiology and Pathogenesis

The etiology and pathogenesis of anencephaly are unknown. There appear to be three major conflicting explanations for its occurrence.

According to one view, the neural tube, either in whole or in part, simply never closed, accounting for the continuity between the vascular areas and the surrounding normal skin. It is difficult in these circumstances to visualize the normal "hiving off" of the neural crest and the formation of choroid plexus tissue.

According to another theory, the tube closes, but develops secondary defects or clefts, which are not necessarily in the midline. The edges of these clefts are characterized by neurectodermal proliferation, and healing is prevented by the interposition of mesenchymal or amniotic tissues. Such clefts have been described in human embryos at the 11- to 12-somite stage, and since this theory allows for closure and possible separation of the neural tube from overlying ectoderm, it seems more in keeping with the meningeal proliferation, choroid plexus formation, and normal peripheral nervous system that are usually present in these cases.

A third explanation is that anencephaly might result from rupture of a normally closed, normally constituted neural tube because of CSF secretion and increased pressure. On such a basis it is difficult to see how the entire neuraxis could be split, since one short rupture would relieve the internal pressure. In any event, it seems unlikely that CSF secretion begins before the eighth week. By this time, neural arches in the cervical and upper thoracic region are well formed in cartilage (and they are complete in all regions by the tenth week). Since vascularization of the CNS does not begin until the seventh week, luminal fluid present prior to this time has diffused from the mesenchymal extracellular space (the normal mechanism for nourishing the CNS at this stage).

On the whole, the possibility that secondary defects of greater or lesser degree may develop in a normally closed neural tube, presumably as a result of unexplained local cell necrosis, fits the pathological observations better than the other suggestions. However, the problem cannot be regarded as solved.

Spina Bifida

In spina bifida the cranium and its contents are usually normally formed, but defects are present in the spinal cord and its coverings, most commonly in

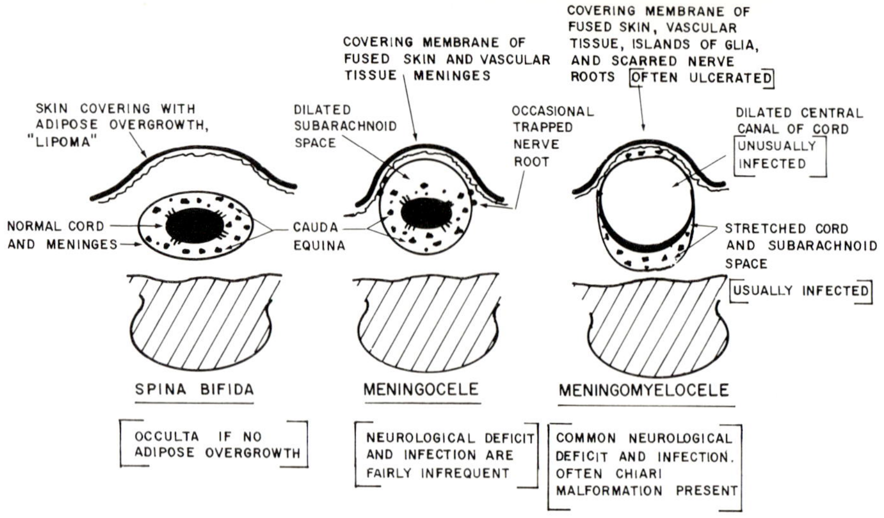

Fig. 19-2. The three major types of posterior spina bifida.

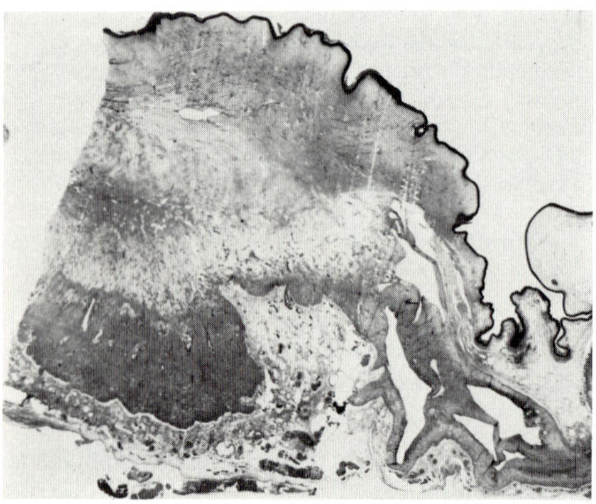

Fig. 19-3. Part of the covering membrane of a meningomyelocele, covered in intact epidermis and subcutaneous tissue (top). A mass of neurectodermal tissue containing neurons and astrocytes (bottom left), and meningeal tissue with large vascular spaces (bottom right) are both present. (H & E, X8.)

the lumbosacral region (Fig. 19-2). Like anencephaly, with which it is occasionally associated, the lesion is somewhat more common in females, probably shows seasonal variation in incidence, and is more common in families low on the socioeconomic scale. The most severe and most unusual type of spina bifida is a segmental rachischisis (myeloschisis) similar to that previously described, but not associated with anencephaly. More commonly, spina bifida is associated with at least an initial skin covering, even though it may be secondarily ulcerated and deficient.

Meningomyelocele

In meningomyelocele, the central canal of the cord is distended, and the wall of the sac includes distorted cord tissue, nerve roots, meninges, subcutaneous tissue, and skin (Figs. 19-2, 19-3), usually with considerable inflammation. Central nervous system infection is common, even in the absence of overt rupture. Since the lumbosacral enlargement is usually involved, these patients have neurological deficits involving sphincters and lower limbs, and their prognosis is poor. It is made even worse by frequent association with Arnold-Chiari deformity (see Arnold-Chiari and Dandy-Walker Malformations, below).

Meningocele

In meningocele, the spinal cord is intact, but there is dilatation of the subarachnoid space associated with deficiency of (usually) lumbosacral vertebral arches. Nerve roots may be involved in the wall of the sac, but the neurological deficit is much less than in meningomyelocele; there may be no functional abnormality. Risk of infection is less severe, and these patients often can be successfully treated by surgery.

Spina Bifida Occulta

In spina bifida occulta, both cord and meninges are normal, the only defect being failure of neural arch closure in one or more lumbosacral vertebrae. Such a

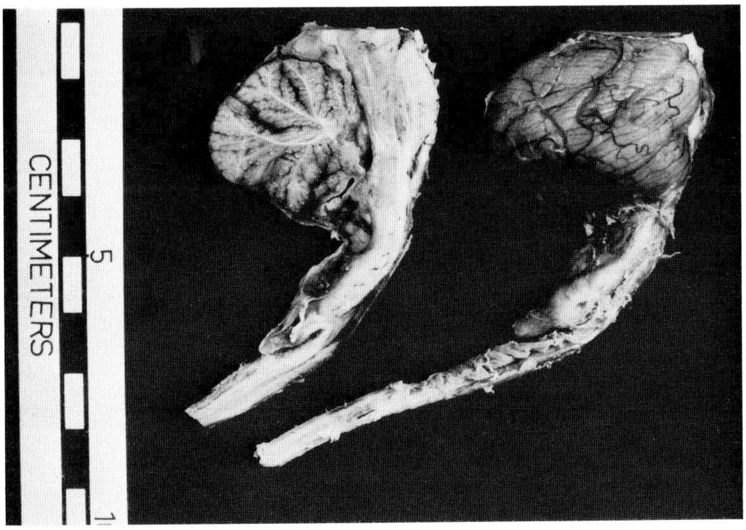

Fig. 19-4. Arnold-Chiari type II deformity. (Left) Sagittal section. (Right) Lateral view. Note the small cerebellum, pons, and medulla, tongues of malformed cerebellar tissue below the notch produced by the foramen magnum, and the overlap of caudally displaced medulla and spinal cord.

defect may be an incidental discovery on x-ray examination, or it may be marked by an overlying localized or diffuse lipoma. Occasionally, spina bifida occulta is associated with splitting of the cord (diastematomyelia), each half having one dorsal and one ventral horn and an individual pial investment, but sharing a common arachnoid and dura; there may be a median bony spur or fibrous band.

Anterior Spina Bifida

The term *spina bifida,* used without qualification, means posterior spina bifida (Fig. 19-2), a failure of closure of neural arches. More rarely, anterior spina bifida occurs, in which one or more vertebral bodies are divided by a median fibrous septum, representing persistent adhesions between the neural tube and fetal gut through the notochord, sometimes associated with a neurenteric cyst (that is lined by gastric or intestinal mucosa) in the spinal canal or with other anomalies (split notochord syndrome).

Etiology and Pathogenesis

Neither the etiology nor pathogenesis of spina bifida is known, although there is said to be a seasonal incidence. Pathogenesis of meningomyelocele could be the same as for anencephaly, although it is clear from the frequency of myelocele and spina bifida occulta that an independent meningeal and mesenchymal defect can also exist.

Arnold-Chiari and Dandy-Walker Malformations

Not necessarily related in etiology or pathogenesis, both the Arnold-Chiari deformity and the Dandy-Walker syndrome involve malformation of the cerebellum as a major feature, with either a decrease (Arnold-Chiari) or an increase (Dandy-Walker) in the size of the posterior fossa. Both are frequently associated with severe hydrocephalus.

Arnold-Chiari Deformity

The Arnold-Chiari deformity is commonly graded from I to III, with increasing severity. Type II is the most common (Fig. 19-4).

Type I. The medulla is partially or almost completely displaced downward into the spinal canal, and elongated processes from the inferior margin of the cerebellum pass down on its dorsal aspect as far as the atlas or axis. These processes show sclerosis or softening, with polygyria. Localized loss of Purkinje's and internal granular cells is frequently observed, but the remainder of the cerebellum is normal. The condition may be asymptomatic, or it may be associated with unilateral or bilateral pareses of the medullary cranial nerves or (rarely) may cause mild hydrocephalus.

Type II. The posterior fossa is markedly reduced in size, the tentorium is flat instead of vaulted upward, and the medullary displacement into the spinal canal includes the foramina of Magendie and of Luschka. Since the cervical cord is less displaced than the medulla, there is an S-shaped bend where the lower medulla overlaps the cord. Upper cervical nerve roots have to pass upward instead of horizontally to reach their intervertebral foramina, and the lower cranial nerves are even more elongated than in type I. The cerebellum, pons, and medulla are reduced in size, the pons frequently showing a midventral depression housing the basilar artery. The cerebellar processes are bound by fibrous adhesions to the medulla, and the cisterna magna is absent.

Changes may also be seen at a higher CNS level,

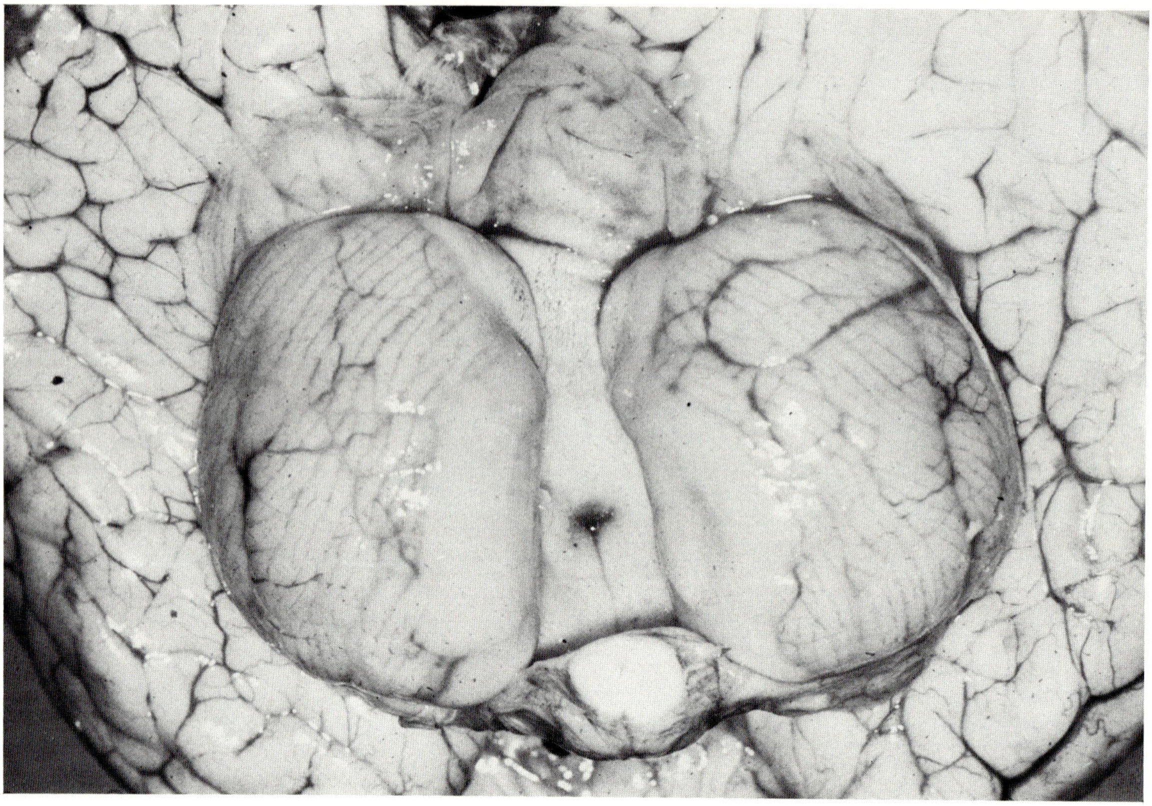

Fig. 19-5. Dandy-Walker syndrome viewed from the caudal aspect. The fourth ventricle is large and distorted, and the lower end of the aqueduct is clearly seen. There is no inferior or posterior vermis, and the membrane that closed the large fourth vermis has been reflected upward (top of photograph).

including beaking of the collicular plate, forking of the aqueduct, squeezing together of the thalami with a large massa intermedia, and ectopic gray matter in the walls of the lateral ventricles. Because of the displacement of the fourth ventricle into the spinal canal and the extensive meningeal fibrosis, there is usually severe hydrocephalus, and there may be dilatation of the central canal of the cord (hydromyelia) and frequently meningomyelocele. Radiologically, type II malformation is associated with enlargement of the foramen magnum, a flattened posterior fossa floor, and grooving of the posteromedial petrous temporal bone by the anterior edge of the cerebellum.

Type III. The posterior fossa is even smaller than in type II, and there is a dorsal midline defect in the occipital bone or upper cervical vertebrae, with a projecting subcutaneous encephalocele containing the cerebellum and sometimes the occipital poles.

Pathogenesis. The pathogenesis of the Arnold-Chiari deformity is obscure. Originally thought due to tethering of the lower end of the cord with traction on the neuraxis, this theory became untenable because the displacement of the medulla is considerably more than that of the cord, as previously noted. It has been suggested that there is disproportion between the growth of the brain and of the skull vault, leading to caudal displacement of the entire brain. This might explain the changes in the thalami and midbrain, as well as the hypoplasia of the posterior fossa and its contents. The frequent association of hydromyelia and meningomyelocele suggests that additional anomalies in the roof of the fourth ventricle, sufficient to prevent the outward permeation or flow of CSF, are present at 8 to 10 weeks, fluid being forced down the central canal of the cord and causing dilatation where the vertebral arches close last in development (lumbosacral region).

Dandy-Walker Syndrome

The Dandy-Walker syndrome is characterized by a large posterior fossa and upward displacement of the lateral sinuses, which can frequently be seen on transillumination of the head. The cerebellar hemispheres and superior vermis are normally developed (Fig. 19-5), but the posteroinferior vermis is replaced by a thin membrane attached to the lower margin of the fourth ventricle and the posterior margins of the hemispheres, composed of ependyma, fibrillary glia, and pia-arachnoid. The foramen of Magendie is therefore absent, and the severity of hydrocephalus appears to depend on the degree of patency of the foramina of

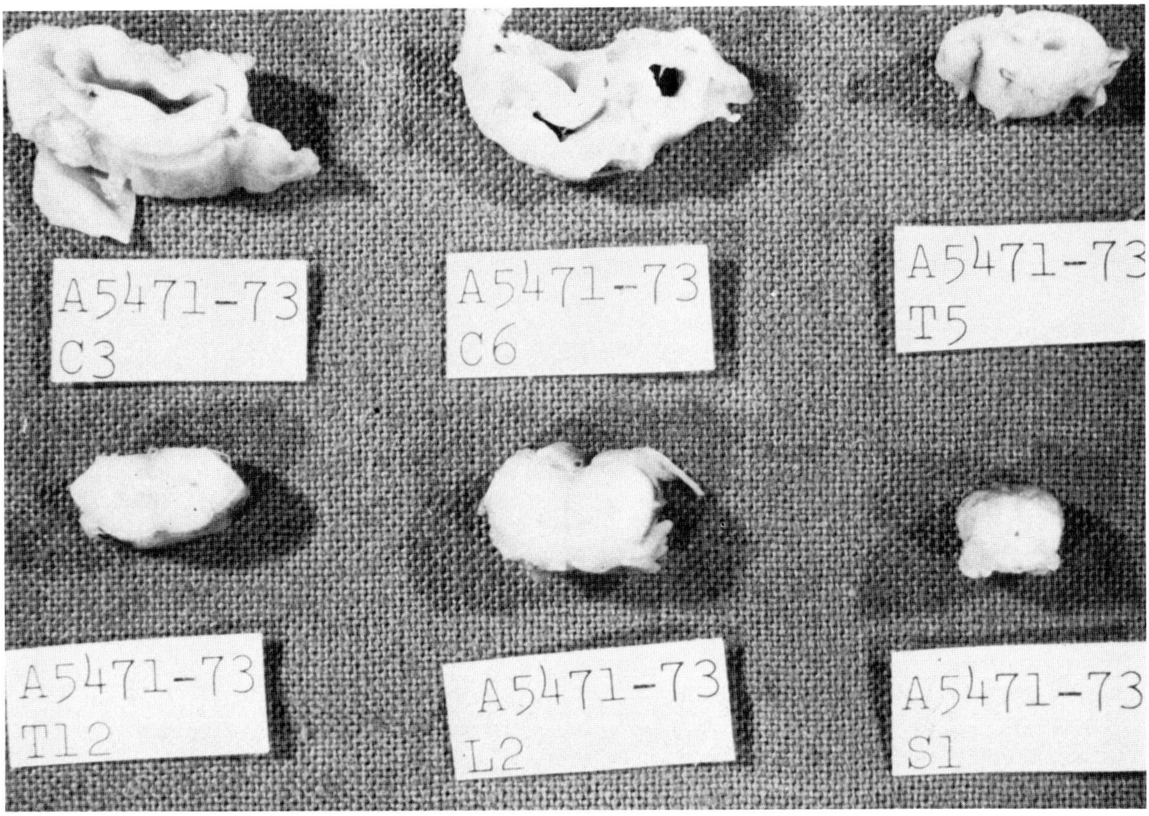

Fig. 19-6. Syringomyelia involving the cervical and upper thoracic cord. The cavity was large (having collapsed in fixation), and the H-shaped section is not seen. The lower cord is intact.

Luschka. Occasional associations are absence of the corpus callosum, occipital encephalocele, and somatic malformations that may involve cervical vertebrae (Klippel-Feil syndrome).

These patients may show hydrocephalus at birth or during infancy. It is usually less severe, and the ultimate prognosis is better, than in the Arnold-Chiari deformity. A few cases do not present until later childhood, with such features of a posterior fossa mass as headache, vomiting, cranial nerve palsies, nystagmus, ataxia, and spasticity. These symptoms may first be noticed after head injury and may be episodic in nature.

Excision of the membrane is not always effective in relieving hydrocephalus, and a shunting procedure is then required. The reason for this is unknown. Almost as difficult to explain are patients in whom hydrocephalus does not develop in spite of the presence of a membrane and apparent stenosis of the foramina of Luschka. Presumably, CSF is lost by permeation through the membrane and to some degree by ventricular absorption (see p. 363).

Syringomyelia and Syringobulbia

Syringomyelia is a tubular dilatation of the cord over several segments that is not due to simple distention of the central canal (hydromyelia). It may be associated with syringobulbia, in which there are slitlike cavities in the medulla or, rarely, in the pons and midbrain. The clinical onset is usually in young adults (20 to 30 years of age), and the disease is slowly progressive, rarely causing death unless the brain stem is involved.

Syringomyelia

In syringomyelia the cord is swollen, with normal meninges, and contains a cavity filled with clear yellow fluid, extending from about the second cervical segment to the midthoracic region (Fig. 19-6). Characteristically, the cavity involves the dorsal parts of the anterior and the entire posterior horns and crosses the midline dorsal to the central canal, forming an H-shaped cross section. The dorsal horn extensions may reach the cord surface. In severe cases there is little residual gray matter except the tips of the anterior horns, and the white matter is compressed to a narrow peripheral band. Occasional midline dorsal and ventral extensions occur through the sites of bilateral fusion of alar and basal plates.

In subacute cavities the wall shows degenerating glial and neural elements with loss of myelin and a spongy appearance, apparently due to transudation of fluid. Chronically, there is gliomesenchymal fibrosis

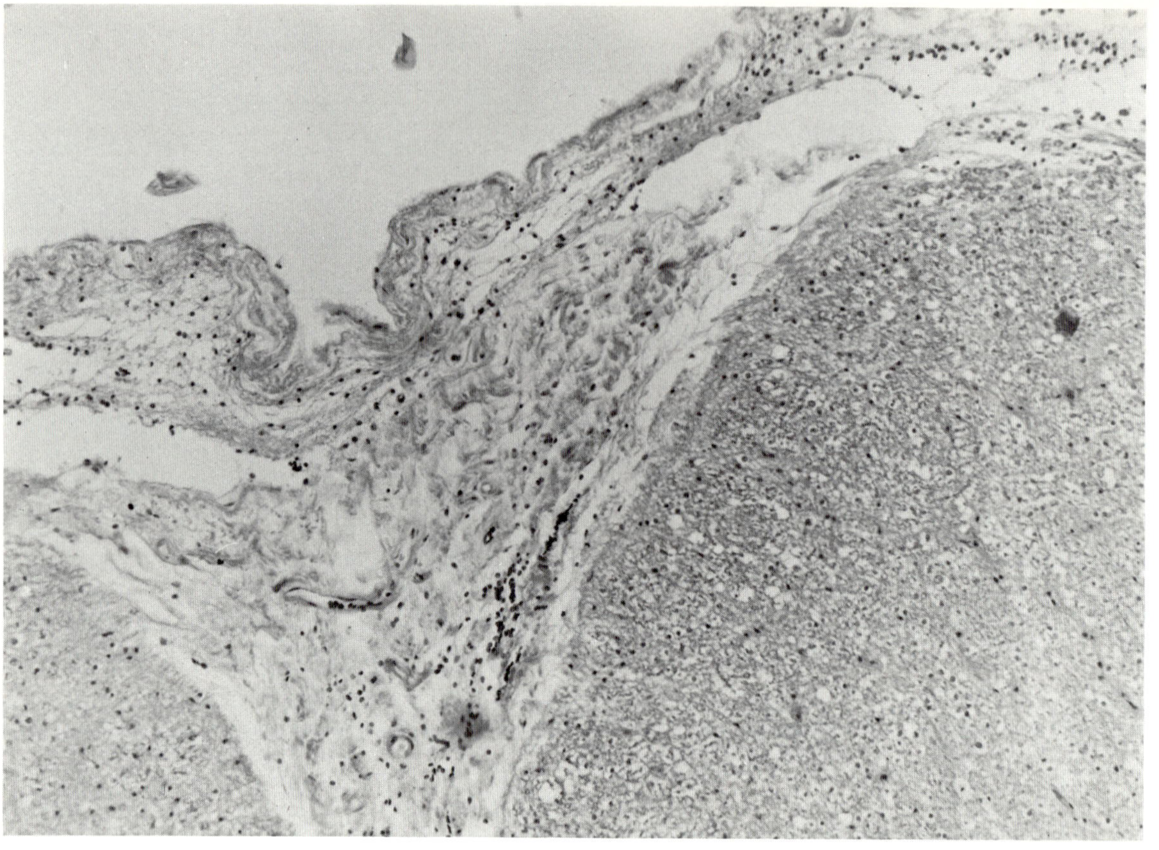

Fig. 19-7. Wall (lining) of syringomyelic cavity, showing gliomesenchymal membrane and almost-normal surrounding white matter (H & E, X115 before 5% reduction).

(Fig. 19-7), often with vessels crossing the cavity and often with incorporation of the central canal and a few areas of ependymal lining. Similar changes may follow the absorption of blood from traumatic hematomyelia or in the presence of an astrocytoma, but primary syringomyelia is not neoplastic.

Post-traumatic syringomyelia usually occurs in the thoracic or lumbar regions, with some cases probably due to absorption of a blood clot and others of unknown origin. Lacerations of the cord, with CSF infiltration during coughing, straining, or other increases of central venous pressure have been postulated and might be particularly damaging if post-traumatic arachnoid adhesions prevented upward transmission of the increased pressure.

The secondary changes induced by syringomyelia include interruption of decussating pain and temperature fibers in the anterior gray commissure and sometimes also damage to the spinocerebellar fibers, either by destruction of the cells of origin or at decussation. Less frequently, there is interference with the pyramidal tracts or posterior columns, apparently by compression.

Syringobulbia

Syringobulbia usually involves the medulla and has several forms. A slit passing toward the fifth spinal nucleus between hypoglossal and dorsal vagal nuclei (and not always communicating with the fourth ventricle) may damage the fasciculus solitarius and fibers running from the ambiguous nucleus to the vagus and from the gracilis and cuneate nuclei to the medial lemniscus. A midline slit in the raphe, often lined by ependyma, interrupts vestibular fibers decussating to the medial longitudinal fasciculus and may produce nystagmus. A cleft between the pyramids and inferior olives may interrupt rootlets of the twelfth nerve (usually unilaterally) or may damage the pyramidal fibers.

Etiology and Pathogenesis

Neither the etiology nor the pathogenesis of idiopathic syringomyelia is understood. The condition is rarely familial. It may occasionally be associated with basilar impression (platybasia) and spina bifida and is thought to be developmental – because of the type of changes occasionally seen in the brain stem rather than because of those observed in the cord. It might represent an instability of the lines of fusion between

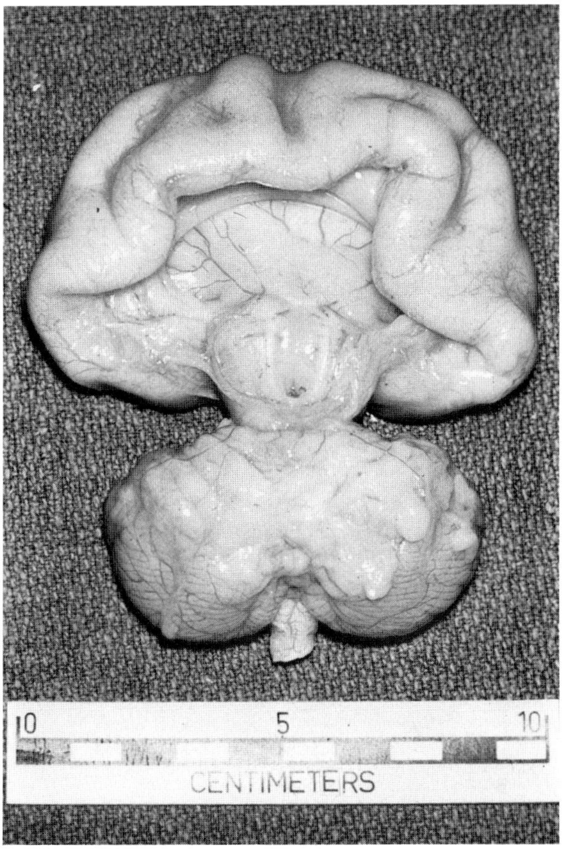

Fig. 19-8. Dorsal view of brain in holoprosencephaly, showing relatively normal cerebellum and brain stem; the upper end of the aqueduct is clearly visible. Diencephalic gray masses are small, and the cortical mantle is present only as an undivided mass that occupied the floor of the anterior and part of the middle fossae. The patient had a single nostril and other facial malformations, but two eyes were present.

the two alar and the two basal plates, manifesting itself earliest in the cervical region because this is the region of greatest mobility. This would not account for the relative infrequency of dorsal and ventral midline extensions. However the process begins, it is thought to progress by the transudation of fluid from spinal cord vessels, associated with episodic increased central venous pressure such as occurs with coughing or straining.

Holoprosencephaly

The term *holoprosencephaly* covers a wide spectrum of abnormalities, of which the most constant feature is absence of the olfactory tracts and bulbs — whence the alternative name of arhinencephaly. It is obviously due to teratogenic agents acting early, since the olfactory evaginations appear during the fifth and sixth weeks. In the majority of cases, the etiological agent is unknown, but a small proportion associated with multiple somatic malformations are due to trisomy 13–15 (D_1 trisomy).

The most extreme holoprosencephaly is characterized by a midline orbit containing a single eye, varying facial and nasal malformations (including a fleshy proboscis above the eye, a single nostril and nasal cavity), median cleft palate, and failure of development of the central upper lip (philtrum). The undivided hemisphere (Fig. 19-8) is represented by a horseshoe-shaped mass in the anterior fossae; basal ganglia are fused in the midline, and the olfactory tracts and bulbs are absent. The thalamus, cerebellum, and brain stem are usually normal, except for the absence of descending cortical fibers. Even in this extreme form the cribriform plates are present, and small olfactory nerve fibers can be found. The pituitary gland may be deficient, displaced, or absent. Patients may survive for weeks or months, presumably because of the normal diencephalic and brain stem structures. In less severe cases, the facial and orbital structures may be normal, while the hemispheres show variable failure of midline separation. Olfactory tracts and bulbs are invariably absent, and there may be callosal agenesis.

Agenesis of the Corpus Callosum

Absence of the corpus callosum may occur as an isolated malformation, the roof of the third ventricle being distended dorsally to form an interhemispheric cyst. The anterior horns of the lateral ventricles are short and slitlike, the septum pellucidum is absent, and the two halves of the fornix are widely separated. In some cases the anterior commissure appears larger than normal. The convolutional pattern on the medial aspect of the hemispheres is altered, the cingulate gyrus being replaced by a series of fissures radiating from the edge of the ventricle. The calcarine and parieto-occipital fissures do not become joined. In many cases a rounded longitudinal bundle of myelinated fibers (Probst's bundle) is present above and parallel to the fornix; where a part of the callosum is absent, Probst's bundle is present only in that region. Occasionally, absent corpus callosum is associated with other interhemispheric abnormalities, such as a meningioma or lipoma, and in a few cases, ectopic gray matter is found in the walls of the lateral ventricles.

The etiology is unknown, and hereditary factors have rarely been noted. Only rarely is it associated with polymicrogyria or other changes in the vascular territory of the anterior cerebral vessel, so it is unlikely to be of vascular origin. The lamina terminalis is usually considered to be a roof-plate derivative and this is unique in giving rise to neural structures (the anterior commissure and at least part of the corpus callosum). Callosal fibers appear during the third month in the upper part of the lamina and neighboring fused areas of the medial hemispheric wall; by the fifth month, a miniature adult structure is present.

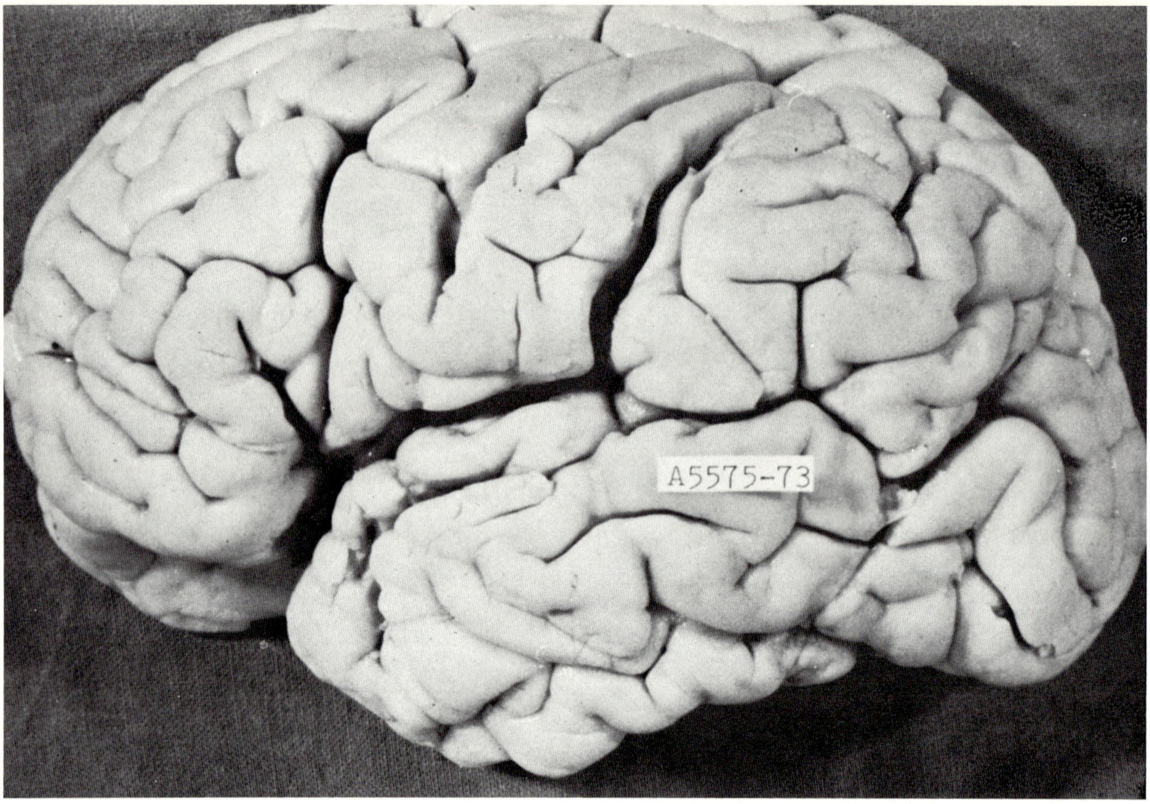

Fig. 19-9. Brain of patient with trisomy 21 (Down's syndrome), showing shortening of the frontal and occipital poles and hypoplasia of the superior temporal gyrus.

Since some cases of callosal agenesis are accompanied by varying degrees of hypoplasia of both the anterior and hippocampal commissures, the condition may represent failure of normal development of the lamina terminalis (median telencephalic structures). The dorsal prolongation of the third ventricle is thought to be secondary to callosal agenesis rather than a feature of the primary defect.

Central Nervous System Malformations Associated with Chromosomal Abnormalities

The best-recognized chromosomal abnormalities associated with CNS malformations are the autosomal trisomies, notably trisomies 13-15, 17-18, and 21. The occasional association of holoprosencephaly with trisomy 13-15 has already been discussed.

Down's Syndrome

The most common condition associated with autosomal trisomy is Down's syndrome (due to trisomy 21 or, occasionally in familial cases, translocation involving 21 and one of the 13-15 group). Patients with multisystem anomalies usually die in infancy or childhood, whereas those with only minor somatic stigmata may survive, mentally retarded, into middle age. The normal, rapid neurological development of the first two years is almost absent, but many mongoloid patients eventually reach the intellectual level of a 6- to 8-year-old child.

The postnatal growth of the brain is slow, and it does not reach adult weight until the age of 4 to 6 years. The frontal and occipital lobes are short, and frequently the superior temporal gyrus is reduced (Fig. 19-9). The cerebellum and brain stem remain small in proportion to the rest of the brain – somewhere between the 6% of the normal neonate and the 12% of the adult. Minor abnormalities of gyral configuration may be present, and there is occasional pachygyria (see p. 355).

The cortical architecture is abnormal, the cells being closely packed, presumably as a result of failure of dendritic development, and normal lamination may be difficult to discern. Myelination, especially of subcortical fibers, is late, giving rise to the impression that the cortex is unusually wide. Fibrillary gliosis may be seen in the white matter. In mongoloid adults there is tendency for senile plaques and neurofibrillary tangles to develop early (see Chap. 24); these appear ultrastructurally identical with those in aging and in Alzheimer's disease. The decreased cerebellar weight indicates a reduction of the middle lobe and may cause the frequent hypotonia.

Numerous biochemical abnormalities have been reported in Down's syndrome, most of them minor variations, and none has been generally confirmed. Leukocyte alkaline phosphatase and other enzymes, often concerned with glucose and galactose metabolism, are at high levels. These patients seem to be more readily depleted of vitamin B_6 (e.g., by administration of the antagonist deoxypyridoxine) than control subjects. The administration of 5-hydroxytryptophan has been reported as occasionally reducing the degree of hypotonia.

Other Chromosomal Abnormalities Associated with Central Nervous System Disease

Trisomy 18 is also associated with mental impairment. About 20% of patients show CNS malformations, usually involving the cerebral or cerebellar cortex. Agenesis of the corpus callosum, meningomyelocele, and even holoprosencephaly have been reported. Abnormalities of gyral pattern or lobar proportions vary from patient to patient, and minor architectural defects often involve the hippocampus, inferior olivary nuclei, and lateral geniculate bodies. None of these changes is specific for trisomy 18.

There appears to be a relationship between deletion of the short arm of chromosome 5, a constellation of somatic malformations, failure to thrive, a weak mewing cry (cri du chat syndrome), and severe mental retardation. The brains show micrencephaly, but no other distinct defects have been reported.

Cortical Dysplasias

Micrencephaly

Underdevelopment of the cerebral cortex and white matter is the main factor reducing brain weight in micrencephaly (arbitrarily, a brain weight of less than 900 g in the adult). There may be a familial form with autosomal recessive inheritance, in which the brain weighs 500 to 600 g and the gyral pattern is simplified. The cortex shows minor architectural anomalies, with persistent arrangement of neurons in radial columns, but subcortical structures are normal. Many micrencephalic brains show calcification, which is often severe in the basal ganglia, deeper layers of the cortex, and dentate nucleus; mineral is apparently being deposited in or near vessel walls. In these cases there is often enlargement of the lateral ventricles and patchy demyelination of the cerebral white matter and brain stem. Lesser degrees of micrencephaly are often found in mental retardates with no substantial histological abnormality.

Macrencephaly

Macrencephaly is a rare condition, which may result from the accumulation of abnormal material, as in the storage diseases (see Chap. 20), or from accumulations of hamartomatous nodules and abnormal cells, as in the phakomatoses (see p. 358). Only rarely does it represent a generalized, approximately proportionate increase of all elements, with or without minor architectural changes. The brain weighs over 1600 g. Some of these patients are of normal or high intelligence.

Porencephaly

Porencephaly is an omnibus term for any large hemispheric defect of prenatal (occasionally postnatal) origin. Prenatal porencephaly may present without evidence of destructive and reparative processes, in the form of slitlike spaces passing symmetrically from the lateral ventricles toward the brain surface. This condition may be of genetic origin, or it may represent localized effects of agents such as viruses, acting early in fetal life to destroy cells without causing any reactive changes. All other porencephalies, either prenatal or postnatal, show clear evidence of a destructive process, with ulegyria, scarring, calcification, and sometimes hemosiderosis, and presumably represent prenatal injury occurring somewhat later (see Chap. 17).

Extreme prenatal porencephaly, in which the hemispheres are represented by glial-meningeal membranous sacs with visible cortex only along the superomedial margins and at the base, is termed *hydranencephaly.* Its etiology is equally speculative, with intrauterine infections and vascular lesions possible. In many such cases the major brain vessels are small, but probably this is secondary to reduced demand and not a causative lesion. Many cases of porencephaly and hydranencephaly probably originate during the fourth or fifth months, since the cerebellum and inferior olives often show minor concomitant malformations.

Pachygyria (Macrogyria)

In pachygyria, there is a simplified gyral pattern, with a reduction in secondary and tertiary gyri and increased depth of the cortex. It is usually associated with micrencephaly and enlargement of the lateral ventricles. In extensive cases only the sylvian, parieto-occipital, calcarine, central, and occasionally the olfactory sulci are present. However, the abnormality is often confined to bilateral areas around the central sulcus (resulting in spastic diplegia) or even to a single small area (often with hemiplegia). If only one or two broad gyri are present and other cortical areas are

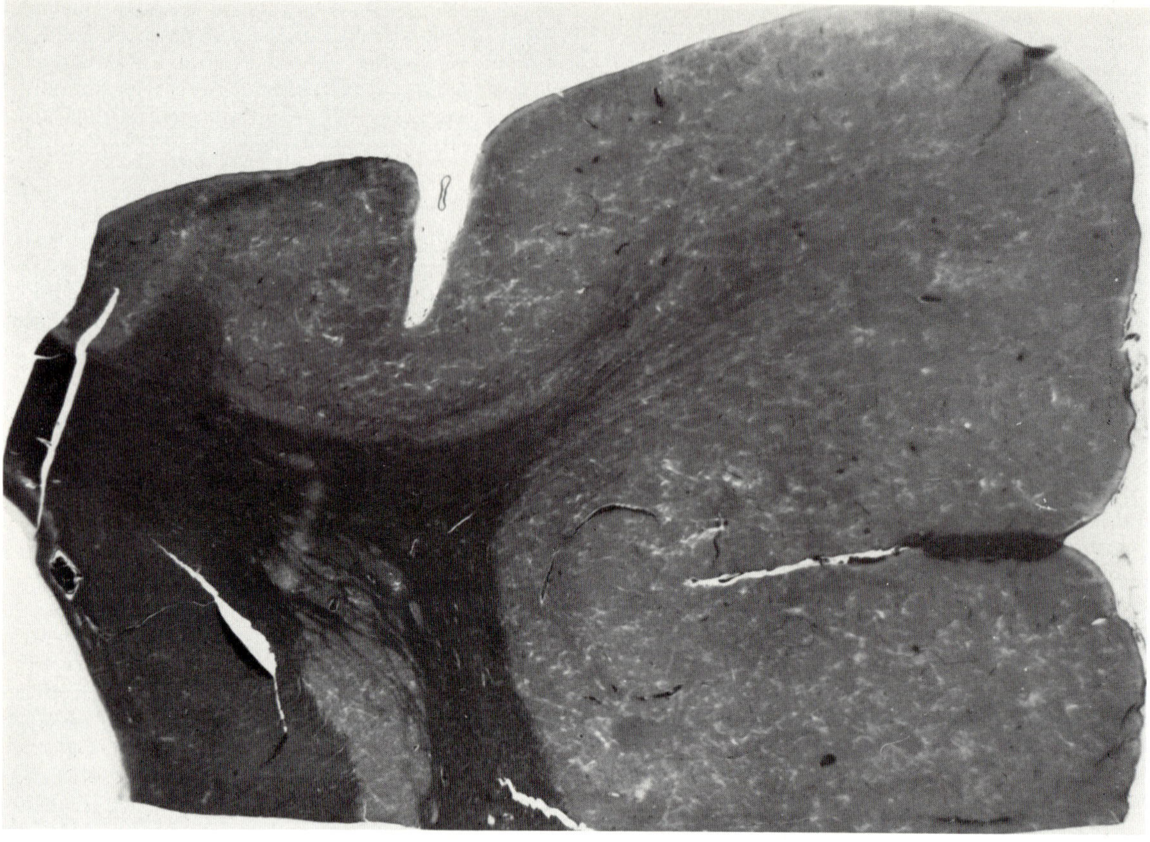

Fig. 19-10. Section from cerebral cortex showing pachygyria. Bundles of radiating myelinated fibers may be seen in the deeper layer (upper right). An irregular mass of ectopic gray matter is present deep to the cortex. (Myelin-H & E, ×8.)

normal, there may be a superficial resemblance to tuberous sclerosis (see p. 359). Associated anomalies of the cerebellum and inferior olives may occur.

Seen microscopically, the cortex shows three layers: A normal molecular layer is present at the surface. Deep to this layer is a thin, irregular band of densely packed neurons, often largely pyramidal, which are irregularly orientated and not laminated. The major part of the thickened cortex is the deepest (third) layer, consisting of neurons in radial columns, separated by bundles of myelinated fibers (Fig. 19-10) that fan out among the cells. The underlying hemispheric white matter tends to be thin.

The condition appears not to be due to altered cell proliferation in the germinal matrix but to arrested migration. The usual interpretation is that the molecular and underlying thin cell layers represent incomplete normal cortex, whereas the deep layer represents somewhat immature cells that have failed to migrate through the cells formed earlier (see Chap. 2). Since neurons begin to reach the cortical surface at about the tenth week of gestation, and the cortex is well formed and stratified by the sixth month, pachygyria probably results from a defect in migration toward the end of this period. The etiology is unknown in most cases.

Polymicrogyria

Polymicrogyria often accompanies micrencephaly. Although the gyri are abnormal and broad, their

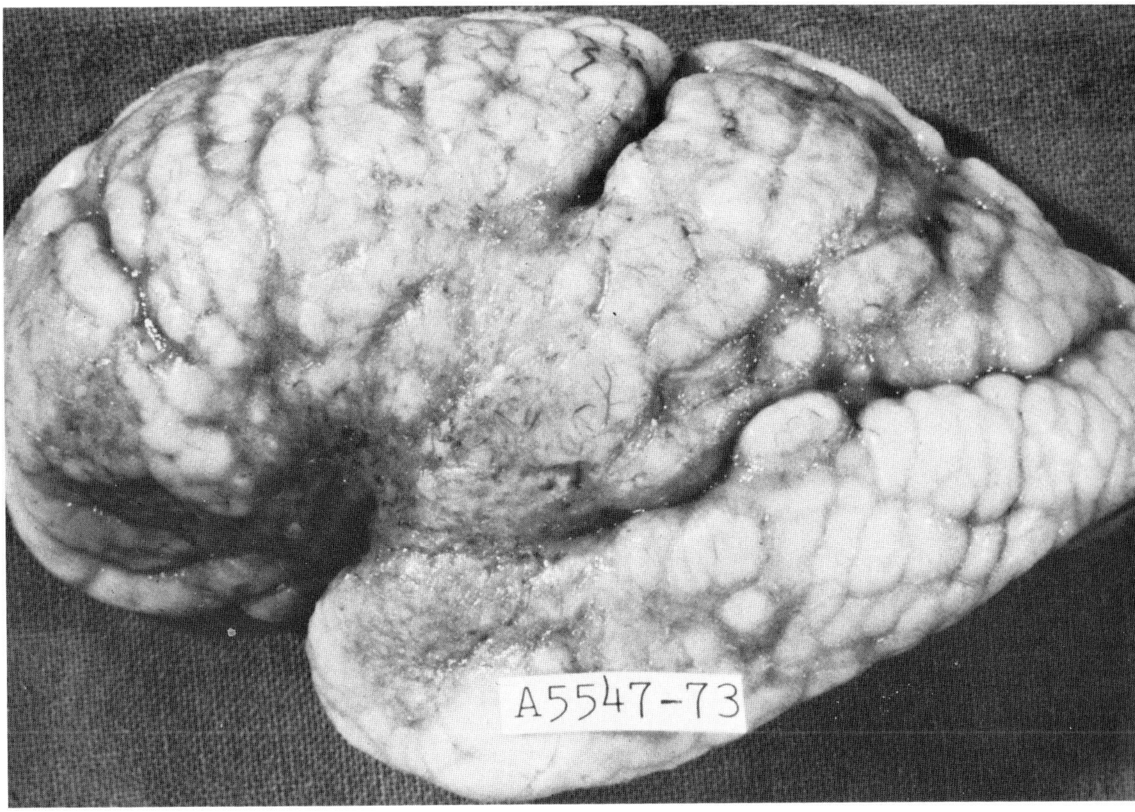

Fig. 19-11. Polymicrogyria involving the lateral surface of the cerebral hemisphere.

surfaces appear wrinkled or pitted like pigskin, and not smooth as in pachygyria. Polymicrogyria may involve the entire hemisphere except for the cingulate, hippocampal, and calcarine areas (Fig. 19-11), but more frequently occurs as small patches, often in the region of the sylvian fissure or parietal cortex, when it may be associated with spastic diplegia or hemiplegia. The lateral ventricles are usually enlarged, and there may be associated anomalies of the cerebellum and inferior olivary nuclei.

Histological examination shows that the apparently broad, flat gyrus is actually composed of small, irregular microgyri whose lateral walls have fused. This is shown by the presence of a molecular layer that dips irregularly into the cortex (Fig. 19-12), partially fused to its neighbor and partially separated by a leptomeningeal layer containing vessels. Deep to the molecular layer, and following its convolutions, is an irregular, thick neuronal band, often divided by a horizontal myelinated zone to form a four-layered cortex. The superficial cellular layer represents the incomplete normal cortex. Though similar in pathogenesis, polymicrogyria is probably of later origin than pachygyria, secondary sulcus formation having occurred, although secondarily obliterated. In either pachygyria or polymicrogyria there may be nodules of apparently normal gray matter, up to 2 cm in diameter, in the walls of the lateral ventricles. Histologically, these resemble basal ganglia rather than cortex, and their origin is not clear.

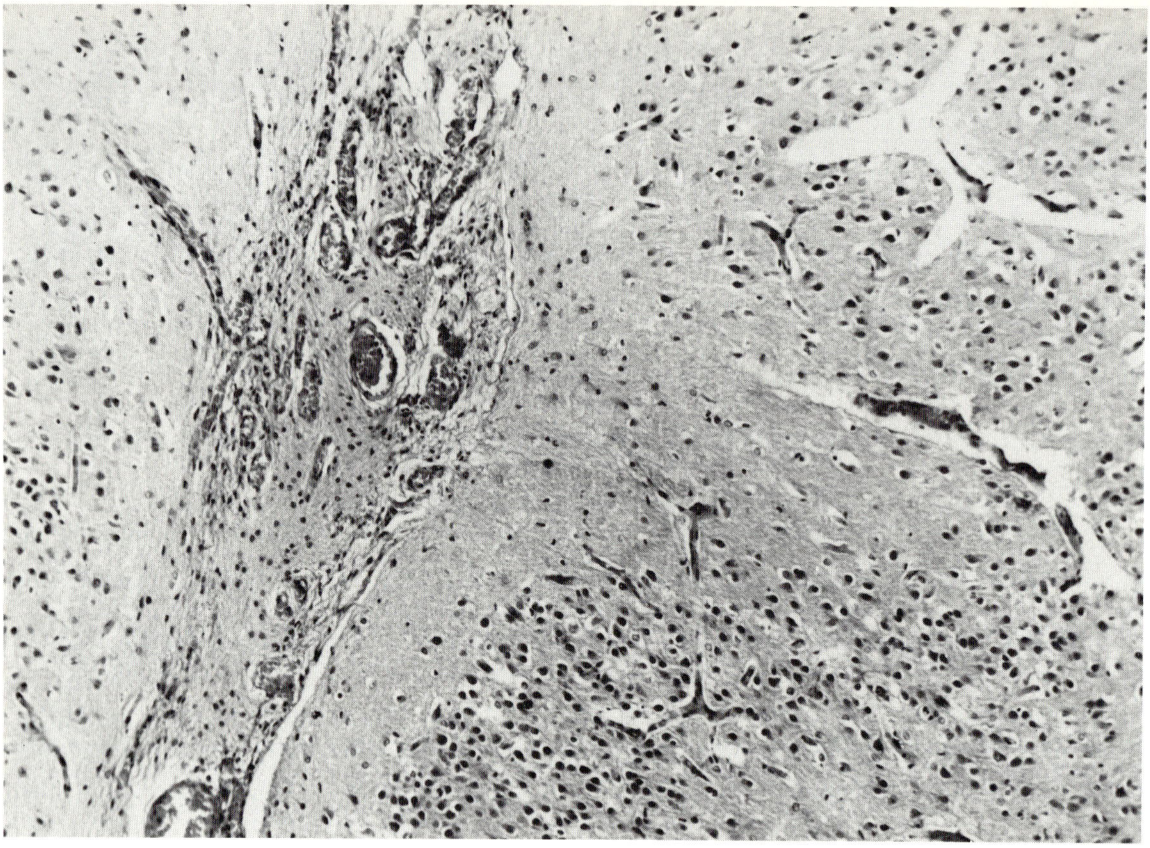

Fig. 19-12. Section from polymicrogyric cortex. The sulcus on the left shows partial obliteration by meningeal gliosis, and to its right side the molecular layer dips into the cortex and distorts neuronal stratification. (H & E, X115 before 5% reduction.)

Malformations of the Aqueduct

Malformations of the aqueduct are frequently associated with the development of hydrocephalus. In many cases they are the only lesions found, although they occasionally occur as part of the Arnold-Chiari deformity or other more extensive lesions.

Aqueductal Stenosis. This is a narrowing of part or all of the aqueduct (distinct from the normal mild constrictions that occur at the levels of the middle superior colliculus and intercollicular sulcus), not accompanied by abnormal gliosis. Some cases show sex-linked transmission, but the majority appear to be sporadic.

Aqueductal Forking. This condition may be an incidental finding, in which case one or more of the channels forms a functionally adequate communication between the third and fourth ventricles. However, it is frequently associated with hydrocephalus, in which case both the dorsal and the ventral channels are small and tortuous, with variable intercommunication. Small midline ependymal nests may also be present, but there is no abnormal fibrillary gliosis. Some of these cases are associated with deformities of the colliculi or oculomotor nuclei or with spina bifida.

Aqueductal Gliosis. In aqueductal gliosis (Fig. 19-13), the outlines of an originally adequate aqueduct are frequently seen as an irregular ring of small ependymal nests. Within this ring are severe fibrillary gliosis and a residual lumen of varying size that is unlined, or incompletely lined, by ependyma. This change is really subependymal gliosis in a vulnerable situation. Similar concomitant changes are often found in other parts of the ventricular system (where they do not obstruct CSF flow). Aqueductal gliosis is usually associated with hydrocephalus, which may be absent at birth. In occasional cases of aqueductal gliosis there is a septum, usually at the caudal end, due to fusion of subependymal granulations across the lumen. It is possible that the lesion represents a reaction either to infection or hemorrhage in the ventricular system.

Neurectodermal Dysplasias (Phakomatoses)

The neurectodermal dysplasias include at least five diseases in which malformations, often of hamartomatous nature, involve the CNS and skin and sometimes other organs. The term *phakomatosis* derives

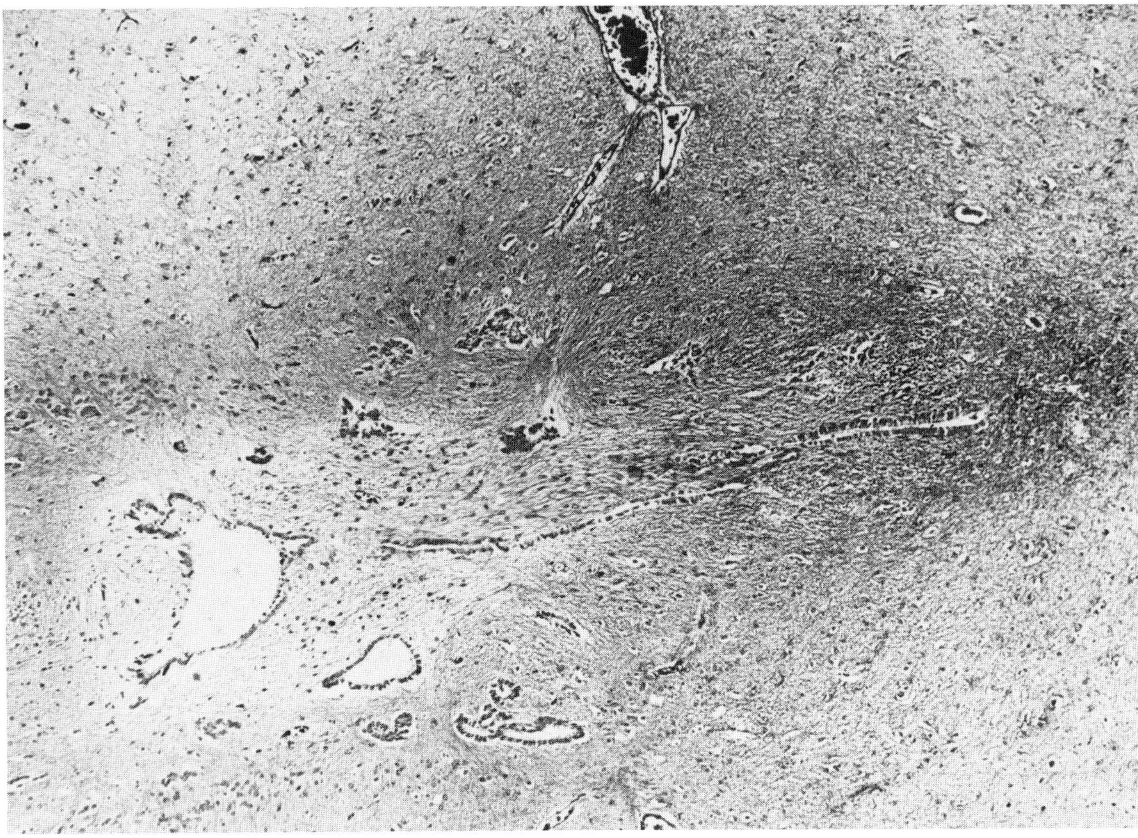

Fig. 19-13. Aqueductal gliosis. Section showing irregular small ependymal nests and a slitlike midline lumen, with loose intervening glial tissue and dense surrounding fibrillary gliosis (darker areas). (Holzer's stain, X75 before 5% reduction.)

from *phakoma,* the small retinal nodule of tuberous sclerosis, the most common of the phakomatoses. In most phakomatoses, dominant inheritance is involved in at least a proportion of cases; others appear to be sporadic, possibly because of the existence of clinically inapparent formes frustes in other members of the kinship. Mental retardation is common and often there are other CNS symptoms.

Tuberous Sclerosis

Tuberous sclerosis is characterized by the presence of dysplastic astrocytes and neurons, both diffusely in the CNS (although much less common in the brain stem and spinal cord) and also grouped as tubers, which are most noticeable in the cortex where they appear as broad, often dimpled areas, pale in color and firm in consistency. Similar nodules may be present in the basal ganglia and thalamus and often project into the lateral ventricles as strings of small beads that have been likened to candle gutterings.

Giant bizarre multinucleate cells, both astrocytes and neurons, are seen on histological examination, especially within the tubers, and there is severe fibrillary gliosis, both diffusely and in the focal lesions. Deposition of calcium and iron may occur, particularly in the ependymal areas. Neoplastic transformation is rare and usually takes the form of a bizarre-looking, but relatively slow-growing and well-circumscribed subependymal astrocytoma. Occasionally, a diffuse astrocytoma of more malignant character occurs.

These patients have seizures, sometimes occurring at birth, and show severe mental retardation. Miscellaneous lesions occur in other parts of the body. In the skin, adenoma sebaceum occurs on the face, usually at puberty, characterized by overgrowth of sebaceous glands and of vascular and connective tissue. Subungual fibromas, consisting of fibrous and angiomatous tissue, are frequent. Retinal nodules often occur and resemble those in the CNS histologically. The heart may show diffuse or focal areas of "rhabdomyomatous" tissue (actually hamartoma rather than neoplasm); the focal lesions are usually less than 1 cm in diameter. The kidneys may show rounded, yellowish-white nodules up to 2 cm in diameter, which consist of connective tissue, fat, and numerous vessels. Lesions have also been described in the liver, lung, duodenum, thyroid, adrenal, ovary, and bone. Inheritance appears to be dominant, with a high mutation rate.

Neurofibromatosis (von Recklinghausen's Disease)

Von Recklinghausen's disease most commonly involves the peripheral nervous system, but occasionally the CNS shows the major lesions, and in these patients the skin lesions are often inconspicuous. Peripheral neurofibromatosis is characterized by cutaneous areas of hyperpigmentation or depigmentation (including café au lait spots), skin hemangiomas, and either focal or diffuse (plexiform) tumor formation in peripheral nerves, neurofibromas being more common than neurilemomas and distinctly liable to become malignant.

Central nervous system involvement is most commonly manifested by acoustic neurilemomas, often bilateral, and meningiomas that may be multiple. Spinal nerve root tumors include neurofibromas and neurilemomas. In the CNS, there is often diffuse proliferation of astrocytes, and sometimes of oligodendroglial cells, which show a tendency to neoplastic transformation much more often than in tuberous sclerosis. Some patients develop multifocal, infiltrating, anaplastic astrocytomas or, less often, relatively low-grade midline pilocytic astrocytomas. Patients with CNS involvement are severely mentally retarded. Inheritance is similar to that of tuberous sclerosis.

Sturge-Weber Syndrome

In Sturge-Weber syndrome angiomatous malformations are invariably present in the skin above the eye and frequently in the retina and the meninges of the occipital and adjacent areas on the same side. The malformed vessels are difficult to classify as either veins or arteries, since they have thick fibrous walls that usually lack both muscle and elastic tissue and show a tendency to early calcification. Since penetrating vessels are also involved, layers I to III of the cortex tend to be partly replaced by crystalline material that contains calcium but little iron. The cutaneous lesion approximately, but not exactly, corresponds to the distribution of the ophthalmic division of the fifth nerve. Patients frequently have contralateral hemiparesis and epilepsy and are severely retarded mentally. Characteristic calcification can be seen radiologically by the end of the second year.

Von Hippel-Lindau Disease

In only about 20% of patients is von Hippel-Lindau disease familial. The disease is characterized by hemangioendotheliomas in the cerebellum and retina. Lesions in the posterior fossa may be multiple, but they are rare above the tentorium. These patients may have renal adenomas and cysts of the pancreas and kidney. It should be noted that a majority of hemangioendotheliomas occurring in the cerebellum are single, isolated lesions, unassociated with von Hippel-Lindau disease. Only the much rarer patients with multiple CNS hemangioendotheliomas are usually examples of von Hippel-Lindau disease.

Neurocutaneous Melanosis

Neurocutaneous melanosis is a rare condition that is frequently associated with mental retardation. The skin shows extensive irregular areas of hyperpigmentation, and there is massive proliferation of the melanin-forming cells normally present (in small numbers) in leptomeninges. Malignant melanoma develops in many of these patients, and they die early in childhood.

HYDROCEPHALUS

In normal clinicopathological usage, the term hydrocephalus is not applied to all increases in CSF volume. Thus, enlargement of the subarachnoid space, whether due to cerebral atrophy or to arachnoiditis with localized cyst formation, is *not* hydrocephalus. Similarly, although dilatation of the ventricular system that is secondary to atrophy of the brain (and therefore usually associated with widening of the subarachnoid space) has been called "hydrocephalus ex vacuo," the term is liable to mislead and should *not* be used. *True hydrocephalus is an enlargement of all or part of the ventricular system (Fig. 19-14), due to production of CSF at a rate greater than the rate of removal.*

This is commonly associated with an increase in intraventricular pressure and, if it originates before birth or in infancy, with a marked increase in head circumference. However, it is now clear that a progressive ventricular expansion can occur that is not secondary to brain atrophy, is relieved by the creation of an artificial pathway for evacuation of the CSF (shunting), but in which intraventricular pressure is normal. This condition may be termed *normal-pressure* or *occult* hydrocephalus.

Pathogenesis

It is generally accepted that active secretion of CSF occurs only from choroid plexuses (see Chap. 4), although during its passage through the ventricular system and over the surface of the brain, changing ion concentrations suggest that diffusion of brain extracellular fluid adds to the total volume. It is also generally accepted that CSF enters the subarachnoid space through the fourth ventricular foramina, and that almost all of it passes upward through the tentorial notch to be absorbed in the lacunae of the superior sagittal sinus through the arachnoid villi and arachnoid (pacchionian) granulations. Thus, hydrocephalus may result from the following:

1. *Overproduction of CSF,* either by active secretion from the choroid plexuses or by an unduly large accession of ECF. It appears possible that rare cases of choroid plexus papilloma are associated with hydrocephalus, perhaps due to overproduction of CSF. However, the possibility of obstruction of flow cannot be excluded. Excess ECF has not been implicated, and it is more likely that the normal flow (ECF to CSF) is reversed in hydrocephalus, absorption of fluid into CNS vessels being perhaps an attempted compensatory mechanism.

2. *Obstruction along the normal routes of CSF flow.* Such obstruction will result in a damming up of

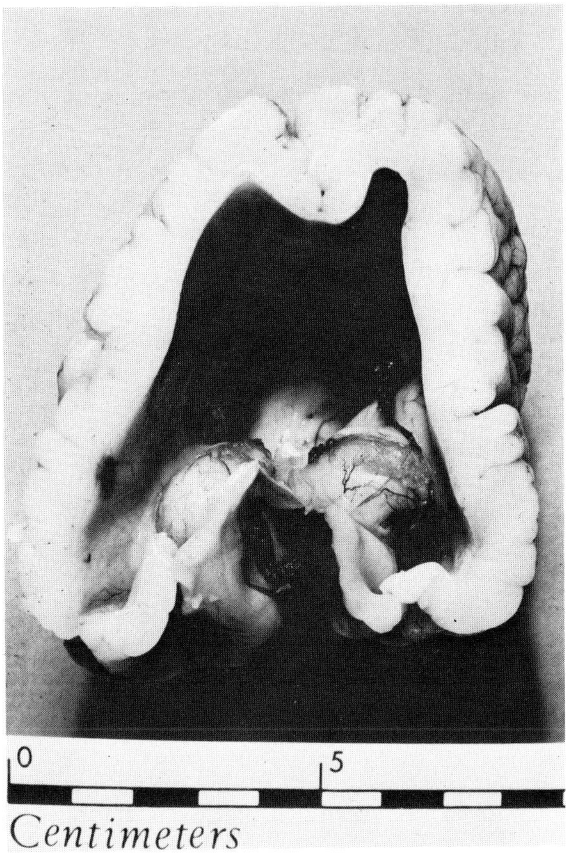

Fig. 19-14. Moderately severe hydrocephalus, viewed from behind the thalamus. The lateral ventricles form a single cavity, and the septum pellucidum has disappeared. The corpus callosum is thin, but a reasonable cortical mantle remains. This patient had congenital aqueductal stenosis.

CSF and ventricular dilatation. Common sites for such obstruction are:

a. *At the foramina of Monro,* associated with a third ventricular tumor such as colloid cyst or, less frequently, with a neoplastic or inflammatory lesion obstructing only one foramen and causing unilateral hydrocephalus. Obstruction due to a colloid cyst (acute hydrocephalus) is an occasional cause of sudden, unexpected death in adults. There is no dilatation of the aqueduct or enlargement of the fourth ventricle.
b. *At the aqueduct.* This may be due to many of the malformations noted in the preceding section and, much less frequently, to other lesions, such as a brain stem glioma, a lesion behind the collicular plate compressing the brain stem (pineal tumor, hemangioma, or lipoma), or following ventricular infections or hemorrhage, debris being deposited within the aqueduct and subependymal gliosis often provoked.
c. *In the fourth ventricle.* This is a relatively unusual cause, not often seen in the neonatal period. However, in childhood, a majority of CNS tumors involve the hindbrain, particularly the cerebellum. A medulloblastoma, ependymoma, astrocytoma, or hemangioendothelioma may compress the fourth ventricle, or actually invade it, and obstruct CSF flow. Brain stem tumors, such as pontine glioma, are unusual causes of hydrocephalus.
d. *At the fourth ventricular foramina.* This may occur as a result of these foramina (notably the foramen of Magendie) to open, as a result of displacement of the medulla into the cervical spinal canal, or as a result of fibrosis of the meninges in the foraminal area. Hydrocephalus due to such obstruction may be observed in the Arnold-Chiari and Dandy-Walker malformations. However, in the majority of cases, meningeal fibrosis is present in the absence of malformation (Fig. 19-15), and it has been speculated that such cases might be associated with intrauterine or early postnatal infections or hemorrhage. There is usually little clinical or pathological support for this supposition, but it remains a possibility, largely by analogy with adult post-traumatic and similar hydrocephalus.
e. *In the subarachnoid pathways.* Such obstruction might be due to a primary failure of the pathways to form, or to secondary fibrosing changes occurring in them. If the subarachnoid space were formed by the pressure of CSF dissecting through the meninges after the opening of the foramina, it would follow that if the foramina failed to open, the subarachnoid space would not exist. It has recently been shown that the subarachnoid space is present in such cases, and thus its formation is an intrinsic property of leptomeningeal tissue. The most vulnerable areas are around the foramina and between the tentorium and midbrain, since these are the narrowest regions. Cases of hydrocephalus associated with meningeal thickening and adhesions in these areas have been reported,

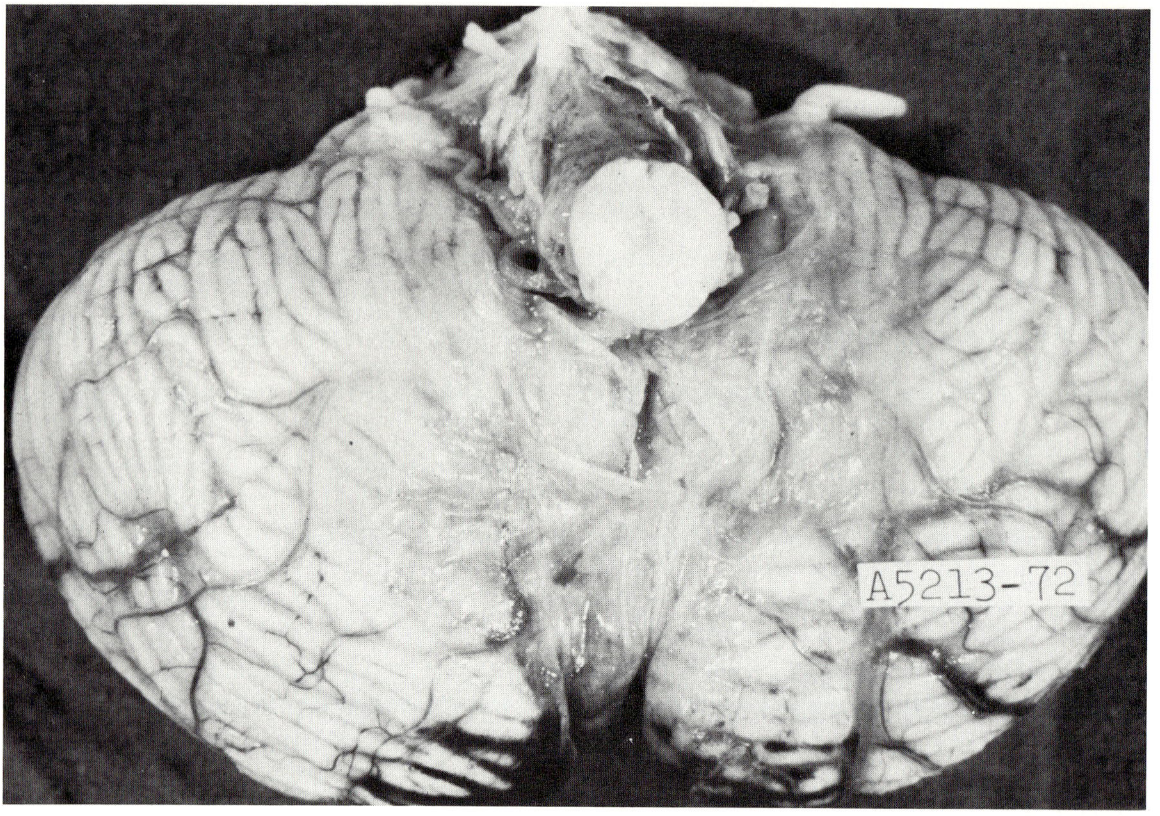

Fig. 19-15. Thickening and moderate fibrosis of leptomeninges in the region of the foramina of Magendie and Luschka. This patient had moderately severe hydrocephalus, with onset in the first year of life.

and in some there was a clear history of meningitis, subarachnoid hemorrhage, or head injury. However, similar changes have been reported in congenital and infantile hydrocephalus, again leading to speculation that intrauterine infection or hemorrhage, or birth hemorrhage, might be responsible.

3. *Failure of CSF absorption at the arachnoid villi and granulations.* If CSF were not adequately absorbed hydrocephalus would naturally develop, and there do not appear to be any totally effective alternative absorptive mechanisms to the villi and granulations. Experimentally, hydrocephalus can be produced by the injection of particulate agents, which are assumed to block the canaliculae in the villi and prevent fluid absorption, but there is no clear evidence of any similar mechanism in clinical cases. Furthermore, possibly because of recanalization, subsequent development of hydrocephalus has not been reported in patients surviving superior sagittal sinus thrombosis. A few cases have been reported in which there appears to have been congenital absence or hypoplasia of arachnoid villi associated with hydrocephalus. This might seem to be a distinctly unusual clinical entity merely because it has not often been sought.

It is apparent that there is a large number of potential causes for hydrocephalus. However, overproduction and failure of absorption of CSF appear to be rare, whereas many cases demonstrate some degree of blockage somewhere along the route of CSF flow. Nonetheless, even in congenital and infantile hydrocephalus there is a proportion of cases in which no convincing obstruction or other cause is detected, and the pathogenesis in these cases is completely obscure. The same may be said for the normal-pressure hydrocephalus occasionally seen in adults.

Only a part of the ventricular system may be distended, depending on the site of blockage. Obstruction of one foramen of Monro leads to enlargement of only one lateral ventricle, whereas obstruction in the third ventricle causes symmetrical dilatation of both lateral ventricles (and usually the third as well, since it is the site of the causative lesion). In obstruction of the aqueduct there is symmetrical dilatation of the lateral ventricles and widening of the third, and dilatation of the aqueduct is added in obstruction of the fourth ventricle. However, obstructions further along the direction of flow, either at the foramina or in the subarachnoid space, dilate the entire ventricular system.

Investigative Techniques

Dye Tests. Hydrocephalus has been divided into communicating and noncommunicating forms. In the former, the CSF, or a large part of it, is presumed to reach the subarachnoid space and ultimately be absorbed, so that dye injected into the ventricles can be detected in lumbar CSF, plasma, or urine within a relatively short time. In noncommunicating hydrocephalus there is little or no passage of CSF to the subarachnoid spaces, absorption of dye into the blood (presumably via brain vessels) is slow, and excretion in the urine is both retarded and prolonged.

Although dye tests are now rarely performed, they serve to draw attention to the fact that failure of CSF absorption is never absolute, and that hydrocephalus usually consists of a retarded, rather than a totally obstructed, CSF circulation. This is particularly true when the site of obstruction is in the subarachnoid space, when the upward flow over the hemispheres, although reduced, is never completely cut off. In addition, there is probably increased absorption of CSF through the vessels of the brain itself, and these two factors – incompleteness of obstruction and increased absorption into brain vessels – undoubtedly account for the clinically nonprogressive nature of some cases of hydrocephalus in the absence of effective therapy.

Radioiodinated Serum Albumin. A useful diagnostic aid in the investigation of hydrocephalus is intrathecal (or intracisternal) injection of serum albumin labeled with ^{131}I (radioiodinated serum albumin [RISA]), followed by lateral and anteroposterior scanning for isotope activity. Following intrathecal injection in the normal patient, activity is detectable in the region of the basal cisterns and sylvian fissure at about 4 hours. At about 24 hours, there is marked accumulation over the upper hemispheres, and by 48 hours, only minimal diffuse activity remains. Normal patients do not show asymmetry or persistent local accumulations, and their ventricles are not visualized. So far, the method appears to have been principally of value in the communicating types of hydrocephalus, with the major abnormal feature having been visualization of the ventricles, possibly due to increased transventricular absorption.

Radiology. Additional methods of investigation include echoencephalography to estimate the width of the third ventricle (a width over 7 mm probably indicates hydrocephalus). This is particularly useful as it can be repeated and used to follow progress after shunting procedures.

It has been suggested that hydrocephalus might also be assessed on anteroposterior plain films by comparing the maximal width of a lateral ventricle with half the skull width. The normal ratio is less than 0.3, and ratios larger than 0.33 are considered to indicate hydrocephalus. This index does not always correlate with the results of RISA injection, which when normal in the presence of a high index perhaps indicates a compensated state, with a reduction both in production and absorption of CSF. The technique has not been extensively tested.

Pathophysiology of Cerebrospinal Fluid Flow

Clinical observations in steady-state hydrocephalus indicate compensatory mechanisms for increased intraventricular pressure, the nature of which has been the subject of a considerable number of investigations.

Effects of Raised Intraventricular Pressure

Anticipated hydrodynamic effects of raised intraventricular pressure might include the following:

1. *Compression of the choroid plexuses,* with reduction of their blood supply and a possible decrease in active secretion of CSF. Experimentally, this does seem to occur, with a 50% decrease in fluid production for each pressure rise of 130 to 140 mm H_2O reported by some investigators.

2. *Increase in the effects of pulse pressure transmitted from the choroid plexuses,* because raised intracranial pressure compresses the cerebral veins, which are the best available damping mechanism to absorb the pulsation. The beneficial effects of shunting, even from the ventricular to the subarachnoid space, may be partially attributable to this reduction in ventricular pulsation, the shunt tube itself acting as a damping mechanism. If, as seems probable, pulsation is a significant factor leading to ventricular dilatation, its reduction may be one of the most significant contributions made by shunting procedures.

3. *Possible increase in reabsorption by choroid plexuses.* On theoretical grounds this appears unlikely, since the choroid plexus is an actively secreting membrane, and alterations in pressure gradient are likely to affect only passive flow. Colloidal matter injected into the ventricles of hydrocephalic animals may be found in vesicles within the choroid plexus epithelium, but this may represent either a specific reabsorptive response or, equally, a degenerative phenomenon.

4. *Increased transependymal absorption.* As noted in Chapter 4, normally there appears to be flow from the extracellular to the CSF compartments. However, the ependyma is not an absolute barrier to fluid flow in either direction, and, under normal pressures, slight penetration of the ependymal membrane by large molecules has been demonstrated. With increased intraventricular pressure, it seems possible that bulk flow might be established from the ventricular to the extracellular spaces, with increased fluid absorption into cerebral venules. It has been shown that the water concentration within about 1 mm of the ependymal surface is increased in experimental chronic hydrocephalus, and that RISA is returned to the bloodstream largely through the straight sinus in such animals (indicating absorption into the deep cerebral circulation) and not through the superior sagittal sinus, as in control animals.

5. When the fourth ventricle is closed by a thin membrane, as in the Dandy-Walker syndrome, increased hydrostatic pressure may cause *permeation of fluid through this membrane* (which does not contain continuous cell junctions), so that some CSF could still leave the ventricles.

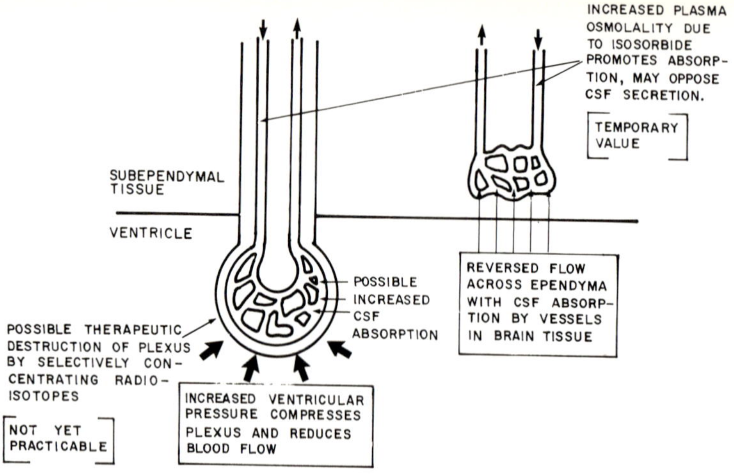

Fig. 19-16. Some naturally occurring and therapeutic attempts to balance CSF production and absorption (by decreasing production) in hydrocephalus. Therapeutically, CSF shunting remains the only really feasible procedure and occasionally allows time for natural absorption to reach and maintain a balance with production (compensated hydrocephalus) even after the shunt tube is removed.

6. *Ventricular dilatation,* which tends to be self-perpetuating since the total force exerted is equal to pressure times area, and the area increases with the dilatation.

Many of the preceding effects might be regarded as compensatory (Fig. 19-16), either reducing production or increasing absorption of CSF.

Other methods of decreasing CSF production might include administration of acetazolamide (see Chap. 4) or selective destruction of the choroid plexuses by radioactive isotopes. Experimentally, the radionuclide ^{198}Au causes plexus necrosis following intraventricular injection; it has a half-life of 2.7 days and a penetrating range of 0.4 mm. It is not considered sufficiently safe for human experimentation, and the search for more suitable isotopes continues. Prior to operation, the oral administration of 45% isosorbide is said to reduce intracranial pressure.

Normal-Pressure (Occult) Hydrocephalus

While plausible mechanisms have been proposed for ventricular dilatation in the presence of raised intraventricular pressure, cases of primary ventricular dilatation with normal pressure are difficult to explain. Marked ventricular visualization follows the administration of intrathecal RISA in cases of normal-pressure hydrocephalus, which indicates that the hydrocephalus is communicating in type, and perhaps due to transependymal absorption. However, there is also a marked delay in clearing RISA from the subarachnoid space, indicating circulatory or absorptive defect. The RISA test appears useful in distinguishing normal-pressure hydrocephalus from secondary hydrocephalus due to brain atrophy, as in Pick's or Alzheimer's disease. In these diseases the ventricles are not visualized, and clearance of radioisotope from the cranial cavity is normal or only slightly delayed.

Hydrocephalus following Head Injury or Subarachnoid Hemorrhage

The RISA test has also proved useful in confirming the suspected nature of hydrocephalus following trauma or subarachnoid hemorrhage. It has been widely assumed that the early hydrocephalus often seen in these patients is due to extensive blockage of the subarachnoid space with blood or other debris, whereas in those in whom a permanent progressive hydrocephalus develops, blockage is due to reactive fibrosis of the subarachnoid space. The RISA test shows delayed passage of isotope over the cerebral hemispheres and accumulation in the parasagittal regions in more than 75% of cases, presumably due to temporary blockage of the arachnoid villi by debris, including precipitated protein and red cells. In about 30% of patients the ventricles are visualized, presumably indicating reflux of CSF from the cisternal to the ventricular system and increased absorption across the ependyma.

Morphological Changes in Hydrocephalus

Progressive hydrocephalus in early life causes expansion of the head with separation of sutures, but this does not occur in adult hydrocephalus. Progressive dilatation of the ventricles is accompanied by thinning of the hemispheres, which is more severe in the white matter than the gray. There is widening and blunting of the lateral angle of the lateral ventricle, so that the distance between the corpus callosum and the caudate nucleus is increased, and the callosum itself usually becomes thinned and the septum pellucidum perforated.

Affected white matter shows diminution in oligodendroglial and astroglial cells, but during the stage of active expansion, small accumulations of gitter cells are present deep to the ependyma. The ependymal lining of the ventricle becomes incomplete, due to the marked increase in surface area. Thinning of the cortex ultimately occurs and is most marked dorsally, where it is not buttressed by the basal ganglia.

There may be marked dilatation of the third ventricle, with bulging of its floor and erosion of the clinoid processes, and although histological changes are difficult to detect in the hypothalamus, there may be clinical indications of hypothalamic dysfunction.

Clinicopathological Correlation

Since maximum dilatation of the ventricle occurs in the anterior horns and involves the frontal lobes, psychomotor retardation and inattentiveness may be seen in children. Involvement of the posterior frontal lobe may cause spasticity that is more marked in the legs than in the arms, but evidence of hypothalamic-pituitary dysfunction is rarely seen (in the form of infantilism or precocious puberty). Sphincter incontinence usually develops early. In adult hydrocephalus, similar changes occur, both in the obstructive (e.g., post-traumatic) and normal-pressure forms. There may be headache, impairment of memory and concentration, sixth nerve palsy, failing vision, spastic gait, and incontinence.

In normal-pressure hydrocephalus, clinical deterioration frequently occurs a few days after pneumoencephalography, associated with a transient increase in ventricular size. This has been attributed somewhat vaguely to a displacement of CSF into the basal system or, more simply, to an increase in total volume of intracranial contents. It is also possible that air in the ventricles interferes with transependymal absorption, thereby causing a temporary decompensation of CSF flow.

BIBLIOGRAPHY

Allan, L. D., Ferguson-Smith, M. A., Donald, I., Sweet, E. M., and Gibson, A. A. M. Amniotic fluid alpha-fetoprotein in the antenatal diagnosis of spina bifida. *Lancet* 2:522-525, 1973.

Banerji, N. K., and Millar, J. H. D. Chiari malformation present in adult life – Its relationship to syringomyelia. *Brain* 97:157-168, 1974.

Blackwood, W., McMenemey, W. H., Meyer, A., and Russell, D. S. (Eds.). *Greenfield's Neuropathology.* London: Arnold, 1963.

Davson, H. *Physiology of the Cerebrospinal Fluid.* London: Churchill, 1970.

Duncan, D., and Hild, W. Embryogenesis of the Nervous System. In J. Minckler (Ed.), *Pathology of the Nervous System.* New York: McGraw-Hill, 1968. Vol. 1, pp. 77-90.

Emery, A. E. H., and Burt, D. Amino-acid composition of amniotic fluid in central nervous system malformations. *Lancet* 1:970-971, 1973.

Emery, J. L., and MacKenzie, M. Medullo-cervical dislocation deformity (Chiari II deformity) related to neurospinal dysraphism (meningomyelocoele). *Brain* 96:155-162, 1973.

Gardner, W. J., Smith, J. L., and Padget, D. H. The relationship of Arnold-Chiari and Dandy-Walker malformations. *J. Neurosurg.* 36:481-486, 1972.

Gilles, F. H., and Davidson, R. I. Communicating hydrocephalus associated with deficient dysplastic parasagittal arachnoid granulations. *J. Neurosurg.* 35:421-426, 1971.

Glanville, E. V. Genetics and Neuropathology. In J. Minckler (Ed.), *Pathology of the Nervous System.* New York: McGraw-Hill, 1968. Vol. 1, pp. 372-380.

Greitz, T. V. P., Grepe, A. O. L., Kalmer, M. S. F., and Lopez, J. Pre- and post-operative evaluations of cerebral blood-flow in low-pressure hydrocephalus. *J. Neurosurg.* 31:644-651, 1969.

Halsey, J. H., Jr., Allen, N., and Chamberlin, H. R. The morphogenesis of hydranencephaly. *J. Neurol. Sci.* 12:187-217, 1971.

Klosovsky, B. N. Hydrocephalus. In J. Minckler (Ed.), *Pathology of the Nervous System.* New York: McGraw-Hill, 1968. Vol. 1, pp. 456-462.

Lichtenstein, B. W. Hamartomas and Phakomatoses. In J. Minckler (Ed.), *Pathology of the Nervous System.* New York: McGraw-Hill, 1971. Vol. 2, pp. 1897-1906.

Milhorat, T. H., Hammock, M. K., and di Chiro, G. The subarachnoid space in congenital obstructive hydrocephalus. Parts I and II. *J. Neurosurg.* 35:1-15, 1971.

Minckler, J. Syringomyelia. In J. Minckler (Ed.), *Pathology of the Nervous System.* New York: McGraw-Hill, 1971. Vol. 2, pp. 1943-1946.

Ogata, J., Hochwald, G. M., Cravioto, H., and Ransohoff, J. Distribution of intraventricular horseradish peroxidase in normal and hydrocephalic cat brains. *J. Neuropath. Exp. Neurol.* 31:454-463, 1972.

Oosterhuis, H. J. G. H., and van der Schoot, J. B. RISA cisternography as a routine procedure in neurological patients. *J. Neurol. Sci.* 13:209-226, 1971.

Padget, D. H. Neuroschisis and human embryonic maldevelopment. *J. Neuropathol. Exp. Neurol.* 29:192-216, 1970.

Sahar, A. The effect of pressure on the production of cerebrospinal fluid by the choroid plexus. *J. Neurol. Sci.* 16:49-58, 1972.

Scharenberg, J. Neurofibromatosis. In J. Minckler (Ed.), *Pathology of the Nervous System.* New York: McGraw-Hill, 1971. Vol. 2, pp. 1906-1916.

Williams, B. Is aqueductal stenosis a result of hydrocephalus? *Brain* 96:399-412, 1973.

Mental Retardation

20

Mental retardation is a manifestation, not a disease entity. In most cases the etiological factors are not yet clearly defined. It may be observed from birth, with either failure or delay in normal neurological development, or it may take the form of intellectual and motor regression, usually beginning in infancy or early childhood after a period of overtly normal progress. While it may be an isolated phenomenon, it is often associated with other manifestations of central nervous system dysfunction, including epilepsy and motor disorders of pyramidal or extrapyramidal type.

Just as mental retardation cannot be defined on an etiological or pathogenetic basis, clinical definition of the borderline between normal and retarded intellectual function is indefinite. To a considerable extent, it is a product both of the individual's ability and the demands of society. Severe mental retardates, incapable of elementary self-help, would clearly be nonviable in a society that was not closely cohesive or lacked either the inclination or the surplus resources to maintain them. Even in compassionate societies, mental retardation of severe and moderate grades represents a massive economic drain. The lack of self-criticism and self-inhibition that characterizes even minor grades of retardation leads to crime and delinquency and represents an additional major challange to society. Thus, although not clearly definable on any etiological, clinical, or (as will be seen) morphological basis, mental retardation is of the greatest medical and social significance.

Statistics on the incidence of mental retardation are not reliable, since the condition is not sharply demarcated from normal intelligence and thus the cutoff point is of necessity arbitrary and likely to vary from society to society, according to the demands imposed. Except in specific disease entities (such as inborn errors of metabolism), which make up only a very small proportion of cases, the evidence for a genetic factor is indefinite. It has been stated that approximately 1% of the general population in Western society is mentally retarded, that the parents and siblings of an index case have a significantly higher incidence of retardation (about 3.5 to 5.0%), and that consanguinity is three times higher in the parents of retardates than of controls. None of these figures is well established. At best, they suggest a genetic background for a minority of patients.

Etiological Factors

As already intimated (see Chap. 19), there is no sharp separation of the minor structural changes sometimes found in the brains of retardates from overt malformations of the CNS. Whether any particular agent produces malformation or mental retardation is largely dependent on the time of its activity (within the range from conception to the second postnatal year), its intensity, and other factors that were discussed in the preceding chapter. For this reason, it is not proposed to recapitulate here the list of suspected etiological factors that account for the great majority of cases of retardation. It is, however, necessary to add some rare disorders associated with retardation, but rarely (if ever) with CNS malformation, presumably because they act late in fetal life or postnatally. Although they will be discussed at some length for their academic interest, diseases based on chromosomal or metabolic errors are a tiny minority of all cases of retardation.

The first such group includes the numerous anomalies of sex chromosomes. The most common disorder in this group is that of the phenotypic females who have three or more X chromosomes (XXX, XXXX, and XXXXX) and show mild to severe mental retardation and short stature, but are usually not malformed. Phenotypic females with four or five X chromosomes show more severe retardation. In Turner's syndrome (XO), which also shows a female phenotype, there is rarely retardation, although there may be specific cognitive defects. In Klinefelter's syndrome (usually XXY) the phenotypically male patients tend to show psychological rather than intellectual abnormalities, but patients with the phenotype of Klinefelter's syndrome who have additional X chromosomes (e.g., XXXXY) are often retarded. Males with phenotype XYY are rarely retarded, although there are said to be increased criminal tendencies among them. The pathogenesis of retardation in these patients with chromosome abnormalities is unknown.

A second group of disorders, each rare but cumulatively not insignificant, are inborn errors of metabolism involving amino acids, sphingolipids, and occasionally other substances. Treatment is rarely available, and all these diseases are progressive, so that the patients rarely live to reproductive age. They are therefore inherited as autosomal recessives, the responsible genes surviving because heterozygotes are clinically normal, though they may show biochemical abnormalities, especially under stress. Rarely, these conditions may be sex-linked recessive diseases. Since they are genetically determined, the enzyme defect or deficiency probably dates from conception; however, a large majority of such infants appear normal at birth. This may be because abnormal metabolites are cleared across the placenta, and essential substances the fetus cannot make are available in the maternal circulation. Particularly with respect to sphingolipid metabolism, activity of the absent, deficient, or defective enzymes might be minimal during the fetal period and only manifestly absent postnatally, when there should be a spurt of myelination, which, of course, fails to occur.

Other conditions that may be associated with mental retardation (but not CNS malformation) include toxic agents, such as pure oxygen, ingestion of lead, and lack of iodine. A majority of congenital cretins remain severely retarded in spite of treatment.

The Morphological Substrates of Mental Retardation

One or another type of CNS abnormality can be detected by the naked eye or light-microscopic examination (i.e., following a well-performed routine autopsy) in a majority of retardates, although there is a proportion in which changes have not been found. This proportion varies considerably from author to author within the range of 10 to 40%. Such wide variation is presumably due to the marginal nature of many changes, which necessitates close familiarity with the architecture of the CNS, particularly of the cortex, and comparison with the same brain regions in age-matched controls. This is a time-consuming, meticulous procedure that is frequently impossible within the budgetary limitations of a service laboratory.

When routine investigation does not disclose abnormalities, it is reasonable to presume that the causes of retardation are either metabolic or at the structural level of the neuronal processes, which consists largely of the ramifications of dendrites occurring during the first year or two of postnatal life and the concurrent formation of synaptic connections. Study of synapses involves electron microscopy and will probably not yield convincing results until the range of normal variation (in numbers, situation, and morphology) has been more fully explored. There are currently no methods for visualizing the dendritic tree of even one neuron in its entirety, and it is only possible to assess the overall bulk of dendritic tissue indirectly by such methods as noting the packing density of neuronal cell bodies. It is often reported that in mental retardation the cell bodies in the cortex are close together and preserve the radial (columnar) arrangement that is normal only early in development, but is disrupted by later dendritic growth.

A problem of equal magnitude is the reporting of primary "abnormalities" that are really normal age variations in the brain, artifactual changes due to processing, staining, or postmortem autolysis, or secondary changes (particularly common in the brains of mental retardates) due to infection, trauma, and epilepsy. Such nonspecific changes have frequently been reported, but it would seem better to state simply that nothing significant has been found. Some possible reasons why this may be the case have been noted in the preceding paragraph.

In the 60 to 90% of cases in which definite abnormalities are found, these are widely variable and are usually not specific for mental retardation. Probably the most common finding is some degree of micrencephaly, often associated with abnormalities of gyral pattern and cortical architecture (see Chap. 19). Other types of malformation may be found, though not all malformations cause retardation. Also common, especially in cases associated with epilepsy or motor abnormalities, are areas of hypoxemic or ischemic destruction and gliosis involving the cortex, white matter, basal ganglia, and thalamus, or minor changes such as status marmoratus and status lacunaris (see Chap. 17). These brains may also show varying diffuse or focal gliosis and scattered mineralization of vessels or neurons.

Another change in mental retardation, which is common in those rare inborn errors of metabolism involving amino acids, is a vacuolation (status spongiosus) involving gray or white matter or both. *Status spongiosus* is merely a descriptive term, and the appearance might be produced by vacuolation of any CNS structure (e.g., myelin sheaths, astrocytic processes) or by focal dilatation of the extracellular space. Only electron microscopy can differentiate these types of vacuolation, and this has usually not been done. The somewhat more specific findings in the sphingolipidoses are considered later, but they, too, are only an insignificant fraction of the total number of cases.

RADIATION AND MENTAL RETARDATION

There is ample clinical and experimental evidence that irradiation of the immature CNS may lead either to overt malformation or to retardation that is usually associated with micrencephaly. As for any other teratogenic agent, the effect produced depends largely on gestational age, and while clinical experience is in full accord with this concept, it is most readily illustrated by the effects of irradiating fetal rats in utero. Rats irradiated before the eighth day following conception either produce normal offspring or abort. Over the next one to two days, radiation produces either severe forebrain defects, absence of the eyes, optic nerves, and tracts, or midline defects, including failure of callosal formation, dorsal prolongation of the third ventricle, and dilatation of the lateral ventricles. Eleven to 20 days after conception (total gestation period about 21 days) radiation produces micrencephaly with dilatation of the lateral ventricles and a decrease in the thickness of the hemisphere walls, cerebellar hypoplasia, cellular and myelin abnormalities of the cortex, ectopic gray matter, and sometimes agenesis of the corpus callosum.

Human experience has come from irradiation of uterine tumors and other pelvic radiation, and from the effects of atomic bomb explosions. About one-third of the infants whose mothers receive pelvic radiation during pregnancy have CNS anomalies, most often consisting of micrencephaly and associated ocular defects (including pigmentary degeneration of the retina and cataracts), and many are mentally retarded. Experience with the effects of atomic bomb explosions suggests that the seventh to fifteenth weeks of gestation represent the most vulnerable period, and there is a clear association between the irradiation and micrencephaly and mental retardation in the offspring. Micrencephaly was seen following irradiation as late as the end of the sixth month.

From experimental studies, it appears that the neuroepithelial cells of the germinal matrix and cerebellar external granular layer are the most radiosensitive; they die within a few hours after exposure to 100 rads. As with other teratogenic agents, areas with a high mitotic rate have a high vulnerability, and loss of these germinal cells must cause neuronal deficit. More mature neurons may not be killed, but their future development is stunted, so that later growth failure of the dendrites is to be anticipated. Irradiation has also led to failure of myelination in the irradiated areas, associated with loss of oligodendroglial cells or their precursors, which appear to be radiosensitive. Although irradiation of the fetal CNS causes *direct* radionecrosis, the brain at this stage is resistant to *indirect* effects, such as those apparently mediated through the vessels that require a latent period for their development (see Chap. 25).

Further discussion of the mechanisms of radiation damage should be sought in special texts, but it may be noted here that radiation destruction of the fetal CNS is not associated with damage to DNA or with abnormal mitoses, but is an example of acute cell death, associated with breakdown of plasmalemma and organelles, swelling of mitochondria, and activation of lysosomes. Less severe irradiation may, however, be associated with delayed cell death, the cell being apparently normal until mitotic division takes place.

MALNUTRITION AND MENTAL RETARDATION

Although it is difficult to make a definite correlation, both experimental data and clinical evidence (in underdeveloped countries) are beginning to point overwhelmingly to the possibility that generalized dietary insufficiency (as opposed to deficiency of any specific factor) leads to delayed and possibly permanently impaired mental development. Appreciation of this fact has been delayed because in Europe and North America it is unlikely to occur. Maternal and infant malnutrition in these areas is currently insignificant compared with that epidemic in Africa, South America, and India.

Animal experimentation is valuable, because to some extent the associated factors in human society correlated with low socioeconomic status are not operative in the experimental situation. There remains suggestive evidence, even in the laboratory, that changes in the amount of handling of newborn animals, such as might readily occur with alterations in laboratory setup, litter size, or frequency of feeding, have a direct effect on behavioral development. In human society, such factors are likely to vary with socioeconomic status. In rats, either malnutrition or environmental stimulus deprivation causes increased emotionality (including increased sexual drive), which is associated with a lower body weight, lower brain weight, delay in myelination, reduction in dendritic branching, and reduced brain levels of acetylcholinesterase. Perhaps stimulus deprivation gives the animal reduced opportunities to learn to respond, whereas malnutrition, by inhibiting structural maturation, actually prevents the animal from learning to respond. Although the effects on behavior are maximal during the actual period of malnutrition, there is probably also permanent impairment of learning ability.

Because it is virtually impossible to alter the diet without other significant environmental changes, attempts to reproduce such work in underfed children are difficult. Retrospective analyses from several countries have associated a past history of severe malnutrition (marasmus) with a statistical reduction in intelligence. Underfed children are apathetic and lethargic. These features tend to disappear with rehabilitation, but it is probable that the earlier in infancy the malnutrition, the more permanent the final impairment. Autopsy studies have suggested that marasmic children's brains show a reduced number of neurons and delay in myelination. The chemical constitution of any myelin present is normal, and the defect presumably lies in the level of oligodendroglial metabolic activity. Malnutrition during the first 12 to 15 months delays cell division, and its effects are in part irreversible; later malnutrition interferes with cell growth and may be at least in part recoverable.

Electron-microscopic studies in starved infant rats have shown increased packing density of neurons and decreased total volume of neuropil in the cortex, but normal concentrations of synapses. Thus, there is a decrease in total synapses proportional to the decrease in neuropil volume — as much as 40%. No structural changes were seen. The DNA, protein, and RNA content of the brain were all reduced, the DNA reduction indicating fewer cells, since cell DNA is constant. These changes are very similar to those reported in hypothyroidism.

It is apparent that both experimentally and clinically there is association between malnutrition and impaired mental development. However, it is less clear whether this is a direct association, or whether malnutrition is acting in concert with other environmental factors that accompany poverty, notably, a reduction in environmental stimuli, including affection. These factors might operate directly on the CNS or through the endocrine system.

INBORN ERRORS OF AMINO ACID METABOLISM

The association between disorders of amino acid metabolism (usually with abnormal levels of amino acids in the blood and urine) and mental retardation is undoubted. What the mechanism of this relationship may be is essentially unknown, and no assistance has so far been forthcoming from morphological CNS

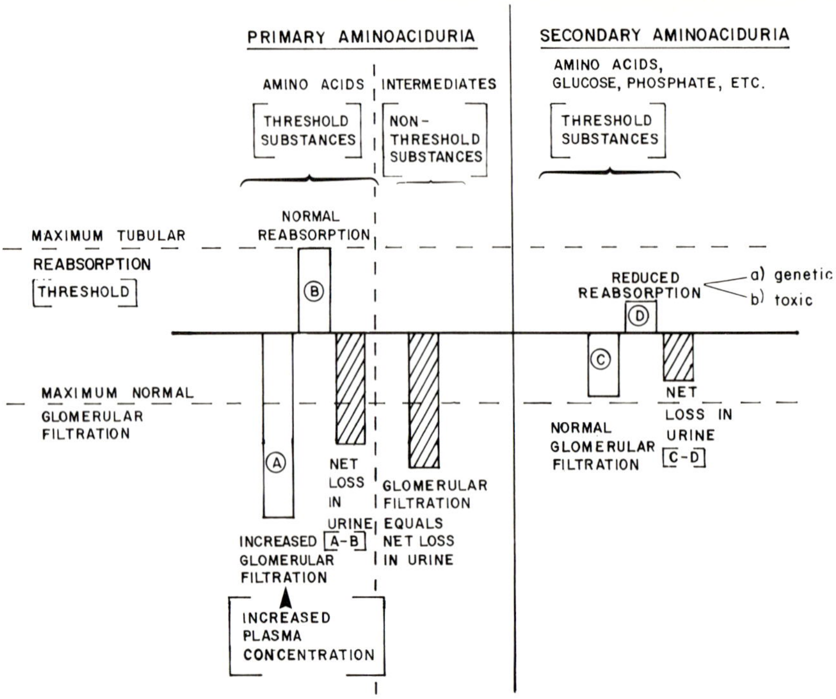

Fig. 20-1. Schematic illustration of the differences between primary and secondary aminoaciduria. For details, see text.

studies in affected patients. In disease, amino acids in the blood may be low, normal, or high, and in many diseases there are accumulations of intermediary metabolites, which are either present in normal plasma in very small quantities or are normally confined to the intracellular fluid. Possible mechanisms of the toxic action on the CNS include:

1. Amino acid deficiency, specific or generalized.
2. Competition for blood-brain barrier transport by an amino acid present in excess, reducing the transfer of others that are equally necessary.
3. Direct toxic effects of intermediate metabolites that are normally absent or present in insignificant quantities.

Types of Aminoaciduria

Aminoaciduria is a constant feature of this group of diseases (Fig. 20-1) although it does not affect all amino acids equally. It may be *primary* (with normal renal tubular function), in which amino acids overflow into the urine because they are present in excess of the reabsorption threshold and intermediate metabolites overflow because they are normally absent from the plasma and therefore have no reabsorptive mechanism. *Secondary aminoaciduria* is associated with abnormal renal tubular transport, which may either be the essential feature of the disease (possibly associated with similar transport defect in other organs, including the gut and CNS) or may be due to toxic factors, as in galactosemia, Wilson's disease, or heavy-metal poisoning.

Because there are separate transport mechanisms for groups of amino acids, the secondary aminoacidurias are usually characterized by excessive loss of only one group. In the renal tubules there seem to be separate mechanisms for the basic amino acids (lysine, arginine, and ornithine) and cystine, for the acidic amino acids (glutamic and aspartic acid), for the imino acids and glycine, for monocarboxylic acids other than glycine, and for beta amino acids. There may be two systems for amino-acid transfer: one of high specificity but low capacity and the second, just described, of group specificity but capable of much more rapid transfer.

Genetics

Probably all aminoacidurias are genetically determined (except for some secondary types due to exogenous toxins) and exhibit autosomal recessive transmission. While the general concept of one gene to one enzyme remains valid, at any given gene locus there may be several alleles, each perhaps changing only one amino acid of the whole enzyme sequence. There may thus be several defective variants of a single enzyme, with the efficiency of each varying according to the closeness of the relationship of the abnormal amino acid to the active site of the enzyme. Effective enzyme activity is therefore not an all-or-none phenomenon

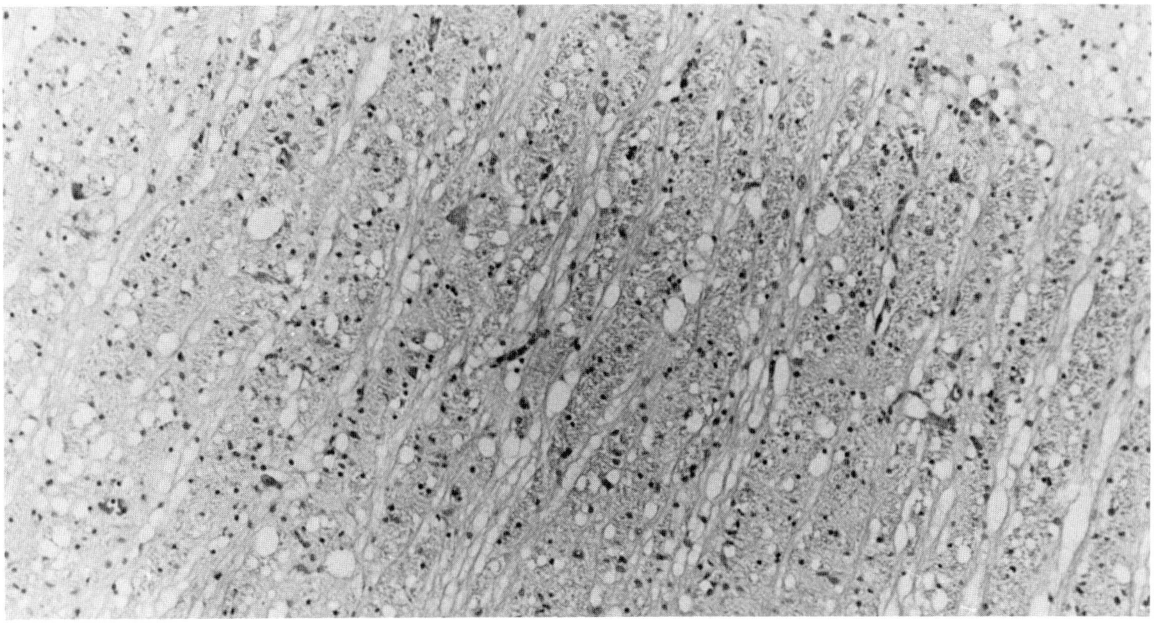

Fig. 20-2. Mild brain stem spongiosis, apparently due to swelling of myelin sheaths, in a patient with an aminoaciduria (hyperglycinemia). (H & E, X300.)

and may reach as high as 20% of normal in patients with a fully developed clinical syndrome. Since only a single case of a single kinship of the rarer aminoacidurias is known, autosomal recessive transmission has not been rigorously proved in all types of aminoaciduria.

Morphological Changes in the Central Nervous System

Some aminoacidurias have been delineated only on a clinical and biochemical basis, and morphological studies are lacking. Where there are such studies, as in phenylketonuria, CNS changes have proved to be mild or moderate and often equivocal. Occasional examples of malformation, such as micrencephaly or foci of microgyria, have been reported, but so few that they are probably coincidental. (However, if metabolic defects were not compensated by placental function, it is conceivable that inborn errors of metabolism might be associated with minor malformations.) Since changes are minor, caution in interpretation is mandatory. It is essential that the brains be well processed to avoid postmortem and processing artifacts as far as possible, and that adequate comparison be made with age-matched control subjects. The latter is especially important, since one of the major effects appears to be delay of myelination, which is normally an active process during the first two years of life. Similarly, there may be fibrillary gliosis, and it is important to know that in certain parts of the CNS, notably the brain stem, moderate numbers of glial fibrils are normal, but that they vary in quantity with age.

The following changes have been reported in the brain (the cord has been little examined) in aminoacidopathies:

1. *Pallor of myelin,* presumably because of a delay in myelin formation diffusely in the hemispheres and elsewhere. No myelin breakdown products or stored materials are present, but there may be diffuse fibrillary gliosis disproportionate to the myelin deficit. There is no convincing evidence that the chemical composition of any myelin present is abnormal.

2. *Status spongiosus* has been commonly reported, and although artifactual changes may contribute, it appears to be a genuine phenomenon. It is often most marked at the junction of the cortex with underlying white matter (arcuate fibers) and in the brain stem (Fig. 20-2), especially in the central tegmental tract from midbrain to inferior olives. The ultracellular location of these vacuoles has in most cases not been determined.

3. In disorders of the urea cycle and some forms of tyrosinosis, Alzheimer type II cells may be found, as in hepatic failure (see Fig. 11-12). These conditions are frequently associated with increased serum ammonia, which may be responsible for the astrocytic changes (see Chap. 11).

4. Delayed neuronal migration and maturation appear probable, though they are not yet confirmed by adequate control material. Thus, in the normal full-term neonate it is usual to find neuroblasts scattered through the hemispheric white matter, and in premature infants the radial arrangement of neurons in the cortex may be emphasized by the paucity of dendrites.

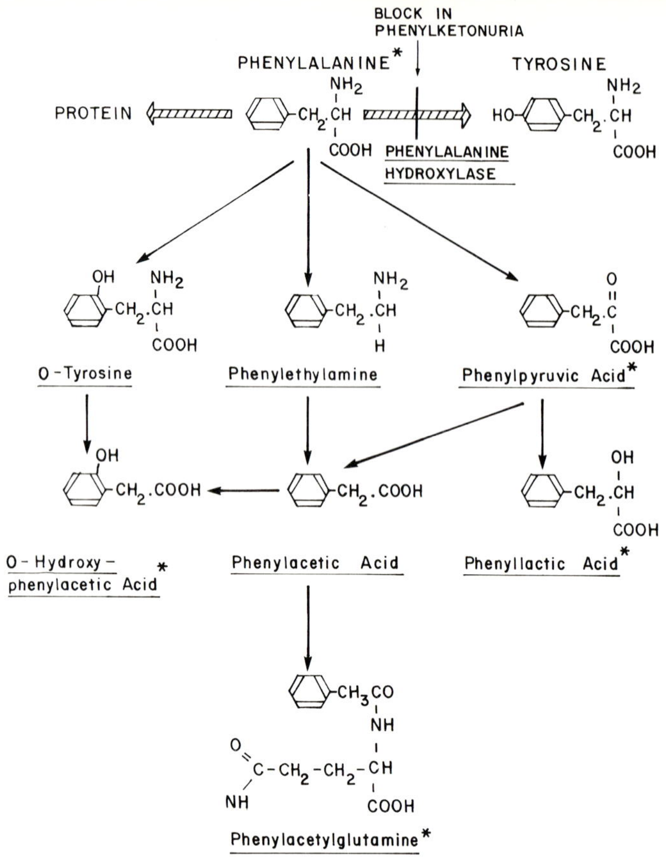

Fig. 20-3. The biochemistry of phenylketonuria (PKU). Cross-hatched arrows indicate major routes of normal metabolism. If conversion to tyrosine is blocked, metabolism of phenylalanine follows the other paths indicated (= increased urinary excretion).*

Biochemical Changes

In some patients with amino acid abnormalities a definite enzyme deficiency has been identified by biochemical determination. In others, the deficiency has been inferred but not tested. In still others (especially where transport mechanisms are involved), the nature of the defect is unknown. The following brief notes present some major findings.

Phenylketonuria

In phenylketonuria (PKU), profound mental retardation may be accompanied by epilepsy, hyperreflexia, hyperkinesia, and tremor, and patients show diminished pigment in hair and iris and sometimes an eczematoid rash. The condition is a confirmed autosomal recessive trait, occurring about once per 10,000 live births. The heterozygotes are of normal intelligence. A mild decrease in brain weight may be noted. The enzyme lacking is phenylalanine hydroxylase (Fig. 20-3), which normally converts phenylalanine to tyrosine. Phenylalanine therefore accumulates in the blood, reaching levels of 50 to 100 mg per 100 ml (normal, 1 to 2 mg per 100 ml, but in neonates the enzyme may be physiologically deficient and levels of 3 to 5 mg per 100 ml may occur in the first few days of life). Excess phenylalanine is diverted to other metabolic pathways, forming intermediates that cannot be completely metabolized. These intermediates are excreted in the urine along with phenyl-

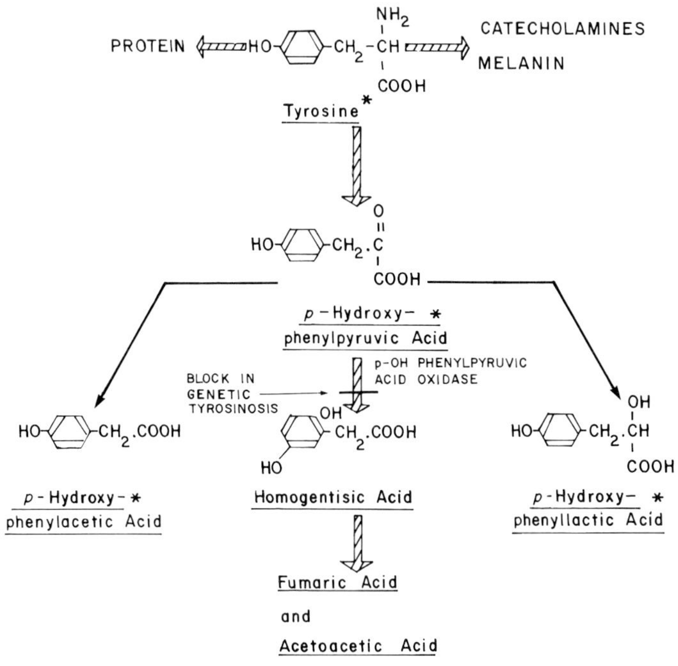

Fig. 20-4. The biochemistry of genetic tyrosinosis. Cross-hatched arrows indicate normal metabolic pathways. If conversion to homogentisic acid is blocked, pathways analogous to those in PKU are followed (= increased urinary excretion).*

alanine itself. One of them, phenylethylamine, is thought to be toxic to the CNS. Excessive blood phenylalanine may competitively inhibit transport of other amino acids into the CNS. There is reduction in the formation of tyrosine and interference with tryptophan metabolism (possibly by competition for the enzyme L-aromatic amino acid [dopa] decarboxylase). Blood levels of serotonin and catecholamines and urinary levels of vanillylmandelic acid (VMA) and 5-hydroxyindoleacetic acid (5-HIAA) are therefore reduced, and deficiency of neurotransmitters might cause or contribute to retardation. If a pregnant patient has blood phenylalanine higher than 20 mg per 100 ml, there may be fetal brain damage; conversely, patients born to normal mothers are usually normal at birth, or at most show a low birth weight.

Tyrosinosis and Related Disorders

High plasma and urine levels of tyrosine accompany raised excretion of *p*-hydroxylated derivatives of phenylpyruvic, phenyllactic, and phenylacetic acids and sometimes of methionine. This condition may be a true inborn error of metabolism (Fig. 20-4), with a deficiency of *p*-hydroxyphenylpyruvic acid oxidase preventing formation of homogentisic acid. Tyrosine is then metabolized along paths parallel to those of phenylalanine in PKU. Often, tyrosinosis is secondary to neonatal hepatic disease or renal tubular defects involving excretion of amino acids, phosphate, glucose, K^+, and HCO_3^-. The brain may show Alzheimer type II astrocytes, presumably associated with liver dysfunction, and surviving patients are usually mentally retarded. Possibly related is Smith-Strang disease, also called oasthouse disease from the odor of the urine, which contains excess tyrosine and other amino acids; the enzyme defect has not been established.

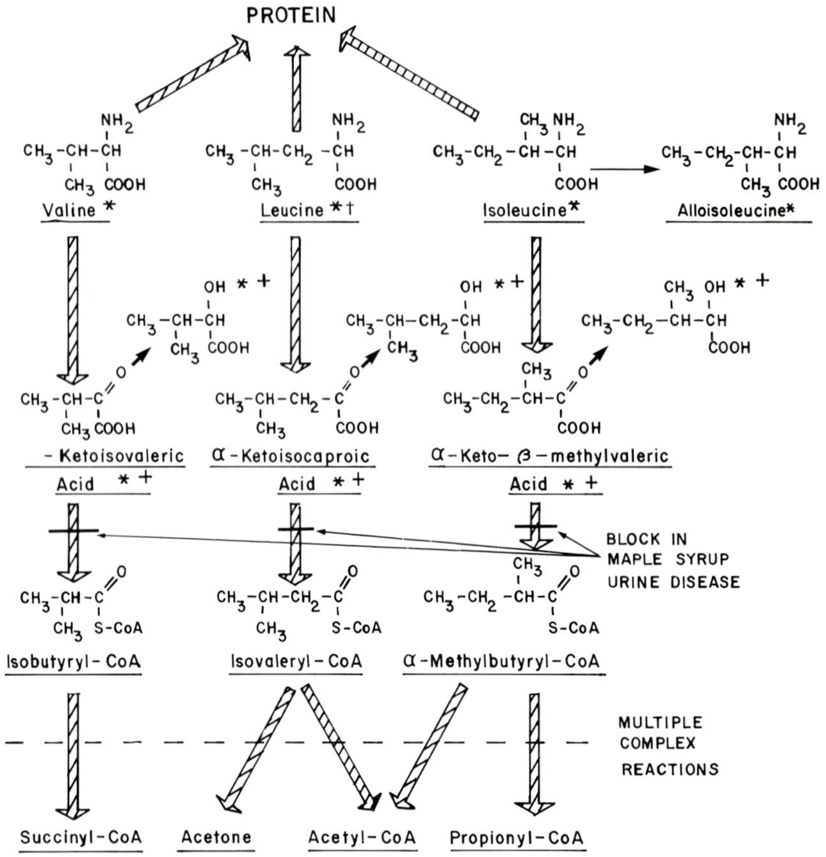

Fig. 20-5. The biochemistry of maple syrup urine disease (= increased urinary excretion; + = may cause characteristic odor; † = may cause severe hypoglycemia, increased insulin secretion). The metabolism of branched-chain amino acids normally follows the cross-hatched arrows. The abnormal organic acids formed may be responsible for the urine odor.*

Maple Syrup Urine Disease

Also named for the odor of the urine, maple syrup urine disease is a rare condition (Fig. 20-5) in which the branched-chain ketoacids derived from valine, leucine, and isoleucine cannot be linked to coenzyme A, and there is a block in oxidative decarboxylation. The three keto acids and the amino acids themselves are excreted in the urine. Patients may present in the first few days of life with feeding difficulties and convulsions and often die early. In those who survive, mental retardation is prominent, and the enzyme which oxidatively decarboxylates branched-chain keto acids is reduced rather than absent.

Hyperprolinemia and Hydroxyprolinemia

Hyperprolinemia and hydroxyprolinemia are extremely rare. Several different enzyme deficits are known to exist in these disorders (Fig. 20-6). *Hyperprolinemia type I* (deficiency of proline oxidase) is associated with mild mental retardation and occasional renal disease. *Hyperprolinemia type II* (deficiency of Δ'-pyrroline-5-carboxylic acid dehydrogenase) shows higher blood proline levels, and mild retardation is present. *Hydroxyprolinemia* (deficiency of hydroxyproline oxidase) shows a twenty- to fifty-fold increase in blood hydroxyproline levels — of some interest since hydroxyproline is only present in collagen, yet in this condition collagen metabolism is normal, and dietary intake minimal. The patients show mental retardation.

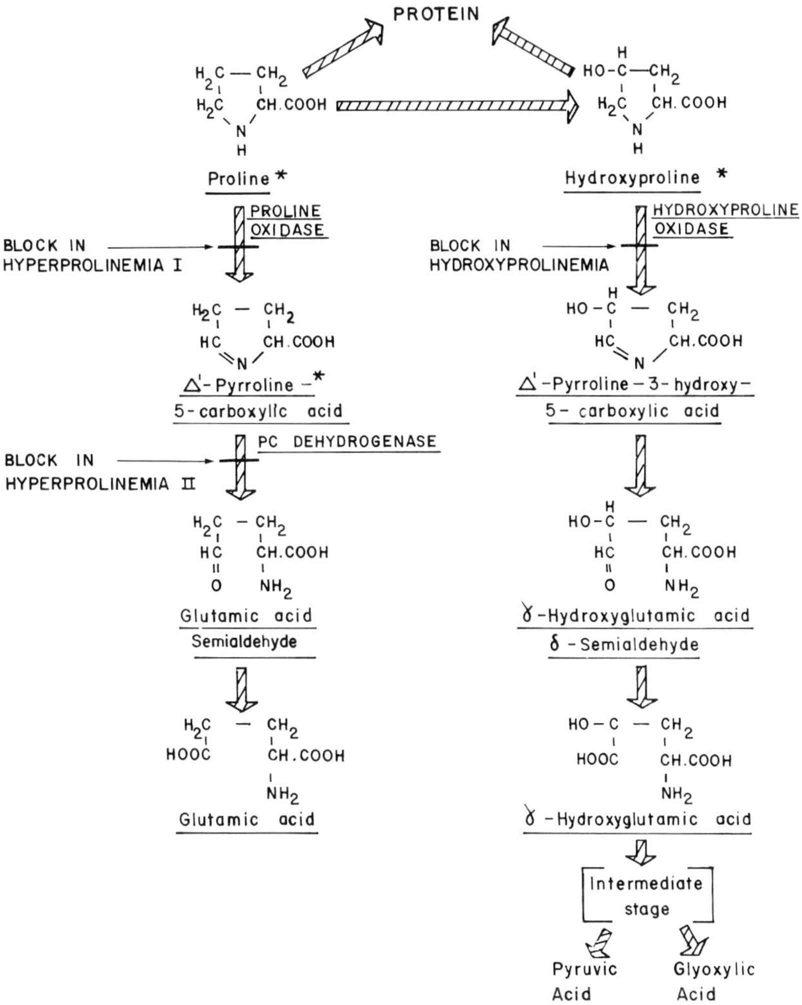

Fig. 20-6. The biochemistry of hyperprolinemia and hydroxyprolinemia (= increased urinary excretion, often of both proline and hydroxyproline, as they share reabsorptive system). Normal metabolism (cross-hatched arrows) may be prevented at one of three sites (see text), causing increased excretion of preceding compounds in the metabolic pathway, but no significant use of alternative routes.*

In *familial iminoaciduria* there is a renal transport defect; blood levels of proline and hydroxyproline are normal, but urinary excretion is excessive. Some of these patients are mentally retarded.

Histidinemia

Histidinemia is usually due to deficiency of histidase (Fig. 20-7), so that normal histidine metabolism cannot occur. Histidine, and imidazole derivatives of pyruvic, lactic, and acetic acids, occur in the urine, and formiminoglutamic acid (FIGLU) is not excreted. Although the abnormal pathways seem analogous in histidinemia and PKU, levels of blood histidine are less because of lower intake and better renal clearance; mental retardation does not invariably occur.

Another enzyme defect beyond FIGLU (absence of cyclohydrolase or formiminotransferase) causes raised serum folic acid and mental retardation.

Homocystinuria and Cystathioninuria

Patients with homocystinuria may show somatic abnormalities and mental retardation associated with seizures, and they are susceptible to thromboembolic

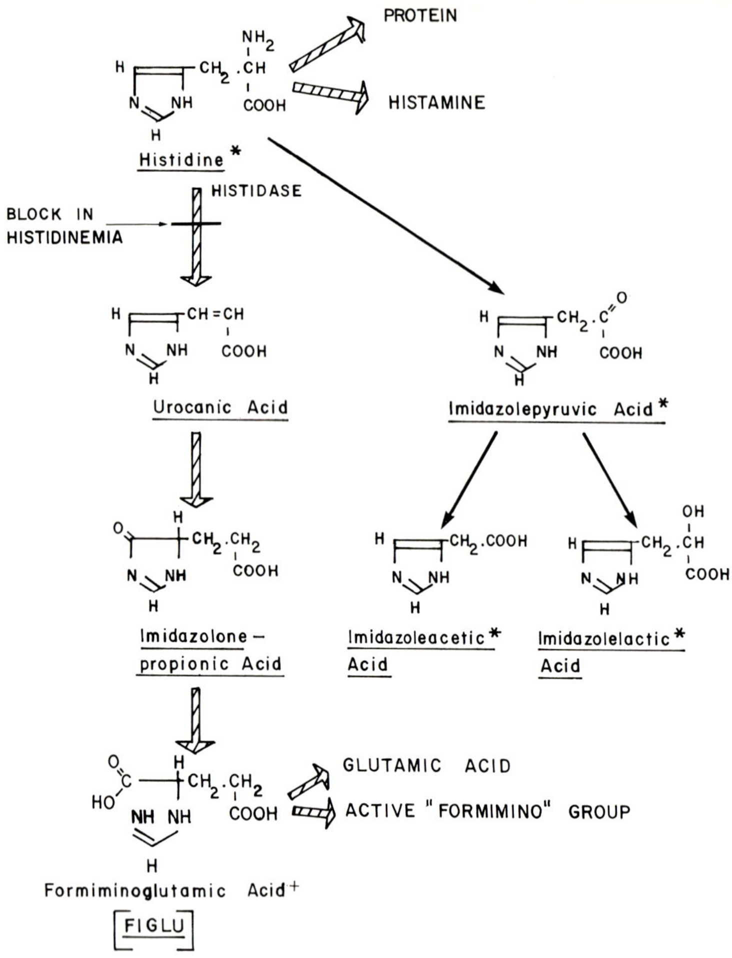

Fig. 20-7. The biochemistry of histidinemia (= increased urinary excretion; + = decreased urinary excretion). Normal metabolism (cross-hatched arrows) is blocked by lack of histidase, and alternative routes analogous to those in PKU are followed.*

accidents in youth. The defective enzyme in homocystinuria is cystathionine synthetase (Fig. 20-8), normally present at least in the liver and brain. Cystathionine synthesis is reduced and homocysteine accumulates, some being oxidized to homocystine (found in blood and urine) and some remethylated to methionine (raised in blood). The thromboembolic accidents are due to increased platelet adhesiveness, related to homocystine accumulation.

In cystathioninuria the deficient enzyme is cystathioninase (Fig. 20-8), and cystathionine is cleared to the urine without plasma accumulation. There is little mental retardation in this condition.

Hyperglycinemia

Several forms of hyperglycinemia, in which glycine accumulates in the body fluids and urine, are associated with retardation.

Some present as a neonatal ketosis simulating maple syrup urine disease, the urine containing methylethylketone, acetone, and longer-chain ketones (suggesting a defect in carboxylation of propionyl-CoA to methylmalonyl-CoA). Survivors are severely retarded.

The nonketotic form is characterized by lethargy, seizures, and other CNS signs during the first weeks

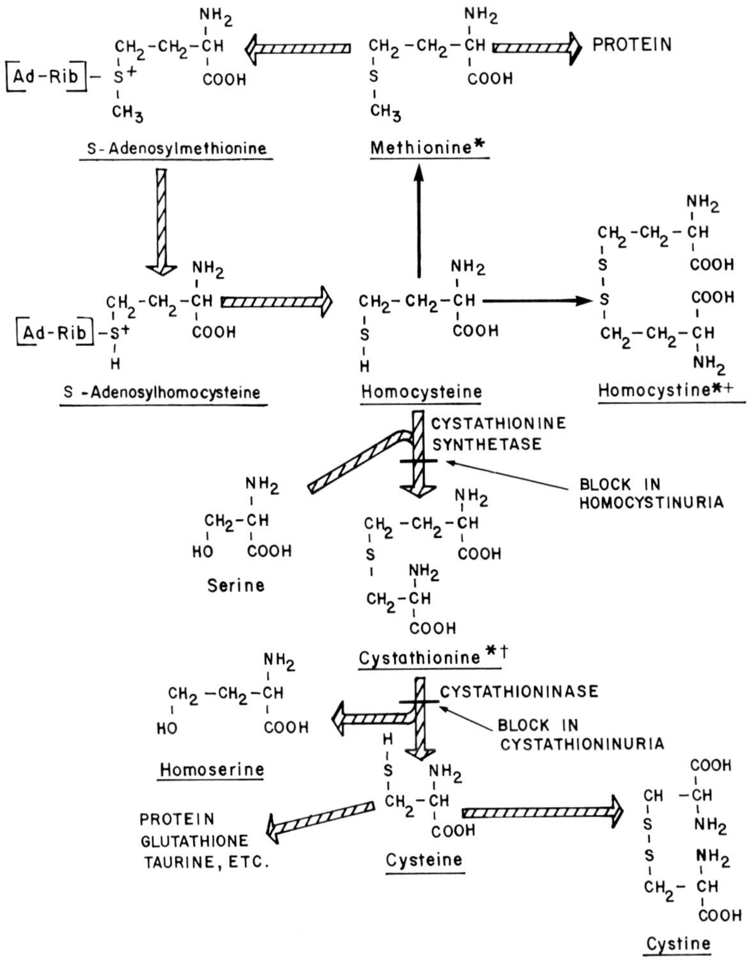

Fig. 20-8. The biochemistry of homocystinuria and cystathioninuria. Normal methionine metabolism (cross-hatched arrows) may be blocked at one of two sites, causing backing up and excretion of preceding compounds (homocysteine appearing as its anhydride, homocystine) (= increased urinary excretion in homocystinuria; + = increased blood levels in homocystinuria; † = increased urinary excretion in cystathioninuria).*

of life, and surviving patients are severely retarded. Several enzyme defects, including a defect in glycine oxidase, are known to be implicated.

A rare and unexplained metabolic error, often associated with mental retardation, is *hypersarcosinemia,* in which sarcosine (N-methylglycine) is raised in the plasma and urine.

Carnosinemia

Carnosinemia is associated with increased plasma levels of β-alanylhistidine dipeptide (carnosine), normally split by an enzyme, carnosinase. Patients with this condition are mentally retarded and frequently have seizures.

Disorders of the Urea Cycle

The combination of ammonia and carbon dioxide to form carbamoyl phosphate and its subsequent conversion to citrulline by combination with ornithine are not yet confirmed in the CNS, the necessary enzymes being absent or of low activity. The remainder of the cycle can be carried out in cerebral tissue.

At least five enzymes in this cycle may be genetically defective (Fig. 20-9), including argininosuccinase,

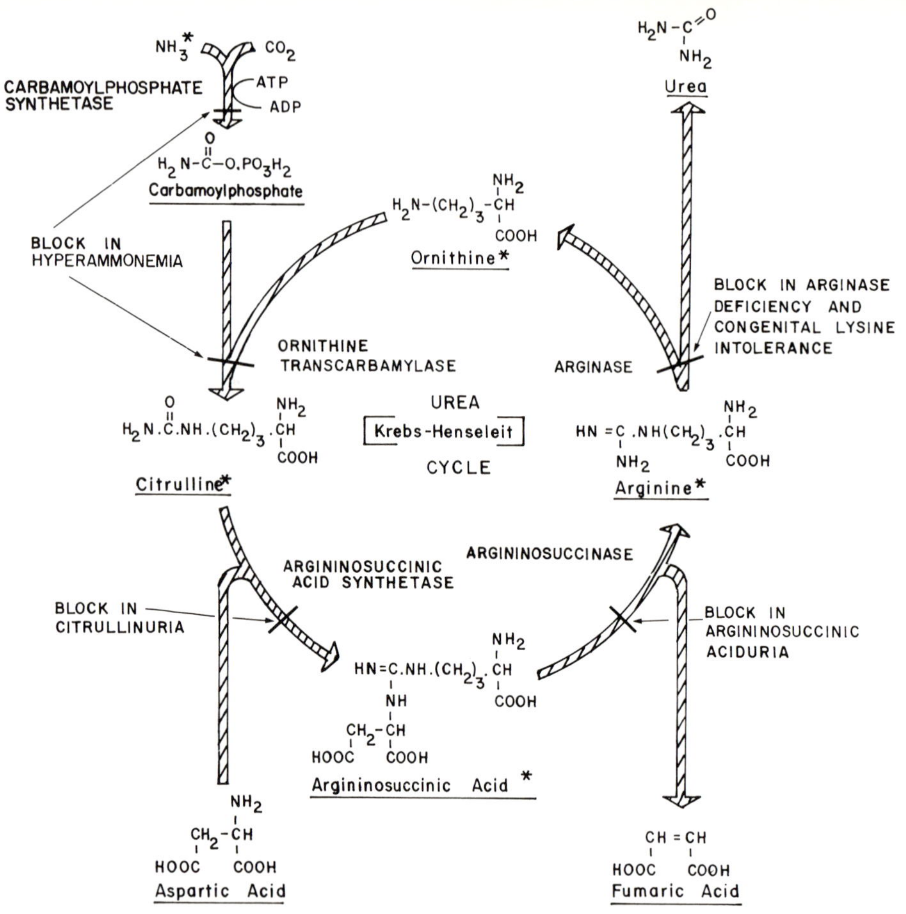

Fig. 20-9. The biochemistry of disorders of the urea cycle (= may be raised in urine and blood, depending on the side of block [ammonia usually raised]). Urea formation normally follows the cross-hatched arrows, but genetically determined blocks may occur at several stages (see text).*

argininosuccinic acid synthetase, ornithine transcarbamylase, carbamoyl phosphate synthetase, and arginase. Intermediate metabolites behind the block are increased in the blood and frequently in the urine, but blood urea is surprisingly normal. Patients have continuously or intermittently raised blood levels of ammonia, which possibly is responsible for the neurological deficit, as in hepatic encephalopathy. In argininosuccinicaciduria, levels of argininosuccinic acid may be higher in CSF than in plasma, and the enzyme defect may be localized or incomplete, especially in view of the adequate formation of urea. Arginase may be inhibited by lysine, and if metabolism of the latter is depressed, as in congenital lysine intolerance, the biochemical features of arginase deficiency appear, with increases in lysine, arginine, and ammonia in the blood. Patients with any of these disorders may show mild to severe mental retardation, and Alzheimer type II astrocytes are found in the CNS.

Possibly related defects are *ornithinemia* (normal urea cycle enzymes but increased serum ammonia), and *saccharopinuria* (block of the main catabolic pathway from lysine to glutaric acid).

Renal Tubular Aminoacidopathies

In *Hartnup disease,* patients often present with mental retardation, cerebellar ataxia, and skin rash. There

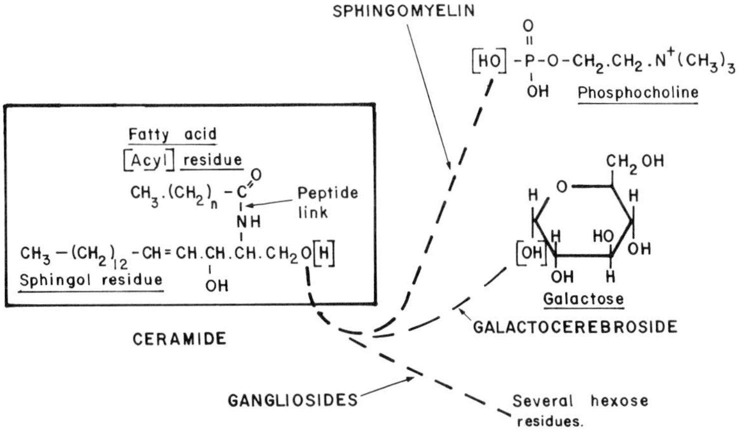

Fig. 20-10. Structure of sphingolipids. All share ceramide (boxed), which is formed from sphingol and a fatty acid. Substituents on the terminal hydroxyl group of ceramide are varied, producing sphingomyelin, cerebroside, or gangliosides.

is massive aminoaciduria, involving only the group of neutral amino acids, in the presence of low or normal blood levels. Since the same transport defect is present in the gut, amino acid absorption (especially tryptophan) is reduced, and there is growth retardation. Many of the symptoms may be due to tryptophan deficiency and lowered levels of nicotinamide, causing pellagra-like features. (The very rare genetic blocks of tryptophan metabolism also show nicotinamide deficiency.)

In *Lowe's syndrome* (oculocerebrorenal syndrome), patients show progressive renal tubular defects, congenital cataracts, hypotonia, and mental retardation.

Cystinuria has been reported in association with mental retardation, mongolism, and limb-girdle muscular dystrophy.

Renal tyrosinosis was mentioned previously.

DISORDERS OF SPHINGOLIPID METABOLISM (SPHINGOLIPIDOSES)

Structure and Metabolism of Brain Lipids

Major Groups

The sphingolipids are based on sphingol (sphingosine), a long-chain alcohol synthesized in the brain from glucose and serine. Sphingol has a terminal hydroxyl group, through which it may form linkages with organic phosphates or hexose derivatives, and an amino group, through which it forms an amide linkage with a long-chain fatty acid; the combination of sphingol and a fatty acid residue is ceramide (Fig. 20-10). The fatty acid (acyl) residue varies from 16 to 26 C, but is frequently either stearic acid (18 C) or lignoceric acid (24 C). Sphingol and the sphingolipids occur in all tissues, and genetic errors of ceramide formation are not known (perhaps they are lethal in utero).

Phospholipids (Fig. 20-11) consist of a diglyceride (glycerol with two acyl residues) combined with phosphate derivatives of choline, ethanolamine, serine, or inositol. If one of the acyl residues is substituted by a β-unsaturated fatty aldehyde, the compound is a plasmalogen. Free (unesterified) cholesterol is another major brain lipid. Metabolic errors involving CNS phospholipids or cholesterol are extremely rare.

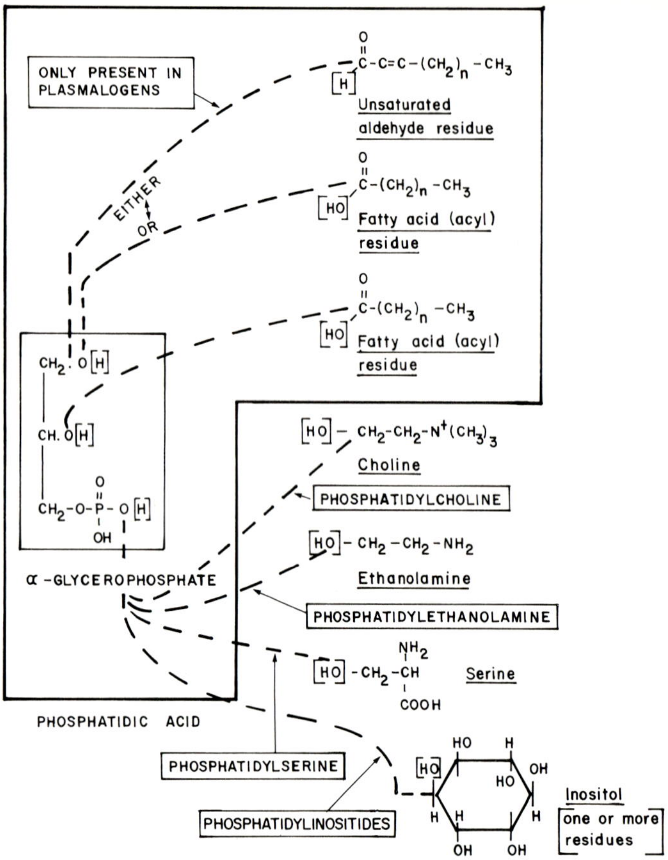

Fig. 20-11. Structure of phospholipids. All share a nucleus of α-glycerophosphate and either two acyl or an acyl and an aldehyde residue (phosphatidic acid, boxed). Various substituents in a hydroxyl group of the phosphate moiety produce several types of phospholipids.

Structure and Synthesis of Sphingolipids

Sphingolipids are derived from ceramide by substitution in the terminal hydroxyl group. If the substituent is phosphatidylcholine, the resulting group of lipids (which differ according to the acyl residue) are the *sphingomyelins,* which occur in high concentration in the CNS. If the substituent is a single hexose residue, the compound is a *cerebroside* – glycocerebroside in most parts of the body, but specifically galactocerebroside in the CNS. If the substituent is a chain of hexose or hexose-derived residues, substances collectively known as *gangliosides* are formed in the brain. In other tissues the most important such substance found is globoside from the red cell envelope. (Some authors restrict the use of the term *ganglioside* to compounds that include sialic acid and would exclude globoside.)

In neutral gangliosides the substituent residues include glucose, galactose, and N-acetylgalactosamine; in acidic gangliosides, N-acetylneuraminic acid (sialic acid) is added to these. Gangliosides may be designated by the letter G, followed by an alphanumeric subscript (Fig. 20-12). The first part of the subscript is M, D, or T, denoting respectively one, two, or three sialic acid residues. The second is 1, 2, or 3; 1 denoting four neutral hexose residues, 2 denoting three, and 3 denoting two (if there is only one residue the compound is a cerebroside, and sialic acid is not present).

In cerebrosides, but apparently not in gangliosides, the hexose residue may be conjugated with sulfate, forming sulfatides (sulfated cerebrosides) that show metachromasia with suitable staining techniques. Acidic gangliosides may also show metachromasia, but of less marked degree.

The CNS freely synthesizes sphingomyelin, cerebrosides, and gangliosides, appropriate groups being transferred to ceramide by a nucleotide carrier – cytosine diphosphate for choline, cytosine monophosphate for sialic acid, and uridine diphosphate for other hexose derivatives (glucose, galactose, and N-acetylgalactosamine) – with the aid of appropriate enzymes.

Breakdown of Sphingolipids in the Sphingolipidoses

Despite the number of enzymes involved, known genetic errors of sphingolipid metabolism seem rarely to involve the formation of sphingolipids, but rather

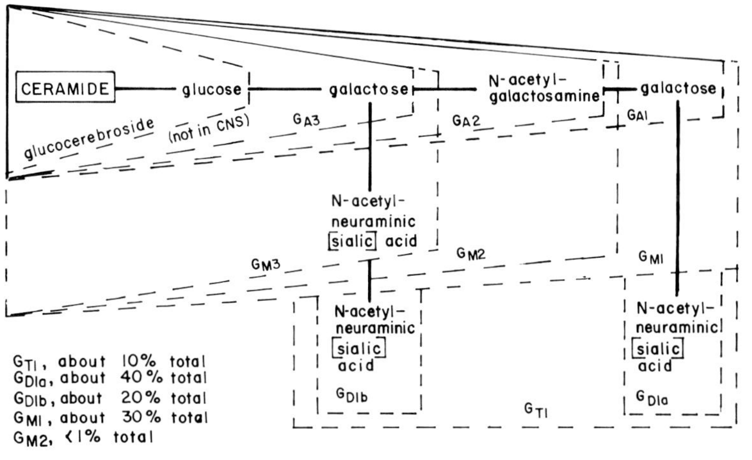

Fig. 20-12. The structure and nomenclature of gangliosides. For explanation, see text.

their degradation by hydrolysis, normally carried out by enzymes (collectively termed hydrolases), one or more of which appear to be deficient. Gangliosides are the most frequently affected, breakdown involving the sequential removal of hexose or hexose-derived residues. Failure of breakdown leads to ganglioside storage in the CNS, which may be an isolated phenomenon, may occur in association with visceral (especially reticuloendothelial) storage of neutral ceramide hexosides (especially globoside), or may occur in association with abnormalities of acid mucopolysaccharide metabolism in other tissues.

Acid mucopolysaccharides consist of very long chains of hexose or hexose-derived residues, including two present in gangliosides (galactose and N-acetylgalactosamine), as well as N-acetylglucosamine and two acidic derivatives (glucuronic and iduronic acids). Mucopolysaccharides may also be sulfated, making them particularly acidic and metachromatic.

Where defects of ganglioside and mucopolysaccharide metabolism are associated, it is tempting to look for deficiency of a single enzyme (hydrolase) that might account for the failure of breakdown of both components. However, this has yet to be fully confirmed for any of these diseases. Enzyme chemistry has become extremely complicated since recognition that enzyme defects may be total or partial, quantitative or qualitative, localized or generalized, and that isoenzymes exist that catalyze the same reaction, but often at different rates and under different conditions. In some diseases, no enzyme deficiency has yet been defined.

Classification

Classification of the sphingolipid disorders is difficult and is in the process of active change. The ultimate classification will presumably depend on a definition of the defective or deficient enzyme (or enzymes), and the sites of this deficiency (which need not involve all tissues). This objective is not within sight, and even when an enzyme has been declared defective, work is still in progress to determine which of its isoenzymes is affected, how severe the deficiency is (not always 100%), and which tissues are affected. Lack of β-galactosidase activity has been associated with distinct disease entities, clearly implying differences in the type and location of deficiencies that have yet to be defined.

Currently, therefore, these diseases are classified largely on the chemical nature of the stored materials in various tissues. Unfortunately, this material may vary from tissue to tissue, is frequently mixed with other components, may be removed inadvertently by techniques now in use in routine laboratories, or may not be detected by generally available staining or other methods. Many histological techniques are imprecise; lipid stains stain most compound lipids, even if with varying intensity; the PAS reaction stains glycolipids irrespective of their chemical constitution; and the alcian blue reaction determines acidic radicals of varying strength, according to the pH at which the reaction is carried out.

However, by a combination of the *clinical features* of the disease, the *type and location of morphological changes,* the *histochemical reactions,* and the *enzyme deficiency (where known),* it has been possible to define groups pragmatically and isolate some of the more common entities. A small group (dysmyelinating diseases) is apparently associated with quantitative defects in the assembly of myelin lamellae, sometimes with prominent storage of metabolites in CNS white matter, but lack of storage in neurons and late (probably secondary) involvement of gray matter. These will be considered separately on p. 390 et seq. The following comments apply only to the storage diseases, in which a prominent feature is the retention of metabolites within neurons of the central and

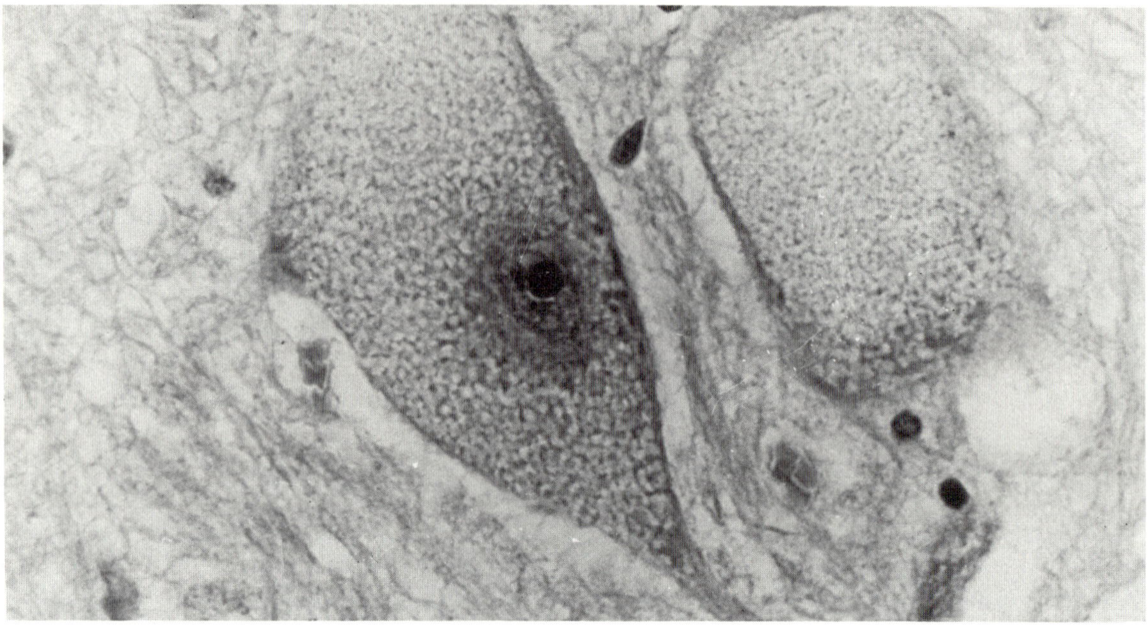

Fig. 20-13. Neuron distended with glycolipid (anterior horn cell in Tay-Sachs disease). (H & E, ×750.)

peripheral nervous systems, within other cells (especially of the reticuloendothelial system), or both. Three major groups may be distinguished.

Sphingolipid Storage Diseases (Lipidoses)

Sphingolipids are stored in large quantities either in neurons or viscera or occasionally in both. A classic example of CNS lipid storage is Tay-Sachs disease; Neimann-Pick disease is a classic example of predominantly visceral storage. Clinically, morphologically, and to some extent histochemically similar is a group of usually postinfantile diseases, in which lipofuscin and a colorless substance related to it (ceroid) are stored, usually in neurons, with less in the viscera. Although the stored material is not clearly a sphingolipid, the clinicopathological resemblances are very close, and, until recently, such cases were considered as juvenile or adult variants of Tay-Sachs disease.

Mucopolysaccharidoses

The constant feature in the mucopolysaccharidoses is the presence of excessive amounts of mucopolysaccharide (glycosaminoglycan) in tissue and urine. Three types are usually associated with mental retardation, and in two others it occurs occasionally. Neuronal damage correlates with retardation and consists of the storage of mixed gangliosides, not of mucopolysaccharide. Additional pathological changes may be seen in the CNS because of mucopolysaccharide accumulation in mesenchymal tissues.

Mucolipidoses

In the mucolipidoses, a very rare group of disorders, ganglioside is stored in neurons, ganglioside or sulfated cerebroside is stored in viscera, and mucopolysaccharide accumulates in the mesenchymal tissues and urine. In two excessively rare varieties, hexose residues are derivatives of either fucose or mannose, normally present only in trace amounts.

Morphology and Histochemistry of Lipid Storage Diseases

It is not necessary to consider morphological changes in these sphingolipid disorders disease by disease. One or more of four groups of changes (effects of lipid or mucopolysaccharide storage in the CNS or extraneural tissues respectively) can be assembled, to derive the morphology from knowledge of the nature and site of storage.

Neuronal Lipid Storage

Neurons, if involved at all, are affected in all areas, including the PNS, though with marked regional variations. Cortical pyramidal cells are usually severely affected, followed with decreasing frequency by the large cells of the basal ganglia and thalamus, the motoneurons (Fig. 20-13) and large reticular neurons of the brain stem and cord, and the basal pontine cells. Purkinje's cells are inconstantly affected, and storage is difficult to detect in small cells, especially those of the internal granular layer. Involved neurons are moderately to severely enlarged and rounded, show

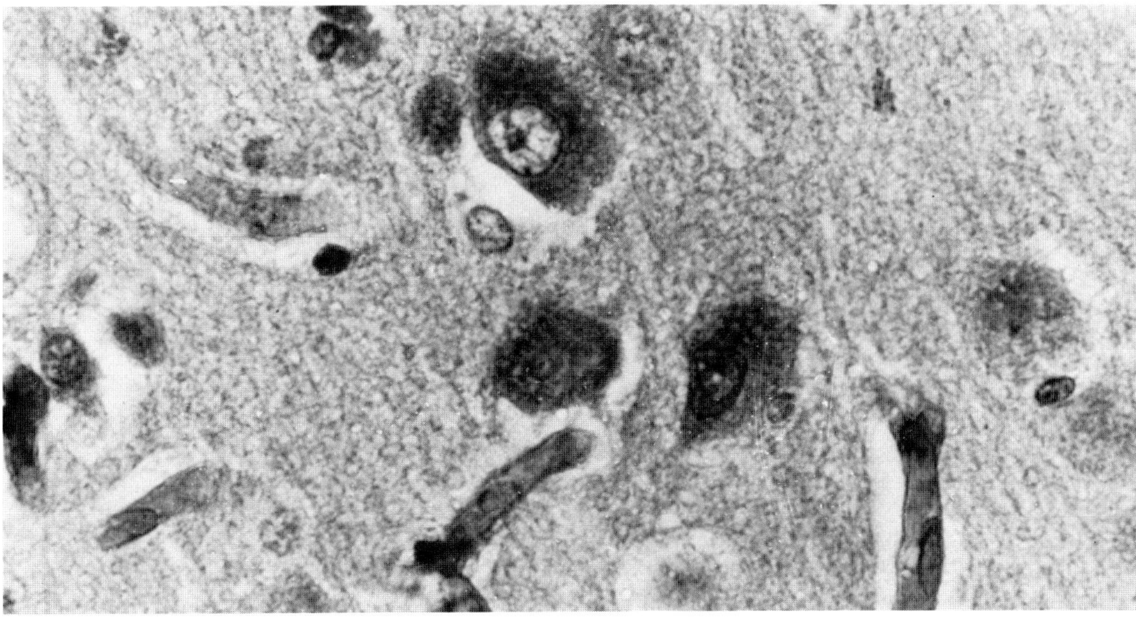

Fig. 20-14. Neurons distended with glycolipid (cortex in Tay-Sachs disease). (PAS, frozen section, X750.)

partial or complete loss of Nissl bodies, and an eccentric nucleus, often in the axon hillock.

Much of the cell is occupied by granular or vacuolar deposits, staining of which depends on the method of processing. During paraffin-embedding, much lipid is dissolved out, unless, as is often the case, it is protein-bound. Thus, frozen section is advisable in histochemical investigation (Fig. 20-14). *Ganglioside,* the most frequently present, is PAS-positive (hexose component), reacts with stains for compound lipids (Luxol Fast Blue, Sudan Black), but only weakly with those for simple lipids (Scharlach R, and others), and if rich in sialic acid, is slightly metachromatic and stains with alcian blue. *Sphingomyelin* stains with compound lipid stains, but is negative with the others, as it lacks hexose derivatives. *Ceroid-lipofuscin* may show some pigmentation in the unstained state, is autofluorescent, PAS-positive, and demonstrable by lipid stains, but is negative with alcian blue.

The stored material may extend into at least the major dendrites and is occasionally seen in astrocytes. Electron microscopy in most lipidoses shows material in membrane-bound vesicles, possibly derived from lysosomes, in the form of lipid lamellae of varying configuration. In ceroid-lipofuscin, storage material may not be membrane-bound. Although neurons appear remarkably tolerant to distention, they finally degenerate and die, and other CNS changes appear to be largely secondary.

Early in the disease, while neurons are still present and enlarged, brain weight is normal or even slightly high, and only minimal fibrillary gliosis is present. As neurons progressively disappear, there is a secondary loss of their axons and myelin sheaths; a few gitter cells may be seen, especially in the white matter, containing myelin breakdown products (see Chap. 21). There is astrocytic hyperplasia and hypertrophy, with moderate to severe fibrillary gliosis, often seen

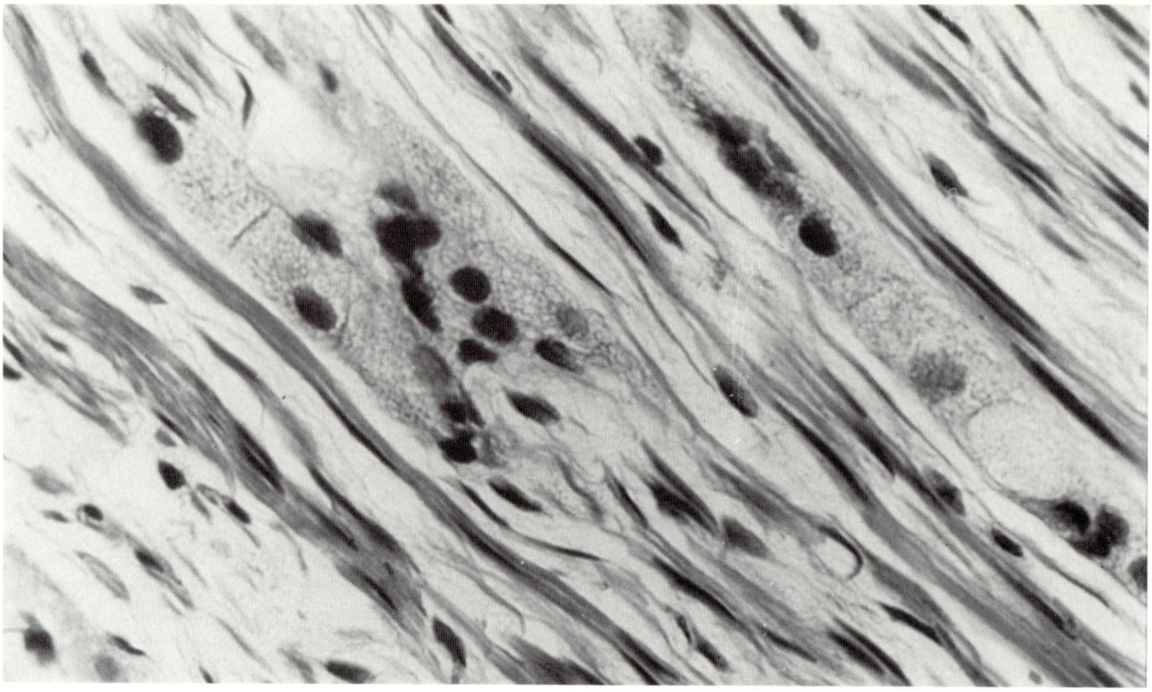

Fig. 20-15. Neurons of the myenteric plexus distended with ganglioside (Tay-Sachs disease, appendix biopsy). (H & E, X750.)

more in the white than in the gray matter. The brain becomes shrunken and reduced in weight, the sulci slightly widened, and the ventricles symmetrically dilated. The cerebellum may be less affected than other areas.

Extraneural Lipid Storage

Apart from PNS neurons (Fig. 20-15), most visceral storage is in large macrophages of the reticuloendothelial system, although parenchymal cells, such as those of the liver and kidney, may occasionally be involved. The liver and spleen are frequently enlarged and the lymph nodes prominent and firm, although generalized lymphadenopathy is rarely severe.

Macrophages of the spleen, lymph nodes, bone marrow, and liver (Kupffer's cells) are converted into foam cells, about 20 to 100μ in diameter, usually with a vacuolar (Fig. 20-16) or granular appearance, although their cytoplasm occasionally appears striated. Enlargement may cause atrophy of adjacent parenchymal elements, such as lymphocytes in the spleen and nodes, and cords of hepatic cells. Staining reactions are generally as in CNS neurons, although the glycolipids stored are not gangliosides but other ceramide-hexose derivatives, which do not give a positive alcian blue reaction because they do not contain sialic acid.

Extraneural Mucopolysaccharide Storage

Abnormalities of mucopolysaccharide metabolism are associated not only with increased concentrations in tissue and urine, but also with skeletal and soft-tissue malformations, the pathogenesis of which is not clear. Periosteal and bony thickening, with persistence of primary (woven) bone, leads to the typical facies associated with Hurler's syndrome (gargoylism) and its variants and often causes deafness and persistent nasal discharge. Vertebral involvement may be associated with various abnormalities, including "beaking" of the bodies, especially in the lumbar region. The cardiac valve rings and cusps may be thickened by accumulation of mucopolysaccharide, both intracellularly and extracellularly, and changes may extend into the aorta. Thickening may also be seen in the perichondrium, around joints, and in the interstitial tissue of muscle and peripheral nerves. There is an increased mucopolysaccharide content in renal convoluted tubules.

In the mucolipidoses (rather than the mucopolysaccharidoses), more severe visceral involvement may be seen, with accumulation of mucopolysaccharide in cardiac muscle, hepatic parenchymal cells (Fig. 20-17), and epithelial cells of the renal glomeruli. Because of the difficulty in retaining mucopolysaccharide in sections, visceral accumulation may be apparent as vacuoles that often fail to give any positive staining reactions, and its presence before processing is merely inferred.

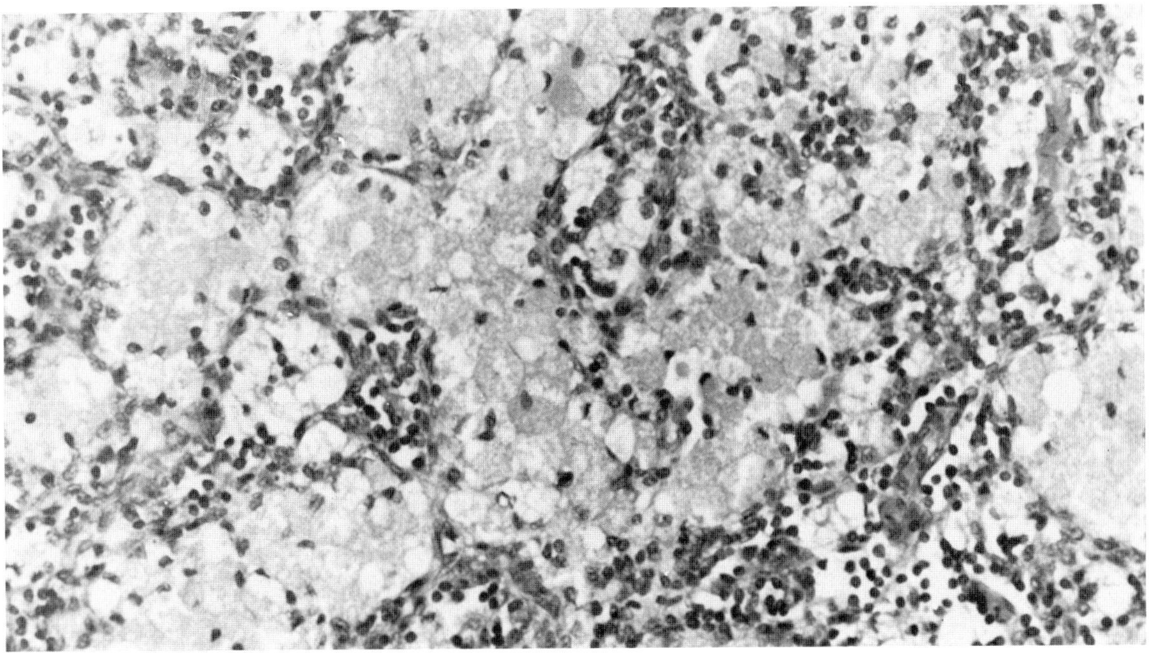

Fig. 20-16. Enlarged lymph node, showing distended foam cells (Niemann-Pick disease, sphingomyelin removed in processing). (H & E, ×750.)

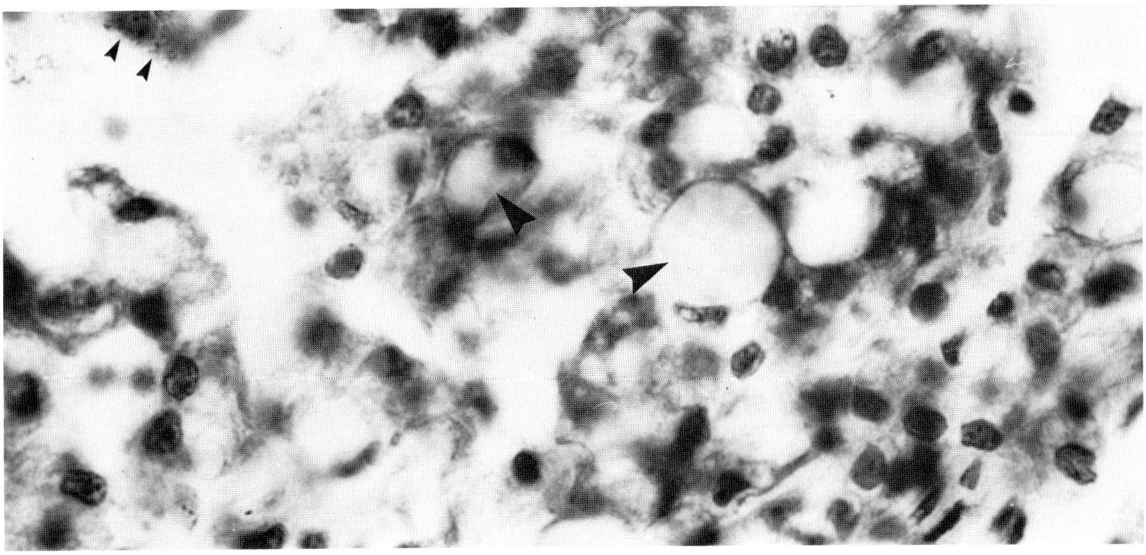

Fig. 20-17. G_{M1} gangliosidosis, in which acid mucopolysaccharide is stored in liver parenchymal cells (large arrows). Stained material in Kupffer's cells (small arrows) is much more stable and is probably glycolipid. (Alcian blue, ×750.)

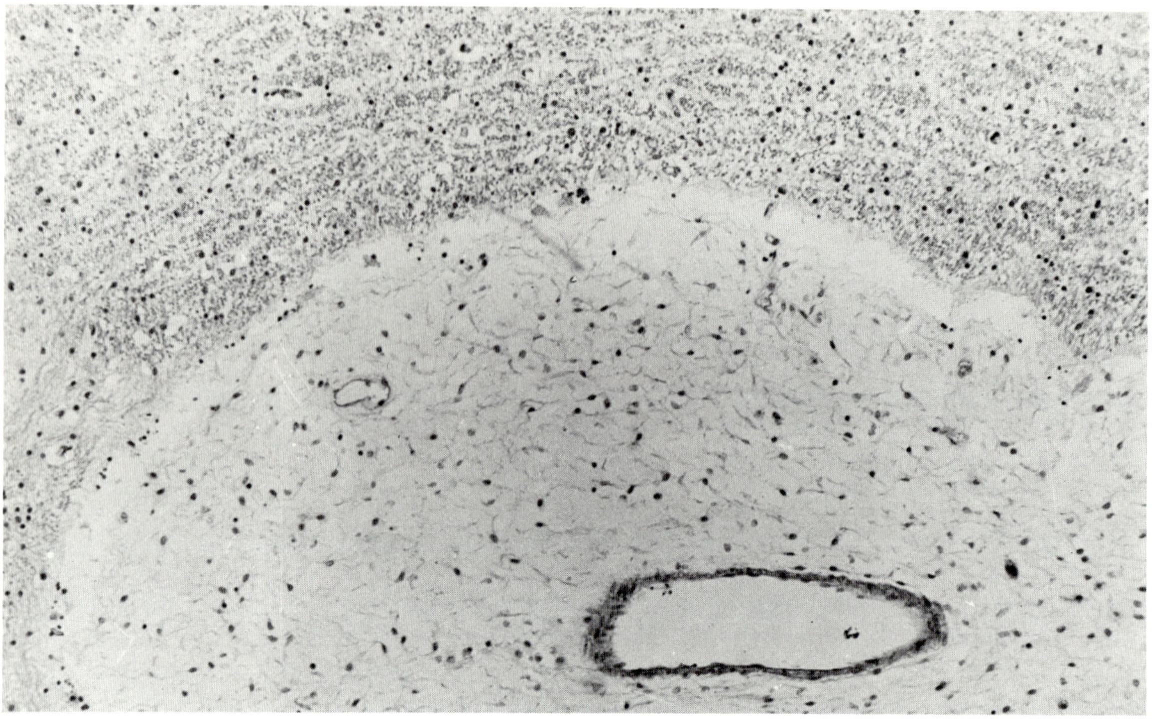

Fig. 20-18. Hurler's syndrome. Section of cerebral hemisphere, showing extreme dilatation of perivascular spaces in white matter. (H & E, ×115.)

Central Nervous System Mucopolysaccharide Storage

Mucopolysaccharide storage in the CNS involves mesenchymal (vascular) and meningeal tissues. The meninges are thickened and opaque, and there may be some hydrocephalus, presumably due to obstruction of CSF flow. Leptomeningeal cells are hypertrophied, often appear free in the subarachnoid spaces, and contain mucopolysaccharide. This change extends along perforating vessels into the brain and may cause widening of the perivascular spaces (Fig. 20-18), apparent on gross examination as small cysts, most noticeable in the hemispheric white matter.

Both in CNS and elsewhere, mucopolysaccharides are particularly labile and difficult to retain in processed tissue. Fibroblasts and other cells frequently appear vacuolated, but do not give mucopolysaccharide staining reactions, and even in frozen sections there is considerable loss and rapid diffusion, so that localization is often in doubt. When tissue is better preserved by special fixatives, mucopolysaccharide gives a positive alcian blue reaction and negative reactions for lipid. It often appears as granules in mesenchymal (Fig. 20-19) and meningeal cells, with diffuse staining of varying intensity, both intracellularly and extracellularly.

Enzyme Deficiencies in the Lipid Storage Diseases

Enzyme deficiencies are not necessarily total, and in many conditions there is a spectrum of disease, acute infantile cases being associated with virtually complete deficiency and juvenile or adult cases with a lesser degree of deficiency, sometimes localized to certain tissues.

Tay-Sachs Disease (G_{M2}-Gangliosidosis)

Tay-Sachs disease (G_{M2}-gangliosidosis) is an infantile (occasionally congenital) disease, with neuronal storage of sphingolipid and occasional involvement of other tissues such as the spleen and liver. Electron microscopy shows concentrically laminated bodies in the neurons, bounded by membranes and about 1.0 to 1.5μ in diameter (membranous cytoplasmic bodies). Chemical examination shows a marked increase in ganglioside G_{M2} in the CNS, with lesser increases in the spleen, liver, and renal tubular cells. Normally, G_{M2} is less than 1% of brain ganglioside, but may be as high as 90% in this condition. Phospholipid, cerebroside, and cholesterol are also increased in the neurons.

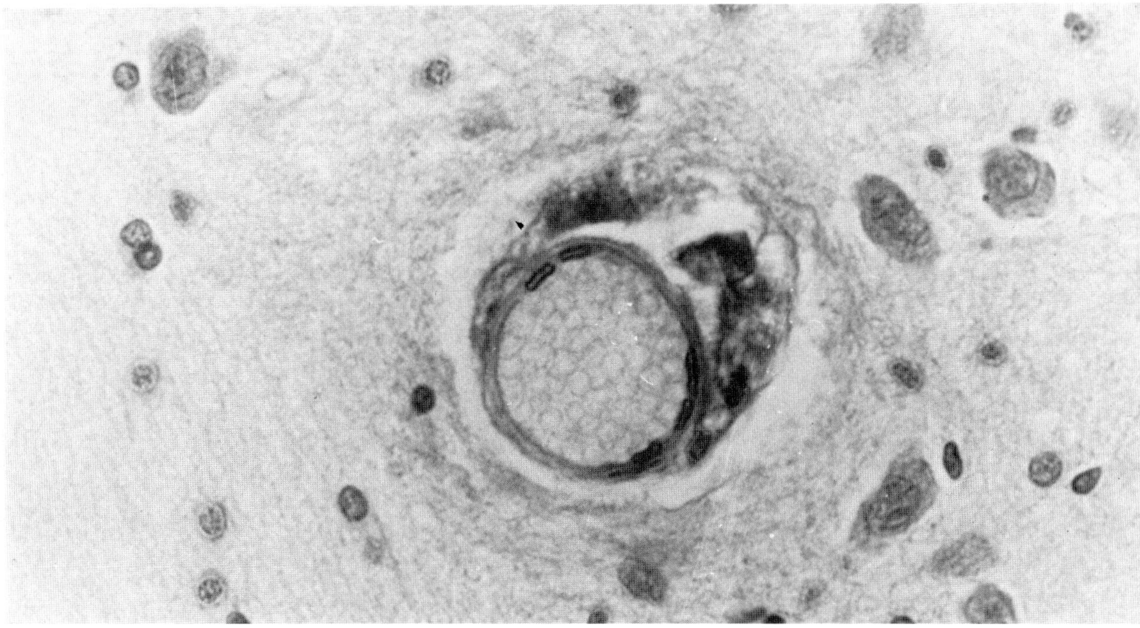

Fig. 20-19. Hurler's syndrome, showing acid mucopolysaccharide in adventitial cells of small vessel. Much of the material is lost in almost any type of processing. (Alcian blue, X750.)

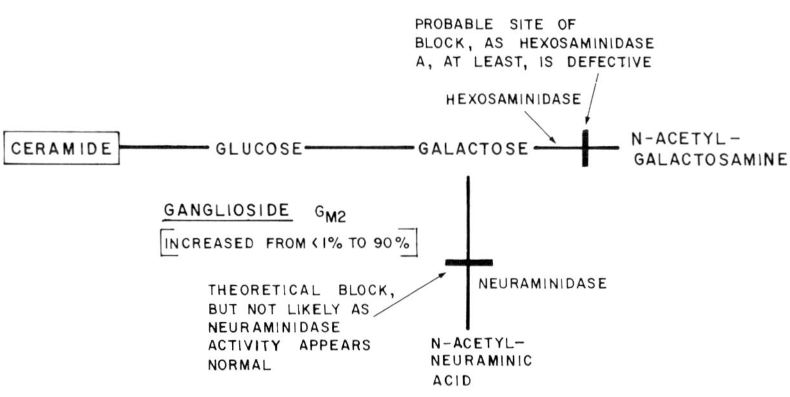

Fig. 20-20. Postulated biochemical defect in Tay-Sachs disease (deficiency of hexosaminidase A).

There is probably a deficiency of hexosaminidase (Fig. 20-20), which has two isoenzymes (A and B); isoenzyme A is absent in cases restricted to the CNS, and both isoenzymes in cases with visceral involvement (globoside being the major visceral sphingolipid). Partial deficiency of hexosaminidase A is associated with a late infantile or juvenile variant. The enzyme can be estimated in amniotic fluid for prenatal diagnosis, and after birth, specialized laboratories can demonstrate enzyme deficiency in blood cells or fibroblasts.

A more presumptive diagnosis depends on cerebral, rectal, or appendiceal biopsy, with identification of ganglioside storage in neurons. This is not specific for Tay-Sachs disease unless the ganglioside is identified as G_{M2}. Rare examples of isolated CNS storage of other gangliosides (G_{D3}, G_{DIa} or G_{M3}) are known.

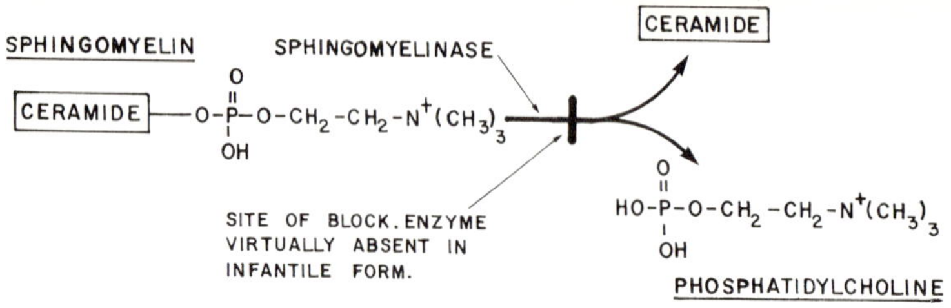

Fig. 20-21. Postulated biochemical defect in Niemann-Pick disease (deficiency of sphingomyelinase).

The last is of interest as showing deficiency of a biosynthetic enzyme (G_{M3}-UDP-N-acetylgalactosaminyl transferase) rather than hydrolase deficiency as in the other gangliosidoses.

Niemann-Pick Disease

In typical Niemann-Pick disease, there is a sphingomyelinase deficiency (Fig. 20-21), so that phosphatidylcholine cannot be split off from sphingomyelin. In infantile cases (which are a minority), the enzyme is absent, and there is both visceral and neuronal storage of sphingomyelin, with mental retardation. Patients with late infantile or later onset show incomplete enzyme deficiency and usually only visceral involvement. Electron microscopy shows concentric lipid lamellae resembling those seen in Tay-Sachs disease.

In variants of Niemann-Pick disease, visceral histiocytes are seen that contain granules staining a deep grayish-blue with Giemsa stains (sea-blue histiocytes); the enzyme defect is unknown. The stored material appears to be largely sphingomyelin, but a faint PAS-positive reaction indicates admixture. These variant cases may also be infantile or juvenile and seen to be associated with abnormalities of vertical eye movement.

Diagnosis of Niemann-Pick disease is by visceral or brain biopsy with demonstration of sphingomyelin or, better, by estimation of sphingomyelinase activity in leukocytes or skin fibroblasts.

Gaucher's Disease

Only the acute infantile form of Gaucher's disease involves the CNS, and the disease is more commonly confined to visceral (largely reticuloendothelial) storage. Storage cells are 20 to 100μ across, and though some appear granular or vacuolar, others show a striated appearance. The stored material is largely protein-bound glucocerebroside (kerasin), the enzyme glucocerebrosidase being absent (in the infantile form) or reduced. Since the normal CNS cerebroside contains galactose, not glucose, it is possible that, in the rare infantile cases, the glucocerebroside present in the CNS derives from gangliosides.

Diagnosis depends on biopsy and, if possible, enzyme determination in leukocytes or skin fibroblasts.

Lactosylceramidosis is an even rarer storage disease involving the CNS, with storage of a dihexoside, ceramide-glucose-galactose. This is one of the conditions with a deficiency of β-galactosidase.

Fabry's Disease

Fabry's disease is a rare condition that usually presents at puberty with multiple skin lesions (angiokeratomas) and storage of ceramide trihexoside in reticuloendothelial cells. The stored material is ceramide-glucose-galactose-galactose, and ceramide trihexosidase is absent or reduced. The CNS is rarely involved.

Ceroid-Lipofuscinosis

As already stated, ceroid-lipofuscinosis is not a sphingolipid storage disease, but is clinically and often morphologically indistinguishable from such diseases.

Most postinfantile variants of Tay-Sachs disease are now reclassified into this group, stored materials being autofluorescent and PAS-positive lipids resistant to paraffin-embedding. Ceroid is nonpigmented, lipofuscin is golden-yellow or brownish in color, and the two are present in varying proportions. The enzyme deficiency is unknown. Depending on the age at onset, mental retardation or dementia may occur. Electron microscopy shows bodies that have been described as "curvilinear profiles," "fingerprints," or "granular osmiophilic deposits." The viscera may be involved in a few cases. Neuronal destruction and distention are less than in Tay-Sachs disease, and secondary changes are therefore less marked.

Mucopolysaccharidoses

Some of the mucopolysaccharidoses are associated with mental retardation and neuronal storage of ganglioside. Retarded patients usually have either type I (gargoylism, or Hurler's syndrome), type II (Hunter's syndrome), or type III (Sanfilippo's syndrome). Type II is unusual in that it is a sex-linked rather than an autosomal recessive disease. The skeletal changes are most marked in type I and least in type III, and there may be cardiac involvement. The neuronal stored material appears to be largely mixed gangliosides, but other lipids are also present. Neuronal destruction and secondary changes are

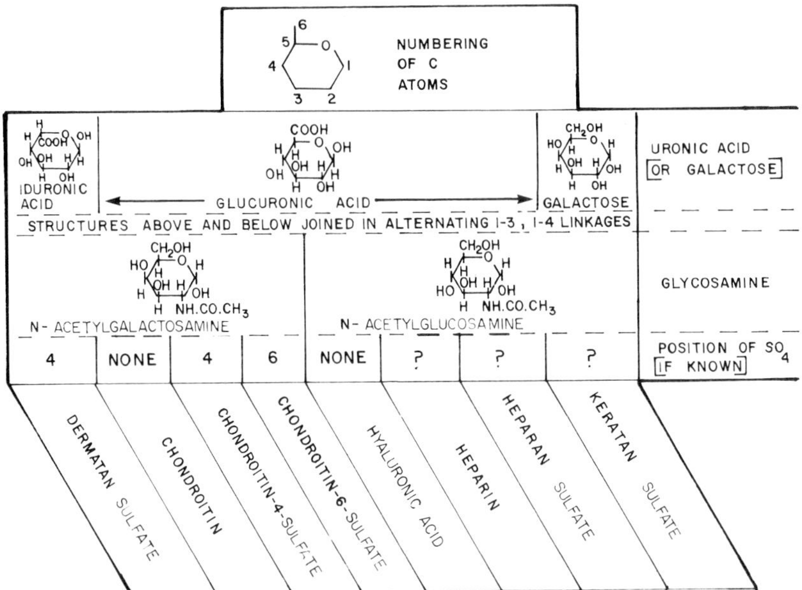

	DERMATAN SULFATE	CHONDROITIN	CHONDROITIN-4-SULFATE	CHONDROITIN-6-SULFATE	HYALURONIC ACID	HEPARIN	HEPARAN SULFATE	KERATAN SULFATE
NORMAL URINE	(+)		+	+			(+)	
HURLER	++		+	+			++	
HUNTER	++		+	+			++	
SANFILIPPO	(+)		+	+			++	
MORQUIO	(+)		+	+			(+)	++
SCHEIE	++		+	+			(+)	

Fig. 20-22. Structure of acid mucopolysaccharides and urinary excretion in normal persons and patients with mucopolysaccharidoses. Urinary excretion (if any) is graded semi-quantitatively from (+) to ++.

usually mild or moderate. Electron microscopy shows membrane-bound granules, with transverse striations (zebra bodies). The mucopolysaccharide (Fig. 20-22) stored in extraneural tissue and meninges is largely dermatan and heparan sulfates in types I and II and heparan sulfate alone in type III. Diagnosis is largely clinical.

Determination of urinary mucopolysaccharide must be quantitative, since urine normally contains chondroitin 4- and chondroitin 6-sulfate, with small amounts of dermatan and heparan sulfates as well. In mucopolysaccharidosis, total excretion is increased about tenfold, and while chondroitin sulfates are still present, they are now minor components, the major ones being those previously listed.

The enzyme deficiencies involved are generally unknown, although in some cases, β-galactosidase is reduced. Tissue culture suggests that hydrolase deficiencies may be specific to each type, since in fibroblast cultures from one variant, serum from another may correct the metabolic defect; work in this area is still in an experimental stage. It is not clear whether the same enzyme deficit prevents normal mucopolysaccharide and ganglioside metabolism, whether separate but related enzymes are involved, or even whether accumulation of mucopolysaccharide in the neurons might cause lysosomal activation and nonspecific lipid accumulation.

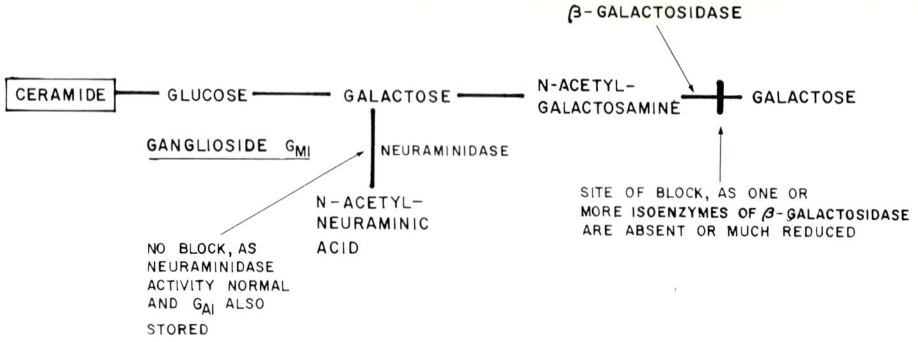

Fig. 20-23. Postulated biochemical deficiency in G_{M1} gangliosidosis (deficiency of β-galactosidase). (G_{A1} = asialoganglioside, lacking NANA.)

Mucolipidoses

The best-known of the mucolipidoses, G_{M1} gangliosidosis, usually presents in infancy with skeletal changes as in Hurler's syndrome, congestive cardiac failure, and rapid neurological deterioration. Neurons are distended by G_{M1} and asialo-derivatives, and the viscera store G_{M1} and keratan sulfate. All three isoenzymes (A, B, and C) of β-galactosidase are usually absent (Fig. 20-23). However, in a mild variety of the disease, mainly confined to the CNS, isoenzyme A is preserved.

Rarer mucolipidoses are associated with α-fucosidase deficit and storage of fusose-containing glycolipids in the CNS and liver; or with deficiency of α-mannosidase with similar features; or with deficiency of all isoenzymes of arylsulfatase (A, B, C), with storage of ganglioside in neurons, sulfated cerebroside in the white matter, and sulfated cerebroside and mucopolysaccharide extraneurally (these latter cases are related to metachromatic leukodystrophy, which is discussed below).

Laboratory diagnosis depends on analysis of biopsied material, tissue culture, and other methods available only in specialized laboratories.

Leukodystrophies

Although sphingolipidoses, the leukodystrophies are morphologically distinct, involving primarily the white matter of the CNS (and less obviously, the PNS) and unaccompanied by significant neuronal or visceral storage. The principal defect appears to be that myelin is not adequately formed or maintained *(dysmyelination).* These diseases differ pathogenetically from the demyelinating (myelinoclastic) conditions considered in the next chapter, in which normally formed myelin is destroyed. The failure of proper myelin formation is most obvious in the hemispheric white matter and progressively less apparent in the cerebellum, brain stem, cord, and PNS. Subcortical arcuate fibers may be relatively normal. Axons survive without a myelin sheath for varying periods, but ultimately are reduced in number, and there is diffuse fibrillary gliosis, with considerable firmness of the brain, symmetrical ventricular dilatation, and thinning of white matter.

Since axon loss and secondary degenerative changes in the gray matter are late, the onset of mental retardation and epilepsy is delayed relative to onset in other sphingolipidoses. It is not clear whether the disease primarily involves the myelin sheath or its parent oligodendroglial cell. In some cases, oligodendroglia appear fewer, but this is difficult to assess even in normal infancy, since there are intermediate forms between astrocytes and oligodendroglia, and the number of oligodendroglia varies with the degree of myelination from region to region.

Krabbe's Disease (Globoid Leukodystrophy)

Krabbe's disease occurs in young infants. There is little or no myelination in the hemispheres, except in the subcortical fibers, and no accumulation of sudanophilic breakdown products. Astrocytic hypertrophy and fibrillary gliosis in the white matter are associated with clusters of globoid cells in recently affected areas; these tend to disappear later. The round multinucleate globoid and smaller epithelioid cells are often perivascular. They contain intensely PAS-positive (Fig. 20-24) material, which also stains as lipid. Electron microscopy shows cytoplasmic stacks of single and paired lamellae that appear to be almost pure galactocerebroside (normal CNS cerebroside). Since total galactocerebroside in the white matter is not raised, it seems that normal quantities are synthesized but fail to become incorporated in myelin. A deficiency of enzyme (galactocerebroside β-galactosidase) allows the material to accumulate.

The globoid cells are presumably derived from macrophages. In experimental changes produced by injections of galactocerebroside, storage cells show microvilli and cell bridges, suggesting that cell fusion might occur. Galactocerebroside is said to be stored in oligodendroglial cells and astrocytes, but these do not fuse. Minor involvement of the PNS may occur, with occasional segmental demyelination and typical inclusions in Schwann's cells and histocytes.

Metachromatic Leukodystrophy

In addition to the generalized morphological features, in metachromatic leukodystrophy there is both intracellular and extracellular white matter storage of sulfatide (cerebroside sulfate) in spherical structures, 30 to 40μ in diameter. Stored material (Fig. 20-25)

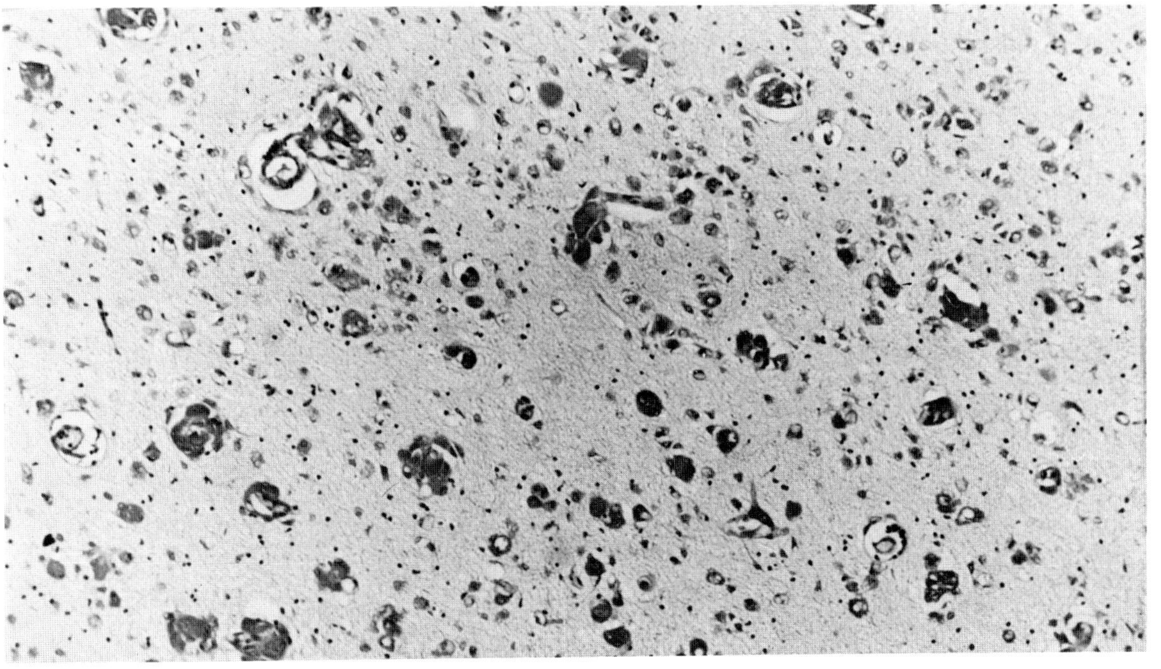

Fig. 20-24. Section showing stored material in the white matter in Krabbe's disease (globoid leukodystrophy). Note the characteristic globoid cells. (PAS, ×115.)

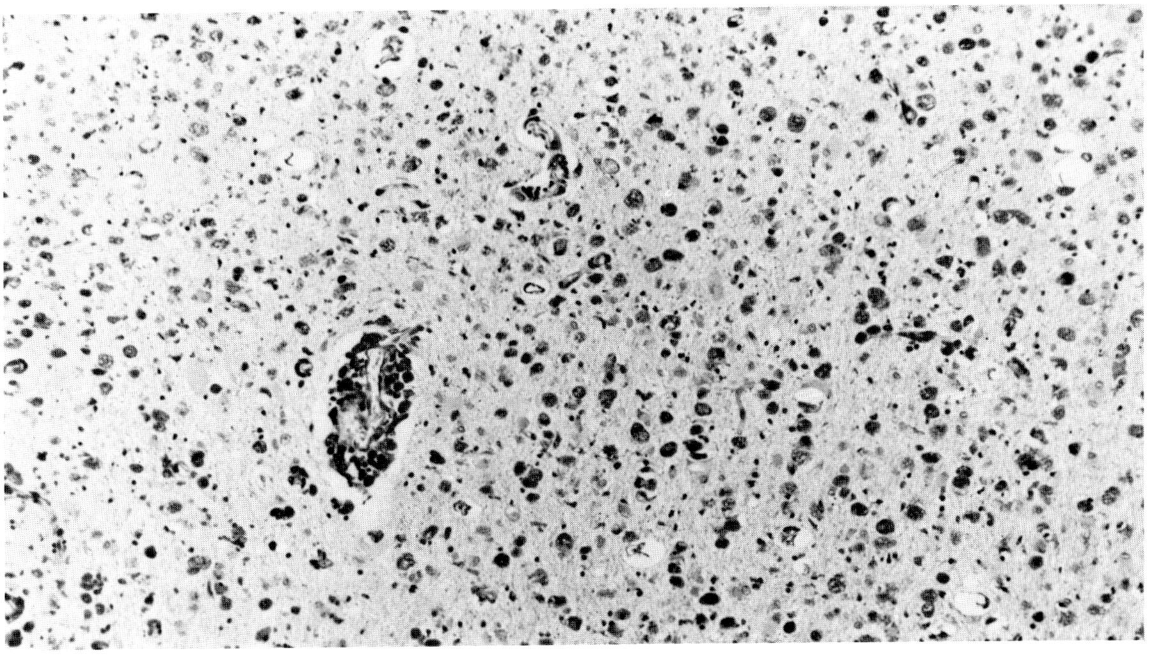

Fig. 20-25. Section showing stored granular material, some extracellular, in metachromatic leukodystrophy. (PAS, ×115.)

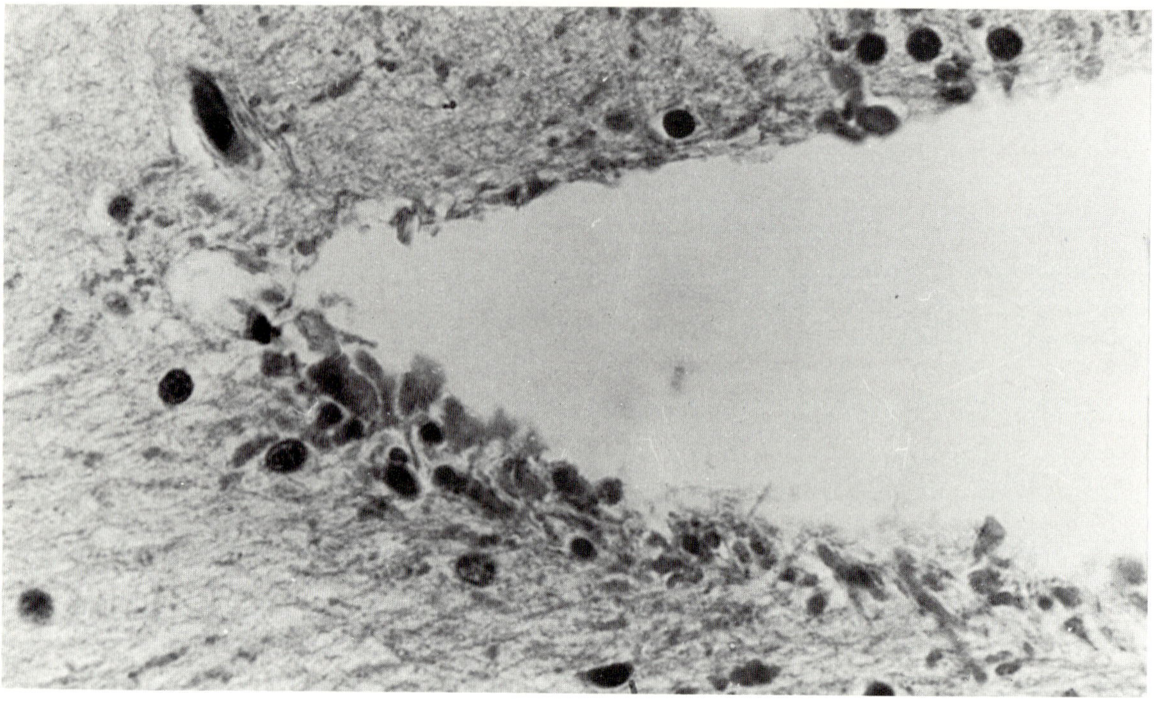

Fig. 20-26. Section showing prominent glial fibrils and masses in Alexander's disease. (H & E, ×750.)

is PAS-positive, stains as lipid, and is strongly metachromatic. The PNS is more commonly involved than in Krabbe's disease, and segmental demyelination and remyelination, with accumulation of metachromatic granules, can usually be seen in nerve biopsy material. Although storage visible with the microscope is confined to white matter, there is increased content of cerebroside sulfate throughout the CNS, in the liver and kidney, and in the urine. Deficiency of one isoenzyme (A) of arylsulfatase is reported.

Other Leukodystrophies

Leukodystrophies other than the globoid or metachromatic type are less clearly definable. They do not show storage of specific materials, and their enzyme deficiencies are unknown.

In *neutral fat leukodystrophy* there are accumulations of sudanophilic lipids. This condition is difficult to distinguish – if indeed it is separate at all – from diffuse cerebral sclerosis (see Chap. 21).

Pelizaeus-Merzbacher disease is a frequently sex-linked recessive condition of early postnatal onset and slow progression. Myelin sheaths may be scarce or even absent, and there is no stored material. At least in some instances, oligodendroglia have been reported as absent or as large and immature for the age of the patient. Juvenile and adult variants exist, in which the number of myelin sheaths remains subnormal, either diffusely or focally. Beyond its genetic determination, nothing is known of the etiology or pathogenesis of this disease. Its differentiation from Seitelberger's disease, Lowenburg-Hill disease, and other entities is probably premature.

In *Alexander's disease* the brain is often enlarged, at least in the early stages, and diffuse deficiency of myelin is associated with rarefaction and cavitation of the white matter and extremely prominent thick astrocytic fibrils (Rosenthal fibers), especially beneath the pia (Fig. 20-26) and ependyma.

In *Canavan's disease,* inadequate myelination is associated with spongiosis of the deep cortex and

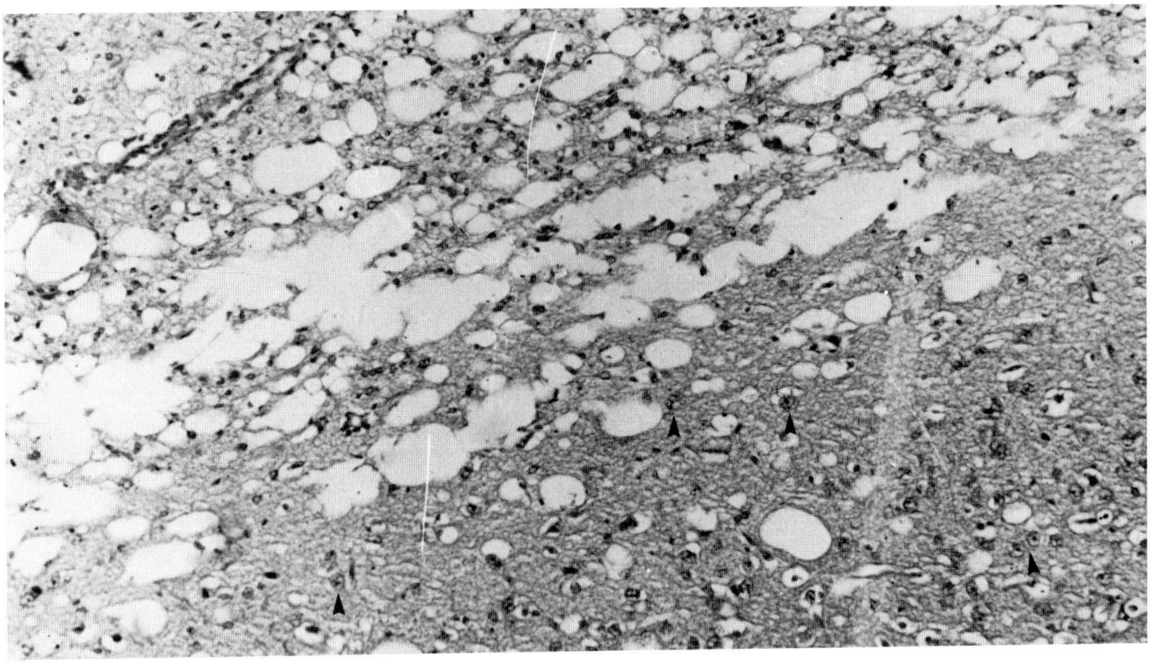

Fig. 20-27. Section at junction of cortex and white matter showing spongiosis and hypertrophied astrocytes (arrows) in Canavan's disease. (H & E, X115.)

adjacent white matter (Fig. 20-27) and cells resembling Alzheimer type II astrocytes, especially in the cortex. Although such features suggest an aminoacidopathy with interference in ammonia metabolism, no such association has yet been described.

For details of these conditions, an appropriate text should be consulted.

OTHER DISORDERS ASSOCIATED WITH MENTAL RETARDATION

Many other genetic errors of metabolism, as well as familial or sporadic disorders without a known biochemical substrate, are associated with retardation. The interested reader is referred to appropriate textbooks, but a few of the more common or interesting ones are considered here.

Inborn Errors of Metabolism

Glycogenosis

There are at least seven types of glycogenosis (Fig. 20-28), with subvarieties. Glycogenosis may produce CNS symptoms including mental retardation, either because of neuronal storage of glycogen (in type II, Pompe's disease; occasionally, in type III, Forbes' disease) or by repeated episodes of severe hypoglycemia (type I, Gierke's disease, or the rare type VII, glycogen synthetase deficiency). Most show autosomal recessive transmission, and some of the rarer types have more than one enzyme deficit, or different enzyme deficits within a single kinship.

In Pompe's disease, lysosomal α-glucosidase (acid maltase) is absent, and storage of glycogen occurs in virtually all tissues, notably in the brain, liver, heart, and skeletal muscle. The CNS morphology resembles that in other storage diseases, neurons being massively

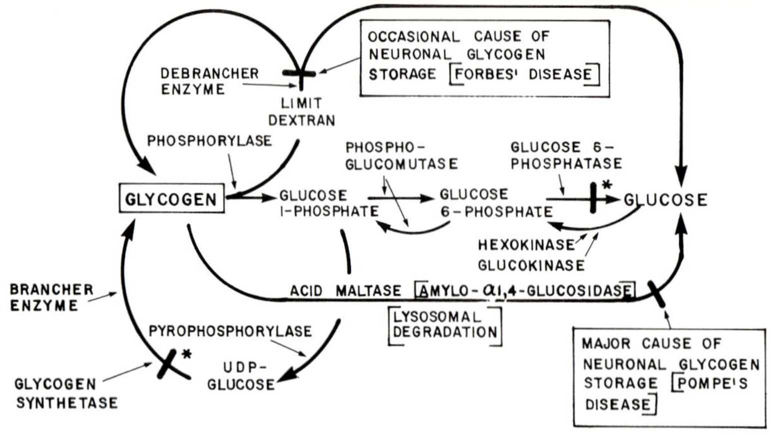

Fig. 20-28. The biochemistry of the glycogenoses. One of several sites of block may cause CNS damage due to storage of normal or abnormal glycogen or to recurrent hypoglycemia (= recurrent hypoglycemia may cause brain damage).*

distended with PAS-positive, lipid-negative material, removed by diastase. Neuronal destruction, less rapid than in the sphingolipidoses, ultimately occurs, leading to the secondary changes already described. Neuronal accumulation of glycogen is said to occur occasionally in type III glycogenosis (Forbes' disease, absence of debrancher enzyme) and in glycogen synthetase deficiency and type I (Gierke's) glycogenosis.

Galactosemia

Galactosemia, with absence or deficiency of galactose 1-phosphate uridyl transferase (Fig. 20-29), shows accumulation of galactose and galactose 1-phosphate. If the enzyme is absent, the neonatal disease is characterized by progressive liver failure, hemorrhage, and convulsions. Patients with an incomplete defect survive longer, but with subsequent retardation, cataracts, and renal tubular defects; the last lead to loss of glucose, amino acids, and protein in the urine. Alternative pathways synthesize sufficient uridine diphosphogalactose (UDP-galactose) (for myelin and mucopolysaccharide synthesis) from UDP-glucose.

Surviving patients may improve because of lower dietary galactose (reduction in milk and milk products) and postnatal development of alternative metabolic pathways. The toxic factor appears to be galactose 1-phosphate, which inhibits the interconversion of glucose 1-phosphate and glucose 6-phosphate and may compete for cell uptake of glucose. The retention within cells of osmotically active metabolites such as dulcitol may be responsible for cataracts. The brain in surviving patients may be reduced in size, have neuronal loss with secondary changes, and sometimes show Alzheimer type II astrocytes.

Hypoglycemic Disorders

Hypoglycemic disorders may be associated with mental retardation, as in association with glycogenosis and possibly galactosemia. Hypoglycemia may be due to hereditary fructose intolerance (fructosemia), in which reduced activity of fructose 1-phosphate aldolase and fructose 1, 6-diphosphate aldolase blocks glycolysis. It may be associated with abnormally high release of insulin (as by leucine), abnormal tissue response to insulin, or failure of response to glycagon. Mental retardation is an inconstant feature, presumably depending on the frequency, duration, and severity of hypoglycemic episodes.

Refsum's Disease

Refsum's disease is characterized by peripheral neuropathy, retinitis pigmentosa, muscular atrophy, skeletal and skin changes, and occasional mental retardation. The CNS shows excess sudanophilic material, most marked in the pallidum and substantia nigra. The tissues contain excess phytanic acid derived from the plant content in the diet. Due to a defect in α-oxidation of fats, phytanic acid becomes incorporated in myelin, apparently decreasing its stability. Dorsal-root ganglion cells in culture, treated with phytanic acid, show progressive granular degeneration of cells and degeneration of some myelin sheaths. The PNS myelin appears more susceptible than CNS myelin, perhaps accounting for the striking peripheral neuropathy.

Hyperuricemia

Hyperuricemia (Lesch-Nyhan syndrome) involves the CNS early, with pyramidal and extrapyramidal symptoms and frequently retardation. The increase in blood uric acid is often associated with renal calculi, but the blood-brain barrier is rather impermeable to uric acid, and the mechanism of the CNS defect is

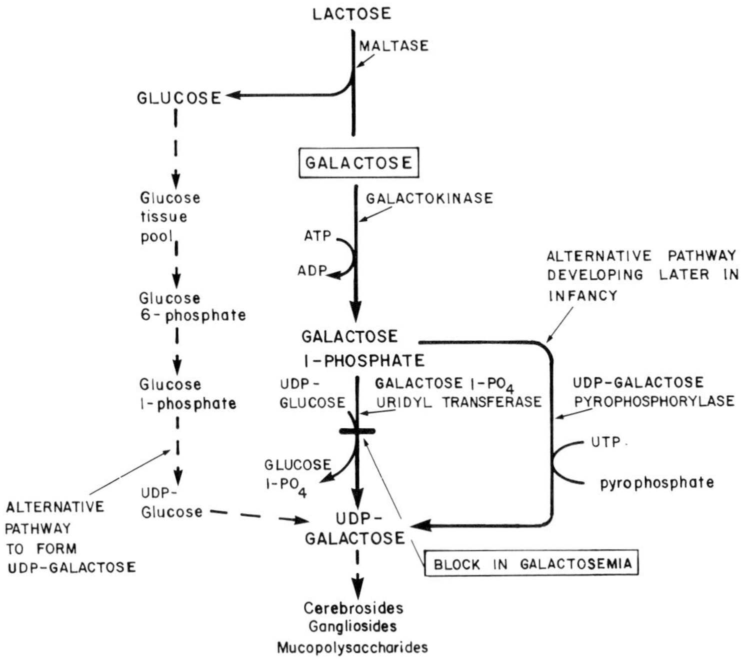

Fig. 20-29. The biochemistry of galactosemia. Alternative pathways prevent deficiency of UDP-galactose and after infancy also reduce accumulation of toxic galactose 1-phosphate.

unclear. The brain is small, with nonspecific neuronal loss and gliosis. The condition is an abnormality of purine metabolism (deficiency of hypoxanthineguanine phosphoribosyltransferase).

Organic Acidurias

The organic acidurias have only recently been studied by such techniques as gas chromatography, although it has long been known that accumulation of organic acids can cause convulsions, lethargy, and coma. The organic acidurias, like the aminoacidurias, form a genetically heterogenous group, with those affected often showing mental retardation. The two groups overlap to some extent, since maple syrup urine disease (see p. 374) owes its toxicity to accumulation of organic acids, one of which (α-ketoisocaproic acid) is thought to inhibit pyruvate decarboxylase. In general, these disorders are due to failure to oxidize organic acids, some of which are normal intermediate metabolites for amino acid catabolism, and multiple enzyme defects have been identified. The apparent frequency of these disorders may increase because of the availability of adequate analytical methods of diagnosis.

Other Considerations

Many other metabolic errors are occasionally associated with retardation, and the list lengthens year by year. Usually, there is accumulation of intermediate metabolites, but an unusual patnogenesis is the frequent association of retardation with nephrogenic diabetes insipidus, due to the altered water and electrolyte metabolism that accompanies hypertonicity and vascular stasis. (An interesting hypothesis is that retardation in these cases is apparent rather than real, learning being interrupted by the practically continuous necessity to be at the tap or the toilet!)

Disorders Awaiting Classification

A large number of common neurological diseases, familial or sporadic, without a recognized biochemical basis, may be associated with retardation. These include the degenerative diseases occurring in childhood (see Chap. 24), rare craniofacial anomalies such as acrocephalosyndactyly (Apert's disease), and muscular dystrophy, especially of the myotonic variety.

In addition, there are numerous syndromes of minor extraneural and occasionally neurological malformations associated with retardation. Perhaps the best documented is the de Lange's syndrome, in which mental retardation is associated with dwarfism, a low anterior hairline, continuity of the eyebrows across the midline, an "antimongolian" slant to the eyes, and often a small, rounded head (micrencephaly and brachycephaly). In a number of syndromes, neurological dysfunction (frequently retardation) is associated with lack of plasma β-lipoprotein and acanthocytosis, but this complicated group of disorders is still in the process of analysis.

BIBLIOGRAPHY

Albers, R. W., Siegel, G. J., Katzman, R., and Agranoff, B. W. *Basic Neurochemistry.* Boston: Little, Brown, 1972.

Austin, J. H. Globoid (Krabbe) Leukodystrophy. In J. Minckler (Ed.), *Pathology of the Nervous System.* New York: McGraw-Hill, 1968. Vol. 1, pp. 843-858.

Brady, R. O. Cerebral lipidoses. *Annu. Rev. Med.* 21:317-334, 1970.

Brady, R. O., Tallman, J. F., Johnson, W. G., Gal, A. E., Leahy, W. R., Quirk, J. M., and Dekaban, A. S. Replacement therapy for inherited enzyme deficiency. *N. Engl. J. Med.* 289:9-14, 1973.

Carpenter, S., Karpati, G., Wolfe, L. S., and Andermann, F. A type of juvenile cerebromacular degeneration characterized by granular osmiophilic deposits. *J. Neurol. Sci.* 18:67-87, 1973.

Crome, L., and Stern, J. *Pathology of Mental Retardation* (2nd ed.). Edinburgh: Churchill/Livingstone, 1972.

Dekaban, A. S., and Herman, M. M. Childhood, juvenile and adult lipidoses: Are these different nosological entities? *Arch. Pathol.* 97:65-73, 1974.

Guazzi, G.-C., and van Bogaert, L. Metabolic Diseases of the Central Nervous System. In G. H. Bourne (Ed.), *The Structure and Function of Nervous Tissue.* New York: Academic, 1969. Vol. 3, pp. 383-439.

Jervis, G. A. Phenylketonuria. In J. Minckler (Ed.), *Pathology of the Nervous System.* New York: McGraw-Hill, 1971. Vol. 2, pp. 1280-1284.

Kalckar, H. M., Kinoshita, J. H., and Donnell, G. N. Galactosemia: Biochemistry, Genetics, Pathophysiology and Developmental Aspects. In G. E. Gaull (Ed.), *Biology of Brain Dysfunction.* New York: Plenum, 1973. Vol. 1, pp. 31-88.

Kornfeld, M. Generalized lipofuscinosis (generalized Kufs' disease). *J. Neuropathol. Exp. Neurol.* 31: 668-682, 1972.

Mahler, H. R., and Cordes, E. H. *Biological Chemistry* (2nd ed.). New York: Harper & Row, 1971.

Martin, J.-J., and Schlote, W. Central nervous system lesions in disorders of amino-acid metabolism. *J. Neurol. Sci.* 15:49-76, 1972.

McIlwain, H., and Bachelard, H. S. *Biochemistry and the Central Nervous System.* Edinburgh: Churchill/Livingstone, 1971.

Milunsky, A., and Littlefield, J. W. The prenatal diagnosis of inborn errors of metabolism. *Annu. Rev. Med.* 23:57-76, 1972.

Moses, S. W., and Gutman, A. Inborn errors of glycogen metabolism. *Adv. Pediatr.* 19:95-169, 1972.

Neufeld, E. F., and Barton, R. W. Genetic disorders of mucopolysaccharide metabolism. In G. E. Guall (Ed.), *Biology of Brain Dysfunction.* New York: Plenum, 1973. Vol. 1, pp. 1-30.

Neville, B. G. R., Lake, B. D., Stephens, R., and Sanders, M. D. A neurovisceral storage disease with vertical supranuclear ophthalmoplegia, and its relationship to Niemann-Pick disease. *Brain* 96:97-120, 1973.

Roizin, L., and Kaufman, M. A. Dyslipidoses. In J. Minckler (Ed.), *Pathology of the Nervous System.* New York: McGraw-Hill, 1971. Vol. 2, pp. 1284-1314.

Schochet, S. S., Jr. Neuronal Inclusions. In G. H. Bourne (Ed.), *The Structure and Function of Nervous Tissue.* New York: Academic, 1972. Vol. 4, pp. 129-177.

Stoffel, W. Sphingolipids. *Annu. Rev. Biochem.* 40:57-82, 1971.

Suzuki, K., and Suzuki, K. Disorders of Sphingolipic Metabolism. In G. E. Gaull (Ed.), *Biology of Brain Dysfunction.* New York: Plenum, 1973. Vol. 2, pp. 1-73.

Towbin, A. Organic causes of minimal brain dysfunction. *J.A.M.A.* 217:1207-1214, 1971.

Towbin, A. Mental Retardation. In J. Minckler (Ed.), *Pathology of the Nervous System.* New York: McGraw-Hill, 1972. Vol. 3, pp. 2612-2626.

White, A., Handler, P., and Smith, E. L. *Principles of Biochemistry* (4th ed.). New York: McGraw-Hill, 1968.

Winick, M., and Coombs, J. Nutrition, environment and behavioral development. *Annu. Rev. Med.* 23:149-160, 1972.

Winick, M., and Rosso, P. Effects of Malnutrition on Brain Development. In G. E. Gaull (Ed.), *Biology of Brain Dysfunction.* New York: Plenum, 1973. Vol. 1, pp. 301-317.

Zeman, W. Studies in the neuronal ceroid-lipofuscinosis. *J. Neuropathol. Exp. Neurol.* 33:1-10, 1974.

Diseases of Myelin

21

The term *diseases of myelin* is used here in a restricted sense, since virtually all central nervous system disease to some extent involves myelin damage. Any focal lesion, such as an infarct, abscess, or tumor, in destroying the brain parenchyma necessarily destroys myelin. However, there are diseases in which damage to myelin is the most prominent morphological change (though not necessarily primary), and these may conveniently be considered in three groups.

Dysmyelinating Diseases

In dysmyelinating diseases, myelin either is not formed, is inadequately formed, or cannot be maintained in a stable state. The defect in myelin formation is apparently the primary feature in these conditions. Many of these diseases are associated with inborn errors of metabolism involving sphingolipids or amino acids or perhaps undetermined defects in oligodendroglial metabolism. Usually, these are disorders of infancy or childhood with a severe enzyme defect (leukodystrophies), although dysmyelination cannot be excluded in adults with a less complete enzyme deficit. The leukodystrophies (Chap. 20) frequently are associated with mental retardation.

Myelinoclastic Diseases (Primary Demyelination)

In the myelinoclastic diseases, myelin appears to be initially formed in the normal amount and to be of normal chemical and physical configuration. The disease attacks mature myelin sheaths, oligodendroglial cells responsible for their maintenance, or both; there are two categories of such change:

1. Clinically most important is the *idiopathic group,* of which the etiology and pathogenesis are uncertain and which includes multiple sclerosis, diffuse cerebral sclerosis of infancy and childhood, and some intermediate and variant forms. These diseases will be considered in some detail.

2. Other primary attacks on myelin at least are associated with a known etiological agent, even though their pathogenesis is uncertain. This group includes the perivenular demyelination that occasionally follows certain infections or immunizations (Chap. 23), demyelination associated with vitamin-deficiency diseases, especially of the B group (Chap. 22), and disorders of the extracellular space, as in chronic edema (Chap. 13). These diseases are dealt with in other chapters, as noted.

Secondary Demyelination

In secondary demyelination, destruction of myelin is often the most prominent gross and histological feature following loss of axons in the CNS. This secondary demyelination, analogous to wallerian degeneration in the PNS, may be seen in the CNS in various forms:

1. It is a prominent feature of some degenerative diseases (the spinocerebellar group of atrophies), in which it is often limited to specific tracts in the cord and brain stem (see Chap. 24).

2. Diffuse demyelination of the hemispheres may be associated with severe cortical neuronal loss, as in some of the dementias (see Chap. 24).

3. Ascending or descending degeneration is best seen in the spinal cord, secondary to focal lesions causing axonal destruction. In transection of the cord, ascending axons above the lesion and descending axons below it are cut off from their respective nerve bodies and incapable of survival. Degeneration of the myelin sheath, which tends to have a tractal distribution, follows necrosis of the severed portion of the axon.

It should not be inferred that there is a sharp distinction between the occurrence of primary and of secondary demyelination. Many diseases that exert a profound primary effect on myelin also cause some axonal or neuronal loss (e.g., diphtheria toxin, vitamin deficiencies) and therefore cause mixed primary and secondary degeneration. (The same is applicable to the PNS, where segmental [primary] demyelination by no means excludes concomitant axonal damage with secondary myelin changes.) Nonetheless, somewhat separate sequences of events are involved in the two processes, and it is convenient to discuss them separately, bearing in mind that they are not mutually exclusive.

STRUCTURE, COMPOSITION, AND BREAKDOWN OF MYELIN

The morphology and function of myelin have been considered in Chapters 2, 3, and 4. It suffices to recall here that myelin is arranged in segments (internodes) along the medium-sized and larger axons of the CNS and PNS, separated by bare areas, the nodes of Ranvier, at which the axon is open to the extracellular space. Each internode consists of a spirally wrapped lamella with the number of turns related to the diameter of the axon, derived from the plasmalemma of the oligodendroglial cell, and connected to it.

Each myelin lamella represents two plasma membranes; fusion of the cytoplasmic surfaces constitutes the major dense line, and fusion of the outer surfaces constitutes the minor dense (intra-period) line. In mature myelin there is neither cytoplasm nor extracellular space, except that at the paranodal extremities and inner and outer edges, and possibly also at the incisures of Lanterman, a little oligodendroglial cytoplasm may persist. The normal plasma membrane has protein on the inner and outer surfaces corresponding to the electron-dense lines, either in fibrillar or tightly linked globular form, and it is presumed that the major and minor dense lines represent this protein component. The protein and lipid constitution of myelin need not be identical with that of the oligodendroglial plasma membrane, although it presumably bears some similarity to it. Under normal conditions, myelin is a stable structure and the half-life of its components is long.

Myelination in the human CNS starts at about the fourth or fifth intrauterine months, but is not complete until the second postnatal year. The formation of myelin sheaths is thought to start at a critical axonal diameter (about 0.3μ in the CNS) and to be directed by the rate of axonal thickening, so that the final thickness is equal to, or slightly less than, the radius of the axon itself. The mechanism of expansion to accommodate continuing growth of the axon remains unclear. "Slippage" of the myelin layers one on another, with growth at the inner edge, has been proposed, but interstitial growth by the intercalation of protein and lipid molecules seems a more probable explanation. The incisures of Lanterman, which are infrequent in the CNS, do not appear in the sheaths of axons less than about 2μ in diameter. The formation of myelin appears to start near the neuronal cell body and extend distally, and its onset is signaled by a local increase in numbers of oligodendroglial cells, probably derived from undifferentiated precursors with astrocytic or oligodendroglial potentialities. Increased glial oxidative and hexose monophosphate shunt activity and raised concentration of brain lipids, including cholesterol esters, are present.

Chemical Composition of Central Nervous System Myelin

The only confirmed components of mature myelin are lipids and proteins.

Lipids

There are three major groups of lipids, and all can be freely synthesized in the CNS:

1. *Cholesterol* and possibly minute quantities of related steroids, synthesized from acetylcoenzyme A as in other tissues, constitute the most numerous lipid molecules in myelin. This cholesterol is unusual (in the human organism) in existing in free (non-esterified) form.

2. *Glycerol-derived phospholipids* derive from phosphatidic acid (Figs. 20-11 and 21-1), which consists of glycerol combined with two fatty acid (acyl) residues and a phosphoric acid residue. One or more of the following substances may be attached to the phosphoric moiety: choline, forming phosphatidylcholine (lecithin); ethanolamine, forming phosphatidylethanolamine; serine forming phosphatidylserine; or inositol (usually with additional phosphate groups), forming the phosphatidylinositides. Derived from phosphatidyl compounds are *plasmalogens,* in which an unsaturated long-chain fatty aldehyde is substituted for one acyl residue. These compounds can apparently be synthesized by cytidine triphosphate (CTP) activation, either of the phosphatidic acid or of the substituent group, the combination eliminating cytidine monophosphate (CMP) or cytidine diphosphate (CDP) and inorganic phosphate.

3. *Sphingolipids* are based on the amino alcohol sphingol (sphingosine), which forms an amide linkage with an acyl residue, producing a ceramide. From ceramide derive (Figs. 20-10 and 21-2) sphingomyelin, cerebroside, sulfatide, and the varied group of gangliosides (see Chap. 20). Gangliosides do not appear to be a significant constituent of myelin, but are present in higher concentration in gray matter, where they are incorporated in the neuronal and axonal plasmalemma.

Besides these major components of myelin in the CNS, there are numerous minor components, involving many different combinations of glycerol or sphingol with fatty acid residues on the one hand and hexose residues and phosphoryl compounds on the other. Their specific functions are unknown. Some are of particularly complex structure and may include sequential glycerol residues, as in the cardiolipins. In the CNS in general, acyl residues vary in chain length from 12 C to 26 C (usually even-numbered), may contain an α-hydroxy group, and may be saturated or unsaturated. The acyl chains in myelin are usually long (20 C or longer) and saturated, which may enable especially close packing. No lipid is known to be unique to myelin, but the polyphosphatidylinositides come close to it. Myelin is relatively deficient in phosphatidylcholine and phosphatidylethanolamine.

The lipid structure of myelin is complex, but the molar ratios of some major lipids appear to be as follows: cholesterol, 10; phosphatidylethanolamine, 4 (including much plasmalogen); cerebroside (including sulfatide), 3; phosphatidylserine, 2; phosphatidylcholine, 2; and sphingomyelin, 1. Lipids make up 70 to 75% of the dry weight of myelin, the remainder being protein. Although polyphosphatidylinositides do not appear in the preceding list and are probably present in small quantities, they appear to serve a uniquely important function which will be mentioned subsequently.

It is generally assumed that the acyl and sphingol chains are arranged radially in the myelin lamella, with attached hydrophilic groups adjacent to the

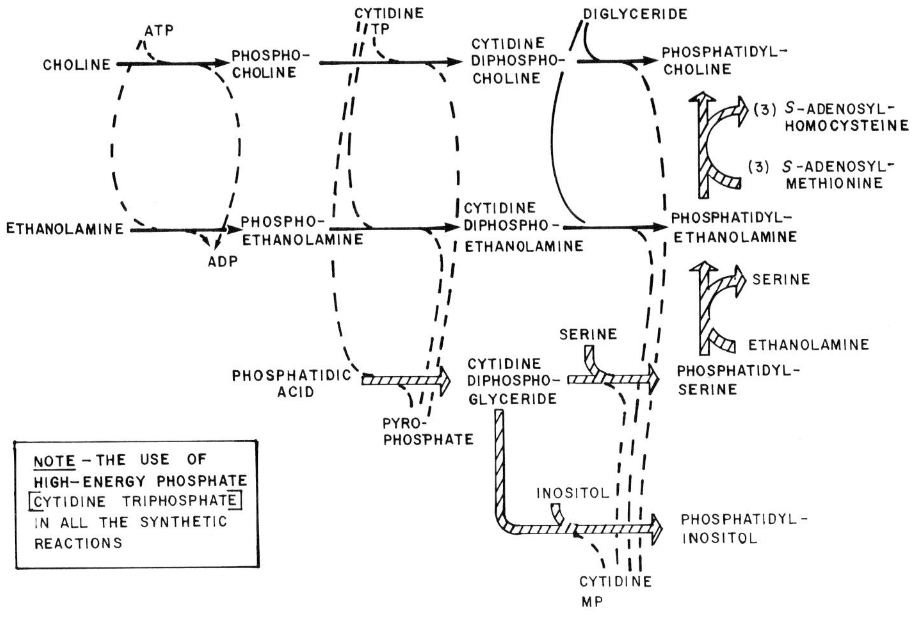

Fig. 21-1. Synthesis of phospholipids. The cross-hatched arrows represent main pathways.

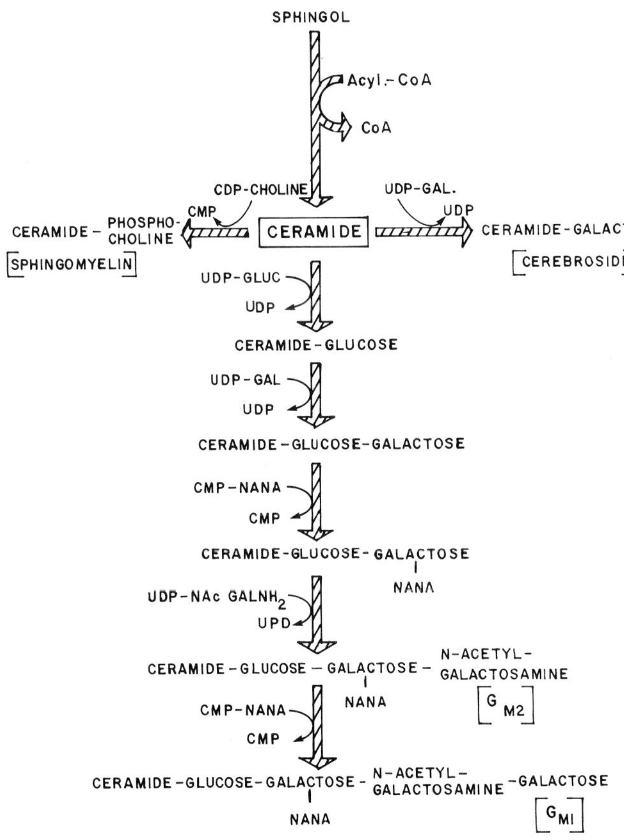

Fig. 21-2. Synthesis of sphingolipids. The starting point is the sphingol-fatty acid compound ceramide. In further reactions the nucleotides serve as carriers rather than as energy sources. NAc = N-acetyl galactosamine.

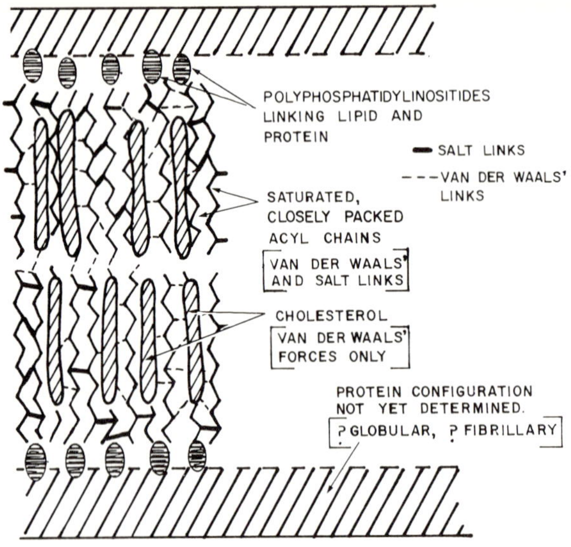

Fig. 21-3. Factors in the stabilization of the myelin sheath. For details, see text.

protein layers. Stabilization of lipid configuration is assisted by the long-chain saturated nature of the acyl residues, and probably there is cross-linking by divalent ions such as Ca^{++} (see Chap. 3).

Structural Proteins

Of the dry weight of myelin, 20 to 30% is protein. The difference between the amount of protein in central and peripheral myelin seems to be more marked than differences with respect to other constituents. It was observed early that during paraffin embedding, a reticular network developed within peripheral myelin sheaths, presumed to be of a protein nature and termed *neurokeratin.* The intervening empty spaces were presumably due to lipid droplets formed and dissolved out during fixation and processing. Neurokeratin resists lipid solvents and the action of most proteolytic enzymes, including trypsin. It appears to be less significant in CNS myelin, which shows only a slight reticular network.

The major protein in CNS myelin (proteolipid), while also resistant to most proteolytic enzymes, has the relatively unusual feature of lipid solubility. It is thought that much of the polyphosphatidylinositide in myelin is associated with this protein and perhaps maintains its tertiary spatial configuration with a nonpolar (hydrophobic) outer surface. Both this proteolipid and neurokeratin show a high content of tryptophan and a slow rate of turnover. Small amounts of neurokeratin are present in the CNS, both in the gray and white matter and therefore are not necessarily localized to myelin. Since proteolipid is the major myelin protein in the CNS, it makes up much of both the major and minor dense lines.

A second major protein (or group of proteins) present both in CNS and PNS myelin is considerably richer in both acid and basic amino acids, the overall result usually being an acid-soluble basic protein of relatively low molecular weight (under 16,000) and tryptophan content. This basic protein also contains polyphosphatidylinositides, and these compounds may be a major component in linkages between protein and lipid in myelin and largely responsible for its stability. The basic protein (or one of the group of basic proteins) appears to contain the major antigenic determinant for myelin and to be responsible for the experimental immunological myelin diseases, experimental allergic encephalomyelitis (see p. 410), and experimental allergic neuritis in the PNS.

It is apparent (Fig. 21-3) that much of the stability of myelin in a radial direction is due to polyphosphatidylinositides, which link protein to lipid and may also participate in protein-protein linkages. Stability in the longitudinal and tangential directions depends on protein linkages and also on the molecular (van der Waals) forces between acyl residues.

Enzymes

In spite of its apparent inertness and generally low metabolic turnover, myelin shows enzyme activity. There are neutral and acid proteinases that when deinhibited may play a significant role in myelin breakdown. Little is known of lipase activity.

At least two hydrolases, if not unique to myelin, are highly concentrated in it. These are 2′-2′-cyclic adenosine monophosphatase (AMPase) and a cholesterol hydrolase active at pH 7.2. Cyclic AMPase and cerebroside have been used as markers for myelin in CNS tissue.

Myelin Breakdown (Myelinoclasis)

Although a distinction is made between primary and secondary myelin degeneration, and there are certain differences between them in both the CNS and PNS, the distinctions and differences are largely based on concomitant circumstances (the degree [if any] of axonal damage, and whether oligodendroglia or Schwann's cells are maintaining myelin); the actual process of breakdown is closely similar in all situations and occurs in two consecutive (although slightly overlapping) phases.

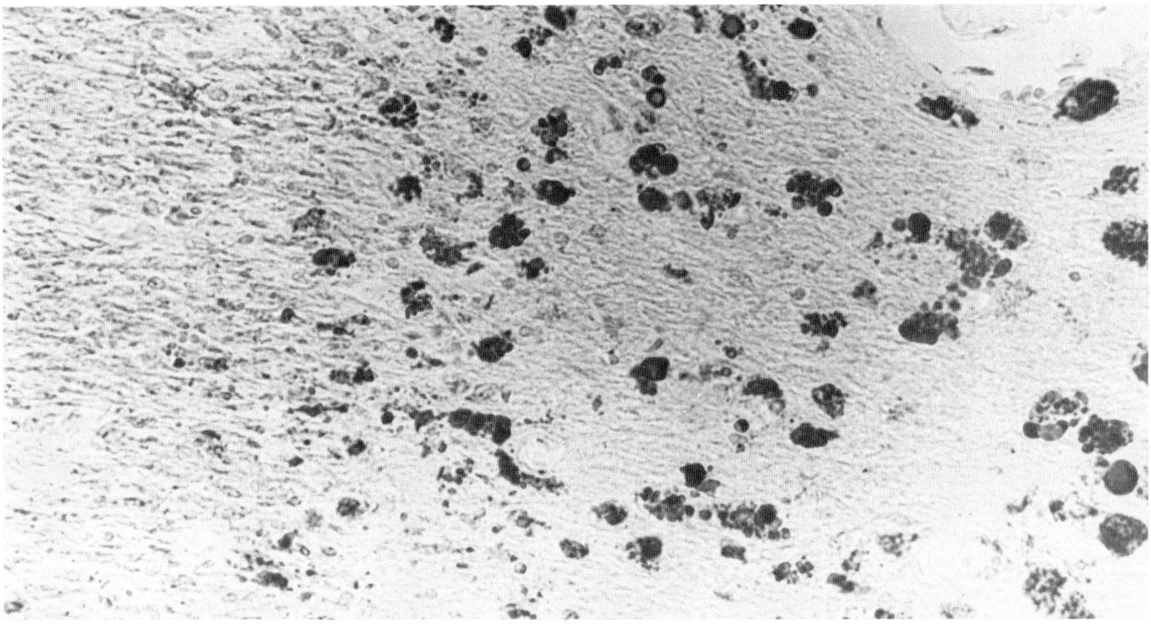

Fig. 21-4. Accumulation of myelin breakdown (abbau) products at the edge of a multiple sclerosis plaque, showing neutral fat, much of it in gitter cells. (Scharlach R, ×300.)

First Phase: Physical Disaggregation

The *first phase* is physical disaggregation of the myelin sheaths, which occurs both longitudinally (so that internodes split up into a chain of closed myelin *ovoids,* or *figures*) and radially, with splitting along major and minor dense lines, often primarily in the latter. Splitting at the minor dense line is always a feature of myelinoclasis, and since this is probably the location of the basic protein susceptible to proteinases, it may be that hydrolysis of this protein is a necessary precursor of myelin disaggregation; there are reports of early loss of basic protein in different types of myelinoclasis.

A rare exception to this preliminary physical disaggregation has been reported in experimental allergic encephalomyelitis (and possibly in multiple sclerosis) and occurs when lymphocytes (sensitized to encephalitogenic protein) produce minute focal zones of myelin lysis spreading concentrically from the cell, which is situated at the external surface of the myelin sheath.

Second Phase: Chemical Degradation

The *second phase* of myelin breakdown is chemical degradation, in which possibly the earliest event is hydrolysis of the basic protein, as has been noted. However, since lysis of proteins yields freely diffusible peptides and amino acids, which are not readily susceptible to demonstration, attention has been directed to the products of lipid breakdown.

Granules and vacuoles of lipid (abbau products) appear at about the sixth to tenth day following myelin damage and may be readily recognized by their staining reactions. Formation of neutral fat from glycerol and acyl residues, and of cholesterol esters from cholesterol, gives a positive reaction with Scharlach R or similar stains (Fig. 21-4). The liberated lipid is doubly refractile and intensely bright

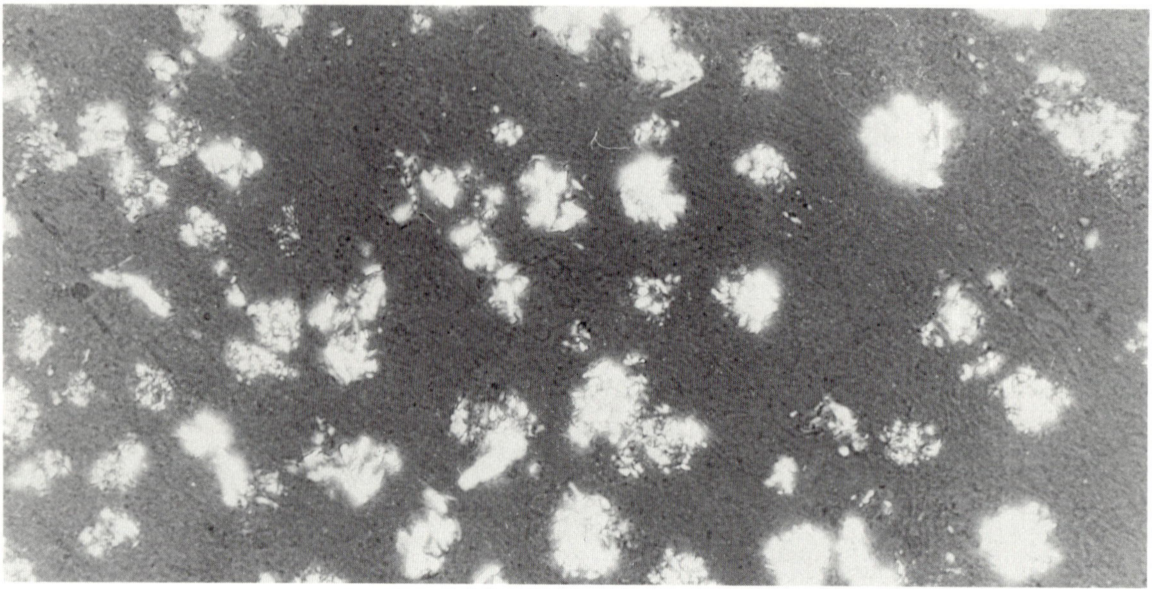

Fig. 21-5. Accumulation of abbau products as in Figure 21-4, showing large amounts of cholesterol esters as needle-like structures. (Polarized light, X300.)

when viewed with polarized light (Fig. 21-5). Glycolipids (presumably largely cerebroside) give a positive PAS reaction, and (like myelin itself) the breakdown products stain as compound lipids with such dyes as Luxol Fast Blue and Sudan Black B. These materials are phagocytized in the CNS largely by macrophages derived from the blood and activated microglia. There may be minimal phagocytosis by astrocytes, and even some uptake of antigenic determinants by sensitized lymphocytes where autoimmune mechanisms are involved. In the PNS, macrophages and Schwann's cells are both phagocytic, and in wallerian degeneration secondary to peripheral axonal degeneration the myelin ovoids and figures containing axonal debris may be enveloped by Schwann's cell cytoplasm prior to the beginning of chemical degradation.

These reaction products are usually maximal at about three to six weeks and disappear over the succeeding weeks or months, depending on the size of the demyelinated area. Presumably, in part, they are removed by macrophages entering the blood, which is a slow process, since these cells are often found accumulated around small vessels. Further degradation may also occur in situ by continuing hydrolytic action.

The degree of accumulation of abbau products depends on the rate and quantity of degeneration. If the process is slow and diffuse, as in the secondary hemispheric demyelination that accompanies gradual cortical neuronal loss in degenerative disease, only a few perivascular cells containing neutral fat may be found. On the other hand, when myelinoclasis involves large numbers of fibers simultaneously (as in ascending or descending degeneration or active plaques of multiple sclerosis), massive accumulations of doubly refractile material, staining with neutral fat and other stains, are seen.

Enzyme activity intrinsic to the myelin sheath can no longer be distinguished by the time phagocytic hydrolases have become active, but there is evidence that a rise in myelin proteinase activity precedes, or is concurrent with, the physical disaggregation stage. Presumably, much of this activity represents unmasking of the native myelin proteinases, although in secondary degeneration, proteolytic activity may originate in the degenerating axons.

Immunology of Myelin

Apparently the most antigenic component of myelin is the basic protein itself (encephalitogenic protein) or some fraction of it that contains an antigenic determinant. Injection of this protein with adjuvant provokes both cell-mediated and humoral autoimmunity. It is possible that other myelin proteins may also be antigenic, or that myelin lipids may act as haptens. However, so far little experimental work has been done on other possible factors, nor has it been suggested that any might have clinical significance.

The myelin membrane is derived from that of the oligodendroglial cell and may share with it some antigenic determinants. Antimyelin antibodies added to myelinated tissue cultures seem to exert a direct effect both on myelin and on a proportion of oligodendroglial cells, which show (apparently) irreversible swelling and necrosis. If the immune serum is removed and replaced by normal serum, such cultures usually remyelinate, suggesting that some cells — either oligodendroglia or cells capable of so differentiating — have survived. Astrocytes and oligodendroglia share a precursor cell, and gel-diffusion techniques following injections of heterologous whole-brain tissue have shown an organ-specific but not species-specific antibody that can be seen by immunofluorescence to react with myelin, oligodendroglial cells, and astrocytes. This is presumably not antibody to encephalitogenic protein, since it reacts with both peripheral and central myelin. The relationship of antimyelin antibodies to other CNS and PNS antibodies requires further clarification.

MULTIPLE SCLEROSIS AND ITS VARIANTS

Multiple sclerosis is the most common and clinically important of the primary demyelinating diseases and has been the subject of incalculable amounts of epidemiological, clinical, biochemical, microbiological, and immunological research. Nonetheless, its etiology is still unknown, and its pathogenesis is imperfectly understood. It is a disease of the CNS, not involving peripheral nerves, with a very variable distribution of lesions, so that clinical symptomatology is protean. Long tract, brain stem, cerebellar, and optic tract signs and symptoms are common. Characteristic of the disease is its insidious onset and relapsing, prolonged course (in most cases), often beginning in young adult life. Mental capacity is often substantially unimpaired, and seizures are unusual. Although the onset is insidious and symptoms often initially temporary, there is a steady downhill trend, with superimposed exacerbations that are frequently precipitated by trivial infection, emotional stress, trauma, or other nonspecific incidents.

Clinical Variants

Clinical variants of multiple sclerosis occur, depending on the distribution of major lesions. In *neuromyelitis optica* (Devics's disease) the lesions principally involve the spinal cord and visual pathways. In one form (not the only form) of *transverse myelitis,* in which the patients present with a complete functional "transection" of the cord, the lesions appear to be similar to those of multiple sclerosis.

Occasionally, multiple sclerosis begins in childhood, often precipitated by a banal infection, and then tends to run a subacute rather than chronic course, with a shorter duration and relatively little tendency to remission.

Relationship of Diffuse Cerebral Sclerosis and Multiple Sclerosis

Diffuse cerebral sclerosis (often called Schilder's disease, although this term has now become ill defined) is a progressive childhood condition, often clinically indistinguishable from the dysmyelinating diseases (leukodystrophies) with which it was originally confused. Unlike multiple sclerosis, which has a low familial incidence (less than 5%), diffuse cerebral sclerosis is said to be often familial, though older data must be regarded as unreliable, since in the past a clear distinction between diffuse cerebral sclerosis and dysmyelinating diseases could not be made. In spite of the younger age at onset and generally unremitting course, the lesions of diffuse cerebral sclerosis are histologically similar to those of multiple sclerosis, and an increasing number of cases seem to represent transitional forms, both the lesion distribution and the clinical picture being intermediate between those of diffuse cerebral and multiple sclerosis. Even some of the typical childhood cases tend to progress in bursts, though these are not punctuated by true remissions. Baló's disease (concentric sclerosis), a morphological variant of multiple sclerosis (see p. 405), may also occur in a mixed form with diffuse cerebral sclerosis.

A small proportion of otherwise typical diffuse cerebral sclerosis patients, all male and usually children, show adrenal insufficiency that may precede clinical CNS dysfunction. Adrenocortical atrophy is associated with ballooned cells in the fascicular and reticulate zones. The eosinophilic cytoplasm of these cells contains granules or striations. The cells are weakly PAS-positive and lipid-positive, but the nature of the included material is not known. It is possible that adrenal insufficiency is a precipitating factor for the CNS disease, or that there is an associated genetic factor (possibly sex-linked).

Composition of Myelin

Chemical analysis of brains from patients with diffuse cerebral sclerosis, multiple sclerosis, Baló's disease, and neuromyelitis optica shows the same changes in lipid composition as in secondary degeneration (myelinoclasis), the accumulation of abbau products depending on the tempo of the disease. While this has been used as one argument for the essential identity of these conditions, it merely represents the only possible mode of chemical breakdown for myelin, irrespective of etiology.

Morphology of Multiple Sclerosis and Allied Diseases

Because of the problematical nature of this group of diseases, morphological changes will be discussed first as a basis for considering theories of etiology and pathogenesis.

Gross Appearances

External examination may reveal no changes or, in long-standing cases, generalized shrinkage of the brain with sulcal widening and increased firmness. Where the cord has been severely involved, segments may be shrunken and firm, and flattening of the posterior columns above such lesions (ascending degeneration) may be observed in some patients.

On sectioning, the characteristic lesion seen is a sharply circumscribed, regular or irregular area (plaque), frequently but not necessarily in white matter, in which myelin has been destroyed. These plaques vary in size from a few millimeters to several centimeters or may even include most of the cerebral

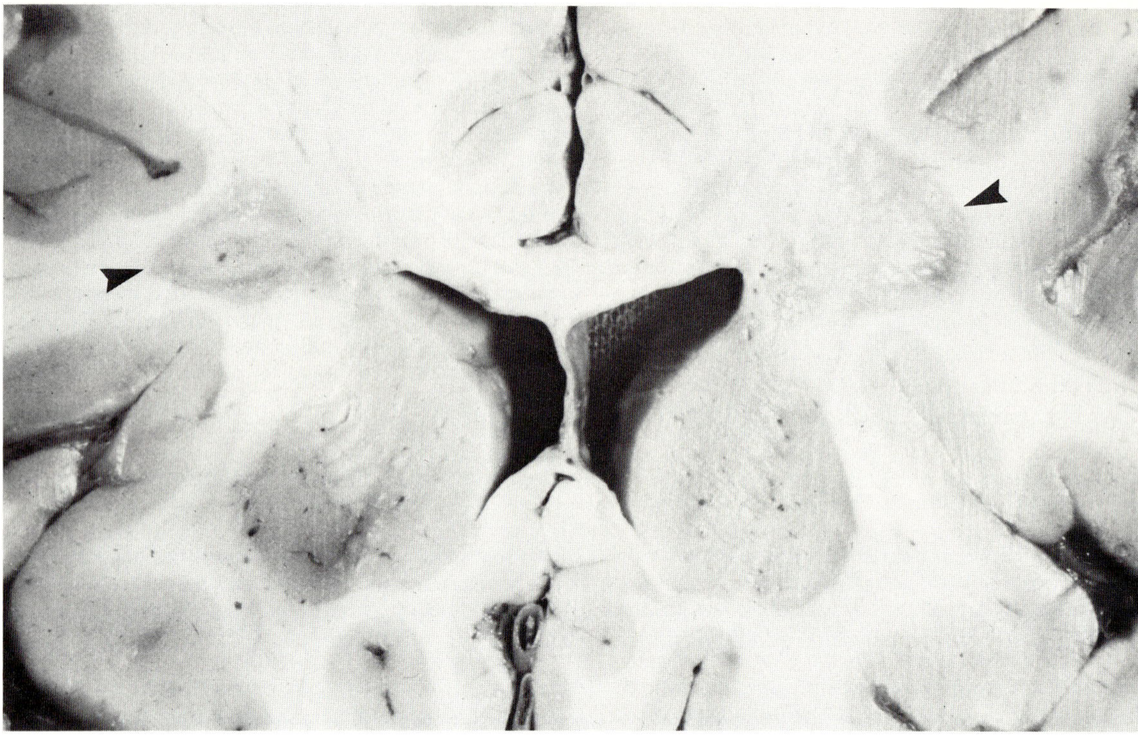

Fig. 21-6. Periventricular demyelination in multiple sclerosis (arrows).

white matter. Old plaques are retracted below the cut surface and are slightly yellowish; larger ones may show cystic gliosis. More recent plaques, which tend to be smaller, are grayish or slightly hyperemic and do not show retraction. Old and new plaques are often found in the same brain. Except by coincidence, plaques are not confined to specific gray or white areas, but are distributed independently of the structural boundaries in the brain and often show some tendency to be symmetrical.

In advanced cases, there is almost always involvement of periventricular white matter (Fig. 21-6) extending laterally and upward from the angles of the lateral ventricles and frequently prominent around the occipital and temporal (less often the frontal) horns. Semicircular or crescentic lesions are often seen in the subcortical white matter (Fig. 21-7). Scattered lesions occur elsewhere in hemispheric white matter and also in deep gray matter, where they are less readily seen because there is less myelin. There is frequently complete or partial involvement of the optic nerves, chiasm, and tracts. Lesions are frequently seen in the cerebellar white matter, often subcortical, as in the cerebral hemispheres, and they are also seen in the brain stem, where they frequently (but not necessarily) reach either the ependymal or pial surface.

Spinal cord lesions are common and are usually wedge-shaped, based on the pia, one to several segments in length, and most prominent in the posterior and lateral white columns. They may involve the central gray matter, which occasionally appears necrotic. Secondary demyelination is sometimes associated with the spinal cord lesions, but since axons are spared for a long time, even in old gliotic

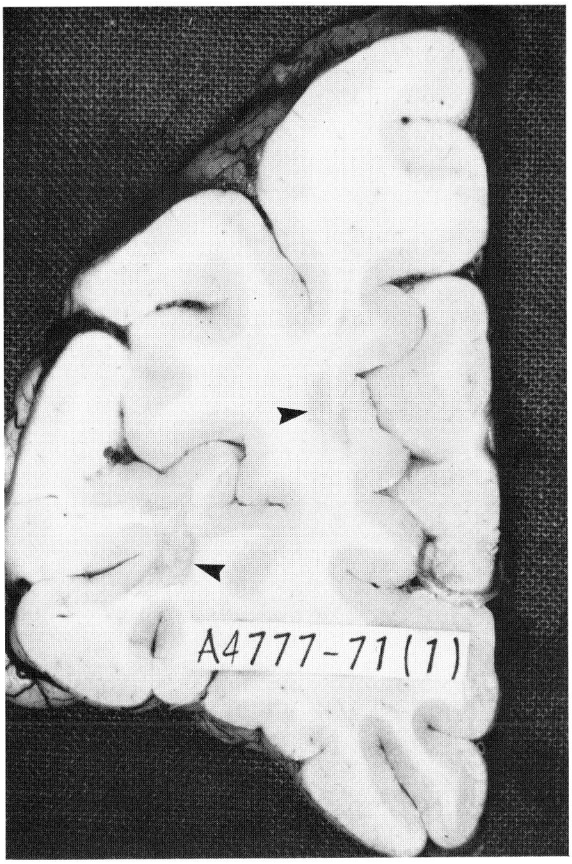

Fig. 21-7. Typical subcortical plaques in multiple sclerosis (arrows).

plaques, it is not commonly seen until late in the disease.

Neuromyelitis Optica. In this condition the most constant lesions are in the visual pathways (optic nerves, chiasm, and tracts), and in the spinal cord where they may cause functional "transection." Careful search usually discloses typical plaques elsewhere in the CNS.

Transverse Myelitis. As already noted, some forms of transverse myelitis appear to be related to multiple sclerosis; in such cases, not only white but also gray matter shows degenerative and necrotic changes (Fig. 21-8). However, a careful search usually discloses typical plaques in other parts of the neuraxis.

Diffuse Cerebral Sclerosis. In classic diffuse cerebral sclerosis, there is extensive, often virtually complete demyelination of the cerebral hemispheres without lesions in other parts of the CNS. Lesions tend to be most marked in occipital white matter, and unlike typical multiple sclerosis, spare the subcortical (arcuate) fibers. In transitional forms between diffuse cerebral and multiple sclerosis, the lesions of diffuse cerebral sclerosis may be less extensive and are associated with typical plaques in other areas. In Baló's concentric sclerosis, hemispheric white matter is the site of a series of concentric rings of demyelination, with zones of apparently normal myelination interposed. The pathological appearance of Baló's concentric sclerosis and diffuse cerebral sclerosis may occur in the same patient.

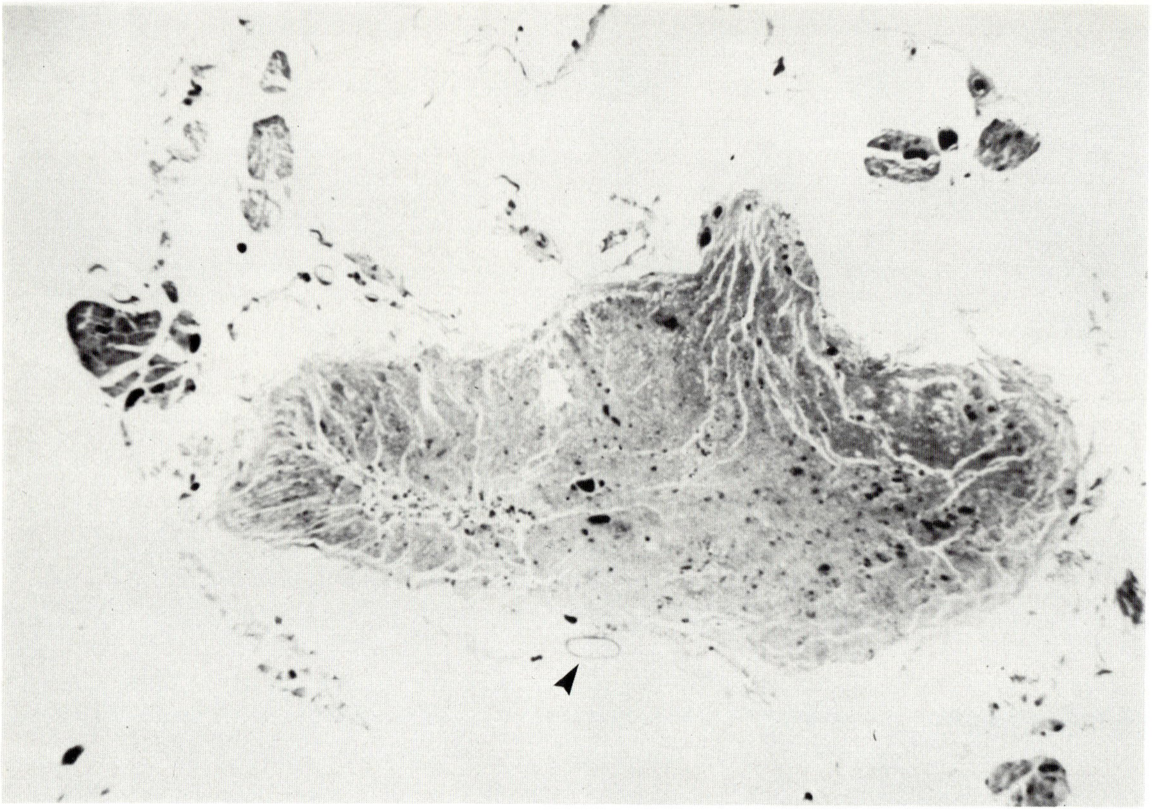

Fig. 21-8. Transverse myelitis. Section through upper thoracic cord, showing total destruction. The anterior spinal artery is indicated by an arrow and is the only means of orientation. This patient had a few small multiple sclerosis plaques at other cord levels and in the brain stem. (H & E, ×10.)

Microscopic Appearances

Characteristics of the Plaque. Microscopically, the hallmark of multiple sclerosis and all its variants is focal, total, sharply defined demyelination (plaques), (Figs. 21-9, 21-10), with loss of oligodendroglial cells from the plaques at an early stage. If demyelination is active, gitter cells containing abbau products with typical staining reactions (see p. 401) are present, especially at the periphery, suggesting centrifugal, concentric, progressive growth. Perivascular cuffing with lymphocytes, macrophages, and occasional plasma cells may be seen, but is not prominent in adults. A large majority of the axons in the plaques are intact or merely show slight beading (Fig. 21-11), and this accounts for the absence of secondary ascending or descending degeneration in relation to most plaques in the cord.

Even in early lesions, hyperplasia and hypertrophy of astrocytes is prominent (Fig. 21-12), and fibrillary gliosis occurs early, the fibers usually being orientated parallel to persistent axons — a pattern described as isomorphic. In older lesions, and in the central parts of large active plaques, fibrillary gliosis is profound, and there is usually a clear reduction in the numbers of axons, although some invariably persist. In the largest lesions with almost total axonal destruction, fibrillary gliosis may be inadequate to occupy the defect, and cystic gliosis develops. Where plaques involve gray matter (e.g., the cortex, basal ganglia, or brain stem), the neurons usually show mild degenerative changes or appear normal.

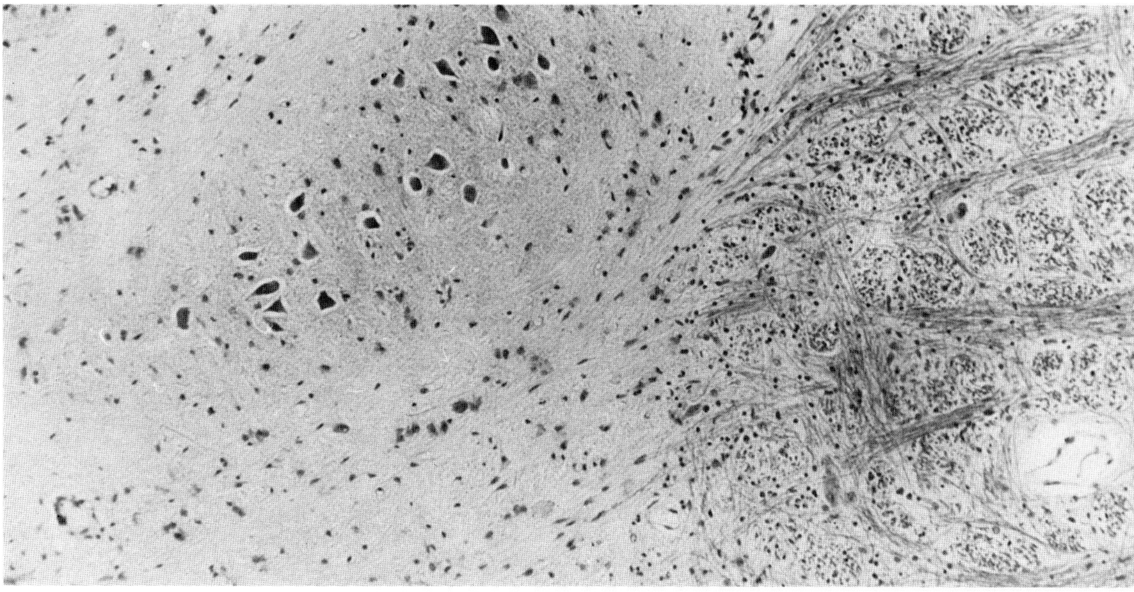

Fig. 21-9. Edge of multiple sclerosis plaque in the brain stem, showing survival of neurons in the lesion and the abrupt cut-off of myelin sheaths. There is virtually no inflammatory exudate. (Luxol-gallocyanin, ×115.)

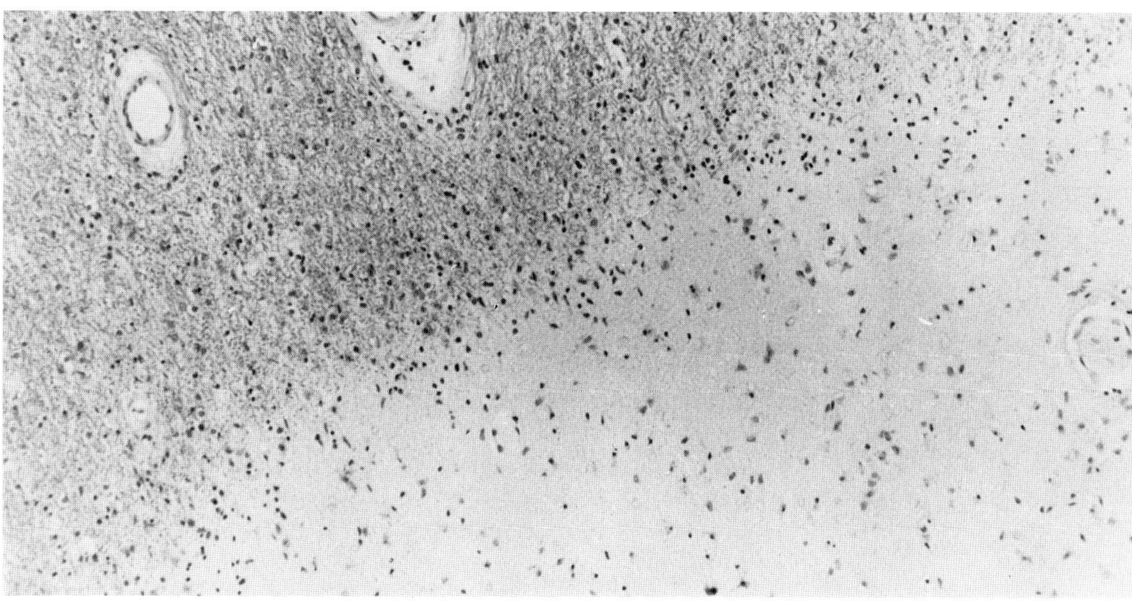

Fig. 21-10. Edge of multiple sclerosis in white matter, showing abrupt cessation of myelin, disappearance of oligodendroglial cells, and a minimal lymphocytic infiltration along the edge of the lesion. (Luxol-gallocyanin, ×115.)

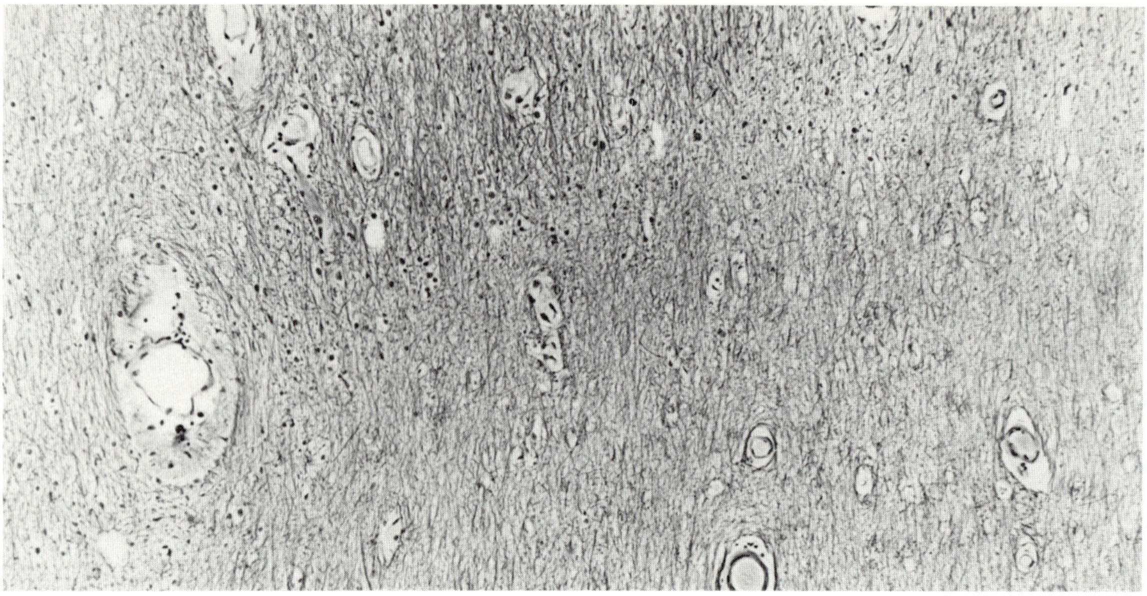

Fig. 21-11. Edge of multiple sclerosis plaque (plaque is below and to the right) showing persistence of axons but disappearance of oligodendroglial cells. (Holmes silver, ×115.)

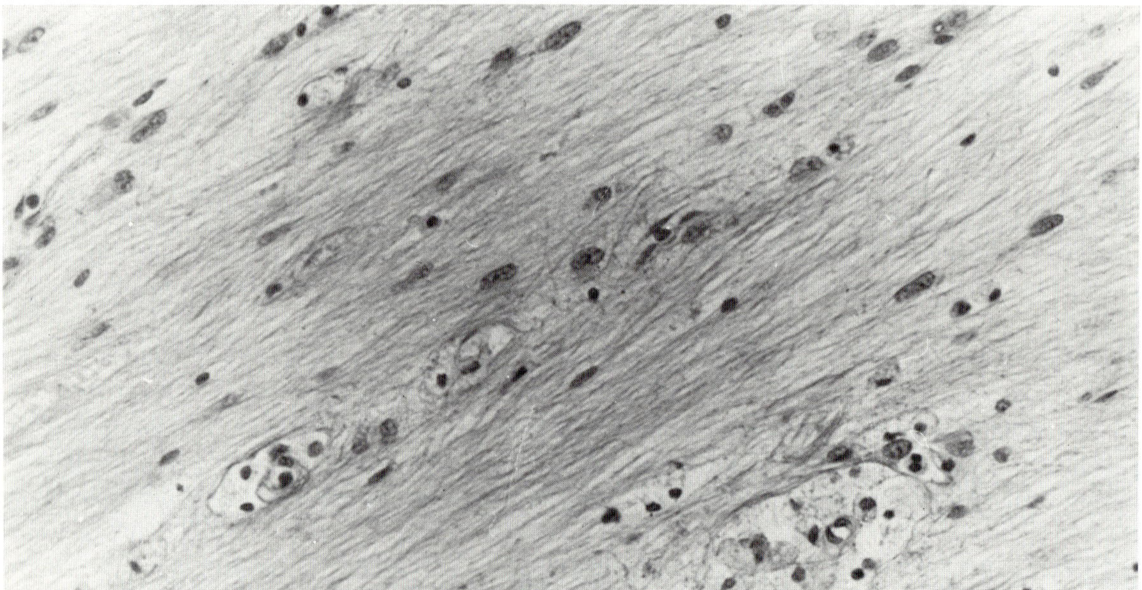

Fig. 21-12. Multiple sclerosis plaque in corpus callosum, showing virtual disappearance of oligodendroglial cells, absence of myelin, a few gitter cells with foamy cytoplasm around vessels, and astrocytic hyperplasia. The overall architecture is well preserved. (Luxol-gallocyanin, ×300.)

A feature commonly disclosed on staining for myelin, but not apparent on naked eye examination, is the presence of *shadow plaques* with partial demyelination, some normal sheaths persisting with a relatively slight astrocytic reaction; these presumably represent the earliest stage in plaque development. Such plaques are usually centered on a vessel, characteristically a venule. However, larger, grossly visible plaques, formed either by progressive growth or by confluence of smaller lesions, do not show such a perivascular relationship. Where lesions extend to the ependymal or pial surface, associated vessels are at the edge and not the center and are subependymal or emergent cortical veins.

Necrosis. In otherwise typical cases of multiple sclerosis – and perhaps more often in the spinal cord gray matter than elsewhere – lesions occasionally become necrotic, with a marked perivascular mononuclear exudate, and then involve neurons, axons, and astrocytes, as well as the oligodendroglial cells and myelin.

Electron Microscopy. This has so far contributed little to the understanding of multiple sclerosis, partly because of the difficulty in ensuring that any biopsy includes a plaque, and partly because of the minute size of tissue samples. Abnormal twisted structures, possibly derived from neurofilaments and similar to those seen in Alzheimer's disease, aging, and human slow virus infections, have been described both in presynaptic and post-synaptic structures of the cortex, but their specificity remains uncertain. Myelin beyond the areas of plaque formation appears morphologically normal.

Changes in Clinical Variants. The histology of multiple sclerosis variants is essentially similar, with only the distribution and extent of the lesions differing. In the occasional subacute forms of juvenile-onset multiple sclerosis, there is usually evidence of a more rapid tempo (accumulation of abbau products) and more pronounced perivascular mononuclear exudate than in the adult disease. In neuromyelitis optica and transverse myelitis, necrosis involving the gray matter of the spinal cord is often unusually prominent and is associated with inflammatory changes.

Other Laboratory Observations in Multiple Sclerosis

Brain Tissue

Chemical analysis of brains from multiple sclerosis patients has not yielded any valuable information. As has been noted, the lipid breakdown products are typical of myelinoclasis and differ in no respect from wallerian degeneration. Scattered reports of early loss of basic protein and increased proteinase activity, even in apparently normal areas of myelin, merely indicate the expected mode of myelin breakdown and are probably in no way specific for multiple sclerosis.

Cerebrospinal Fluid

The cerebrospinal fluid is clear and colorless and shows only a slight increase in mononuclear cells, rarely exceeding 25 per cubic millimeter. Neutrophils are not seen. Protein is often raised, but there is a considerable overlap between normal control subjects and patients with multiple sclerosis. In 50% of patients the level is less than 50 mg per 100 ml, although occasional levels as high as 200 mg per 100 ml have been reported. The colloidal gold reaction yields a first-zone or mid-zone reaction, each in about 20% of cases.

Electrophoresis shows an excess of gamma globulin (largely IgG, but including some IgA and IgM). This rise is partly a diffuse increase in the gamma globulin peak, but also includes a few discrete, slowly moving bands, thought to be derived from clones of lymphocytes possibly resident within the CNS. This concept is supported by the differences found in the ratios of heavy to light chains between gamma globulin in the CSF and in the same patient's serum. Slightly increased concentrations of gamma globulin have even been reported within CNS tissue, and the albumin-globulin ratio is often decreased. Levels of CSF complement seem to be reduced in some cases.

Etiology and Pathogenesis of Multiple Sclerosis

Epidemiology

Epidemiological studies show an overall pattern of incidence of multiple sclerosis, the significance of which is not clear. In general, the incidence is low in tropical regions, increases northward and southward to a maximum at about 45 to 50 degrees from the equator, and thereafter is relatively constant. Superimposed on this general gradient are unexplained foci of high prevalence, as in northern Scotland and Scandinavia, and of low prevalence, as in Japan. About 5% of cases of multiple sclerosis are familial, but a similar incidence is not infrequently found even in infectious disease.

Lack of any significant genetic basis is suggested by migration studies from South Africa and Israel. The incidence in Britain is considerably higher than in South Africa, but if British residents emigrate to South Africa before the age of 14 to 15, their subsequent incidence is that of the host country; if they migrate as adults, their subsequent incidence is that of the resident British population. Similar studies in Israel, which has received large influxes of Jews both from North European countries (high incidence) and from Afro-Asian countries (low incidence) show that migrants who enter Israel below the age of 14 to 15 show a uniform incidence of multiple sclerosis, irrespective of their country of origin. It might be concluded that, whatever the etiological factor, it is operative in the future patient in childhood, so that removal from a high-risk zone prior to puberty dramatically reduces subsequent incidence.

Multiple sclerosis does not correlate well with socioeconomic status, tending, if anything, to be more frequent in the higher socioeconomic groups. In spite of the overall geographical incidence, it does not correlate with specific climatic factors. There is tentative evidence of an inverse correlation with efficiency of sanitation, compatible with a hypothesis that children exposed to poor sanitary facilities acquire resistance to multiple sclerosis, whereas with good sanitation the repeated, early subclinical contacts with a possible infectious agent do not occur. Data such as these suggest an environmental and possibly an infectious factor, but give little hint as to its nature.

The Possible Role of Infection

The possible association of multiple sclerosis with infection has been considered for some time, perhaps in part due to the increase in gamma globulin levels in CSF and, to a lesser extent, in serum. This interest has been heightened by the discovery of slow virus CNS diseases in animals and man (see Chap. 23). So far, however, there is little to suggest that infection per se causes multiple sclerosis, although it might act as a precipitating factor. Neither cultural nor morphological studies have yielded significant results, although there are scattered reports of structures resembling a paramyxovirus (possibly measles) and one report of isolation of measles virus from the CNS of patients with multiple sclerosis. Although this is scanty evidence, it cannot be disregarded because of the sampling problems in multiple sclerosis brains. These include the minute size of electron microscopic specimens necessary for detection of virus-like structures, the difficulty of locating a plaque in biopsy material, and the possible presence of virus only in the young plaques but not elsewhere. Persistent CNS infection cannot be ruled out, although the balance of evidence currently is against it.

Indirect serological evidence includes many patients with multiple sclerosis with raised antibody titers to several viruses (usually measles, but also some parainfluenza and influenza virus strains). Such increases are not invariable and are only marginal in comparison with those in subacute sclerosing panencephalitis, in which measles virus is known to persist in the CNS. The variety, inconstancy, and marginal degree of these increases might better be interpreted as evidence for altered immunological responsiveness than as evidence for infection.

The Possible Role of Autoimmunity

A number of findings indicate that an immunological process might be concerned in the etiology or the perpetuation of multiple sclerosis. These include raised CSF gamma globulins, variable statistical abnormalities in specific antibody levels (see above), the perivenular nature of some early lesions, and the frequent precipitation of the juvenile subacute form, and of remissions in the adult form, by trivial, often nonspecific infections. In the absence of a recognized infectious agent, a basis for these phenomena has been sought in the concept of autoimmunity, and the findings in multiple sclerosis have been compared and contrasted with those in experimental allergic encephalomyelitis (EAE). To understand the comparison further, a short account of EAE is necessary.

Experimental Allergic Encephalomyelitis. This condition develops when experimental animals are inoculated intradermally with whole-brain homogenate, white matter, myelin basic protein (encephalitogenic protein), or its polypeptide antigenic determinant, in each case mixed with Freund's adjuvant. Intense proliferation of cells in regional lymph nodes draining the inoculated area is followed seven to eight days later by a peak of circulating mononuclear cells containing newly synthesized DNA.

A few days after these cells appear in the blood, CNS changes occur, especially in the cord, medulla, and cerebellum. These changes are characterized by perivascular mononuclear cuffing (around veins and venules) and a zone of tissue necrosis in which demyelination is conspicuous. Seen electron-microscopically, myelin near some of the mononuclear cells undergoes focal lysis, with dissolution of the lamellae. Through these gaps, phagocytic cells attack and gradually destroy the sheaths, becoming transformed into lipid macrophages (gitter cells) in the process. Concurrently, myelin is broken down by vesiculation along the minor and major dense lines, followed by phagocytosis, frequently starting at the nodes of Ranvier (features not specific for EAE). Autoradiographic studies show that only a few of the mononuclear cells present are labeled and might be presumed to contain antibody, and it is in the vicinity of these cells that myelinolysis occurs. Oligodendroglial cells also undergo swelling and necrosis, and axons and astrocytes may be attacked.

Experimental allergic encephalomyelitis can be passively transferred to another animal by mononuclear cells, but not by serum. However, EAE serum contains a *gliotoxic antibody* which causes demyelination of CNS or PNS tissue cultures that is associated with severe oligodendroglial and possibly astroglial damage. In addition, specific *antimyelin antibody* may sometimes be present. This is not necessary for the development of EAE, and indeed, in high concentration, it appears to have a protective rather than a toxic action, presumably by combining with antigenic sites and preventing their being attacked by sensitized lymphocytes. The animals exhibit a delayed-type skin reaction to encephalitogenic protein, and this protein is capable of causing lymphoblastic transformation of lymphocytes (sensitization).

The gliotoxic antibody titer correlates, at least in monkeys, with the severity of the induced disease, and since it may be found in the serum of recipients after lymphocyte transfer, it is possible that EAE tissue damage is caused in part, or even largely, by circulating complement-dependent gliotoxic antibody produced by the transformed lymphocytes, as well as by the cells directly.

In summary, EAE is an autoimmune disease exhibiting both cell-mediated and humoral immunity, although the relationships between gliotoxic and specific antimyelin effects, both humoral and cellular, require further clarification.

Comparison of Multiple Sclerosis with Experimental Allergic Encephalomyelitis. Such a comparison clearly indicates that these two conditions are not the results of identical processes. EAE is an acute or subacute (or occasionally hyperacute and hemorrhagic) process without remission, characterized by prominent invasion of the CNS by transformed and other mononuclear cells, nonspecific perivascular destruction, and a clear mode of induction. Multiple sclerosis, on the other hand, is almost always a chronic, remitting process, characterized by a much more selective destruction, involving myelin and oligodendroglia only, and with no known inducing factors. However, relatively little is known of the immunogenic properties of nervous tissue. Although there may well be others, at least two complement-dependent antibodies are known. One, antimyelin antibody, is specific for myelin and oligodendroglia, and the other (gliotoxic antibody) also affects other elements of cultured CNS tissue.

It is a reasonable hypothesis that, in contrast to EAE, in which the mode of induction leads to predominant formation of gliotoxic antibody, naturally occurring multiple sclerosis may be associated largely with antimyelin antibody, partly accounting for the different pathological changes.

Antibodies to Central Nervous System in Multiple Sclerosis. Antibody has been demonstrated by immunofluorescence in the CNS of a few cases of multiple sclerosis; with complement, it is attached to myelin, oligodendroglia, and astrocytes at the plaque edges (as well as to PNS myelin). It is not clear whether this is similar to the gliotoxic antibody of EAE, or whether it represents an antimyelin factor exhibiting a cross reaction between oligodendroglia and astrocytes. This might not be surprising in view of their common cellular origin and might explain the profound and apparently disproportionate astrocytic hyperplasia, hypertrophy, and fiber formation by sublethal damage to the astrocytes.

Multiple sclerosis sera may contain antimyelin antibody that, when added to tissue cultures, causes lysis of myelin and swelling and destruction of a proportion (not all) of the oligodendroglial cells. The myelin destruction is principally initiated by vesicle formation and separation at the minor dense line, the presumed site of encephalitogenic protein, and not by the local lysis associated with transformed lymphocytes. Unfortunately, antimyelin antibodies in serum are not detectable in all cases; they tend to increase in frequency and titer with chronicity and to be more obvious during relapses. More unfortunately, they are not limited to multiple sclerosis, but occur in other CNS diseases (especially motoneuron disease) and occasionally in normal persons. It has not yet been possible to make a distinction between the quantity or type of antibody in these various conditions.

Patients with multiple sclerosis have a uniformly negative delayed-type skin test reaction to encephalitogenic protein, suggesting that cell-mediated immunity plays a minor part in the process. This conclusion is supported by the relatively small number of mononuclear cells in the CNS (although they are presumably sufficient to account for the oligoclonal globulin of the CSF).

Remitting clinical features often occur in these patients, and it is possible that they are associated with an antisynaptic effect, seen when either the patient's or EAE serum is added to electrically active nerve tissue. This antisynaptic factor has not been identified, but appears to be separate from antimyelin antibody and probably also from gliotoxic antibody.

Possible Role of Infection in the Induction of Autoimmunity. The mode of induction of autoimmunity, if it is a primary phenomenon as is now generally believed, is unknown. Epidemiological data, together with serological studies, at least raise the possibility of an infection, probably viral, in the initiation of the disease process. Paramyxoviruses such as measles, which derive their envelope from the plasmalemma and might incorporate antigenic determinants from the plasmalemma within that envelope, might well be responsible for bringing encephalitogenic protein and immunologically competent cells into contact outside the CNS, after which the process could be self-perpetuating. The lymphocytes from multiple sclerosis patients occasionally show transformation in the presence of brain extract or encephalitogenic protein, although this phenomenon is not restricted to such patients.

In children with acute viral infections – including, but not exclusively, measles – the "sensitivity" of lymphocytes to encephalitogenic protein is markedly raised. This does not indicate common antigenic determinants, since the protein sensitivity rapidly drops off after the acute infection, whereas measles or other viral sensitivity does not. Thus, such results need not imply a "resident" virus in the CNS that maintains lymphocyte sensitivity, but would be equally in favor of a temporary viral infection initiating autoimmunity and subsequent banal infections causing nonspecific increased lymphocyte sensitivity or "irritability" and relapses in clinical condition, which, as already noted, are often associated with increased titers of antimyelin antibody.

It is reported that multiple sclerosis patients show a higher proportion of human lymphocyte antigens HL-A 1, 3, 7, and 18A than in the general population. HL-A antigens may be related to resistance to viral infections, but the significance of this in relation to multiple sclerosis remains to be assessed.

Conclusions

Thus, although the etiology and pathogenesis of multiple sclerosis remain undetermined, a plausible case can be made for its being an autoimmune process, possibly initiated by transient CNS infection with paramyxovirus or other organisms, resulting in lymphocyte sensitization, mainly to basic protein. Differing from EAE, this sensitization seems to express itself principally in terms of a complement-dependent antimyelin antibody that causes oligodendroglial and myelin destruction around venules (initially), and possibly (by antigenic cross reaction) stimulates astrocytes to disproportionate reactivity. Diffusion of antimyelin antibody within the CNS is relatively slow, and as the titer drops the disease becomes relatively quiescent, only to be reactivated by further lymphocyte stimulation due to nonspecific infections. Small numbers of transformed lymphocytes persist both peripherally and in the CNS and produce oligoclonal gamma globulin.

SECONDARY MYELIN DEGENERATION

As already noted, breakdown either of central or peripheral myelin begins with configurational changes in the myelin lamellae (the physical stage of disruption), followed by chemical degradation, the products of which are phagocytized by available cells. Following axonal loss in the CNS, degeneration of myelin sheaths ensues that is analogous to wallerian degeneration in the PNS. The changes are first observed within 24 to 48 hours and consist of splitting of the myelin, mainly along the minor dense lines, probably associated with increased proteolytic activity, and accompanied by increased water content and loss of basic protein. By three days, changes are visible under the light microscope and consist of irregular swelling and beading of the myelin sheaths, with shrinkage that causes widening of the nodes. The axon also shows irregularity of contour and fragmentation, following which the myelin sheath itself fragments, frequently at the same level as the axon, forming a chain of spherical, elliptical, or granular bodies, often containing fragments of axons (digestion chambers). These axonal remnants appear to undergo proteolysis within their myelin coating, presumably due to lysosomal and myelin proteinases. This process is complete by about 10 days and is more rapid in the larger fibers. Products of chemical degradation are detectable about 6 to 10 days after axonal damage.

The major role in phagocytosis is played by macrophages, some of which may be microglia or resident perivascular cells, but many of which undoubtedly come from the circulating blood. These cells begin to appear 4 to 10 days after axonal damage, between and within the disintegrating sheaths, and may undergo local mitotic activity. The phagocytic phase may be as short as three to six weeks or last for three to four months, depending on the quantity of myelin products to be removed. It is accompanied by mild to moderate reactive astrocytosis and fibrillary gliosis. A role for astrocytes and oligodendrocytes in the removal of breakdown products has been suggested, but evidence that this occurs on any significant scale is slight.

The loss of axons is accompanied by degeneration and disappearance of their terminal presynaptic processes, which begin to swell as early as 24 hours after injury. After 3 days they are enlarged, granular, and often clearly visible under the light microscope. They disintegrate completely within 10 days.

BIBLIOGRAPHY

Adams, C. M. W., and Leibowitz, S. The General Pathology of Demyelinating Diseases. In G. H. Bourne (Ed.), *The Structure and Function of Nervous Tissue.* New York: Academic, 1969. Vol. 3, pp. 309-381.

Duboid-Dalcq, M., Schumacher, G., and Sever, J. L. Acute multiple sclerosis: Electron microscopic evidence for and against a viral agent in the plaques. *Lancet* 2:1408-1411, 1973.

Field, E. J. Role of viral infection and autoimmunity in the etiology and pathogenesis of multiple sclerosis. *Lancet* 1:295-297, 1973.

Hirano, A. The Pathology of the Central Myelinated Axon. In G. H. Bourne (Ed.), *The Structure and Function of Nervous Tissue.* New York: Academic, 1972. Vol. 5, pp. 73-162.

Kies, M. W. Experimental Allergic Encephalomyelitis. In G. E. Gaull (Ed.), *Biology of Brain Dysfunction.* New York: Plenum, 1973. Vol. 2, pp. 185-224.

Lampert, P. W. Fine Structural Changes of Myelin Sheaths in the Central Nervous System. In G. H. Bourne (Ed.), *The Structure and Function of Nervous Tissue.* New York: Academic, 1968. Vol. 1, pp. 187-204.

Liebowitz, U. Multiple sclerosis: Progress in epidemiologic and experimental research. *J. Neurol. Sci.* 12:307-318, 1971.

Link, H. Oligoclonal immunoglobulin G in multiple sclerosis brains. *J. Neurol. Sci.* 16:104-114, 1972.

McAlpine, D., Lumsden, C. E., and Acheson, E. D. *Multiple Sclerosis — A Re-appraisal* (2nd ed.). Baltimore: Williams & Wilkins, 1972.

McMurray, W. C., and Magee, W. L. Phospholipid metabolism. *Annu. Rev. Biochem.* 41:129-160, 1972.

Peters, G. Multiple Sclerosis. In J. Minckler (Ed.), *Pathology of the Nervous System.* New York: McGraw-Hill, 1968. Vol. 1, pp. 821-843.

Poser, C. M. Diseases of the Myelin Sheath. In J. Minckler (Ed.), *Pathology of the Nervous System.* New York: McGraw-Hill, 1968. Vol. 1, pp. 767-821.

Raine, C. S., and Bernstein, M. B. Experimental allergic encephalomyelitis: An ultrastructural study of experimental demyelination in vitro. *J. Neuropathol. Exp. Neurol.* 29:177-191, 1970.

Rose, A. S. Multiple sclerosis. A clinical and theoretical review. *J. Neurosurg.* 41:279-284, 1974.

Seil, F. J. Multiple sclerosis — current etiological concepts. *Calif. Med.* 116:25-33, 1972.

Stoffel, W. Sphingolipids. *Annu. Rev. Biochem.* 40:57-82, 1971.

Vaughn, J. E., and Skoff, R. P. Neuroglia in Experimentally Altered Central Nervous System. In G. H. Bourne (Ed.), *The Structure and Function of Nervous Tissue.* New York: Academic, 1972. Vol. 5, pp. 39-72.

Weiner, L. P., Johnson, R. T., and Herndon, R. M. Viral infections and demyelinating diseases. *N. Engl. J. Med.* 288:1103-1111, 1973.

Wickremesinghe, H. R., and Yates, P. O. Immunological properties of normal neural tissues. *J. Neurol. Sci.* 15:225-242, 1972.

Wolman, M. Myelin Structure, Ultrastructure and Degeneration. In J. Minckler (Ed.), *Pathology of the Nervous System.* New York: McGraw-Hill, 1968. Vol. 1, pp. 758-767.

Vitamin-Deficiency Diseases

22

Pure vitamin-deficiency diseases are rarely seen in clinical practice and are often difficult to induce experimentally, either in human subjects or animals, because of the ubiquitous distribution of many vitamins and their frequent association in the same foods. Vitamins are deficient in patients with severe malnutrition, and the deficiency of one particular factor may occasionally dominate the clinical picture and produce overt CNS disease. Probably partly as a result of concurrent malnutrition, but possibly also due to metabolic effects, chronic alcoholism is also associated with CNS disease, either definitely due to vitamin deficiency or suspected of so being. Much more rarely, genetic errors of metabolism or membrane transport may produce features of vitamin deficiency (see Chap. 20).

The CNS is dependent for its functional and structural integrity on a continuous high energy supply almost entirely derived from carbohydrate (see Chap. 13) and therefore is particularly susceptible to deficiencies of vitamins of the B group. Deficiency of some B-group vitamins is associated with damage to oligodendroglial cells and myelin, in both the central nervous system and peripheral nervous system, in spite of the relatively low metabolic rate of white matter. This may be in part due to the association of these vitamins, particularly thiamine, with the hexose monophosphate shunt, essential to produce reduced nicotinamide-adenine dinucleotide phosphate for lipid synthesis. Neuropathological changes are most clearly recognized with deficiencies of thiamine, nicotinic acid, pyridoxine, and cobalamin. Other deficiencies are not yet conclusively associated with CNS disease.

THIAMINE DEFICIENCY

Thiamine, probably in the form of its diphosphate (pyrophosphate, TDP) is an essential coenzyme of the hexose monophosphate shunt (transketolase), for the conversion of pyruvate to acetylcoenzyme A and the conversion of α-ketoglutaric acid to succinyl-CoA. In addition, it may have a yet undefined role in membrane function. Thiamine deficiency might therefore be expected at least to reduce utilization of pyruvate, slow the tricarboxylic acid cycle, and reduce the supply of $NADPH+H^+$. Normal CNS tissue contains about 1 ppm thiamine (which is high in comparison with the amount in other tissues), about 70% as the diphosphate and about 10% each as free thiamine, monophosphate, and triphosphate. In thiamine deficiency, the brain retains thiamine better than most other tissues, but metabolic defects ultimately develop. These include (in vitro) accumulation of pyruvate and lactate, reduction of acetate, citrate, and α-ketoglutarate, reduced acetylcholine synthesis, and substantial loss of transketolase activity. About half the total brain thiamine is necessary just to maintain pyruvate oxidation, so there is little safety margin.

It is generally accepted that beriberi and Wernicke's encephalopathy are associated with thiamine deficiency in man, and in the former there is usually a clear dietary deficiency. A role for thiamine deficiency is suspected in several diseases often associated with alcoholism or malnutrition (alcoholic neuropathy, central pontine myelinolysis, and Marchiafava-Bignami disease) and in subacute necrotizing encephalopathy, a disease of infancy and childhood that histologically resembles Wernicke's encephalopathy.

Beriberi

Beriberi occurs mainly in the tropics of the Far East, but occasionally in other tropical areas, particularly in association with famine or prisoner-of-war conditions. Peripheral neuropathy, which may be associated with cardiac lesions and congestive failure, begins in the legs and arms but may even extend to the cranial and autonomic nerves and nerve roots; evidence of CNS disturbance is rare. Histologically, the nerves show degeneration of axons and myelin, so that myelin loss is both secondary (wallerian) and primary (segmental).

Wernicke's Encephalopathy

Wernicke's encephalopathy is frequently associated with a peripheral neuropathy and is manifested by alterations of consciousness, frequently associated with ataxia, nystagmus, and visual involvement. In chronic cases, Korsakoff's psychosis may develop. Blood pyruvate levels may be raised. Lesions are present in the hypothalamus (especially in the mamillary bodies) (Fig. 22-1) and the periaqueductal and periventricular gray matter; less consistently, they

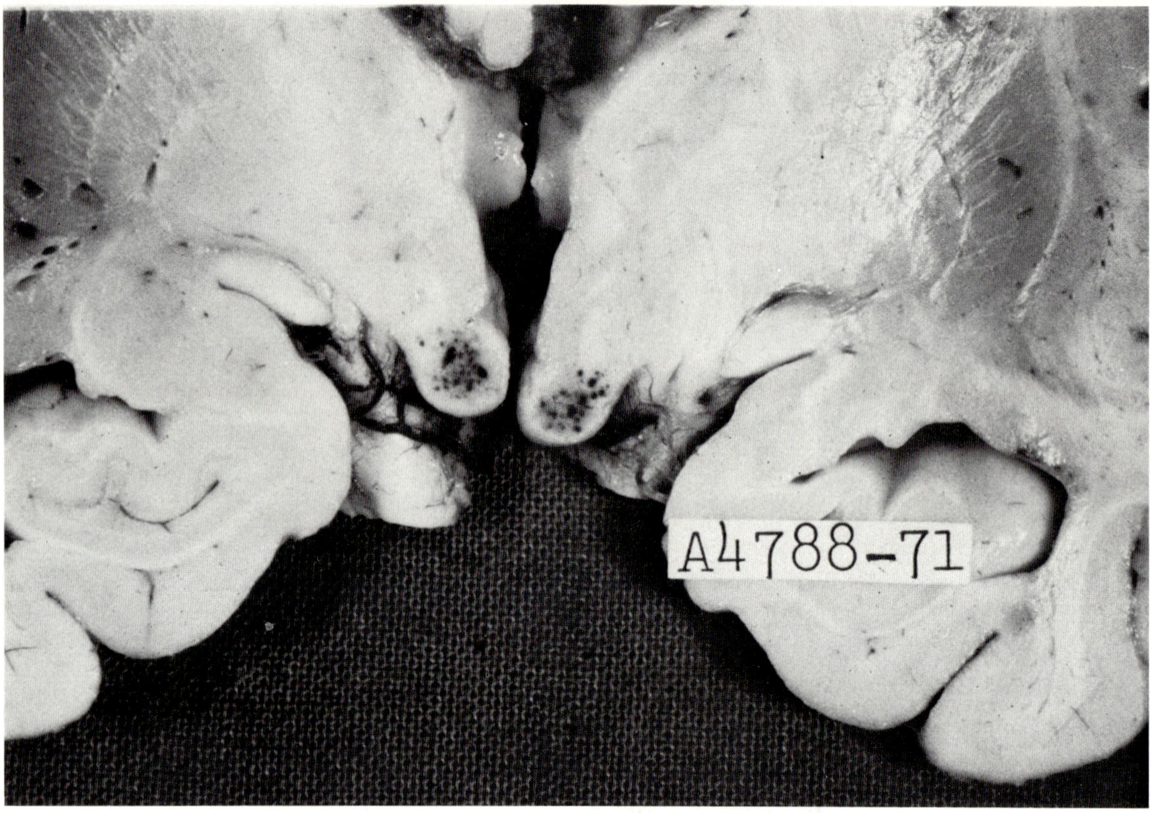

Fig. 22-1. Wernicke's encephalopathy, showing petechial hemorrhages in the mamillary bodies.

involve the inferior colliculus, vestibular nucleus, and dorsal nucleus of the vagus nerve.

Prominent proliferation and thickening of capillary endothelium occurs, sometimes associated with perivascular petechiae (Fig. 22-2). While there is severe demyelination and loss of oligodendroglial cells, the neurons and axons appear relatively resistant, and there is little microglial or astrocytic reaction. Coarse vacuolation or spongiosis is often prominent, due both to an increase in the extracellular space and to swelling and vacuolation of oligodendroglial cytoplasm.

Wernicke's encephalopathy is most frequently associated with alcoholism, severe malabsorption, persistent severe infections, or chronic disorders of water and electrolyte balance. In the Far East, it occurs acutely in infants because of thiamine deficiency in breast milk and is colloquially called "breast milk intoxication."

Subacute Necrotizing Encephalopathy

Subacute necrotizing encephalopathy is the current term for a condition occurring in infants and children that histologically resembles Wernicke's encephalopathy, although it is not necessarily subacute or necrotizing. The brunt of the disease falls on the hypothalamus and the periaqueductal and periventricular regions (Fig. 22-3), although the mamillary bodies are often spared, and petechiae are rarely seen. However, it is frequently much more extensive, often involving the basal ganglia, thalamus, other areas of

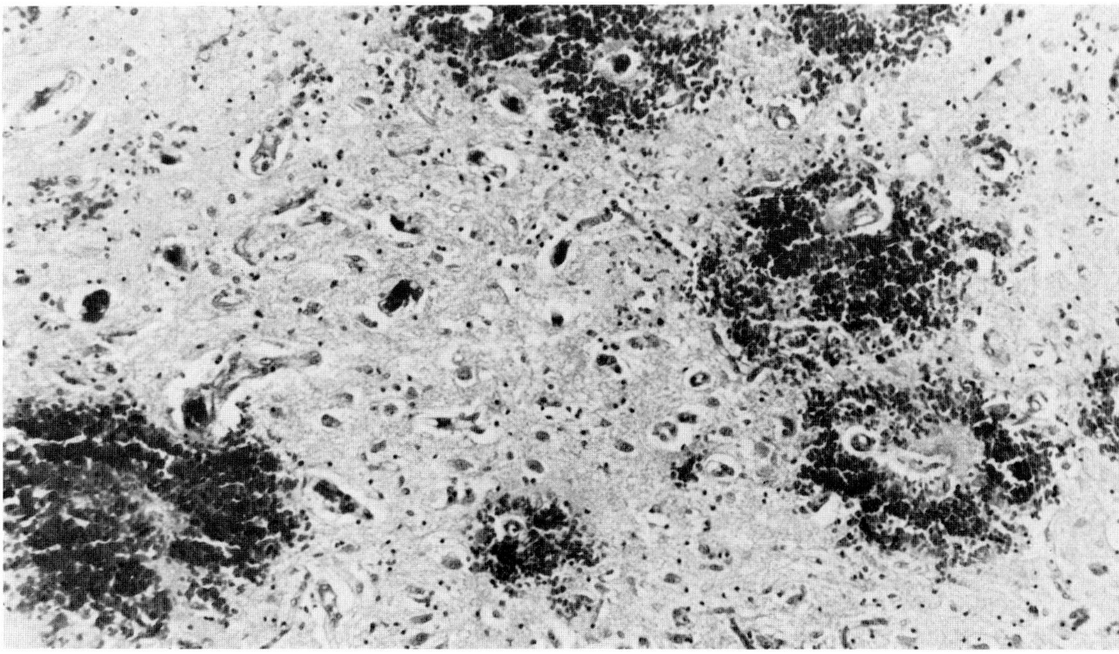

Fig. 22-2. Wernicke's encephalopathy, showing perivascular petechiae and prominence of capillaries. (H & E, X115.)

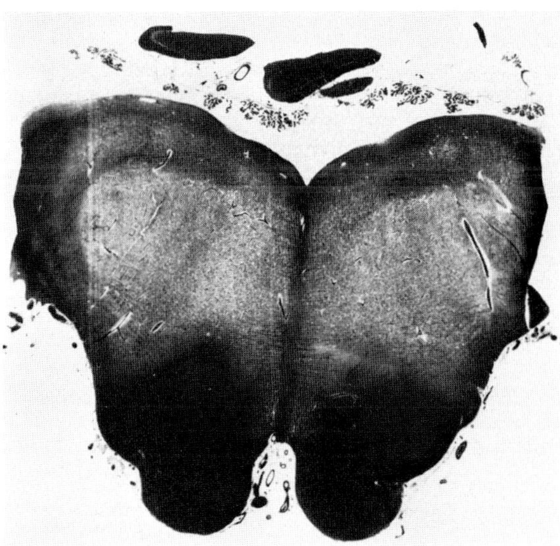

Fig. 22-3. Infantile necrotizing encephalopathy. Section at pontomedullary junction, showing symmetrical rarefaction (which involved the whole brain stem and deep cerebral structures). (Weil's stain, X 6.)

the brain stem, and the posterior columns of the cord. In all areas the histological changes are similar to those described for Wernicke's encephalopathy except for the lack of perivascular hemorrhage (Fig. 22-4).

There is no evidence of dietary deficiency of thiamine, nor is there any clinical response to vitamin administration. Almost half the reported cases have been familial, with an increased incidence of consanguinity in the parents, suggesting a possible autosomal recessive mode of inheritance. In this condition, there appears to be inability to convert TDP to thiamine triphosphate (TTP), which is reduced from its usual proportion of about 10% to less than 0.1% of total thiamine. Thiamine triphosphate is synthesized from TDP and adenosine triphosphate (ATP) by a phosphotransferase that is said to be inhibited by the blood, urine, and cerebrospinal fluid of some patients. However, the function of TTP in the CNS is unknown.

Central Pontine Myelinolysis

A possible relationship of central pontine myelinosis to thiamine deficiency is suggested by its occasional concurrence with Wernicke's encephalopathy in the same brain and by similar associations, including alcoholism and malnutrition. However, there is no direct evidence of thiamine deficiency, and there have been no reports of patients responding to administration of the vitamin. The condition occurs in alcoholism, malnutrition, metastatic carcinoma, chronic infections, neoplasms of the reticuloendothelial system, and immunosuppression for renal transplantation. Diagnosis is usually made postmortem, since there are no clear clinical correlates; some mental changes are often noted.

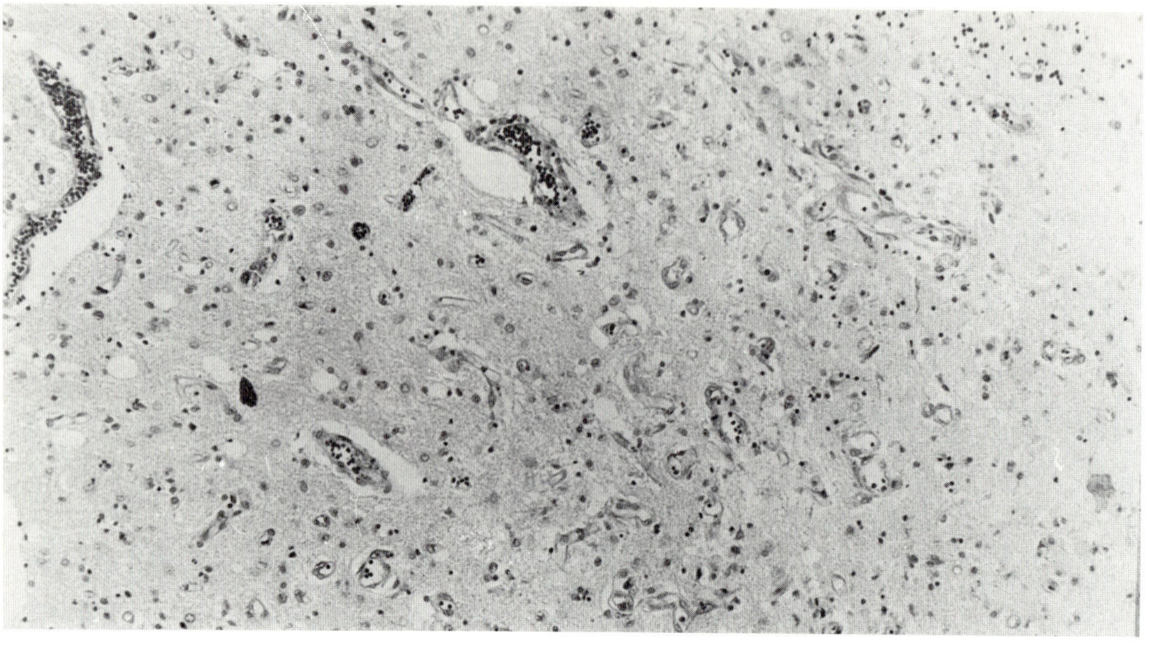

Fig. 22-4. Infantile necrotizing encephalopathy, showing apparent proliferation of capillaries and moderate spongiosis. (H & E, X300.)

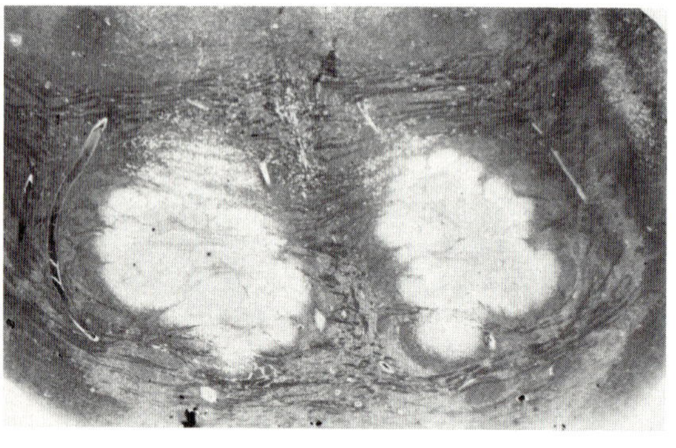

Fig. 22-5. Central pontine myelinolysis, showing symmetrical demyelinating lesions in the basal pons. (Luxol-H & E, X5.)

Characteristically, there is a central, usually symmetrical lesion in the basal pons (Fig. 22-5), which microscopically shows demyelination and loss of oligodendroglial cells, and occasional neuronal and axonal damage with glial reaction. The center of large lesions may become cystic, and Alzheimer type II cells are frequently present, presumably due to the concurrence of liver disease. A possible immunological basis has been hypothesized because a few cases are associated with immunosuppression or reticuloendothelial neoplasms, and numerous plasma cells were noted in one case. The condition is somewhat rare.

Marchiafava-Bignami Disease

Marchiafava-Bignami disease may also occur concurrently with Wernicke's encephalopathy and therefore has been tentatively attributed to thiamine deficiency. The majority of patients so far reported have been Italian and unduly fond of wine, but neither of these characteristics is essential for the development of the disease. However, in all the reported cases, the patients have been either alcoholic or severely malnourished. Clinically, these patients show a nonspecific dementia that is difficult to correlate with the pathological lesions, which include single or confluent areas of necrosis in the medial corpus callosum, often starting rostrally and leading to callosal atrophy. Similar lesions are occasionally found in the anterior commissure, middle cerebellar peduncles, hemispheric white matter, and optic chiasm.

As in central pontine myelinolysis, the lesion appears to be a primary attack on the oligodendroglial cells and myelin, although at such a slow tempo that there is no accumulation of myelinoclastic products and only minimal microglial or astrocytic reaction.

NICOTINIC ACID DEFICIENCY

Nicotinic acid is a component part of nicotinamide-adenine dinucleotide (NAD) and nictotinamide-adenine dinucleotide phosphate (NADP) and is integrally linked with energy metabolism and lipid synthesis. It is not clear how much needs to be preformed in the diet, since it may be synthesized by bacteria in the gut and probably also (in man) from tryptophan in the tissues. The deficiency disease pellagra, associated with a diet largely of maize, is indirectly due to tryptophan deficiency. However, features of pellagra may develop in the absence of dietary deficiencies. This may occur in some cases of carcinoid syndrome, in which up to 60% of tryptophan, instead of 1%, is diverted to serotonin; in Hartnup disease, in which there is deficiency of tryptophan transport in the gut; occasionally in other inborn errors of metabolism, such as phenylketonuria and maple syrup urine disease, in which conversion of tryptophan to nicotinic acid is reduced by unknown mechanisms; and in prolonged isoniazid therapy, which interferes with the pyridoxine coenzymes needed for the synthesis of nicotinic acid from tryptophan.

The CNS symptomatology of pellagra includes spasticity, ataxia, extrapyramidal disorders, and psychoneurotic changes that may progress to dementia. Occasionally, convulsions are seen. In addition, these patients may exhibit retrobulbar neuritis, polyneuritis, erythematous and atrophic skin lesions, glossitis, diarrhea, and anemia.

On pathological examination, pellagra of the CNS is seen to be characterized by widespread swelling and central chromatolysis of the neurons, which tends to spare the seventh and twelfth cranial nerve motoneurons and Purkinje's cells. Although this resembles the axonal reaction (see Chap. 10), it seems more likely to be on a direct metabolic basis. Little glial reaction occurs. Pellagra may be associated with demyelination of the posterior and lateral white columns of the cord and the anterior and posterior roots, peripheral demyelination being both segmental and associated with axonal loss. These demyelinating lesions are not always present in pellagra and may be due to deficiency of some other dietary factor.

Central nervous system concentrations of NAD and NADP are maintained better than those of most other tissues in acute nicotinic acid deficiency. The neurometabolic alterations in pellagra are not understood.

PYRIDOXINE DEFICIENCY

Pyridoxine is a generic term for a group of closely related compounds, namely, pyridoxol, pyridoxal, pyridoxamine, and their phosphates. In tissues the vitamin is usually found as pyridoxal and pyridoxamine phosphate. It is involved in transamination, the formation of serotonin, the decarboxylation of glutamic acid to gamma-aminobutyric acid, and sphingol metabolism.

Experimentally, deprivation of pyridoxine causes convulsions, and the convulsant action of hydrazines, oximes, and hydroxylamines may be due to their interference with pyridoxine-dependent reactions. Pyridoxine deficiency is probably responsible for some infantile convulsions, the normal daily requirement being about 1.5 mg. However, a small group of infants, apparently on a genetic basis, require much higher daily intakes (up to 15 mg), at least in the early years of life and are termed *pyridoxine-dependent.* Unless their diet is adequately supplemented, severe and intractable convulsions ensue (see Chap. 18).

COBALAMIN (VITAMIN B_{12}) DEFICIENCY

Although usually either dietary or due to malabsorption, vitamin B_{12} deficiency may be seen in prolonged treatment with anticonvulsants, such as phenobarbital and diphenylhydantoin. Its role in the CNS is unclear. It is necessary for the conversion of methylmalonyl-CoA to succinyl-CoA, and patients with a deficiency excrete increased amounts of methylmalonic, propionic, and acetic acids. It is also involved in protein, RNA, and carbohydrate metabolism.

Cobalamin deficiency is usually associated with megaloblastic (pernicious) anemia, and the CNS complication is *subacute combined degeneration.* Its appearance is not related to the degree of anemia, from which it differs in responding only to vitamin B_{12} and not to folic acid. Clinically, the disease progresses over weeks or months, with mixed spastic and ataxic paraplegia, often associated with hypesthesia that is more marked in the legs than the arms, and peripheral trophic lesions. Mental changes and seizures are occasional complications.

Lesions involve the white matter of the cord and are often most severe in the midthoracic region, where they appear to spread from the centers of the posterior column on each side, from the pial surface immediately ventral to the dorsal horns, and from the anterior median fissure, even involving the fasciculi proprii. Above this level the posterior columns and the spinocerebellar tracts show ascending degeneration (secondary demyelination); below, the corticospinal fibers show descending degeneration. Secondary central chromatolysis of the thoracic nucleus of Clarke may occur. Early lesions appear to involve mainly oligodendroglial cells and myelin; later, axons are involved, producing the ascending and descending degeneration noted above. Microglial and astrocytic reactions vary from mild to moderate. Variable myelin and axonal changes are seen in the peripheral nervous system, but it is not clear whether these are directly due to vitamin B_{12} deficiency or to some other factor. Occasional small demyelinated foci are present in the hemispheric white matter.

OTHER VITAMIN DEFICIENCIES

There is no clear evidence of human CNS disease resulting from deficiencies of other members of the B group of vitamins, or of vitamins A, C, or D.

It has been suggested that the peculiar neuroaxonal swelling (neuroaxonal dystrophy) seen in the gracilis and cuneate nuclei, and occasionally in other areas, in infants suffering from severe malabsorption may be due to deficiency of vitamin E. In rats on a chronically E-deficient diet, there is said to be terminal degeneration of afferent axons, also involving the posterior columns and posterior roots — a possibly analogous finding. In growing chicks maintained on a vitamin E-deficient diet, an acute condition known as *nutritional encephalomalacia* develops, characterized by necrosis, capillary proliferation, and reactive changes, especially in the cerebellum. There appears to be no corresponding human disease.

BIBLIOGRAPHY

Goebel, H. H., and Zur, P. H.-B. Central pontine myelinolysis. *Brain* 95:495-504, 1972.

Löken, A. C. Ethyl Alcohol. In J. Minckler (Ed.), *Pathology of the Nervous System.* New York: McGraw-Hill, 1971. Vol. 2, pp. 1671-1678.

Montpetit, V. J. A., Andermann, F., Carpenter, S., Fawcett, J. S., Zborowska-Sluis, D., and Giberson, H. R. Subacute necrotising encephalopathy. *Brain* 94:1-30, 1971.

Poser, C. M. Demyelination in the central nervous system in chronic alcoholism: Central pontine myelinolysis and Marchiafava-Bignami's disease. *Ann. N. Y. Acad. Sci.* 215:373-381, 1973.

Scheck, S. A. Central Pontine Myelinolysis. In J. Minckler (Ed.), *Pathology of the Nervous System.* New York: McGraw-Hill, 1968. Vol. 1, pp. 859-861.

Infectious and Immunological Diseases

23

The central nervous system and the cerebrospinal fluid are normally sterile, and there is no evidence that any cells originating from the neurectoderm or the neural crest are immunologically competent. However, neural crest cells, including at least Schwann's cells and cells of the leptomeninges, are capable of phagocytosis (and probably of digestion of organisms), like macrophages derived from the reticuloendothelial system. Since there are no antibody-forming cells in the CNS, and the normal blood-brain and blood-CSF barriers are almost impermeable to protein, only minimal amounts of gamma globulin are present, derived from the plasma. The relative immunological sequestration of the CNS depends entirely on an intact barrier system. If this is damaged by inflammation or other vascular factors, plasma proteins and leukocytes enter the brain and cord as readily as any other tissue, and both inflammation and autoimmunization may occur. The latter phenomenon is infrequent, although the effective antigenicity of CNS tissue has been adequately demonstrated experimentally in experimental allergic encephalopathy (see Chap. 21).

In addition to leptomeningeal cells, a number of phagocytes are resident in the CNS as microglia and adventitial cells, derived from the reticuloendothelial system during vascularization of the brain in midfetal life. *Phagocytosis* can thus occur within the CNS in at least three types of cells, which cannot be morphologically distinguished in an inflammatory process: these are leptomeningeal cells, microglial cells, and macrophages or histiocytes derived from the adventitia or blood. *Antibody formation* within the CNS, however, can only take place in cells of the lymphocytic series directly derived from the blood across an abnormal barrier system.

Infection of the CNS may take place by one of several alternative routes:

1. *Via the bloodstream (hematogenous).* This is by far the most frequent route, with CNS infections occurring during dissemination of organisms in the bloodstream, such as occurs in the early stages of many infectious processes.

2. *By direct access from the environment.* Such infections are usually associated with skull fracture and tearing of the dura. Occasionally, they follow infections of the scalp, organisms passing through venous channels in the skull. More rarely, they follow surgical procedures, especially if the brain tissue is already devitalized by trauma or ischemia.

3. *From infected cavities adjacent to the cranium.* These cavities include the middle ear and mastoid air cells, frontal and other sinuses that are open to the nasal cavity, and the nasal cavities and nasopharynx themselves. Most CNS infections result from inflammation and infection spreading through and involving the intervening bones and dura; because of the reaction to such inflammation, the infections tend to be localized, with the production of cerebral abscesses and local meningitis. It appears unlikely, although not completely disproved, that retrograde spread of common organisms occurs through the contiguous lymphatic and subarachnoid channels around the olfactory nerve fibers.

4. *Along the axons of motor or sensory nerves.* This intracytoplasmic spread into the CNS appears only to be important in respect to rabies virus. It is considered unlikely that poliovirus reaches the CNS in this manner, but this possibility has not been totally excluded.

A very large range of viral, rickettsial, bacterial, fungal, protozoal, and metazoal organisms can cause CNS infection, some of them having worldwide distribution and others being geographically restricted by the habitats of insect vectors, by animal reservoirs, or for unknown reasons. In the more prosperous parts of the world, some important CNS infections (such as poliomyelitis and syphilis) have become rarer because of adequate control or therapeutic procedures. However, this rarity is dependent on a society's being organized and affluent and would be rapidly reversed in the event of social or economic breakdown.

Central nervous system infections can be classified by etiological agent or by the distribution (and therefore the clinical symptomatology) of the resultant inflammatory and secondary changes. Thus, changes may be virtually confined to the meninges (*meningitis*) or to the CNS parenchyma (*encephalitis* if only the brain is involved; *myelitis* if only the cord is involved; *encephalomyelitis* if both are involved, which occurs more often), or both the meninges and the parenchyma may show inflammatory changes. Changes in the brain and cord may be widespread,

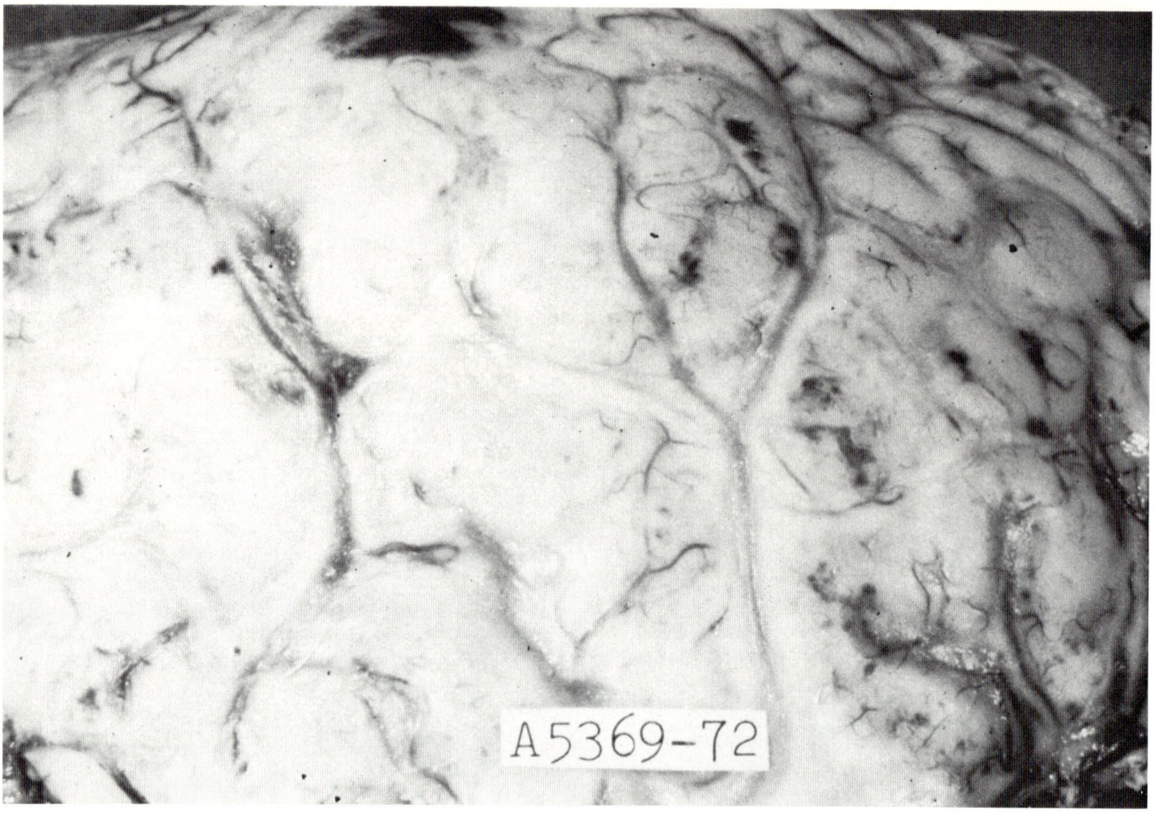

*Fig. 23-1. Purulent leptomeningitis, showing accumulation of pus in sulci. Small petechial hemorrhages are also present, associated with thrombosis of the arterioles and venules (*Hemophilus influenzae *meningitis).*

although even infections may show a preference for certain areas; or they may be localized to one or more macroscopic areas, often as cerebral abscesses. In this chapter, a combined etiological-topographical classification is used on a purely pragmatic basis, to try and bring together diseases that are clinically similar.

MENINGITIS (LEPTOMENINGITIS)

A wide range of viruses, bacteria, fungi, and protozoa may produce meningitis, so that the clinical picture may be acute, subacute, or chronic, self-limiting or progressive. Correspondingly, the histological appearances may be predominantly neutrophilic, mononuclear, or granulomatous, and differ in no essential respect from lesions due to the same organism in other parts of the body. Pus or granulomatous lesions occur especially at the base of the brain, but may be widespread in the sulci (Fig. 23-1).

Meningitis is an inflammation of the subarachnoid space, its bounding membranes, and its extensions, of which the most prominent are those surrounding penetrating arteries and emerging veins of the brain. Although this space is in free continuity with the ventricular system, in many cases the outward flow of CSF seems sufficient to prevent the appearance of identifiable lesions in the ventricles. However, an infection of the ventricular system, either arising from a focus in the choroid plexus or the subependymal regions, almost inevitably means a concomitant meningitis.

The site of the original lesion in meningitis is unclear. It has been suggested that it may be due to primary foci either in the brain or the choroid plexuses, but this has not been substantiated by careful examination in the majority of cases, although it is of course possible that a small primary lesion could be missed even by the most intensive search. On the other hand, there appear to be few, if any, subarachnoid capillaries from which organisms might escape directly into the subarachnoid space. Whatever the origin, the vast majority of cases of meningitis are not accompanied by encephalitis, except insofar as limited cuffing of the penetrating arteries and veins, and sometimes a very modest astrocytic hyperplasia in the molecular layer of the cortex, may be seen. There is a breakdown of the blood-CSF barrier, but not of the blood-brain barrier, with escape of inflammatory cells, organisms, and plasma proteins into the CSF.

The nature of the hematogenous cells (e.g., neutrophils, lymphocytes) depends on the infecting organism, but they are invariably mixed with what appear to be free phagocytic cells, often containing ingested organisms and probably derived from the leptomeninges themselves, as well as from the blood. If the infection persists, these cells manifest their capacity to form reticulin and collagen fibers in the subarachnoid space, so that an adhesive (fibrous) arachnoiditis may result.

Acute meningitis, with appropriate antibiotic treatment as indicated, often resolves completely, and long-term sequelae are rare. Improperly treated, or naturally chronic, meningitis may have several complications, frequently associated with fibrosis. These include communicating postmeningitic hydrocephalus, infiltration or compression of cranial or spinal nerve roots by contracting scar tissue, and the formation of arachnoid cysts that may produce the symptoms of a space-occupying lesion. Uncommonly, meningitis is associated with vasculitis in the subarachnoid space and areas of infarction due to thrombosis of small or (rarely) large arteries.

Normal CSF contains less than 5 mononuclear cells per cubic millimeter and has a protein content of 15 to 40 mg per 100 ml, with no globulin. It is a clear and colorless fluid with a sugar content approximately 10 mg per 100 ml below that of the blood and a chloride content of 720 to 750 mg per 100 ml. In meningitis, these values are altered to a varying extent, depending on the organism and duration. In acute purulent meningitis, cell counts may be as high as 6000 to 10,000 per cubic millimeter (the cells are mostly polymorphonuclear), and protein may reach 50 to 500 mg per 100 ml, frequently including globulin and fibrinogen; the latter may form a translucent clot if the CSF is allowed to stand. Turbidity depends largely on the cell count. Cerebrospinal fluid sugar is reduced, as compared with a simultaneous blood sugar, though it is not clear whether it is consumed by leukocytes, organisms, or both. Chloride is often reduced to 650 to 680 mg per 100 ml, though values lower than this are said to be characteristic of tuberculous meningitis. Such changes may not be a primary feature of meningitis, but may be due to vomiting, dehydration, or electrolyte imbalance.

Viral Meningitis

Viral or benign aseptic meningitis is a relatively innocuous, self-limiting condition, presumably associated with the presence of virus in the subarachnoid space. Moderate increases in CSF cell count and protein content and some depression of CSF glucose are noted; the cells are mononuclear, except in the very earliest stages, when (as in most virus infections in most situations) there is a transient polymorphonuclear response. Viral meningitis may be an isolated clinical finding or may be associated with skin rashes, chest pain, upper respiratory infections, or other relatively banal symptoms.

These cases are usually due to enteroviruses such as coxsackieviruses A and B, echovirus, or reovirus. Occasionally, viral meningitis may follow an acute specific disease such as mumps, when it is possibly a hypersensitivity phenomenon.

Acute Purulent Meningitis

Acute purulent meningitis is a bacterial meningitis that may be associated with any pyogenic organism (Fig. 23-2), either as an isolated clinical finding or with septicemia. Focal meningitis, but less often diffuse, may also occur if organisms from the sinuses, mastoid air cells, middle ear, or nasopharynx invade the cranial cavity. In diffuse meningitis, the commonest associated organisms are *Escherichia coli* (especially in the neonatal period), *Hemophilus influenzae* (especially in children), *Neisseria meningitidis* (meningococcus), and *Diplococcus pneumoniae* (pneumococcus).

The CSF shows high protein and moderate to extreme cellularity, many of the cells being neutrophils. Sugar and chloride are moderately reduced, and the fluid may be opalescent or turbid, depending on the cell count. Numerous intracellular and extracellular organisms are usually present, and culture is often successful.

With antibiotic therapy the prognosis is good and sequelae are uncommon. However, *H. influenzae* meningitis may cause antemortem thrombosis of small penetrating vessels and local superficial or penetrating infarcts (Fig. 23-3).

Fungal Meningitis

Many fungi are capable of infecting the subarachnoid space and meninges. Some are recognized pathogens that produce systemic mycoses in which CNS involvement is a predominant or frequent occurrence; these include *Cryptococcus, Coccidioides* (Fig. 23-4), and *Histoplasma.* Others, such as *Actinomyces, Nocardia,* and hyphal fungi like *Mucorales,* may involve the meninges from adjacent cavities. Meningitis associated with miliary cerebral and generalized visceral abscesses may occur in debilitated patients, in patients with uncontrolled diabetes, in patients on massive corticosteroid therapy or receiving broad-spectrum antibiotics, or in those with immunological deficits or receiving immunosuppressive drugs. The opportunistic pathogens include *Candida.*

Fungi cause a subacute infection in which large numbers of both neutrophils and macrophages are present, and the characteristic organisms can usually be found on histological examination. *Cryptococcus* is seen histologically as an oval or round, thick-walled organism about 15μ across, which may show a single bud and is surrounded by a refractile, gelatinous capsule. *Coccidioides* appears in the exudate as a thick-walled, round structure, 20 to 200μ across, which contains granular material or 2 to 5μ spores. Textbooks of mycology should be consulted for details.

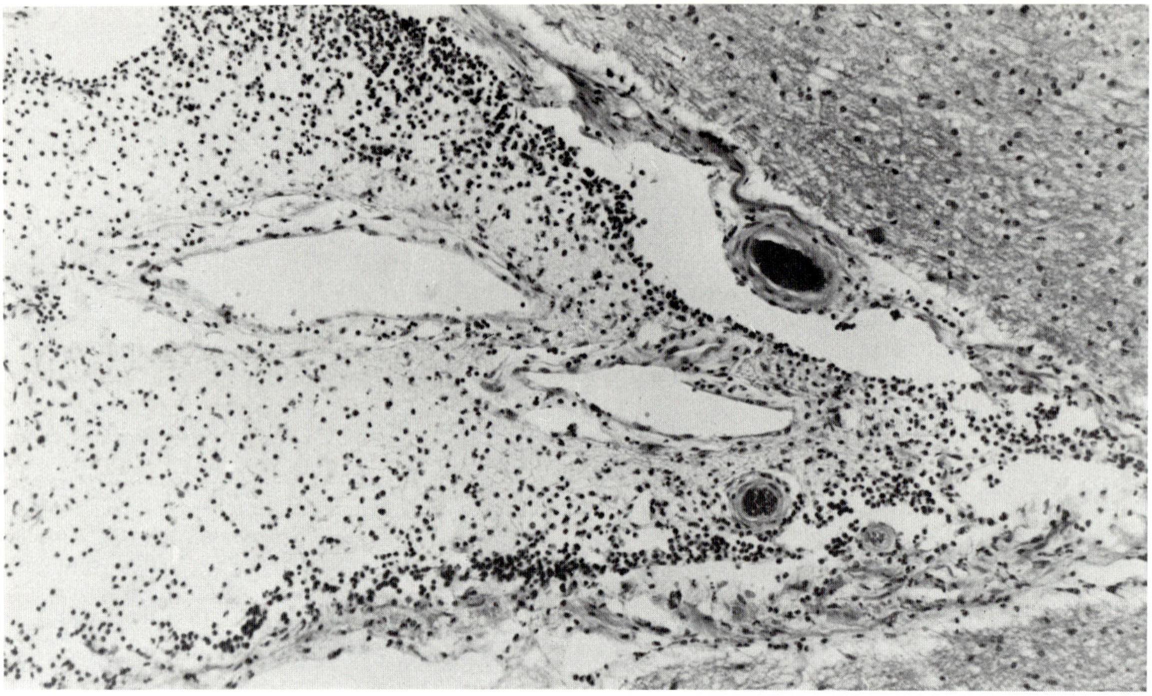

Fig. 23-2. Purulent leptomeningitis, with accumulation of neutrophils and macrophages (Escherichia coli *meningitis). Note the lack of involvement of underlying brain. (H & E, X115.)*

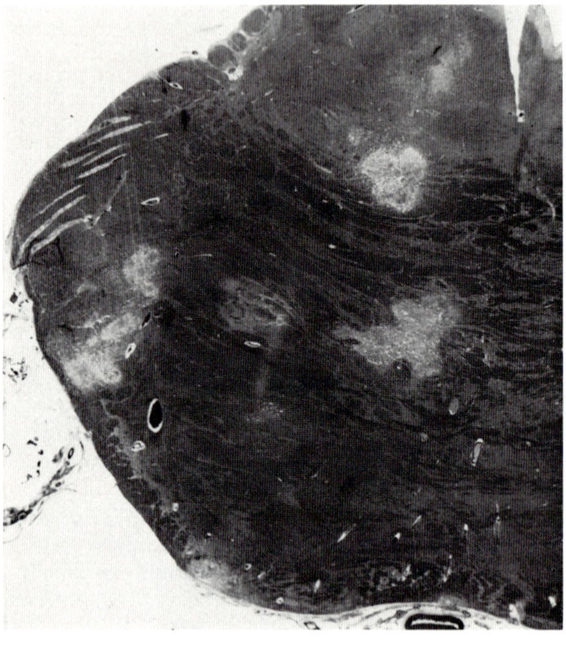

Fig. 23-3. Microinfarcts produced in the basal pons by a thrombosing leptomeningitis (same case as in Fig. 23-1). (Myelin, X8.)

Tuberculous Meningitis

Tuberculous meningitis usually occurs in children and may be due to either the human or bovine form of *Mycobacterium*. As is the case with all forms of meningitis, its mode of access to the meninges is unknown. Direct spread from the brain, spread from foci in the choroid plexus, or direct hematogenous infection might occur. Certainly, cerebral and plexus foci occur, but it cannot be proved that they antedate the meningitis.

The histological picture is typical of tuberculosis. There may be granulomas up to 2 or 3 mm in diameter, frequently paravascular, and sometimes showing central caseation and Langhan's giant cells. Diffuse lymphocytic and macrophage exudate is also present, especially in the perivascular spaces, and there may be moderate diffuse fibrosis (Fig. 23-5). Vessels may show mononuclear inflammation of the wall and occasional antemortem thrombus, with small, superficial, wedge-shaped infarcts. Though small, these may cause considerable damage if, for example, they involve the cerebrospinal fibers in the cerebral peduncle or emerging cranial nerve roots.

The CSF shows pleocytosis up to 1000 mononuclear cells except in the earliest stage, moderately raised protein with some globulin, and often a fibrin clot if fluid is allowed to stand. Sugar is reduced and chloride is usually below 600 mg per 100 ml. Such low CSF chloride is said to be strongly indicative of tuberculous meningitis and to be helpful if the diagnosis cannot be confirmed by culture or direct smear (but see p. 421). Hydrocephalus or cranial nerve palsies may develop, and tuberculous meningitis has a less satisfactory prognosis than most of the other forms of meningitis.

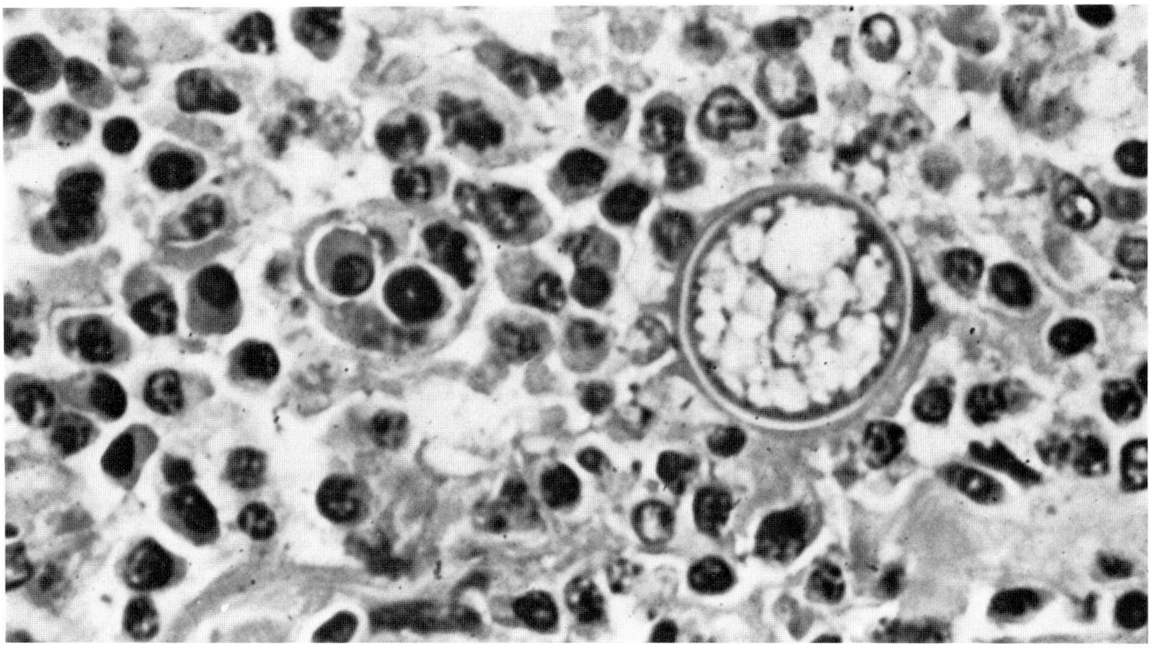

Fig. 23-4. Meningeal coccidioidomycosis. Note the subacute exudate and the organism with endospores. (H & E, ×750.)

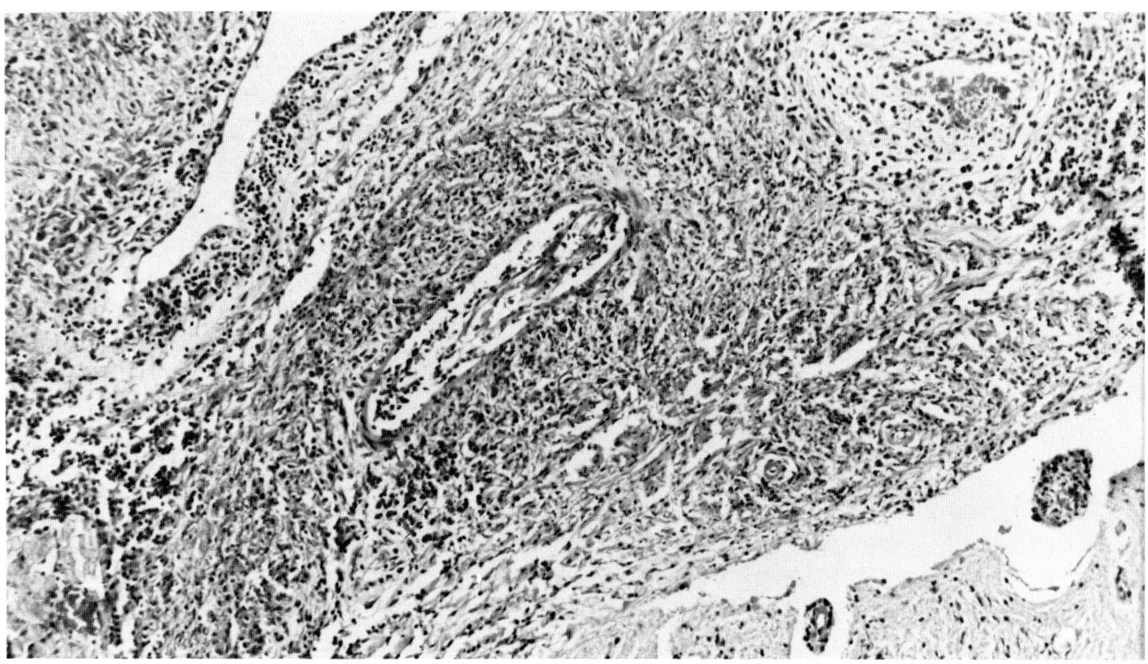

Fig. 23-5. Meningeal tuberculosis. Note the dense, fibrosing, chronic exudate and epithelial cells. No well-formed granulomas are seen, as is often the case. Diagnosis is confirmed by bacterial staining and culture. (H & E, ×115.)

Syphilitic Meningitis

Whereas the other forms of meningitis usually occur in isolation, the syphilitic form is usually accompanied by parenchymal involvement, either in the form of cortical inflammation or posterior column demyelination (tabes). Acute syphilitic meningitis may occur in the secondary stage, with a subacute exudate of lymphocytes and plasma cells. Usually, the chronic form is seen as a concomitant of tertiary syphilis, associated with lymphocytic, plasma-cell, and macrophage exudate, formation of granulomas with central necrosis (gummas), and vascular changes, including endarteritis with severe narrowing. The condition tends to extend into the perivascular parenchyma, or interstitially into cranial or spinal nerve roots. The CSF shows up to 2000 mononuclear cells, with a moderate increase in protein and a positive globulin test. Reactions for the albumin-globulin ratio, such as the colloidal gold test, usually show a first-zone or midzone reaction. Positive CSF serology is obtained in 90% of cases.

BACTERIAL OR FUNGAL ENCEPHALITIS

Except in syphilitic infection, *diffuse* bacterial or fungal invasions of the brain occur only secondary to open head injury, associated with ischemic or traumatic brain damage that is too massive to be amenable to adequate debridement. Widespread infection of devitalized brain, often with a mixed flora including *Clostridia,* is sometimes termed *cerebritis.* Such a development accentuates an already gloomy prognosis. On the other hand, *localized* infections of the brain are frequent with open brain injury, especially if penetrating; metallic, bony, or other fragments frequently prove to be contaminated with environmental organisms. In the majority of such cases, either debridement apparently sterilizes the CNS or a local abscess forms that is amenable to surgical and antibiotic treatment. Thus, the prognosis in this type of encephalitis is good as far as the infection is concerned.

Focal pyogenic or other infections of the brain in the absence of trauma, due to either bacteria or fungi, are relatively common and run the gamut from the myriad miliary lesions associated with septicemia or pyemia to one or a few large abscesses usually associated with infection elsewhere in the body, but without persistent, detectable septicemia.

Miliary Abscesses

Miliary abscesses are usually associated with septicemia or pyemia, with debilitation and attenuation of the defense mechanisms, or commonly with both. Septicemia or pyemia may occur in association with bacterial endocarditis, puerperal infection, lung abscess, suppurative thrombophlebitis, or other infective processes. Causes of debilitation or impaired defense mechanisms include malnutrition, extreme fatigue, cachexia, diabetes, carcinomatosis, administration of broad-spectrum antibiotics (resulting in altered gut flora and fungal overgrowth), immunosuppression associated with transplantation procedures, leukemia and lymphoma, or a primary immunological deficit. Responsible organisms include *Streptococcus* of the *viridans* type, enterococci, and other bacteria, as well as opportunistic fungi such as *Candida* and *Actinomyces* (Fig. 23-6).

Since these lesions are frequently terminal, they are usually seen in the acute stage in the CNS and elsewhere. Vessels may contain infected thrombus and show vasculitis, which in some cases results in localized dilatations of the vessel wall (mycotic aneurysm). There is perivascular destruction of brain parenchyma, with dense infiltration by neutrophils, macrophages, and moderate numbers of lymphocytes. Organisms can sometimes be demonstrated by suitable staining. Microglia in the region are frequently activated, showing rod-shaped or irregular twisted nuclei, and a narrow zone of edema surrounds the lesions. If they have been present for more than a week or two, astrocytic hyperplasia and even early fibrillary gliosis may be seen, together with capillary proliferation at the periphery, associated with an increase in reticulin fibers and later in collagen fibers.

Brain Abscess

The typical brain abscess presents clinically as a focal lesion and is usually subacute or chronic. Occasionally, several such lesions may be present, with correspondingly decreased amenability to surgical treatment. A solitary brain abscess (Fig. 23-7) is not associated with debilitation or immunological deficiency, but in most cases is associated with a detectable infection elsewhere in the body that presumably acts as a primary focus, either by causing transient bacteremia or pyemia or by spreading directly to the CNS. The major associations of cerebral abscess are endocarditis or lung disease (blood-borne spread) or craniofacial infections (direct spread). Some cerebral abscesses occur in which no primary lesion can be detected.

The peak incidence in the blood-borne group is in middle age or somewhat later, although persons of any age may be affected, since a single abscess is occasionally associated with septicemia, congenital heart disease, or septic emboli. Abscesses resulting from direct spread bear some topographical relation to the primary focus. Thus, those associated with frontal sinus infection are in the frontal lobe; those associated with nasopharyngeal infection are also in the frontal lobe, but are located more inferiorly; and those associated with otitis media or mastoiditis are in the temporal lobe or cerebellum. In many cases these infections apparently spread by producing ischemic necrosis and infection of the bone, necrosis of the dura, localized chronic leptomeningitis, and finally involvement of the adjacent brain. However, some abscesses associated with a primary craniofacial infective focus are present in the hemispheric white matter; the intervening bone, dura, leptomeninges, and often the cortex appear grossly and histologically normal. The explanation of these cases is difficult, although some at least may involve retrograde venous spread, with or without septic thrombophlebitis that

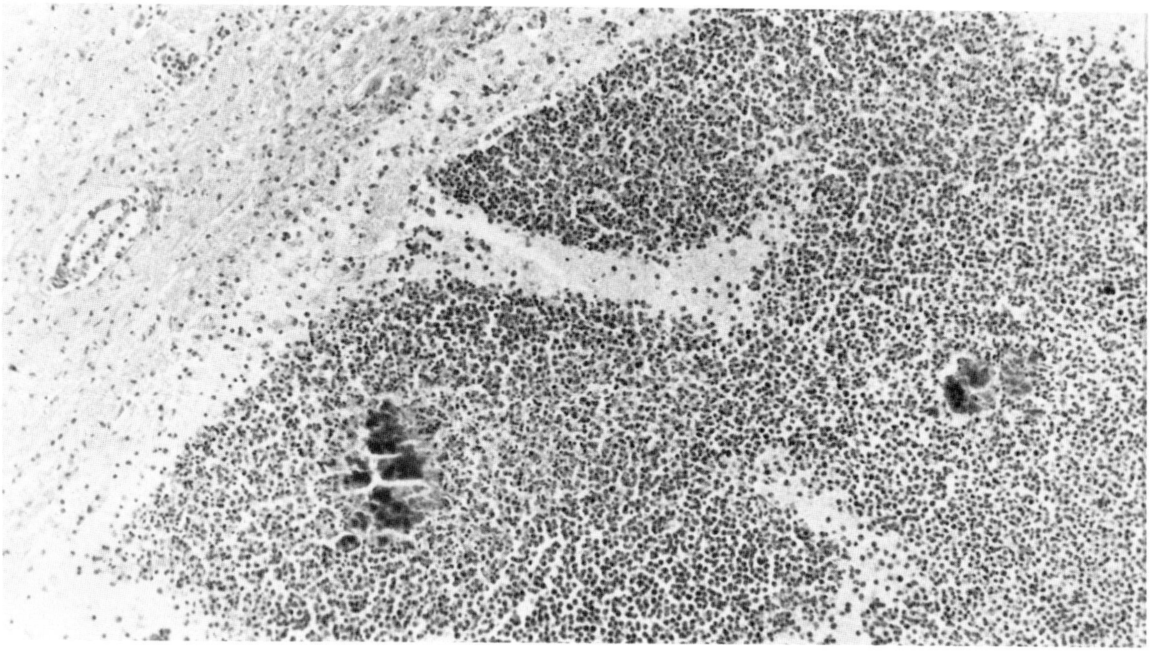

Fig. 23-6. Actinomycotic abscess (one of many) in a patient with Hodgkin's disease. (H & E, ×115.)

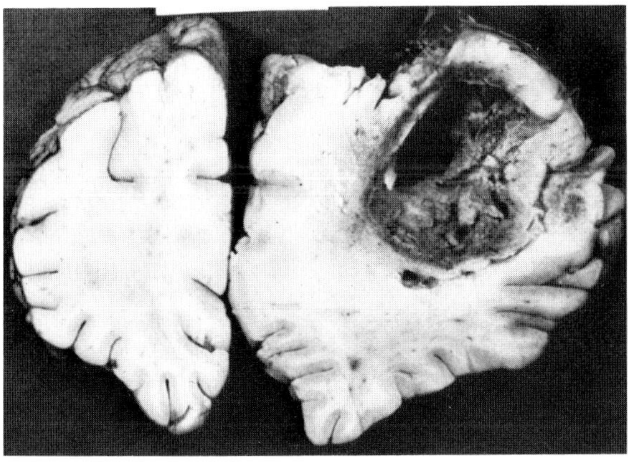

Fig. 23-7. Solitary brain abscess (subacute) in the left frontal lobe, associated with suppurative lung disease.

may have resolved at the time of examination. On culture, about 15% of brain abscesses are sterile. The organisms usually found include staphylococci, streptococci, *H. influenzae,* or, in local spread, various fungi.

An acute or subacute cerebral abscess consists of an area of purulent necrosis of the brain that is relatively poorly demarcated and includes debris derived from the brain and polymorphonuclear leukocytes. The adjacent brain shows infiltration of acute and chronic inflammatory cells, numerous gitter cells, and marked capillary hyperemia and proliferation. A wide zone of edematous white matter surrounds the abscess.

In more chronic cases the debris has become delimited by an abscess wall of varying thickness and rigidity. The inner layer of this wall usually still contains acute and chronic inflammatory cells, although the latter may predominate. The outer layer consists of mesenchymal and glial elements; the former are usually preponderant. The early capillary proliferation has regressed, but perivascular cells have laid down large numbers of interlacing reticulin and collagen fibers (Fig. 23-8). Mild to moderate astrocytic reaction occurs with fibrillary gliosis, but this often contributes relatively little to the abscess wall, which is mainly collagenous. The surrounding brain shows a mild astrocytic reaction and fibrillary gliosis, but little edema. Although infective organisms usually persist in these abscesses, they are relatively well encapsulated, and the lesions can frequently be removed surgically with antibiotic cover.

Syphilis

Invasion of the CNS by *Treponema pallidum* occurs during the secondary phase of syphilis, associated with (clinical or subclinical) acute meningitis with

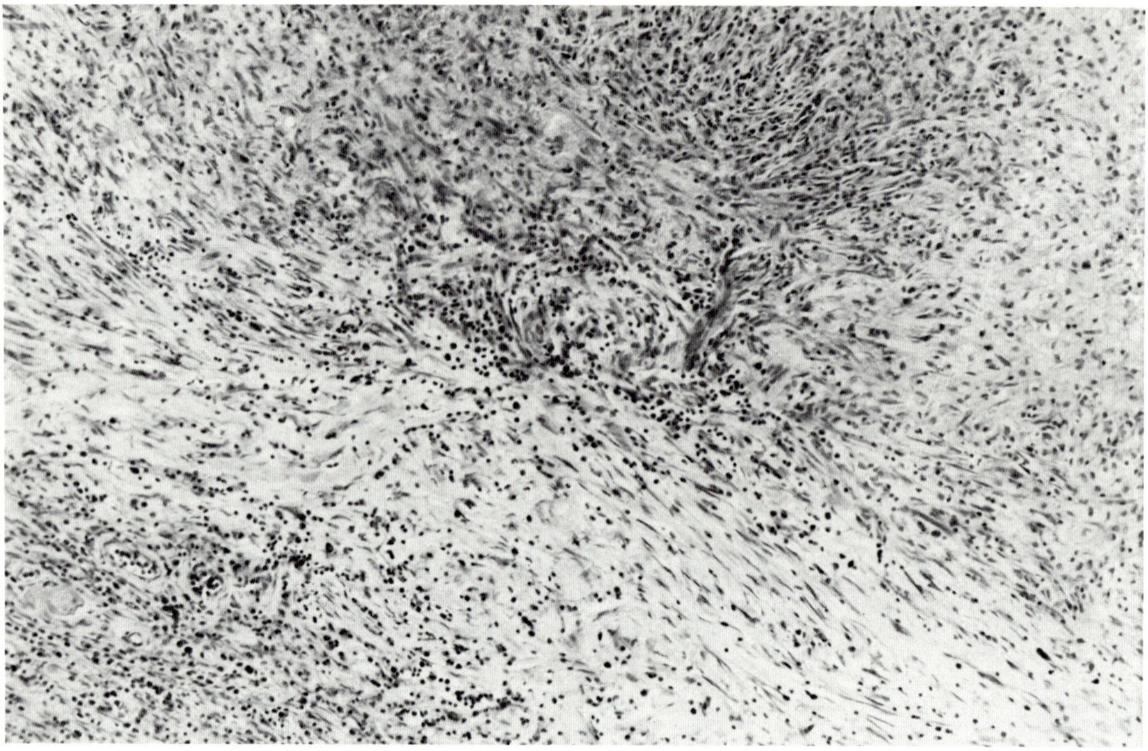

Fig. 23-8. Part of the wall of a chronic abscess, showing capillary and fibroblastic proliferation and moderate lymphocytic infiltration. Astrocytes are conspicuously absent. (H & E, X115.)

lymphocytic and plasma-cell exudate. The later manifestations include meningovascular syphilis, tabes dorsalis, and general paralysis of the insane. The lesions of meningovascular syphilis were discussed on p. 424.

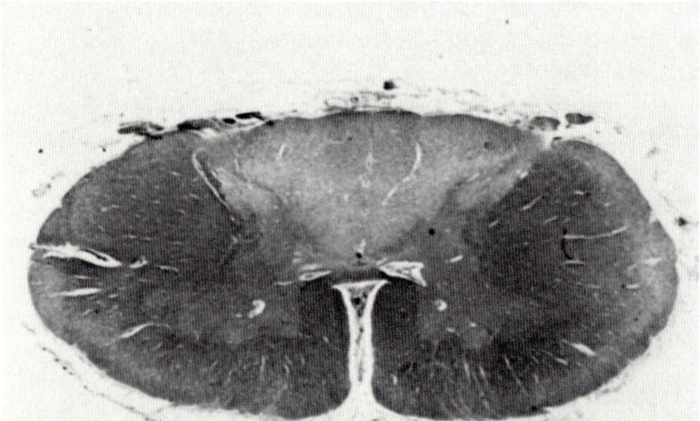

Fig. 23-9. Tabes dorsalis. The cord shows flattening, due to atrophy and demyelination of posterior columns. (Myelin, X8.)

Tabes Dorsalis

In tabes dorsalis there is moderate thickening of the cord meninges, which is more marked dorsally. The cord appears flattened ventrodorsally, due to posterior-column atrophy (Fig. 23-9). The dorsal roots, especially in the lumbosacral region, are thin compared with the (normal) ventral roots, but dorsal root ganglia show little gross change. Histologically, there is loss of myelin in the posterior columns, especially along their lateral borders, but in more advanced cases this is virtually complete and is accompanied by profound fibrillary gliosis. Oligodendroglial cells are lost early. Both segmental and secondary demyelination are seen in the posterior roots (Fig. 23-10), but are rarely total, the largest fibers being the most affected. Cranial sensory nerves may show similar changes.

There is no agreement as to the presence or absence of lesions in the dorsal root ganglia themselves, and the pathogenesis of tabes dorsalis has not been elucidated. It is possible that the earliest lesions are in the dorsal roots proximal to the ganglia, with secondary loss of posterior-column fibers. Ischemic change in the posterior roots, due to meningeal fibrosis that would first affect the larger myelinated fibers, is a plausible but speculative cause. *T. pallidum* is not present in these lesions.

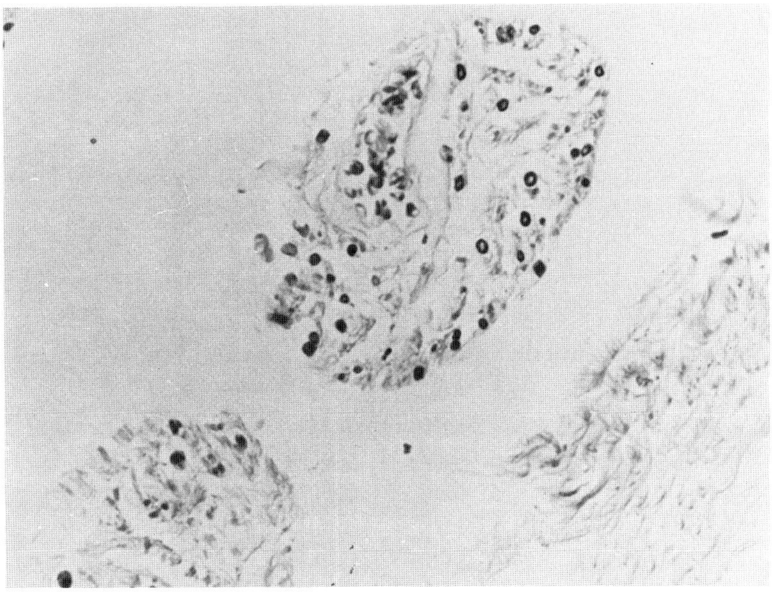

Fig. 23-10. Tabes dorsalis, showing almost complete demyelination and shrinkage of posterior roots. (Myelin, X300.)

General Paralysis of the Insane

General paralysis of the insane is essentially a disease of the cerebral cortex. The brain is shrunken and firm, and the meninges are opaque and often adherent. Mild to moderate convolutional atrophy is present, especially in the frontotemporal areas, and the ventricles are symmetrically dilated, with their lining roughened by subependymal gliosis.

Histologically, the lesions are best seen in the cortex, putamen, and hypothalamus. They consist of severe loss and degeneration of nerve cells, such that the normal cortical layers cannot be recognized. The affected areas show astrocytic reaction and fibrillary gliosis (implying conversion of protoplasmic to fibrillary astrocytes), and the cortical vessels show perivascular cuffing, with mononuclear cells and some endarteritis. Microglial cells show reactive changes characterized by elongation of their nuclei, frequently at right angles to the surface (rod cells) and some enlargement of cytoplasm, but do not progress to typical macrophages.

Unlike tabes dorsalis, the lesion is a direct infection, and numerous organisms can be demonstrated either around vessels, diffusely, or in small aggregates.

VIRAL AND RICKETTSIAL ENCEPHALITIS

Unlike bacteria or fungi, both viruses and rickettsiae are frequently associated with diffuse encephalitis involving all parts of the neuraxis. Although diffuse in this sense, with multiple lesions, histologically each lesion is small and often perivascular. Occasionally, preferential localization in limited areas of brain and cord is noted, but the reasons for this are unknown.

Grossly, the brains usually show swelling, hyperemia, and petechiae on the external and cut surfaces; occasionally, no gross abnormalities are apparent.

General Histological Features

Viral Encephalitis

Histologically, the viral encephalitides are associated with diffuse vascular dilatation, and there may be focal exudation of serum, perivascular hemorrhage, or acute arteritis. Perivascular cuffing is seen, with a few neutrophils in the early stages, rapidly replaced by mononuclear cells, apparently mainly lymphocytes. If there is total destruction around the vessel, some gitter cells may appear later. Focal and diffuse microglial proliferation occurs in relation to the peri-

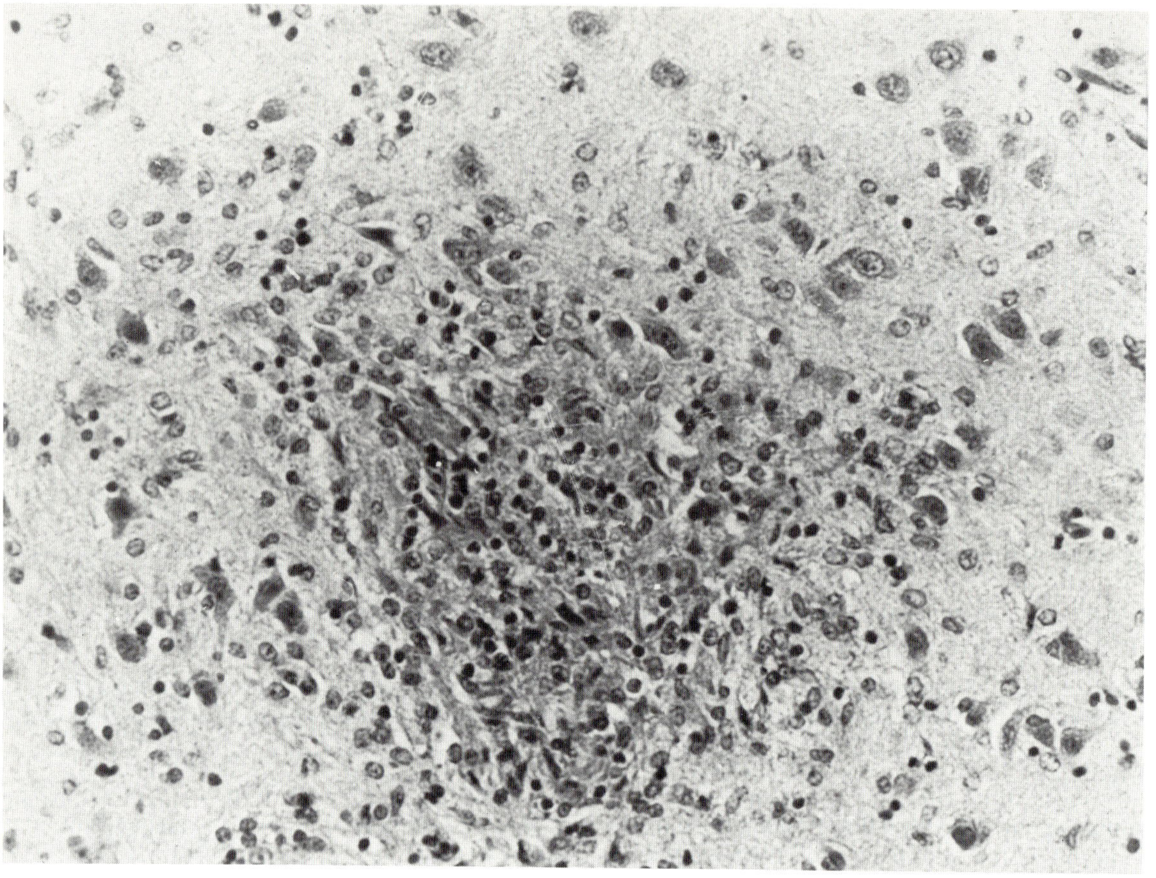

Fig. 23-11. Focal lesion in thalamus in case of western equine encephalomyelitis. The center shows tissue destruction, and there is lymphocytic and macrophage exudate. (H & E, ×300.)

vascular lesions; such proliferation may also be seen in the form of glial nodules, not necessarily related to vessels, which tend to be larger and to show some central tissue destruction if situated in the gray matter (Fig. 23-11). Diffuse neuronal changes are frequently seen, but often bear little topographical relationship to the sites of inflammation. These neuronal changes vary from central chromatolysis, through various forms of degeneration, to either irreversible cell swelling or pyknosis. (In chronic viral diseases, neurofibrillary tangles may occasionally be seen.) Astroglial reaction is relatively slight, and fibrillary gliosis is minimal.

Larger areas of tissue rarefaction, with loss of all cellular and formed elements except the mesenchymal framework, are occasionally seen, but are a minor feature in most cases.

In some viral diseases, intranuclear inclusions are present and are classified either as type A, which fill the nucleus except for a chain of chromatin granules at the periphery and are usually eosinophilic, or type B, which may be multiple and no larger than nucleoli and do not disrupt the chromatin pattern. Type A inclusions are specific for viral infection, but the significance of type B inclusions is less certain.

Rickettsial Encephalitis

Rickettsial infections show similar gross and histological features, although hemorrhage is occasionally

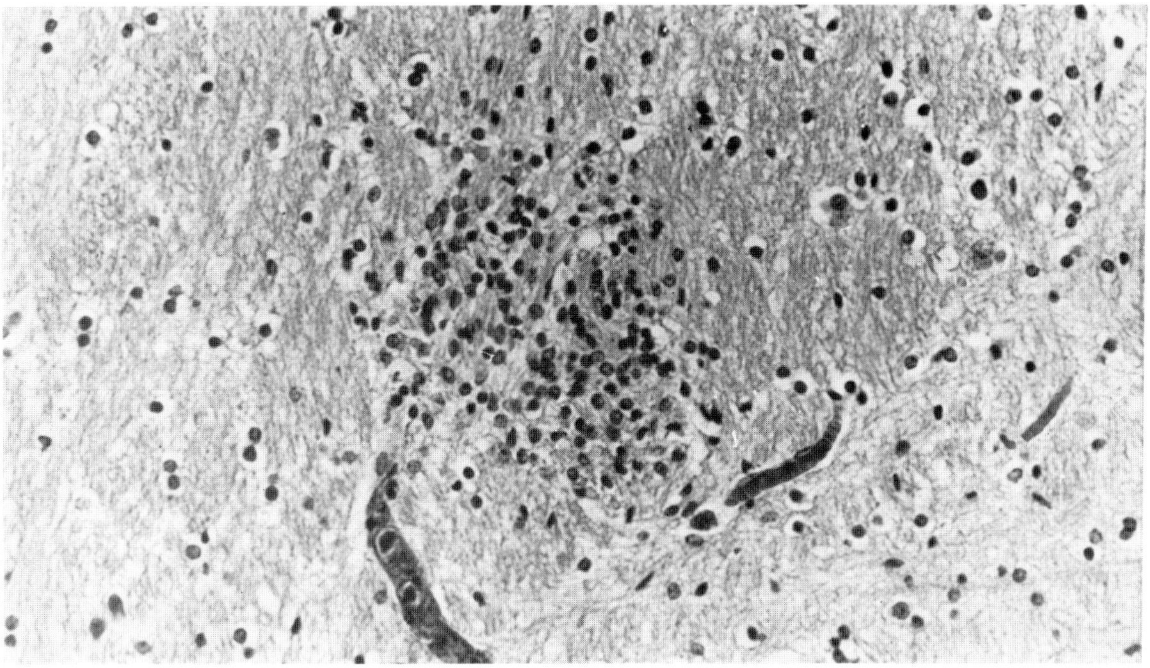

Fig. 23-12. Typical rickettsial glial nodule (from a case of scrub typhus). (H & E, X300.)

prominent. The vessels show marked swelling and proliferation of the endothelium and adventitia, associated with intracellular organisms. Antemortem thrombus may be seen, and neutrophils may be present in the thrombus, vessel wall, and adjacent parenchyma. Similar changes may be seen in the meninges. The perivascular exudate usually includes many macrophages, together with lymphocytes and a few polymorphonuclear leukocytes.

Glial nodules (Fig. 23-12) are a prominent feature, although it is not certain whether they are independent of vessels or represent perivascular aggregates in which the vessel is not apparent in the plane of section. In any event, they are loose or compact collections of macrophages, lymphocytes, and microglial cells, up to about 150μ across, the more chronic showing a mild peripheral astrocytic reaction. Nodules are more common in the gray matter and especially in the brain stem. Rickettsiae may be found in the microglial cells.

Generalized parenchymal changes include mild to moderate nonspecific degeneration of neurons, with a slight microglial and astrocytic reaction; the myelin and oligodendroglia usually appear normal. In patients who survive, the small parenchymal nodules form minute gliomesenchymal scars.

Poliomyelitis

Poliomyelitis is a somewhat atypical virus infection of the CNS and shows the following differences from the general description of the viral encephalitides that has been given:

1. Gross changes are confined to hyperemia of the anterior horns and cranial motor nuclei, with occasional minute areas of necrosis and petechiae. In chronic cases there is thinning of the anterior roots.

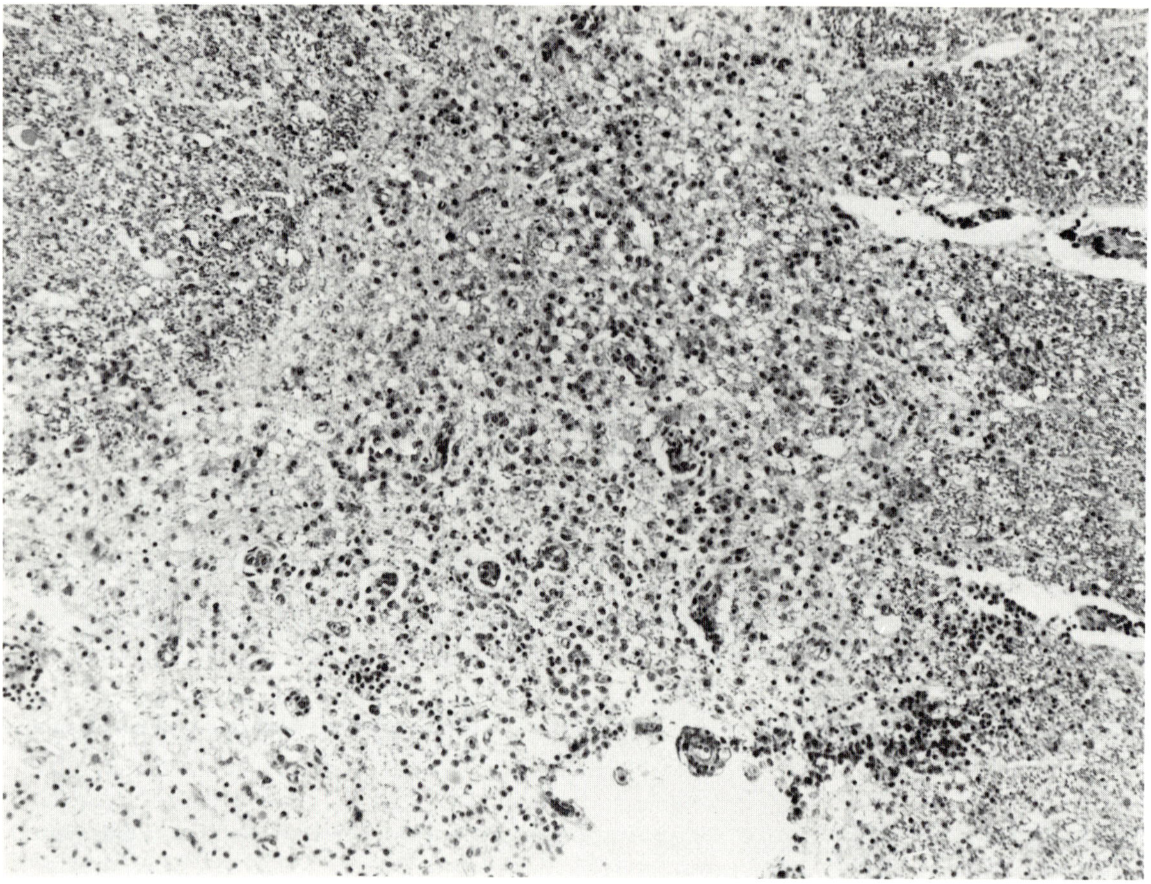

Fig. 23-13. Anterior horn in subacute poliomyelitis. The entire gray matter is necrotic, but the surrounding white matter is virtually intact. No neurons have survived, and the neutrophilic exudate has by now been replaced by lymphocytes. Many gitter cells are present. (H & E, X75.)

2. The inflammatory exudate shows unusual prominence and persistence of polymorphonuclear leukocytes, which are only replaced by mononuclear cells after several days.
3. Because of the localization, the major attack is on motoneurons (Fig. 23-13), with consequent loss of motor axons and denervation atrophy of muscle.
4. No type A inclusion bodies are present.
5. In addition to the invariable major changes noted, there may be some perivascular cuffing in the sensory gray matter of the spinal cord and brain stem, as well as rare neuronal degeneration with little inflammatory change in the motor cortex, deep nuclei of the cerebellum, thalamus, and hypothalamus.

Virtually all cases of poliomyelitis are due to poliovirus, which exists in three apparently unvarying antigenic types with worldwide distribution. Very rare cases of poliomyelitis are due to other enteroviruses (coxsackievirus group). Poliovirus enters the body by either respiratory or oral routes and multiplies in the tonsils (leading to a brief pharyngeal secretion of virus about one week after infection) or in the lymphoid tissue of the large intestine (leading to fecal excretion of the virus, often for many months). Viremia 5 to 10 days after the initial infection may be subclinical or may produce a nonspecific respiratory infection. In a *very small minority* of cases, the virus localizes in the CNS, producing the changes just described. The distribution of these changes led to the hypothesis that poliovirus enters the CNS by retrograde axoplasmic flow in motor axons, but this is unsubstantiated and does not account for the frequent minor histological changes in other areas. In the small proportion of cases in which paralysis occurs, it starts 10 to 15 days after infection.

Electron microscopy shows detachment of ribosomes from the granular endoplasmic reticulin, leading to loss of organization of the Nissl bodies, together with severe loss of organelle membranes and an increase in large glycogen granules (the latter are also seen in the neighboring astrocytes). Smaller granules of RNA appear on both sides of the nuclear envelope, presumably representing viral synthesis, and in the

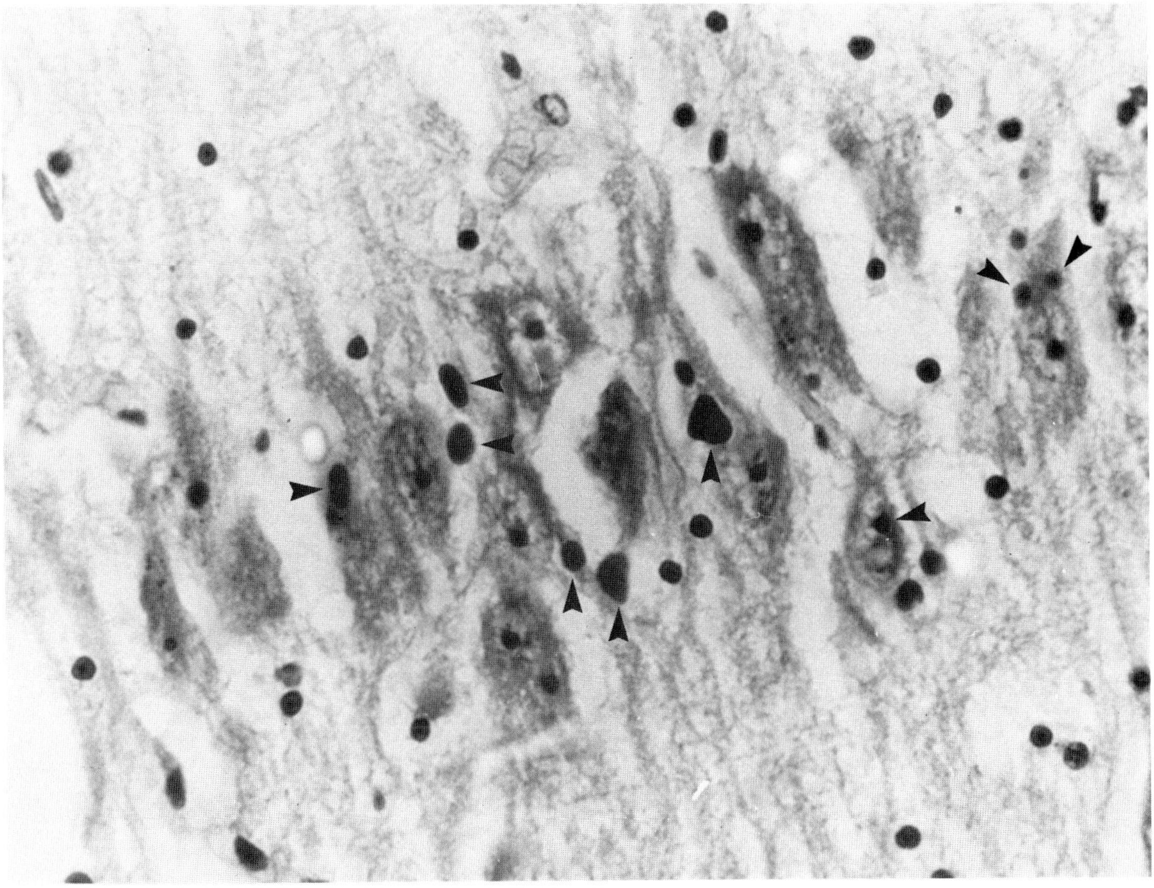

Fig. 23-14. Section of hippocampus, showing the deeply stained, generally rounded Negri bodies of rabies encephalitis (arrows). (PAS, ×750.)

late stages form crystalline arrays. Some nerve cells recover from the earlier stages. Irreversibility is probably marked by loss of organelle membranes and ribosomes and destruction of mitochondria.

Rabies

The gross changes in the brain in rabies are slight and as noted in the general description. Microscopically, changes are seen in the cord, brain stem, and hippocampus; the neocortex is relatively unaffected. As in many viral diseases, the areas of neuronal degeneration and of severe inflammatory change often appear spatially dissociated. The microscopic appearance in rabies differs from the general description given previously in one major respect, namely, the presence of Negri bodies in about 70% of neurons in the affected areas (Fig. 23-14). These are round or oval, eosinophilic, dense, well-defined bodies, single or multiple within a given cell, and especially prominent in the large cells of the hippocampus and Purkinje's cells. Their nature is unclear, but they appear to represent cytoplasmic deposition of unknown material on a core of virus nucleic acid.

The rabies virus is almost always acquired by bites, but in heavily infected areas (such as in caves inhabited by bats), it possibly can be inhaled as a particulate suspension. It appears to proliferate in regional lymph nodes and thereafter to reach the nervous system by autonomic or somatic peripheral nerves, the time required increasing with the length of the path. Thus, the latent period after bites on the foot is considerably longer than after bites on the face. Axoplasmic passage of the virus has been demonstrated by severing limb nerves, which effectively prevents the virus from reaching the CNS in spite of the persistence of the lymph node focus and an intact blood supply.

Herpes Encephalitis

Herpes simplex encephalitis exists in two clinical contexts. The first is neonatal infection, probably acquired from the mother's genital tract during delivery, with typical CNS and disseminated visceral focal necrotizing lesions that show type A inclusions. The second is an isolated herpes encephalitis without visceral dissemination and occurring up to at least middle age.

Herpes encephalitis of the latter type differs from

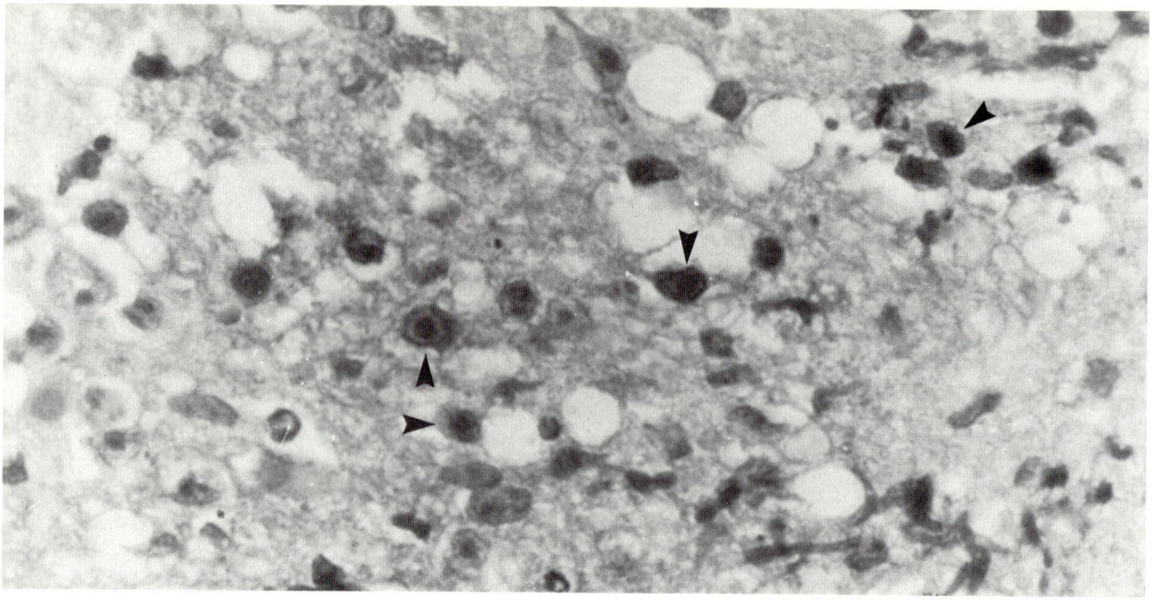

Fig. 23-15. Herpes simplex encephalitis. Section from necrotic area near insula, showing several type A intranuclear inclusions (arrows), apparently in oligodendroglial cells. (H & E, X750.)

the general description of the viral encephalitides in the following ways:

1. In some cases the brain shows generalized swelling and hyperemia, but in many the gross lesions are focal, on one or both sides, and more severe in the insula and opercula, frequently showing confluent hemorrhage. Indeed, these focal lesions may present as neurosurgical problems.
2. In all cases the changes are most prominent in the cerebral cortex, with less involvement of the cerebellum and brain stem; in focal cases they may be virtually confined to the insular and opercular regions.
3. These lesions are frequently more hemorrhagic than other types of viral encephalitis.
4. The presence of type A eosinophilic, intranuclear inclusions is mandatory for the diagnosis. They occur in neurons and oligodendroglial cells (Fig. 23-15); type B inclusions may be seen in astrocytes.

Similar cases, usually confined to the insular and opercular area, have been described in the absence of virological or serological proof of herpes infection. These are usually termed *inclusion body encephalitis,* but it seems highly probable that most or all of them are due to herpesvirus.

The virus of herpes simplex is not normally a hazard to life, and many people carry a latent infection that produces cold sores in association with acute respiratory tract infections. The cause of occasional localization in the CNS is unknown. The virus is one of the DNA group, new virus being synthesized in the nucleus, inducing cytoplasmic protein that enters the nucleus and surrounds viral DNA to form a nucleocapsid. The nucleocapsids then derive an envelope from the nuclear membrane and are released by budding through the plasmalemma. Infection presumably reaches the CNS during a period of viremia and spreads within the CNS from cell to cell. This is a tentative conclusion, but is supported by the frequent occurrence of grouped cells showing intranuclear inclusions.

Herpes Zoster

Although in herpes zoster the major lesions are in the PNS, the CNS is also involved. The histological changes resemble those given in the general description of the viral encephalidites. It differs from typical viral encephalitis in the following respects:

1. Histologically, lesions are seen in the dorsal root ganglia, corresponding posterior roots, and dorsal horn and are frequently unilateral.
2. Because of the damage to dorsal root ganglion cells, atrophy of the dorsal roots and peripheral mononeuritis occur, associated with posterior-column axonal loss. Secondary demyelination may be seen in associated peripheral nerves and the posterior column.
3. Type A inclusion bodies have been reported in both dorsal root ganglion neurons and satellite cells and occasionally in sympathetic ganglia at the same level.

The varicella-zoster virus is related to that of herpes simplex, both being DNA viruses largely synthesized in the nucleus. It differs from herpes simplex virus in that few of the newly formed virus particles are released from the cell, presumably accounting for the strict localization of the condition.

Arbovirus Infections

A considerable number of arboviruses are pathogenic to man and involve the CNS. In general, their gross and histological features are typical of those given in the general description of the viral encephalitides. In none of them are type A inclusion bodies found. Although preferential involvement of different areas of the neuraxis has been reported, these do not seem to be uniform except in the case of Russian spring-summer encephalitis, in which changes may be largely confined to the cord and precentral cortex and therefore may be confused with poliomyelitis.

The term *arbovirus* comes from *ar*thropod-*bo*rne, indicating that some arthropod, usually a mosquito, tick, or mite, acts as an intermediate host, the diseases usually being acquired by bites from these insect vectors. Several types of arbovirus severely affect horses, resulting in a condition termed *equine encephalitis.* However, the horse, like man, is not a normal part of the virus life cycle. The best known of the arbovirus infections are transmitted by various species of mosquitos and include eastern, western, and Venezuelan equine encephalomyelitis, St. Louis encephalitis, Japanese B encephalitis, yellow fever, dengue fever, and others. A number are tickborne, including Russian spring-summer encephalitis and its many variants. In North America, the arbovirus infections of the CNS likely to be encountered include eastern, western, and Venezuelan equine encephalomyelitis, St. Louis encephalitis, Powassan encephalitis, Colorado tick fever, and California encephalitis. In Europe most of these infections appear to be variants of Russian spring-summer encephalitis, which has its focus in Siberia, but extends into Eastern Europe. These variants include louping ill in the United Kingdom. Mortality is variable. Eastern equine encephalomyelitis has a death rate in excess of 50% and is particularly common in children. Japanese B encephalitis has a mortality of 25 to 50% and St. Louis encephalitis and western equine encephalomyelitis, a mortality of 2 to 15%. Other arbovirus infections appear to carry a lower mortality. Yellow fever and dengue fever do not involve the CNS except incidentally.

Seen electron-microscopically, all the arboviruses show approximately similar changes, although the virus particles are variable in size. Twenty-four hours after intraperitoneal injection in mice there is enlargement of the extracellular space around CNS vessels and virus particles are present within the vessel lumens, on both sides of the vascular basement membrane, and in extracellular spaces. A little later, all cell types appear to become infected, with the exception of endothelial cells. Small, rounded nucleoids, presumably nucleic acid, appear in the cytoplasm, either free or attached to distended membranous structures. These migrate to the plasmalemma and other membranes, and evaginate as a "bud," so that each new virus particle consists of a central nucleoid covered by an envelope derived from the plasmalemma or other membrane. This envelope retains its three-layered structure, but shows numerous external projections. Invaded cells are destroyed, thus liberating more particles from cytoplasmic vacuoles and the nuclear envelope. Studies using a variety of Russian spring-summer encephalitis (also in mice) showed more glial than neuronal invasion, associated with a marked tendency to astrocytic proliferation.

Subacute Sclerosing Panencephalitis

Subacute sclerosing panencephalitis (SSPE) is a diffuse CNS disease that usually occurs in children and young adults and has a total course of 3 to 12 months, although a few patients survive longer. The CSF is normal, except for an increase in gamma globulin giving a first-zone colloidal gold curve.

Morphological Changes

The general description of the gross and histological features of viral encephalitis previously given is *not* applicable to SSPE, in which all areas of the CNS are extensively involved by grossly visible, irregular areas of demyelination and necrosis (Fig. 23-16). There is perivascular infiltration with lymphocytes and plasma cells, accumulation of gitter cells in necrotic and demyelinated areas, and prominent plump hyperplasia of astrocytes (Fig. 23-17), with moderate to intense fibrillary gliosis. Demyelination is widespread, but is usually incomplete even within the areas involved. However, it is inappropriate to regard this as a demyelinating disease, since it is associated with generalized tissue damage and necrosis. Nerve cells show

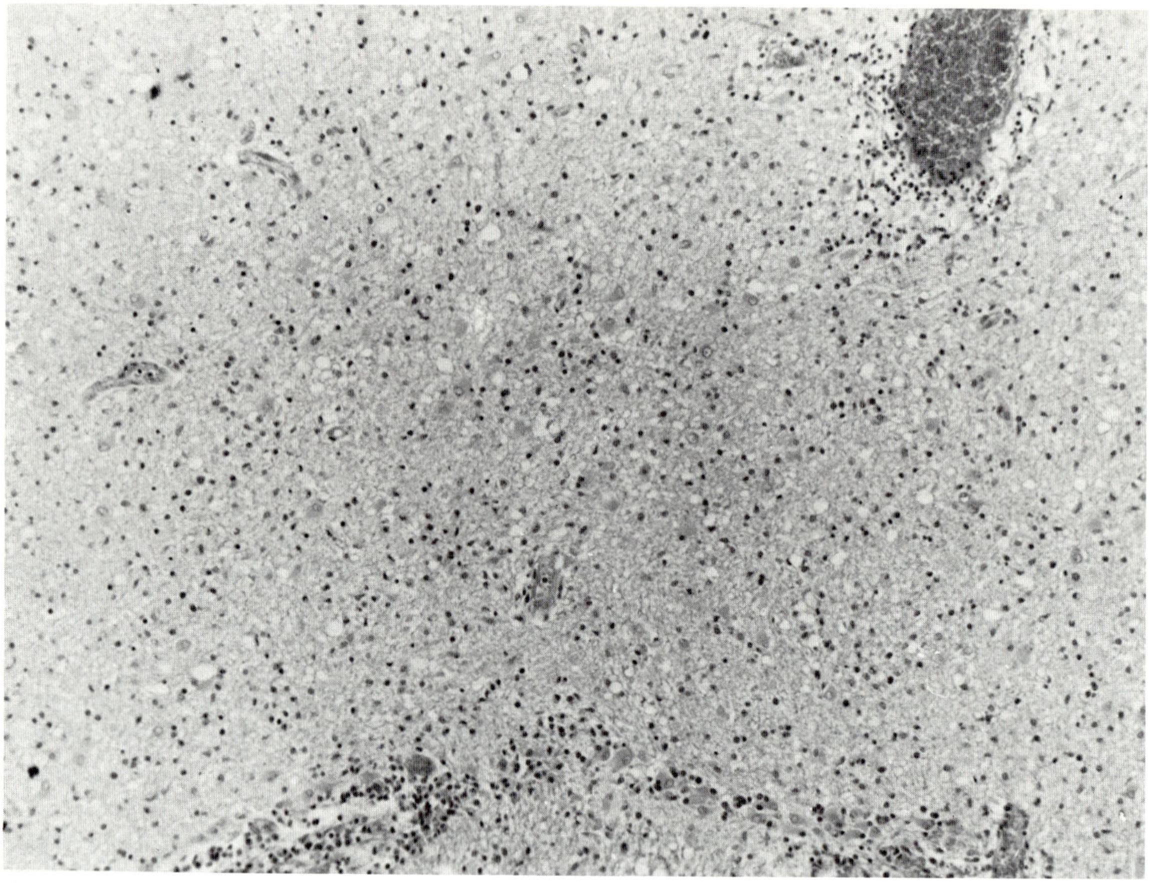

Fig. 23-16. SSPE. General view, showing cuffing, spongiosis, lymphocytic infiltrate, and astrocytic hyperplasia. (H & E, X115.)

degenerative and frequently necrotic changes. A variable proportion of neurons, oligodendroglia, and occasionally other cells contain type A eosinophilic intranuclear inclusions (Fig. 23-18), sometimes associated with irregular inclusions of variable size in the cytoplasm.

Relationship to Measles Infection

Most, but not all, of these patients give a history either of previous exposure to or vaccination against measles, and serum levels of measles antibody are extremely high, frequently continuing to rise during the disease to levels exceeding those found in patients convalescing from an acute attack of measles. Antibody is also present in the CSF. Measles antigen itself can be readily demonstrated in the CNS by immunofluorescent techniques, staining both intranuclear and intracytoplasmic inclusion bodies. Electron microscopy shows particles in neuronal cell bodies and axons, as well as in neuronal and glial nuclei, that are morphologically compatible with measles virus.

In spite of almost conclusive evidence that measles virus is responsible for SSPE, it has only recently been isolated from brain tissue. Infected cells show increased concentrations of RNA and protein but reduced DNA, presumably due to enlargement and accumulation of RNA virus particles. The nucleocapsid of measles virus contains a core of RNA with a protein capsid derived from cytoplasm, but is not infective unless it acquires a third component, the envelope from the plasmalemma. Immunofluorescent studies have shown antigen, antibody, and complement within the plasmalemma of infected cells and also in the outer lamellae of myelin sheaths.

The serum of these patients appears not to contain antimyelin or gliotoxic antibodies, and there is no evidence for an autoimmune component. The condition is regarded as a partially suppressed (by circulating antibody), persistent measles virus infection of the CNS, with the virus spreading directly from cell to cell because myxoviruses tend to cause cell fusion and thereby enable transfer without exposure to antibody.

A few recent reports have suggested that papovavirus may also be present in SSPE, but it is difficult to see what essential function it might serve in the maintenance of measles virus infection.

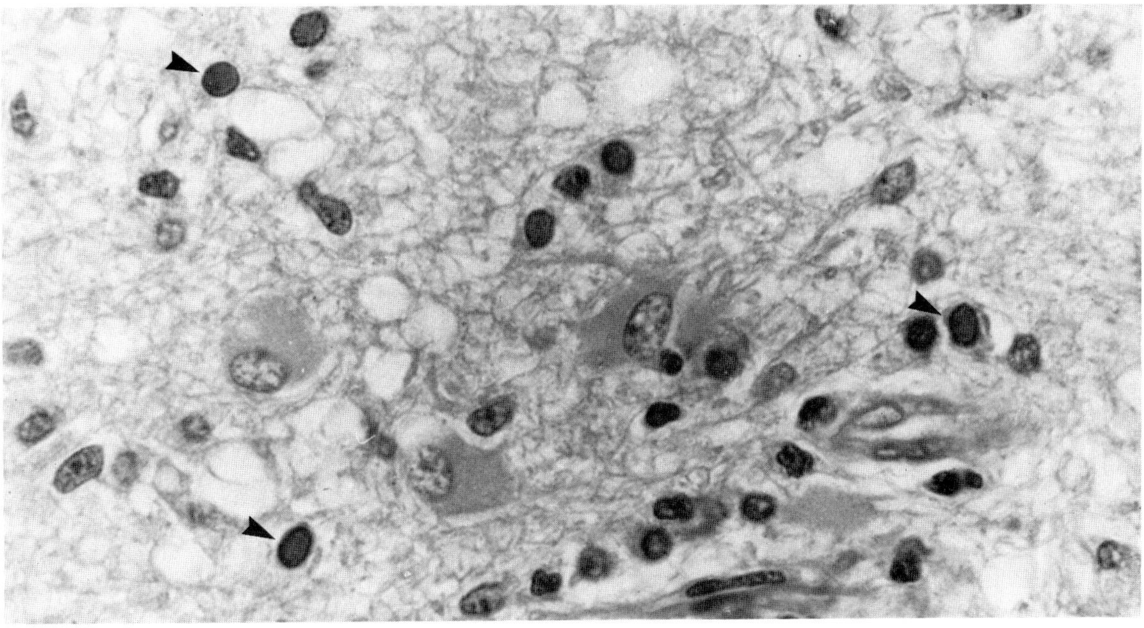

Fig. 23-17. SSPE showing hyperplastic astrocytes, cuffing of small vessel, and oligodendroglial intranuclear inclusions (arrows). (H & E, ×750.)

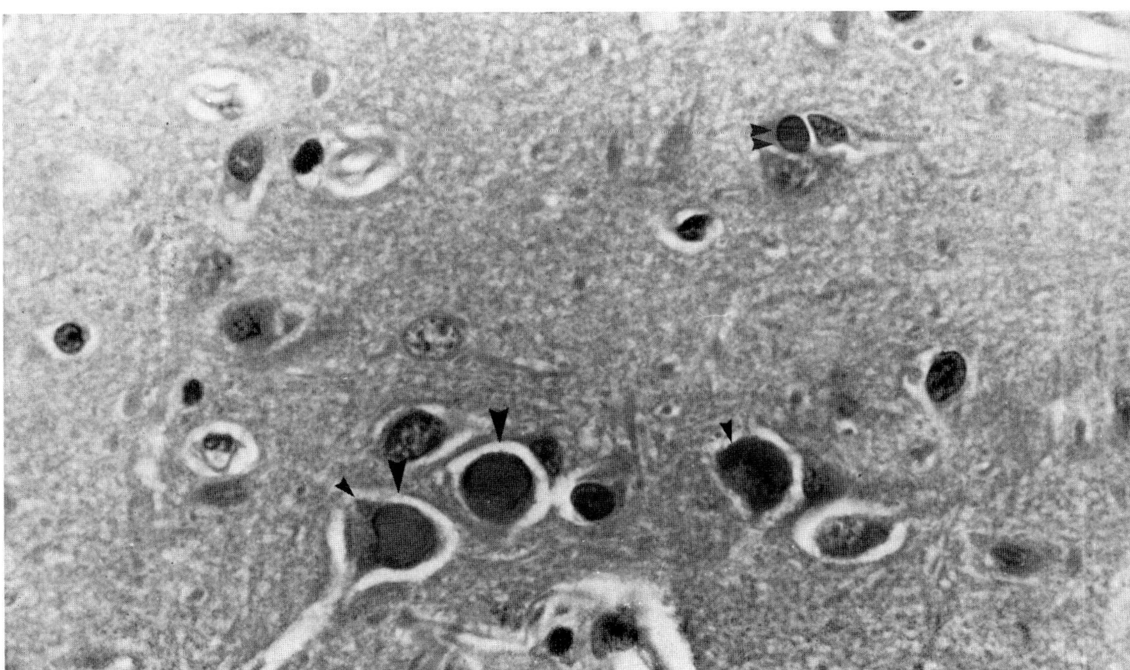

Fig. 23-18. SSPE. Two neurons showing large intranuclear inclusions (large arrows). Two cells also show cytoplasmic inclusions (small arrows). An oligodendroglial cell with intranuclear inclusion is also seen (double arrow). (H & E, ×750.)

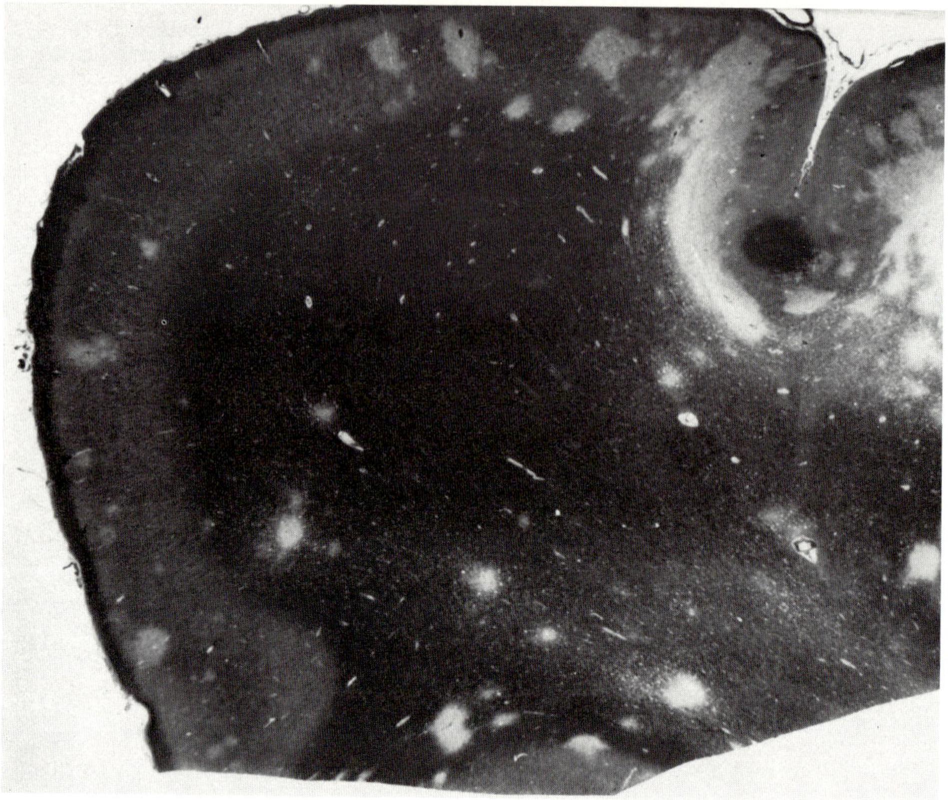

Fig. 23-19. PMLE. Section showing scattered and confluent areas of demyelination. (Myelin, X8.)

Subacute sclerosing panencephalitis should be distinguished from the occasional measles encephalitis complicating a typical acute attack of measles, in which similar inclusion bodies may be seen within the CNS.

Papovavirus Infection: Progressive Multifocal Leukoencephalopathy

Progressive multifocal leukoencephalopathy (PMLE) occurs in a variety of conditions in which it might be supposed that immunological reactivity was altered or reduced. These include neoplasms of the reticuloendothelial system (Hodgkin's disease, leukemia, lymphosarcoma), sarcoidosis, severe cachexias, as in chronic tuberculosis and carcinomatosis, diffuse collagen disease, corticosteroid therapy, and the use of immunological suppressants. A few cases have been reported with no detectable associated disease. It occurs in adult patients as an afebrile, progressive condition, usually lasting three to twelve months, but occasionally as long as five years. The CSF is normal.

The gross and histological features of this disease do *not* correspond to the general description of the viral encephalitides. The major features are as follows:

1. Grossly, there are irregular areas of apparent demyelination or necrosis in white matter, with occasional extension into the gray matter (Fig. 23-19).
2. Histologically, there are multiple, often confluent circular areas of oligodendroglial and myelin loss, with retention of fairly normal axons. Some lesions appear to be perivenular, and in all there is lymphocytic cuffing of vessels (Fig. 23-20).
3. Although oligodendroglial cells are largely lost from the demyelinated areas, at the periphery they frequently show nuclear enlargement, with the nuclei containing type A eosinophilic inclusions.
4. Astrocytes within and adjacent to the lesions show remarkable hypertrophy and hyperplasia, with bizarre, large, hyperchromatic nuclei (Fig. 23-21). Multinucleate cells and abnormal mitotic figures are often seen.

Thus, this disease combines two striking features: a perivenular type of demyelination, possibly suggesting an autoimmune mechanism (as seen in experimental allergic encephalomyelitis and multiple sclerosis), and type A intranuclear inclusions, suggesting a viral infection. Virus-like particles, present in the nuclei of oligodendroglial cells only, appear to belong to the SV40-polyomavirus group of papovaviruses. Several viruses of this group may be inhabitants of human

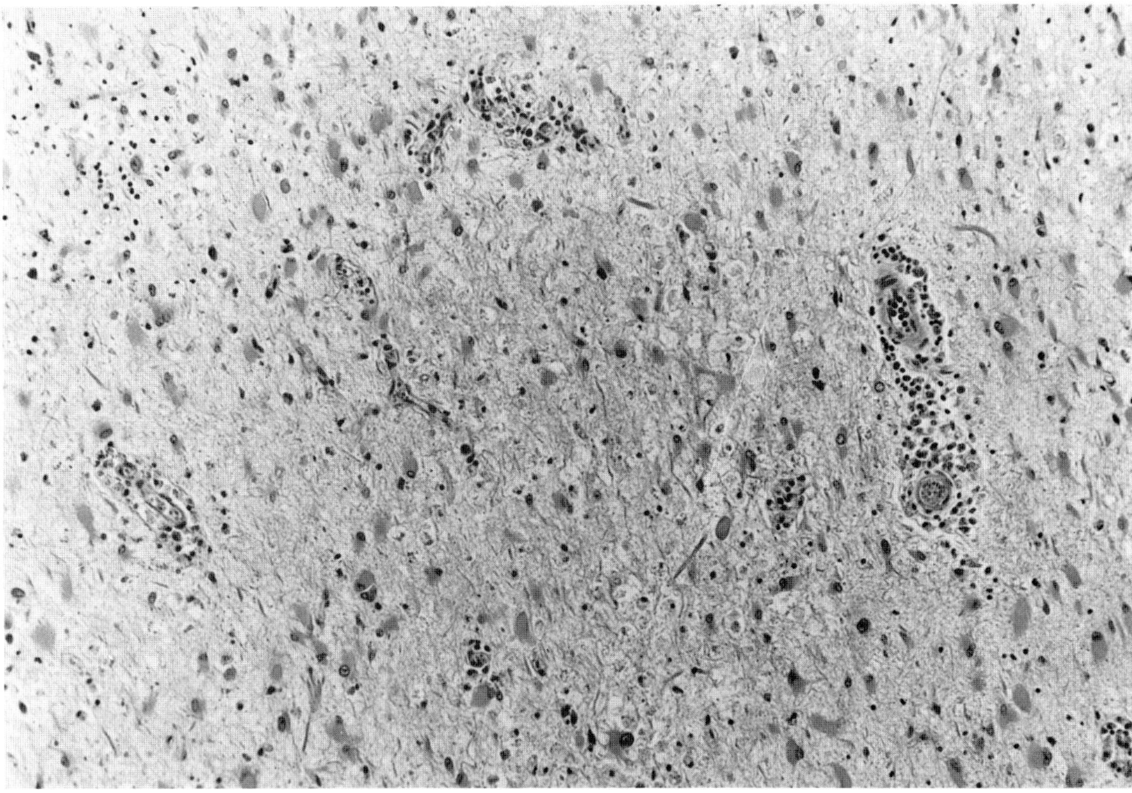

Fig. 23-20. PMLE showing cuffing, demyelination, and prominent astrocytic hyperplasia. (H & E, ×115.)

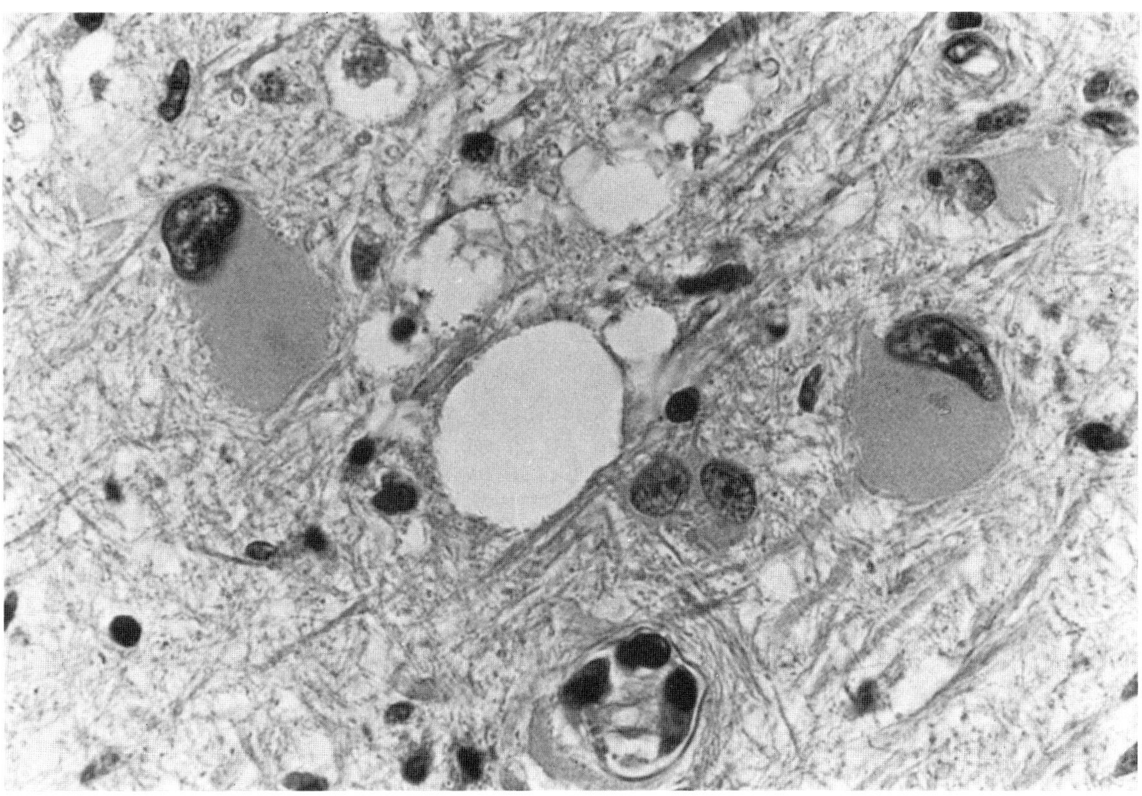

Fig. 23-21. PMLE showing bizarre astrocytic hyperplasia. (H & E, ×750.)

tissues, but not of the CNS. The pathogenesis is presumably diffusion of the virus from small vessels (which would explain the perivenular distribution followed by virus localization selectively in oligodendroglia). Demyelination is an inevitable consequence of oligodendroglial destruction. Since CNS virus is present (peripheral to the demyelination), since there is little or no inflammatory component, and since many patients have impaired immunological responses, the disease may be regarded as an opportunistic virus infection of oligodendroglia associated with impaired immunological defenses. The demyelination due to oligodendroglial disease, and the perivenular distribution due to the hematogenous source of the virus, combine to simulate the appearances of autoimmune disease, for which there is no other evidence.

Rickettsial Encephalitis

The general gross and microscopic appearance of the rickettsial encephalitides closely resemble those of viral encephalitis, a major difference being that type A inclusions are never found in the rickettsial diseases, but the organisms themselves may be seen in endothelial, adventitial, and microglial cells. Perhaps the most significant morphological variant occurs in Rocky Mountain spotted fever, in which there is a tendency to inflammation and thrombosis of larger vessels, which may cause areas of infarction.

The rickettsial diseases are conveyed by a variety of lice, ticks, and mites, with the additional possibility of inhalation in the case of Q fever. In North America the major rickettsial diseases are typhus (transmitted by lice), Rocky Mountain spotted fever (transmitted by ticks), Q fever (transmitted by ticks and perhaps by inhalation), and rickettsialpox (transmitted by mouse mites). In Europe the main diseases are typhus and murine typhus (louse or rat flea), Mediterranean (boutonneuse) fever (dog tick), trench fever (louse), and Q fever. Other rickettsial diseases with other vectors occur elsewhere. One of these, namely, scrub typhus, was of considerable importance in the Far East during World War II. Of the diseases mentioned, typhus, murine typhus, Rocky Mountain spotted fever, and scrub typhus have moderate to high mortality, and their neuropathological features are well investigated and closely similar in all cases. It is presumed that changes in the other conditions are at least qualitatively similar, though probably less severe.

PROTOZOAL AND METAZOAL DISEASES

Many of the protozoal and metazoal diseases fall more properly into the field of tropical medicine and, despite their considerable economic importance and academic interest, cannot be considered here for reasons of space. Many parasitic diseases may involve the CNS following dissemination in the bloodstream. However, such involvement is frequently subclinical. This is often the case in trichinosis or schistosomiasis, in which variable numbers of CNS granulomas containing remnants of larval forms or ova are seen. However, in other such diseases, including cysticercosis and echinococcosis, expanding cystic CNS lesions can occur that either function as space-occupying lesions, produce focal symptomatology (including convulsive episodes), or occasionally rupture into the ventricular system or subarachnoid space, producing daughter cysts and ultimately obstructing CSF flow.

Malignant tertian malaria (due to *Plasmodium falciparum*) may produce acute neurological symptoms, including alteration of consciousness and coma, because of widespread synchronous schizogony occurring in the cerebral capillaries and obstructing blood flow. Petechial hemorrhages and small glial nodules may be noted. This complication does not occur in other types of malaria.

Amebic dysentery (due to *Entamoeba histolytica*) usually produces abscesses in the liver and lung, but may involve the brain, producing single or multiple ragged, necrotic areas in which vegetative amebae may be demonstrated by suitable stains. Recently, a free-living ameba *(Naegleria)* has been associated with severe meningitis, usually following swimming or diving in water contaminated by the organism. The portal of entry may be the lymphatic-subarachnoid space anastomoses that surround olfactory nerve filaments, apparently used only by this organism.

These are but a few of the diseases that may be endemic in temperate areas or may be seen in visitors returning from the tropics. Many other tropical infections and infestations may involve the CNS. In any patient with CNS disease of an unusual type and a history either of close association with animals or residence in other parts of the world, parasitic infections and infestations should be considered and the appropriate texts consulted.

SLOW VIRUS INFECTIONS

Slow viruses appear particularly to persecute Icelandic sheep, who have at least three such diseases, two of them involving the CNS: visna and scrapie (rida). Their range has since been extended from Iceland to the tropics and from sheep to potatoes, mink, man, and (at least experimentally) other higher primates, including the chimpanzee.

Slow viruses (also termed *latent* or *temperate viruses)* involving the CNS have the following features in common:

1. They are transmissible by cell-free injections of infected brain tissue to suitable experimental animals.
2. The incubation time between injection and clinical manifestation of the disease varies from months to years.
3. They all have a regularly progressive, protracted, ultimately fatal clinical course.
4. Pathological changes are confined to the CNS (with the possible exception of liver involvement in Creutzfeldt-Jakob syndrome in man, and the reticuloendothelial system in experimental animals).

5. With the exception of visna in sheep, the basic CNS changes are vacuolar presynaptic and postsynaptic neuronal degeneration with reactive gliosis.

Visna has aroused interest because of some similarities with multiple sclerosis. Transmitted experimentally from sheep to sheep by intracerebral inoculation of cell-free infected brain tissue, the disease has an incubation period during which the CSF shows pleocytosis, with an increase in gamma globulin. The histological appearance of the disease more resembles that of experimental allergic encephalitis than of multiple sclerosis, with a total perivenular necrosis not confined to oligodendroglial cells and myelin, prominent near the ependyma, and associated with inflammatory change. The agent is said to be an RNA virus that forms syncytia in cell culture. Its histological appearance is not a good model of multiple sclerosis because of the nonselective nature of the perivenular damage. Attempts to isolate slow virus from brains involved by multiple sclerosis have so far failed.

The other natural animal CNS diseases associated with slow viruses are scrapie, which affects sheep and goats, and mink encephalopathy. The two viruses involved appear to be closely related. In the case of the mink infection, the virus is transmitted by the ingestion of infected meat. The mode of natural transmission of scrapie is not established, but it appears not to require direct animal-to-animal contact. It has been transmitted to goats, mice, rats, hamsters, gerbils, mink, and, more recently, monkeys, suggesting that it may be the agent from which the mink encephalopathy virus developed.

The human diseases so far associated with slow virus are Creutzfeldt-Jakob syndrome and kuru, and they present interesting analogies to the animal diseases. In kuru, as in mink encephalopathy, infection is transmitted by the ingestion of infected meat (ritual cannibalism), and this must be one of the rare situations where the imposition of Western social values has actually resulted in a decrease, rather than an increase, in disease among native populations. Creutzfeldt-Jakob syndrome, like scrapie, has a totally unknown mode of transmission, and there is suggestive evidence in both diseases of at least a genetic predisposition, inherited as an autosomal recessive trait. A proportion of cases of Creutzfeldt-Jakob syndrome are familial. Just as the virus of mink encephalopathy probably developed from scrapie virus, it seems possible that the virus of kuru developed from that of Creutzfeldt-Jakob syndrome, due to the congenial circumstances in which it found itself.

The nucleic acid portion of these animal and human viruses appears to be unusually small and either tightly bound to, or incorporated in, fragments of plasmalemma, producing an unusual degree of resistance to ultraviolet irradiation, heat, and many other inactivating agents. If first treated with agents expected to be lytic to plasma membranes, the resistance of the virus to inactivating agents is considerably reduced. Membrane-binding not only protects the virus against many agents, but apparently also makes it difficult to recognize electron-microscopically, since virions have not so far been reported, although the presence of irregular membrane fragments is characteristic of presumably virus-infected cells. Recent work suggests that certain plant RNA viruses are also very stable in crude suspension, but much more susceptible to inactivation when purified.

So far, all attempts to prepare antibody of any type, in any species, with or without the use of adjuvant, appear to have been unsuccessful, presumably either because the association of virus with plasmalemma masks its antigenic determinants, or because its determinants are the same as those of the membrane with which it is incorporated, so that potential antibody-producing clones are inhibited. The viruses can be maintained in tissue cultures of brain cells in such a state that cell-free extracts of these cultures are infective to suitable experimental animals. Indeed, the infected cells actually appear to grow better, suggesting a cell-stimulating effect resembling the marked glial reaction seen in Creutzfeldt-Jakob syndrome and kuru (and also in multiple sclerosis). Filtration studies suggest that the infective unit size for scrapie is 270 to 470 A for kuru, and that for Creutzfeldt-Jakob virus it is 1000 to 2200 A.

Microscopic Changes in Slow Virus Central Nervous System Disease

The histological picture of slow virus disease varies from area to area in different diseases. In sheep scrapie, lower centers such as the medulla are frequently most affected. In both kuru and Creutzfeldt-Jakob syndrome, the changes are widespread, but are often most marked in the cerebellum in the former and the cerebral cortex in the latter. However, irrespective of distribution, the microscopic changes are similar in all three diseases and include the following:

1. Vacuolation (Fig. 23-22), occurring within the cell bodies, dendrites, and axons of neurons (status spongiosis).
2. Nonspecific changes such as central chromatolysis and accumulation of lipochrome in neurons.
3. Intense hypertrophy, hyperplasia, and fibrillary gliosis of astrocytes, sometimes associated with accumulation of lipochrome pigment.
4. Histologically normal oligodendroglial cells, microglial cells, and vessels and no inflammatory exudate.
5. Frequent or infrequent appearance of stellate plaques, staining centrally as amyloid and virtually identical with the senile plaques of Alzheimer's disease.

Eventually, neurons degenerate and disappear with their axons, so that in long-standing cases there is some secondary demyelination associated with neuronal loss. Little if any change is seen in the CSF at any stage of the disease, and there is no histological or other evidence for autoimmune response.

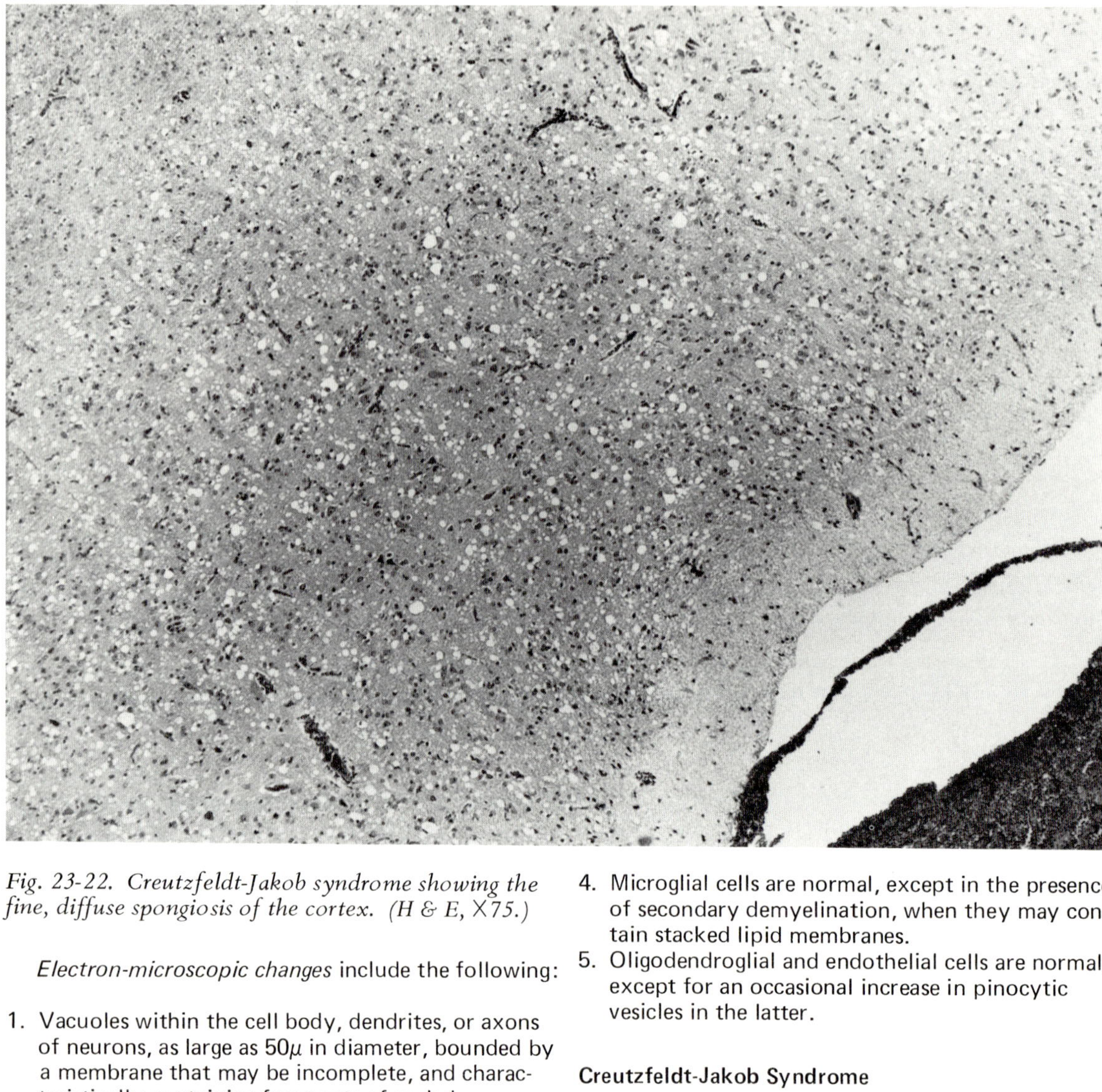

Fig. 23-22. Creutzfeldt-Jakob syndrome showing the fine, diffuse spongiosis of the cortex. (H & E, X75.)

Electron-microscopic changes include the following:

1. Vacuoles within the cell body, dendrites, or axons of neurons, as large as 50μ in diameter, bounded by a membrane that may be incomplete, and characteristically containing fragments of curled-up membrane, either filling the vacuoles or at least near the edges. Sometimes, the central part contains granular material.
2. Extruded processes of cytoplasm surrounded by plasma membrane (which may be ruptured) are present in both neuronal and astroglial cells, and adjacent processes may appear to fuse, forming a syncytium. Curled membrane fragments are usually present at sites of rupture.
3. Although astrocytes may show extruded processes, they do not exhibit vacuolation; nonspecific reactive changes, including glial fiber formation and pigment granules, are usual.
4. Microglial cells are normal, except in the presence of secondary demyelination, when they may contain stacked lipid membranes.
5. Oligodendroglial and endothelial cells are normal, except for an occasional increase in pinocytic vesicles in the latter.

Creutzfeldt-Jakob Syndrome

Creutzfeldt-Jakob syndrome is a subacute CNS dysfunction affecting either sex, usually starting between 40 and 60 years of age and lasting about a year. A few cases are familial. Anxiety, intellectual and speech deterioration, and disturbances of gait are followed by pyramidal and extrapyramidal dysfunction, with myoclonic and epileptic seizures. The EEG changes are nonspecific.

Grossly, the brain may appear normal or show slight sulcal widening, and histological changes are diffuse in the cortex and basal ganglia, with variable involvement of the thalamus, cerebellum, brain stem, and cord. Light- and electron-microscopic changes are as previously described, except that senile plaques are unusual.

The disease has been successfully transmitted to chimpanzees and other monkeys. The latent periods vary from months to years, and the histological changes in these animals are the same as in the human patients, but are sometimes more florid. Successfully transmitted cases, of which at least one was familial, have tended to show a shorter clinical course and less involvement of motor neurons, and it has been suggested that the cases usually grouped as "Creutzfeldt-Jakob syndrome" may include two separate entities: subacute spongioform encephalopathy, which is transmissible, and a true Creutzfeldt-Jakob syndrome, which is not. However, there appears to be no clear clinical or pathological distinction. Since no antigen has been isolated, there is no information as to the presence of antibody in Creutzfeldt-Jakob syndrome.

Among 41 patients with Creutzfeldt-Jakob syndrome, 9 have had clinical liver disease, with histological changes including inflammation of the portal tracts, necrosis of liver cells, and centrilobular atrophy. It is not known whether this is an incidental or significant association; inflammation of the portal tracts is not an unusual finding in middle-aged and elderly people, but it is not often associated with clinical hepatic dysfunction.

Kuru

Kuru is a disease found in certain New Guinea tribes that formerly practiced ritual cannibalism. With the abolition of this custom over the last 15 to 20 years it has disappeared in children, suggesting a direct causal relationship. The brain in kuru may be grossly normal or may show mild frontal or cerebral atrophy. There are widespread histological changes of a general type. In the cortex, they are virtually confined to Golgi type II (granular) cells, but are more widespread in the cerebellum, pons, thalamus, and basal ganglia. Plaques are often seen in the cerebellar cortex and are occasionally seen elsewhere.

Kuru can be transmitted by cell-free filtrates to chimpanzees and other monkeys. Experimental animals show more severe changes than those in the human disease, with particular involvement of the cerebral cortex. Some affected neurons show diffuse or well-defined, spherical, argentophil bodies resembling those found in Pick's disease, which possibly are a reaction to axonal or dendritic injury.

INTRAUTERINE AND INTRANATAL INFECTIONS

Infectious diseases may be present in newborn infants or may develop after birth within the normal incubation period for the disease in question. Presumably, such cases are accounted for by the ability of many virus diseases to infect the placenta, or cross it from the maternal to the fetal circulation, or both. Such infections are uncommon but there is clinical evidence that poliovirus, arbovirus (especially western equine encephalomyelitis), herpesvirus, and coxsackievirus (causing infantile encephalomyocarditis) may cross the placenta in the last few days of pregnancy. Alternatively, during passage through the birth canal, herpesvirus infection may be acquired from maternal genital tract lesions. Such infections may be manifested as disseminated neurovisceral herpes or as herpes encephalitis that is often restricted to the hemispheres, both showing numerous type A intranuclear inclusions in all affected organs.

At least four organisms, namely, rubella virus, cytomegalovirus, *Toxoplasma gondii,* and *Treponema pallidum,* are known to cross the placenta and damage the developing fetus at a much earlier stage of pregnancy. It is possible that other organisms may also do so, but the evidence for this is tenuous.

Rubella Virus Infection

A rubella infection that may be mild or even clinically inapparent in the mother may cross the placenta in the first trimester and cause severe congenital defects in the fetus, particularly involving the CNS, heart, eyes, and internal ears. Such infections usually occur only in mothers who have not themselves had rubella or been immunized against it and in whom a period of viremia therefore develops preceding the appearance of protective (humoral) antibody. During this period, rubella lesions may be established in the placenta, or the virus may cross the placenta and establish itself in the fetus.

As a result of this infection, the mother produces transient IgM antibodies, rapidly followed by IgG antibodies, which are thought to cross the placenta from the fourth month to term. The fetus itself is incapable of immunological response until late in gestation, when it acquires the ability to synthesize IgM antibodies. Cord blood therefore contains IgG of maternal origin and IgM of fetal origin; not until the first year after birth does the infant produce its own IgG. In spite of the presumed passage of maternal IgG across the placenta from the fourth month onward (assuming infection in the first trimester), rubellavirus persists in the fetus and is almost invariably detectable throughout the neonatal period or, in infants with malformations, up to two or three years after birth.

As in the case of any teratogenic agent, the first trimester appears to be the most critical period. Maternal rubella developing later than this is not usually associated with malformation, although it may cause low birth weight, perhaps due to general reduction in cell division. The CNS malformations associated with rubella infection are varied and include micrencephaly, polymicrogyria, cerebellar dysplasia, and agenesis of the corpus callosum. Studies of infected abortuses indicate that the virus destroys actively dividing cells, which are not replaced, but without inflammation or other reactive changes. This may account for the low birth weight. The CNS malformations are usually of the type associated with failure of division or migration of neuroepithelial and neuroblastic cells.

In addition to, or instead of, malformations, there may be a *rubella encephalopathy,* with focal, noninflammatory cystic degeneration, usually involving the white matter and germinal matrix, but sometimes involving the basal ganglia and thalamus. These changes may be associated with hyperplasia of vessel walls, leading to focal ischemia, and chronic mononuclear meningitis may be present. Because these reactive changes are mild, they may indicate a somewhat later intrauterine infection.

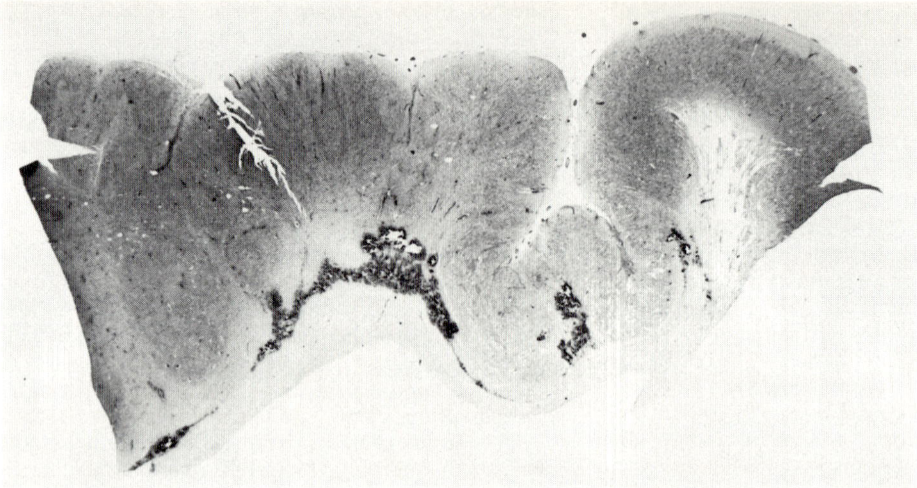

Fig. 23-23. Paraventricular calcification in infant brain, probably due to intrauterine cytomegalovirus infection. (H & E, X6.)

Cytomegalovirus Infection

Cytomegalovirus apparently may cross the placenta at any time during pregnancy and be associated with CNS malformations produced during the second trimester (e.g., micrencephaly, polymicrogyria). It appears to involve the periventricular areas, including the germinal matrix. Later fetal infection may be associated with prematurity and low birth weight, and general neurovisceral involvement without malformation may be seen in stillborn or premature infants. Small granulomas, containing enlarged cells with or without the characteristic intranuclear and intracytoplasmic inclusions, may be found in all parts of the CNS, especially, adjacent to the ventricles, and they frequently show calcification (Fig. 23-23). It is not clear whether the inclusion-bearing cells are astrocytes or microglia. Hydrocephalus or seizures may develop in surviving infants, who may ultimately become mentally retarded.

Toxoplasmosis

Toxoplasma gondii may attack nonimmune pregnant women, producing either no symptoms or a mild illness with lymphadenopathy. During the ensuing parasitemia, focal lesions of the placenta and invasion of the fetus may occur. As in cytomegalovirus infection, the effects depend on the time of fetal involvement. Infection during the second trimester causes micrencephaly, microphthalmia, cataracts, and optic atrophy. Later infection frequently leads to prematurity, with generalized neurovisceral infection, and neonatal jaundice, hepatosplenomegaly, anemia, rash, seizures, and frequently hydrocephalus develop. Survivors may be permanently affected, with mental retardation and convulsions. The whole spectrum of changes closely resembles that seen in cytomegalovirus infections.

At whatever period the fetus becomes infected, cord blood contains antibody derived both from the mother (IgG) and from the fetus (IgM); a high titer is usually present in the mother and a rising titer in the infant. In theory, chronic subclinical maternal infection might cause transmission to the fetus. However, there appear to be no reports of the condition in siblings, so it is probably only during the parasitemia of the initial maternal infection that the fetus can be infected.

Grossly, the brain shows focal, yellow, depressed lesions in the cortex, with meningeal opacities from pinpoint size to about 20 mm across. Less often, deeper lesions, particularly in the periventricular region, may become calcified and cause hydrocephalus. Histologically, focal necrotic lesions are seen in gray and white matter, with a mixed gliomesenchymal reaction at the edges. Early deposition of calcium is seen, both diffusely in the lesions and in degenerating neurons. Separate from the necrotic lesions are small granulomas consisting of epithelioid cell foci with or without lymphocytes. Subependymal granulations and mononuclear meningitis are common. Organisms may not be found or are identified as cysts, 15 to 20μ across, in the host cells, with a thin wall, produced jointly by the host and the parasite; they contain clusters of ovoid or fusiform organisms 2 to 5μ in

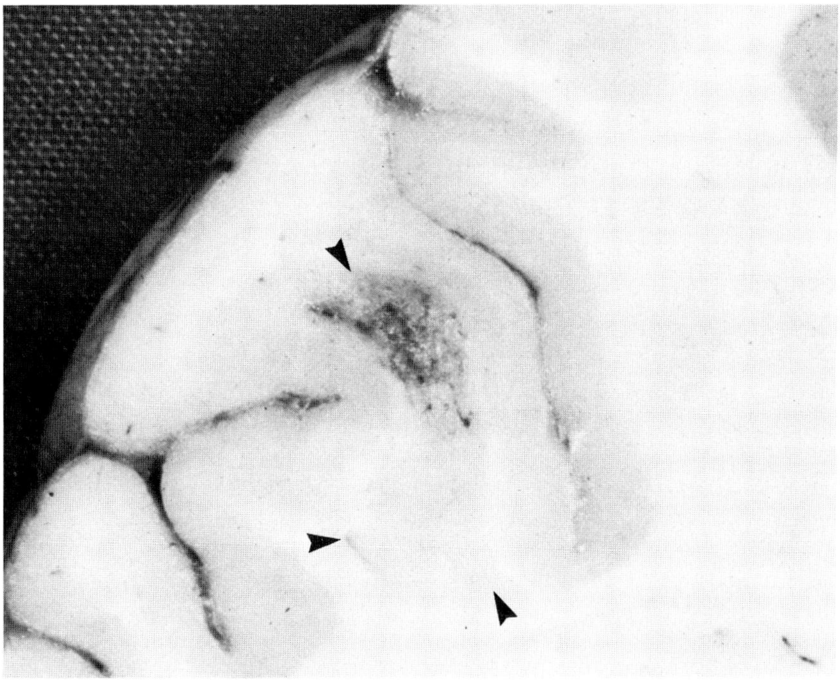

Fig. 23-24. ADEM. One of many demyelinating and sometimes necrotic lesions (arrows) found in a young adult male following a nonspecific respiratory infection 13 days previously, with acute deterioration and coma. Thus, this case has some features of ADEM but in others more resembles AHLE (see text).

length. Single extracellular parasites may be seen, but they are difficult to distinguish from debris or calcified granules.

Syphilis

Congenital syphilis is probably acquired transplacentally, between the fourth and seventh months of pregnancy, and is not usually associated with CNS malformations. If other features, such as mucocutaneous rash or hepatosplenomegaly, lead to a suspicion of syphilis, mononuclear cells will be found in the CSF in about 50% of cases, and, after the first few weeks, serological findings in the blood and CSF will be positive. However, symptoms are rare at birth: the manifestations, which may include any seen in the acquired form of the disease, develop in childhood or adult life. The neuropathological changes are identical with those in the acquired form.

DISEASES PROBABLY INVOLVING AUTOIMMUNITY

The existence of occasional cerebral complications following acute specific diseases and certain immunization procedures after a latent period of 10 to 21 days has long been recognized. These complications are often referred to as *postinfectious* or *parainfectious encephalopathy,* and fall into three groups.

Post-Rabies Encephalitis

The perivenular demyelination and acute inflammatory exudate that may complicate rabies immunization is unique. The histological features correspond to those of experimental allergic encephalomyelitis (see Chap. 21), presumably because post-rabies immunization encephalitis is due to the presence of brain tissue in many of the rabies vaccines that have been used. Except for the absence of an adjuvant, the etiology and pathogenesis of post-rabies immunization encephalopathy are therefore identical with that of experimental allergic encephalomyelitis, and the condition is presumed due to cell-mediated autoimmunity and gliotoxic antibody. In a few of these patients, plaque-like lesions develop that have a distribution and histological appearance similar to that of multiple sclerosis, the major difference being that the postimmunization disease is progressive and monophasic, in contrast to the remitting character of multiple sclerosis.

Acute Disseminated Encephalomyelitis and Acute Hemorrhagic Leukoencephalopathy

A second group is rather similar, in that it is characterized by areas of perivenular demyelination and tissue destruction (Fig. 23-24) associated with a mononuclear perivascular exudate (Fig. 23-25). Thus histologically it resembles experimental allergic encephalitis and post-rabies immunization encephalopathy, the fundamental difference being that there has been *no* challenging injection of CNS tissue.

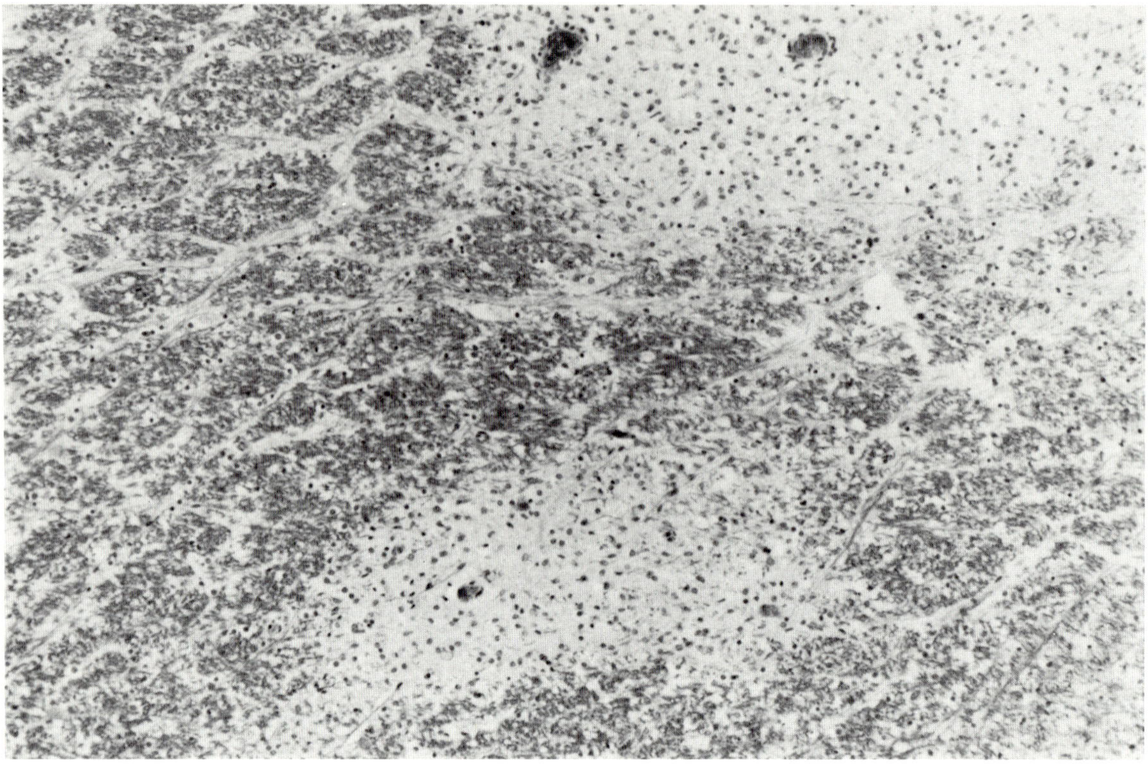

Fig. 23-25. ADEM. Same case as in Figure 23-24. Perivenular tissue destruction with gitter cells and a few lymphocytes. (Myelin, X115.)

The usual form of this disease, *acute disseminated encephalomyelitis* (ADEM), is rare under the age of 2 years. It is an occasional late complication of primary vaccination (after two years) and of measles and rubella infections. Changes are most severe in the brain stem and cord, but may occur in any part of the CNS. There are no inclusion bodies, nor is there other evidence of direct virus invasion in any of these cases.

Probably allied to ADEM is a more acute condition, *acute hemorrhagic leukoencephalopathy* (AHLE), which instead of following a specific exanthem or vaccination procedure, tends to be preceded by nonspecific upper respiratory tract infection. It differs in the presence of severe vascular injury, with massive exudation of fibrin, neutrophils, and red cells, resembling the hyperacute form of experimental allergic encephalitis. Again, there is no evidence for the presence of virus in the CNS.

Both ADEM and AHLE are presumed to be autoimmune phenomena, probably cell-mediated. The nature of the initial challenge is unknown.

Other Postinfectious or Postimmunization Encephalopathies

The third group of postinfectious CNS complications, which is considerably more common than either of the preceding types, has much less characteristic pathological findings. The brain may show edema, congestion, perivascular hemorrhages, and minimal perivascular lymphocytic cuffing, associated with acute neuronal degeneration. This condition can occur at a younger age than the other types. It may be associated with primary vaccination under the age of 2 years, revaccination, smallpox, pertussis, scarlet fever, and occasionally other immunization procedures. As in the preceding groups, the occurrence of the complication is separated from the acute phase of the disease by a latent interval averaging 10 to 14 days, and there is neither morphological nor any other evidence of direct virus infection of the CNS.

However, the resemblance of the nonspecific changes to those of the viral encephalitides already described may be noted. The likelihood of this being an autoimmune phenomenon is perhaps reduced by the lack of specific histological features and by the fact of its occurrence in very young infants, in whom immunological mechanisms are poorly developed. Perhaps these cases represent viral infections of the CNS in which the presence of virus has not been detected — a possibility that requires further investigation.

BIBLIOGRAPHY

Alvord, E. C., Jr. Hypersensitivity States Affecting the Nervous System. In J. Minckler (Ed.), *Pathology of the Nervous System.* New York: McGraw-Hill, 1972. Vol. 3, pp. 2246-2260.

Berry, R. G., and Alpers, B. J. Bacterial Encephalitis. In J. Minckler (Ed.), *Pathology of the Nervous System.* New York: McGraw-Hill, 1972. Vol. 3, pp. 2362-2375.

Bodian, D. Poliomyelitis. In J. Minckler (Ed.), *Pathology of the Nervous System.* New York: McGraw-Hill, 1972. Vol. 3, pp. 2323-2344.

Carpenter, S., and Lampert, P. W. Postinfectious Perivenous Encephalitis and Acute Hemorrhagic Leukoencephalitis. In J. Minckler (Ed.), *Pathology of the Nervous System.* New York: McGraw-Hill, 1972. Vol. 3, pp. 2260-2269.

Gadjusek, D. C. Spongiform virus encephalopathies. *J. Clin. Pathol.* [Suppl.] 25:78-83, 1971.

Gadjusek, D. C., and Gibbs, C. J., Jr. Subacute and Chronic Diseases Caused by Atypical Infections with Unconventional Viruses in Aberrant Hosts. In *Perspectives in Virology.* New York: Academic, 1973. Vol. 8, pp. 279-311.

Gibbs, C. J., Jr., and Gadjusek, D. C. Isolation and characterization of the subacute spongiform virus encephalopathies of man: Kuru and Creutzfeldt-Jakob disease. *J. Clin. Pathol.* [Suppl.] 25:84-96, 1971.

Gibbs, C. J., Jr., and Gadjusek, D. C. Cell-Virus Interactions in Slow Infections of the Nervous System. In F. O. Schmitt and F. G. Worden (Eds.), *The Neurosciences. Third Study Program.* Cambridge, Mass.: MIT Press, 1974. Pp. 1025-1041.

Jenis, E. H., Knieser, M. R., Rothouse, P. A., Jensen, G. E., and Scott, R. M. Subacute sclerosing panencephalitis: Immunoultrastructural localization of measles-virus antigen. *Arch. Pathol.* 95:81-89, 1973.

Johnson, R. T., and Gibbs, C. J. Koch's postulates and slow infections of the nervous system. *Arch. Neurol.* 30:36-38, 1974.

Kirschbaum, W. R. Jakob-Creutzfeldt Disease. In J. Minckler (Ed.), *Pathology of the Nervous System.* New York: McGraw-Hill, 1971. Vol. 2, pp. 1410-1419.

Lampert, P. W., Gadjusek, D. C., and Gibbs, C. J., Jr. Subacute spongiform encephalopathies. *Am. J. Pathol.* 68:626-646, 1972.

Melnick, J. L., and Richardson, L. S. Slow Viruses. In J. Minckler (Ed.), *Pathology of the Nervous System.* New York: McGraw-Hill, 1972. Vol. 3, pp. 2968-2974.

Moore, M. T. Meningitis. In J. Minckler (Ed.), *Pathology of the Nervous System.* New York: McGraw-Hill, 1972. Vol. 3, pp. 2375-2411.

Narayan, O., Penney, J. B., Johnson, R. T., Herndon, R. M., and Weiner, L. P. Etiology of progressive multifocal leukoencepahalopathy: Identification of papovavirus. *N. Engl. J. Med.* 289:1278-1282, 1973.

Nieberg, K. C., and Blumberg, J. M. Viral Encephalitides. In J. Minckler (Ed.), *Pathology of the Nervous System.* New York: McGraw-Hill, 1972. Vol. 3, pp. 2269-2323.

Norris, F. H. An ultrastructural study of herpes simplex virus encephalitis. *J. Neuropathol. Exp. Neurol.* 31:611-623, 1972.

Reynolds, D. W., Stagno, S., Hosty, T. S., Tiller, M., and Alford, C. A. Maternal cytomegalovirus excretion and perinatal infection. *N. Engl. J. Med.* 289:1-5, 1973.

Roos, R., Gadjusek, D. C., and Gibbs, C. J., Jr. The clinical characteristics of transmissible Creutzfeldt-Jakob disease. *Brain* 96:1-20, 1973.

Schober, R., and Herman, M. M. Neuropathology of cardiac transplantation. *Lancet* 1:962-967, 1973.

Schochet, S. S., Jr. Neuronal Inclusions. In G. H. Bourne (Ed.), *The Structure and Function of Nervous Tissue.* New York: Academic, 1972. Vol. 4, pp. 129-177.

Verhaart, W. J. C. Encephalopathy in Reticuloses (Progressive Multifocal Leukoencephalopathy). In J. Minckler (Ed.), *Pathology of the Nervous System.* New York: McGraw-Hill, 1968. Vol. 1, pp. 1061-1064.

Wiener, L. P., Johnson, R. T., and Herndon, R. M. Viral infections and demyelinating diseases. *N. Engl. J. Med.* 288:1103-1111, 1973.

Wolf, A., and Cowen, D. Perinatal Infections of the Central Nervous System. In J. Minckler (Ed.), *Pathology of the Nervous System.* New York: McGraw-Hill, 1972. Vol. 3, pp. 2565-2611.

Degenerative Diseases

24

Degeneration in the strict histological sense implies reversible changes occurring within a cell, irrespective of their etiology. However, the term *degenerative diseases* used in respect to the CNS has an entirely different meaning, since the changes that occur are neither morphologically nor functionally reversible. Since it covers such a wide spectrum of clinical manifestations and CNS localization of changes, the group is hard to define. However, all the entities to be discussed fulfill the following criteria:

1. The primary disease involves the neuron itself — either the perikaryon with resulting cell loss or primarily the axon (most readily seen as demyelination of long tracts).
2. Changes in astrocytes or oligodendroglial cells are secondary responses to cell loss or degeneration of myelin.
3. There are no inflammatory changes; microglia remain essentially unaltered and leukocytes and macrophages are absent.
4. The areas of attack are selective and represent functional units in the gray or white matter or both (thus, they differ from inflammatory, vascular, or demyelinating processes that transgress the boundaries of functional areas within the CNS).
5. Clinically, the degenerative disorders are chronic or subacute in duration, many of them being relentlessly progressive and shortening life. Death frequently occurs as a result of marasmus or intercurrent infection.

Because a salient feature of many of these diseases is either an insidious loss of neurons accompanied by no other change than mild fibrillary gliosis, or a gradual "dying back" of axons with secondary loss of myelin, it has been suggested that they represent a shortening of neuronal or axonal life-span compared to that of the patient, with the reasons unknown; the term *abiotrophy* has been used to describe the process. Alternatively, since an individual disease tends to be confined to certain systems within the central nervous system, the generic term *system diseases* may be encountered. Neither appears to offer any significant advantage over the more commonly used *degenerative diseases.* However, they emphasize some of the most important features just outlined.

At least some cases of any individual disease within this group show a familial incidence, and there are examples within the group of autosomal dominant, autosomal recessive, and sex-linked recessive inheritance. However, some cases of each disease entity are sporadic. Thus, each clinicopathological entity is associated with more than one mode of inheritance, as well as with sporadic occurrence. In this respect the group is much less clear-cut than the group of inborn errors of metabolism involving the CNS or even the phakomatoses. However, progress is being made in determining the biochemical basis of a few of these diseases, and slow virus infection may be found to account for others (Creutzfeldt-Jakob syndrome was often included in this group). *Degenerative* is no longer synonymous with *idiopathic.*

Classification

A further justification for considering the degenerative disorders in one chapter is the considerable overlap that exists between the various types (Fig. 24-1). While it is possible to pick out a few well-defined entities that constitute perhaps 90 to 95% of all cases in the group, there remains a significant residue of disorders that exhibit clinical and pathological features intermediate between more typical forms, which considerably complicates classification. In this chapter, only the best defined and most common nosological entities will be considered, with passing reference made to intermediate forms where appropriate. Pursuing this somewhat arbitrary course, the degenerative diseases may be considered in four clinical categories (though it will be appreciated that these are not mutually exclusive).

1. *Dementia.* In this group, the brunt of pathological changes is borne by the cerebral cortex, especially the frontotemporal regions. The changes seen are frequently an exaggerated form of those associated with aging of the brain, and the diseases to be described are Alzheimer's disease (presenile and senile dementia) and Pick's disease. The rare Parkinson-dementia complex and Alper's disease (a doubtful entity with lesions not confined to the cortex, occurring in infants and young children and compatible with an ischemic or hypoxemic origin) are not considered.

2. *Extrapyramidal disorders.* These are associated with abnormal involuntary movements (dyskinesias)

++ = usually severely affected; + = usually moderately affected; ± = slightly or inconsistently affected	CEREBRAL CORTEX	CEREBRAL WHITE MATTER	CAUDATE / PUTAMEN	PALLIDUM	THALAMUS	HYPOTHALAMUS	SUBSTANTIA NIGRA	SUBTHALAMIC NUCLEUS	RED NUCLEUS	BASAL PONS	INFERIOR OLIVES	CEREBELLUM	BRAIN STEM	PROPRIOCEPTIVE TRACTS	MOTOR TRACTS	CORD GRAY MATTER
ALZHEIMER'S DISEASE	++	±														
PICK'S DISEASE	++	+	+	±												
HUNTINGTON'S CHOREA	+	±	++													
DYSTONIA MUSCULORUM DEFORMANS			++?													
WILSON'S DISEASE			++													
HALLERVORDEN-SPATZ SYNDROME	±			++	±		++	±	±				± [grac. cun.]			± [post.]
PARALYSIS AGITANS (PRIMARY)						±	++			±	±	±	+ [pig. nuc.]			
OLIVOPONTOCEREBELLAR ATROPHY			±				±			++	++	++		±		± [lat.]
CEREBELLO-OLIVARY ATROPHY											++	++				
CEREBELLAR ATROPHY												++				
FRIEDREICH'S ATAXIA	± [4,6]											±	+ [coch. S.ol.]	++	+	
MOTONEURON DISEASE	± [4,6]												+ [mot. nuc.]		++	++ [ant.]
INFANTILE SPINAL MUSC. ATROPHY																++ [ant.]
OTHER SPINAL MUSC. ATROPHY																+ [ant.]

Fig. 24-1. The distribution of shrinkage and gliosis in some of the degenerative diseases (4,6 = areas 4 and 6 of cortex; grac.cun. = gracilis and cuneate nuclei; pig.nuc. = pigmented brain stem nuclei; coch. S.ol. = cochlear nuclei and superior olives; mot.nuc. = motor nuclei of cord and brain stem; lat., post. = lateral and posterior columns of cord; ant. = anterior horns).

and frequently with alterations in muscle tone. The most severe neuronal loss is in various components of the basal ganglia. The disorders to be considered include paralysis agitans (parkinsonism), hepatolenticular degeneration (Wilson's disease), Huntington's chorea, dystonia musculorum deformans, and the Hallervorden-Spatz–neuroaxonal dystrophy group. Kernicterus is not included, since it represents a cytotoxic anoxia (see Chap. 17), and Sydenham's chorea is excluded because it is an increasingly rare complication of rheumatic fever and, in any case, has no generally agreed morphological substrate.

3. *Ataxic disorders.* These are the spinocerebellar degenerations in which demyelination is often a prominent component, involving afferent proprioceptive fibers of the spinal cord and associated nuclei and afferent sources to the cerebellum such as the pontine and inferior olivary nuclei, together with the deep nuclei and cortex of the cerebellum. Considered under this heading are Friedreich's ataxia, cerebello-olivary degeneration, olivopontocerebellar disease, and cerebellar atrophy.

4. *Motoneuron disorders.* These present clinically as muscular weakness and wasting with clinical features of motoneuron disease (in the cord, brain stem, or both) but not of peripheral neuropathy. Major pathological changes affect motor nuclei of the brain stem and cord, but the Betz's cells and other large pyramidal cells of cortical areas 4 and 6 may also be reduced, with demyelination of the pyramidal tracts. Diseases to be considered in this group include spinal muscular atrophy (infantile, juvenile, and other variants) and motoneuron disease, including amyotrophic lateral sclerosis.

It is apparent that few parts of the CNS are immune from degenerative disease. Involvement of the thalamus and hypothalamus is, however, extremely rare, though thalamic neuronal loss has been reported in the areas related to damaged cortex (trans-synaptic degeneration). Upper motoneuron lesions (cortical areas 4 and 6) do not occur on their own, but may be associated with disorders in groups 3 or 4 above. Autonomic dysfunction on a degenerative basis rarely occurs as an isolated lesion (Shy-Drager syndrome), but may be the presenting feature in variants of paralysis agitans (parkinsonism) or of olivopontocerebellar disease.

The appropriate classification of *progressive supranuclear palsy,* which is characterized by progressive paralysis of vertical eye movements among other clinical features, remains unclear, although lesions are widely distributed in the brain stem, cerebellum, and sometimes in the diencephalon and closely resemble

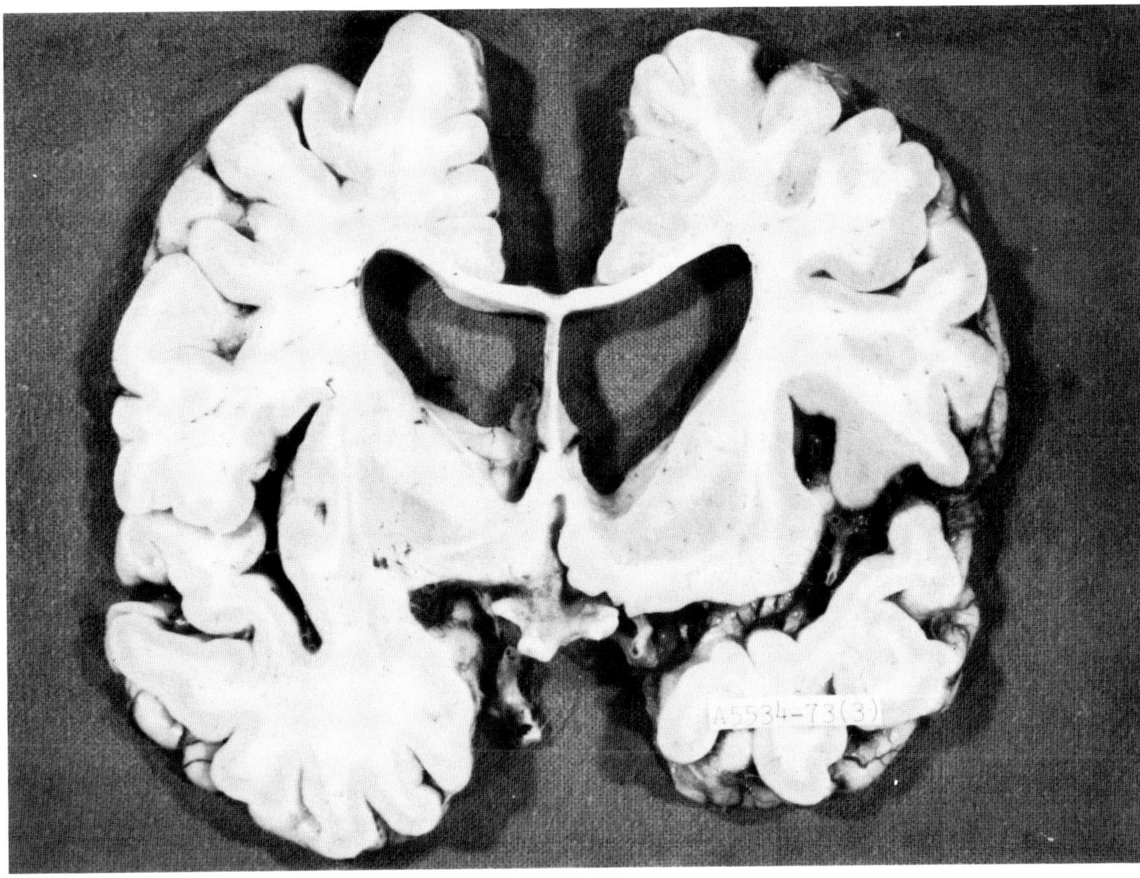

Fig. 24-2. Some of the manifestations of shrinkage in a mild example of Alzheimer's disease. Note the widened sulci, dilatation of lateral ventricles, flattening of caudate nuclei, and reduction in white matter and corpus callosum.

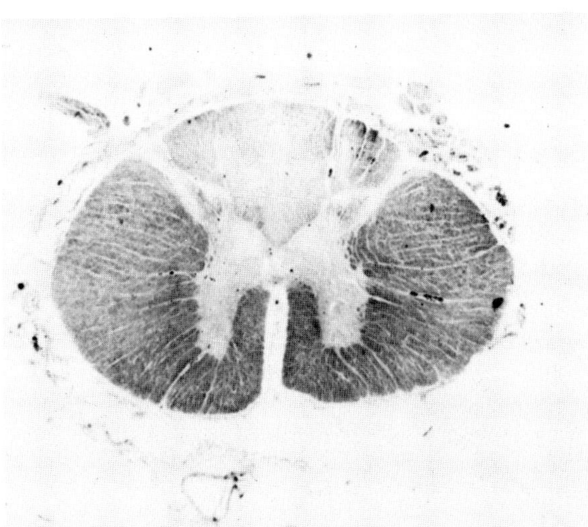

Fig. 24-3. Demyelination of the posterior columns, probably secondary to degeneration of the proximal processes of dorsal root ganglion cells, in a case of Friedreich's ataxia. (Myelin, X5.)

those associated with aging and Alzheimer's disease. It is difficult to relate this disorder to any of the preceding groups.

General Morphological Characteristics

Certain morphological features may be regarded as common to the degenerative disorders. Each disease is an insidious, slowly progressive process of neuronal or axonal loss, accompanied by entirely nonspecific reactions on the part of the glia. Minor peculiarities of individual diseases will be considered under the appropriate heading.

Gross Appearances

Gross changes in the affected areas consist of shrinkage and usually a moderate increase in firmness due to reactive gliosis. This shrinkage (Fig. 24-2) may be manifested by such changes as mild to moderate decreases in brain weight, widening of cortical sulci, flattening of the heads of the caudate nuclei, or decrease in the cross-sectional area of cord white matter. If the primary change is in long tract axons, secondary demyelination (Fig. 24-3) will also be a prominent gross feature accompanying or preceding shrinkage and sclerosis. Degenerative diseases only rarely show cystic gliosis, though it is occasionally seen in the basal ganglia in hepatolenticular degeneration (see p. 466).

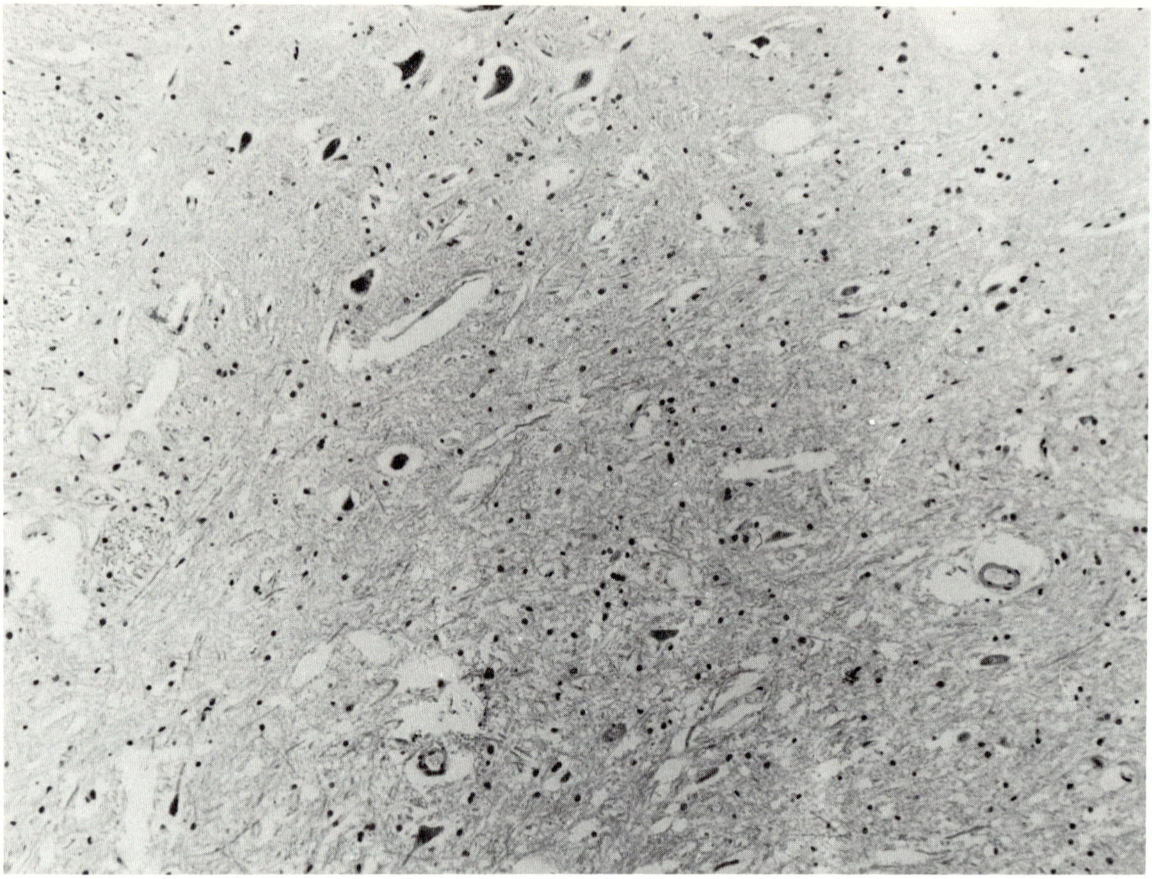

Fig. 24-4. Severe neuronal loss, with remaining neurons shrunken and sclerotic. Anterior horn from a case of spinal muscular atrophy. (H & E, X115.)

Microscopic Appearances

Primary Lesion in Gray Matter. The primary histological lesion in affected gray matter is reduction in the number of neurons (Fig. 24-4). Those that remain may appear normal or show such nonspecific changes as sclerosis or swelling. Since the tempo of these diseases is slow, neuronophagia is rarely seen. Peculiarities of the individual diseases are merely superimposed on this general picture of cell loss and nonspecific degeneration. Associated with loss of neurons (including, of course, their dendritic and axonal processes), a mild to moderate astrocytic hypertrophy or even hyperplasia may be apparent, associated with fine fibrillary gliosis (Fig. 24-5). Oligodendroglial and microglial cells and vascular elements appear normal. Secondary demyelination of varying degree must be present, but in hemispheric white matter is usually mild and accompanied by slight fibrillary gliosis. Oligodendroglia are not significantly reduced, presumably because they are responsible for the maintenance of myelin internodes on several different axons and do not become redundant until each of these has been destroyed.

Primary Lesion in White Matter. The change in primarily affected white matter is gradual distoproximal "dying-back" of axons, accompanied by secondary demyelination. Because of the extreme slowness of the process, accumulation of abbau products is not seen, and, as previously noted, the loss of oligodendroglial cells is late, death often occurring before tractal degeneration and demyelination are complete. Degeneration is accompanied by mild astrocytic hypertrophy and fibrillary gliosis orientated in the direction of the tract (isomorphic gliosis).

Since there is evidence that the integrity of the axon depends almost entirely on its cell body and not on oligodendroglial cells, it might be supposed that disappearance of axons must reflect dysfunction of the perikaryon. While this is probably true, reduction in the numbers of perikaryons in these cases (as in dorsal root ganglia) is less marked and much later than tractal degeneration; however, there might be disordered axoplasmic flow.

Role of Trans-Synaptic Degeneration. Particularly in the spinocerebellar group of diseases, two or more in a functional chain of neurons may show degeneration. This could be regarded either as a primary change, simultaneously affecting both neurons, or as trans-synaptic degeneration. Thus, degeneration of the dorsal roots may be associated with loss of

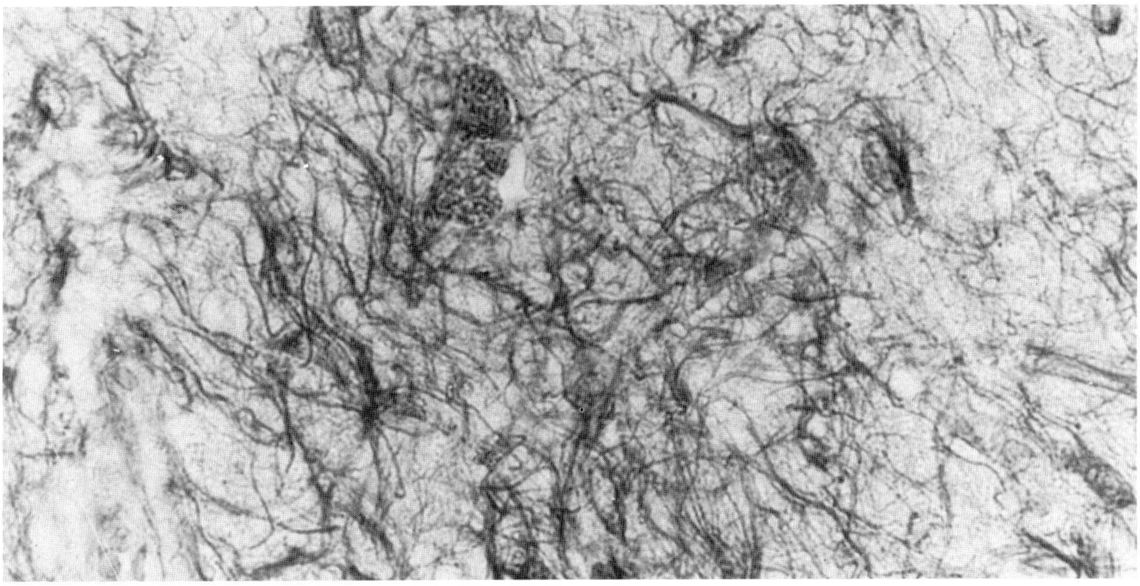

Fig. 24-5. Moderate astrocytic hyperplasia and fibrillary gliosis characteristic of degenerative disease. Substantia nigra from a case of paralysis agitans. (Holzer's stain, ×750.)

neurons, probably trans-synaptic, in the thoracic nucleus of Clarke and with demyelination of the spinocerebellar tracts. The situation in cerebello-olivary and olivopontocerebellar degeneration is less simple, since pontine and olivary afferents to the cerebellar cortex synapse principally with granular and Golgi cells, which in turn project to Purkinje's cells. If, as it appears, Purkinje's cell loss is considerably more severe than loss from the internal granular layer, the strict concept of trans-synaptic degeneration is not applicable. However, cell loss from the closely packed granular layer might be greater than appreciated. Thus, the problem is unresolved.

DEMENTIA

There are very many causes of dementia, including infections, juvenile- or adult-onset metabolic errors involving the CNS, alcohol and other (generally hypothetical) toxic agents, psychoactive drugs, and perhaps even diffuse vascular insufficiency associated with small-vessel disease (arteriolosclerosis). Some of these are acute or subacute conditions, and CNS changes are widespread, without topographical limitation.

To be considered here are two chronic conditions, Alzheimer's disease and Pick's disease, in which there are major changes in the cerebral cortex. These changes conform to the general pattern outlined in the introductory section, with the addition of some specific types of change in the neuronal cell bodies and neuropil. These latter changes are similar to those seen in aging brains, even when intellectual capacity remains normal. A brief discussion of aging changes therefore precedes a description of the two diseases.

Aging in the Central Nervous System

Gross Appearances

From the end of the fourth decade there is a general decline in brain weight averaging 5 to 10% by the age of 70 and 16 to 18% by the age of 80 (a decrease to averages of 1170 g in the male and 1060 g in the female). Because of individual mature-weight variation, the ratio of brain weight to skull volume would be a better indication of atrophy, but is impracticable in a service hospital context. Since atrophy mainly affects the hemispheres, an increase in the ratio of cerebellum plus brain stem weight to total brain weight, normally about 12%, may be a helpful indication of early atrophy. The decrease in weight is accompanied by a slight widening of the cerebral sulci, least marked in the occipital region, and symmetrical dilatation of the lateral ventricles, apparently due more to a decrease in volume of white matter than of cortex. All areas of gray matter become darker and even slightly brownish, due to the accumulation of lipofuscin pigment (see Fig. 10-7).

Microscopic Appearances

Neurons tend to decrease in size, have small dark nuclei, and lose Nissl substance. They accumulate lipofuscin pigment. (In certain areas, such as the dentate and inferior olivary nuclei, prominent accumulations of lipofuscin are normal by middle age.) There may be mild neuronal loss, especially of cortical pyramidal cells, but this is generally a subjective impression unless accompanied by neuronophagia, which rarely occurs. In general, aging changes are

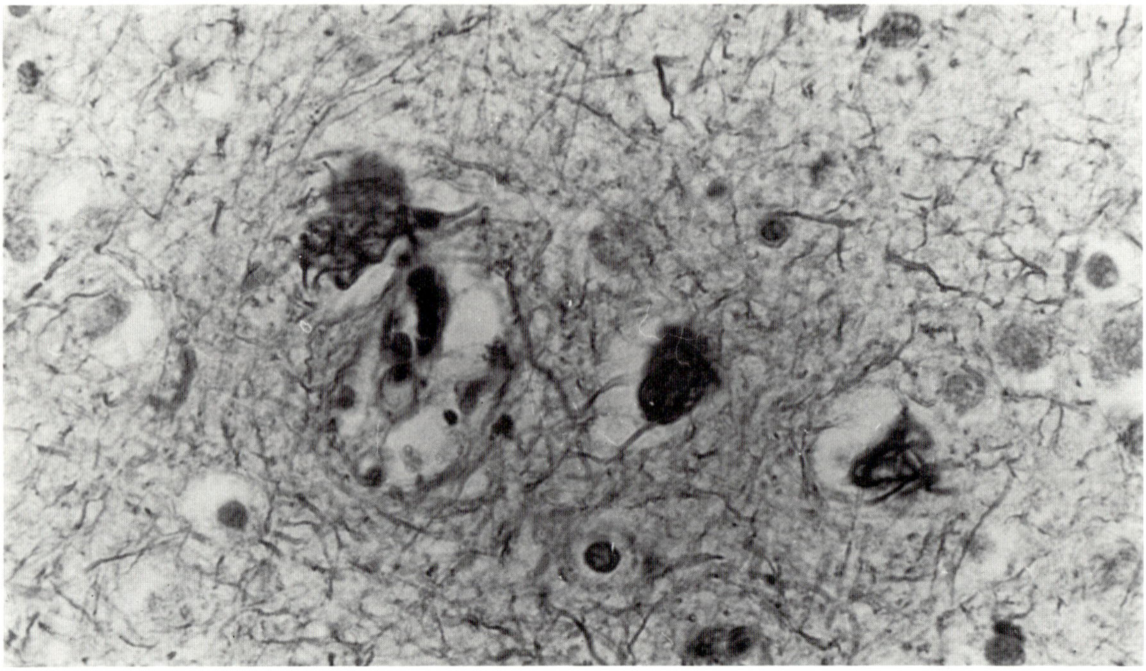

Fig. 24-6. Clumping of neurofibrils in the cortical neurons to form neurofibrillary tangles, often hiding the nucleus. From brain of a normally intelligent woman, age 93. (Silver, X750.)

much less marked in the phylogenetically ancient parts of the brain such as the hypothalamus and brain stem.

Apart from the accumulation of lipofuscin pigment, the changes seen electron-microscopically are indefinite, but are said to include shrunken mitochondria, fragmentation of the Golgi complex, and clumping of nuclear chromatin. Uncommonly, small numbers of neurons, usually cortical pyramidal cells, show apparent clumping of neurofibrils (Fig. 24-6) to form argyrophilic skeins that surround or displace the nucleus. These neurofibrillary tangles will be discussed subsequently.

Astrocytes tend to change from protoplasmic to fibrillary form, and there may be a mild diffuse increase in glial fibers, some of which are thick and bizarre, forming spirals, rings, or other unusual forms. Oligodendroglial, microglial, and ependymal cells do not exhibit visible changes.

Senile Plaques. Small, rounded areas of degeneration of the neuropil may be seen, particularly in the cerebral cortex (Fig. 24-7), and appear under light microscopy to consist of granular debris, with or without a homogenous hyaline central core. If a core is present, it stains positively for amyloid. While these areas of degeneration (senile plaques) can be seen on sections stained with hematoxylin and eosin, they are better visualized by a silver stain or the periodic acid-Schiff (PAS) technique. Their nature is discussed on page 455.

Lipofuscin. The accumulation of lipofuscin pigment is not peculiar to neurons, but occurs in other tissues, notably in cardiac muscle. It is yellowish-brown and autofluorescent, gives a positive reaction with PAS and any lipid stain, is usually acid-fast and stains by silver impregnation methods. Iron is pres-

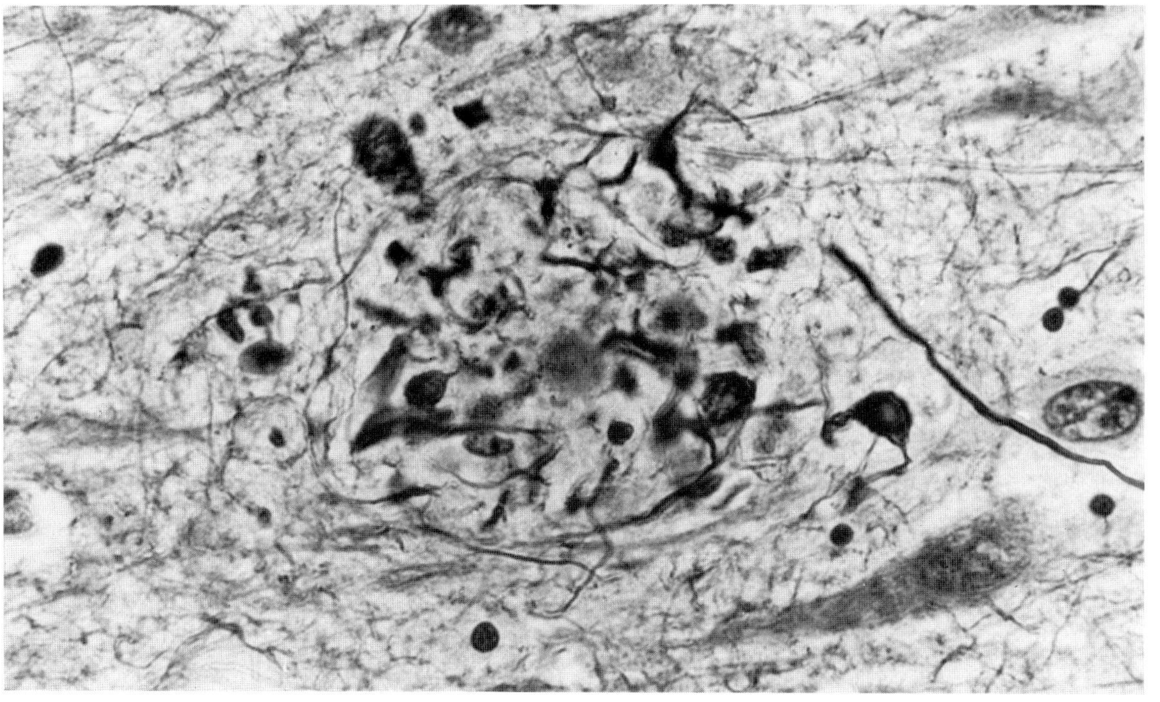

Fig. 24-7. Focal area of degeneration in the neuropil of the cortex, showing distorted argyrophilic processes of uncertain origin and a small, homogenous amyloid core. This is the so-called senile plaque. (Silver, X750.)

ent, but not demonstrable by the Prussian blue reaction. The granules contain acid phosphatase but no mitochondrial (oxidative) enzymes, and appear on electron-microscopic examination as dense, irregular, finely granular bodies. The origin of lipofuscin is unknown, and its alternative designation as "wear-and-tear pigment" merely indicates its association with aging.

Occasional Changes in Parenchyma. Whereas senile plaques and neurofibrillary tangles are not rare in the aging cortex, especially the hippocampus, much less common aging changes have been described in other areas. These include *spheroids,* which are rounded silver-staining bodies, probably situated in axons, in the gracilis and cuneate nuclei (Fig. 24-8), and occasionally in other areas. These are discussed under Hallervorden-Spatz syndrome (see p. 465). Small, rounded, intracytoplasmic inclusions (Lewy bodies) are occasionally found in the substantia nigra. These are discussed under paralysis agitans (see p. 460). Recently, small eosinophilic bodies, round or oval and 4 to 8μ in length, in the cytoplasm of thalamic neurons have been described. Rounded extracellular bodies in the neuropil, differing from senile plaques in their smaller size, hyaline appearance, and location (corpora amylacea), occur especially just beneath the pia and ependyma. Their origin is unknown.

Changes in Blood Vessels. Changes in the vessels of the brain and cord also occur with advancing age. The internal elastic lamina may show thinning, fraying, and even fragmentation beginning about the age of 45 to 50. Replacement of smooth muscle by collagen occurs from the age of 60 on, so that walls become thick and fibrous and may appear hyaline. Mineral deposits occur especially in arterioles, with a predilection for certain areas, notably the pallidum and the dentate nucleus.

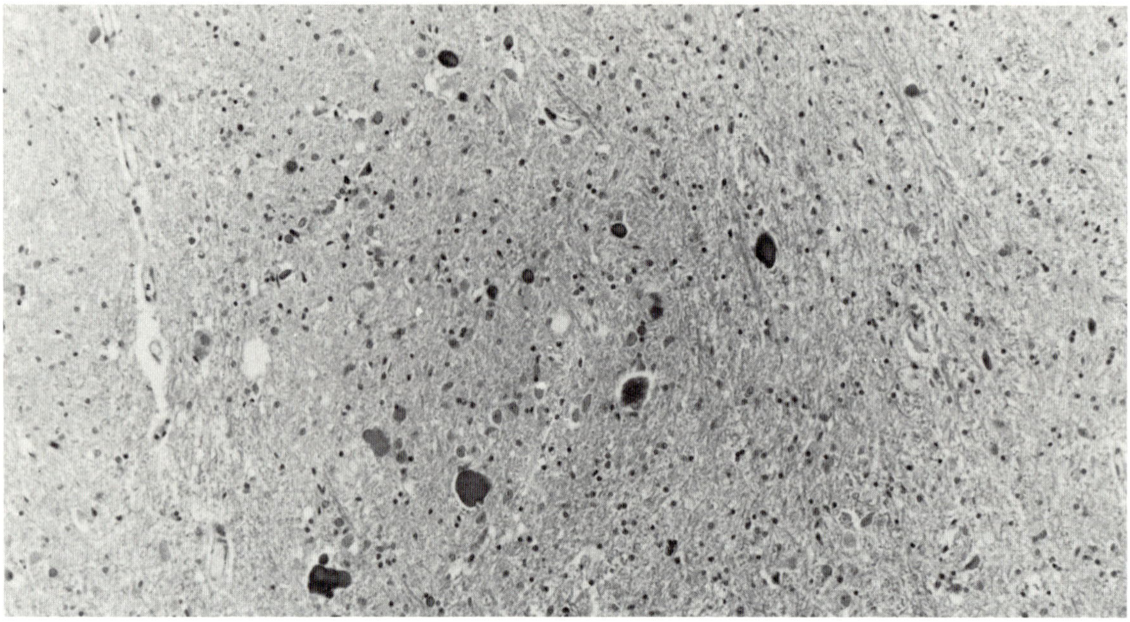

Fig. 24-8. Homogenous, irregularly rounded swellings, probably of axonal origin (axonal dystrophy) in the gracilis nucleus of a 77-year-old man without other features of CNS abnormality. (H & E, X115.)

Some hyaline material staining as amyloid occurs in the media, adventitia, and even in the periadventitial spaces of small intracerebral vessels. (Amyloid may also be deposited in larger meningeal vessels, when it is usually restricted to the media.) Deposition of amyloid in senile plaques and in aging cerebral vessels bears no relation to generalized amyloidosis, although the staining properties of the material and its fibrillary appearance on electron microscopy are identical in the two conditions.

Alzheimer's Disease (Presenile and Senile Dementia)

The term *Alzheimer's disease* was originally applied only to presenile dementia, arbitrarily defined as dementia with onset before age 65. The disease is more common in women than men, and although it usually becomes apparent between 50 and 60, has been described in young adults and even children. A syndrome with identical clinical and morphological features occurs after age 65 (senile dementia), and there is no evidence to suggest that these cases are not all the same disease, irrespective of age of onset. A few are familial, but most are sporadic, and there is no clear genetic basis.

The usual duration is two to five years, with the disease terminating in emaciation and intercurrent infection. A prominent, early feature is progressive memory failure (particularly of short-term memory), sometimes accompanied by restlessness and hallucinations, and progressing through a phase of confusion to complete dementia. Alzheimer's disease is only occasionally associated with focal features such as cortical blindness, impairment of pyramidal or extrapyramidal motor function, or seizures.

Morphological Features

Gross Appearances. Loss of brain weight is moderate to severe, with weight often reduced to under 1000 g, with diffuse sulcal widening that is usually most marked in the frontotemporal cortex and less extreme than the typical "knife-edge" appearance seen in Pick's disease. Moderate meningeal thickening occurs, especially superolaterally. Sections show a reduction in cortical thickness, with lesser involvement of the hemispheric white matter, and moderate symmetrical ventricular dilatation.

Microscopic Appearances. Neuronal loss is largely confined to the cerebral cortex. It is often most severe in Sector H_1 and the subiculum of the hippocampus, and the pyramidal cell layers (III and V). Astrocytic hypertrophy and fibrillary gliosis are moderate, and the swollen astrocytes may contain pale yellow pigment. Myelin loss is mild, and no abbau products accumulate. Residual cortical neurons may show excess lipofuscin and other nonspecific degenerative changes. In addition, there are three histological changes that are particularly marked in, but not specific for, Alzheimer's disease. Two of them (neurofibrillary tangles and senile plaques) are to a much smaller extent concomitants of normal aging; the third, granulovacuolar degeneration, is described under Pick's disease (p. 458).

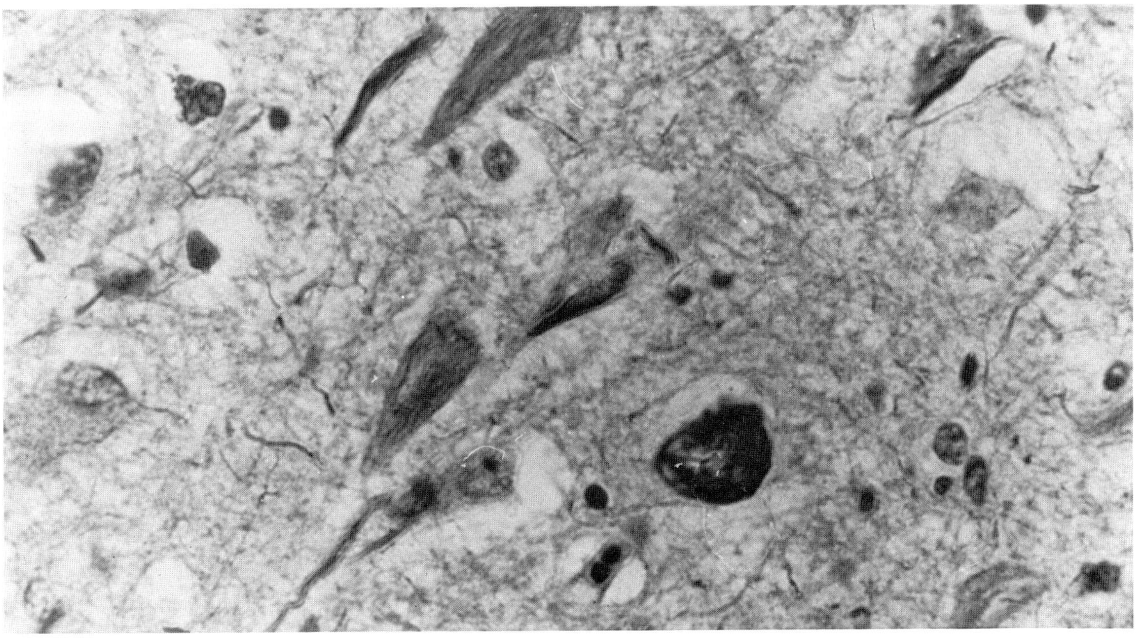

Fig. 24-9. Alzheimer's disease, showing thickening of neurofibrils in all hippocampal neurons and a prominent tangle. (Silver, X750.)

Structure and Origin of Neurofibrillary Tangles

Neurofibrillary tangles occur mainly in cortical pyramidal neurons, often in almost all the surviving cells. They are especially frequent in Sector H_1 and the subiculum of the hippocampus (Fig. 24-9). The early, prominent memory loss in these patients may possibly be associated with this involvement of the limbic system. The tangles consist of coarse, irregular fibers (within the cytoplasm of the perikaryon and occasionally extending into the apical dendrite) which stain densely with silver.

Electron-microscopically, they are seen to consist of clusters of regular tubules, each of which appears twisted or constricted at intervals of 800 A. The tubules are 200 to 220 A at their widest and about 100 A at the constrictions. Cross sections show a wall about 50 A thick and made up of 10 to 13 subunits, with a central 40-A dot. The tubules are not separated from cytoplasm by any membrane and are unconnected with cell organelles. Since the content of neurofilaments remains normal, whereas that of microtubules is markedly reduced, it is presumed that the abnormal structures are of microtubular origin. If axoplasmic flow is dependent on microtubules (see Chap. 3), it is probable that flow is interfered with in the presence of tangles.

These structures are not specific for Alzheimer's disease, since they occur in small numbers in normal aging and are seen in postencephalitic paralysis agitans (mainly in the brain stem), progressive supranuclear palsy (also in the brain stem), and the Parkinson-dementia complex of Guam. They appear identical in all these conditions.

Changes induced in nerve cells by colchicine, vincristine, or aluminium phosphate or found occasionally in sporadic motoneuron disease consist of aggregations of fibers about 90 to 100 A in diameter and are not the same as neurofibrillary tangles.

Recent reports suggest that synaptic terminals may be enlarged in the vicinity of senile plaques in Alzheimer's disease and contain tubules or vesicles 200 to 350 A wide, with a wall 45 to 90 A thick. These also differ from neurofibrillary tangles and appear to be derived by dilatation of endoplasmic reticulum or possibly from microtubules or synaptic vesicles. It is not yet clear whether or not this change is specific for Alzheimer's disease.

Structure and Origin of Senile Plaques

Senile plaques in large numbers (Fig. 24-7) are characteristic of Alzheimer's disease (at all ages). From 10 to 150μ in diameter and initially round, they may coalesce to irregular shapes. They are seen most frequently in the cortex and basal ganglia and less often in the substantia nigra, amygdala, hypothalamus, and periaqueductal gray matter.

An early plaque appears to consist of degenerating presynaptic and postsynaptic terminals together with unidentified cell processes. These terminals are distended by twisted tubules (neurofibrillary tangles), dilated tubules (probably from endoplasmic reticulum), densely stained bodies apparently derived from mitochondria, and low-density, membrane-bound vesicles of uncertain origin. The structureless core

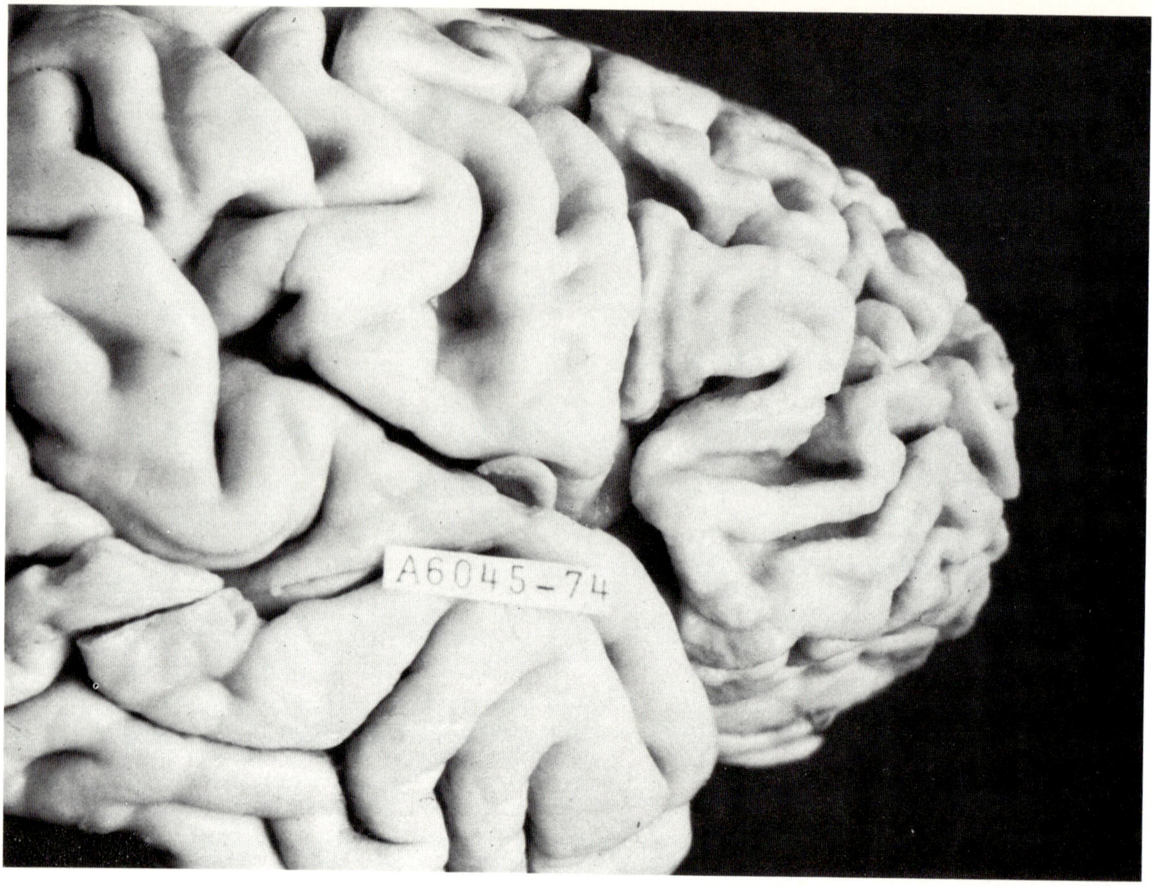

Fig. 24-10. Pick's disease, showing severe convolutional atrophy of the frontal pole and of the anterior part of the superior temporal gyrus.

develops early and has the staining reactions and electron-microscopic appearance of amyloid. Some plaques, presumably the oldest, consist almost entirely of amyloid. Plaques exhibit variable oxidative and hydrolytic enzyme activity, depending on their content of mitochondria and lysosomes.

Pick's Disease

Pick's disease is a much rarer type of presenile dementia than Alzheimer's disease. Like Alzheimer's disease, it is more common in women. It usually begins in middle age and runs a course of 2 to 10 years, with symptomatology generally similar to that of Alzheimer's disease, though early memory loss may be less conspicuous. A few cases show a familial pattern consistent with autosomal dominant inheritance.

Morphological Features

Gross Appearances. Gyral atrophy tends to be more localized than in Alzheimer's disease (Fig. 24-10) and characteristically more severe, the affected gyri having a knife-edge configuration. However, many patients with Pick's disease die before this degree of atrophy has developed. About 55% of patients show both frontal and temporal atrophy, extending as far as the precentral gyrus and tending to spare the posterior part of the superior temporal gyrus (auditory area). Most of the remaining 45% have either frontal or temporal atrophy, but in rare cases the inferior parietal lobule is involved, alone or in association with frontal atrophy. About 65% show asymmetrical cortical atrophy, usually greater on the left. Sections show moderate shrinkage of the hemispheric white matter, with sclerosis. Involvement of the basal ganglia is common, the caudate, putamen, and pallidum being affected in decreasing order of frequency.

Microscopic Appearances. Neuronal loss, astrocytic hyperplasia, and fibrillary gliosis are largely confined to the obviously shrunken areas (Figs. 24-11, 24-12), the remainder of the cortex being almost normal. Secondary myelin loss and astrogliosis of white matter are more marked than in Alzheimer's disease, and there are neuronal loss and astrocytic reaction in the basal ganglia in many cases. Of the residual cortical neurons, many show nonspecific

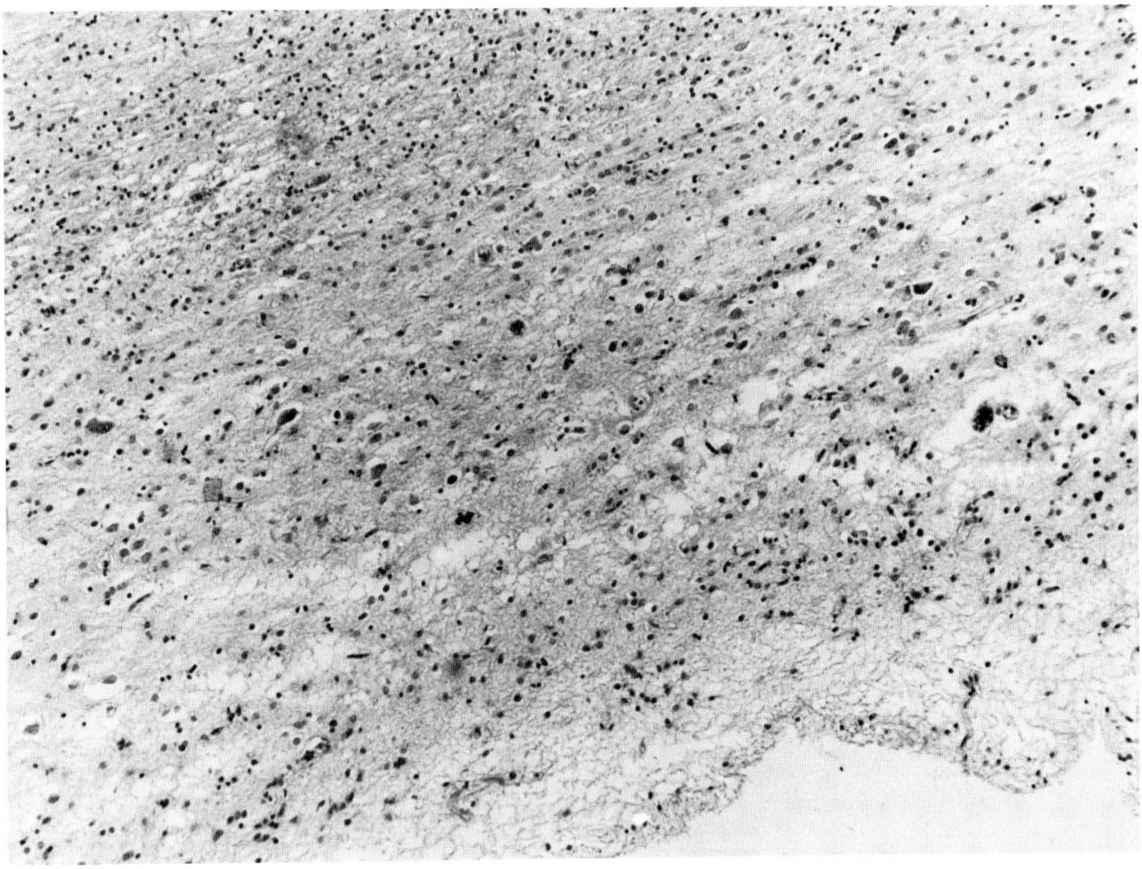

Fig. 24-11. Full thickness of cortex in Pick's disease (abnormal area), showing neuronal loss, disorganization, and thinning. (H & E, X75.)

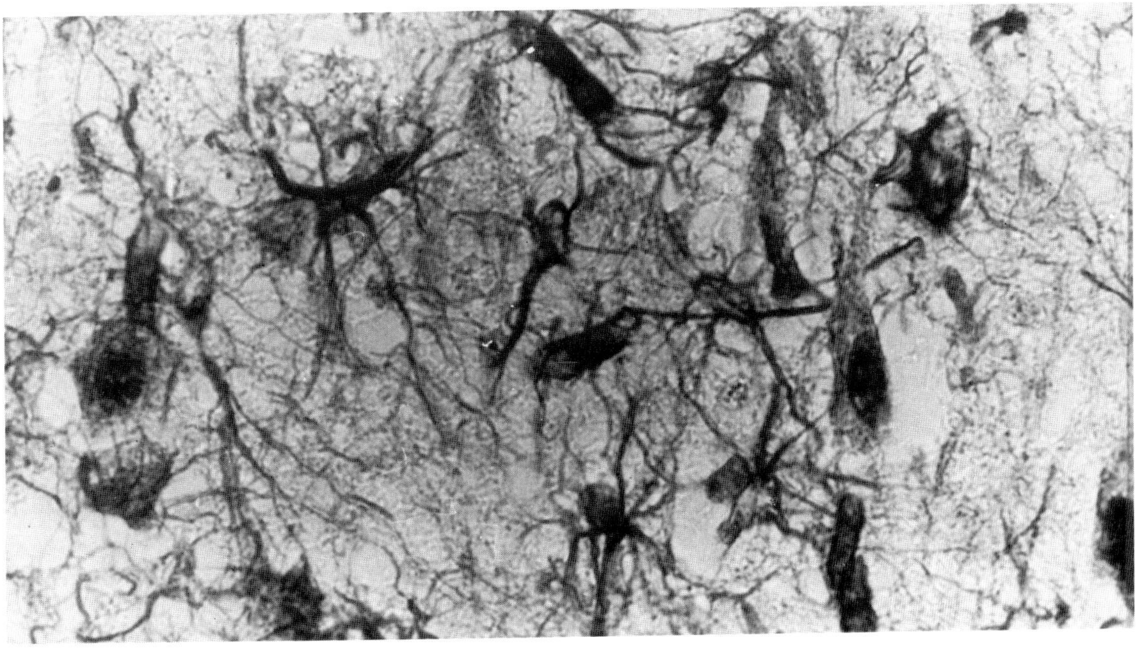

Fig. 24-12. Pick's disease, astrocytic hyperplasia and fibrillary gliosis of affected cortex. (Holzer's stain, X750.)

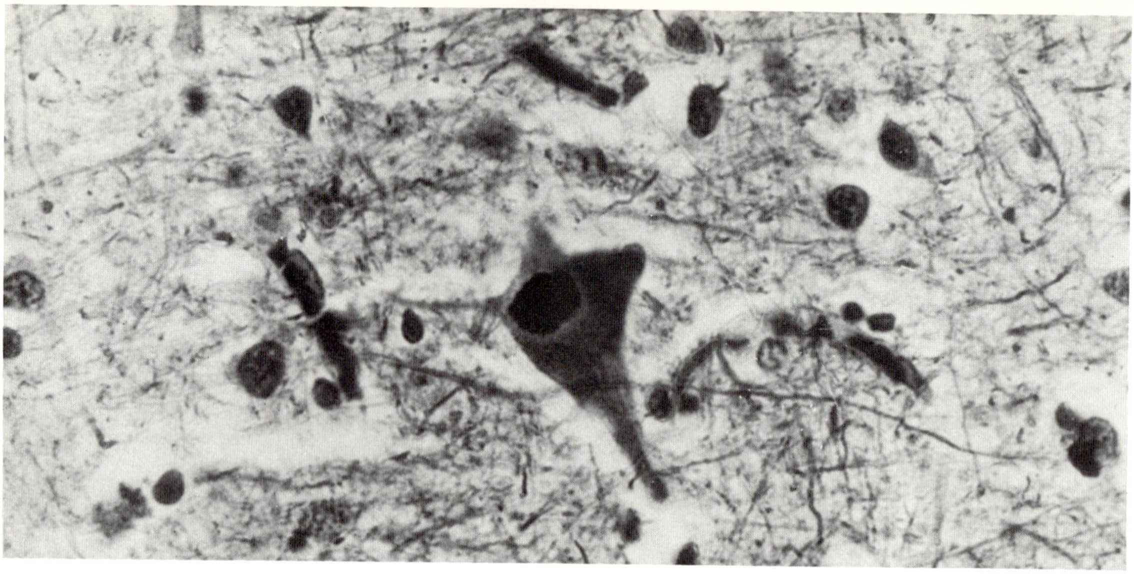

Fig. 24-13. Pick's disease. Prominent argyrophilic inclusion in cortical neuron. (Silver, ×750.)

atrophy, but a few become rounded and swollen, with displacement of the nucleus toward the apical dendrite and either diffuse cytoplasmic argyrophilia or a well-defined (Fig. 24-13), silver-positive inclusion (Pick cells). Another neuronal change, *granulovacuolar degeneration,* is seen in both Alzheimer's and Pick's disease, the affected cells showing small (5μ) vacuoles in the perikaryon or dendritic base (Fig. 24-14), each with a central 1μ granule that stains with hematoxylin or silver. The cells are swollen and degenerating, and the change is confined to the hippocampus. Neurofibrillary tangles and plaques may be seen in Pick's disease, but are confined to the atrophic cortex and absent from normal areas.

EXTRAPYRAMIDAL DISORDERS

The extrapyramidal motor system originates in a wide area of the cortex and in subcortical gray masses (the basal ganglia) and exerts its influence on motoneurons through the reticular formation (see Chap. 7). Extensive investigation has clarified neither the overall function of the system nor the individual functions of its component nuclei, but frequent involvement in disease processes makes the latter of considerable clinical importance.

Unlike other groups of degenerative diseases, a little is known about the biochemical effects of some extrapyramidal disorders. At least one, paralysis agitans, can be partially improved by medication. Paralysis agitans may also be ameliorated by destructive lesions deep within the hemispheres, but in so many varying locations that the results have to some extent confused rather than clarified normal function.

Overlap between this and other groups of degenerative diseases includes the frequent occurrence of dementia in Huntington's chorea (and probably intellectual deterioration in paralysis agitans), frequent involvement of the basal ganglia in Pick's disease, and the occasional association of paralysis agitans with degeneration involving the autonomic or cerebellospinal systems.

Paralysis Agitans (Parkinsonism)

Paralysis agitans, or parkinsonism, is a syndrome of diverse etiology, the patients usually having rigidity, tremor, and poverty of movement (akinesia). A description of these characteristics follows.

1. *Rigidity* is increased muscle tonus that affects even opposing muscle groups (abolition of reciprocal inhibition) (Chap. 7), with constant uniform resistance to passive movements. Thus, it differs from spasticity that is due to exaggeration of postural stretch reflexes, and can be overcome by extreme passive movement, which invokes the clasp-knife reflex (lengthening reaction). Rigidity could be due to hyperactivity of alpha motoneurons, gamma motoneurons, or interneurons. There is some indirect experimental evidence that it is due to hyperactivity of interneurons. Lack of reciprocal inhibition is compatible with such a hypothesis.

2. *Tremor* is of two types. *Resting tremor,* 3 to 6 cycles per second (cps), is not (under experimental conditions) associated with lesions of the basal ganglia (including the substantia nigra), but is only seen when cerebellar efferent fibers are interrupted. It appears to originate in the lateral ventrolateral thalamic nucleus and be transmitted via the cortex. *Action tremor,* at 6 to 12 cps, is an exaggeration of physiological tremor, the origin of which is unknown.

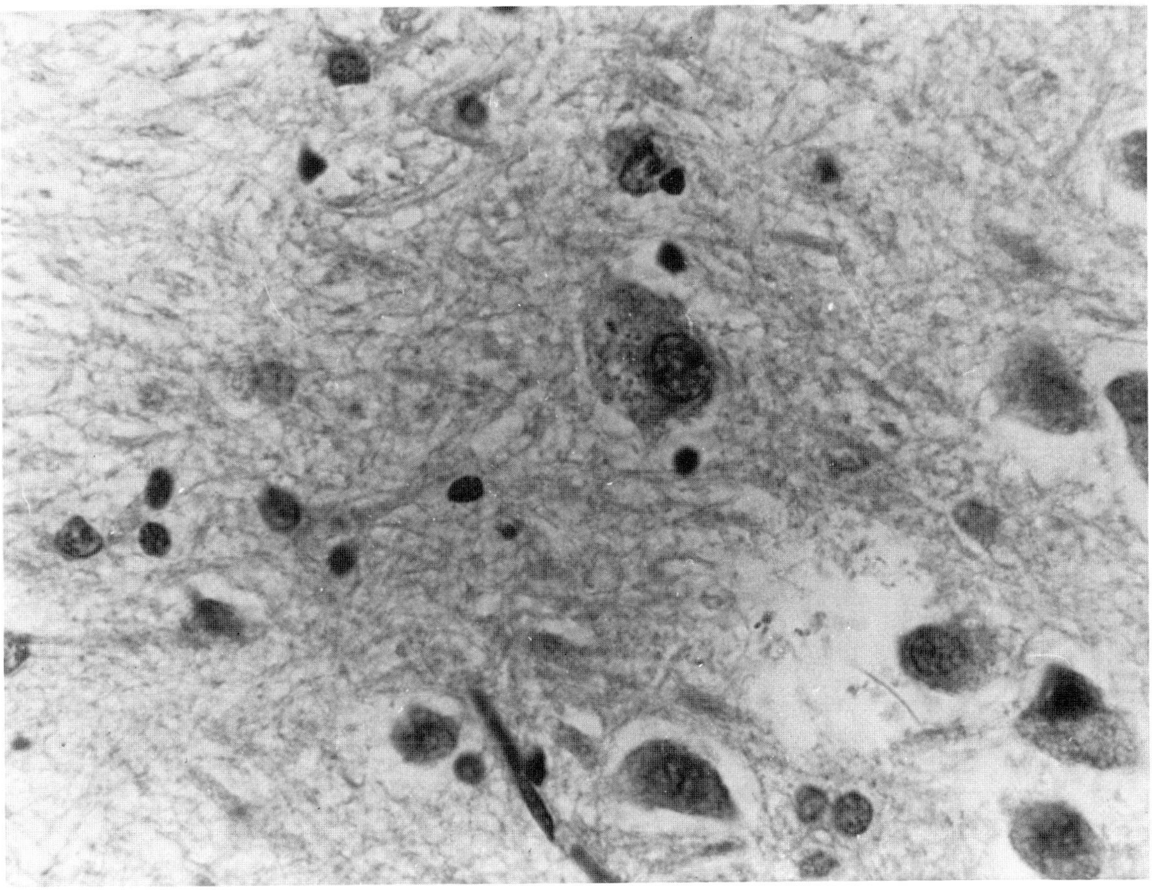

Fig. 24-14. Pick's disease. The neuron near the center shows cytoplasmic vacuoles each with a small central dot (granulovacuolar degeneration, also seen in Alzheimer's disease). (Silver, ×750.)

The superposition of rigidity and tremor produces the characteristic "cogwheel" sensation felt when passively moving the limbs of a parkinsonian patient.

3. *Akinesia* is independent of rigidity and may progress clinically in its absence. Little is known of its origin except that lesions of the substantia nigra in monkeys may reduce voluntary movement. Levodopa medication, which usually raises brain dopamine, is the only treatment that effectively reduces akinesia. It seems reasonable to speculate that akinesia may be a direct effect of reduced substantia nigra activity, and therefore is not responsive to surgical destructive lesions; rigidity and tremor, however, represent release phenomena that might respond to surgical lesions in their nuclei of origin or efferent tracts.

Classification

The only type of paralysis agitans that, strictly speaking, belongs in this chapter is the *idiopathic* variety. However, there are many forms of *secondary* or symptomatic paralysis agitans, including the following:

1. Postencephalitic (especially following encephalitis lethargica, although few of these patients have survived to the present day)
2. Atherosclerotic
3. Post-traumatic
4. Drug-induced, including such agents as reserpine, phenothiazines, haloperidol, and methyldopa
5. Rare and miscellaneous associations, including carbon monoxide poisoning, manganese poisoning, intracranial tumors, and anoxia

Paralysis agitans may be associated with olivopontocerebellar atrophy, with the Parkinson-dementia complex seen in Guam, or with orthostatic hypotension and other evidences of autonomic disorder. In some of the latter cases, autonomic dysfunction may be the presenting feature, and in many apparently classic cases of paralysis agitans, there may be such autonomic changes as segmental esophageal spasm, gastroesophageal reflux, large bowel atony and megacolon, or bladder dysfunction.

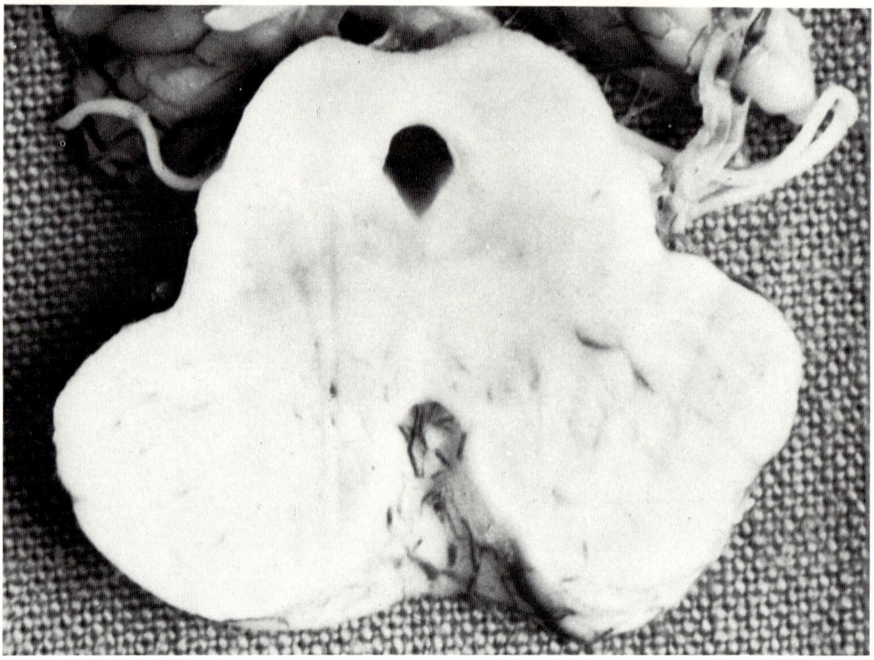

Fig. 24-15. Paralysis agitans (idiopathic). Section of midbrain, showing disappearance of the grossly pigmented bands of substantia nigra.

Morphological Features of Idiopathic Paralysis Agitans

The morphological substrate of idiopathic paralysis agitans is reasonably uniform, although changes in the secondary forms are extremely variable.

In the idiopathic disease (Fig. 24-15), there is neuronal loss and fibrillary gliosis, largely confined to the substantia nigra, involving the caudal more than the rostral areas. This causes depigmentation of the substantia nigra, usually the only gross change. Many neurons disappear, leaving clumps of melanin free in the neuropil, but in some, intracytoplasmic inclusions *(Lewy bodies)* are present. These are round, hyaline eosinophilic bodies, often concentrically marked (Fig. 24-16); one or more may be present in a neuron. Occasionally, they appear free in the neuropil, presumably following neuronal loss. Similar bodies, usually with less neuronal loss, are seen in other pigmented brain nuclei, including the locus ceruleus and some neurons of the dorsal vagal nucleus.

Much less constantly, lesions involving the striatum and pallidum have been reported, including loss of myelinated striopallidal bundles, reduction in fibers of the ansa lenticularis, and mild neuronal loss and gliosis in both divisions of the pallidum. The explanation of such changes is not clear, since cell loss has not been reported in the caudate and putamen. Reduction in pallidal neurons has been regarded as trans-synaptic degeneration secondary to loss of nigropallidal fibers, but such fibers represent only a part of the input to pallidal neurons. Nigrostrial fibers are presumably of at least equal importance, but there is no significant striatal cell loss.

Morphological Features of Secondary (Symptomatic) Paralysis Agitans

Postencephatic Paralysis Agitans. In postencephalitic (secondary) paralysis agitans, multiple gliomesenchymal scars are seen throughout the CNS, especially in the substantia nigra. Nigral cell loss may be even more severe than in the idiopathic form, but neurons that are still present accumulate neurofibrillary tangles, especially in patients under the age of 60. Originally described following an epidemic of encephalitis lethargica, postencephalitic parkinsonism also occurs after Japanese B encephalitis.

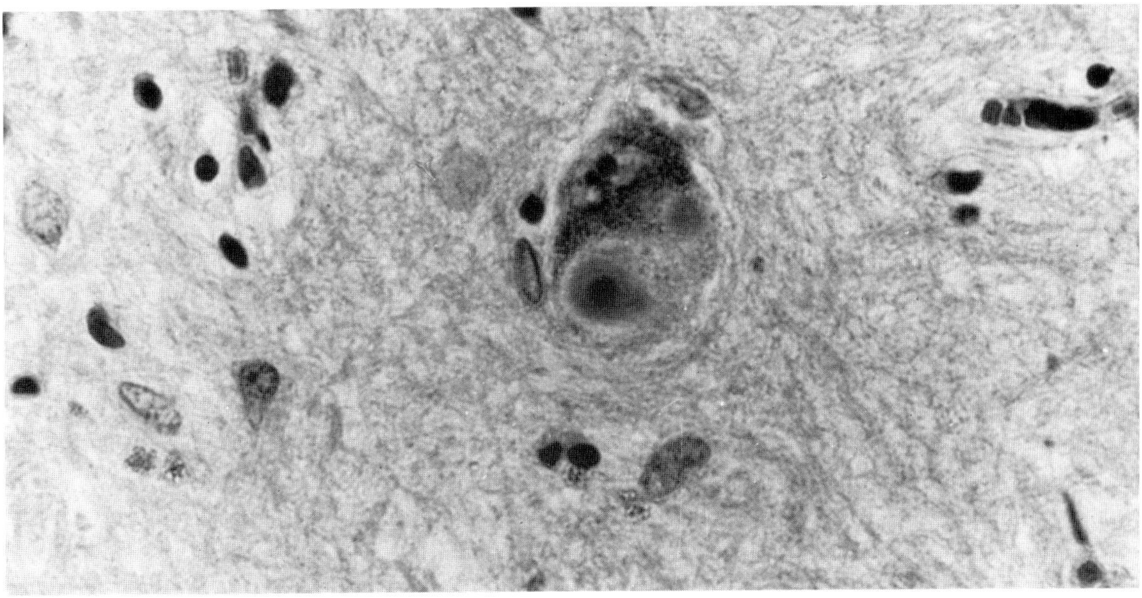

Fig. 24-16. Paralysis agitans (idiopathic). The neuron in the substantia nigra shows two Lewy bodies, one with a denser center, and a reduction of melanin. Astrocytic nuclei show reactive changes. (H & E, X750.)

Parkinson-Dementia Complex. In the peculiar Guam form of the disease, associated with dementia and amyotrophic lateral sclerosis, brain changes are widespread, as might be assumed from the clinical picture, with neurofibrillary tangles in almost all areas, but no plaques or Lewy bodies.

Toxic and Atherosclerotic Paralysis Agitans. Paralysis agitans associated with carbon monoxide or manganese poisoning or with senile vascular changes shows widely variable pathological changes, involving the striatum, pallidum, and substantia nigra in varying degrees.

Relationship of Pathological Changes to Symptomatology

Because of the wide variability of the morphological changes in these many forms of parkinsonism or parkinsonism-like syndromes, there is no consensus as to where the primary lesion might be. Thus, even though patients with the idiopathic disease respond to replacement therapy for the dopamine that is lost with nigral cells, it could still be argued that nigral degeneration itself was secondary to some other lesion. However, it seems reasonable to make the following generalizations: *first,* that idiopathic paralysis agitans can be regarded as a primary degeneration of the pigmented nuclei, especially the substantia nigra, directly resulting in reduction of voluntary movement and loss of dopaminergic inhibition of the caudate, putamen, and pallidum. Rigidity and tremor arise somewhere within the circuitry of the basal ganglia, thalamus, and cortex because of this loss of inhibition. *Second,* other forms of paralysis agitans that are secondary to vascular lesions, toxins, or generalized brain disease are not in all cases clinically identical (not all of the three cardinal features may be present). They show a wide variety of deep hemispheric lesions that do not necessarily involve the substantia nigra. The whole group is in need of much more intensive clinical and pathological correlation.

Pathogenesis of Idiopathic Paralysis Agitans

Restricting further discussion to idiopathic paralysis agitans, it will be assumed (in the absence of morphological evidence to the contrary) that the primary change (Fig. 24-17) is neuronal loss of the pigmented nuclei, the most massive loss being in the substantia nigra, although changes in other structures, such as the dorsal vagal nucleus, may be associated with autonomic dysfunction.

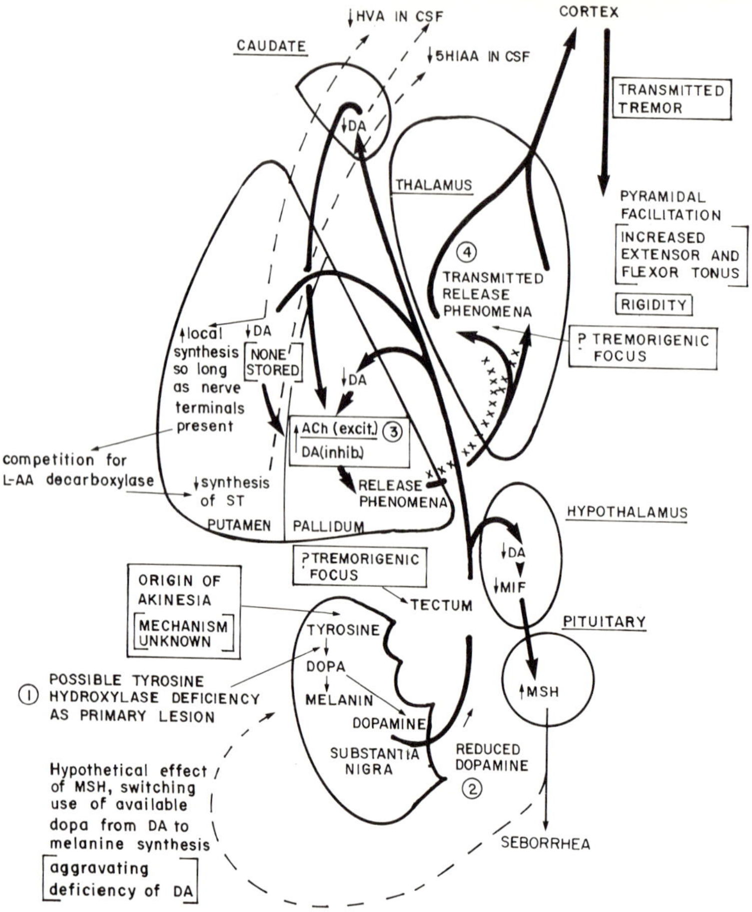

Fig. 24-17. The sequence (1-4) of biochemical abnormalities in idiopathic paralysis agitans. The reduction of dopamine (DA) formation in the substantia nigra upsets the excitatory-inhibitory balance of acetylcholine (ACh) and DA in the striatum in favor of the ACh (excitatory). Release phenomena are probably conveyed via the pyramidal fibers. XXXXXX = areas of surgical attack (no relief of akinesia). MIF = melanocyte stimulating hormone inhibiting factor; MSH = melanocyte stimulating hormone; for other abbreviations, see text.

Reduction of Striatal Dopamine Due to Loss of Nigrostrial Fibers. Major efferent fibers from the substantia nigra run to the pallidum, caudate, and putamen of the same side. They pass through the ventromedial tegmentum, lateral hypothalamus (presumably in the median forebrain bundle), and anterior limb of the internal capsule, to reach the target nuclei. These neurons are dopaminergic, and loss of substantia nigra cells severely reduces the dopamine content of the caudate nucleus and putamen, though not affecting the pallidum as severely. Dopamine (DA) loss is more severe in the putamen than in the caudate; perhaps the former is more closely connected to the caudal two-thirds of the substantia nigra, which bears the brunt of the primary disease.

Changes in Striatal Dopamine Metabolism. As a corollary of reduction of dopamine in the caudate and putamen, there is reduced homovanillic acid (HVA) in the CSF. This reduction is less than expected (i.e., the HVA-DA ratio is increased), suggesting partial biochemical compensation, at least in the early stages, with dopaminergic terminals still present in the striatum synthesizing and releasing more DA (which is converted to HVA), but storing very little. Patients with high CSF levels of HVA show relatively low levels of 5-hydroxyindoleacetic acid (5-HIAA), suggesting reduced serotonin (ST) metabolism, perhaps because of competition for L-amino acid (L-AA) decarboxylase. Striatal levels of serotonin are reduced, although less than those of dopamine.

Effects of Levodopa Administration. Attempts to ameliorate the symptoms of paralysis agitans by administration of DA are unsuccessful since it does not cross the blood-brain barrier, but administration of levodopa has proved effective, particularly in patients with severe akinesia in whom surgery is ineffective. Levodopa readily enters the CNS and is decarboxylated to DA in the striatum. The rate-limiting tyrosine hydroxylase is bypassed using this drug, but to be effective it must virtually saturate L-amino acid decarboxylase throughout the tissues.

Patients with very advanced disease show no response to levodopa, presumably because degeneration of presynaptic terminals is so severe that insufficient striatal decarboxylase is available, and little or no DA is formed. The drug is also relatively ineffective in early cases where CSF HVA is high, possibly because available decarboxylase is already being fully utilized.

Effects of Anticholinergic and Other Drugs. Before the advent of levodopa, anticholinergic drugs were used and perhaps helped to create a balance. The dopaminergic inhibitory terminals in the caudate nucleus and putamen were reduced by the disease and the cholinergic excitatory fibers were depressed by the drug. The therapeutic effect of amantadine, an RNA inhibitor intended as an antiviral agent, is unexplained.

Effects of Surgical Treatment. Surgical treatment is ineffective against akinesia, since the only possible beneficial result of tissue destruction is the abolition of release phenomena, thought to include both tremor and rigidity. Surgical lesions abolish tremor in about 99% of cases and rigidity in about 90%, but, unfortunately, recurrences are not uncommon. For detailed consideration of the areas of surgical attack, the reader is referred to appropriate textbooks, However, attention has generally been focused on feedback pathways leading to the cerebral cortex, including the medial pallidum, ansa lenticularis, and ventrolateral thalamic (cerebellar and pallidal relay) nucleus; lesions in the latter also interrupt cerebello-cortical pathways, but it is not known whether or not this is of any significance.

Postulated Primary Role for Deficient Tyrosine Hydroxylase Activity. A recent hypothesis suggests that the primary defect in the substantia nigra is a failure of tyrosine hydroxylase activity, so that tyrosine cannot be converted to dopa. Early compensatory events include depletion of nigral neuromelanin (which contains DA as well as dopa), leading to the observed changes in the substantia nigra. Lack of DA affects hypothalamic as well as striatal functions, melanocyte stimulating-hormone inhibiting factor (MIF) secretion being reduced and melanocyte-stimulating hormone (MSH) formation raised (confirmed by raised plasma levels in paralysis agitans, and increased incidence of seborrhea in this disease).

Since MSH exacerbates paralysis agitans (and MIF is said to reduce drug-induced tremors in animals), a condition of positive feedback is attained, the initial biochemical defect causing paralysis agitans and increased MSH and the MSH exacerbating the symptoms. At present, this must be regarded as unproved.

Huntington's Chorea

Huntington's chorea is another of the more common extrapyramidal degenerative diseases, usually beginning during the fourth or fifth decade of life, with the duration varying from 5 to 30 years and the sex incidence equal. In many cases there appears to be autosomal dominant inheritance. The condition is characterized by involuntary choreiform movements and mental deterioration (dementia). In most cases chorea presents first, but occasionally mental changes may precede it. It is one of the purest examples of a degenerative or abiotrophic process, since neither plaques, neurofibrillary tangles, Lewy bodies, nor other specific histological changes are seen, but only the general features described in the introductory section.

Morphological Features

Gross Appearances. Major atrophy involves the caudate and putamen (Fig. 24-18), being least in the inferior part of the caudate head and most severe in the posterior two-thirds of the putamen. The normal projection of the basal ganglia into the anterior horns of the lateral ventricles is flattened, or the ventricular surface may even become concave, a change readily visible on a pneumoencephalogram. Grossly visible atrophy of the cortex, mainly involving the frontal lobe but sometimes extending to the region of the sylvian fissure, may be noted.

Microscopic Appearances. The caudate and putamen (Fig. 24-19) show severe neuronal loss, particularly involving the small cells, and the large ones may show sclerosis and increased lipofuscin. Astroglial hypertrophy and hyperplasia, with moderate fibrillary gliosis, are more marked than in many other diseases of this group, so that the number of nuclei is often increased in spite of the severe neuronal loss. A similar uncomplicated cell loss with minimal astroglial change is seen in involved cortex, particularly in the deeper layers, and there may be associated partial demyelination and gliosis of frontal white matter. Neuronal loss and gliosis in the pallidum and subthalamic nucleus, though infrequent, may occasionally be severe. Since the frontotemporal cortex and basal ganglia may also be involved in Pick's disease, clinical confusion occasionally occurs, although the histological changes are different.

Dopamine Metabolism

The levels of DA and HVA are normal or minimally reduced in Huntington's chorea, and considering the marked striatal neuronal loss, this presumably indicates an unduly high amount of dopamine per striatal neuron. It is therefore of interest that administration of levodopa aggravates Huntington's chorea, and that drugs such as reserpine and the phenothiazines, which precipitate symptoms of paralysis agitans, may ameliorate Huntington's chorea, presumably by reducing the amount of dopamine in the striate body. It might be speculated that there is overinhibition of the striate body in this disease, in contrast to deinhibition in paralysis agitans, but it is unclear how this produces choreiform movements.

Dystonia Musculorum Deformans (Torsion Dystonia)

Torsion dystonia is a rare condition, usually involving children and characterized by writhing movements and prolonged periods of distorted posture like

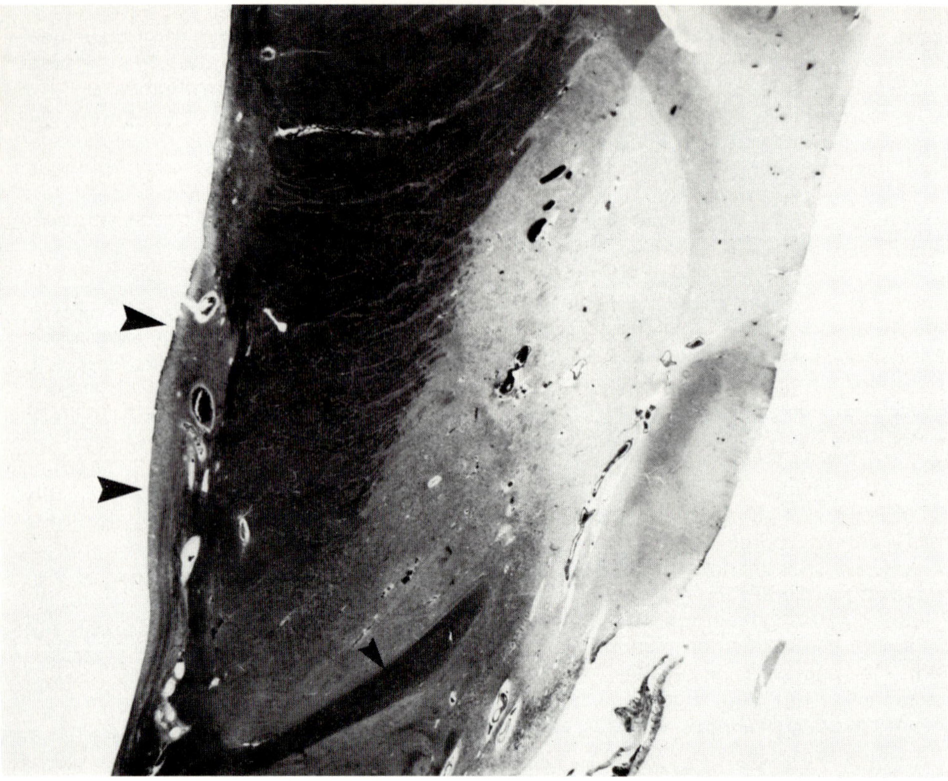

Fig. 24-18. Huntington's chorea. Transverse section at the level of anterior commissure (small arrow), showing atrophy of caudate (large arrows) and flattening of the putamen. (Myelin, X5.)

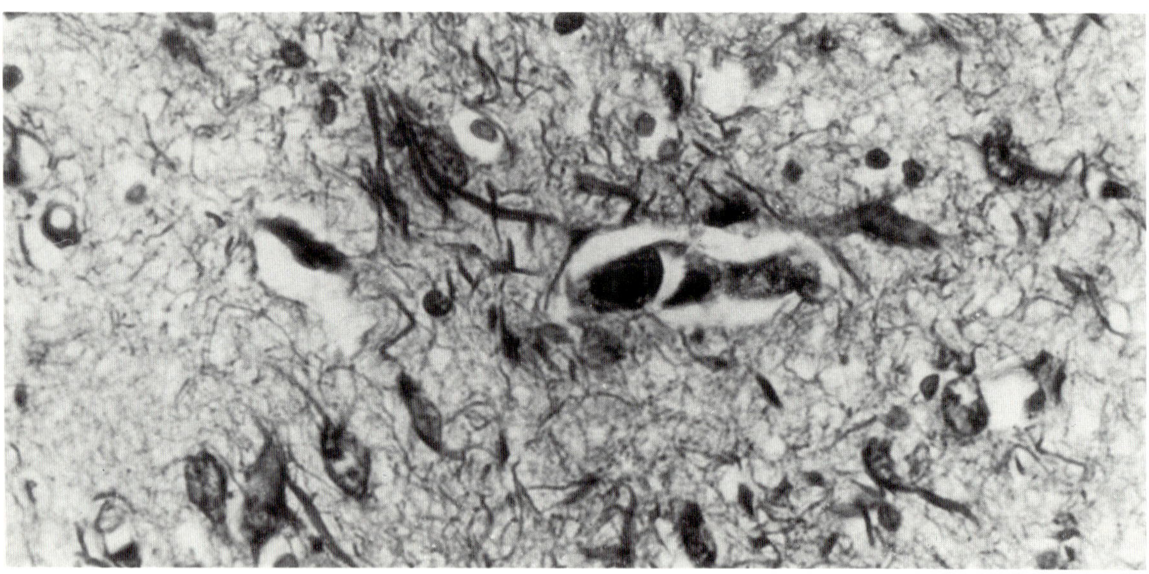

Fig. 24-19. Huntington's chorea. Section showing one sclerotic neuron, several astrocytes with plump reactive nuclei, and mild fibrillary gliosis. (Holzer's stain, X750.)

paralysis agitans, it may occur as a primary or as a secondary phenomenon; in the latter case, it is associated with tumor or infarcts of the basal ganglia, encephalitis, hepatolenticular degeneration, Hallervorden-Spatz syndrome, or other conditions. Patients with the primary disorder may exhibit autosomal dominant or autosomal recessive inheritance; most of the latter are Jewish. There are some clinical differences between the two forms. Plasma levels of dopamine β-hydroxylase are higher in the autosomal dominant group than in the autosomal recessive group or in control subjects, and there are other reports of altered catecholamine metabolism (e.g., symptomatic improvement with levodopa, reduced HVA in CSF). The significance of these observations remains to be worked out.

Very few cases of the primary disease have had adequate pathological study. However, it appears that the disease is largely confined to the basal ganglia and is a simple degeneration, with loss of both large and small neurons from the caudate nucleus, putamen, and pallidum (in varying portions), astrocytic hyperplasia, hypertrophy and fibrillary gliosis, demyelination of striopallidal fibers and efferent fibers from the pallidum, and inconstant changes in other areas.

Hallervorden-Spatz Syndrome and Neuroaxonal Dystrophy

Hallervorden-Spatz syndrome is a rare affliction, usually starting during the second or third decade and resulting in death before the age of 30. A few cases are familial, but the mode of inheritance is not clear. It is characterized by progressive rigidity that involves the legs more than the arms and is often accompanied by abnormal movements, including chorea, athetosis, or torsion dystonia. If the face, tongue, and palate are involved, the patients have dysarthria and dysphagia. Dementia is common, but seizures are unusual.

Morphological Features of Typical Hallervorden-Spatz Syndrome

Gross Appearances. The brain is usually of normal size, and the characteristic feature is rusty-brown discoloration of the pallidum and substantia nigra, not associated with gross atrophy.

Microscopic Appearances. Microscopically, a brownish, granular or globular pigment is seen, especially in the cytoplasm and processes of astrocytes, deposits of iron are present in granular or diffuse form in the neuropil, and small mineralized concretions may be found. The pallidum and substantia nigra show slight to moderate neuronal loss. The cells that remain are often pale and swollen. Fragmentation and loss of myelin are most marked in the pallidum, and globular axonal swellings (spheroids), which may contain lipofuscin, are present. The swelling of neurons and axons may actually enlarge the pallidum and substantia nigra, a condition of pseudohypertrophy. Mild astroglial reaction with minimal fibrillary gliosis is seen. In a few cases, spheroids are seen in the gracilis and cuneate nuclei.

Infantile and Congenital Variants

Occasional patients present during the first or second year of life in whom *gross* pigmentation of the pallidum and substantia nigra is slight or absent. Nonetheless, microscopic changes in these two areas are just as described above. In addition, there is widespread spheroid formation, which is associated with partial demyelination and pseudohypertrophy and may affect the cortex, thalamus, subthalamic and red nuclei, cerebellar white matter, tegmentum of the brain stem, and dorsal horns in the cord. The mode of spheroid formation is unclear, but it seems to be accompanied by axonal fragmentation and homogenization of neuronal cell bodies.

More recently, a condition known as *infantile neuroaxonal dystrophy* has been reported, the patients showing CNS dysfunction at birth, with psychomotor retardation and death within a few years. Grossly, the brains are normal, and no pigmentation is seen; however, spheroid formation is widespread and severe. There may be increased neutral fat, especially in the pallidum, perhaps associated with dysmyelination or myelinoclasis.

Classification

Originally described as separate diseases, there seems little reason to doubt that Hallervorden-Spatz syndrome and infantile neuroaxonal dystrophy form a single nosological entity, the extent, and to some degree the type, of histological change varying with age of onset. The childhood onset cases of Hallervorden-Spatz syndrome form an intermediate type. The etiology and pathogenesis are completely unknown.

Spheroids are not specific for this disease, since they may be seen in the gracilis and cuneate nuclei of aging brains and also (usually confined to the same areas) in the brains of infants with malnutrition due to cystic fibrosis of the pancreas or congenital biliary atresia. Experimentally, they may be associated with vitamin E deficiency, but up to now this has shed no light on the human disease.

Hepatolenticular Degeneration (Wilson's Disease)

Hepatolenticular degeneration is a chronic disease that usually starts during the second decade, though occasionally in the first, third, or fourth decade. Its duration is about 3 to 10 years. The main pathological changes are in the basal ganglia and the liver, although liver disease occasionally remains subclinical for the entire course. The onset of CNS symptomatology may follow febrile jaundice. Patients with advanced disease may have ascites, a large, firm spleen, and ankle edema, and there is usually secondary renal aminoaciduria. Pigmented rings around the cornea (Kayser-Fleischer rings) are often seen. The CNS features include progressive rigidity and coarse tremor of the limbs, spasticity of the face, mouth, and pharynx, leading to dysarthria and dysphagia, and often late-onset dementia.

Morphological Features

Gross Appearances. Externally, the brain often appears normal, but sections show a "sinking-in" of the insular cortex, associated with marked shrinkage of the striate body, particularly its middle third. The caudate and putamen have a brown or brick-red color, depending on the duration of fixation, and there is often cavitation or cystic gliosis of the putamen, which may extend into the caudate (and very rarely to the thalamus or red nucleus).

Microscopic Appearances. There is reduction of large and small neurons in the caudate nucleus and putamen, with secondary loss of striopallidal fibers. Infrequently, neuronal loss is seen in the subthalamic or in the dentate nucleus, where it may be associated with secondary demyelination of the superior cerebellar peduncle. Although there is marked hyperplasia of astrocytes, as in other degenerative diseases, these cells also reflect the coexistent liver disease and appear as typical Alzheimer type II cells (see Chap. 11). Multinucleated hyperchromatic (Alzheimer type I) cells are rare and occasionally absent. The type II cells are widely distributed throughout the CNS, particularly in areas where protoplasmic astrocytes normally predominate. A peculiar cell type, which appears specific for Wilson's disease, is the Opalski cell, present in the pallidum rather than in the caudate nucleus or putamen. It is a large, oval or round cell with a central nucleus and granular or finely foamy cytoplasm, presumably derived from the microglia. Its significance is unclear.

The pigmentation around the cornea is due to a row of brownish granules in Descemet's membrane that stain positively for copper, but not for iron or melanin. The liver shows multilobular cirrhosis, with brownish granules in the parenchymal cells.

Changes in Copper-Binding Plasma Proteins

The disease appears to be associated with, but not necessarily due to, reduction or absence of a specific alpha globulin (ceruloplasmin), normally responsible for binding copper; some copper therefore remains loosely attached to plasma albumin. Other copper-binding globulins appear to be present in normal amounts, and about 40% of the serum copper remains loosely albumin-bound, compared with a normal 5%.

This albumin-bound fraction is readily taken up by proteins in the brain and liver or excreted in the urine and is presumed to be toxic to tissues. An occasional patient with hepatolenticular degeneration has shown normal levels of ceruloplasmin, and the siblings of patients may lack ceruloplasmin but have no signs of disease. Deficiency of the globulin may be on a genetic basis, but is probably only one factor involved in the development of hepatolenticular degeneration.

SPINOCEREBELLAR DEGENERATIONS

The spinocerebellar degenerative disorders are further examples of "pure" degeneration. Unlike the preceding groups, the primary effect often seems to be axonal, leading to centripetal degeneration toward the perikaryon ("dying-back"). Primary degeneration of the cell body may also occur. Following axonal loss, demyelination of tractal distribution results, and it has been argued that these diseases might be *primarily* demyelinative, with axonal degeneration as a *secondary* result. There is no conclusive and little suggestive evidence for this, and the frequent association of both long tract and nuclear involvement and some overlap with degenerative processes in other disease groups (e.g., motoneuron, autonomic) make primary neuroaxonal disease a more logical possibility. However, the question has not been finally resolved.

The etiology is of course unknown, but in many cases there is a strong familial association, with evidence of autosomal recessive, sex-linked recessive, or autosomal dominant inheritance; there are also sporadic cases. However, there is little correlation of the type of inheritance with the age of onset or clinical presentation, except for the expected tendency of the recessive cases to present at an earlier age (14.7 years in Friedreich's ataxia, compared with about 36 years for cases of dominant inheritance).

The spinocerebellar degenerations may occur in exclusively spinal, exclusively cerebellar, or mixed forms, but are always associated with movement disorders, including ataxia and sometimes spasticity. They do not fall into mutually exclusive "sets," and intermediate forms abound, as well as linkages with degeneration elsewhere in the CNS (e.g., dementia, basal ganglion disease, amyotrophic lateral sclerosis, optic atrophy, deafness) or even in other systems (e.g., myocardial degeneration, cataract, telangiectasia). However, clusters of patients with a more or less uniform distribution of lesions are recognized and will be described, though dissociation between symptomatology and discoverable lesions at autopsy is often marked. Classification therefore tends to be on the basis of autopsy examination, and it must be assumed that physiological dysfunction resulting in clinical deficiencies can appreciably precede the development of morphological changes discoverable at autopsy. In a few cases, external factors, such as infection, alcoholism, or trauma, may precipitate clinical awareness of the disease, but it seems improbable that they are etiological factors.

The tempo of these diseases is so slow that abbau products are not seen, but they are nonetheless progressive and do not remit. Cases of cerebellar involvement tend to be of later onset than cases of spinal involvement and are less often associated with abnormalities outside the CNS. On the other hand, they are more often associated with extrapyramidal disorders, spasticity, optic atrophy, and other CNS changes.

Friedreich's Ataxia

Friedreich's ataxia usually presents in children, or at least in patients below the age of 20, and is strongly familial. It is associated with pes cavus, ataxia, clumsiness, dysarthria, nystagmus, loss of deep tendon reflexes, and absent vibration sense. Some

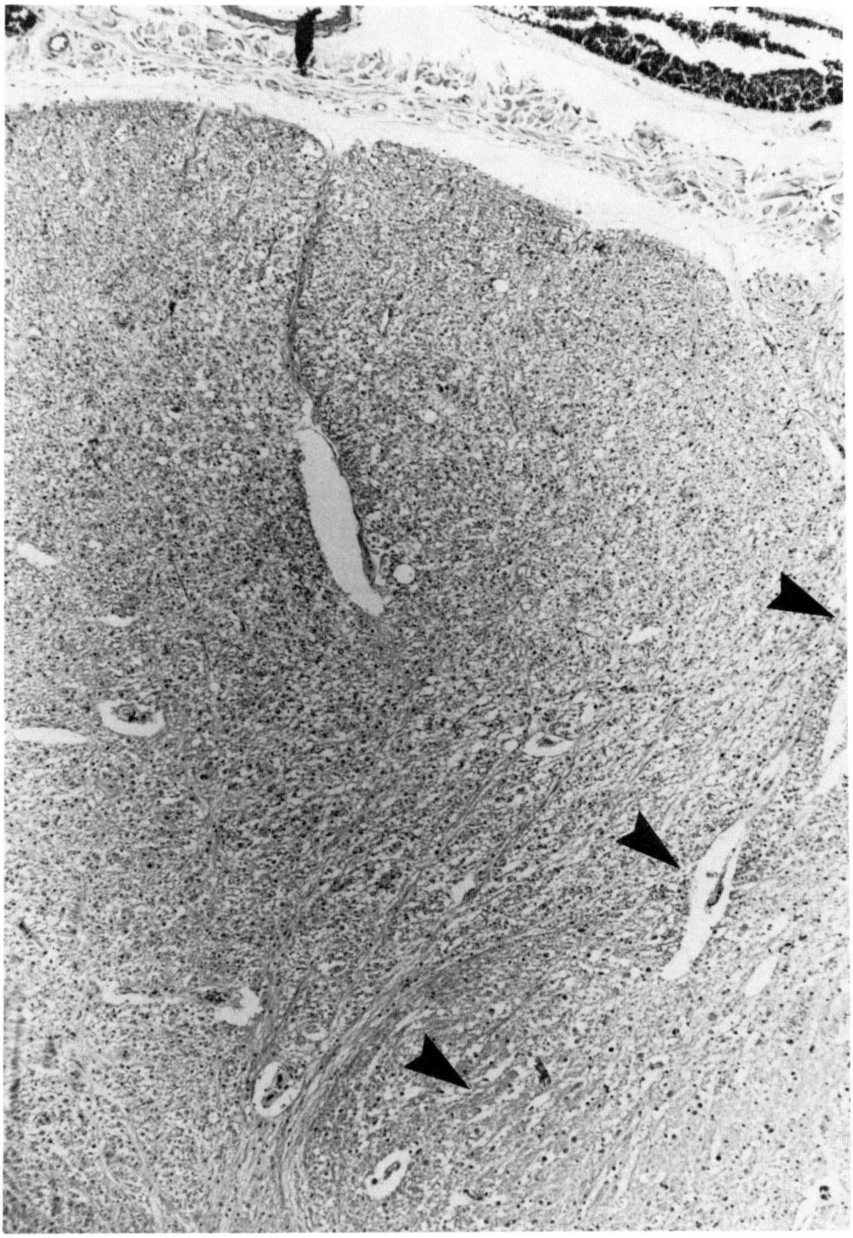

Fig. 24-20. Friedreich's ataxia. The posterior columns (left and top), normally the darkest part of the cord with myelin stains, are considerably demyelinated and little darker than the adjacent dorsal horn (arrows, lower right corner). (Myelin, ×75.)

patients show muscle-wasting (including peroneal muscular atrophy), dementia, myocarditis, and cardiorespiratory failure. Of the patients with a familial history, about 40% appear to have autosomal dominant inheritance and 60% recessive inheritance.

As noted, recessive inheritance is associated with earlier onset and occasionally a shorter course. The disease is said to present earlier in successive generations *(anticipation)* and may disappear from a pedigree in about three generations.

Morphological Features

Gross Appearances. Grossly, changes are confined to the cord and nerve roots, both of which appear shrunken and firm.

Microscopic Appearances. There is gradual loss of neurons, particularly the larger ones, from the dorsal root ganglia, resulting in the disappearance of large myelinated fibers from the posterior roots and posterior columns (Fig. 24-20). The thoracic nucleus of

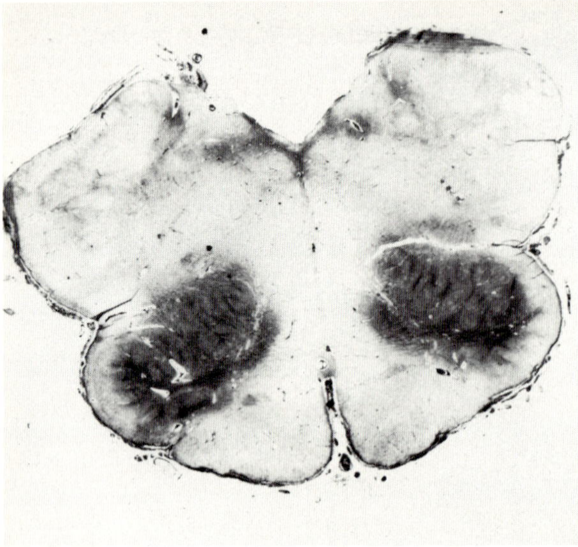

Fig. 24-21. Olivopontocerebellar atrophy. Shrinkage and gliosis of inferior olives. (Holzer's stain, ×6.)

Clarke is usually severely affected, and there is loss of fibers from both spinocerebellar tracts. Partial fiber loss from the lateral corticospinal tracts is also noted, and there may be a corresponding neuronal deficit in motor and premotor cortex.

To this characteristic picture of Friedreich's ataxia may be added inconstant areas of demyelination or neuronal loss in many parts of the CNS. Optic atrophy and retrobulbar neuritis may be associated with visual impairment; sclerosis of the ventral cochlear nuclei and superior olives may be associated with progressive deafness. There may be minor Purkinje's cell loss and dentate atrophy, with shrinkage of the superior cerebellar peduncle; very occasionally, other parts of the brain stem, substantia nigra, pallidum, or ventrolateral column of the thalamus may be involved. Although demyelination of peripheral nerves has rarely been reported, it must be assumed that loss of dorsal root ganglion cells leads to loss of their peripheral processes. Sometimes, an interstitial proliferation of Schwann's cells may occur, resembling hypertrophic interstitial neuropathy.

Occasional non-neural lesions include interstitial myocarditis, with atrophy or hypertrophy of fibers. Skeletal muscle may show variable denervation atrophy if anterior horn cells are affected, the histological picture often showing neuropathic and apparent myopathic features. This resembles *peroneal muscular atrophy* (Charcot-Marie-Tooth disease), which is also heredofamilial and often occurs in kinships that include typical Friedreich's ataxia. It may be part of the spectrum of Friedreich's ataxia rather than a distinct entity.

Clinical Variants

There are other variants of Friedreich's ataxia. In *Biemond's disease* the main feature is loss of dorsal column sensation (vibration and position sense), with ataxia resembling tabes dorsalis. In *hereditary spastic ataxia,* pes cavus is absent and ataxia severe. The patients also have increased deep tendon reflexes and extensor plantar responses. In *hereditary spastic paraplegia* there is neither pes cavus nor ataxia, the patients showing weakness, increased tendon reflexes, and extensor plantar responses. There may be associated dysarthria, wasting of distal musculature, and optic atrophy.

The findings of the few autopsies that have been carried out in such cases suggest that the pathological changes are indistinguishable from those of Friedreich's ataxia. Presumably, the variation in symptomatology depends on the relative dysfunction in different long tracts and, as previously noted, this dysfunction may be poorly correlated with morphological changes.

Olivopontocerebellar Atrophy

Olivopontocerebellar atrophy may be familial or sporadic. The average age of onset is at 35 to 40 years, although affected children have been recorded. Patients show generalized ataxia and often have associated symptoms, depending on the extension of degeneration in the CNS.

Morphological Features

Gross Appearances. Grossly, severe, usually symmetrical shrinkage of inferior olives and basal pons is seen, associated with moderate diffuse atrophy of the cerebellum and sclerosis of all involved areas (Figs. 24-21, 24-22, 24-23).

Microscopic Appearances. There is marked neuronal loss that is apparently due to a process of shrinkage and simple atrophy. In the basal pons this is associated with shrinkage and demyelination of the middle cerebellar peduncles, and in the inferior olives, with loss of some internal arcuate fibers and partial demyelination of the inferior cerebellar peduncle. Such severe loss of afferent fibers causes shrinkage and demyelination of the cerebellar white matter, except in the vermis and flocculonodular lobe, whose afferent fibers are from other sources. The cerebellar cortex shows moderate loss of Purkinje's cells and usually of internal granular cells, although it is rare for either to be complete. Little change is seen in the roof nuclei and superior cerebellar peduncle.

Clinical Variants

This pure form of the disease is not often seen, and major or minor associated CNS changes are frequent. Especially in the familial cases, any or all of the features of Friedreich's ataxia may be present. In other cases there is neuronal loss with gliosis (but no Lewy bodies) in the striate body or substantia nigra, usually with the clinical features of paralysis agitans. Still others, with idiopathic postural hypo-

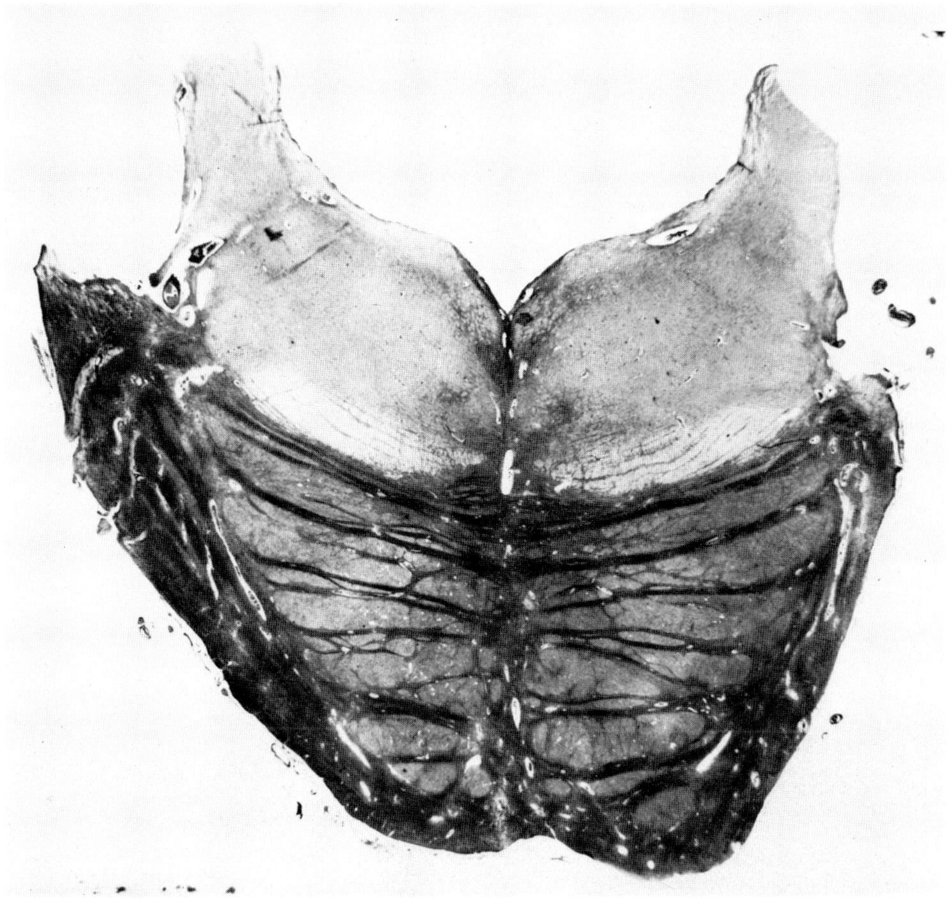

Fig. 24-22. Olivopontocerebellar atrophy. Shrinkage and gliosis of basal pons. (Holzer's stain, X6.)

tension and other autonomic dysfunction, are associated with severe cell loss from the intermediolateral (sympathetic efferent) columns of the thoracic cord.

Cerebello-Olivary Degeneration

Cerebello-olivary degeneration may be sporadic or familial. The usual onset is at age 40 to 50, but it occasionally occurs later. It is very slowly progressive and does not shorten life. Patients show ataxia of gait and clumsiness; later, dysarthria and intention tremor may develop.

Atrophy and sclerosis of the cerebellum may involve any part, including the vermis and the flocculonodular lobe. Atrophy of the inferior olives is often most marked dorsally. Microscopic changes are usually confined to the inferior olives and cerebellar cortex, with neuronal loss and moderate to severe fibrillary gliosis. Purkinje's cells are usually more affected than the internal granular layer. Because the middle cerebellar peduncles are spared, there is less shrinkage and demyelination of the cerebellar white matter, and the dentate nuclei, other root nuclei, and the superior cerebellar peduncles are normal. Only rarely are other CNS areas involved (in contradistinction to olivopontocerebellar atrophy). This may be of value in making an otherwise difficult clinical distinction, the presence of pyramidal, extrapyramidal, or other atypical features pointing strongly to olivopontocerebellar rather than cerebello-olivary disease.

Cerebellar Cortical Degeneration

Cerebellar cortical degeneration usually occurs in patients over 40, and a familial history is exceptional. Childhood cases are extremely rare. These patients are mentally normal and in the early stages tend to report an ataxia affecting first the legs and then the arms — both early in the course of the disease. Skeletal changes are absent. There is no sensory loss, nystagmus, or change in tendon reflexes. The etiology is unknown, although it may be associated with alcoholism (probably only a precipitating factor) or with carcinomatosis (see p. 470).

Grossly, the brain may appear normal, or there may be some reduction in size and increase in the consistency of the cerebellum, which is more marked

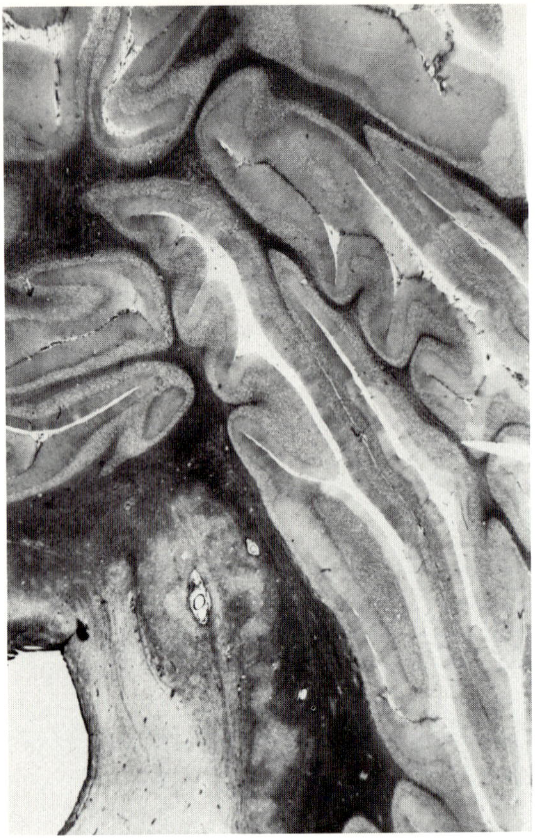

Fig. 24-23. Olivopontocerebellar atrophy. Transverse section of cerebellum, showing gliosis of the molecular layer and white matter. (Holzer's stain, X6.)

anteriorly and superiorly, especially in the vermis, and decreases posteriorly and laterally. Loss of Purkinje's cells (Fig. 24-24) varies from moderate to virtually total loss, with prominent astrocytic (Bergmann's cell) nuclei, but often little fibrillary gliosis. Occasional changes in the inferior olives include neuronal loss, gliosis, and increased lipofuscin pigment, but it is arguable whether these represent retrograde trans-synaptic degeneration or are a primary feature of the disease. Cells of the internal granular layer may appear normal, show a tendency to clumping *(conglutination)*, or be reduced in number.

Rare cases of cerebellar cortical degeneration in infancy may be associated with dementia or with telangiectasia of the skin and conjunctiva and deficiency of gamma globulin (Louis-Bar syndrome). In the Marinesco-Sjögren syndrome, cerebellar or spinocerebellar ataxia is associated with cataracts and mental and physical retardation.

Degeneration Associated with Carcinoma

Apart from direct invasion of the CNS by metastasizing carcinoma, a statistical association has become apparent between many types of tumor and degenerative changes in the CNS, which often resemble (both in distribution and histological characteristics) the spinocerebellar degenerative diseases. Of course, such lesions do not develop in the overwhelming majority of patients with carcinoma, so that the carcinoma itself is not a sufficient cause. Since similar changes may be associated with alcoholism and other toxic and nutritional diseases, especially involving the cerebellum, it appears probable that certain factors external to the CNS, including carcinoma, are merely precipitants of degenerative disease, possibly in patients with a genetic predisposition. Some carcinomatous encephalopathy has been associated with changes resembling Wernicke's encephalopathy. The interpretative problem is complicated by the liability of the cerebellar cortex to severe autolytic change.

While most of these carcinomatous encephalopathies are associated with tumors of the lung or female genitalia, many other associations have been recorded. Changes in the CNS most often consist of Purkinje's cell and internal granular cell loss, followed by partial demyelination of the posterior columns and spinocerebellar tracts. Rarely, the pyramidal tract, subthalamic nucleus, dentate nucleus, inferior olive, vestibular nucleus, medial longitudinal fasciculus, and medial lemniscus may be affected, and even diffuse changes in the cortex with microglial proliferation (particularly in the limbic area) are described. With these rare associations, coincidence cannot be ruled out.

MOTONEURON DISEASES

The motoneuron diseases are a relatively simple group compared with the other degenerative CNS diseases that have been discussed. However, some overlap is already apparent from the fact that lower motoneurons may be involved in the spinocerebellar group. With this exception, patients with motoneuron degeneration fall into two broad categories: the spinal muscular atrophies, in which the corticospinal tracts are not involved, and motoneuron disease, in which they are.

Spinal Muscular Atrophies

In the spinal muscular atrophies, the brunt of the degenerative process falls on lower motoneurons of the spinal cord and brain stem, with secondary degeneration of motor roots and denervation atrophy of the muscles supplied. The concept of clear histological differentiation between denervation atrophy of muscle and myopathic changes is breaking down. The muscle histology in these cases may vary from clear bundle or "sub-bundle" atrophy to a picture that includes hypertrophy with internal muscle nuclei and some evidence of degeneration and regeneration. It appears probable that some cases hitherto regarded as rare adult variants of dystrophy may indeed repre-

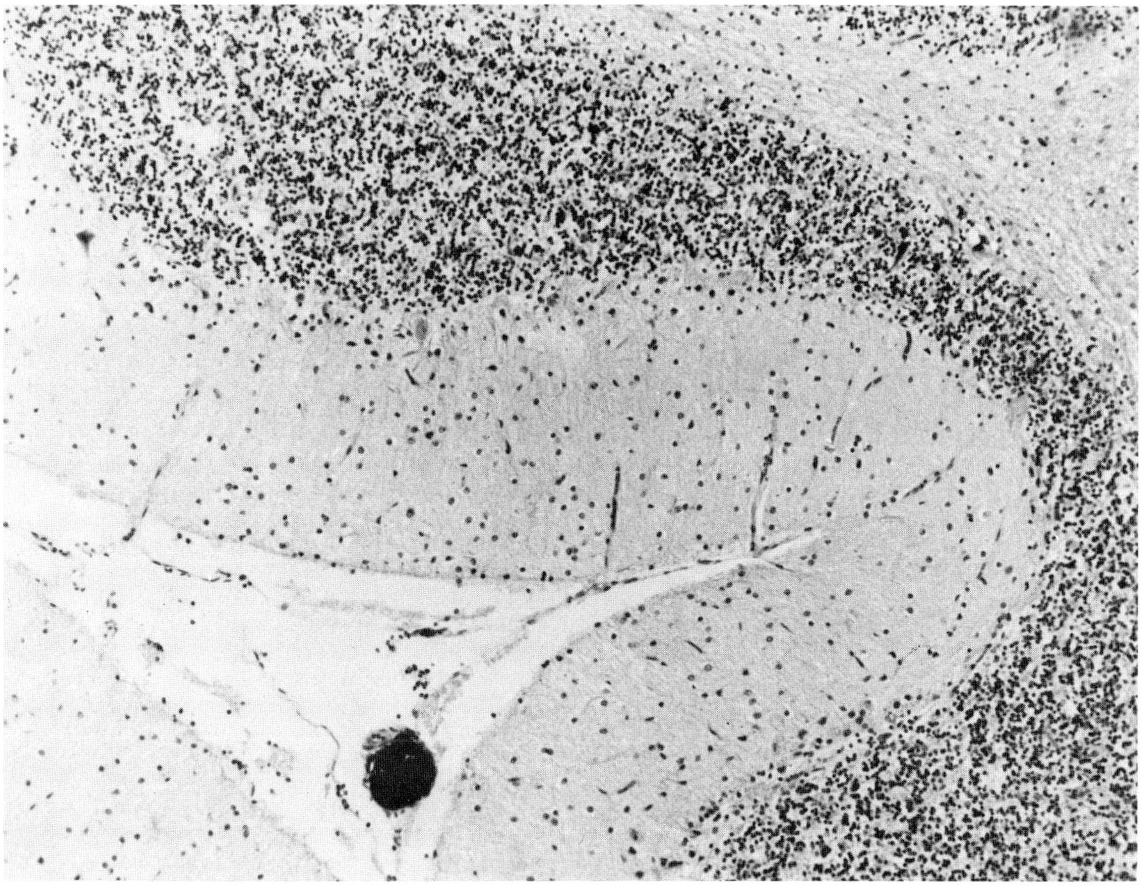

Fig. 24-24. Cerebellar cortical degeneration, showing almost complete loss of Purkinje's cells, with little other apparent change. No etiological factor was determined. (H & E, ×115.)

sent variants of adult motoneuron disease, and they are briefly discussed in the section on chronic spinal muscular atrophies.

Arthrogryposis

Arthrogryposis is a rare condition in which infants are born with two or more joints in a position of absolute fixation and often have other malformations. It is nonprogressive and therefore is not an intrauterine variant of infantile spinal muscular atrophy. In the few cases in which there was adequate examination, the primary changes appeared to be neuronal loss from the anterior horns. This might be due to ischemia or some other local condition rather than being a true degenerative process.

Infantile Spinal Muscular Atrophy (Werdnig-Hoffmann Disease)

This is characterized by rapidly progressive, approximately symmetrical muscle atrophy, with electromyographic or biopsy evidence of denervation. Nerve conduction velocity is normal, and there are no changes in the CSF. The acute condition may be present at birth, and there may have been diminished fetal movement during the third trimester. It is almost invariably apparent by the age of 3 months, and the patients usually die by 30 months. It appears to be inherited as an autosomal recessive condition. The cord shows progressive shrinkage and sclerosis, loss of neurons with mild fibrillary gliosis (Fig. 24-4), and shrinkage and schwannosis of the anterior roots. Similar changes may be seen in the brain stem and cranial motor roots. There may be a genetically distinct later form with onset usually after the age of 6 months and a duration of 4 to 20 years; this form does not exhibit an autosomal recessive pattern. Gross and histological changes are similar.

Juvenile Spinal Muscular Atrophy (Kugelberg-Welander Disease)

In this condition there is slowly progressive, mainly proximal muscle atrophy with onset during childhood or adolescence. About 65% of cases are familial, mostly autosomal recessive, but this group may

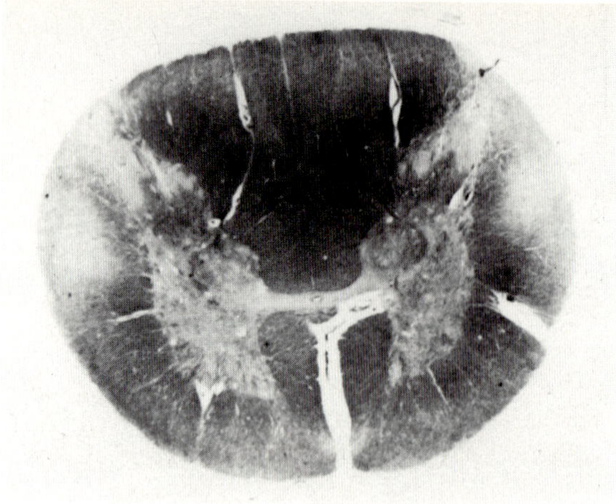

Fig. 24-25. Motoneuron disease. Section of cord at low thoracic level, showing substantial loss of myelin in the region of the crossed cerebrospinal tracts. (Myelin, ×6.)

overlap the subacute infantile spinal muscular atrophies discussed in the preceding section. Electrophysiological and muscle biopsy studies suggest lower motoneuron disease, but little autopsy confirmation is available. Few patients show brain stem involvement. A similar disease of high incidence occurs in a small genetic isolate in southern Japan (Ryukyuan spinal muscular atrophy).

Chronic Spinal Muscular Atrophies

These are a heterogenous group, in which onset may be from infancy to late middle age. Progression is extremely slow. They include sporadic, autosomal recessive, autosomal dominant, and sex-linked recessive conditions. In the past, some may have been diagnosed as muscular dystrophy. There is a distal form that resembles peroneal muscular atrophy except for the lack of sensory change, normal nerve biopsy findings, and normal conduction velocity. Localized facioscapulohumeral, scapulohumeral, and scapuloperoneal forms also exist. Very rarely, there is brain stem involvement.

Motoneuron Disease

Motoneuron disease is a progressive sporadic disorder of adults with involvement of lower motoneurons and denervation atrophy of muscle, almost invariably associated with pyramidal signs at some stage. It has been termed *progressive bulbar palsy, motor neuron disease,* or *amyotrophic lateral sclerosis* (ALS), depending on whether the presenting symptoms are due to loss of brain stem motoneurons, cord motoneurons, or involvement of pyramidal tracts respectively; in any event, all three usually occur before death, with corresponding pathological changes. The disease is almost twice as common in men as in women, except for a hereditary form of ALS (about 5% of the total cases) in which the sex ratio is equal.

Many of those with *hereditary amyotrophic lateral sclerosis* show additional CNS features, including degeneration of the thoracic nucleus of Clarke, partial demyelination of the posterior column and spinocerebellar fibers, and unusual hyaline inclusions in surviving anterior horn cells. These appear to be aggregates of neurofilaments about 90 to 100 A in diameter and are not neurofibrillary tangles. Possibly, this hereditary group is related to the spinocerebellar degenerations, although the latter do not show similar inclusions. Onset is usually after the age of 30, and the average duration is three to five years.

Morphological Features

Gross Appearances. The brain and cord may show little change except for atrophy of the anterior roots and sometimes of the hypoglossal nerve. Occasionally, atrophy of the precentral gyrus, especially of its upper third, may be noted.

Microscopic Appearances. There is loss of fibers and myelin from the cerebrospinal tract (Fig. 24-25), which is more marked distally than proximally and occasionally includes the uncrossed fibers. Demyelination rarely extends above the midbrain level. Occasional loss of myelinated fibers is noted in the spinocerebellar tracts, but posterior columns are normal. Motoneurons in the spinal cord are diminished in number and show nonspecific degenerative changes, including accumulation of lipofuscin pigment and loss of Nissl bodies. Changes tend to be earlier and more severe in the cervical region and later and least severe in the lumbosacral enlargement. In the brain stem, the facial and hypoglossal nuclei are most affected, and those of the ocular muscles are spared. Mild to moderate loss of pyramidal cells, especially of Betz's cells, from areas 4 and 6 may be seen. All affected areas show some fibrillary gliosis. Anterior roots show reduction of large myelinated fibers with little Schwann's cell reaction.

Features resembling motoneuron disease occur in Creutzfeldt-Jakob syndrome, for which there is evidence of a slow virus etiology, and in the Parkinson-dementia complex, also suspected to be of infective origin. Limited transmission experiments and electron-microscopic examinations have failed to suggest a slow virus etiology in the degenerative motoneuron diseases, but this does not exclude the possibility.

BIBLIOGRAPHY

Alvord, E. C., Jr. The Pathology of Parkinsonism. In J. Minckler (Ed.), *Pathology of the Nervous System.* New York: McGraw-Hill, 1968. Vol. 1, pp. 1152-1161.

Bannister, R., and Oppenheimer, D. R. Degenerative diseases of the nervous system associated with autonomic failure. *Brain* 95:457-474, 1972.

Bernheimer, H., Birkmayer, W., Hornykiewicz, O., Jellinger, K., and Seitelberger, F. Brain dopamine and the syndromes of Parkinson and Huntington. *J. Neurol. Sci.* 20:415-455, 1973.

Defendini, R., Markesbery, W. R., Mastri, A. R., and Dufy, P. E. Hallervorden-Spatz disease and infantile neuro-axonal dystrophy. *J. Neurol. Sci.* 20: 7-23, 1973.

Dreese, M. J., and Netsky, M. G. Degenerative Disorders of the Basal Ganglia. In J. Minckler (Ed.), *Pathology of the Nervous System.* New York: McGraw-Hill, 1968. Vol. 1, pp. 1185-1204.

Fahn, S., Libsch, L. R., and Cutler, R. W. Monoamines in the human neostriatum: Topographical distribution in Parkinson's disease and their role in akinesia, rigidity, chorea and tremor. *J. Neurol. Sci.* 14: 427-456, 1971.

Gilman, S., and Barrett, R. E. Hallervorden-Spatz disease and infantile neuroaxonal dystrophy. Clinical characteristics and nosological considerations. *J. Neurol. Sci.* 19:189-205, 1973.

Gumpert, J., Sharpe, D., and Curzon, G. Amine metabolites in the cerebrospinal fluid in Parkinson's disease and the response to levadopa. *J. Neurol. Sci.* 19:1-12, 1973.

Hornykiewicz, O. Dopamine and Its Physiological Significance in Brain Function. In G. H. Bourne (Ed.), *The Structure and Function of Nervous Tissue.* New York: Academic, 1972. Vol. 6, pp. 367-415.

Jervis, G. A. Alzheimer's Disease. In J. Minckler (Ed.), *Pathology of the Nervous System.* New York: McGraw-Hill, 1971. Vol. 2, pp. 1385-1395.

Jervis, G. A. Pick's Disease. In J. Minckler (Ed.), *Pathology of the Nervous System.* New York: McGraw-Hill, 1971. Vol. 2, pp. 1395-1404.

Malamud, N. Infantile Progressive Muscular Atrophy. In J. Minckler (Ed.), *Pathology of the Nervous System.* New York: McGraw-Hill, 1968. Vol. 1, pp. 725-730.

McMenemey, W. H. The Aging Brain. In J. Minckler (Ed.), *Pathology of the Nervous System.* New York: McGraw-Hill, 1971. Vol. 2, pp. 1372-1378.

Netsky, M. G. Degenerations of the Cerebellum and Its Pathways. In J. Minckler (Ed.), *Pathology of the Nervous System.* New York: McGraw-Hill, 1968. Vol. 1, pp. 1163-1185.

Schochet, S. S., Jr. Neuronal Inclusions. In *The Structure and Function of Nervous Tissue.* New York: Academic, 1972. Vol. 4, pp. 129-177.

Schulman, S. Wilson's Disease. In J. Minckler (Ed.), *Pathology of the Nervous System.* New York: McGraw-Hill, 1968. Vol. 1, pp. 1139-1151.

Shuster, S., Burton, I. M., Thody, A. J., Plummer, M., Goolamali, S. K., and Bates, D. Melanocyte-stimulating hormone and Parkinsonism. *Lancet* 1: 463-464, 1973.

Steele, J. C. Progressive supranuclear palsy. *Brain* 95:693-704, 1972.

Wolstenholme, G. E. W., and O'Connor, M. (Eds.), *Alzheimer's Disease and Related Conditions.* Ciba Foundation Symposium. London: Churchill, 1970.

Neoplasms and Developmental Tumors

25

Neoplasms and developmental tumors are considered together because they are both space-occupying lesions that may produce increased intracranial pressure, displacement, compression, or destruction of parts of the brain, with focal symptoms, obstruction of cerebrospinal fluid flow, and other common effects. They are one type of tumor in the strict sense of the word. However, other "tumors" also occur in the central nervous system, some of the more common being hemorrhages, areas of infarction with adjacent edema, and cerebral abscesses. These have been considered in preceding chapters. Neoplasms and developmental tumors may involve any part of the brain or cord, and no age group nor sex is exempt. They must be considered in the initial differential diagnosis of a majority of cases of chronic neurological disease and even of some of acute onset.

Published incidence figures for intracranial and intraspinal neoplasms vary widely according to the particular bias of the reporting center, the age-sex structure and size of the population under consideration, and inclusion or exclusion of metastatic lesions. It has been estimated that up to 10% of neoplasms may be primarily located in the cranial or spinal cavities — a figure that includes not only intrinsic tumors of the CNS (gliomas), but also tumors arising in the pituitary and pineal glands, leptomeninges, nerve roots, and blood vessels. About 50 to 60% of these (representing an incidence of 3 to 8 per 100,000 population) are gliomas; 12 to 18% each are either pituitary tumors or meningiomas; 5 to 10% are neurilemomas of the eighth cranial nerve; and the remainder are rarer neoplasms. There appear to be no accurate figures for the frequency of metastatic tumors in the CNS, although clinically perhaps 20 to 25% of intracranial or intraspinal neoplasms are metastases. The true incidence is higher, since many cases are discovered incidentally at autopsy.

In patients below the age of 15, about 70% of intracranial neoplasms are in the posterior fossa, whereas in older patients, 70% or more are above the tentorium. About 15% of craniospinal neoplasms occur in the spinal canal, the majority being nerve-root tumors, meningiomas, or gliomas. Most gliomas are more common in males, whereas other types of craniospinal neoplasms, notably meningiomas, are more common in females.

EFFECTS OF INTRACRANIAL AND INTRASPINAL NEOPLASMS

In neoplasms outside the CNS, it is generally true that features such as pleomorphism, hyperchromasia, marked mitotic activity, invasiveness, and metastasis correlate with poor prognosis. Thus *benign* as a pathological description is roughly equivalent to the same term used in prognosis. This relationship is not true in the CNS, since a histologically benign tumor may be clinically sinister for one or more of a number of reasons. On the other hand, a histologically malignant CNS tumor is clinically malignant as well. The reasons for the poor prognosis of intracranial neoplasms include the following:

1. Unlike other organs, the entire CNS does not have a uniform function. It contains a number of small irreplaceable areas whose integrity is essential for life to continue (brain stem, hypothalamus). Even a slow-growing, well-differentiated tumor in such regions endangers homeostasis, and surgery may cause additional destructive or irritative lesions. Thus, an important aspect of the prognosis of an intracranial neoplasm is its location.
2. Paradoxically, in areas where vital functions are not threatened (such as the frontal lobes), a neoplasm may expand for a long time without detection. Clinical diagnosis of brain tumors must initially be carried out without the benefit of direct inspection or palpation, which favors the persistence of slowly growing lesions.
3. Because of the bony enclosure, there is little room for any mass to expand without seriously endangering the blood supply of the adjacent CNS or even of the entire intracranial contents. Even a slowly growing neoplasm will ultimately cause a sufficient rise in intracranial pressure to initiate the deteriorating cycle of cerebral ischemia and edema with subsequent death (see Chap. 13).
4. Some (not all) tumors of the CNS produce marked local vasogenic edema (Fig. 25-1), and some become centrally necrotic, leading to hemorrhage within the tumor. Either or both of these factors may summate with the volume of the tumor itself to increase intracranial pressure.
5. Tumors in some locations, notably within the ventricles or posterior fossa, may block CSF flow

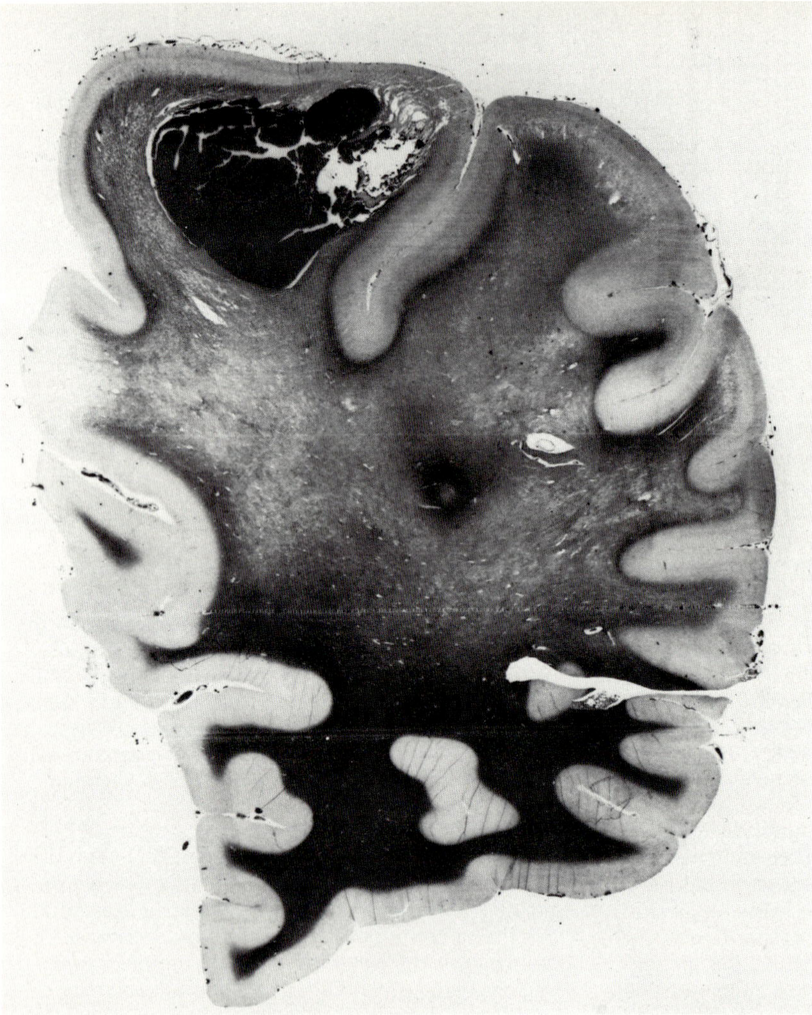

Fig. 25-1. Metastatic melanoma in frontal lobe. The tumor nodule is almost replaced by hemorrhage, and moderate edema affects the upper two-thirds of the white matter. (Myelin, ×1.5.)

and produce noncommunicating, acute or chronic hydrocephalus (see Chap. 19). Occasionally, CSF circulation is impeded by dissemination of the tumor within the ventricular or subarachnoid pathways, but this is relatively uncommon.

Clearly, many more factors must be considered in assessing the prognosis of CNS tumors than is the case with tumors occurring elsewhere. Nonetheless, the malignancy of the neoplasm in the classic sense remains important, since it is related to the speed of deterioration, development of cerebral edema, liability to necrosis, hemorrhage and metastasis in the CSF pathways, and sensitivity to radiation or chemotherapy.

The only effective method of determining malignancy is surgical biopsy, usually combined with resection of as much tumor as is feasible. Occasionally, the diagnosis may be made by cytological examination of the CSF, but the method is not widely practiced or adequately tested, and neoplasms that do not reach the ventricular or pial surface are unlikely to yield CSF cells. Methods for localization of a tumor prior to surgery are not specific for neoplasms, since they depend either on distortion of the intracranial contents (echoencephalography, pneumoencephalography, and angiography) or on localized development of blood-brain barrier deficiencies (brain scan), which occur in many cerebral lesions, including infarcts and abscesses, but may not occur in all neoplasms. Computerized axial tomography (CAT scan) shows promise for more accurate localization of masses of all types.

INTRINSIC CENTRAL NERVOUS SYSTEM (GLIAL) TUMORS

Intrinsic CNS tumors are derived from the neural tube (neurectoderm). (For a brief discussion of the cytogenesis of CNS cells, see Chap. 2.) Primitive neurons (neuroblasts) are the first to differentiate, and the formation of neuroblasts probably continues in man with decreasing tempo up to about the time of birth. The cytogenesis of glial cells is much less clear. Presumably, the ependyma differentiates in situ from the neuroepithelium, and astrocytes and oligodendroglia have a common precursor in the fine bipolar spongioblast, which, unlike the neuroblast, retains its ability to divide during migration. Although spongioblasts have not been recognized in the normal neonatal brain, it is probable that a slightly more differentiated but still bipotential cell remains, giving rise to the large number of oligodendroglia that appear during myelination; it is less certain that this cell contributes throughout life to the astrocytes that proliferate in brain damage. There is much circumstantial evidence pointing to a close relationship between astrocytes and oligodendroglia, including a tendency for the latter to revert to astrocyte-like cells in tissue culture, the observation of intermediate forms with scanty glial filaments on electron microscopy, and the frequent concurrence of the two cell lines in neoplasms. (It has even been suggested that in areas of secondary demyelination, oligodendroglia may be converted to astrocytes.)

The nomenclature of brain tumors is confusing, one reason being the uninhibited use of the suffix *-blastoma* for anaplastic tumors of varying type. This suffix should be reserved for tumors derived from incompletely differentiated fetal cells (blast cells), but except for the medulloblastoma, such tumors are exceedingly rare in the CNS. In common usage the suffix has come to mean a markedly dedifferentiated or anaplastic tumor (e.g., glioblastoma, ependymoblastoma) or even tumors with a type of architecture resembling a postulated stage of cell maturation (astroblastoma). These anaplastic tumors are pleomorphic and frequently bizarre, occur in all age groups, but are more common in adults, and are almost certainly derived from mature glial cells by a process of anaplasia or dedifferentiation. By contrast, the true *blastomas* show cellular uniformity, often have architectural features recapitulating the fetal tissue, and are presumably directly derived from fetal cells that are not completely differentiated. They occur chiefly in infants and children. A major reason for the confusion may be that both groups are biologically aggressive, tend to grow rapidly and metastasize within CSF pathways, and carry correspondingly gloomy prognoses.

Neoplasms of Fetal Central Nervous System Cells

The most primitive of the fetal cell tumors is the *medulloepithelioma,* which is either congenital or occurs before the age of 5. Such tumors are located in a hemisphere or adjacent to the ventricular system. They show irregular cleftlike lumens with an internal limiting membrane, lined by columnar epithelium that rests on delicate mesenchymal stroma. They clearly recapitulate the histology of the primitive neural tube. Foci of differentiation to neuroblasts, neurons, ependymal cells, astrocytes, and oligodendroglia have been reported.

Slightly more differentiated are the rare cerebral *neuroblastomas,* which resemble their counterparts in the peripheral nervous system, often showing poorly formed perifibrillary rosettes and occasional neuronal differentiation. A few childhood cases of *pineoblastoma* and very rare examples of true *ependymoblastoma* occurring near the ventricular system have been reported, both showing a uniform cellular picture resembling the corresponding fetal cells and metastasizing widely in the CSF.

Probably related to the spongioblast are the polar *spongioblastoma* and the *astroblastoma,* both rare hemispheric tumors occurring under the age of 20 and located near the ventricles. Each has its own entirely uniform histological picture: in the former, bipolar, spindle-shaped cells are arranged in parallel groups separated by delicate mesenchyme; in the latter, unipolar plump cells are arranged in pseudorosette formations around vessels. (These rare true astroblastomas are distinct from the perivascular rosettes, separated by a loose matrix, seen as one component of an astrocytoma that varies in microscopic appearance in different areas examined, but is often termed *astroblastomatous.*)

Medulloblastoma

The *medulloblastoma* is the only true fetal tumor of the CNS (except for the retinoblastoma) that is common. These tumors occur only in the cerebellum (Fig. 25-2), tending to be midline in younger children and hemispheric in older children and young adults. The term *medulloblastoma* is distinctive and firmly entrenched, although the "medulloblast" is not a recognized cell type in fetal development. They are thought to arise from neuroepithelial cells of the rhombic lip, many of which migrate over the surface of the developing cerebellum to form the external granular layer (which gives rise to the internal granular layer by migration); others remain in the lip area or roof of the fourth ventricle and migrate through the cerebellum to form Purkinje's and possibly other cells. Glial cells of the cerebellum are presumably also derived from these neuroepithelial elements.

The medulloblastoma is usually a rounded, well-defined tumor (less vascular than the ependymoma), which may be confined to the cerebellum, transgress the fourth ventricle, or even invade the brain stem. Seen histologically (Fig. 25-3), it consists of closely packed, hyperchromatic, round or oval nuclei, often with relatively few mitotic figures, and is sometimes difficult to distinguish from an anaplastic ependymoma, which may occur in the same location in children. (Typically, the ependymoma has larger, elliptical nuclei that are slightly less dark-staining, and it is also more vascular.)

Medulloblastomas may form true rosettes with an internal limiting membrane that suggests their neuroepithelial origin, perifibrillary rosettes indicative of early neuroblastic differentiation, or small areas of delicate, parallel, bipolar cells that suggest spongioblastic differentiation. They are therefore commonly considered to be bipotential tumors, supporting their origin from neuroepithelial cells and their truly blastomatous nature.

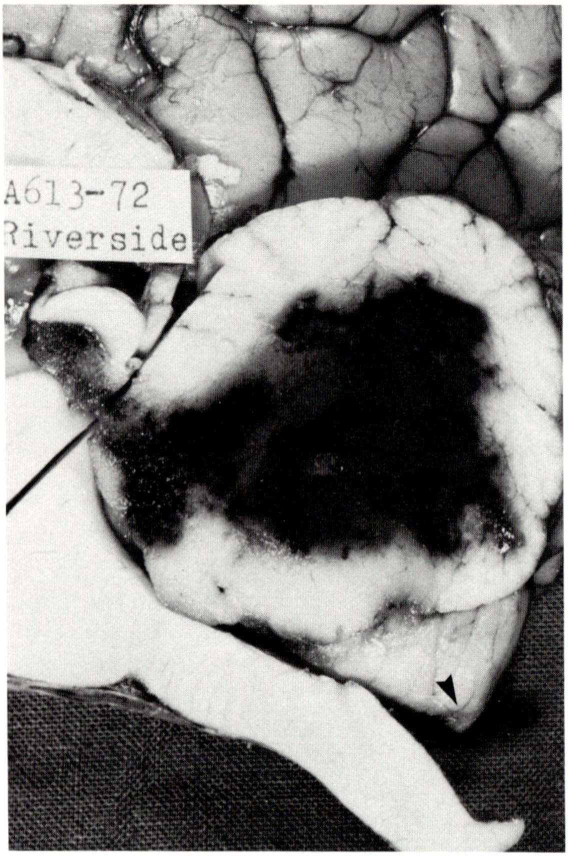

Fig. 25-2. Medulloblastoma from the cerebellum, invading the roof of the fourth ventricle and along the aqueduct. Normal cerebellum can be seen above. Much of the tumor is hemorrhagic. The medulla is flattened, and severe tonsillar herniation (arrow) is present.

Some, especially those in the cerebellar hemispheres in older patients, invade the leptomeninges and provoke a profound collagenous and reticulin-forming reaction (Fig. 25-4), to produce the *desmoplastic medulloblastoma,* previously termed *cerebellar sarcoma.* This change does not alter the gloomy prognosis, since the tumor is invasive, difficult to remove in its entirety, and freely metastasizes in the CSF pathways.

Seen electron-microscopically, the cells have no particular distinguishing characteristics: They contain moderate numbers of microtubules, but this is of little help in differentiating them from ependymomas.

General Features of Dedifferentiated (Nonfetal) Gliomas

Nomenclature

Gliomas that do not exhibit peculiarly fetal characteristics have presumably arisen from mature CNS cells by anaplasia (dedifferentiation) of varying degree and may therefore be simply classified as *astrocytomas, oligodendrogliomas,* or *ependymomas.*

Since astrocytomas are by far the most common, and since a high proportion of them are markedly anaplastic, the anaplastic astrocytoma is a common neoplasm. It is a histologically malignant glioma exhibiting considerable pleomorphism and mitotic activity, and often termed *glioblastoma multiforme.* Many authors retain this term; some use it descriptively but others consider it to be an entirely separate entity from the anaplastic astrocytoma. However:

1. Many glioblastomas contain less anaplastic areas that are recognizably astrocytic and are presumably highly anaplastic astrocytomas.
2. There appears to be no clinical, biological, or morphological discontinuity between anaplastic astrocytomas with marked mitotic activity, typical pleomorphic "glioblastomas," and tumors exhibiting both types of tissue.
3. There is no evidence from electron microscopy or tissue culture studies that would preclude glioblastomas from being merely anaplastic astrocytomas (the bizarre features seen are no greater than may be observed in undifferentiated carcinomas).
4. Their very pleomorphism almost certainly precludes their having arisen from undifferentiated (fetal) cells, and "glioblasts" are not a recognized precursor cell.

Until more compelling evidence is adduced, it appears reasonable to equate the terms *glioblastoma multiforme* and *anaplastic astrocytoma,* recognizing that the former is redundant, but is likely to persist for a long time in the literature with a descriptive, not a cytogenetic, connotation.

The terms *ependymoblastoma, oligodendroglioblastoma, spongioblastoma,* and *astroblastoma* are also still currently used to describe particularly anaplastic varieties of tumor. This usage should not be allowed to obscure the existence of true fetal neoplasms, discussed in the preceding section.

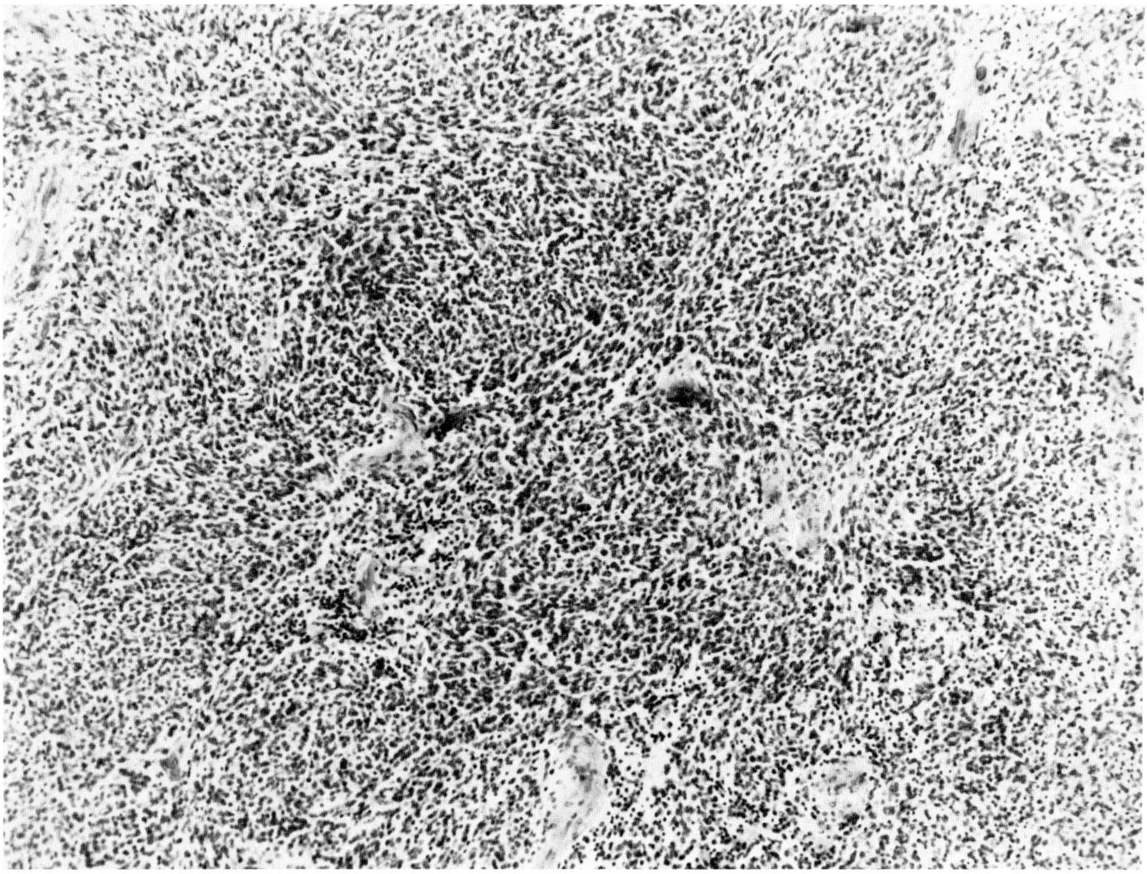

Fig. 25-3. Medulloblastoma, showing closely packed, uniform, small cells. (H & E, ×115.)

Etiology and Pathogenesis

Nothing is known of the etiology or pathogenesis of human gliomas, and there is little evidence of genetic predisposition, since familial cases are rare.

Experimental Induction of Gliomas

Experimentally, gliomas can be induced by radiation, chemical carcinogens, or oncogenic viruses. As in teratogenesis, the results are highly variable from species to species. However, they vary to a greater extent with the agent used, and are less time-dependent, than is the case in induction of malformations. Chemical carcinogens may be implanted in the CNS or administered intravenously or transplacentally. Recently, interest has centered on compounds of the nitrosourea type, which cause malformations and cerebral neoplasms in fetal rats, mainly gliomas in neonatal animals, but a mixture of glial and mesenchymal tumors in adults. The glial tumors may be pleomorphic or show chiefly astrocytomatous, oligodendrogliomatous, or ependymomatous growth. They tend to be concentrated in the region of subependymal germinal cells (subependymal plate), perhaps because this is the area of greatest mitotic activity.

Oncogenic CNS viruses include Rous sarcoma virus and human adenovirus, the former producing astrocytomas (some resembling human "glioblastoma") in dogs. Dogs also suffer from spontaneous astro-

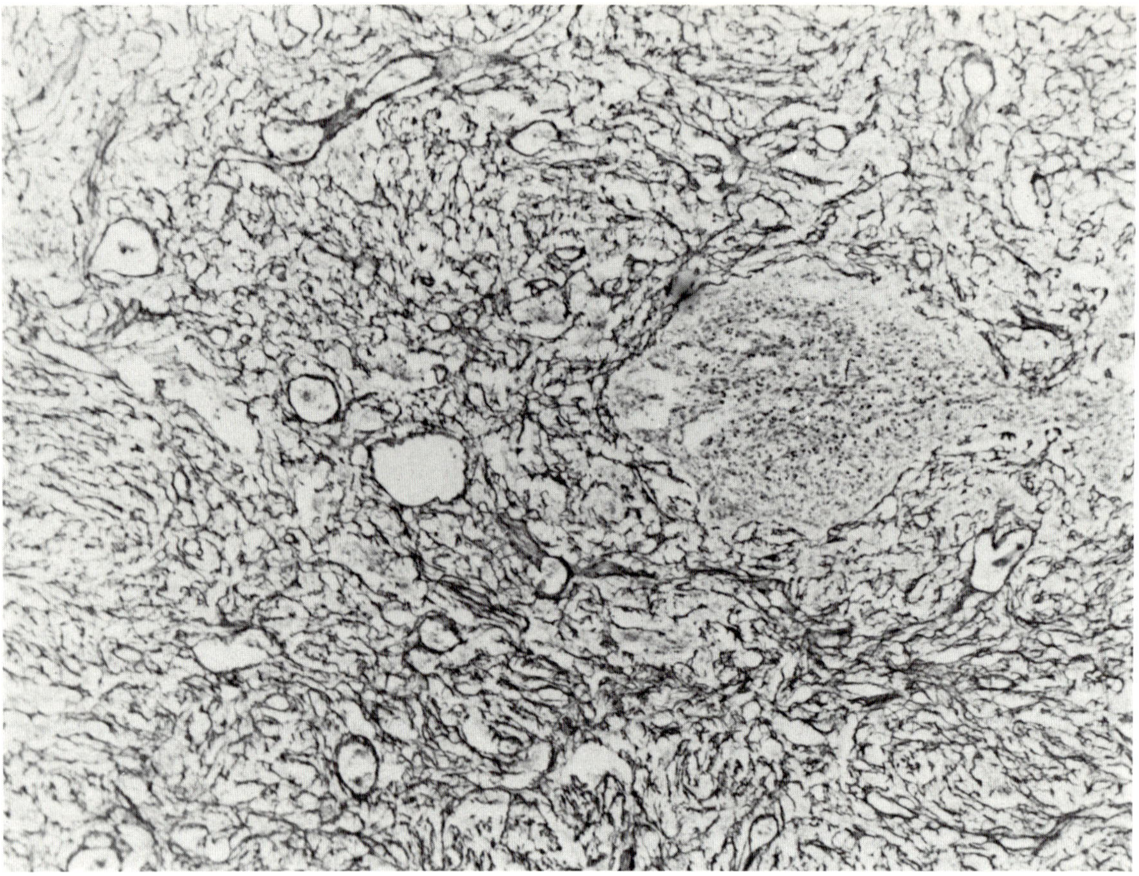

Fig. 25-4. Desmoplastic medulloblastoma. Thin cords and occasional clumps of cells are separated by the complex reticulin network, as in Figure 25-3. (Reticulin, ×115.)

cytomas, and both these and the experimental variety show changes in the vessels. Instead of nonfenestrated capillaries characteristic of the normal CNS, areas with fenestrations closed by a single unit membrane, or unclosed, have been demonstrated. Both abnormalities are permeable to substances of large molecular weight such as ferritin and plasma protein. Similar gaps have been demonstrated in human anaplastic astrocytomas, probably forming the basis of the barrier deficiency present in many such tumors.

Neoplasms induced in hamsters by human adenovirus type 12 are medulloepitheliomas or ependymomas, again tending to occur in the walls of the lateral ventricle. Indispensable and fascinating as such work is in the long term, it does not appear to offer immediate prospects for the prevention or improved therapy of human gliomas.

Biochemistry

Work on the chemical composition and metabolism of brain tumors has been largely confined to the much more common astrocytomas. The lipid content appears to be constant, irrespective of the degree of anaplasia, and resembles that of immature brain, particularly in the presence of desmosterol, which is normally coverted to cholesterol by desmosterol reductase. Presumably, gliomas have insufficient amounts of this enzyme. Astrocytomas contain only trace amounts of gamma-aminobutyric acid and N-acetylaspartic acid, confirming that these are products of neuronal rather than of glial metabolism. Transfer RNA in glial tumors shows increased methylation, possibly proportional to the degree of anaplasia, which may reflect a fundamental defect in neoplastic tissue.

The oxidative enzyme pattern of gliomas resembles that of the immature brain, with a fetal lactic dehydrogenase isozyme pattern and increased concentrations of lactate and glucose 6-phosphate. Comparison of mouse ependymoma and normal mouse brain shows decreases in adenosine triphosphate (ATP) and creatine phosphate (CrP) in the tumor, but increases in lactate, adenosine diphosphate (ADP), and adenosine monophosphate (AMP). Anaerobic incubation shows a greater accumulation of lactate than can be accounted for by loss of hexose, indicating an alternative source of energy (possibly pentose nucleic acids, since their diester bond has an energy comparable to that of the terminal phosphate in ATP). Increased hydrolase activity is associated with areas of degeneration.

Astrocytomas and oligodendrogliomas have approximately the same content of the brain-specific acid protein S100 as does normal white matter, confirming its suspected localization in glial cells. Medulloblastomas and normal gray matter contain less S100, and so do highly anaplastic astrocytomas. In astrocytomas, the concentration of S100 may bear an inverse relationship to survival time. There is presently no conclusive evidence for the existence of a specific glioma antigen or for the production of antiglioma antibodies by the reticuloendothelial system.

Cell Kinetics

The rate of tumor growth depends on the balance between production of new cells by proliferation and loss of cells by autolysis or from ischemia or other causes. In many tumors outside the CNS, cell loss appears to vary between 70 and 95%, so that the actual time required for a tumor to double its size is much longer than calculated from its rate of mitotic activity. Preliminary studies in human anaplastic astrocytomas suggest a cell loss rate of about 85% and a possible doubling in volume about every six weeks. As can be seen histologically, especially in less anaplastic tumors, many tumor cells are nonproliferating at any given time and are therefore less susceptible to chemotherapeutic agents.

Growth and Metastasis

Both experimental oncogenesis and tissue-culture studies have stressed the significance of the environment on the form taken by tumor cells and on their architectural arrangement, which has led to the concept of primary, secondary, and tertiary structures.

1. *Primary structures* are intrinsic and not subject to modification by the host or the environment. They include such features as rosettes, palisading, and whorl formation, which occur even in tissue culture.
2. *Secondary structures* are dependent on the preexisting neural elements and include the elongated shape of tumor cells in myelinated tracts, aggregation of cells around neurons, and larger aggregations at the CNS interfaces, as around vessels or beneath the ependyma or pia.
3. *Tertiary structures* are associated with such degenerative changes as hemorrhage, necrosis, and scarring.

Remarkably, even the most anaplastic gliomas rarely invade vessels, and when they do, it is usually following surgical intervention, with tumor nodules in the operative scar and occasional extraneural metastasis. No explanation for the vascular impermeability to gliomas is available, but since it appears to break down following surgery in some cases, it may represent yet another facet of the blood-brain barrier. The rarity of generalized metastases following surgery and their virtual nonoccurrence without surgery suggest that there may be additional factors, such as inability to adapt biochemically to other situations, or failure of vascular stroma induction, which prevent extraneural spread. Invasion of the meninges is common and is often followed by dissemination within the CSF spaces.

The Blood-Brain Barrier in Gliomas

As has been noted, vessels in some experimental tumors show both fenestrations and gaps that would readily permit the passage of large molecules and the bulk flow of plasma into the extracellular space. Although few observations of such vascular changes have been made in human material, the presence of an enlarged extracellular space containing light amorphous material (probably plasma protein) is well documented. While it is difficult to reconcile such observations with any role for the barrier system in preventing vascular invasion, they have obvious significance in relation to the development of cerebral edema. This is most widespread and most marked in relation to highly anaplastic astrocytomas (glioblastomas), and it is in these tumors that vascular damage is most intense and the extracellular spaces are widest. Such spaces exist both between individual tumor cells and between cells and the basement membrane; and as in experimental cerebral edema (see Chap. 12), fluid can extend considerable distances from a small focus of vascular damage, even involving an entire hemisphere.

The success of tumor localization by scanning, such as the use of technetium isotopes, is dependent on the material's escaping from the vessels and remaining in the extracellular space after they have been flushed clear. Occasional failures to demonstrate tumor may therefore be due not to poor vascularity, but to relatively intact tumor vessels.

Barrier damage may be necessary to permit the ingress of chemotherapeutic agents, such as intravenous methotrexate, particularly since most such drugs are water-soluble and ionized. In a study on experimental mouse ependymoma, tritiated methotrexate was concentrated most heavily in tumor cells in the center of the neoplasm, but less so at the edge. However, it was virtually absent from normal brain cells, except those adjacent to the lesion. This distribution may depend more on damage to the barrier system than on specific uptake of methotrexate by tumor cells.

Although administration of corticosteroids postoperatively seems to reduce cerebral edema, it is unknown whether or not its effects are only on the barrier system. (A further possible rationale for their use following tumor removal is their reported growth-inhibiting, or even cytotoxic, effects on anaplastic astrocytomas in tissue culture. These effects vary with the cell strain and the corticosteroid used, and it is uncertain whether or not they are of clinical significance.)

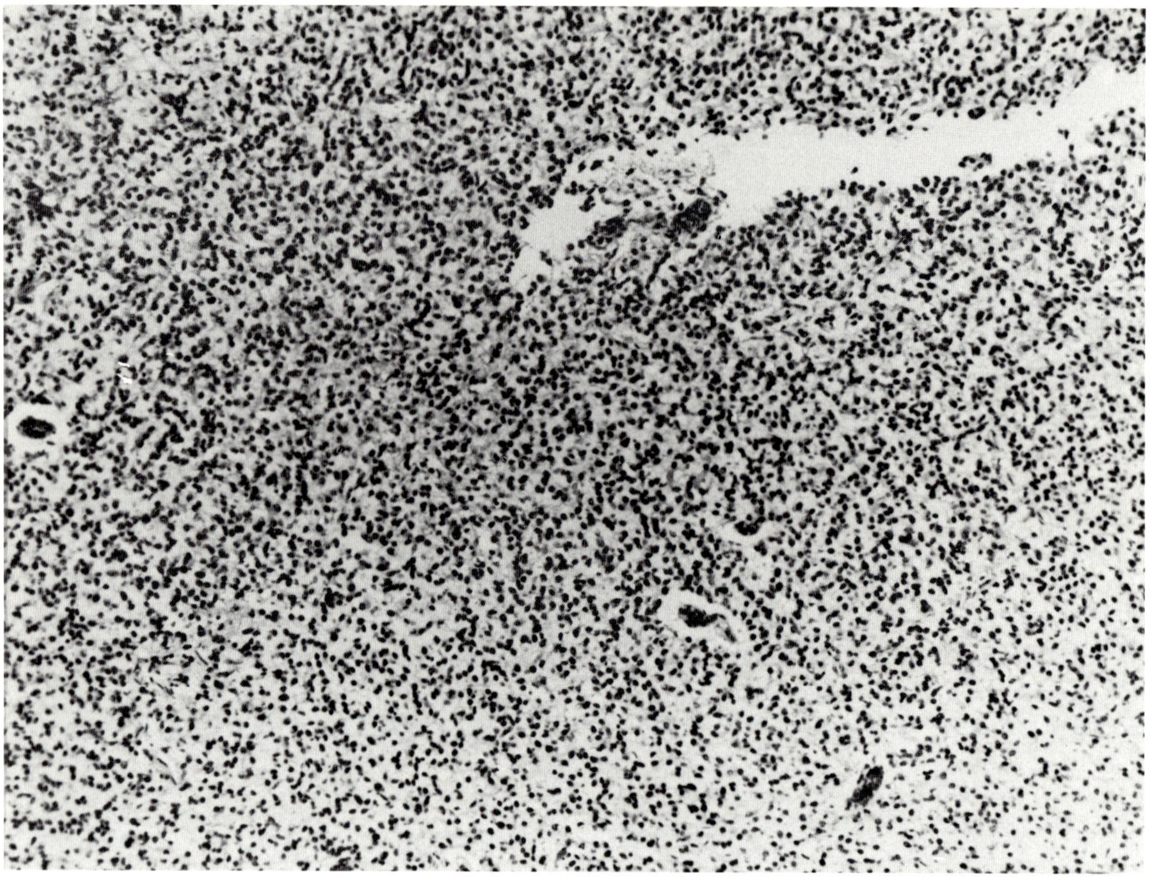

Fig. 25-5. Astrocytoma of protoplasmic type, well differentiated (grade I). (H & E, ×115.)

Astrocytoma (Including Glioblastoma)

Astrocytomas are tumors with widely variable degrees of anaplasia, occurring in any part of the CNS and derived from mature astrocytes. Non-neoplastic astrocytes may be protoplasmic or fibrillary in the normal brain or gemistocytic in the reactive phase (see Chaps. 2 and 10), and tumors with only slight anaplasia may correspond to any, or a mixture, of these types. With moderate to severe anaplasia and with increasing pleomorphism and mitotic activity, the distinction is lost. These anaplastic tumors are the more common.

A grading system is often used to make the degree of anaplasia more objective. In this system, grades I and II indicate increasing pleomorphism, but no (detectable) mitotic activity, whereas grades III and IV indicate mitotic activity, the latter often corresponding to glioblastoma multiforme.

Relationship of Grading to Appearances of Tumor

The cells in a *grade I* tumor (Figs. 25-5, 25-6) differ little from normal astrocytes (protoplasmic, fibrillary, or gemistocytic), but are more closely packed. The limits of the tumor may be impossible to define grossly and even may be difficult to determine microscopically. Central areas may show microcystic degeneration that ultimately coalesces to grossly visible cysts. *Grade II* tumors are grossly somewhat

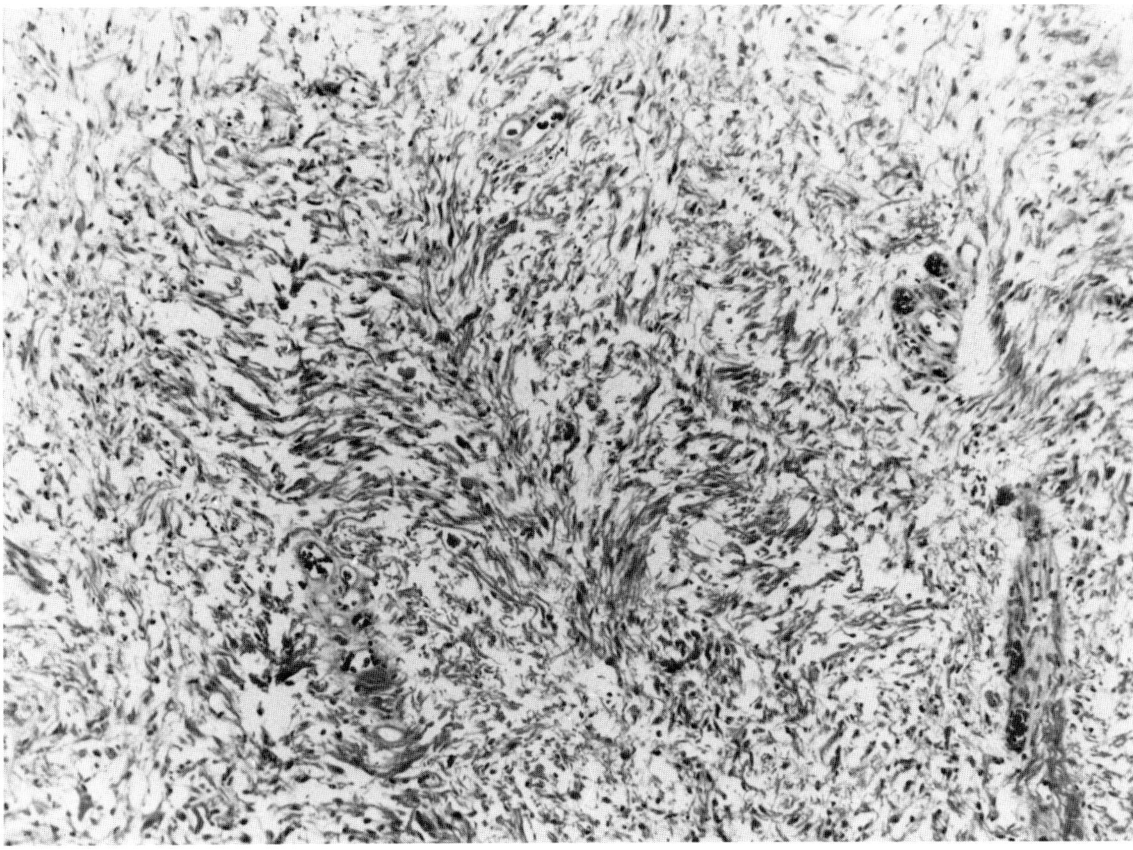

Fig. 25-6. Astrocytoma of fibrillary type from optic chiasm of a child, well differentiated (grade I). (H & E, ×115.)

better defined, with nuclei more closely packed and variable in size, shape, and staining (Figs. 25-7, 25-8).

Grade III tumors show closely packed, hyperchromatic, sometimes pleomorphic nuclei, with scanty mitotic activity. Vessels within such tumors may show moderate adventitial thickening and endothelial hyperplasia; central areas may show ischemic necrosis with cavity formation. In *grade IV* astrocytomas, cellularity is again high, and mitotic activity is moderate to extensive. The degree of pleomorphism is variable, some tumors appearing uniform (Fig. 25-9) and others showing large, multinucleate cells (Fig. 25-10), often with bizarre nuclei containing cytoplasmic invaginations. Vascular hyperplasia, with adventitial changes so severe that it sometimes mimics fibrosarcoma or may even be independently malignant (producing a "gliosarcoma"), is prominent. These tumors undergo extensive necrosis and hemorrhage, the latter occasionally producing an intracerebral hematoma.

Electron-Microscopic Appearances

Seen electron-microscopically, increasing anaplasia is characterized by more and more irregularity of the nucleus, with clumping and margination of chromatin. Nuclear "inclusions" seen on light microscopy are usually invaginations of cytoplasm into the highly irregular nuclei. The cell outline also becomes irregular, and the extracellular space is wide and frequently contains collagen fibers. Numerous glial filaments in the cytoplasm remain a feature even of markedly anaplastic tumors.

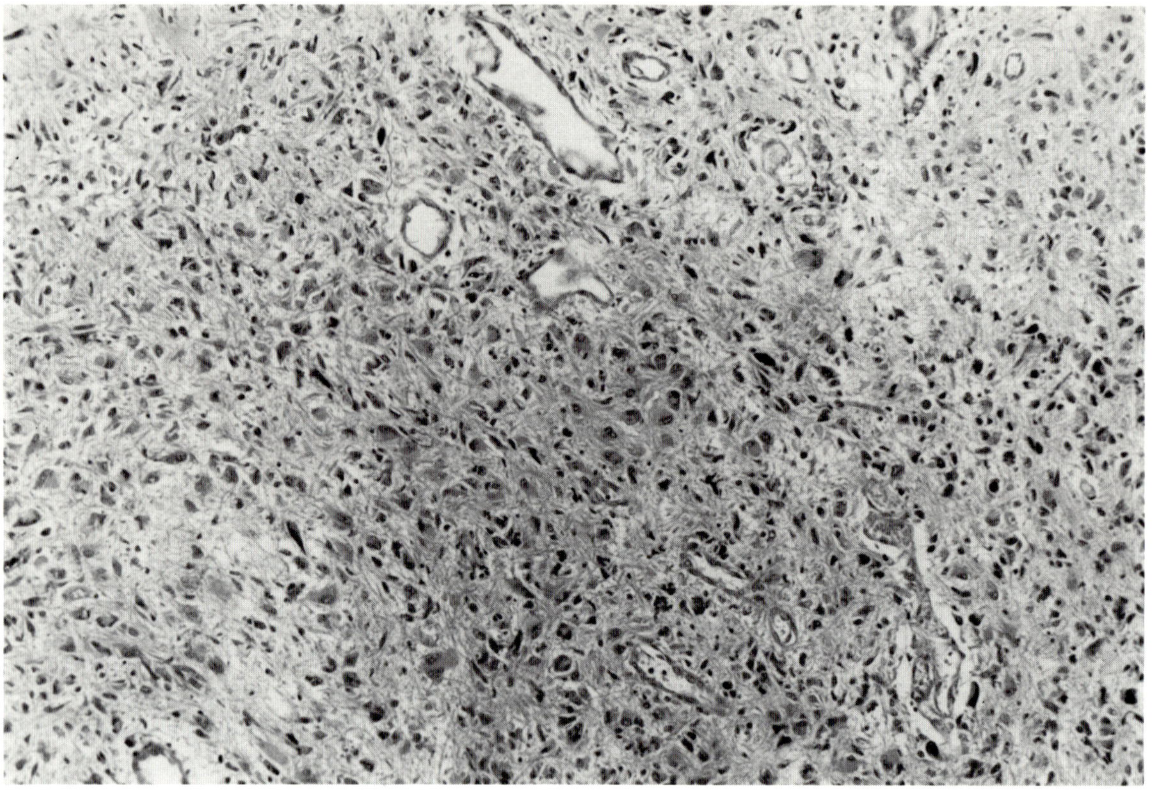

Fig. 25-7. Astrocytoma of gemistocytic type, showing moderate pleomorphism and hyperchromatism (grade II). (H & E, ×115.)

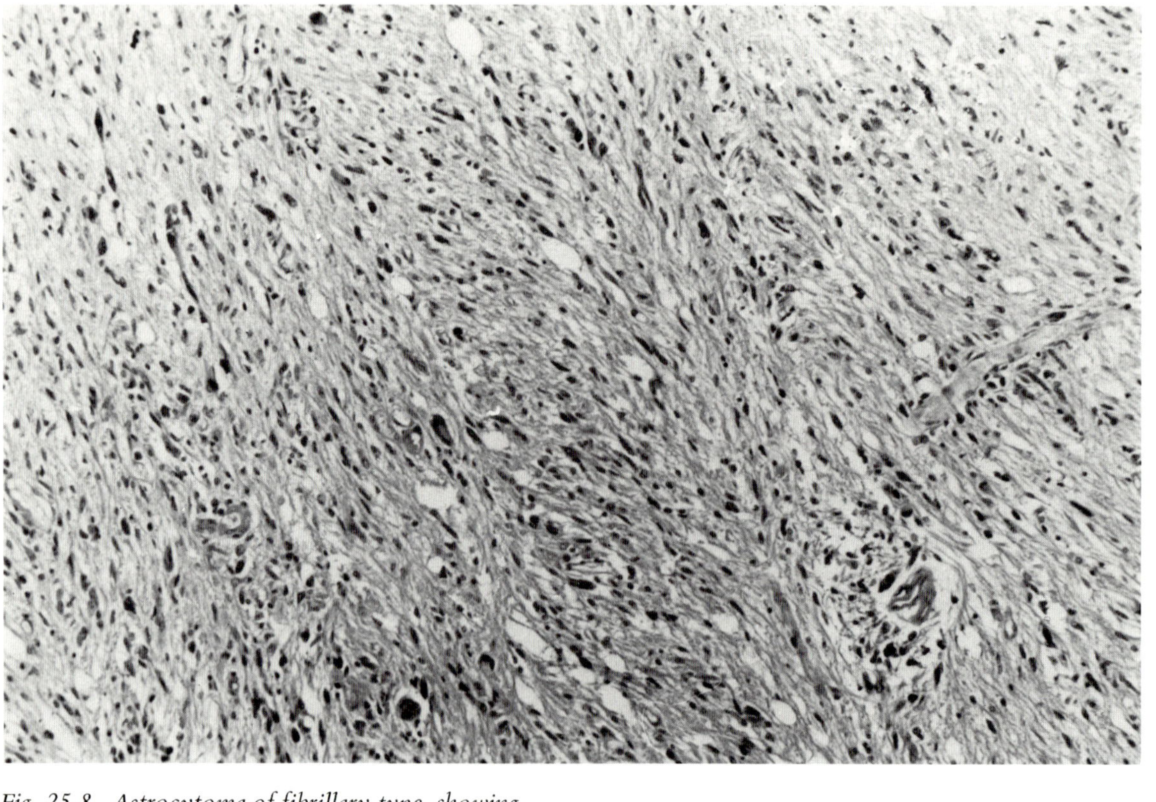

Fig. 25-8. Astrocytoma of fibrillary type, showing moderate pleomorphism and hyperchromatism (grade II). (H & E, ×115.)

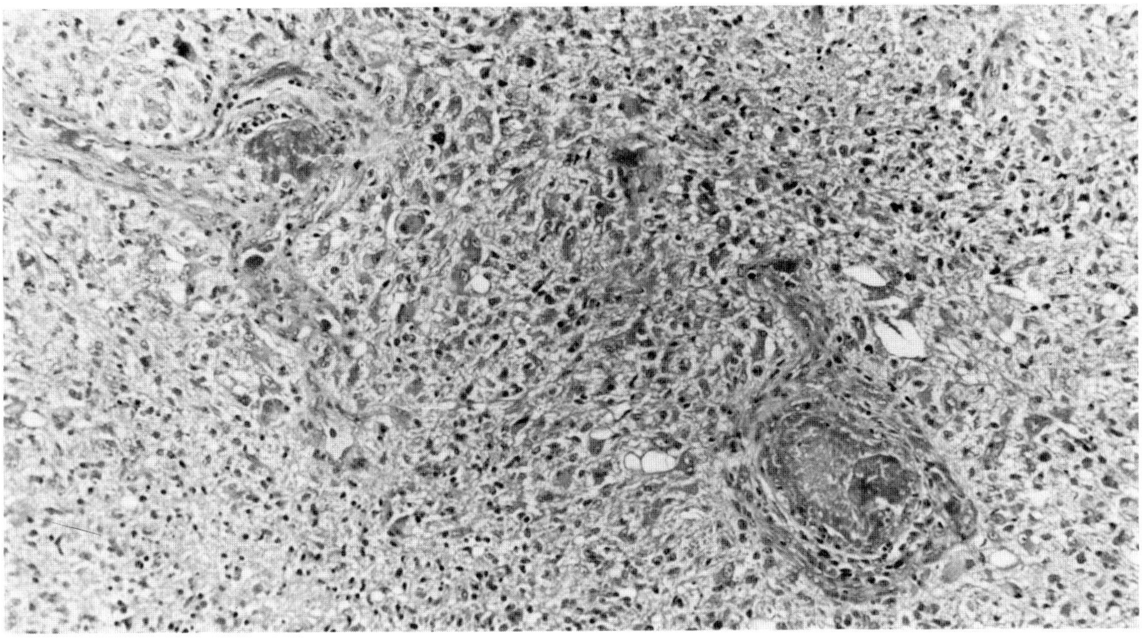

Fig. 25-9. Astrocytoma showing anaplasia, mitotic activity, and moderate vascular hyperplasia (grade IV). (H & E, ×115.)

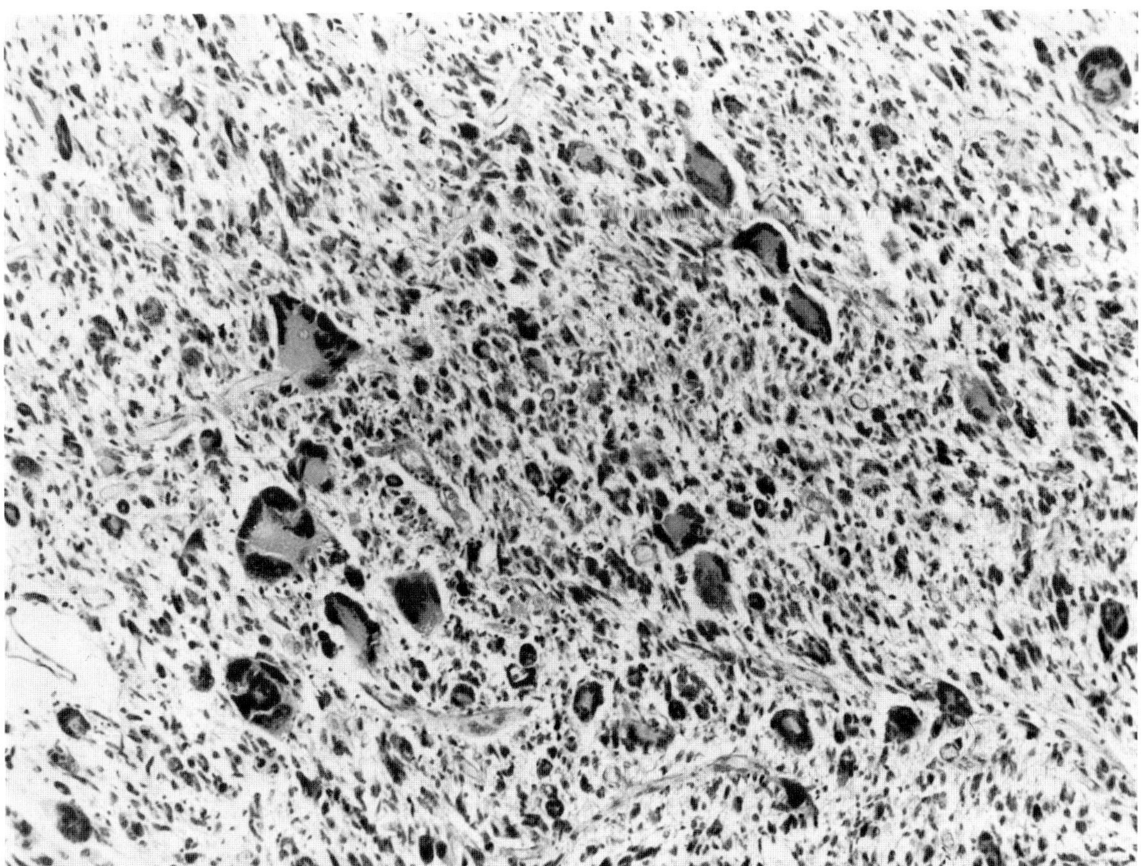

Fig. 25-10. Astrocytoma showing anaplasia with mitotic activity and marked pleomorphism (grade IV, glioblastoma multiforme). (H & E, ×115.)

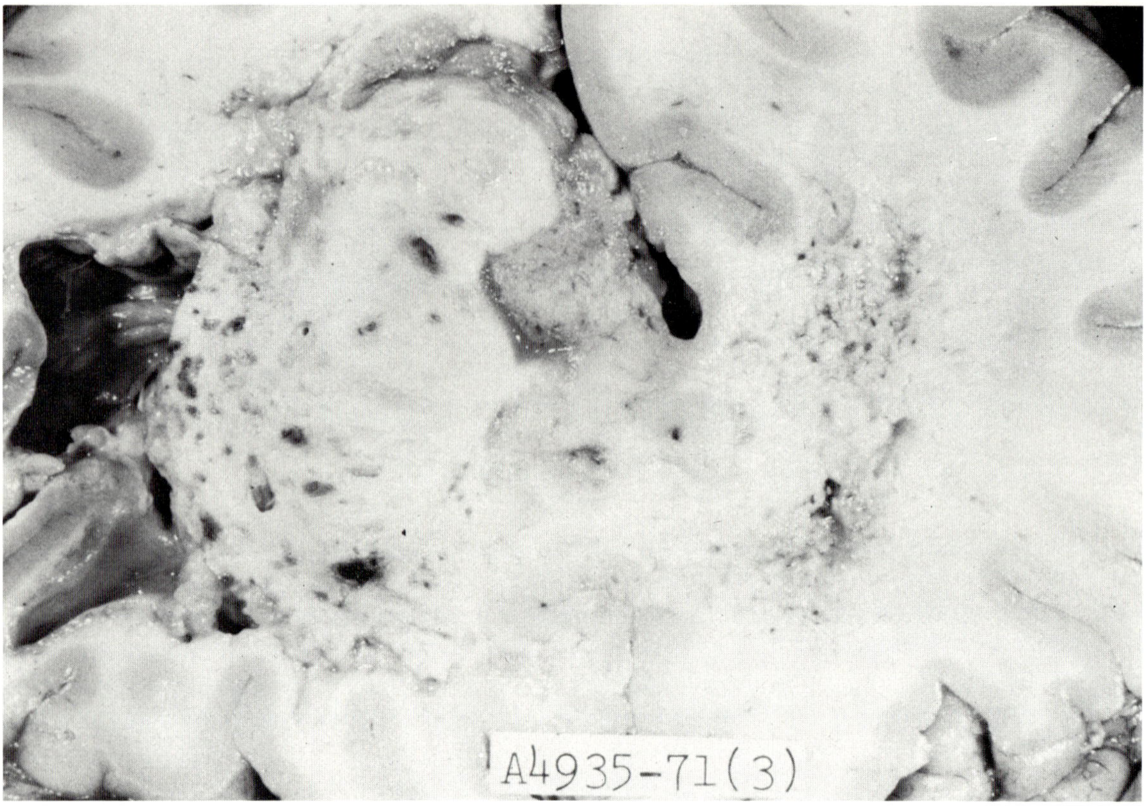

Fig. 25-11. Anaplastic astrocytoma in frontal hemispheres, involving corpus callosum and white matter of both sides. The tumor is cystic and necrotic, but with little hemorrhage.

Tissue Culture

In tissue culture, increasing anaplasia is marked by faster migration of cells and a tendency to shortening and blunting of processes. Malignant astrocytes in tissue culture often show numerous small lateral projections on their cell processes, and with increasing anaplasia these move from the distal parts of processes to proximal parts and the cell body. As previously noted, none of these studies indicates a clear line of demarcation between astrocytomas and glioblastomas.

Distribution

Astrocytomas of the hemispheres may occur at any age, but are much more common in adults, in whom they tend to be anaplastic, with characteristic degeneration, cystic necrosis, and often hemorrhage. They may cross the corpus callosum (Fig. 25-11) to form an approximately symmetrical dumbbell-shaped structure. They usually appear to arise in white matter, although they may pass through the cortex and invade meninges.

Cerebellar astrocytomas occurring in adults are similar to those that have been described above. However, in children, a benign variant, susceptible to surgical removal, is usually found. This *cystic cerebellar astrocytoma* is histologically a grade I tumor, but with a much-enhanced tendency to cyst formation (Fig. 25-12), so much so that a single cyst with only a mural nodule of tumor is sometimes found.

Astrocytomas near the midline usually occur in children, although anaplastic tumors apparently arising in the thalamus are occasionally found in adults. Childhood midline tumors may involve the hypothalamus, optic chiasm (Fig. 25-6), and nerves and are grade I tumors with cells of elongated (piloid) shape due to the parallel fiber bundles of the optic pathways. In spite of their cytologically benign nature and slow

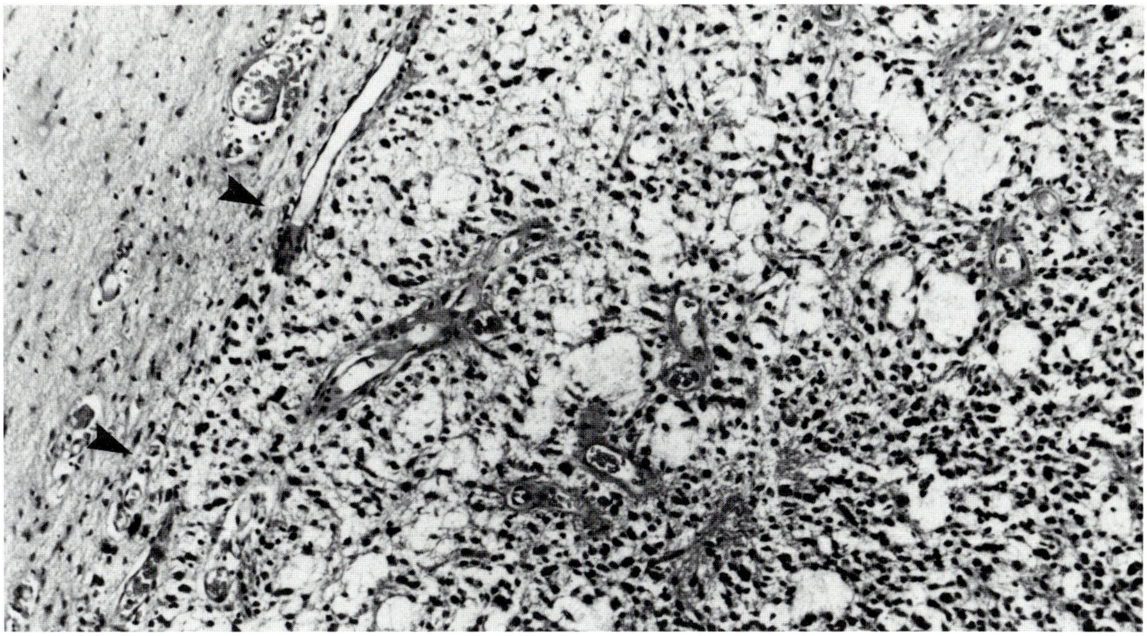

Fig. 25-12. Cystic cerebellar astrocytoma from a child. The tumor is well differentiated, with microcyst formation, and is well demarcated from adjacent cerebellum (arrows). (H & E, ×115.)

growth, they carry a poor prognosis, since they cannot be excised surgically and are not very sensitive to radiotherapy.

Tumors of the brain stem, usually of the pons, also occur principally in children. They are moderately anaplastic and infiltrate widely (Fig. 25-13), often surrounding large numbers of apparently normal neurons and other cells. They cannot be removed, and the response to radiotherapy is variable; the prognosis is ultimately poor.

Oligodendroglioma

Oligodendrogliomas are uncommon and occur in middle-aged and elderly patients, usually in the white matter of one frontal lobe. They spread through the cortex, often presenting beneath the meninges (which they do not usually invade). They arise from mature oligodendroglial cells.

Grossly, they are seen to be ill-defined lesions expanding the white matter, blurring its demarcation from the cortex, and occasionally undergoing cystic necrosis. Because of their characteristic slow growth and location they may grow to a large size without producing disabling symptoms, particularly without focal signs.

Histologically, they appear cellular, with vacuolated cytoplasm and round, uniform darkly stained nuclei resembling those of normal oligodendroglia (Fig. 25-14). They may show small focal areas of calcification, sometimes sufficiently dense to suggest the diagnosis radiologically. They frequently contain foci of apparently neoplastic astrocytes, suggesting that either undifferentiated precursor cells have become neoplastic and are producing both oligodendroglia and astrocytes, or that the oligodendroglia themselves are changing to astrocytic forms, as they frequently do in tissue culture.

On electron-microscopic examination, areas of typical oligodendroglioma show closely packed cells with little extracellular space and uniform, round nuclei. Small numbers of glial filaments are present in the cytoplasm, and miniature processes may be seen clustered between the cells.

In tissue culture, the oligodendroglioma cells, which migrate early, show short, branching processes and an elliptical cell body reminiscent of the form seen on silver-staining (see Chap. 2); they are said to exhibit rhythmic, pulsatile movements. Later, they appear to become astrocytes.

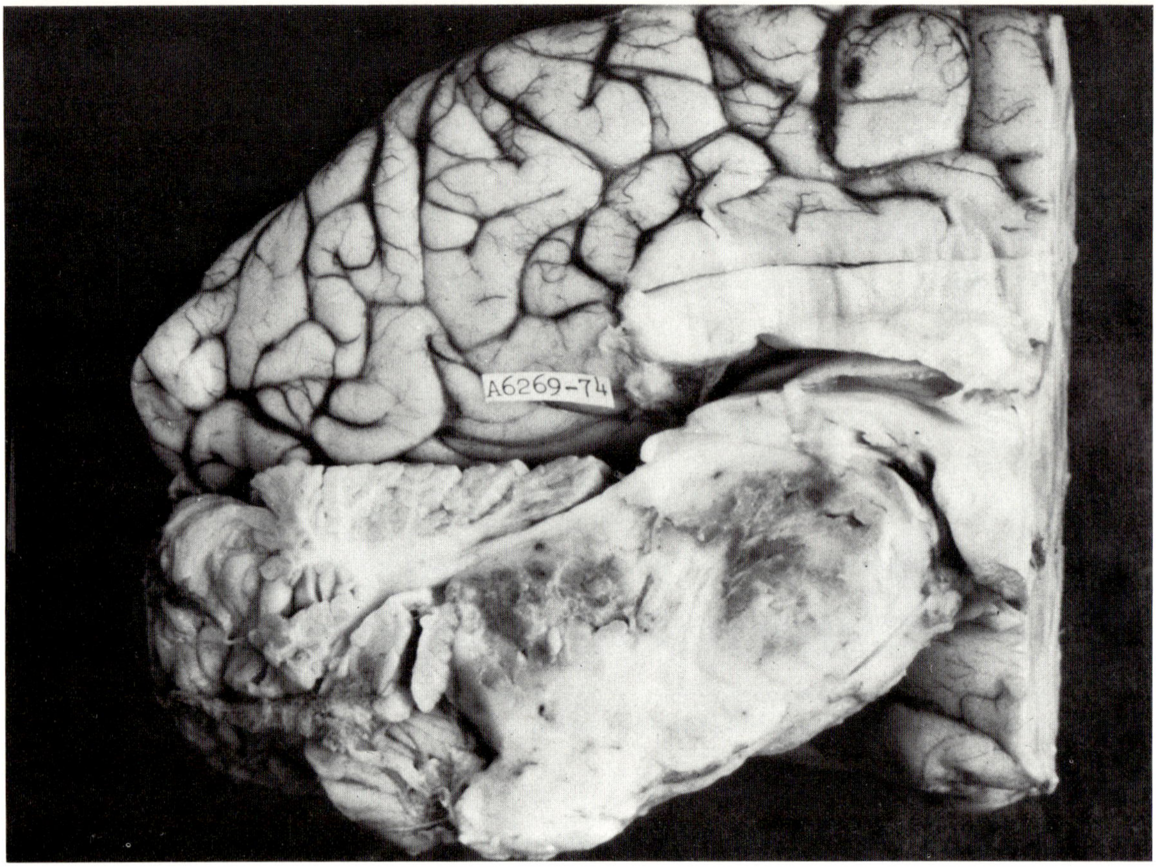

Fig. 25-13. Astrocytoma of pons from a child, showing local infiltration and diffuse, irregular enlargement of the pons.

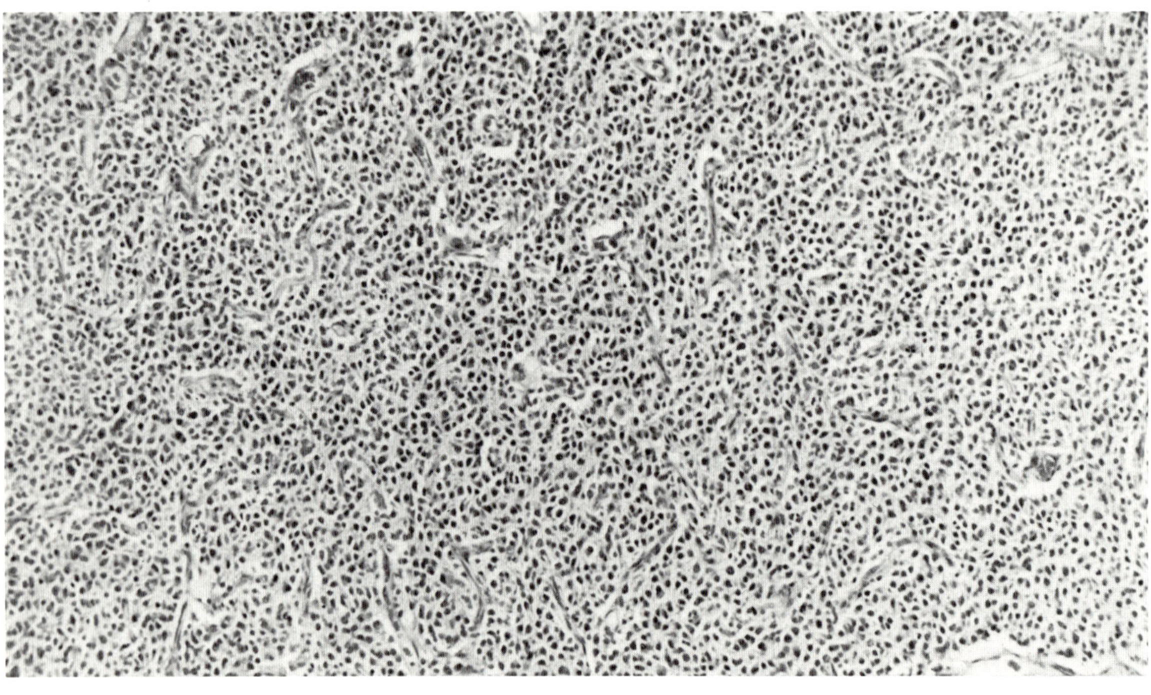

Fig. 25-14. Oligodendroglioma showing small, dark nuclei and pale, often vacuolated cytoplasm. (H & E, ×115.)

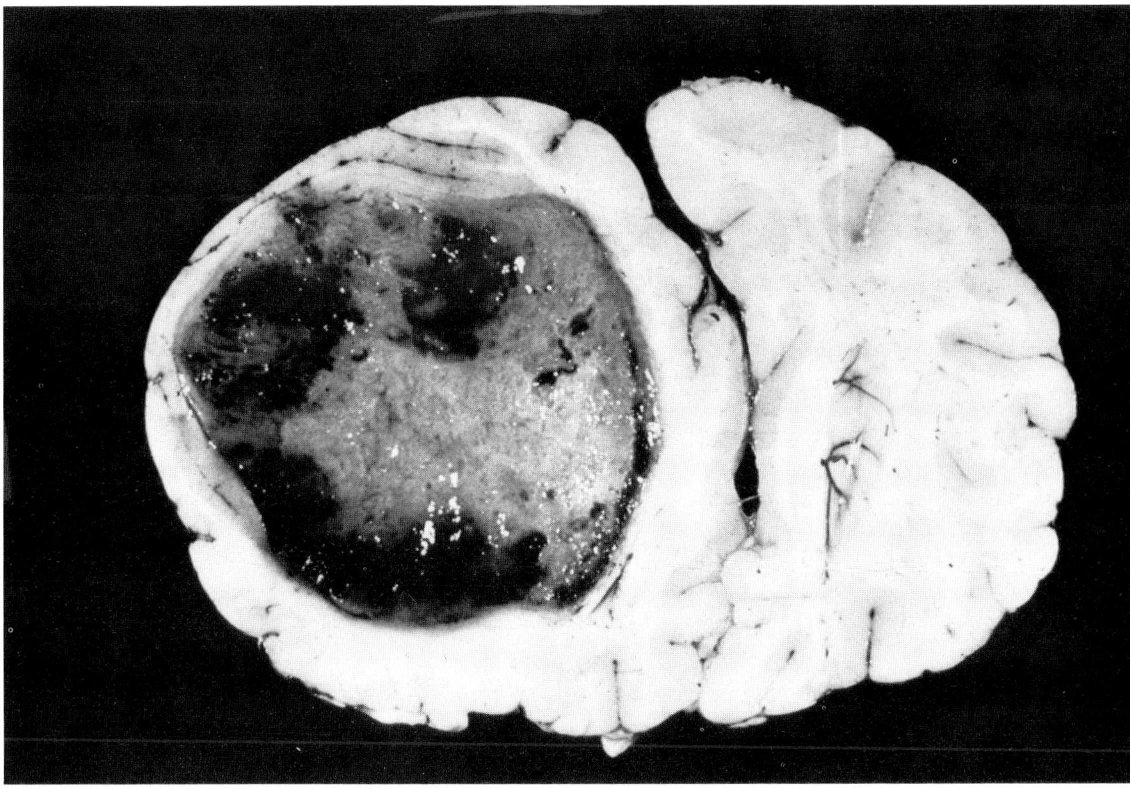

Fig. 25-15. Ependymoma (viewed from behind) distending the left lateral ventricle of a child. The tumor is well defined and is soft and hemorrhagic.

Ependymoma

Ependymomas arise from mature ependymal cells, most frequently occurring in relation to the lateral ventricles or central canal of the cord in adults or to the fourth ventricle in children. Seen grossly, they usually form well-defined vascular tumors within the ventricular cavity (Fig. 25-15) or brain substance.

Some show very little anaplasia and form papillae (Fig. 25-16) and perivascular rosettes in which thin-walled vessels are surrounded by a radial layer of columnar cells with fine cell processes directed toward the vessel wall. More anaplastic ependymomas form sheets of closely packed nuclei, usually elliptical in shape, with a dense chromatin pattern. However, traces of perivascular rosettes or occasional true rosettes with an internal limiting membrane can usually be found on extensive search. These tumors are said to contain blepharoplasts, but this often proves extremely difficult or impossible to demonstrate. The more anaplastic tumors metastasize freely in CSF pathways (Fig. 25-17) and are frequently associated with nodules of metastatic growth on the surface of the cord and among the roots of the cauda equina.

Electron-microscopically, the nature of these tumors can usually be recognized by the presence of microvilli, although these are often distorted and may be packed into small invaginations of the extracellular space into the cell body. Cilia and cell junctions may be seen, and the cytoplasm contains moderate numbers of microtubules. Highly anaplastic ependymomas, however, may show very few of these features, but there may be widening of the extracellular space. Glial filaments are absent or scanty, in contrast to anaplastic astrocytomas.

Choroid Plexus Papilloma

The classification of choroid plexus papilloma is controversial, but it is included here as an intrinsic CNS tumor only on the dual assumptions that the primary overgrowth is of choroid plexus epithelium (an ependymal derivative) rather than of the meningeal stroma, and that it is a neoplasm rather than a hyperplasia or developmental defect. It seems to consist of well differentiated choroid plexus. Such tumors have been implicated as possibly causing hydrocephalus by oversecretion of CSF or obstruction of CSF flow.

Often an incidental autopsy finding, the tumor forms a compact, rounded, intraventricular mass, differing from normal choroid plexus only in its size and tendency to severe stromal vacuolation.

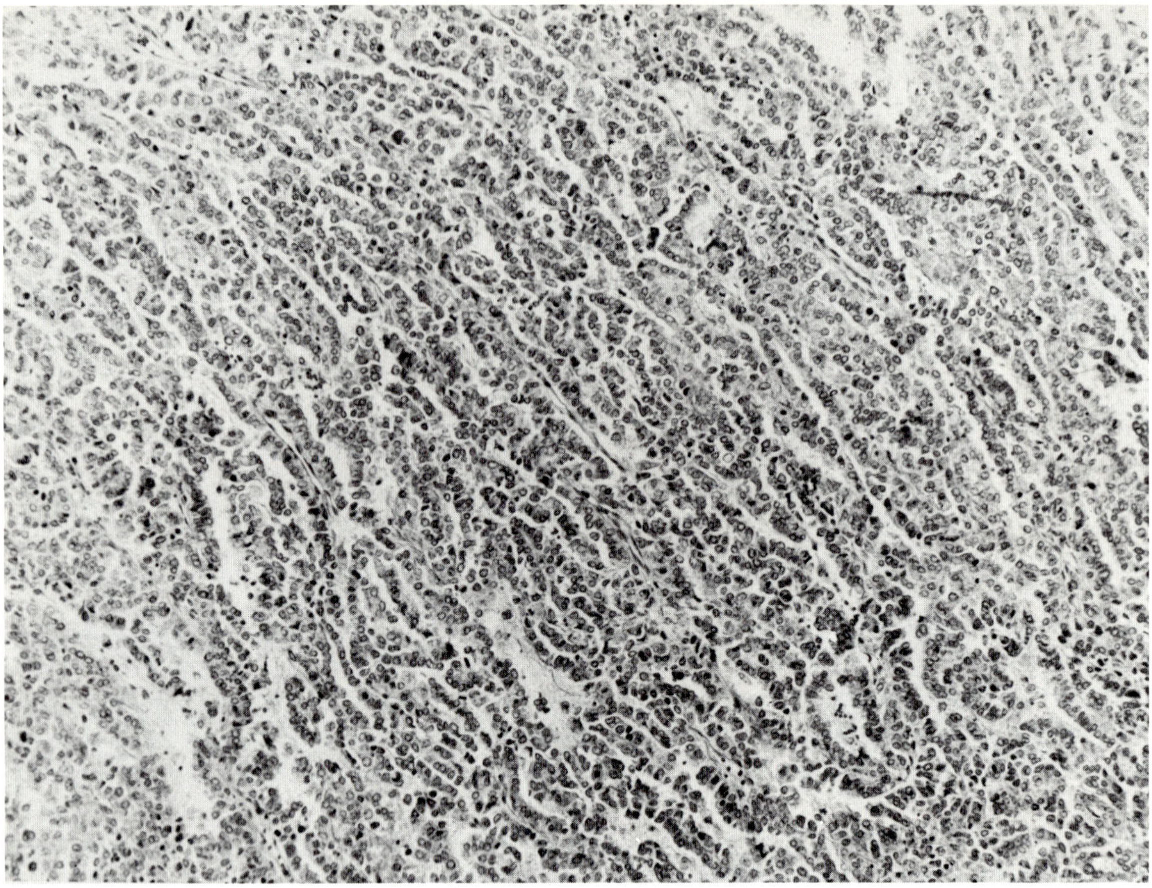

Fig. 25-16. Ependymoma. This example shows a papillary rather than a rosette pattern and thin-walled vessels bearing a layer of irregularly columnar cells. (H & E, X115.)

Radiation Damage to the Central Nervous System

Although many degrees of experimental radiation damage, the slightest of them reversible, have been described, two appear to be of clinical significance: *acute radionecrosis,* which can be produced in normal tissues by doses of radiation considerably larger than the therapeutic dose, and *delayed radionecrosis,* which, although not sharply delineated from the acute process, usually has the following differential characteristics:

1. The radiation dosage employed is within or close to accepted therapeutic levels.
2. Tissue necrosis is selective, and not total as in acute radionecrosis.
3. There is a period of latency, varying from months to years, during which neurological function appears to be entirely normal.
4. There is selectivity for certain regions of the CNS.

Thus, one of the risks of applying therapeutic radiation doses to a neoplasm is the possibility that it may induce delayed radionecrosis in adjacent normal tissues. This danger emphasizes the desirability of a very sharp drop in dosage rate at the edge of the neoplasm. The incidence of delayed radionecrosis is unclear; the reported incidence in the cord, for example, varies from 0.6 to 12.5% (whether irradiation was for spinal or extraspinal lesions is immaterial).

Acute radionecrosis is not usually a clinical problem, since doses far in excess of those used therapeutically are necessary to produce it. It is characterized by nonspecific acute cell necrosis associated with generalized membrane damage, the significant membrane in this case probably being lysosomal. In addition, there is hyperemia, edema, and diapedesis of blood cells, providing clear evidence of massive barrier damage, probably again due to membrane destruction.

Delayed Radionecrosis

Delayed radionecrosis is a recognized complication of radiation for neoplasms in the CNS or adjacent tissue, although why it should occur in a few cases and be absent in the majority is unknown.

Radiation Encephalopathy. This develops acutely after a latent interval of many months, with local or generalized seizures and frequent, sudden stupor or coma. Characteristic lesions involve the white matter

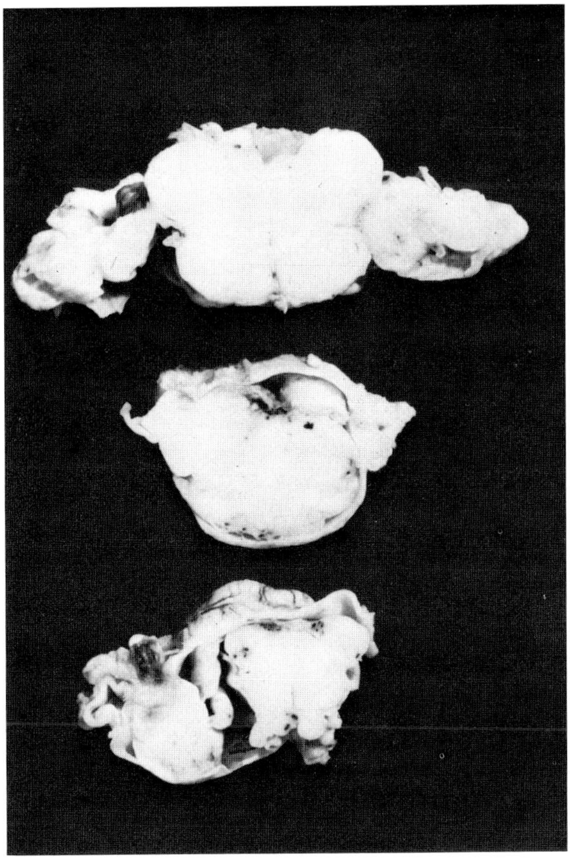

Fig. 25-17. Ependymoma. Nodules of tumor from a primary growth in the lateral ventricle have "seeded" the subarachnoid space and nerve roots around the medulla.

and vary from extensive areas of cystic necrosis (with more or less fibrillary gliosis, depending on survival time), through multiple, relatively discrete demyelinated areas somewhat reminiscent of multiple sclerosis, to a single zone surrounding the site of the tumor.

The susceptible element appears to be the oligodendroglial cell, yet the satellite oligodendroglia in gray matter may be unaffected. This difference might be due to a higher PO_2 in white matter because of the lower rate of metabolism, or to the paucity of mitochondria in interfascicular as opposed to perineuronal oligodendroglia, oxygen being diffusely distributed throughout the cytoplasm instead of concentrated in the numerous mitochondria, as in satellite cells.

In addition to the loss of oligodendroglial cells and myelin, there is evidence of vascular damage, including perivascular hemorrhages and edema and small focal areas of infarction. Vessel walls may be markedly thickened and associated with collagenous scar tissue, and dilated vascular channels (ectasias) are often seen. Astrocytes survive, but frequently in bizarre, hyperchromatic, often multinucleate forms, with increased oxidative enzyme activity.

Lesions are not absolutely confined to white matter and may transgress the overlying cortex. Regional susceptibility has also been reported in the hypothalamus. This may also be related to a particularly high PO_2 due to the extensive blood supply.

Radiation Myelopathy. This has a latent interval varying from a few months to two or three years, probably averaging 9 to 12 months. It may present either with sensory or motor symptoms, usually associated with sphincter dysfunction. Primary changes are limited to the irradiated sections of the cord, but ascending and descending secondary demyelination occur because of axonal destruction. The topography of the lesions is varied, some involving the entire cross section and some localized in white matter, especially the deeper posterior and superficial posterolateral areas. They may be multifocal. Histopathological changes are similar in all respects to those described in the brain.

Latency. The cause of latency in this disastrous complication is unknown. Endothelial cells are mitotically active at a slow rate, and cumulative abnormalities of DNA might account for the vascular changes that are usually present. However, such changes are not invariable, and may be spatially dissociated from the prominent areas of loss of oligodendroglial cells and myelin. Mitotic activity in normal oligodendroglia has not been described.

NEUROENDOCRINE TUMORS

Both the endocrine organs within the craniospinal cavity – the pituitary and pineal glands – are susceptible to neoplasia. Little is known of the function of the normal pineal gland (see Chap. 8), and generalized endocrine disturbances are not associated with pineal tumors. (Precocious puberty, which is reported relatively rarely, might be due to pressure on the hypothalamus, either directly or because of noncommunicating hydrocephalus.) Tumors of the anterior pituitary are among the more common in the cranial cavity and are often associated with endocrine dysfunction, either hypopituitarism due to destruction of the normal glandular tissue by the expanding neoplasm or, less often, overproduction of pituitary hormones by the neoplasm itself. Because of the location of the pituitary gland, its tumors are often associated with visual defects.

Tumors of the Pineal

The term *pinealoma* has confusing connotations, since it has frequently been applied to tumors occurring in the pineal region with a histological structure resembling the seminoma of the testis (dysgerminoma of the ovary), which are in fact teratomas. Such tumors include *ectopic pinealomas,* since they may also occur in the region of the infundibulum and pituitary (see p. 510).

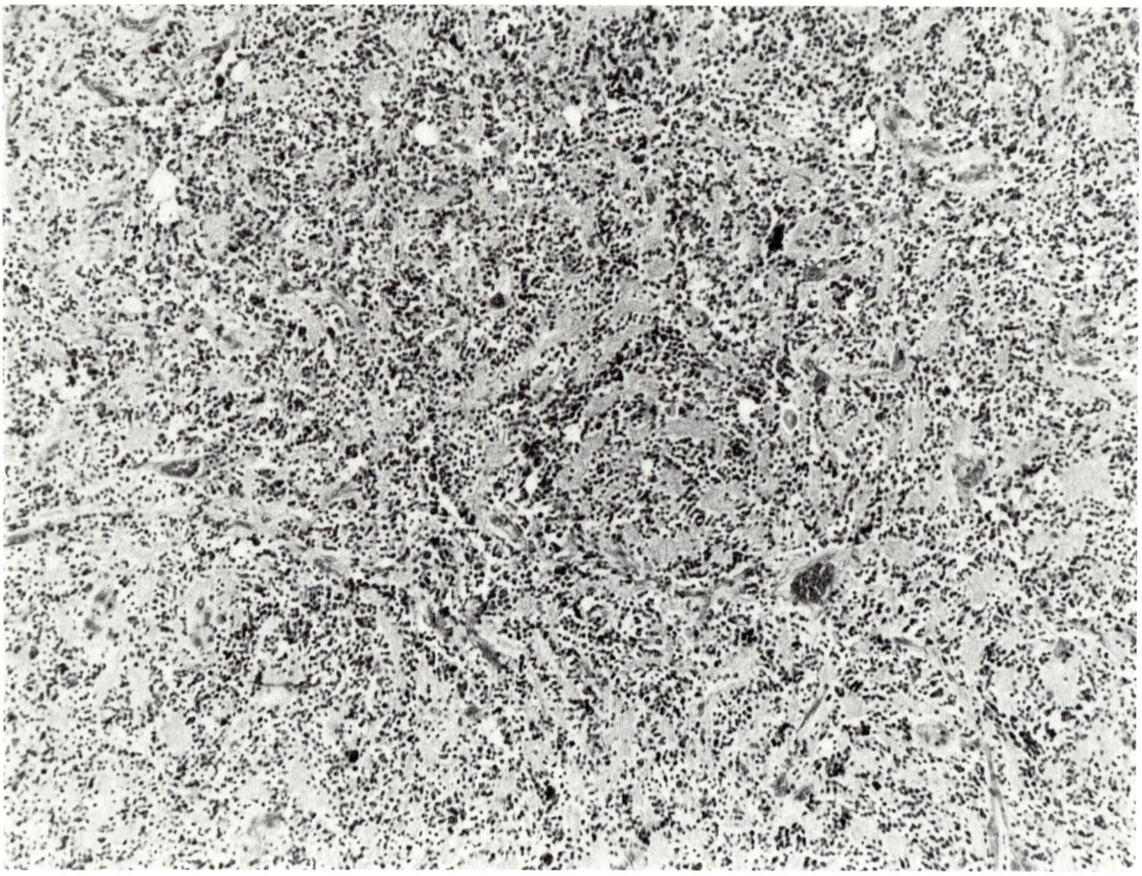

Fig. 25-18. Pinealoma. Often an incidental autopsy finding or a cause of noncommunicating hydrocephalus, it closely recapitulates the structure of the normal gland. (H & E, ×115.)

True pineal neoplasms are rare and include the very unusual *pineoblastoma,* an aggressive embryonal tumor with early, extensive CSF metastasis, and the ordinary *pinealoma (pineocytoma),* presumably derived from mature pineal cells. These tumors are usually noninvasive and slowly growing and may be incidental autopsy findings. Microscopically (Fig. 25-18), they usually resemble the normal pineal gland. A small number of clinically malignant metastasizing tumors are more anaplastic. Locally expanding pinealomas occasionally cause noncommunicating hydrocephalus because of pressure on the midbrain or invagination into the third ventricle.

Tumors of the Pituitary

Except for rare small masses discovered incidentally in the neurohypophysis, pituitary tumors arise in the adenohypophysis and are usually benign, relatively slowly growing, and circumscribed. However, their expansion may erode surrounding bone (including the clinoid processes), cause atrophy or distortion of the optic nerves, chiasm, or tracts, produce pressure on the hypothalamus, or invaginate the third ventricle. Although histologically innocent, these pituitary adenomas tend to infiltrate their capsules as well as adjacent meninges, but only rarely transgress the dura or invade the brain. If capsular and meningeal invasion is extensive, the paradoxical term *malignant*

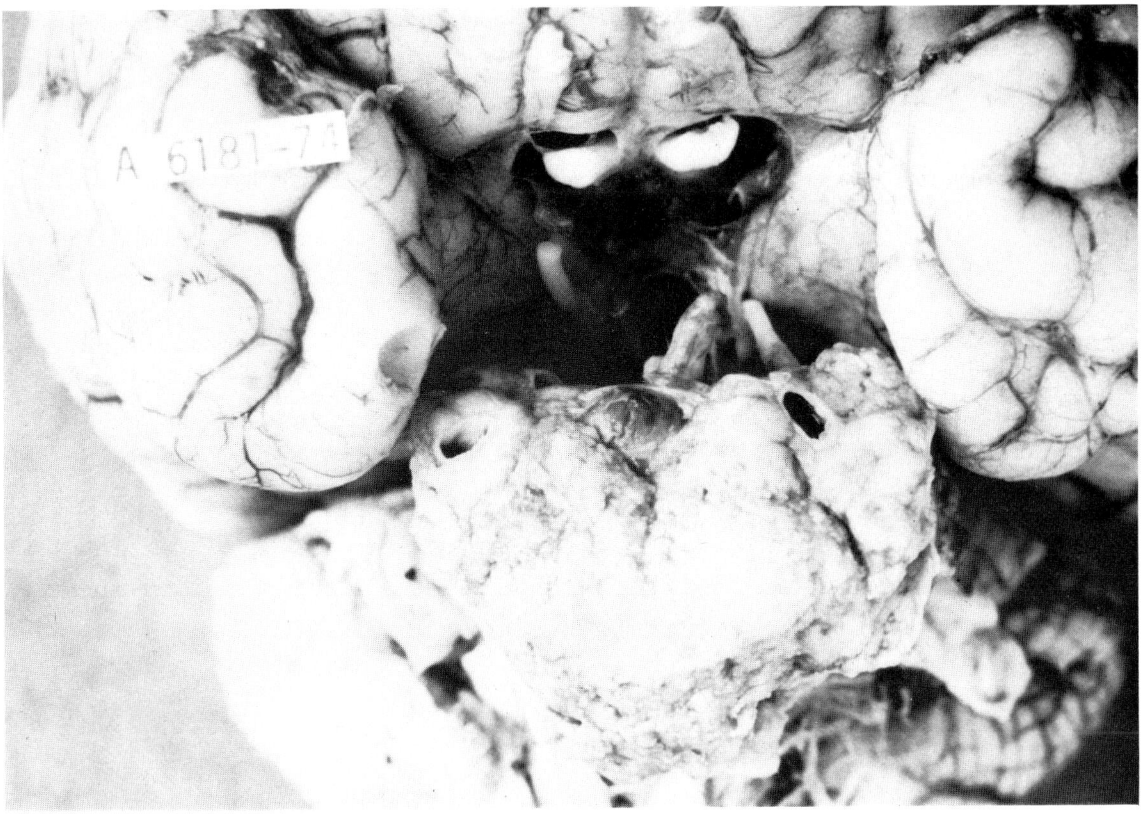

Fig. 25-19. Chromophobe adenoma. This is a large, locally invasive example, which, in spite of being histologically benign, has infiltrated around the carotid arteries, trigeminal nerves, and other structures.

adenoma has been proposed, but this is semantically dubious, and it appears preferable to regard this as normal biological behavior for these tumors. True malignancy, with CNS invasion and occasional metastasis, is very rare.

Chromophobe Adenoma

About 80% of pituitary adenomas appear to be derived from nonsecretory cells. These are the chromophobe adenomas, which are soft, locally invasive, or encapsulated tumors (Fig. 25-19), from pale pink to red, depending on their vascularity, and occasionally showing cystic change or even severe tumor hemorrhage.

The cells are small and polygonal, with uniform, rounded nuclei and pale eosinophilic cytoplasm that is usually nongranular. They are often arranged in diffuse sheets with little stroma (Fig. 25-20), but occasionally a vascular stroma is prominent, and cells may show a papillary arrangement, which in no way alters their biological behavior.

Chromophobe adenomas may cause pressure effects as noted above and may be associated with overt or subclinical hypopituitarism due to pressure on the surrounding normal gland. Reports of Cushing's syndrome associated with chromophobe adenoma indicate that some of these apparently nonsecretory tumors are in fact producing adrenocorticotropic hormone (and possibly melanocyte-stimulating hormone). Occasionally, apparent chromophobe adenomas are associated with acromegaly, indicating secretion

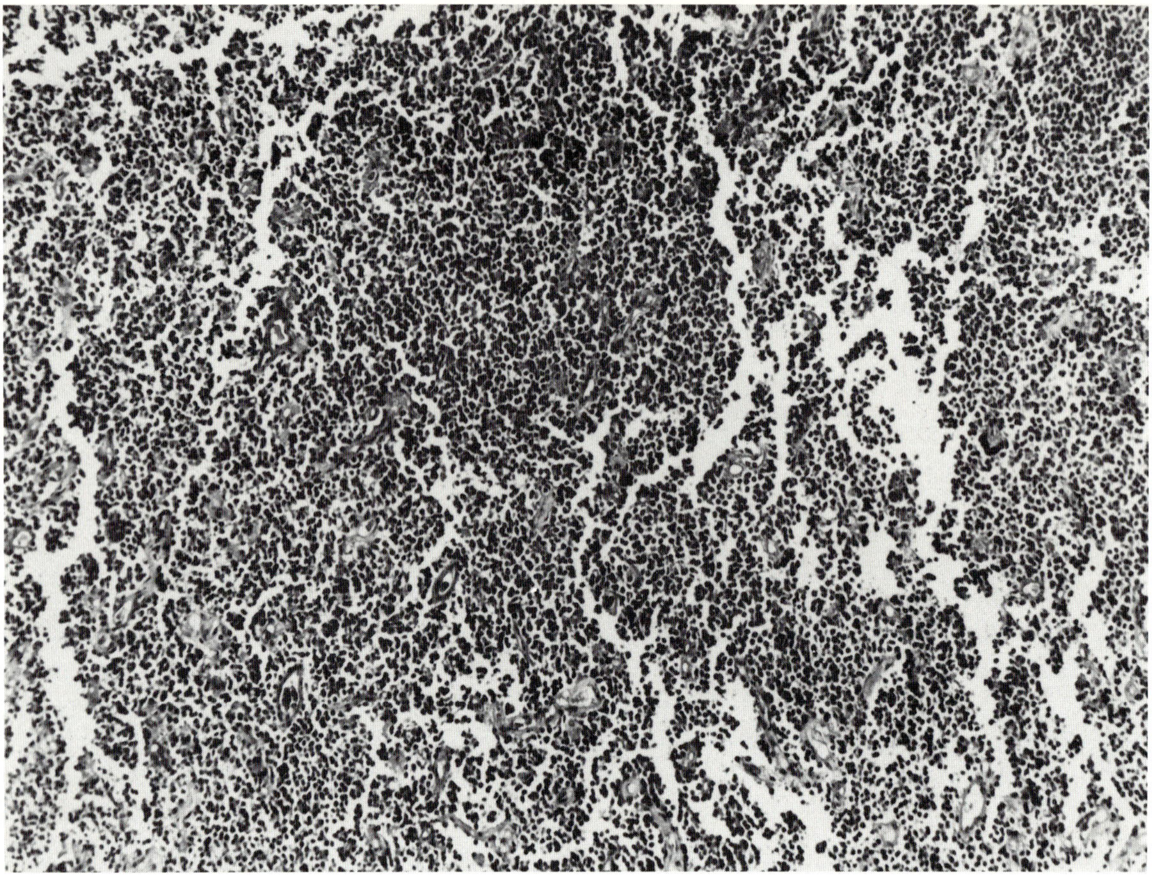

Fig. 25-20. Chromophobe adenoma showing uniform, featureless sheets of small cells with dark round nuclei. (H & E, X115.)

of growth hormone, perhaps related to the not infrequent presence of cells showing a few eosinophilic granules. Nonetheless, the majority of these tumors appear to be truly nonsecretory and presumably derived from chromophobe cells, the exceptional minority indicating only the inadequacies of light-microscopic examination.

Eosinophil Adenoma

Eosinophil adenomas make up most of the remaining 20% of pituitary tumors. Many patients show diffuse somatic tissue hyperplasia or frank acromegaly, indicating that these are functional growth hormone-secreting neoplasms. Seen grossly, they are similar to the chromophobe variety.

Microscopically, they are seen to be cellular, with no characteristic architectural arrangement, and may exhibit more pleomorphism than chromophobe tumors, though still lacking mitotic activity. The cytoplasm shows eosinophilia, and variable numbers of granules are seen.

Basophil Adenoma

Less common than the other two types of pituitary tumors are the basophil adenomas, many of which are incidental autopsy discoveries (Fig. 25-21). They rarely grow to the size of the preceding types, but in proportion to their small absolute numbers, they

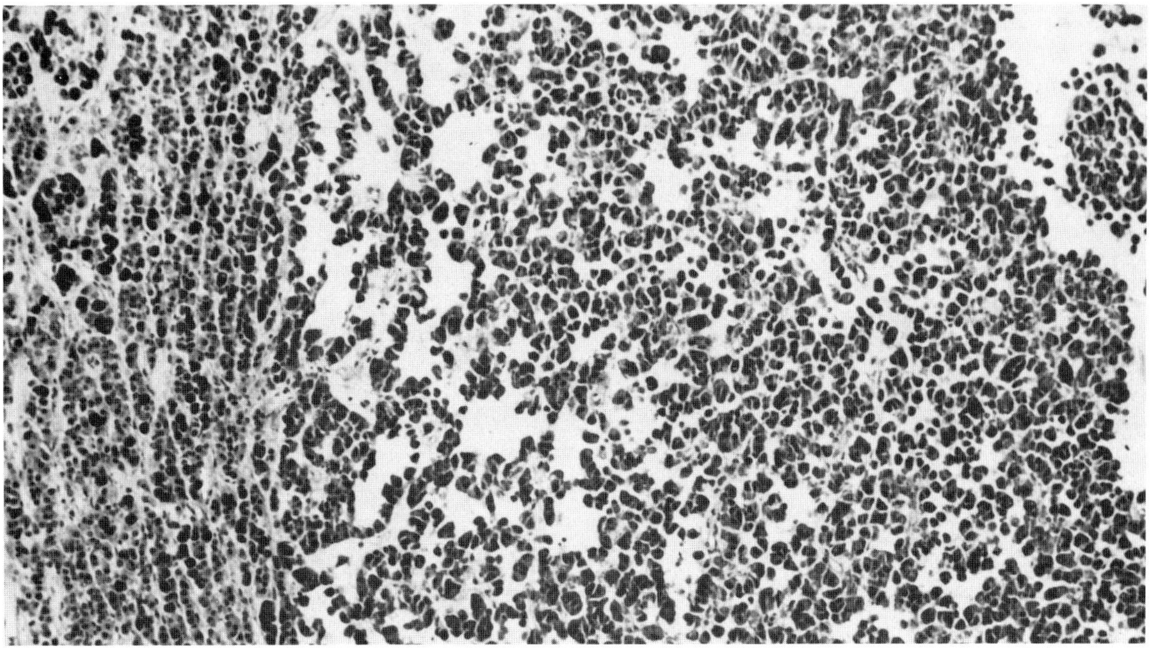

Fig. 25-21. Basophil adenoma discovered incidentally at autopsy. Normal pituitary tissue is seen to the left. (H & E, ×115.)

metastasize relatively often. Polygonal cells in these tumors are randomly arranged, with a scant vascular stroma, and contain basophilic granules.

Most cases of Cushing's syndrome (pituitary basophilism) are not associated with pituitary tumor; in those that are, most of the tumors appear to be chromophobic. It is suggested that in Cushing's syndrome (other than those cases associated with autonomous adrenal adenoma or carcinoma) the primary defect is excessive secretion of (still undiscovered) corticotropin releasing factor, which may be associated only with Crooke's hyaline degeneration in the pituitary or (in decreasing order of frequency) with chromophobe adenoma, basophil adenoma, or rare metastasizing basophilic carcinoma.

NEURAL CREST TUMORS

The neural crest is thought to be the origin of leptomeningeal cells (meningocytes), Schwann's cells, and melanocytes within the cranial and spinal cavities. The meningocytes form the pia, arachnoid, and periadventitial sheaths of penetrating vessels and the arachnoid villi and arachnoidal granulations that invade the dural sinuses. Schwann's cells are present in the cranial and spinal nerve roots. Melanocytes are scattered in the meninges and are often readily seen on the ventral and lateral surfaces of the medulla as a diffuse, brownish-black pigmentation. Benign tumors derived from meningocytes and Schwann's cells are each common within both the cranial and spinal cavities. Tumors of the melanocytes are rare, often multicentric, and highly malignant.

Meningioma

Meningiomas are more common in women than men and usually present at or after middle age. Paradoxically, in view of their leptomeningeal origin, they are usually firmly attached to the dura, which is locally infiltrated by tumor cells. Where possible, they grow as round, sharply defined, expanding lesions, which, if they reach significant size, produce deformity of the brain or cord and cause pressure symptoms such as sensory and upper motoneuron lesions in the cord, or seizures from pressure on the motor cortex.

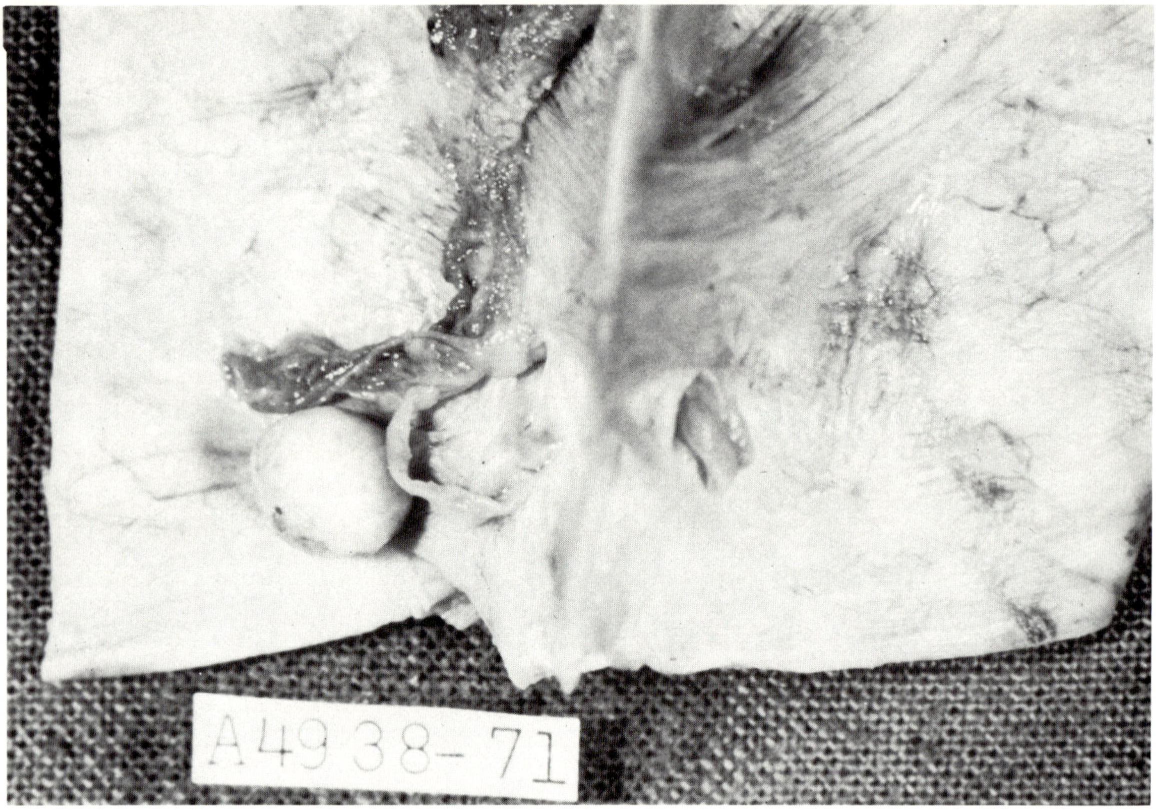

Fig. 25-22. Meningioma showing a rounded mass that is firmly attached near the junction of dura and falx. Larger tumors in this location often cause clinical symptoms.

Attachment to the dura is commonly in the region of the venous sinuses, especially at the root of the falx (Fig. 25-22), along the greater wing of the sphenoid, or at the root of the tentorium in the posterior fossa. Small, often multiple meningiomas are not uncommon as incidental autopsy findings in elderly patients. Especially over the vault, meningiomas may transgress the dura and infiltrate the bone, producing a local area of thickening (meningioma en plaque). Depending on their content of collagen and reticulin, they vary in consistency from soft and fleshy to firm and gritty and only occasionally show areas of necrosis and cyst formation.

Normal meningocytes may form a flat surface epithelium (meningothelium) lining subarachnoid spaces or may be fibroblast-like cells capable of forming reticulin and collagen. A tendency to form epithelial sheets devoid of reticulin, and to form spindle-shaped cells with reticulin production, is manifested in varying proportions in each meningioma. Some tumors consist largely of sheets and clumps of polygonal cells, with uniform, pale nuclei and scanty connective tissue septa that contain the only reticulin. This is the *meningotheliomatous* (misnamed *syncytial*) variety (Fig. 25-23). Others consist of interlacing bundles of parallel spindle-shaped cells, separated by more or less extensive deposits of reticulin and collagen, the *fibrous* meningomas (Fig. 25-24). The *transitional* form includes both meningotheliomatous and fibrous areas, but is characterized particularly by the presence of psammoma bodies (Fig. 25-25), which are small, whorled structures that frequently contain

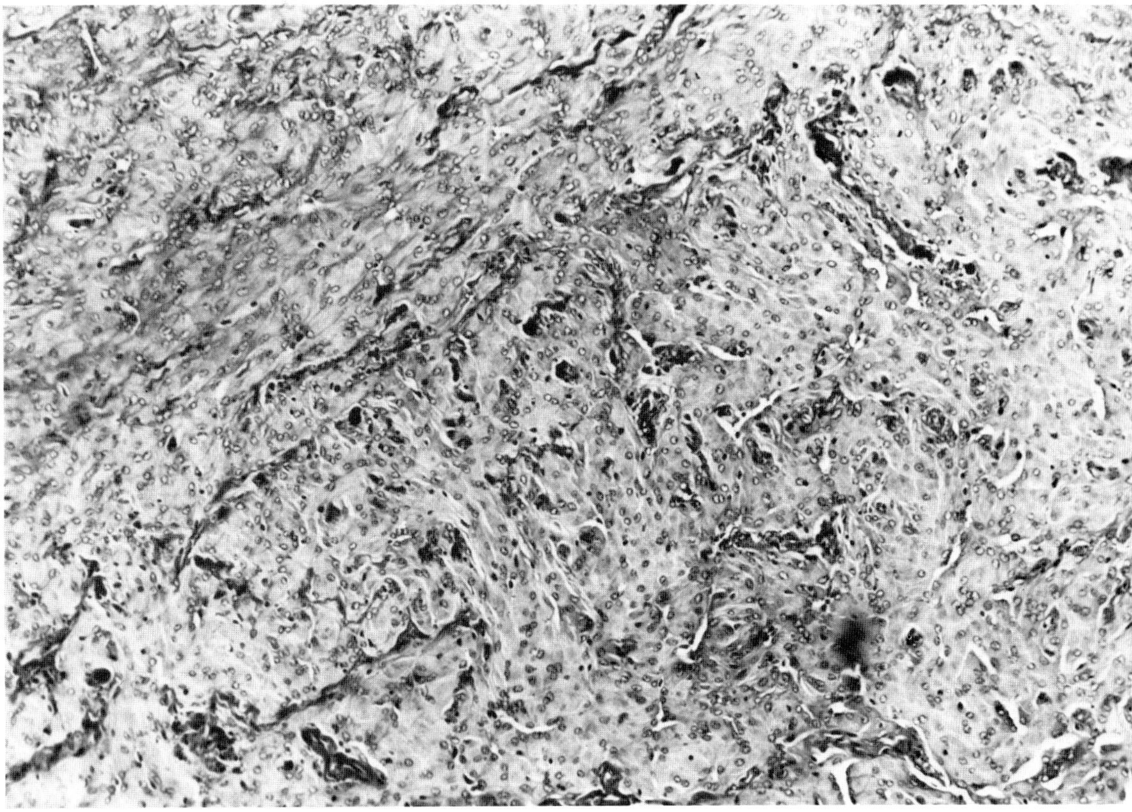

Fig. 25-23. Meningotheliomatous ("syncytial") meningioma, with epithelioid sheets of polygonal cells. (H & E, ×115.)

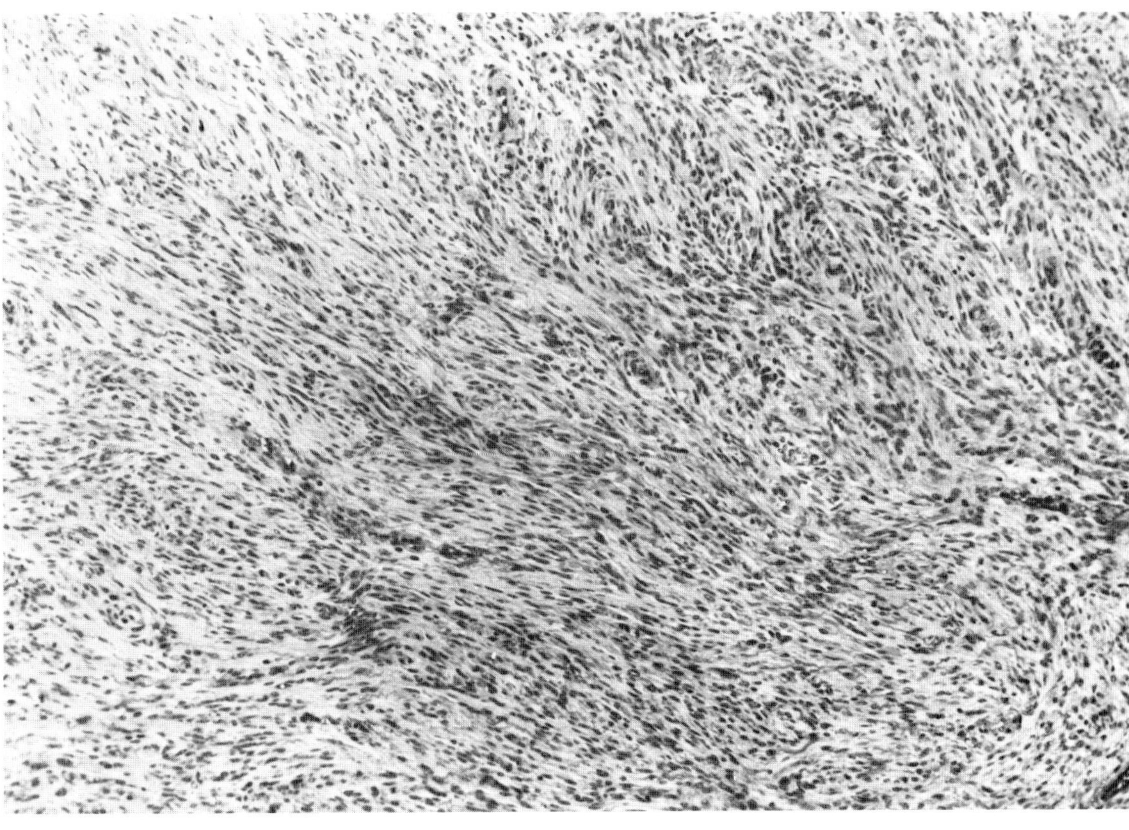

Fig. 25-24. Fibrous meningioma. (H & E, ×115.)

a calcified central area that gives a gritty sensation on cutting.

Whether a meningioma is meningotheliomatous, transitional, or fibrous, the prognosis is similar (usually good if removed before irreversible pressure changes have been produced in the CNS). Like pituitary adenomas, meningiomas show a tendency to infiltrate their capsules and also to invade the dura and overlying bone, which may be thick and hyperostotic. This local aggressiveness is not indicative of malignancy, since these tumors rarely invade the CNS.

Occasional exceptions to the preceding generalizations occur. Rare meningiomas are not situated in the subarachnoid space attached to the dura, but are in the ventricular system, usually the lateral ventricles attached to the choroid plexus or tela choroidea. A few meningiomas exhibit true local malignancy in that they transgress the pia and invade the brain. They frequently show some mitotic activity and greater nuclear pleomorphism than typical meningiomas. Metastasizing meningiomas, however, are exceedingly rare.

Angioblastic Meningioma

A further type of solid tumor firmly attached to the dura (usually above the tentorium) is the angioblastic meningioma. These highly vascular tumors, with a dense, intersecting reticulin network, resemble blood-vessel tumors and differ from true meningiomas also in being more highly cellular, more frequently exhibiting mitotic activity, and often containing large, lipid-laden foamy cells (Fig. 25-26). They do not contain fibrous, syncytial, or transitional areas and show a significant biological difference in that they tend to recur locally after excision.

Their cytogenesis remains uncertain. Some consider them to be hemangiopericytomas and others consider them variant true meningiomas. Although the balance of evidence would appear to favor the former view, the term *angioblastic meningioma* will remain, since both clinically and on gross inspection these tumors are indistinguishable from true meningiomas. Electron-microscopic examination and tissue-culture studies may throw some light on the origin of these neoplasms.

Nerve-Root Tumors

Acoustic Schwannoma

Nerve root tumors are common in the craniospinal cavity, but, remarkably, in the cranium the vast majority are confined to the root of the auditory (vestibulocochlear) nerve and are commonly termed *acoustic schwannomas* (Fig. 25-27). Examples in the facial and glossopharyngeal nerves have been reported. These tumors are usually single. Bilateral acoustic schwannomas generally indicate central Recklinghausen's disease (see Chap. 19).

The acoustic schwannoma is an encapsulated, expanding, slowly growing lesion in the cerebellopontine angle. Patients frequently present with deafness, tinnitus, involvement of adjacent cranial nerves, and cerebellar dysfunction. Although benign tumors, their removal is attended by a risk of damage to adjacent structures (including the brain stem), particularly to the anterior inferior cerebellar artery, which runs on the surface of the pons to the internal auditory meatus before turning upward on the middle cerebellar peduncle. These tumors have the characteristic histological features of schwannomas or neurilemomas, differing only in having a slightly greater tendency to nuclear pleomorphism, which may be a regressive phenomenon and does not imply increased malignancy (Fig. 25-28). Microscopically, they show interlacing coarse bands of collagen and reticulin-like material (probably Schwann's cell basement membrane), with plump irregular spindle-shaped nuclei. These nuclei rarely show palisading (unlike peripheral schwannomas); there is no mitotic activity. Degenerative changes are common, and include mucoid areas, fat-laden macrophages, and conspicuous hyalinization of tumor vessels.

Cord Schwannoma

Cord schwannomas are usually on a posterior root, and their expansion may cause cord or nerve-root compression and enlargement of the intervertebral foramen (in the latter case, they are often dumbbell-shaped, situated partly within and partly outside the spinal canal). They are capsulated benign tumors with a characteristic histological appearance.

Neurofibroma

Neurofibromas either of cranial or spinal nerve roots are rare except in Recklinghausen's disease, and unlike the schwannomas, they share with their peripheral relatives a tendency to malignant change. Histologically, they resemble those occurring on peripheral nerves.

MESENCHYMAL TUMORS

The mesenchymal components of the cranial and spinal cavities include the fibrous dura and its internal limiting epithelium, the vascular system with associated reticuloendothelial cells, and microglial cells scattered through the CNS, particularly beneath the ependyma and the pia. The morphological peculiarities of microglia (see Chap. 2) seem to be dictated by the environment, and they are capable of becoming typical macrophages. Neither the dura nor its internal limiting epithelium appears susceptible to tumor formation. However, tumors of blood vessels and primary reticuloendothelial tumors – the former usually benign and the latter usually malignant – are both moderately common within the cranial cavity.

Capillary Hemangioendothelioma

Capillary hemangioendotheliomas are sometimes termed hemangioblastomas, but there is no evidence that they arise from persistent embryonal cells, and the term may thus be inappropriate. They usually present in young or middle-aged adults. The majority of these tumors are in the cerebellum, with fewer

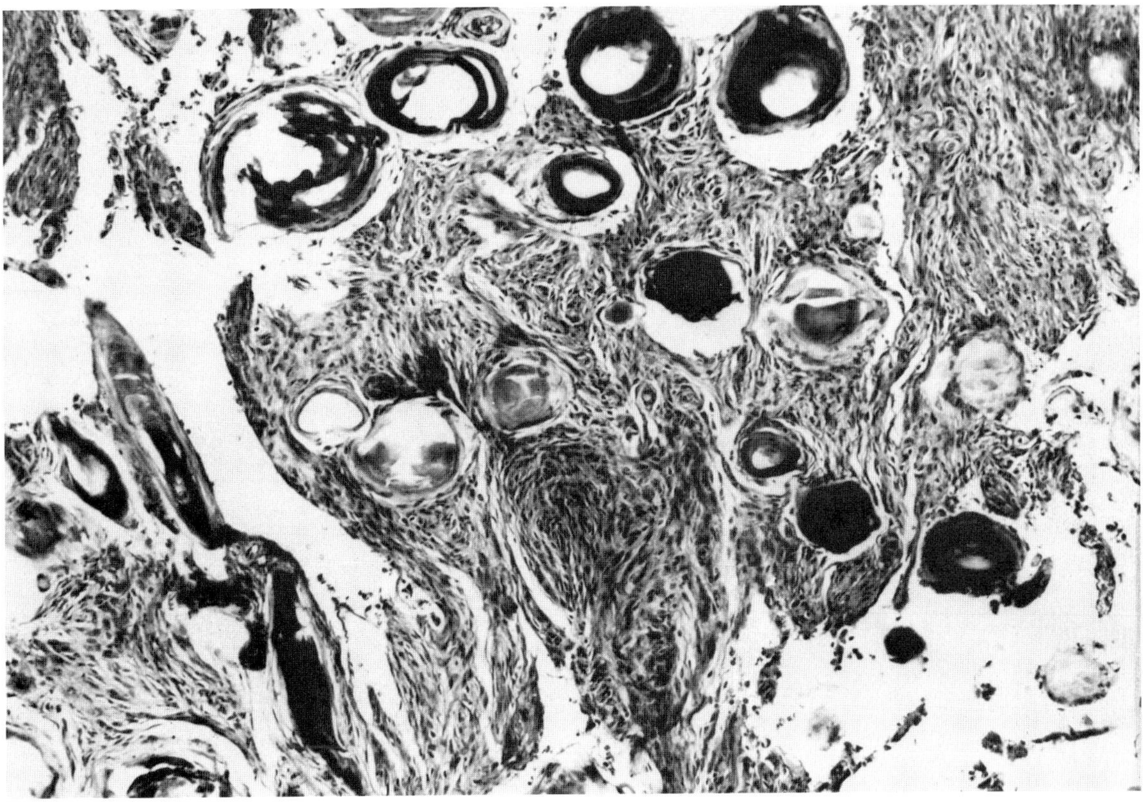

Fig. 25-25. Transitional meningioma, with numerous rounded, mineralized psammoma bodies, which tend to be displaced or fragmented on cutting. (H & E, X115.)

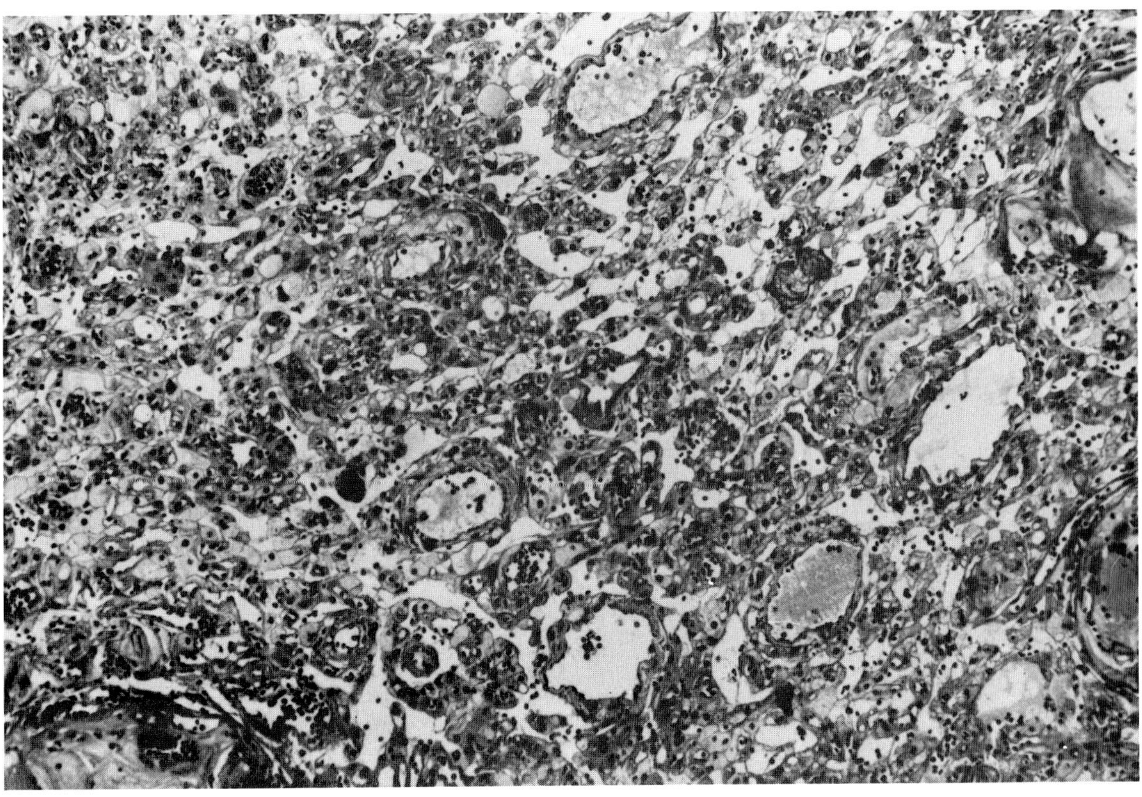

Fig. 25-26. "Angioblastic meningioma," a highly vascular tumor grossly resembling a meningioma, but with few microscopic similarities. Foamy cells may be seen between vessels. (H & E, X115.)

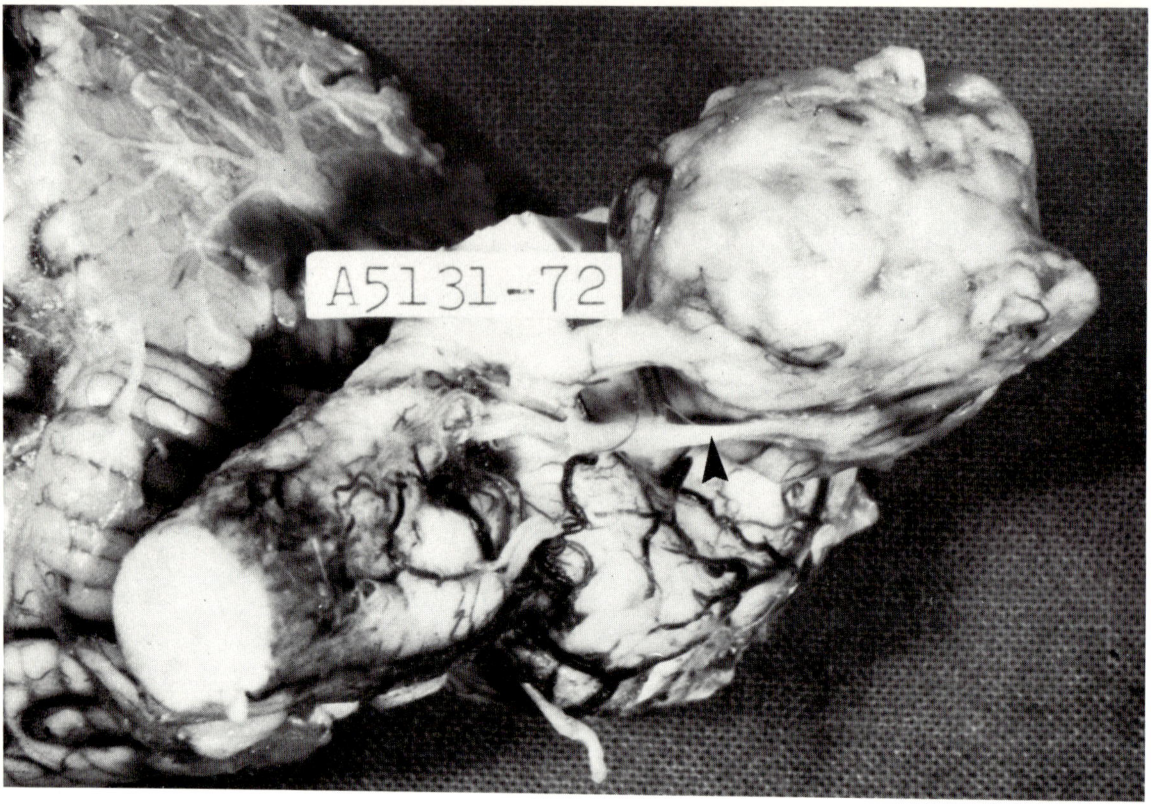

Fig. 25-27. Acoustic schwannoma, showing attachment to the vestibulocochlear (acoustic) nerve and involvement of the facial nerve (arrow) in the capsule.

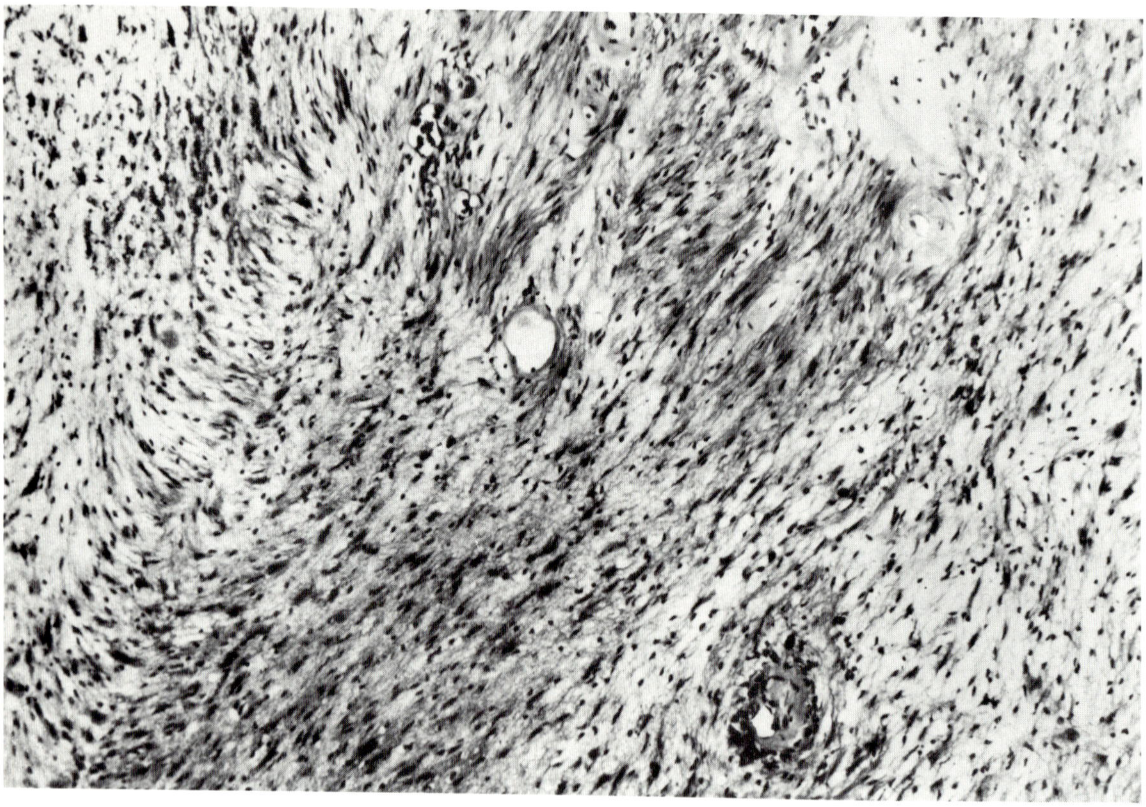

Fig. 25-28. Acoustic schwannoma. These tumors show some nuclear hyperchromatism and pleomorphism, which is apparently innocent, and often mucoid degeneration and foam cells. (H & E, X115.)

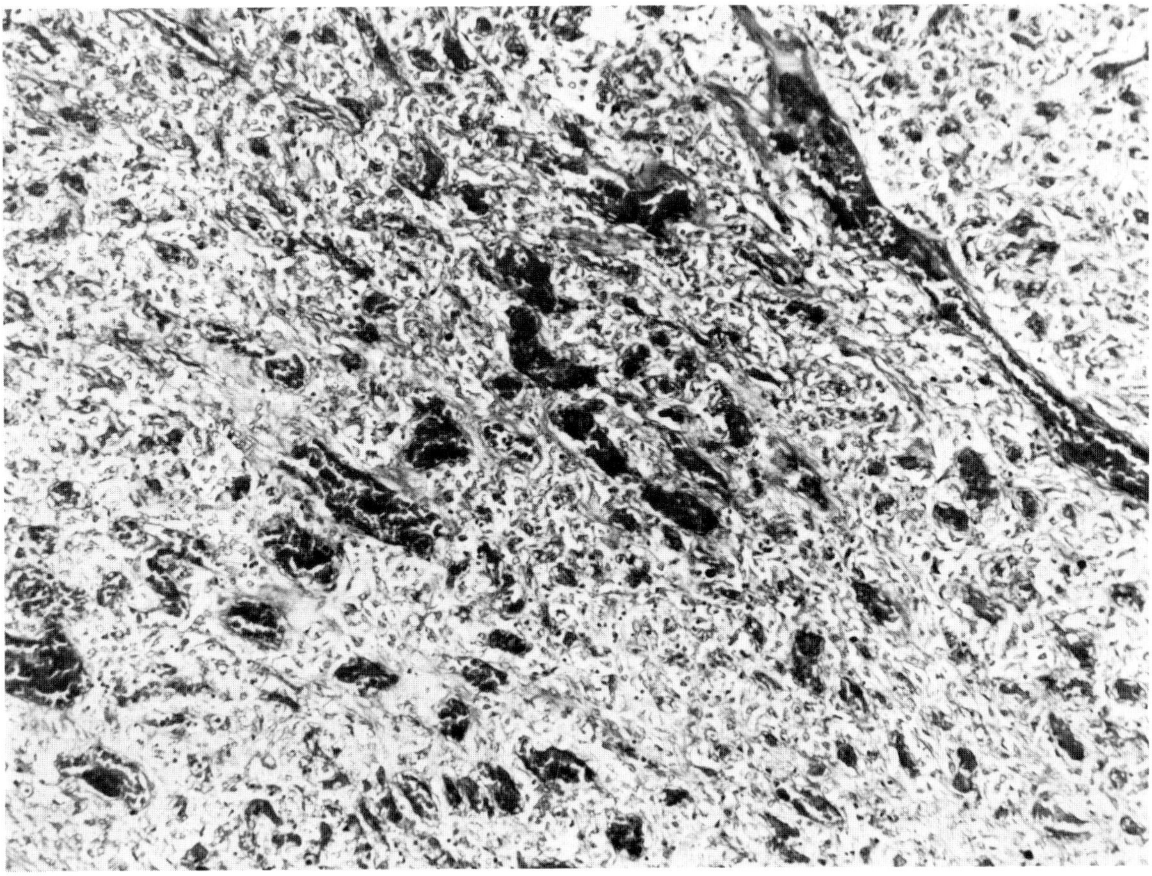

Fig. 25-29. Capillary hemangioendothelioma ("hemangioblastoma") of the cerebellum. Large and small vessels are separated by clumps of polygonal cells. (H & E, X115.)

occurring in the cord. They are exceptional in other areas, unless multiple, as they are in von Hippel-Lindau disease (see Chap. 19).

They are frequently cystic cerebellar tumors, and the neoplasm may be reduced to a small nodule in the wall of a hemorrhagic cyst. Solid tumors are heterogenous on the cut surface, due to areas of old and recent hemorrhage and deposition of fat, and are sharply demarcated from normal cerebellar tissue. Seen histologically, they consist of uniform polygonal or flattened cells, often with vacuolated cytoplasm containing lipid and a dense network of reticulin enclosing clumps of such cells, often with a central lumen, with or without erythrocytes (Fig. 25-29). Nuclei are usually small, dark, and uniform, though large, even bizarre forms are described and apparently do not alter the relatively benign prognosis. However, these tumors are prone to local recurrence.

Reticuloendothelial Tumors

Although the reticuloendothelial system is spread throughout the body, it is not uncommon for hyperplasia or neoplasia to develop focally, with or without later spread to other areas. The CNS is often involved in lymphomas that apparently originate elsewhere in the body. Such CNS involvement is often difficult to treat, since chemotherapeutic agents may fail to cross a relatively intact blood-brain barrier following systemic administration.

Reticuloendothelial Neoplasms Primary in the Brain

There are now many recorded cases supported by adequate autopsy examination in which reticuloendothelial tumors are present only in the CNS and absent elsewhere. Grossly, such lesions may take the form of a single, well-defined tumor (often located anteriorly in a hemisphere) or a more diffuse proliferation, often involving the subarachnoid, perivascular, and periventricular areas (Fig. 25-30).

As in other sites, the distinction between hyperplasia and neoplasia in this group appears unclear, and the histological picture varies from a mixed exudate of reticular cells with lymphocytes, plasma cells, and histiocytes, many of which stain positively with silver (a sign of some functional differentiation), and scanty mitotic activity, to a frank reticulum cell sarcoma (Fig. 25-31), with nuclear pleomorphism, multiple mitoses, and no silver-staining. The former tumors tend to be confined to the perivascular regions, whereas the latter frankly infiltrate the CNS, although often retaining a prominent perivascular component.

Thus, it appears more probable that reticuloendothelial cells in the adventitia, rather than microglial cells, are primarily concerned in the neoplastic process. Probably both are ultimately affected, and these tumors are termed either *reticulum cell sarcomas* or *microgliomas.* The clinical course tends to be rapid, but most patients respond relatively well to radiation, with many three to five year survivals.

Histiocytosis in the Central Nervous System

Solitary pleomorphic tumors resembling histiocytosis may be seen in the infundibular region, or an infundibular mass may be associated with similar lesions elsewhere in the body (Hand-Schuller-Christian variant of histiocytosis X). These tumors grow slowly and present as hypothalamic dysfunction (often diabetes insipidus). They provoke a profound fibrillary reaction in local astrocytes.

Reticuloendothelial Neoplasms Primary in the Meninges

Malignant lesions such as reticulum cell sarcoma may occasionally present as a solitary nodule at the base of the brain. An apparently primary meningeal lymphosarcoma without invasion of the brain or other parts of the body has been described.

Reticuloendothelial Neoplasms Secondary in the Central Nervous System

In disseminated *lymphoma,* the meninges are most commonly involved. This is one of the most common tumors in the epidural fat, where it produces root or cord compression. The dura and leptomeninges may be infiltrated, with involvement of the brain, either along the perivascular spaces or around the infundibulum and optic chiasm.

Leukemia, on the contrary, commonly presents as intracerebral hemorrhage (due either to coagulation disorders or bleeding into proliferations of cells in the brain), although meningeal infiltration may occur.

Cerebral Sarcoma

The vast majority of intracerebral sarcomas belong to the *reticuloendothelial group* previously noted. In addition, it seems probable that a few *malignant meningiomas* may develop sufficient anaplasia so that they microscopically resemble connective-tissue sarcomas. In highly anaplastic astrocytomas, the proliferation of adventitial mesenchyme may be so intense as to simulate a fibrosarcoma. These mixed tumors are often colloquially termed *"gliosarcoma."* A group of cerebellar tumors occurring in children (cerebellar sarcomas) are now considered to be infiltrating medulloblastomas that have provoked an intense leptomeningeal hyperplasia *(desmoplastic medulloblastoma).*

Eliminating the preceding categories, there remains a small group of rapidly growing "connective-tissue" tumors of the cerebral hemispheres, occurring almost entirely in infants and children (and on this ground alone unlikely to have arisen from meningiomas). They grow rapidly and invade the brain, although remaining grossly well demarcated. Histologically, they show local infiltration and resemble sarcomas in other tissue, being termed *fibrosarcoma, spindle cell sarcoma,* and *pleomorphic sarcoma* in ascending order of anaplasia. The cell of origin of such tumors is not clear, and although their properties (including reticulin formation) are compatible with an origin from meningocytes, their age incidence, rapid clinical course, and histological appearance are certainly not characteristic of meningiomas. It is possible that they arise from fibroblasts, presumably situated in the dura.

METASTATIC OR INFILTRATING TUMORS

Metastatic Carcinoma

Since many carcinomas commonly spread through the bloodstream, there is no reason to suppose the CNS exempt from metastasis, particularly as it receives a large proportion of the cardiac output and has a dense capillary bed in many areas. For reasons that are not clear, carcinomas from the bronchus and breast and malignant melanomas most frequently metastasize to the CNS, but virtually any carcinoma may do so. Carcinoma of the bronchus may present as an intracerebral tumor before the primary lesion is detected.

Grossly, a very variable pattern of craniospinal metastases is seen in these tumors. Diffuse meningeal infiltration, which may at first sight resemble meningitis, is not infrequent. A particularly common area for metastatic lesions is the junction of the cerebral cortex and underlying white matter (Fig. 25-32), perhaps on account of the dense capillary plexus, and thus presumably slow rate of flow, in this area. It is not uncommon to find multiple lesions of variable size scattered superficially in the hemispheres. Another common site is the cerebellum, but no areas are exempt, and metastases may be found in white matter, basal ganglia, thalamus, brain stem, cord, and even the pituitary gland. They are usually well demarcated from surrounding normal brain and almost always show central necrosis. In some cases the remaining viable tumor is not grossly recognizable.

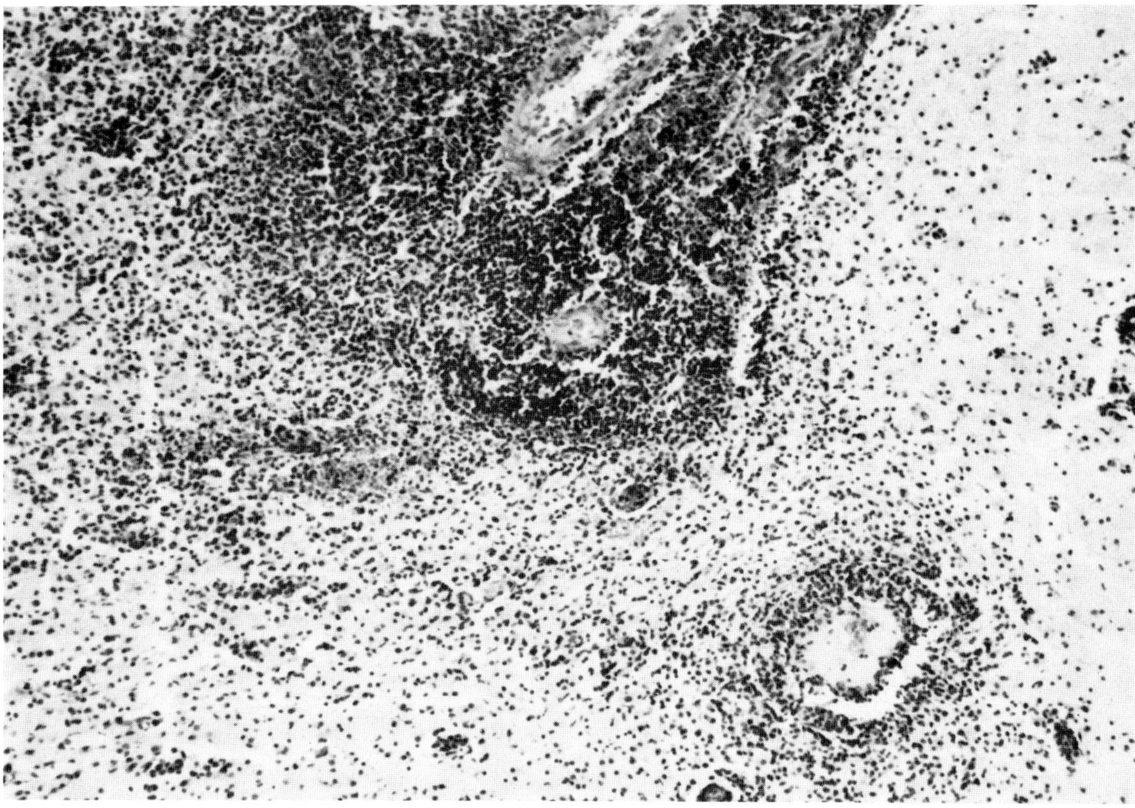

Fig. 25-30. Diffuse reticuloendothelial tumor confined to the CNS, showing subarachnoid, perivascular, and early diffuse infiltration. (H & E, ×115.)

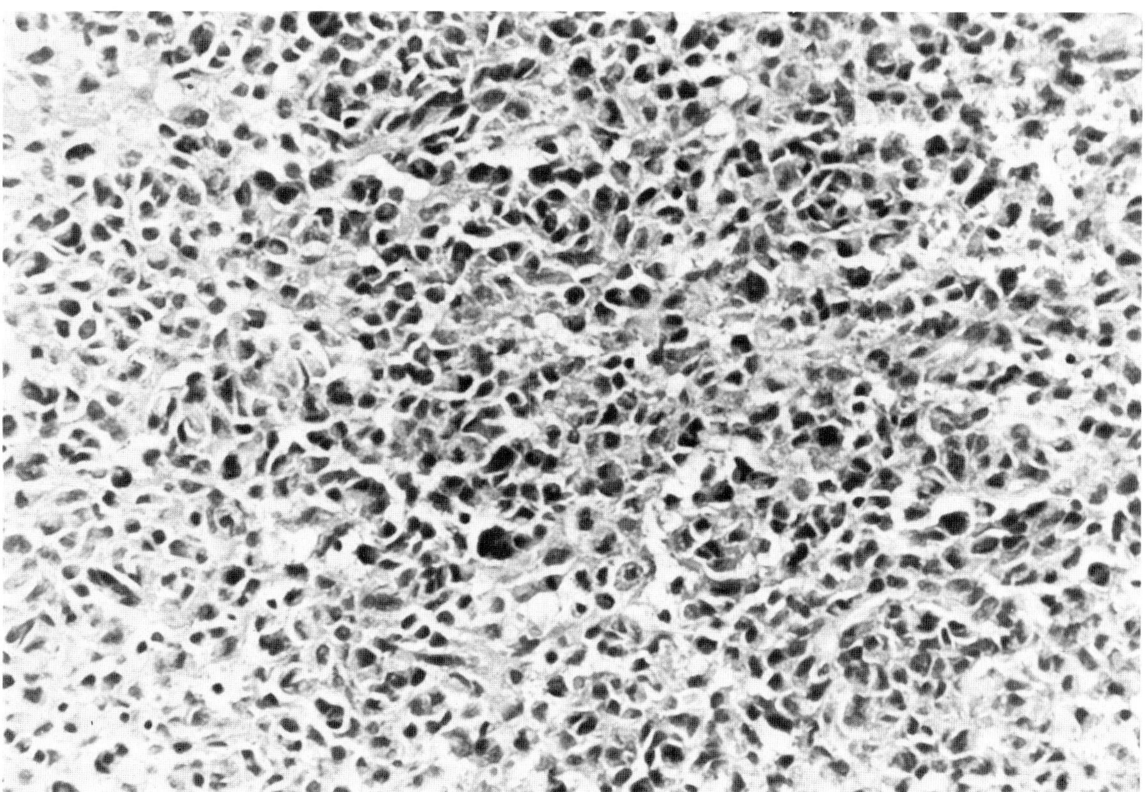

Fig. 25-31. Reticulum cell sarcoma (microglioma), confined to the CNS and diffusely infiltrative (same case as in Fig. 25-30). (H & E, ×300.)

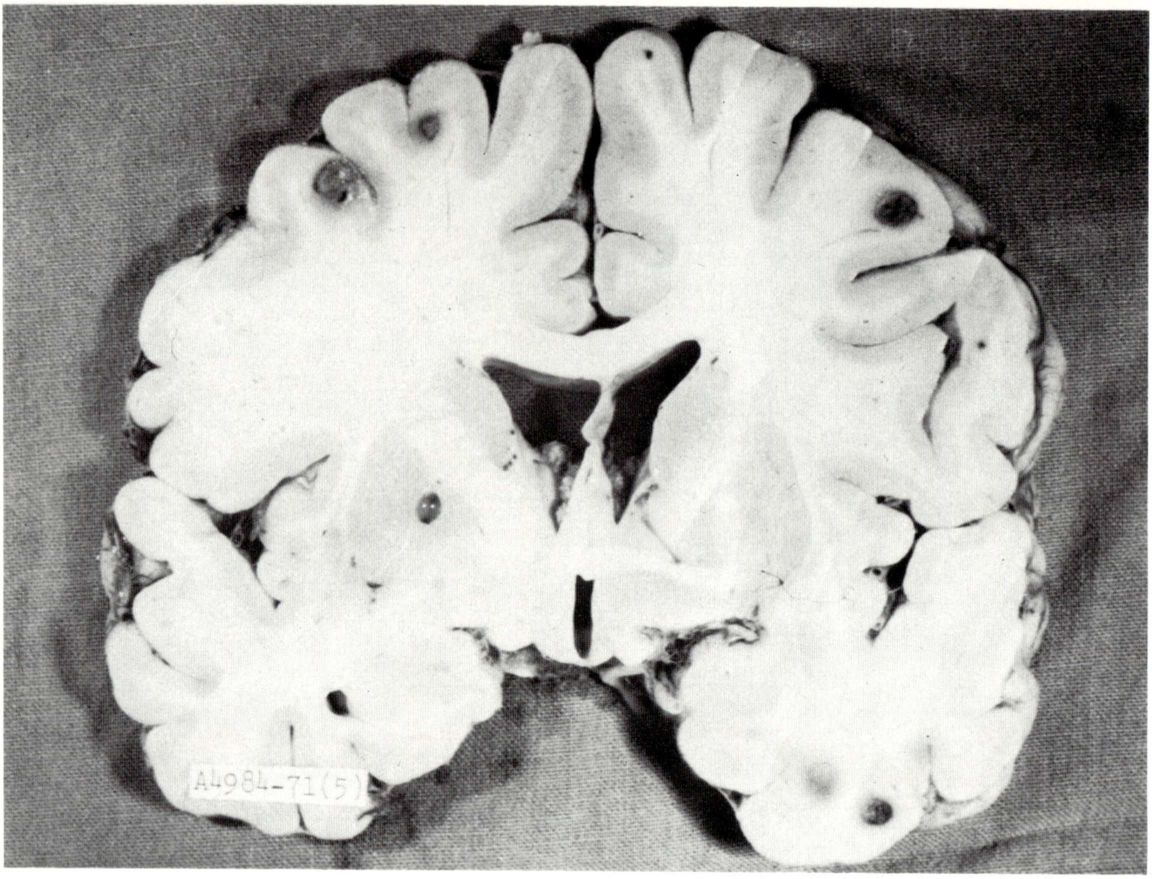

Fig. 25-32. Metastatic breast carcinoma in the brain. Several lesions are situated at the corticocentral junction, and one is situated deep in the right lateral pallidum.

Seen microscopically, the tumor recapitulates the structure of the primary lesion and appears to destroy adjacent brain by growth and compression ischemia rather than by infiltration. The astrocytic reaction is inversely proportional to the speed of metastatic growth. Occasional metastatic lesions, particularly in the cerebellum, may be solitary, but usually several or many are visible on gross examination, and additional foci are seen by microscopy.

Lymphogenous spread does not occur into the CNS since, with the possible exception of the area of the cribriform plate, there are no communications between the lymphatic and subarachnoid systems.

Infiltrating Neoplasms

The intracranial cavity may be directly infiltrated by malignant lesions passing through the bone (Fig. 25-33), such tumors arising, for example, in the parotid gland or nasopharynx.

A lesion peculiar to this area is the *chordoma* (Fig. 25-34), which apparently arises from notocordal remnants entrapped in the sphenoid or basioccipital bones. These malignant tumors expand through the bone and produce symptoms of increased intracranial pressure, or local pressure, at the base of the brain or brain stem. Similar tumors arise from the other end of the notochord in the sacrococcygeal region and may extend into the epidural or subarachnoid spaces around the cauda equina.

Grossly, the tumor appears lobulated and often hemorrhagic, the cut surface showing varying proportions of fibrous tissue, soft gray tumor, and hemorrhage. Microscopically, the cells show uniform, round nuclei and cytoplasm that is often markedly distended by coalescent vacuoles (the contents of which are PAS-positive in frozen section). Large groups of cells are often enclosed by coarse connective tissue septa, and the central areas may completely degenerate. leaving irregular spaces filled with mucin-like material. Although chordomas are only locally invasive, their situation usually precludes complete removal, and the ultimate prognosis is poor.

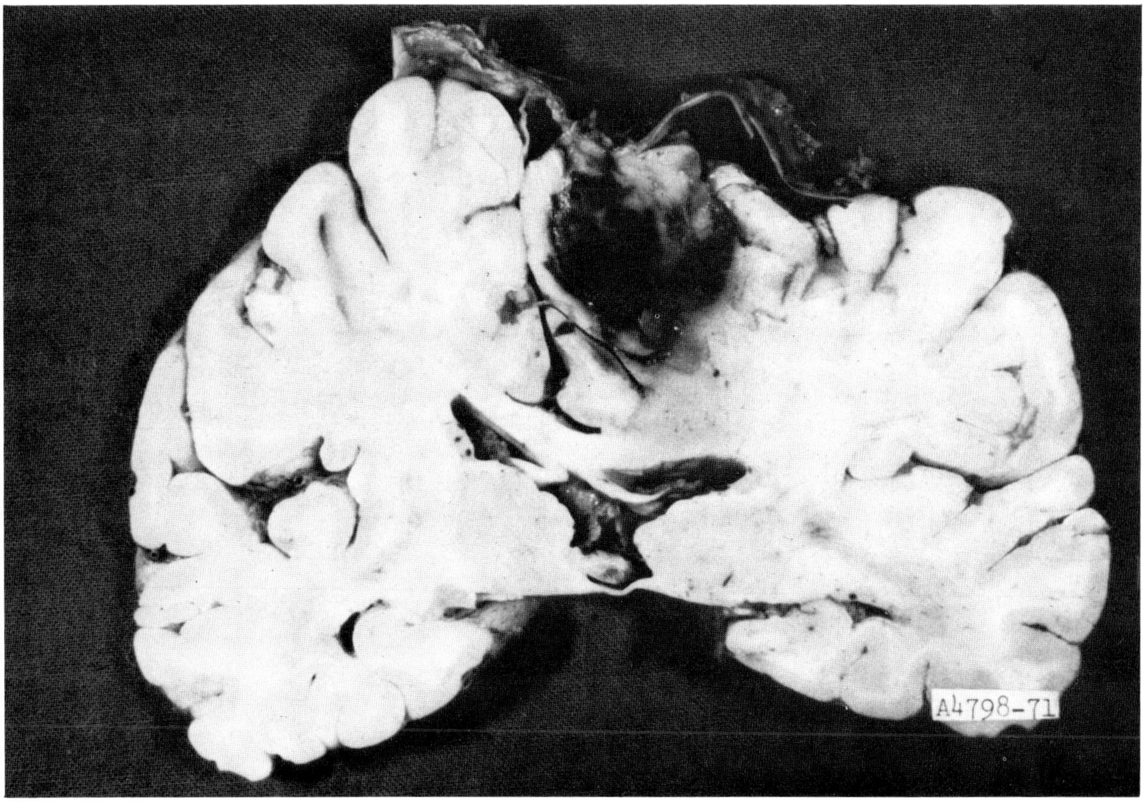

Fig. 25-33. Invasion of the brain by osteogenic sarcoma (in Paget's disease).

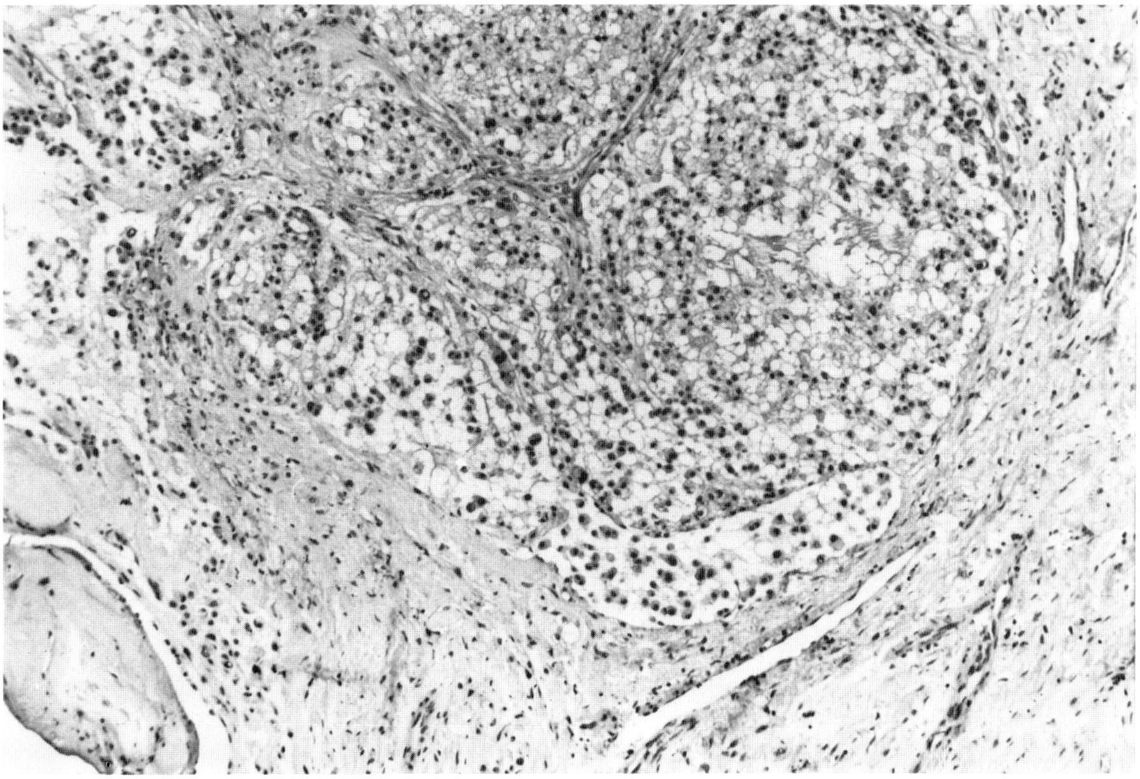

Fig. 25-34. Chordoma. Lesion erupting from the basioccipital bone into the posterior fossa and causing local pressure symptoms. (H & E, ×115.)

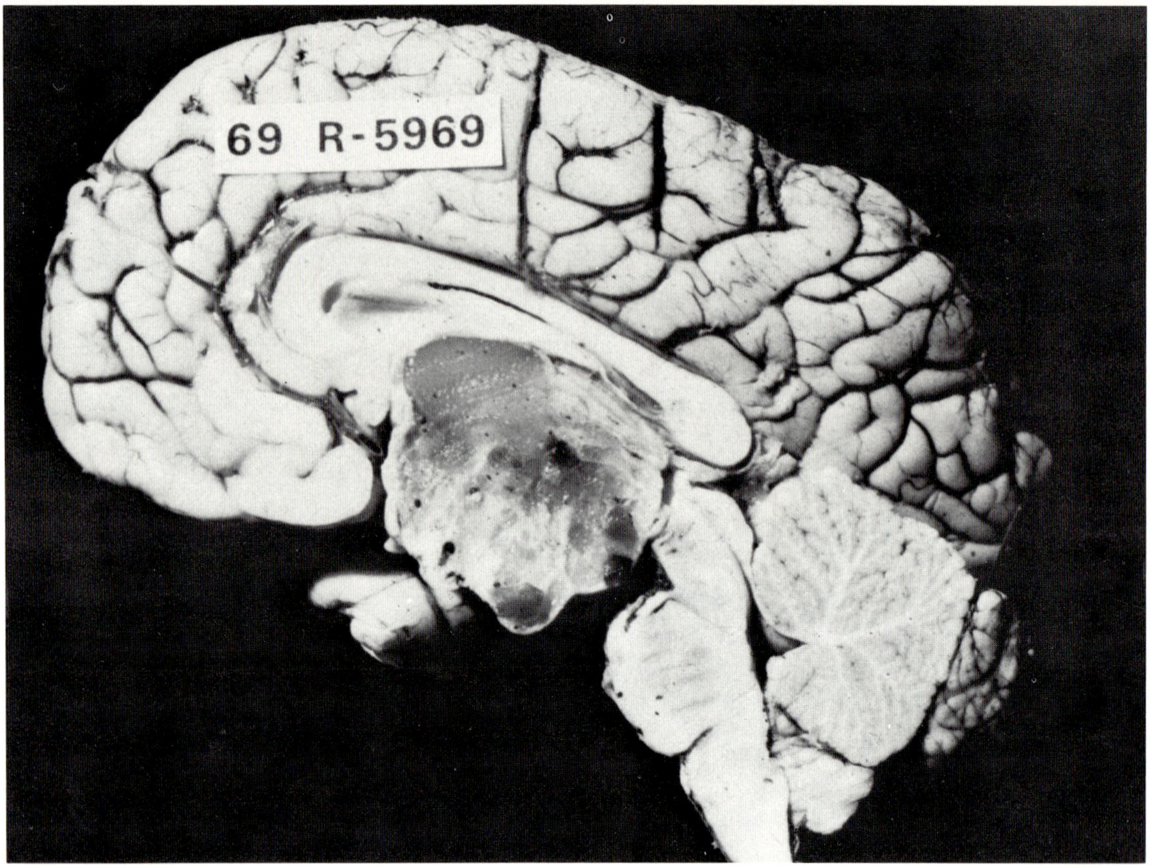

Fig. 25-35. Craniopharyngioma forming a very large cystic mass invaginating the third ventricle.

The brain and cord may also, of course, be infiltrated by tumors arising from other structures within the intracranial and intraspinal cavities, including carcinoma or lymphoma of the meninges and the few invasive examples of meningioma and pituitary adenoma.

DEVELOPMENTAL TUMORS

Most developmental tumors are not true neoplasms, although some examples of teratoma contain malignant infiltrating or even metastasizing components. Craniopharyngioma, epidermoid cyst, colloid cyst, and teratoma (in descending order of frequency) are relatively common, but the others may be regarded as extremely rare. Except for epidermoid cysts, they tend to be midline tumors. Although congenital, they are rarely symptomatic in infancy and make their clinical appearance at any time during the first 20 years or even later. Epidermoid cysts may not become manifest until the fifth to seventh decades.

Craniopharyngioma

Craniopharyngiomas are said to make up 3% of all intracranial tumors, mostly presenting before the age of 20, but an appreciable number up to the fifth and sixth decades. They apparently arise from oral or pharyngeal mucosa, presumably from cell rests incorporated at the time of formation of the adenohypophysis; however, no definite cytogenetic information is available. Originating above the pituitary as suprasellar cysts, they are benign, but often progressively enlarging lesions (Fig. 25-35), which may compress the pituitary, optic chiasm, and other structures at the base of the brain or may completely invaginate the third ventricle, causing hydrocephalus. In such cases, although they do not invade the brain, they may be attached by gliomesenchymal reactive tissue. Otherwise, the external surface is smooth and lobular, and the cut surface shows cysts containing turbid fluid, granular pale areas, yellow fatty deposits, and, not infrequently, mineralization.

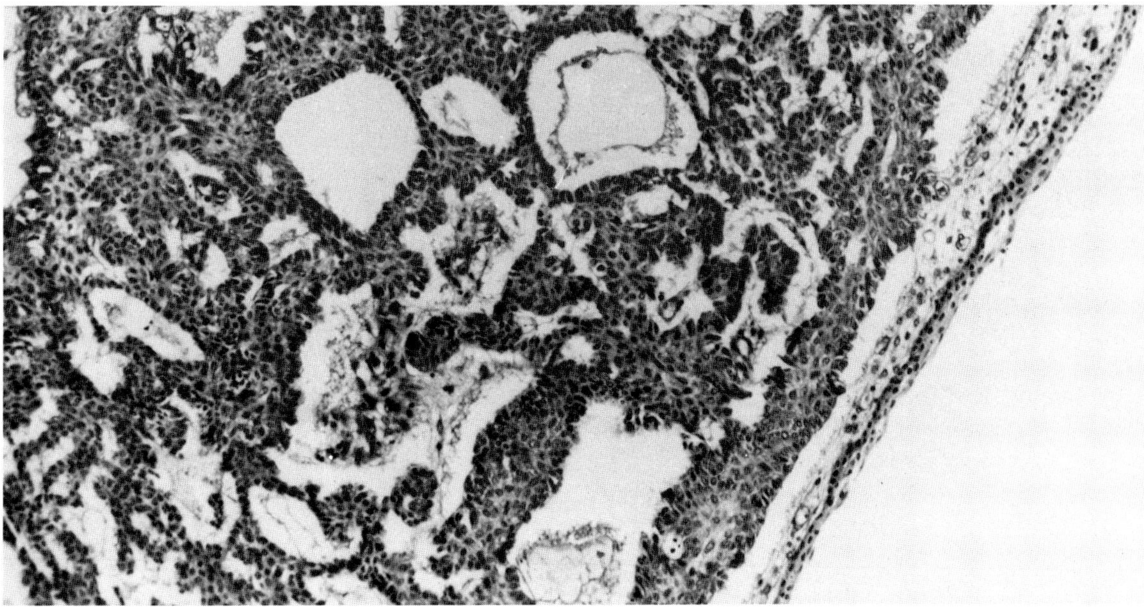

Fig. 25-36. Craniopharyngioma. Fairly solid areas with microcystic change. To the right is the stratified squamous lining of a larger cavity. (H & E, ×115.)

Seen microscopically (Fig. 25-36), some of the cysts are lined by poorly keratinized stratified squamous epithelium. More solid areas consist of sheets of polygonal cells, often exhibiting intercellular bridges, with extracellular microcysts that progressively coalesce to form multilocular cavities lined by one or more layers of cells, presumably merging into stratified squamous epithelium. Extensive areas of scar tissue with hemosiderin and cholesterol deposits, the latter surrounded by foreign-body giant cells, are often present. Because of their location, these tumors are difficult to eradicate and tend to recur locally, but true malignancy and metastasis of these tumors are virtually unknown.

Colloid Cysts

Colloid cysts are rounded masses, 3 mm to 3 cm in diameter, occurring in the third ventricle (Fig. 25-37). They apparently arise from the anterior tela choroidea (e.g., the region of the foramina of Monro). Apart from its slender pedicle, the tumor has no attachment to other tissues. If the tumor is small, it may be freely mobile within the third ventricle.

The colloid cyst is a unilocular cyst, originally lined by a cuboidal or low-columnar epithelium that is sometimes ciliated, although in large cysts this may be difficult to detect. The epithelium rests on a thin, collagenous wall, occasionally bearing external fronds of atrophic choroid plexus. These cysts rarely present until adult life and may be incidental autopsy findings. They are important in that their enlargement may obstruct the flow of CSF through the third ventricle, by occluding either both foramina of Monro or the upper end of the aqueduct. Impaction may occur suddenly, producing acute noncommunicating hydrocephalus with massive tonsillar and uncal herniation, and death may follow within 48 hours. Intermittent or partial obstruction also occurs.

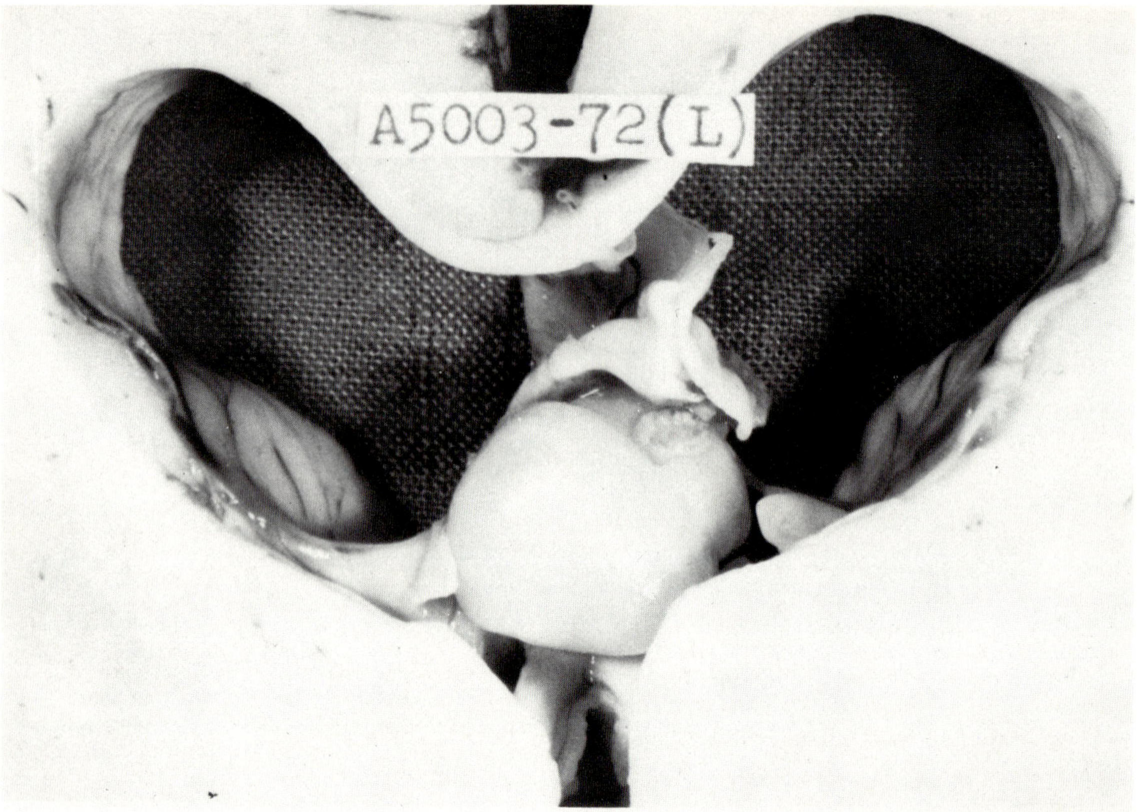

Fig. 25-37. Colloid cyst (viewed from behind) found in a case of rapid, unexpected death in an adult (death within 24 hours of onset of headache). The cyst is blocking both foramina of Monro, and the fornix is stretched over it. The lateral ventricles show considerable enlargement (acute or acute-on-chronic hydrocephalus).

Epidermoid Cysts

Epidermoid cysts make up about 0.5% of intracranial tumors. They may present at virtually any age and differ from most other developmental lesions in often being lateral. Common sites include the cerebellopontine angle and sylvian fissure; others occur in the region of the orbital cortex (Fig. 25-38), in the diploë of the frontal and parietal bones, and near the midline in both the cranial and spinal cavities. They are circumscribed lesions with a well-defined, nodular, often somewhat pearly appearance, and the cut surface may show foci of calcification, cysts full of soft laminated or amorphous material, or dark-brown, oily fluid. They may be multilocular and within the hemispheric white matter may appear to show "budding" (as though forming daughter cavities). Typically, these spaces are lined by keratinized squamous epithelium resting on a thick, often hyaline collagenous layer, but much of the epithelium may be degenerate. Dense scar tissue occurs, with deposits of hemosiderin and cholesterol, the latter with foreign-body giant cells. These lesions are benign, although they may recur following incomplete removal. Occasionally, they rupture or leak into the subarachnoid space and cause granulomatous meningitis.

Teratoma

Making up about 0.2% of intracranial masses, teratomas are characteristically midline tumors with a considerably more sinister prognosis than the developmental lesions previously discussed. Some occur in the

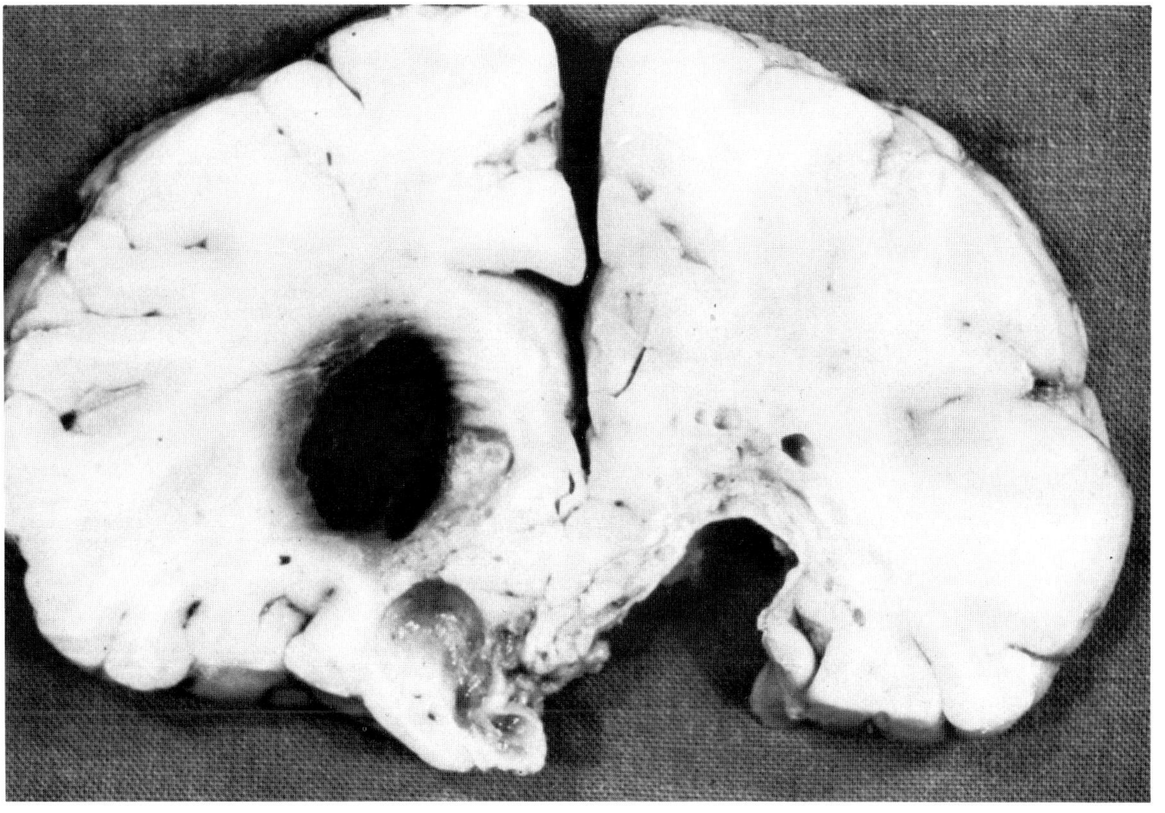

Fig. 25-38. Epidermoid cyst (bifrontal) eroding both frontal lobes from below and causing necrosis (with a hematoma on the right) of adjacent tissue. This middle-aged woman received treatment for major psychosis for many months before the nature of her problem was suspected.

sacrococcygeal area, but the majority are intracranial, usually occurring in the region either of the pineal gland or of the infundibulum and pituitary. The clinical symptoms vary with their location. They usually present under the age of 10 years, but occasionally appear in the second or later decades.

Dermoid Cysts

Dermoid cysts are rare and tend to occur in the midline posterior fossa, with a few in the inferior frontal region. They are cystic or multicystic lesions containing hair and debris, similar to dermoid cysts in other parts of the body except that teeth are somewhat rare. A few contain bone and cartilage, providing a link with the more complex teratomas. As in the case of epidermoid cysts, rupture or leakage may cause chronic granulomatous meningitis, and incomplete removal is followed by recurrence.

Typical Teratoma

Typical teratomas are usually well defined, though often irregular and lobulated. Only rarely are they grossly invasive, although like other lesions at the base of the brain they may invaginate and occupy the third ventricle. The cut surface may show bone or cartilage and is usually in part cystic. Seen microscopically, the tissues include bone, cartilage, varying types of epithelium with more or less organoid formation, and smooth muscle; neural tissues may be present. Uncommonly, there is a malignant component.

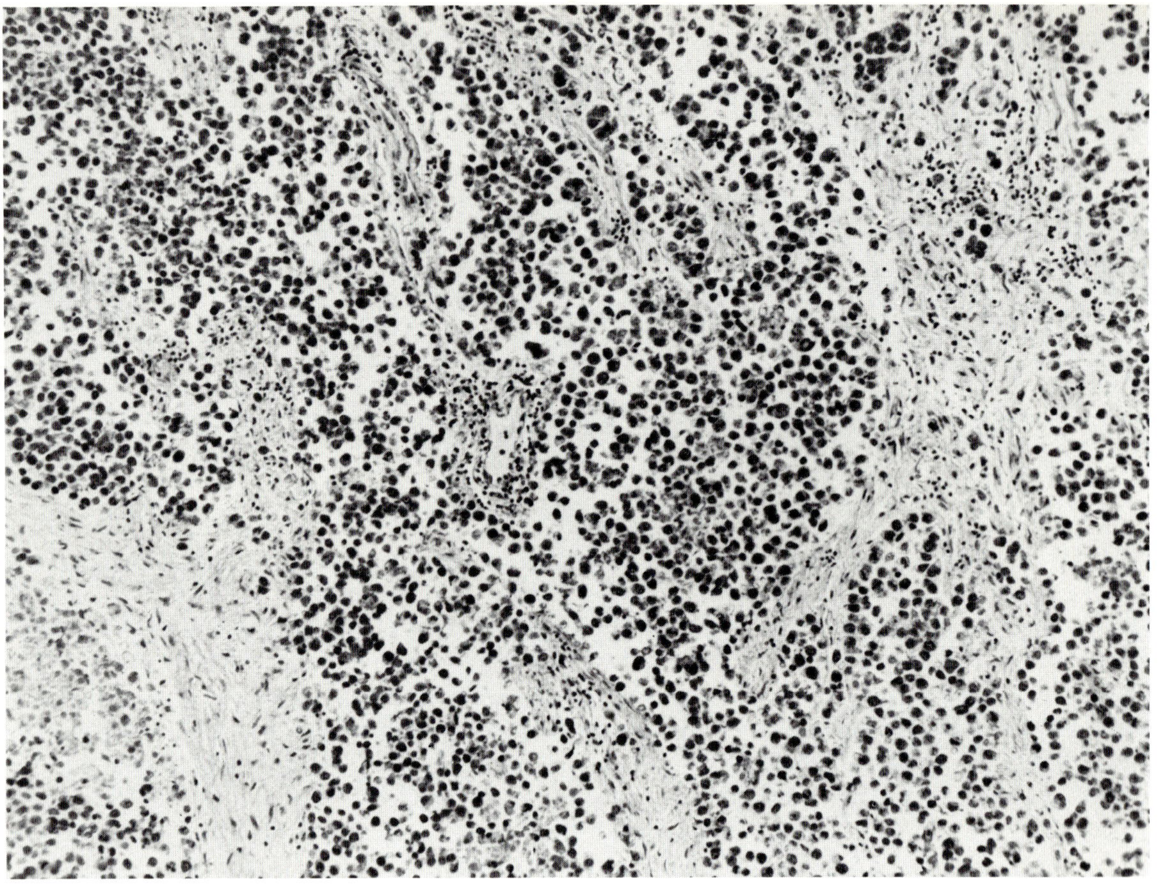

Fig. 25-39. Germinoma or ectopic pinealoma (see Fig. 25-18). Large, hyperchromatic, rounded cells are separated by a stroma containing lymphocytes. (H & E, X115.)

Pineal and Infundibular Tumors

A proportion of tumors in the pineal and infundibular regions show an almost uniform histological picture, considered identical with that of the seminoma or dysgerminoma. These tumors formerly were called "ectopic pinealomas" because their pattern (Fig. 25-39) of large-cell lobules, separated by a mesenchymal stroma containing lymphocytes, was thought to mimic the gradation of cell size seen in a typical pinealoma. However, their pineal origin is no longer accepted, and they are regarded as a distinct variety of CNS teratoma (teratoid tumor or germinoma). The ascription of the origin of such tumors to migrating germ cells, said to be present during fetal life, does not explain their affinity for the regions of the pineal and pituitary glands, but no alternative cytogenetic theories have been proposed. These tumors usually present clinically between the ages of 20 and 35 and are much more common in males. Much of the symptomatology, both in the pineal and infundibular regions, may be explained by mechanical expansion. Any hormonal effect of the tumor itself remains unverified.

Seen grossly, they are either well defined or locally infiltrating in adjacent brain, the tissue being homogenous and grayish-pink on the cut surface. Infundibular tumors may extend into the third ventricle or enlarge the sella. Microscopically, a delicate connective-tissue stroma is seen dividing the tumor into lobules, the stroma itself being infiltrated with moderate numbers of lymphocytes that may extend into the tumor parenchyma. Tumor cells are large and polygonal, with pale, clear, faintly eosinophilic cytoplasm and a rounded central nucleus with a prominent nucleolus. Some mitotic activity may be seen. A few contain frankly teratomatous areas.

Invasion of the brain causes prominent astrocytic and often microglial proliferation. Occasionally, the invasive propensities of these tumors extend to the ventricular and even subarachnoid spaces, but bloodborne metastasis is extremely rare.

Because of their location, surgery is both difficult and hazardous, but the majority appear to be radiosensitive, and three- to five-year survivals occur in patients treated by radiotherapy after biopsy verification of the diagnosis.

BIBLIOGRAPHY

Cravioto, H., and Dart, D. The ultrastructure of "pinealoma" (seminoma-like tumor of the pineal region). *J. Neuropathol. Exp. Neurol.* 32:552-556, 1973.

Currie, S., and Henson, R. A. Neurological syndromes in the reticuloses. *Brain* 94:307-320, 1971.

Haglid, K. G., Stavrou, D., Rönnbäck, L., Carlsson, C.-A., and Weidenbach, W. The S100 protein in water-soluble and pentanol-extractable form in normal human brain and tumors of the human nervous system. *J. Neurol. Sci.* 20:103-111, 1973.

Hoshino, T., Barker, M., Wilson, C. B., Boldrey, E. B., and Fewer, D. Cell-kinetics of human gliomas. *J. Neurosurg.* 37:15-26, 1972.

Jellinger, K., and Sturm, K. W. Delayed radiation myelopathy in man. *J. Neurol. Sci.* 14:389-408, 1971.

Lumsden, C. E. The Study by Tissue Culture of Tumors of the Nervous System. In D. S. Russell and L. J. Rubinstein (Eds.), *Pathology of Tumors of the Nervous System* (3rd ed.). London: Arnold, 1971. Pp. 334-420.

Matakas, F., Cervós-Navarro, J., and Gulotta, F. The ultrastructure of medulloblastomas. *Acta Neuropathol.* (Berl.) 16:271-284, 1970.

Minckler, J. (Ed.) *Pathology of the Nervous System.* New York: McGraw-Hill, 1971. Vol. 2.

Palmer, J. J. Radiation myelopathy. *Brain* 95:109-122, 1972.

Rubinstein, L. J. Cytogenesis and differentiation of primitive central neuroepithelial tumors. *J. Neuropathol. Exp. Neurol.* 31:7-26, 1972.

Rubinstein, L. J. Tumors of the Central Nervous System. In *Atlas of Tumor Pathology.* Washington: Armed Forces Institute of Pathology, 1972. Second series, fascicle 6.

Rubinstein, L. J., and Northfield, D. W. C. The medulloblastoma and the so-called "arachnoidal cerebellar sarcoma." *Brain* 87:379-412, 1964.

Russell, D. S., and Rubinstein, L. J. *Pathology of Tumors of the Nervous System* (3rd ed.). London: Arnold, 1971.

Schaumburg, H. H., Planck, C. R., and Adams, R. D. The reticulum cell sarcoma-microglioma group of brain tumors. *Brain* 95:199-212, 1972.

Schober, R., and Herman, M. M. Neuropathology of cardiac transplantation. *Lancet* 1:962-967, 1973.

Tung, P. P., Hirano, A., and Zimmerman, H. M. *Electron Microscopic Atlas of Brain Tumors.* New York: Grune & Stratton, 1971.

Vuia, O., and Hager, H. Primary cerebral blastomatous reticulosis. *J. Neurol. Sci.* 19:407-423, 1973.

Vuia, O., and Mehraein, P. Primary reticulosis of the central nervous system. *J. Neurol. Sci.* 14:469-482, 1971.

Wilson, C. B. Medulloblastoma. Current views regarding the tumor and its treatment. *Oncology* 24:273-290, 1970.

Zülch, K. J. *Brain Tumors, Their Biology and Pathology* (2nd American ed.). Translated by A. B. Rothballer and J. Olszewski. New York: Springer, 1965.

Psychoses

26

Under normal circumstances, the normal brain effects a synthesis of environmental and internal input with stored experience to produce an appropriate, if not necessarily an optimal, reaction, enabling a person to achieve reasonable social adjustment. However, the functioning of the brain may be affected adversely in many ways. In many of the diseases considered up to this point, focal lesions in recognized neural pathways abolish some aspect of sensory input, integration, or motor performance, sometimes temporarily, but more often permanently. In others, consciousness is reduced or abolished by adverse metabolic factors that can usually be identified with absolute or comparative certainty. In still another group of diseases, the primary manifestation is an apparent failure to develop normal powers of reasoning and memory or a failure of these powers once developed (mental retardation and dementia respectively). In a large majority of such patients, CNS lesions, qualitative or quantitative, can be identified (although not clearly in some instances of mental retardation). Thus, in all these cases of organic deterioration of brain function, morphological factors or systemic metabolic factors can be identified or are assumed.

It is common experience that even in so-called normal people, excessive emotion may interfere with judgment on a temporary basis, although rarely to the point of social maladjustment. In the psychoses, on the other hand, there are disorders of mood, behavior, or thought, apparently spontaneous, so severe as to interfere with environmental and social adjustment on a long-term basis. The degree of this interference varies from patient to patient and during the course of one patient's illness, and its evaluation and diagnosis are to some extent subjective, since they depend on the social expectations of the observer.

A small proportion of the psychoses are associated with organic disease of the brain (e.g., neurosyphilis and other dementias), but the majority occur in the absence of clearly established morphological changes in the CNS and in patients with at least intermittently normal intellectual and motor function. Changes in mood or behavior suggest abnormal function of the archaic core of the brain, including the limbic lobe, hypothalamus, and reticular formation. A somewhat indistinct borderline may be drawn between psychosis proper, in which dysfunction overflows massively from the limbic lobe to the neocortex, and the neuroses, in which neocortical function remains substantially intact in spite of more or less severe subjective emotional abnormality.

By its very nature, the incidence of psychosis and neurosis is difficult to establish, and the most pessimistic estimates would indicate that 10% of the population suffer definite psychiatric disturbance, a further 70% are mildly disturbed but function well, and only 20% are mentally healthy. Nothing could more clearly indicate the subjective nature of the assessment of psychiatric disease than an opinion that 80% of the population are "abnormal" and only 20% "normal."

While classifications of psychiatric disease are somewhat complex, the two major types of psychosis appear to be depression and schizophrenia. *Depressive patients* suffer recurrent attacks of intense and distressing melancholy, which may be accompanied by anxiety and agitation or may be so intense as to obstruct virtually all spontaneous activity. Tentatively, depressive patients may be divided into a *unipolar* group, who do not exhibit periods of intense excitement, or mania, and a *bipolar* group, in whom mania or hypomania alternates with periods of depression. It is probable that this classification is purely pragmatic.

Schizophrenia is characterized by disordered thought processes (unrelated to abnormal intelligence), with a tendency to withdraw into fantasy, and by abnormal and frequently "flattened" emotional reactions. This condition also is subgrouped into chronic (process) schizophrenia, acute (reactive) schizophrenia, and borderline (pseudoneurotic) schizophrenia, depending on the prepsychotic personality, the onset, and the prognosis. As with the depressive patients, this must be an empirical classification because of the absence of knowledge of etiopathogenesis.

Intermediate forms between depression and schizophrenia occur, so that even these terms are descriptive rather than explanatory. Other types of personality defect, which will not be considered, include the *neuroses* (with irrational anxiety and hyperexcitability, which often respond well to drugs such as meprobamate and the benzodiazepines, which inhibit the limbic system and especially the hippocampus), and the *psychopathic personalities* (who exhibit impulsive, irresponsible, antisocial behavior, are relatively devoid of anxiety or guilt in spite of realizing the nature of their actions, and respond poorly to drugs).

Etiology and Pathogenesis

Virtually nothing is known of the etiology or pathogenesis of the psychoses, but there appears to be a genetic predisposition in both the major categories, manifestations of which may vary from spontaneous psychosis to one precipitated by intense, abnormal environmental stress. Evidence for a genetic factor includes moderately high concordance in monozygotic twins, increased frequency of psychosis (and conditions such as alcoholism) in the relatives of affected persons, and the persisting high frequency of psychosis in the children of psychotic parents adopted by (relatively) nonpsychotic foster parents. However, since many cases of both depression and schizophrenia are precipitated by environmental stress, it is apparent that nature versus nurture arguments are no longer relevant — both play their part.

It has been interestingly speculated that the schizoid personality (predisposed to schizophrenia) had survival value in societies organized in small (e.g., family) units, whereas the cyclothymic personality (predisposed to depression or mania) had a similar value in strongly hierarchical societies, where it facilitated adaption to downgrading or upgrading within the hierarchy. Such survival advantages in the presumed heterozygotes would compensate for the development of psychosis in a small number of homozygotes and prevent elimination of the responsible genes.

Among the environmental factors possibly involved are deprivation of affection in early life, faulty patterns of family communication, conflicting models for identification when parents or others in authority have opposing standards, and the interaction of deficient intelligence with environmental stress. Environmental factors (i.e., cultural values) also determine the content of delusions and the rationalizations attached to feelings of guilt (e.g., about sexual fantasies or the death of a relative).

TOPOGRAPHICAL SUBSTRATE OF PSYCHOSES

Because of the clinical and experimental evidence that the limbic system is associated with emotion and mood, it appears probable that dysfunction of this system is a primary factor in the development of psychotic manifestations. It might be expected a priori that such dysfunction would be accompanied by hypothalamic and reticular-system dysfunction — and neuroendocrine and autonomic manifestations indeed occur in psychoses. Since the limbic cortex projects extensively to the neocortex, interference with the functions of the latter, including cognition and appropriate reactions to the environment, might also be expected.

Evidence from Monoamine Localization

Among CNS neurotransmitters, the monoamines (norepinephrine, dopamine, and serotonin) are particularly associated with the reticular formation, hypothalamus, and limbic system (Chap. 3). It is therefore of considerable interest that definite or probable abnormalities of monoamine metabolism have been discovered in some psychoses, and that most of the drugs used in such cases affect monoamine metabolism. These drugs act principally to alter the release, receptor reactivity, reuptake, or catabolism of the transmitters, rather than directly affecting (so far as is known) their synthesis. Their activity is probably centered on the presynaptic terminals of monoaminergic neurons in the hypothalamus and limbic system.

Evidence from Frontal Lobe Surgery

The connections between the limbic system and neocortex have already been discussed (Chap. 5), and there is no conclusive evidence as to which, if any, are of especial importance in the genesis of psychotic symptoms. Morphological examination of brains from psychotic patients has provided little information; frequently, no changes are found. The best available information has come from the neurosurgical procedures carried out to ameliorate the more distressing overt manifestations of psychosis. Because anatomical observations (many connections with the limbic cortex) and clinical findings (such as the effect of tumors in the frontal lobes) have suggested that the frontal cortex may be of particular importance in the psychoses, attempts have been made to isolate it by more or less extensive lesions in the white matter.

Earlier operations were almost total frontal lobotomies, in that virtually all white matter was separated in a vertical plane at the level of the tips of the anterior horns. While some patients showed immediate improvement, many showed serious long-term deterioration, with, for example, the development of seizures and progressive failure of social adaptation. For this reason, and because of the availability of new anatomical knowledge and better techniques, it became the practice to perform less extensive operations. These techniques include the use of freezing, radiofrequency heating, or ultra-short-range radioactive seeds (^{90}Y), which, together with improved stereotactic procedures, have enabled the production of accurately localized small lesions. New anatomical knowledge includes the delineation of two major pathways from the limbic to the frontal cortex, one passing from the white matter of the cingulate gyrus to the medial surface and one passing from the uncus and amygdala to the orbital surface.

Small lesions (up to about 1 cm in diameter) have been placed either in the cingulate gyrus above the anterior callosum to interrupt the former pathway, or in the inferomedial frontal white matter below the head of the caudate nucleus to interrupt the latter pathway, or in both. Although a large series with adequate controls remains to be presented and analyzed, there is little doubt that these operations result in improved clinical status and a low incidence of significant complications. Up to 80% of the patients return to work.

It may be assumed that these two limbic-neocortical connections are of significance in conducting the underlying disturbance to the neocortex, although this gives no indication as to the level at which the disturbance originates. The earlier operations were designed to sever the anterior thalamic radiation (from the medial column of the thalamus to the orbital cortex); the lesion that severs connections between the uncus and orbital cortex also destroys most of these fibers. The lesion in the cingulate gyrus, in addition to interrupting cingulofrontal fibers, transects the classic Papez circuit (see Chap. 5). Stimulation of the amygdala increases anxiety and tension and causes adrenocorticotropic hormone release, and lesions between uncus and orbital cortex appear of particular value in correcting inappropriate emotional responses such as depression, phobia, and anxiety.

Although these circumscribed operations have been used in selected cases of many types, they appear to be of particular value in deeply depressed patients and may be useful in severe obsessive-compulsive neurosis. However, psychosurgery is no longer frequently performed and is likely to diminish in importance with the advances made in drug therapy.

PSYCHOACTIVE DRUGS

In the absence of consistently detectable gross or microscopic CNS findings in the psychoses, it must be presumed that the biological abnormality is at a molecular level. The lack of structural changes and the remitting nature of the disease would argue against metabolic errors involving nucleic acids, protein, or lipid. Substances of more rapid turnover, such as neurotransmitters or ions, might be suspect. Although there is some evidence of ionic imbalance (at least in some patients with depression in whom there is apparent intracellular accumulation of Na^+), and ionic disequilibrium has by no means been excluded, experimental and clinical investigation has been largely directed toward neurotransmitters, particularly the monoamines, which show appropriate CNS localization and are affected by many psychoactive drugs. No significant active role for acetylcholine seems to emerge from the current literature.

Review of Monoamine Metabolism

The monoamines believed to be of importance in the CNS (also see Chap. 3) include two catecholamines, norepinephrine and dopamine, and one indoleamine, serotonin. Separate systems employing these substances have been identified, most of them with cell bodies in the brain stem and a significant distribution to the hypothalamus and limbic system, as well as to other parts of the brain and cord.

Dopamine is manufactured from tyrosine by consecutive 4-hydroxylation by tyrosine hydroxylase (which is rate-limiting) and decarboxylation by L-aromatic amino acid decarboxylase, which is widely distributed, with high levels of activity. Norepinephrine is derived from dopamine by the insertion of a hydroxyl group into the side chain by dopamine-β-hydroxylase, which is thought to be present only in the synaptic vesicles or granules of the appropriate cells. Tyrosine itself, or its 4-hydroxylated derivative (L-dopa), may serve as a source for CNS dopamine and norepinephrine, but the transmitters themselves cannot cross the blood-brain barrier. Serotonin is derived from tryptophan by analogous enzyme actions; first, 5-hydroxylation by tryptophan hydroxylase, which is rate-limiting, and second, decarboxylation by L-aromatic amino acid decarboxylase. Again, tryptophan and 5-hydroxytryptophan can serve as precursors, but serotonin itself does not cross the barrier system.

The degradation of monoamines is largely dependent on two enzymes, monoamine oxidase (MAO) and catechol-O-methyltransferase (COMT), the former situated in the outer membranes of mitochondria and the latter free in the synaptic cytoplasm and extracellular space. Dopamine reacts preferentially with MAO first, and is then 3-methoxylated by COMT to produce homovanillic acid (HVA). Norepinephrine appears to be affected by MAO and COMT in either sequence, producing an unstable aldehyde that may be oxidized to vanillylmandelic acid (VMA) or reduced to 3-methoxy-4-hydroxyphenylglycol (MHPG). Although in the peripheral nervous system VMA appears to be the major end product, there is some evidence that MHPG predominates in the central nervous system. The catabolism of serotonin does not normally involve COMT; an unstable aldehyde produced by MAO is oxidized to 5-hydroxyindoleacetic acid (5-HIAA).

Thus, under normal circumstances, there appear to be four major catabolic products of the monoamines, of which at least the three acids (HVA, VMA, and 5-HIAA) are actively removed by the choroid plexus (and probably also across the blood-brain barrier). All four appear in plasma and urine, but since similar compounds are formed in the PNS and adrenal medulla, the assessment of CNS turnover by plasma or urinary estimations is fraught with danger.

There is considerable evidence for normally minor metabolic pathways that may assume increased importance in the psychoses. Thus, it appears probable that COMT, and possibly other methylating enzymes, using S-adenosylmethionine as a methyl donor, can methoxylate dopamine (and possibly norepinephrine) in the 4 as well as the 3 position, or in both. CNS tissue also contains an N-methyltransferase potentially capable of methylating the amino group in all three transmitters. Another minor pathway involves the action of L-aromatic amino acid decarboxylase and dopamine-β-hydroxylase directly on tyrosine, without previous 4-hydroxylation. This produces tyramine and octopamine, which may be stored in synaptic vesicles, but on release have little or no effect on postsynaptic receptors. They are therefore termed *false transmitters.* If present in quantity, they displace true neurotransmitters from the vesicles, leading to their destruction by MAO and COMT. It is probable that other hitherto unidentified minor pathways of CNS monoamine metabolism exist. The physiological significance, if any, of these pathways remains to be determined, but their possible relationship to the psychoses is the subject of intensive investigation.

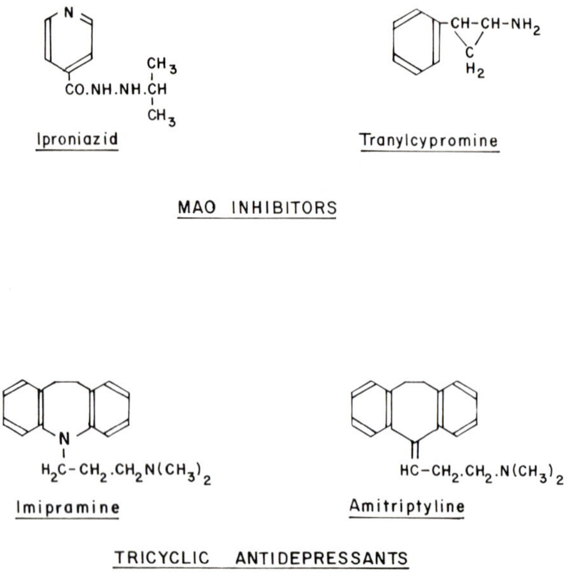

Fig. 26-1. Commonly used antidepressant drugs.

Drugs Used in Depression (Antidepressants)

In this and succeeding sections on drug action, no attempt is made to present a comprehensive pharmacology, for which an appropriate text should be consulted, but rather to correlate, where possible, clinical use of the drug with its effects on monoamine concentration and metabolism within the CNS.

Monoamine Oxidase Inhibitors

Monoamine oxidase inhibitors (Fig. 26-1) reduce the activity of MAO, an important enzyme in the breakdown of all monoamines. The *hydrazine group* is exemplified by iproniazid, but many similar compounds have been synthesized. Although they effectively inhibit MAO, they frequently have severe side effects, due to such inhibition peripherally. A group of *nonhydrazine inhibitors* is exemplified by tranylcypromine, which has the advantage of not only inhibiting MAO, but also being to some extent a direct stimulant, with some structural resemblance to amphetamine.

All MAO inhibitors have disadvantages, among which are relatively slow clinical effectiveness and undesirable side effects, including hypotensive crises. They increase CNS concentrations of dopamine and serotonin, since the first step in the catabolism of these compounds is normally oxidative deamination. They produce a smaller increase in the concentration of norepinephrine, as this can still be inactivated to normetanephrine by COMT alone. Trace amines such as tyramine and octopamine accumulate. Urinary excretion of deaminated metabolites such as HVA, VMA, and 5-HIAA is reduced. It may be noted in passing that there is no clinically effective inhibitor for COMT.

Tricyclic Antidepressants

Tricyclic antidepressants (Fig. 26-1) are three-ring structures (the center ring may contain N), to which a side chain is attached by either a single or double bond. A single bond is present in imipramine and desimipramine, and a double bond is present in amitryptyline and nortryptyline. The side chain in each is identical except for substituents on the terminal N. In imipramine and amitryptyline, both are methyl and these drugs are considered effective in raising serotonin; in desimipramine and nortryptyline, there is only one substituent, methyl, and these drugs are said to raise norepinephrine levels preferentially.

The essential action of these agents, like that of cocaine, appears to be blockade of transmitter reuptake through the presynaptic membrane, prolonging action at the postsynaptic receptor and increasing initial methylation by (extracellular) COMT. The increased excretion of methylated metabolites mimics MAO inhibition. Possibly, serotonin elevates mood and norepinephrine activity promotes psychological drive. In depression with agitation, the concurrent use of a phenothiazine may be helpful.

Stimulants

Stimulants are of less clinical importance than they were before the advent of effective MAO inhibitors and the tricyclic drugs. However, amphetamine and some derivatives may still be used as adjunctive therapy, D-amphetamine probably being most effective, since it has maximal CNS and minimal cardiovascular effects (unlike L-amphetamine). Amphetamine is a sympathomimetic drug (direct stimulant action on the postsynaptic membrane) and perhaps also displaces norepinephrine and other monoamines from storage vesicles, inhibits MAO, and reduces presynaptic reuptake. Displacement of norepinephrine from vesicles or granules may be so rapid as to exceed MAO capacity, and more methylated derivatives are excreted.

Drugs Used in Mania

Episodes of mania or hypomania are usually treated by phenothiazines (see the next section) or by lithium salts.

Lithium appears to have a firm place in the treatment of mania and possibly as a prophylactic, provided that plasma concentration is adequately controlled. Desirable levels of 0.8 to 1.6 mEq per liter

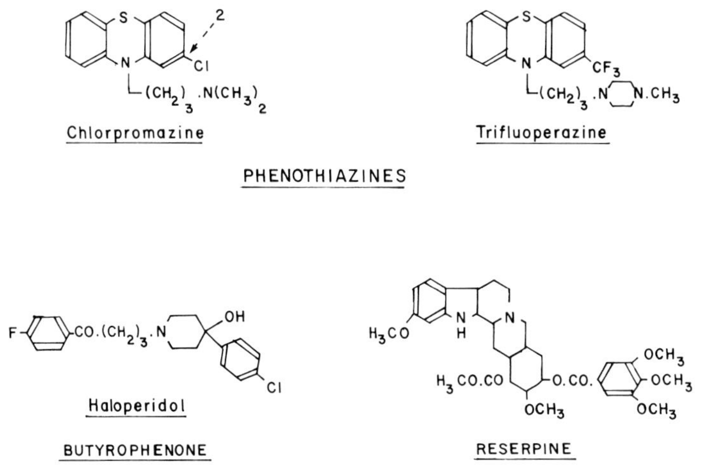

Fig. 26-2. Drugs used in the treatment of schizophrenia.

are usually not achieved for five to eight days, but, once achieved, can be maintained by a single daily dose. Gastrointestinal upset, neuromuscular irritability, and mental confusion are rarely seen with plasma concentrations under 2 mEq per liter. A major disadvantage is its five- to eight-day buildup period, during which patients may need treatment with phenothiazines or other drugs. However, it has less sedative effects and causes less mental obtundity than other agents.

Even less is known of the mechanism of lithium action than of most other psychoactive drugs. The effect may be on the presynaptic membrane, reducing release of monoamines, but whether or not this is associated with changes in intracellular Na^+ concentration and consequent altered membrane potential remains unclear.

Drugs Used in Schizophrenia

Four classes of drugs are commonly used for schizophrenic patients, three of which appear to have similar modes of activity in spite of differing chemical structures. The action of the fourth, reserpine, appears to be distinct.

Phenothiazines and Related Drugs

Like the tricyclic antidepressants, the phenothiazines (Fig. 26-2) are three-ring compounds, but the central ring contains both S and N. There are many phenothiazines, with a minor site of substitution at position 2 on one benzene ring, where short chains that often contain halogen are inserted. The major substitution is on the N and divides phenothiazines into three groups: aliphatic, piperidyl, and piperazine. The piperazine group appears to be the most potent and to produce the least sedative effect. Related to the phenothiazines in activity, but not in structure, are the *thioxanthenes* and *butyrophenones,* of which the best known is haloperidol.

All these drugs have a calming effect in excess of their sedative activity, produce extrapyramidal symptoms as side effects, and do not induce dependence. In spite of extensive investigations, their activity at the synapse is unknown. Actions that have been suggested include blockage of presynaptic reuptake and, in the case of dopamine alone, possible blockage of postsynaptic receptors, since they increase turnover of dopamine in doses that have no effect on norepinephrine or serotonin, and their efficiency in the treatment of schizophrenia runs remarkably parallel to their ability to produce extrapyramidal side effects.

Reserpine

Reserpine (Fig. 26-2) is a complex, naturally occurring alkaloid containing several methoxy groups. In normal persons it causes depression that is associated with depletion of monoamine stores (norepinephrine, dopamine, and serotonin). This is apparently a specific effect on the membrane of the synaptic vesicle or granule, preventing uptake of monoamine and releasing monoamine already present, which is then destroyed by MAO. Release is gradual, and deaminated rather than methylated products are formed. Depression induced by reserpine may be relieved by levodopa, presumably due to formation of dopamine, since if the vesicle or granule membrane is blocked, dopamine-β-hydroxylase may not be available for norepinephrine synthesis.

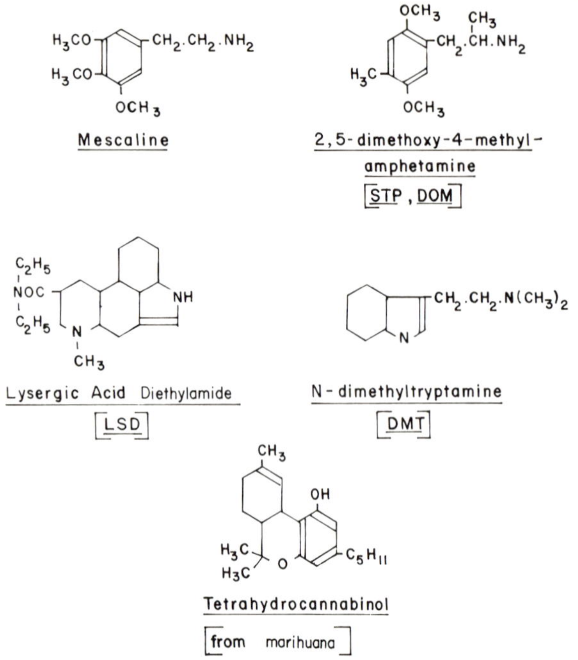

Fig. 26-3. Psychotomimetic drugs.

Psychotomimetic Drugs

Two of the three groups of psychotomimetic (hallucinogenic) drugs (Fig. 26-3) are related to catecholamines or indoleamine, and tolerance to one drug involves cross-tolerance, not only between members of one group, but also between the groups. Related to catecholamines are a group of substances derived from phenylethylamine, such as mescaline (the latter containing 3-methoxy groups), and the substituted amphetamines, such as 2, 5-dimethoxy-4-methylamphetamine (STP, DOM) and 3-methoxy-4,5-methylenedioxyamphetamine (MDA), both of which contain methoxy groups. Related to the indoleamines are lysergic acid diethylamide (LSD) and N-dimethyltryptamine (DMT). The third hallucinogenic group are the cannabinols such as marihuana, of somewhat different chemical structure. The effects of these drugs are still being investigated, but it is known that LSD is a serotonin antagonist (possibly blocking access to postsynaptic receptors) that increases CNS serotonin concentrations, but does not affect norepinephrine and dopamine concentrations or only slightly reduces them.

Experimental Drugs Affecting Monoamine Metabolism

A number of other drugs or synthetic compounds are known to have a significant effect on concentrations of monoamines in the CNS, although they have not yet found general clinical application.

Methysergide and sinanserine apparently inhibit the CNS actions of serotonin and may lead to depression.

The synthetic drug H44-68, which inhibits tyrosine hydroxylase, and the synthetic drug FLA-63, which inhibits dopamine-β-hydroxylase, both reduce CNS concentrations of norepinephrine. H44-68 reduces dopamine as well. Norepinephrine losses due to these drugs are enhanced by chlorpromazine and haloperidol, whereas dopamine loss associated with H44-68 is markedly enhanced by haloperidol, but much less so by chlorpromazine, suggesting that the latter has a direct inhibitory action on dopamine-β-hydroxylase in addition to its blockade of dopamine receptors.

The presence of α-methyltyrosine inhibits tyrosine hydroxylase, and α-methyldopa is thought to inhibit L-aromatic amino acid decarboxylase partially; however, it reduces CNS norepinephrine more by conversion to α-methylnorepinephrine, which displaces norepinephrine from synaptic granules. α-Methylnorepinephrine is another false transmitter; and the displaced norepinephrine is destroyed by MAO.

A specific inhibitor of tryptophan hydroxylase, p-chlorophenylalanine apparently combines irreversibly with the enzyme, whose activity is abolished until new enzyme is synthesized. The action of p-chlorophenylalanine is not associated with tranquilization or depression, but the latter is precipitated by subsequent administration of reserpine.

DEPRESSIVE PSYCHOSIS

Depressive psychosis is a descriptive term and not a nosological entity. It may or may not be complicated by episodic hypomania or mania and may be spontaneous or precipitated by various stresses. Little is known of its etiology, except that it results from an interplay between genetic and environmental factors, apparently including bereavement and emotional deprivation in early life. Extensive and intensive morphological investigation has failed to reveal any substrate. Swelling of oligodendroglial cells has been occasionally described in patients with this psychosis, but this change is so subjective, so liable to be produced by agonal conditions or artifact, and so inconstant that it does not merit serious consideration without further confirmation. Indeed, the only reasonably constant findings in depressive psychosis relate to the concentration and excretion of monoamine metabolites. Even these do not appear uniform in all cases, confirming the probable heterogeneity of this group of diseases.

Biochemical Changes

Monoamine metabolism has usually been studied by examining blood and urine, although an increasing number of reports of CSF changes (and occasionally, of alterations in brain tissue) are appearing. Plasma and urinary changes must be interpreted with considerable caution, since the metabolites estimated represent efflux from both the PNS and CNS, and it is probable that there are significant alterations in peripheral neuromuscular and autonomic activity in depression and mania. Even determinations on CSF or brain tissue are not free from interpretative pitfalls. Low concentrations of monoamines in the brain might imply decreased synthesis, increased breakdown, or both. Increased concentrations in CSF might reflect either increased breakdown with reduction of amine concentration in the brain, or an increased rate of turnover (synthesis and breakdown), with normal tissue concentrations.

Subject to these considerations, a consistent picture nonetheless emerges in depressive psychosis, suggesting decreased turnover of all monoamines associated with depression and increased turnover in periods of mania, with certain exceptions to be noted subsequently. This is the case whether estimations are made of the amines themselves or of various metabolites, including normetanephrine, VMA, MHPG (thought to be the best indicator of CNS activity available in blood or urine), HVA, and 5-HIAA. The major exceptions occur in depressed patients with considerable agitation, in whom metabolite excretion may be at normal levels, with the probably significant exception of MHPG, which is still reduced. In some patients in whom expected alterations are not seen, they can be precipitated by test procedures. Depressed patients with normal urinary levels of norepinephrine frequently show a diminished norepinephrine response to insulin stress. Those with CSF levels of HVA in the normal or low normal range accumulate HVA at reduced rates if active removal of the compound by the choroid plexus is prevented by probenecid. Altered excretion of monoamine metabolites tends to return to normal following effective treatment with MAO inhibitors or tricyclic antidepressants. A similar normalization in patients with mania is produced with α-methyltyrosine although it is less effective therapeutically than lithium.

Peripheral enzyme activity in depressive states appears variable. Circulating levels of MAO have been variously reported as normal or high, but, in any case, tend to increase normally with age beyond 35 years. They tend to be higher in women than men. In bipolar depression, MAO activity has been reported as low, with (correspondingly) high urinary tryptamine and platelet octopamine. Levels of circulating COMT are only depressed in women and tend to be lower in unipolar than in bipolar depression.

Other reported changes in depressive patients, some of them probably secondary to the disease process, include retention of Na^+, which is apparently largely intracellular. However, it might be expected that this will partially depolarize cell membranes, and thus it is difficult to correlate with decreased neurotransmitter effectiveness. High circulating corticosteroid levels have been reported, probably due to an effect of the limbic system on the hypothalamus. An odd alteration in the diurnal rhythm of plasma tyrosine has been described, the levels being lower before noon in depressive patients than in control subjects, but relatively normal at other times. The 24-hour excretion of adenosine 3′:5′-cyclic phosphate (cyclic AMP) is low during episodes of depression and is increased during mania. However, a major part of this change might be associated with altered neuromuscular activity. Tryptophan-loading suggests that in many depressive patients, more tryptophan than normal follows the kynurenine pathway, possibly leading to, or resulting from, deficient serotonin formation.

There seems to be a close association between reduced monoamine turnover and depression on the one hand, and increased monoamine turnover and mania on the other. However, this merely establishes that the clinical phenomena and amine changes are associated in time, but does not prove a causal relationship. Since many noradrenergic, dopaminergic, and serotonergic pathways are themselves considered inhibitory, it is difficult to construct a simple hypothesis. It is not even clear which, if any, monoamine is of greater importance than the others, and current methods are not sufficiently accurate to estimate the balance of monoamines either between themselves or in relationship to acetylcholine or other possible neurotransmitters. At present, it is only possible to record the data and await further elucidation of the structure and function of the reticulohypothalamic-limbic system and the precise mode and site of action of psychoactive drugs.

SCHIZOPHRENIA

The term schizophrenia, like depressive psychosis, probably covers a group of diseases with similar manifestations but different etiologies and exemplifies the variable balance between genetic and environmental causes in precipitating clinical symptomatology. There are no characteristic morphological changes in the brains of depressive patients, but a number of such changes have been reported in schizophrenia. They have been widely variable, but this may simply reflect the impossibility of examining an entire brain in minute detail. Thus, changes found in one study may reflect the topographical area of interest of the investigator and do not exclude concurrent changes elsewhere reported by others. The frequently remitting nature of schizophrenia suggests that morphological changes are secondary and develop late in the disease, but this does not prevent their possibly providing useful information.

Morphological Features Reported in Schizophrenia

Most of the changes reported have involved the cerebral cortex and are variously reported as focal or diffuse, with or without observable reactive astrocytosis and fibrillary gliosis. Neuronal loss from various or all layers and degenerative changes have been reported, the latter including shrinkage (producing dwarf cells) that appears to progress to cell disappearance without neuronophagia. Problems of assessing cell loss and nonspecific neuronal degeneration or necrosis have previously been considered (see

Chap. 20). Changes in subcortical structures have included chromatolysis and increased lipofuscin in neurons of the basal ganglia and cell loss from diencephalic nuclei, both in the thalamus and hypothalamus, with moderate astrocytic reaction and fibrillary gliosis.

None of these observations has been consistent in even a majority of schizophrenic brains, none are specific for schizophrenia, and all might be regarded as incidental, accidental, or artifactual. Nonetheless, they are described by reputable observers, in marked contrast to the virtual absence of change in depressive psychosis, and though their significance cannot be assessed, neither can they be rejected out of hand. An occasional finding has been small glial nodules conceivably associated with the antibrain antibodies that have been reported in serum. There are scattered reports that serum from schizophrenic patients is destructive to embryonal and adult brain cultures, and that lymphocytes from such patients damage human and rat embryonic brain explants. However, evidence for an autoimmune component in schizophrenia is at present not generally accepted.

Scattered reports of changes in extraneural tissues suggest hypoplasia of the cardiovascular system, including the heart, great vessels, vessels in the CNS, and capillaries in the retina. Atrophy of endocrine organs, particularly of the testes or ovaries, also has been described. If there is a real association between somatic changes and schizophrenia, it would seem most likely that they are parallel expressions of genetic constitution rather than either a cause or a result of CNS dysfunction.

Biochemical Changes in Schizophrenia

Whereas the findings in depressive psychosis appear to indicate a generalized decrease or increase of monoamine metabolism, there seems to be no such straightforward relationship in schizophrenia. There are no consistent reports of either decreased or increased monoamines or normal metabolites in the brain, CSF, blood, or urine. Schizophrenia might represent hyperresponsiveness to monoamines in normal concentrations, or the presence of abnormal metabolites acting as neurotransmitters. Two pieces of circumstantial evidence have led investigators in the latter direction: the first is the presence of unusual monoamine metabolites in the urine of many schizophrenic patients; the second is a generic resemblance between the structure of many psychotomimetic drugs (i.e., those that produce hallucinations and other psychotic effects) and normal monoamine neurotransmitters (Fig. 26-4).

Urinary Metabolites: The "Pink Spot"

The presence of a chromatographic "pink spot" in schizophrenic urine has long been noted. This appears to contain, among other products, 3,4-dimethoxyphenylethylamine (DMPEA), a substance that could readily be derived from dopamine by the action of COMT, methoxylating both the 3- and 4-hydroxyl groups (instead of just the usual 3-). However, the pink spot is not entirely DMPEA, but may also include tyramine and possibly methylated derivatives such as monomethyl- and dimethyltyramine. Although there is no direct evidence, the methylated derivatives could be produced by phenol-N-methyltransferase (PNMT), an enzyme that is known to be present in the CNS, although its function is uncertain. While there has been some uncertainty as to the identification of these compounds, there now seems little doubt that they are present in many schizophrenic patients, although so far their excretion does not seem to parallel the intensity of clinical symptoms.

Experimental Studies of Methylation and Methoxylation

The possibility that increased methylation or methoxylation occurs in schizophrenia has led to much experimental work, largely on human volunteers, both schizophrenic and control subjects.

Effects of Methionine on S-Adenosylmethionine Levels in the Brain. The normal methyl donor in mammalian tissue is S-adenosylmethionine, and since little methionine is present in the diet, the methyl donor may be rate-limiting in both methylating and methoxylating reactions. Since N-methylation cannot occur after oxidative deamination by MAO, most of the experimental work has centered on the administration of methionine (or cysteine), together with MAO inhibitors. Such treatment often worsens the clinical condition of schizophrenic patients and is associated with increased urinary excretion of abnormal methylated derivatives of both catecholamines and indoleamines. Experimentally, this procedure raises brain levels of S-adenosylmethionine. Administration of methionine or cysteine alone increases plasma amino acids, including methionine, but these rise to considerably higher levels with the addition of MAO inhibitors.

If the blood-brain barrier selects only the amino acids necessary for current brain metabolism, it appears unlikely that these increased plasma levels would of themselves explain the psychotic disturbances induced, though presumably there is a selective increase in methionine uptake, at least in schizophrenic patients, perhaps indicating a CNS methionine deficiency in this condition. The blood levels of S-adenosylmethionine appear to be the same in schizophrenic patients as in control subjects. Possible small increases in COMT levels, not related to treatment or age, have been reported.

Handling of 3- and 4-Methoxy Compounds in the Brain. Other studies indicate a possible relationship between abnormal brain methoxylation and psychotic episodes. Radioisotope-labeled dopamine administration leads to the presence of labeled DMPEA in schizophrenic urine. Since a 4-alkoxy grouping is constant in catecholamine-related psychotomimetic drugs, studies were made of the physiological formation of methoxy compounds. The results suggest that the normal predominance of 3-methoxy compounds in the CNS is not due to their preferred formation, but rather to earlier demethylation of 4-methoxy compounds. Thus, using DMPEA

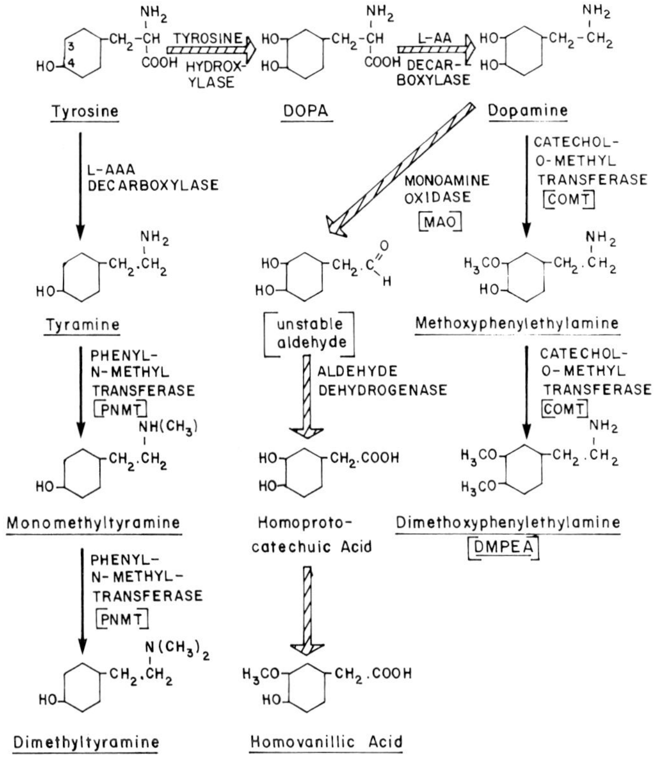

Fig. 26-4. Possible abnormalities of catecholamine metabolism in schizophrenia.

labeled in the 4 position, $^{14}CO_2$ appears in expired air at 5 minutes after administration, reaches a peak at 25 minutes, and rapidly declines thereafter; if labeling is at the 3 position, only small amounts of $^{14}CO_2$ appear, with an ill-defined peak at 30 to 60 minutes. The possibility is raised of a defect of the (unidentified) enzyme that normally demethylates at the 4 position.

Size of Methyl Pool in the Brain. Another study involved determination of $^{14}CO_2$ after the administration of labeled methionine. In control subjects, $^{14}CO_2$ peaked in the expired air at 20 to 30 minutes and then slowly declined, but in schizophrenic patients, excretion at 20 to 30 minutes was lower, but remained steady or even increased slightly over a prolonged period. This seems a clear indication of abnormal methionine metabolism, but does not distinguish between a large pool of methionine and other methylated compounds and a slow turnover in a pool of normal size. Methionine antagonists produce no improvement in schizophrenic patients, but induce psychotic episodes in normal persons, perhaps associated with abnormally reduced methylation.

Relationship of Biochemical Changes to Therapeutic Drug Activity

On the evidence presently available, it seems reasonable to suppose that schizophrenia is associated with some abnormality in the transfer of methyl or methoxy groups to one or more monoamines. To be any more specific than this appears unjustified at the present time.

It is less easy to rationalize even superficially the effect of drugs used in schizophrenia than the effect of those used in depressive psychosis. It has been suggested that phenothiazines increase brain dopamine turnover before they affect other monoamines, and that one function may be blockage of dopamine receptor sites. While this fits the concept of undue CNS sensitivity to monoamines in schizophrenia, it is difficult to relate to possible abnormalities of methyl metabolism, unless it is assumed that methylated amines are themselves excitatory to receptor membranes, and that undue sensitivity is to them rather than to the ordinary neurotransmitters. In fact, the methylated derivatives are not so much abnormal as present in abnormally high quantities. Perhaps the trace amounts in the normal CNS have a neurotransmitter or other physiological function of which we are presently ignorant.

Analysis of the actions of phenothiazines and allied drugs, and of reserpine, is premature, since too little is known either about the drugs themselves, the metabolic abnormality in schizophrenia, or the circuitry of the limbic and allied systems. Phenothiazine has been reported to have different effects at neurons inhibited or excited by norepinephrine: in the former, blocking reuptake and prolonging inhibition; in the latter, combining with the receptor and blocking excitation. This overall inhibitory enhancement, perhaps equally applicable to normal and methylated transmitters, is said to decrease rostral projection (from the limbic system to the neocortex). Physiologically, phenothiazine has been reported to desynchronize efferent activity of the amygdala and hippocampus and reduce sensory input to the reticular formation. Reserpine is presumed to reduce concentrations of monoamines and, like phenothiazines, to decrease rostral projection and reduce reticular sensory inputs. Perhaps reserpine-induced loss of monoamines with predominant action of MAO before COMT reduces N-methylated, if not O-methylated, compounds.

NOTE OF CAUTION

It will be apparent that the presumed biochemistry of the major psychoses is based on fragmentary, even contradictory, clinical and experimental evidence, and it is possible that entirely new concepts will render the work described here irrelevant. The topic is fascinating and, for the more pragmatically minded, of considerable socioeconomic importance, since these patients account for a large proportion of total hospital admissions and tend to remain in the hospital for long periods of time. While the prognosis and outlook of the major psychoses have been improved by recent developments in psychopharmacology, they remain one of the major problems of medicine and society – which is felt to justify this short chapter.

BIBLIOGRAPHY

Abdulla, Y. H., and Hamadah, H. 3′-5′-Cyclic adenosine monophosphate in depression and mania. *Lancet* 1:378-381, 1970

Berger, F. M. Mental disease and drugs affecting it. *Perspect. Biol. Med.* 13:31-44, 1969.

Eisenberg, L. The future of psychiatry. *Lancet* 2: 1371-1376, 1973.

Gershon, S. Lithium salts in the management of the manic-depressive syndrome. *Annu. Rev. Med.* 23:439-452, 1972.

Glen, A. I. M., and Reading, H. W. Regulatory action of lithium in manic-depressive illness. *Lancet* 2:1239-1241, 1973.

Israelstam, D. M., Sargent, T., Finley, N. N., Winchell, H. S., Fish, M. B., Motto, J., Pollycove, M., and Johnson, A. Abnormal methionine metabolism in schizophrenic and depressive states: A preliminary report. *J. Psychiatr. Res.* 7:185-190, 1970.

King, L. J. Chemotherapy of mental depression. *Annu. Rev. Med.* 21:367-378, 1970.

Klerman, G. L. Pharmacotherapy of schizophrenia. *Annu. Rev. Med.* 25:199-217, 1974.

Logan, D. G., and Deodhar, S. D. Schizophrenia, an immunologic disorder? *J.A.M.A.* 212:1703-1704, 1970.

Nieto, D., and Escobar, A. Major Psychoses. In J. Minckler (Ed.), *Pathology of the Nervous System.* New York: McGraw-Hill, 1972. Vol. 3, pp. 2654-2665.

Roizin, L. Histopathologic Observations in Schizophrenia. In J. Minckler (Ed.), *Pathology of the Nervous System.* New York: McGraw-Hill, 1972. Vol. 3, pp. 2670-2677.

Schildkraut, J. J. Neuropharmacology of the affective disorders. *Annu. Rev. Pharmacol.* 13:427-454, 1973.

Schildkraut, J. J. Biogenic amines and affective disorders. *Annu. Rev. Med.* 25:333-348, 1974.

Singer, I., and Rotenberg, D. Mechanisms of lithium action. *N. Engl. J. Med.* 289:254-260, 1973.

Sweet, W. H. Treatment of medically intractable mental disease by limited frontal leukotomy – justifiable? *N. Engl. J. Med.* 289:1117-1125, 1973.

Torrey, E. F., and Peterson, M. R. Slow and latent viruses in schizophrenia. *Lancet* 2:22-24, 1973.

Wender, P. H. Adopted children and their behavior in the evaluation of nature-nurture interaction in the schizophrenic disorders. *Annu. Rev. Med.* 23:355-372, 1972.

Glossary

ACHE	acetylcholinesterase
ACTH	adrenocorticotropic hormone
ADEM	acute disseminated encephalomyelitis
ADH	antidiuretic hormone
ADP	adenosine diphosphate
AHLE	acute hemorrhagic leukoencephalopathy
ALS	amyotrophic lateral sclerosis
AMP	adenosine monophosphate
ARAS	ascending reticular activating system
Arc	periventricular nuclei (arcuate nucleus) of hypothalamus
ATP	adenosine triphosphate
ATPase	adenosine triphosphatase
cAMP	cyclic adenosine monophosphate
CAP	compound action potential
CAT	choline acetyltransferase
CBF	cerebral blood flow
CDP	cytidine diphosphate
CMP	cytidine monophosphate
CNS	central nervous system
COEPS	cortically originating extrapyramidal system
COMT	catechol-O-methyltransferase
CRF	corticotropin releasing factor
CrP	creatine phosphate
CSF	cerebrospinal fluid
CTP	cytidine triphosphate
CVP	central venous pressure
cyclic AMP	adenosine 3′:5′-cyclic phosphate
DA	dopamine
DC	cortical standing potential
DFP	di-isopropyl fluorophosphate
DMPEA	3, 4-dimethoxyphenylethylamine
DNA	deoxyribonucleic acid
DPH	diphenylhydantoin
ECF	extracellular fluid
ECS	extracellular space
EAE	experimental allergic encephalomyelitis
EEG	electroencephalogram
EPSP	excitatory postsynaptic potential
FAD	flavine adenine nucleate
FIF	follicle stimulating hormone inhibiting factor
FIGLU	formiminoglutamic acid
FRF	follicle stimulating hormone releasing factor
FSH	follicle stimulating hormone
GABA	γ-aminobutyric acid
GH	growth hormone
GIF	growth hormone inhibiting factor
GRF	growth hormone releasing factor
5-HIAA	5-hydroxyindoleacetic acid
5-HIOMT	hydroxyindole-O-methyltransferase
HL-A	human lymphocyte antigen
HVA	homovanillic acid
IADH	inappropriate secretion of ADH
ICP	intracranial pressure
IF	inhibiting factor
IPSP	inhibitory postsynaptic potential
LDH	lactic dehydrogenase
LH	luteinizing hormone
LIF	luteinizing hormone inhibiting factor
LRF	luteinizing hormone releasing factor

LSD	lysergic acid diethylamide
MAO	monoamine oxidase
MAP	mean arterial pressure
MHPG	3-methoxy-4-hydroxyphenylglycol
MIF	melanocyte stimulating hormone inhibiting factor
MsI	primary motor area
MsII	supplementary motor area
MSH	melanocyte stimulating hormone
NAc	N-acetylgalactosamine
NAD^+	nicotinamide-adenine dinucleotide
NADH	reduced form of NAD^+
$NADP^+$	nicotinamide-adenine dinucleotide phosphate
NADPH	reduced form of $NADP^+$
NANA	N-acetyl neuraminic acid (sialic acid)
5-OHT	5-hydroxytryptophol
Pco_2	partial pressure of carbon dioxide
P_i	inorganic phosphate
PDS	paroxysmal depolarization shift
PHS	paroxysmal hyperpolarization shift
PIF	prolactin inhibitory factor
PKU	phenylketonuria
PL	prolactin
PMLE	progressive multifocal leukoencephalopathy
PNS	peripheral nervous system
PO	preoptic region of limbic system
Po_2	partial pressure of oxygen
PP	perfusion pressure
PSIP	postsynaptic inhibitory potential
PSP	postsynaptic potential
PV	paraventricular nucleus of hypothalamus
RF	releasing factor
RISA	radio-iodinated serum albumin
RNA	ribonucleic acid
SC	suprachiasmatic region of hypothalamus
SmI	primary somatosensory area
SmII	secondary sensory area (= secondary motor area)
SO	supraoptic nucleus of hypothalamus
SSPE	subacute sclerosing panencephalitis
TDP	thiamine diphosphate (thiamine pyrophosphate)
TRF	thyrotropin releasing factor
TSH	thyroid stimulating hormone
TTP	thiamine triphosphate
UDP-galactose	uridine diphosphogalactose
VM	ventromedial nucleus of hypothalamus
VMA	vanillylmandelic acid

Index

Index